MENTAL HEALTH AND DISASTERS

Since the attacks of September 11, 2001, disaster preparedness and response has developed into a discrete subspecialty in medicine and has become a national health priority. The mental health consequences of disasters are an important area of study. Disasters are associated with substantial short and long-lasting psychological burden, at both an individual and a community level. The range of psychopathologies associated with disaster is broad and includes different types of psychiatric disorders and behavioral problems, including posttraumatic stress disorder, depression, and prolonged grief. This book is the definitive reference on mental health and disasters, focused on the assessment and treatment of the full spectrum of psychopathologies associated with different types of disasters. Considerations about the use of preexisting community-based mental health services, as well as the development and the testing of new treatment programs, are covered in depth. Detailed case studies, incorporating lessons from major disasters such as Hurricane Katrina and the September 11, 2001, terrorist attacks, are included.

Yuval Neria, Ph.D., is Associate Professor of Clinical Psychology at Columbia University, College of Physicians and Surgeons, and Director of the Trauma and PTSD Program at the New York State Psychiatric Institute, New York, New York.

Sandro Galea, M.D., Dr. PH., is Professor of Epidemiology at the University of Michigan School of Public Health and a Research Professor at the Institute for Social Research at the University of Michigan, Ann Arbor, Michigan.

Fran H. Norris, Ph.D., is Research Professor in the Department of Psychiatry at Dartmouth Medical School, Hanover, New Hampshire.

To Mariana, Michal, Oren, and Maya, forever with love (YN);
For Margaret, Oliver Luke, and Isabel Tess, as always (SG);
To my husband, Michael, for his unending support, and
my brother, Fred, for a lifetime of love (FHN).

Mental Health and Disasters

Edited by

Yuval Neria

Columbia University Medical Center, New York, New York

Sandro Galea

University of Michigan, Ann Arbor, Michigan

Fran H. Norris

Dartmouth Medical School, Hanover, New Hampshire

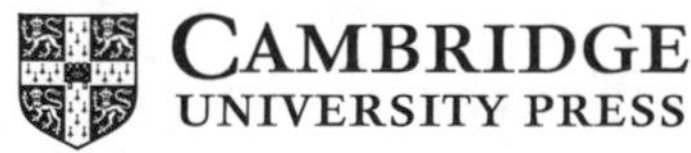
CAMBRIDGE
UNIVERSITY PRESS

CAMBRIDGE UNIVERSITY PRESS
Cambridge, New York, Melbourne, Madrid, Cape Town, Singapore, São Paulo, Delhi

Cambridge University Press
32 Avenue of the Americas, New York, NY 10013-2473, USA

www.cambridge.org
Information on this title: www.cambridge.org/9780521883870

First published 2009

Printed in the United States of America

A catalog record for this publication is available from the British Library.

Library of Congress Cataloging in Publication data
Mental health and disasters / edited by Yuval Neria, Sandro Galea, Fran H. Norris.
p. cm.
Includes bibliographical references and index.
ISBN 978-0-521-88387-0 (hbk.)
1. Disasters – Psychological aspects. 2. Psychic trauma. 3. Mental health.
I. Neria, Yuval. II. Galea, Sandro. III. Norris, Fran H. IV. Title.
BF789.D5M46 2009
616.85′21–dc22 2009009880

ISBN 978-0-521-88387-0 hardback

Contents

PART FOUR: SPECIAL GROUPS

PART FIVE: INTERVENTIONS AND HEALTH SERVICES

PART SIX: CASE STUDIES

Acknowledgments

We are grateful to Sara Putnam, MPH, our Editorial Coordinator, who provided outstanding help in all stages of the work on this book. Without her dedication and attention to detail this project would never have been possible.

Partial support for this book was provided by the SPUNK Fund Inc.

Contributors

Jennifer Alvarez
National Center for Posttraumatic Stress Disorder
VA Palo Alto Health Care System
Menlo Park, California

Ananda B. Amstadter
Department of Psychiatry and Behavioral Sciences
National Crime Victims Research and Treatment Center
Medical University of South Carolina
Charleston, South Carolina

Metin Başoğlu
Section of Trauma Studies
Division of Psychological Medicine and Psychiatry
Institute of Psychiatry, King's College
London, United Kingdom
and
The Istanbul Center for Behavior Research and Therapy (ICBRT / DABATEM)
Istanbul, Turkey

David M. Benedek
Department of Psychiatry
Center for the Study of Traumatic Stress
Uniformed Services University School of Medicine
Bethesda, Maryland

Charles C. Benight
Department of Psychology and the CU: Trauma, Health, and Hazards Center
University of Colorado at Colorado Springs
Colorado Springs, Colorado

George A. Bonanno
Teachers College
Columbia University
New York, New York

Evelyn J. Bromet
Departments of Psychiatry and Preventive Medicine
State University of New York at Stony Brook
Stony Brook, New York

Richard A. Bryant
School of Psychology
University of New South Wales
Sydney, Australia

Barbara Lopes Cardozo
International Emergency and Refugee Health Branch
Centers for Disease Control and Prevention
Atlanta, Georgia

M. L. Somchai Chakkraband
Department of Mental Health
Thailand Ministry of Public Health
Nonthaburi, Thailand

Claude Chemtob
Department of Psychiatry
Mount Sinai School of Medicine
New York, New York

Roman Cieslak
CU: Trauma, Health, and Hazards Center
University of Colorado at Colorado Springs
Colorado Springs, Colorado
and
Department of Psychology
Warsaw School of Social Psychology
Warsaw, Poland

Lauren M. Conoscenti
National Center for PTSD
VA Boston Healthcare System
Boston University School of Medicine
Boston, Massachusetts

Joan M. Cook
Department of Psychiatry
Yale University School of Medicine
National Center for PTSD
West Haven, Connecticut

Judith Cukor
Program for Anxiety and Traumatic Stress Studies
Weill Cornell Medical College
New York Presbyterian Hospital
New York, New York

Carla Kmett Danielson
Department of Psychiatry and Behavioral Sciences
National Crime Victims Research and Treatment Center
Medical University of South Carolina
Ralph H. Johnson Medical Center
Charleston, South Carolina

JoAnn Difede
Program for Anxiety and Traumatic Stress Studies
Weill Cornell Medical College
New York Presbyterian Hospital
New York, New York

Charles DiMaggio
Department of Epidemiology
Mailman School of Public Health
Columbia University
New York, New York

Anja J. E. Dirkzwager
Netherlands Institute for Health Services Research
Utrecht, The Netherlands
and
Netherlands Institute for the Study of Crime and Law Enforcement (NSCR)
Leiden, The Netherlands

Cristiane S. Duarte
Division of Child and Adolescent Psychiatry
Columbia University
New York, New York

Jon D. Elhai
Disaster Mental Health Institute
The University of South Dakota
Vermillion, South Dakota

Diane L. Elmore
Public Interest Government Relations Office
American Psychological Association
Washington, DC

Yael L. E. Errera
Department of Psychiatry
Hadassah University Hospital
Jerusalem, Israel

Julian D. Ford
Department of Psychiatry
University of Connecticut Health Center
Farmington, Connecticut

Carol S. Fullerton
Department of Psychiatry
Center for the Study of Traumatic Stress
Uniformed Services University School of Medicine
Bethesda, Maryland

Sandro Galea
Department of Epidemiology
University of Michigan School of Public Health
Survey Research Center
Institute for Social Research
Ann Arbor, Michigan

Freya Goodhew
University of Adelaide
The Centre for Military and Veterans' Health
Adelaide, South Australia

Neil Greenberg
Academic Centre for Defence Mental Health
King's College
London, United Kingdom
and
Weston Education Centre
London, United Kingdom

Lindsay Greene
Department of Psychiatry
Columbia University
New York, New York

Linda Grievink
National Institute for Public Health and the Environment (RIVM)
Bilthoven, The Netherlands

Michael J. Gruber
Department of Health Care Policy
Harvard Medical School
Boston, Massachusetts

Sumati Gupta
Teachers College
Columbia University
New York, New York

Johan M. Havenaar
Department of Psychiatry
Vrije Universiteit Medical Centre
Amsterdam, The Netherlands

Alesia O. Hawkins
Department of Psychiatry and Behavioral Sciences
National Crime Victims Research and Treatment Center
Medical University of South Carolina
Charleston, South Carolina

Clare Henn-Haase
University of California
San Francisco, California
and
San Francisco VA Medical Center
San Francisco, California

Kimberly Eaton Hoagwood
Department of Psychiatry
Columbia University
New York, New York
and
Child and Adolescent Services Research
New York State Office of Mental Health
Albany, New York

Christina W. Hoven
Departments of Epidemiology and Child Psychiatry
Columbia University and New York State Psychiatric Institute
New York, New York

Sabra S. Inslicht
University of California
San Francisco, California
and
San Francisco VA Medical Center
San Francisco, California

Krzysztof Kaniasty
Department of Psychology
Indiana University of Pennsylvania
and
Opole University
Opole, Poland

Ronald C. Kessler
Department of Health Care Policy
Harvard Medical School
Boston, Massachusetts

Rachel Kimerling
National Center for Posttraumatic Stress Disorder
VA Palo Alto Health Care System
Menlo Park, California

Richard V. King
Department of Health Care Sciences
Southwestern School of Health Professions
Department of Surgery/Emergency Medicine
University of Texas Southwestern Medical Center
Dallas, Texas

Rolf J. Kleber
Institute for Psychotrauma
Diemen, The Netherlands
and
Department of Clinical & Health Psychology
Utrecht University
Utrecht, The Netherlands

Jessica Mass Levitt
Department of Psychiatry
Columbia University
New York, New York

Brett T. Litz
National Center for PTSD
VA Boston Healthcare System
Boston University School of Medicine
Boston, Massachusetts

Maria Livanou
Division of Psychological Medicine
Section of Trauma Studies
Institute of Psychiatry
London, United Kingdom

Katelyn P. Mack
National Center for Posttraumatic Stress Disorder
VA Palo Alto Health Care System
Menlo Park, California

Paula Madrid
National Center for Disaster Preparedness
Mailman School of Public Health
Columbia University
New York, New York

Shira Maguen
San Francisco VA Medical Center
University of California
San Francisco School of Medicine
San Francisco, California

Paul Maguire
Australian National University
Canberra, Australia

Donald J. Mandell
Department of Child and Adolescent Psychiatry
New York State Psychiatric Institute
New York, New York

Charles R. Marmar
University of California
San Francisco, California
and
San Francisco VA Medical Center
San Francisco, California

Andrea R. Maxwell
Department of Epidemiology
University of Michigan School of Public Health
Ann Arbor, Michigan

Shannon E. McCaslin
San Francisco VA Medical Center
San Francisco, California
and
University of California
San Francisco, California

Alexander C. McFarlane
University of Adelaide
The Centre for Military and Veterans' Health
Adelaide, South Australia

Thomas J. Metzler
University of California
San Francisco, California
and
San Francisco VA Medical Center
San Francisco, California

Summer Nelson
Department of Psychology
University of Tulsa
Tulsa, Oklahoma

Yuval Neria
Department of Psychiatry
Columbia University
New York, New York
and
New York State Psychiatric Institute
New York, New York

Elana Newman
Department of Psychology
University of Tulsa
Tulsa, Oklahoma

Thomas C. Neylan
University of California
San Francisco, California
and
San Francisco VA Medical Center
San Francisco, California

Fran H. Norris
Department of Psychiatry
Dartmouth Medical School
National Center for Disaster Mental Health Research
Department of Veterans Affairs National Center for PTSD
White River Junction, Vermont

Carol S. North
VA North Texas Health Care System
Dallas, Texas
and
Departments of Psychiatry and Surgery
Division of Emergency Medicine
University of Texas Southwestern Medical Center
Dallas, Texas

Lawrence A. Palinkas
School of Social Work
University of Southern California
Los Angeles, California

Benjaporn Panyayong
Department of Mental Health
Thailand Ministry of Public Health
Nonthaburi, Thailand

Maria Petukhova
Department of Health Care Policy
Harvard Medical School
Boston, Massachusetts

Betty Pfefferbaum
Department of Psychiatry and Behavioral Sciences
College of Medicine
University of Oklahoma Health Sciences Center
Oklahoma City, Oklahoma

Marleen Radigan
New York State Office of Mental Health
Albany, New York

Beverley Raphael
University of Western Sydney and Australian National University
Australia

James Rodriguez
Department of Psychiatry
Columbia University
New York, New York

G. James Rubin
Department of Psychological Medicine
James Black Centre
King's College
London, United Kingdom

Kenneth J. Ruggiero
Department of Psychiatry and Behavioral Sciences
National Crime Victims Research and Treatment Center
Medical University of South Carolina
Charleston, South Carolina

Ebru Şalcıoğlu
Section of Trauma Studies
Division of Psychological Medicine and Psychiatry
Institute of Psychiatry
King's College
London, United Kingdom
and
The Istanbul Center for Behavior Research and Therapy (ICBRT / DABATEM)
Istanbul, Turkey

Nancy A. Sampson
Department of Health Care Policy
Harvard Medical School
Boston, Massachusetts

Arieh Y. Shalev
Department of Psychiatry
Hadassah University Hospital
Jerusalem, Israel

Bruce Shapiro
Dart Center for Journalism and Trauma
Columbia University
New York, New York

Laura M. Stough
Department of Educational Psychology
Texas A & M University
College Station, Texas

Prawate Tantipiwatanaskul
Department of Mental Health
Thailand Ministry of Public Health
Nonthaburi, Thailand

Warunee Thienkrua
Thailand Ministry of Public Health – U.S. CDC Collaboration
Thailand Ministry of Public Health
Nonthaburi, Thailand

Phebe Tucker
Department of Psychiatry
University of Oklahoma Health Sciences Center
Oklahoma City, Oklahoma

J. Blake Turner
Department of Child Psychiatry
Columbia University and New York State Psychiatric Institute
New York, New York

Robert J. Ursano
Department of Psychiatry
Center for the Study of Traumatic Stress
Uniformed Services University School of Medicine
Bethesda, Maryland

Bellis van den Berg
Institute for Risk Assessment Sciences (IRAS)
Utrecht University
Utrecht, The Netherlands

Peter G. van der Velden
Institute for Psychotrauma (IvP)
Diemen, The Netherlands

Frits van Griensven
Thailand Ministry of Public Health – U.S. CDC Collaboration
Thailand Ministry of Public Health
Nonthaburi, Thailand

Miranda Van Hooff
University of Adelaide
The Centre for Military and Veterans' Health
Adelaide, South Australia

Edward Waldrep
Department of Psychology
University of Colorado at Colorado Springs
Colorado Springs, Colorado

Philip S. Wang
Division of Services and Intervention Research
National Institute of Mental Health
Rockville, Maryland

Simon Wessely
King's Centre for Military Health Research
King's College
London, United Kingdom
and
Department of Psychological Medicine
Weston Education Centre
London, United Kingdom

Leslie H. Wind
School of Social Work
University of Southern California
Los Angeles, California

C. Joris Yzermans
Netherlands Institute for Health Services Research (NIVEL)
Utrecht, The Netherlands

Heidi M. Zinzow
Department of Psychology
Clemson University
Clemson, South Carolina

1 Disaster Mental Health Research: Exposure, Impact, and Response

YUVAL NERIA, SANDRO GALEA, AND FRAN H. NORRIS

1.1. INTRODUCTION

Disasters occur frequently, sometimes in multiple locations at the same time, and although they vary in terms of type, impact, and their consequences, they are often life changing for large numbers of people. Although disaster forecasting has improved in recent decades, many disasters remain unforeseen, and even more disasters continue to exceed the response capacities of the communities that they affect.

A number of large-scale human-made and natural disasters during the past decade have resulted in considerable popular and academic attention being paid to population effects of disasters, particularly in terms of mental health effects. Among these, the Marmara Earthquake in August 1999; the September 11, 2001, terrorist attacks in New York City and Washington, DC; the March 11, 2004, train bombings in Madrid; the London terrorist attacks of July 7, 2005; and Hurricane Katrina in August 2005 all have been studied by several teams of scientists and clinicians and have resulted in a rapidly growing body of knowledge about the mental health consequences of such events.

Building on the work presented in recent volumes in the field (Cameron, Watson, & Friedman, 2006; Neria, Gross, Marshall, & Susser, 2006; Norris, Galea, Friedman, & Watson, 2006; Ursano, Fullerton, Weisaeth, & Raphael, 2007), the goal of this book is to address crucial gaps in our knowledge by reviewing and synthesizing the existing literature on the mental health consequences of disasters, evaluating strengths and shortcomings of past and current methodologies, and suggesting a comprehensive overview of future directions for improved research about the mental health consequences of disasters.

1.2. CONTENT AND STRUCTURE

This book has been organized thematically into seven parts. In PART ONE, two chapters describe the central themes that underpin research about the mental health consequences of disasters. In the first chapter, Beverly Raphael and Paul Maguire provide a comprehensive review of the history of the field of disaster mental health from the 1940s to the present. They present the main topics of the field and discusses key challenges ahead for mental health research. Next, Norris and Wind discuss the challenges involved in studying the impact of disasters, considering the nature of "indirect exposure" to traumatic events, the interplay between the "objective" and the "subjective" domains of exposure, and the "personal" level versus the "collective" level of catastrophic events.

In PART TWO, Psychopathology after Disasters, each chapter summarizes the literature about particular psychopathologies after disasters, considering both the evidence documenting these psychopathologies and the challenges inherent in understanding them. In the first chapter, McFarlane, Van Hooff, and Goodhew review the literature on the prevalence and the etiology of anxiety disorders following disaster. The authors underscore the complexity of anxiety disorders, the interplay between the various conditions, and the methodological shortcomings of some studies that limited our full understanding of anxiety disorders after disasters. The second chapter in this part addresses an overlooked, yet central, domain of concern: physical health problems. Yzermans, van den Berg, and Dirkzwager discuss somatic diseases and disorders in disaster survivors, the differences between symptoms and diseases, and the relationship between psychological problems and physical symptoms. In the third chapter, Van der Velden and Kleber provide a critical review of the evidence regarding changes in the prevalence of use and misuse of substance, alcohol, and cigarettes after disasters of different types and magnitudes. The fourth chapter in this part focuses on two mental health conditions frequently associated with the experience of loss, namely depression and prolonged grief (also known as traumatic or complicated grief). Maguen, Neria, Conoscenti, and Litz suggest that while postdisaster depression has received considerable attention over the years, disaster-related grief, a condition that has been shown to be common and disabling among people who experience loss of attachment figures, remains understudied. The chapter further reviews risk factors for depression and prolonged grief following disaster and current treatments that should be considered. The closing chapter in PART TWO provides a synthesis of the current knowledge of the mental health effects of disaster. Ursano, Fullerton, and Benedek describe the range of psychological sequelae in the wake of disasters, from subsyndromal symptoms of distress, to alterations in behavior, to the development of specific psychiatric disorders, particularly posttraumatic stress disorder (PTSD). They also provide an integrative theoretical framework for understanding and studying postdisaster psychopathology.

PART THREE focuses on key aspects of vulnerability and resilience in the face of disasters. The first chapter, by Bonanno and Gupta, reviews the evidence on the human capacity to cope with adversities. They discuss the conceptual differences between psychological resilience (low levels of disaster-related psychopathology) and recovery (decreased psychopathology over time) and review the available evidence on the correlates of resilience. In the next chapter, Benight, Cieslak, and Waldrep critically review the research that has developed and tested a number of social and cognitive theoretical frameworks predicting mental health consequences of disasters, while providing a cross-theoretical model that depicts the interactions among the major constructs presented. In the last chapter in this part, Kaniasty and Norris offer an extensive discussion about social support during and after disasters, including the differences between received social support, perceived social support, and social embeddedness. Research on the differential role of those constructs and the evidence on support mobilization and support deterioration is systematically assessed.

PART FOUR provides a review of the scientific literature on the key known determinants of the mental health consequences of disasters. The part is focused on the role of gender, race/ethnicity, and age as determinants of mental health after disasters, as well as the mental health consequences of disasters among particular groups, including media personnel and uniformed rescuers. In the first chapter, Kimerling, Mack, and Alvarez address why women have repeatedly been shown to be at increased risk for psychopathology after disaster. In the second chapter in the part, Hoven, Duarte, Turner, and Mandell critically review the literature on postdisaster PTSD among children and adolescents, with a particular focus on the methodological shortcomings of the literature in the area. In the next chapter, Cook and Elmore provide a comprehensive and critical analysis of the evidence of the consequences of disasters among older adults; they also discuss the implications of the available evidence for disaster policy and planning for the needs of the aging population after such events. In the fifth chapter, Hawkins, Zinzow, Amstadter, Danielson, and Ruggiero summarize the evidence on the relations between race/ethnicity and socioeconomic status and mental health outcomes following disasters. Newman, Shapiro, and Nelson review the current knowledge about the role of journalists and the news media during disasters, the evidence about the impact of disasters on the mental health of journalists, and the evidence regarding the impact of media coverage upon the public. In the final chapter in this part, McCaslin, Inslicht, Henn-Haase, Chemtob, Metzler, Neylan, and Marmar focus on the aftermath of disasters among uniformed rescue workers, including police officers and firefighters. As these groups are often required to take part in rescue efforts and recovery, they may find themselves at heightened risk of exposure to high impact trauma and its emotional aftermath.

PART FIVE discusses the science of interventions after disasters, along with the barriers and challenges faced in providing mental health care services after these events. Bryant and Litz summarize the state-of-the-science evidence on mental health interventions after disaster in the immediate and intermediate stages and propose recommendations with regard to the choices clinicians, policy makers, and researchers must make regarding provision of mental health care during this time. This chapter is followed by a review of long-term treatments among adult survivors and rescue workers. Difede and Cukor focus on the scarce evidence base for long-term treatment of the most common outcomes following disaster and the gaps in that knowledge base. Next, Levitt, Hoagwood, Greene, Rodriguez, and Radigan review the literature on postdisaster trauma treatments for children and adolescents and discuss the need to translate efficacious treatments to the community for use in the wake of disasters. Finally, Elhai and Ford provide a critical analysis of utilization of mental health services, barriers to utilization, and specific examples of implementation of mental health services in the aftermath of disasters.

The case studies in PART SIX present detailed explorations of a number of sentinel natural, technological, and human-made disasters, with discussions that integrate many of the observations made in other chapters in the book. Chapters include discussions about the Southeast Asian tsunami, by Lopes Cardozo and colleagues; the Marmara Earthquake, by Başoğlu and colleagues; Hurricane Katrina, by Kessler and colleagues; the Chernobyl nuclear accidents, by Bromet and Havennar; the *Exxon Valdez* oil spill, by Palinkas; the Enschede fireworks disaster, by Van der Velden and colleagues; shooting episodes, by North and King; the Oklahoma City bombing, by Pfefferbaum and colleagues; the September 11th attacks, by DiMaggio and Madrid; the London bombings, by Greenberg and colleagues; and terrorism in Israel, by Shalev and Errera.

PART SEVEN offers concluding remarks about key challenges in research concerned with postdisaster mental health. Galea and Maxwell discuss the methodological challenges that researchers face when they design, implement, and analyze studies aimed at understanding the mental health consequences of disasters. Neria, Galea, and Norris conclude the book by summarizing the evidence about the burden of psychopathology after disasters as presented in various chapters throughout the book, the challenges in assessing psychopathology in these circumstances using established criteria, the limitations of current research, and the extent to which what we have learned thus far has enabled us to predict and anticipate the mental health consequences of future disasters.

REFERENCES

Cameron, R., Watson, P., & Friedman, M. (2006). *Interventions following mass violence and disasters strategies for mental health practice*. Guliford Press. New York.

Neria, Y., Gross, R., Marshall, R., & Susser, E. (Eds.). (2006). *9/11: Mental health in the wake of terrorist attacks*. Cambridge University Press.

Norris, F. H., Galea, S., Friedman, M., & Watson, P. J. (Eds.). (2006). *Methods for disaster mental health research*. Guliford Press. New York.

Ursano, R., Fullerton, C., Weisaeth, L., & Raphael, B. (2007). *Textbook of disaster psychiatry*. Cambridge University Press.

PART ONE

Concepts

2 Disaster Mental Health Research: Past, Present, and Future

BEVERLEY RAPHAEL AND PAUL MAGUIRE

2.1. INTRODUCTION

Insights about disasters inevitably arise from history, social science, and the vast range of attempts to understand the nature of human behavior in such settings. Insights relevant to mental health have been developed more recently, in part because of the evolving nature of both the mental health and disaster fields. In reviewing the development of mental health interest in and research about disasters, there are many seminal studies and publications, building progressively in their contributions to the science of this field. It is impossible here to acknowledge each of these individual projects. Instead, the challenge lies in identifying the core themes of this field, their scientific evolution, their application to the reality of disaster contexts, and what may be required for the future. The themes that will be considered in this chapter have influenced research and practice over the past four to five decades, particularly in recent times. Nevertheless, they require critical examination and development, as do the research methodologies applied, if we are to meet the challenges of the future.

2.2. HISTORICAL BACKGROUND

2.2.1. Early Efforts

The field of disaster mental health research emerged from inquiries into the phenomena associated with the mental health impacts of war. An example, for instance, is Freud's attempts to understand civilization(s) and their discontents, the "traumatic" neuroses, and mourning and melancholia. An early specific focus for mental health in relation to disaster was led by Lindemann's (1944) report on the "Symptomatology and management of acute grief," which brought the mental health aspects to the fore, as did his colleague Adler's (1943) paper about the neuropsychiatric consequences for victims of the Coconut Grove Night Club fire.

Tyhurst (1950) wrote eloquently on individual reactions to community disaster and the natural history of certain psychiatric phenomena, offering new concepts in describing the overlapping phases of impact, recoil, and the post-traumatic period, including recovery. He also discussed the "disaster syndrome" – the period of impact or immediately afterwards where the person is dazed, stunned, unaware, frozen, or wandering aimlessly – which he believed could affect up to 20% to 25% of exposed people. He described it as usually transient, giving way to hyperactivity or appropriate adaptive response. Wolfenstein (1957), in her psychological essay on disaster, continued these phenomenological themes of behavioral responses and their patterns over time. Understanding of phenomena was also carried forth from work such as that of Quarantelli (1954), a sociologist, who described the unlikelihood of panic behaviors. This challenged the popular beliefs of the time that the threat of disaster, or its occurrence, would lead to panic and social disintegration, thus, highlighting the contribution of sociology to informing the mental health understanding of such threats. These early researchers acknowledged the nature of stressors, such as death, destruction, injury and loss, and their significance in relation to the phenomena that might emerge. However, they did not systematically examine specific correlations.

Throughout the 1960s, societal themes were prominent; examinations included *Man and society in disaster* (Baker & Chapman, 1962) *Communities in disaster; A sociological examination of collective stress* (Barton, 1969); and *Organisational behaviour in disaster* (Dynes, 1970). This stream was an important component of analysis, often setting the context for more individualistic analyses devised from psychological research observations. These works also highlighted the importance of the effects of events on communities and societies, the mass response to them, and the interpretations and meaning that followed. The themes had very significant implications, at times reinforcing stigmatized and victim identities and helplessness, and at other times presenting such positive interpretations that the suffering from mental health consequences of disasters seemed to be denied. Critically important in identifying the value of such approaches was Lifton's (1967) study of Hiroshima victims, "Death in life," which portrayed vividly the stressors, the phenomenology, and the social construction of meaning for both those directly affected (Hibakusha) and their communities. He highlighted courage and resilience as well as suffering and stigmatized identity.

2.2.2. The 1970s and 1980s

Mental health aspects of disasters became a more specific focus during the 1970s and 1980s. A valuable review by Kingston and Rosser (1974) drew together some of the impacts of disaster on mental and physical health. In this period, and subsequently, there were many different studies focusing on specific natural disasters: floods, tsunamis, earthquakes, volcanic eruptions, bush and forest fires, cyclones, hurricanes, tornados, storms, and the like. These studies involved population-based epidemiological methods in some instances, in others, reports on selected victim groups. The majority looked for impacts on the health and mental health of the general victim population for example, Abrahams, Price, Whitlock, and Williams, 1976 (floods in Brisbane, Australia); Logue, Hansen, and Struening, 1979 (Hurricane Agnes); Shore, Tatum, and Vollmer, 1985 (Mt. St. Helen's Volcano); or of specific affected subgroups, such as children (Milne, 1977). Also during this time, there were studies of "human-caused" disasters. Perhaps the best example is exemplified by Weisaeth's (1989) detailed studies on the effects of a paint factory explosion and fire, in which using a total population sample he was able to demonstrate a dose-response effect of stressor exposures.

These and many other research reports of this period contributed in significant ways to better understandings of the nature of the particular disaster exposures and their potential implications for mental health in the short and long term. Studies of different disaster contexts and causes – for instance, vehicle crashes, system failures such as mine collapses, chemical accidents, structural and building collapses, and marine incidents – demonstrated that such experiences would be likely to be associated with greater risk to mental health. Scientists noted this could potentially be related to the mass and gruesome nature of the deaths; the deaths of children; levels of personal life threat; bereavements in disaster circumstances that were untimely, unexpected, and traumatic in nature; and the dislocations and associated disruptions of social bonds through evacuations, destruction of homes, and the like.

In addition, research during this period provided greater understanding of the different affected populations and the stressors and mental health outcomes they experienced. The impacts on disaster responders in emergency organizations and the differing "victim" categories among this population, as noted in Taylor and Frazer's (1982) and Jones' (1985) descriptions of the stress of body handling and disaster victim identification, were highlighted. The special needs of children, adolescents, families, and older people were all identified. However, these studies used diverse methods and their findings allowed only limited synthesis.

The use of both sociological and mental health approaches was extended in the multiple studies of the Buffalo Creek Disaster, where stressors such as dislocation from communities, exposure to life threat, gruesome and untimely deaths, loss of loved ones, impacts on children, and disruptions of social bonds were shown to have profound, damaging, and long-term effects. Multiple sociological and clinical research studies on disasters contributed to the development of a comprehensive picture of these processes over time with sociologists, psychologists, and psychiatrists providing diverse contributions (Erikson, 1976; Gleser, Green, & Winget, 1978; Titchener, Kapp, & Winget, 1976). Ochberg, and Soskis (1982 also contributed to the field with recognition of the mental health impacts for victims of political terrorism. These studies placed mental health findings in societal contexts recognizing the powerful social influences in individual experience and outcomes.

In the attempt to develop appropriate responses to the impacts of disasters, manuals were developed, for instance, *Emergency and disaster management: a mental health source book*, which included contributions from many researchers in this field (Parad, Resnick, & Parad, 1976). Cohen and Ahearn's (1980) *Handbook of mental health care of disaster victims* was also influential, particularly in its recognition of the need for a systems approach and engagement with affected communities.

It is important to see the growth of interest in the field of disaster mental health during this time in additional contexts. The implications of psychological trauma were building on top of the understanding of these concepts from World Wars I and II and the detailed examination of the long-term effects of Holocaust trauma by researchers such as Eitinger (1969), Krystal (1968), and Frankl (1984). With Horowitz's conceptualization of Traumatic Stress Syndromes (1976), this focus became very relevant to examining the effects of massively traumatic incidents such as disasters. Findings that Vietnam Veterans suffered significant levels of psychologically traumatic impacts on their mental health and the establishment of the diagnosis of posttraumatic stress disorder (PTSD) in 1980 in DSM-III further focused interest on this syndrome. Studies of disaster in civilian populations provided the opportunity to examine the etiology and evolution of posttraumatic morbidity such as PTSD, as exemplified in McFarlane's (1988) research following an Australian forest fire. While early research distilled the multiple and diverse stressors that may arise with disasters – life threat, loss and bereavement, dislocation, loss of resources – the field of studies, as well as response systems, became almost overwhelmed by the evolving concepts of psychological trauma and traumatic stress as the principal paradigm during the decades from the 1980s onwards.

Nevertheless, up through the mid-1980s, the disaster studies available dealt with a wide range of outcomes, variable methodologies, and provided little systematic research to guide intervention. Thus, the field of disaster mental health could be seen as involving a number of research and response themes. Mass events such as disasters were recognized as potentially having significant impact on mental health and well-being. These outcomes were seen as more severe for those affected by "human-caused" disasters, but affecting all age groups, with children and perhaps minorities being particularly vulnerable. Resilience, capacity for effective response, altruism, courage, and effective actions for recovery were likewise recognized, although poorly operationalized and measured at this time. Though scientists such as psychologists and psychiatrists played an increasing role through their research contributions, the influences of sociologists, so valuable in the early stages, were often not encompassed in the mental health approaches that dominated. Nor were cultural themes and differences adequately incorporated, despite the knowledge that developing countries were more frequently and adversely affected.

Consequently, in the mid-1980s, it became evident that there was a need to promote more collaborative international approaches and potentially shared methodologies (Raphael, 1986). The extent of disasters and their mental health consequences had become matters of interest for world bodies, such as the World Health

Organization (WHO), the United Nations, and numerous nongovernment relief and aid organizations, such as the Red Cross. In this context, an international group of researchers in the field met to draw together suggestions for common research measures that could provide comparable core data so as to allow enough comparisons of findings from diverse disasters, with multiple stressors affecting multiple complex population groups (Raphael, Lundin, & Weisaeth, 1989).

A very important international development through this period involved the establishment of the International Society for Traumatic Stress Studies, which brought together passionate advocates and scientists dedicated to building the knowledge base, the integration of research findings with disaster planning and response. Indeed, these questions of the translation of research to practice and the translation of practice to research remain an issue even today, well exemplified in recent reports on response to mass terrorism events such as September 11th (Neria, Gross, Marshall, & Susser, 2006).

The wish to assist, the psychological impacts on those who were not direct victims, and the convergence of informal helpers, combined to make intervention a priority development. Concepts of psychological first aid and psychological debriefing (Raphael, 1977), counseling for these bereaved (Singh & Raphael, 1981), and psychotherapeutic outreach (Lindy, Green, Grace, & Titchener, 1983) were all implemented, but the limited evaluation highlighted the need for a more informed, systematic set of intervention strategies linked to assessment. However, the model developed by Jeffrey Mitchell (1983), Critical Incident Stress Debriefing, with its structured format for emergency services, was attractive in that it offered clear guidelines of what to do in the face of chaos and uncertainty. This became, as with the traumatic stress paradigm, the principal intervention modality postdisaster, used well beyond the framework for first responders for whom it was originally developed and, as with other disaster interventions described earlier, not subjected to the randomized controlled trial.

2.3. INTEGRATING RESEARCH INTO DISASTER RESPONSE

During the 1990s and beyond, a range of groups attempted to draw together what was known to guide planning and response. The WHO recognized the importance of developing guidelines for disasters as a whole, producing, with the support of researchers in the field, Psychosocial Guidelines for Preparedness and Intervention in Disaster (WHO, 1991). This represented an important contribution from such an authoritative body and gave emphasis to the psychosocial/mental health aspects of response. There was an emerging focus on the disasters and related trauma that occurred in different countries and continents. The *International Handbook of Traumatic Stress Studies* drew together a wide range of studies across nations and catastrophes, demonstrating the complexity and advances in this field, and addressing a more international approach (Wilson & Raphael, 1993). Other processes expanded the knowledge base about disaster mental health during the 1990s, including the increasing quality and numbers of publications such as those of the *Journal of Traumatic Stress* and the work of societies such as the European and International groups of Traumatic Stress Studies. The National Centers for Post Traumatic Stress Disorder and the Child Traumatic Stress Networks in the United States contributed significantly.

A number of studies and conceptualizations started to influence both research and response in the field. Diverse research contributing to the understanding of single disasters, such as the Buffalo Creek Disaster, demonstrated the chronicity of stress syndromes in such circumstances (Green et al., 1990), the range of mental health outcomes and social change, as well as the impact on children. Hurricane Andrew was extensively researched from psychiatric and sociological perspectives (Norris, Perilla, Riad, Kaniasty, & Lavizzo, 1999). Such studies reiterated the importance of social contexts, particularly, social bonds, and support and the buffering effects these may have in the face of adversity (Norris & Kaniasty, 1996). Cultural variables, as well as the background factors of poverty, conflict, and inequity, on which disasters may be superimposed, were increasingly recognized but not consistently researched. New models also became influential, for instance, Hobfoll's (1989) Conservation of resources theory. The volume *Individual and community responses to trauma and disaster: the structure of human chaos* drew together the available knowledge from multiple studies of trauma in workers and communities and integrated it into strategies for response (Ursano, McCaughey, & Fullerton, 1994).

Recognition of "natural" and "human-caused," or technological, disasters, plus their similar and dissimilar impacts was well established, but it was with the Oklahoma City bombing in 1995 that the focus on terrorism as disaster came to the fore. North's extensive studies, following this event, demonstrated the extent of population morbidity amongst survivors (North et al., 1999) and the coping and problems of rescue workers (North, Tivis, McMillen, Pfefferbaum, Cox, et al., 2002; North, Tivis, McMillen, Pfefferbaum Spitznagel, et al., 2002). Extensive studies after this incident highlighted the horrific impacts for children and young people in terms of psychological trauma and bereavement (e.g., Pfefferbaum et al., 1999). This built on the earlier work by Pynoos and colleagues (1987). In addition, studies demonstrated acute and long-term impacts on adults, first responders, and the population more broadly.

Terrorism as a growing reality meant a focus on prevention of such incidents and their mental health consequences, wherever possible, as with preparation for and prevention of natural and other disastrous hazards. There was a need to build on knowledge from other sources, such as chemical spills, naturally occurring epidemics, and nuclear and radiological incidents, such as Three Mile Island (e.g., Bromet, Parkinson, Shulberg, Dunn, & Gondek, 1982). The Sarin Gas Attack in Tokyo in 1995 (Ohbu, Yamashina, Takasu, & Yamaguchi, 1997) demonstrated the reality of chemical attacks and the massive psychosocial as well as physical impacts that they could produce, in the acute and long term, with traumatization and chronic health complaints. The particular implications of such agents for first responders also became a focus. The threat of biological agents of infectious disease was recognized, although there was little research data to inform response and understanding of psychosocial impacts, apart from aspects of HIV/AIDS studies on fear and stigma. Holloway et al. (1997) and DiGiovanni (1999) reviewed such threats and the possibility of mitigation. The notion of the Chemical, Biological, Radiological, and Nuclear (CBRN) terrorism threat built on these reviews in relation to explosive incidents such as bombings, which were for the most part viewed in terms of the psychological trauma of their impact.

Research exploring the factors of such variables that might affect mental health response and outcomes increasingly recognized the multiplicity of variables interacting in diverse ways. With the expansion of disaster research to encompass terrorism, work such as that of the WHO at a global level emphasized the threat of complex emergencies where "disaster" caused by natural events, such as earthquakes, may be superimposed on preexisting, ongoing conflict. Deprivations due to famine, refugee status, or failing states meant multiple ongoing traumatic and other stressors. Thus, the stressor impacts of acute natural disasters were likely to exacerbate many underlying population and individual vulnerabilities. Indeed, such chronic underlying and profound vicissitudes threatening ongoing survival of families and their communities might well be identified as slow disasters, their effects often insidious, uncontrollable. They provide continuing challenges quite different from single acute incidents. The HIV/AIDS epidemic in Africa would be one example of such catastrophe, as would the chronic conflicts in many states, famine, and population displacements, both internal and external.

2.4. THE NEW MILLENNIUM

With the dawning of the year 2000, there were further important research developments aimed, for the most part, at enhancing understanding, preparedness, and response. A number of themes have dominated this field in the new millennium.

2.4.1. Terrorism

Not only was there preparation and planning for potential cyber disasters around the arrival of the new millennium, but preparation to deal with potential terrorism and other disaster types became more scientifically based, evidence-informed, and consensus-driven. For instance, in preparation for the Sydney, Australia, Olympics in 2000, an evidence-based Mental Health Disaster Manual was developed to provide a basis for preparation, education, training, and response should a terrorist or other incident occur (Raphael, NSW Institute of Psychiatry, 2000). This was available online and subsequently extensively used in other international incidents. In late 2000, a consensus conference process was established by Ritchie (personal communication, 2000) to provide evidence-based guidelines for early intervention and response to mass violence. The final face-to-face meeting of this group occurred about 7 weeks after the September 11th terrorist attacks (http://www.nimh.nih.gov/publicat/massviolence.pdf).

The terrorist attacks of September 11, 2001, focused the world's attention on the impacts of such events, including the unpredictability and nature of the attack, which challenged the sense of personal and national invulnerabilities; the role of media and evolving technologies; the ongoing mental and physical health impacts; and the challenges to systems of response to deal with diverse threats and needs. Extensive research followed immediately, dealing with both population and individual mental health impacts with a national survey of stress reactions (Schuster et al., 2001), psychological reactions (Schlenger et al., 2002), a national longitudinal study of psychological responses (Silver, Holman, McIntosh, Poulin, & Gil-Rivas, 2002), psychological sequelae (Galea et al., 2002), and the impacts on children (Hoven et al., 2005) and emergency responders (Difede, Roberts, Jayasinghe, & Leck, 2006). Importantly, despite the shock of this attack, major efforts for outreach and systematic evidence-based interventions occurred and were subject to research and evaluation. The lessons and insights from the numerous research reports following September 11th have been drawn together in a valuable volume by Neria and colleagues (2006). Like other investigations of incidents, such honest reviews and "lessons learned" further inform future planning and response.

That terrorism would be a continuing theme of this decade was evident with the Bali bombing (October 2002), the Madrid bombing (March 2004), the London bombings (July 2005), and the extensive suicide bombings in the Middle East. Research following these incidents provided early indications of high levels of distress, with subsequent studies indicating that this decreased significantly over the following months, although, for some there were ongoing mental health effects, particularly PTSD. Galea, Nandi, and Vlahov (2005) have provided extensive research into the occurrence of PTSD post-disaster, incorporating work post-September 11th as well as major contributions from other settings, including the Madrid train bombings. Neria, Nandi, Arijit, and Galea's paper (2008) has also contributed significantly in expanding knowledge of PTSD after disaster.

The bereaved population has been poorly researched in recent catastrophes in terms of their needs, mental health impacts, and appropriate intervention strategies. Rubin and colleagues (2007) showed the continuing mental health consequences 7 months after the London bombings and the contributing influences of uncertainty and separation from loved ones. At the same time, the government report on "lessons learned" following this incident highlighted the need to provide better support for families who were bereaved and potentially bereaved at such times.

The experience of both trauma and grief and the need for interventions addressing both themes has been increasingly recognized (Litz, 2004; Raphael & Wooding, 2004). An outreach and intervention program after September 11th providing for family members of those killed in the attack showed the value of group support, as seen in other disasters, and the feasibility of a flexible and extensive clinical appraisal, which used the restorative retelling therapy model sessions (Rynearson, 2006) (Shahani & Trish, 2006). Therapeutic intervention with Australian survivors of the 2002 Bali bombings showed the need for outreach to be associated with practical support when needed and to be available over time when those affected were ready (Raphael, Dunsmore, & Wooding, 2004).

Such work with the bereaved needs to recognize the potential impacts of the earliest times where there can be uncertainty about the death, processes of victim identification, desperate searching for reunion with loved ones, lack of any "remains" of the dead persons, spontaneous memorializations, and alternating hope and dread. While resilience is common (Bonanno, 2004), it should not be assumed, and many may often appear resilient and later show delayed response. Complicated or prolonged grief may also appear and can be extensive and disabling, as demonstrated by Neria, Gross, and colleagues (2007). This may require specific interventions (Shear, Jackson, Essock, Donahue, & Felton, 2006).

2.4.2. Review: Taking Stock and Integrating What Is Known

Critical to building the science base to inform response has been a meta-analyses and synthesis in two reports by Norris and colleagues (Norris, Friedman, & Watson, 2002; Norris, Friedman, Watson, Byrne, & Kaniasty, 2002). These reviews showed that there were specific psychological problems, ranging from the symptom spectrum to the criteria for disorders such as PTSD, major depression, and anxiety disorders. Nonspecific distress, general health problems, chronic problems of living, resource loss, and problems particular to young people, particularly regressive problems for younger children and behavioral problems for older, were also noted amongst these findings. Impairment was more likely for those from developing countries and after mass violence as compared to natural or technological disasters. For adults, more severe exposure to stressors, secondary stresses, and diminishing psychosocial resources were associated with more adverse outcomes.

The implications for disaster mental health research were reviewed in the second report, which highlighted greater levels of vulnerability with some threats and some populations. The need for interventions focused on the family context was recognized and for interagency coordination and cooperation. The authors emphasized the importance of designing and testing community-level, population wide (i.e., universal) interventions, and focusing scarce clinical resources in those with greatest vulnerability, such as children, women, and those in developing countries.

Norris' next review (Norris, 2005) updated her findings over the range, magnitude, and duration of effects of disaster on mental health. These further samples were consistent with previous work indicating that impacts were worse in developing countries. PTSD was common (and was frequently the focus of study); however, like most mental health reactions, it decreased over time, although those disasters resulting from mass violence were more likely to be severe in their effects. As previously, these analyses showed that rescue and recovery workers were "likely to be resilient." Norris concluded that "the finding regarding the consequences of experiencing disaster caused by malicious human intent were unequivocal" (p. 11), and those affected were more likely to be severely or very severely impaired. Such findings highlight not only the vulnerabilities often associated with severe and enduring effects on mental health, but also more broadly the impacts on health behaviors, relationships, physical health, and so forth. They also clearly indicate that resilience is frequent, perhaps the norm.

The importance of understanding and addressing children's needs, particularly in family contexts, had been identified – as noted above – by many earlier reports. A valuable volume, *Helping children cope with disasters and terrorism* drew many of the studies in this field together (La Greca, Silverman, Vernberg, & Roberts, 2002). It provided an overview of key issues such as reactions and responses to and assessment and intervention models for natural disasters, human-caused and technological disasters, or acts of violence such as school shootings, hostage-taking, terrorism, war, and community violence. It concluded with emphasis on the development of evidence-based disaster mental health interventions and supportive public policy to address children's needs in such circumstances with emphasis on sustaining families and school environments.

The themes relevant to terrorism and particularly CBRN terrorism continued to strengthen over the early years of this decade. Ursano's group produced important contributions, first in terrorism and disaster generally (Ursano, Fullerton, & Norwood, 2003) and subsequently with the hallmark volume on *Bioterrorism: psychological and public health interventions* (Ursano, Norwood, & Fullerton, 2004). This text provided for the first time important contributions to understanding and building response capacity to this type of threat, potentially more psychologically damaging than other disasters. This was increasingly relevant in view of the potential for bioterrorism, as evidenced by the Anthrax attack after September 11th, possible pandemic influenza, and concerns about chemical, radiological, and nuclear attacks.

Theoretical conceptualization and research about the nature and impact of terrorism have been advanced by researchers such as Shalev (2006) who highlighted the need to extend understanding after incidents such as September 11th and also to explore resilience in the face of "continuous terrorism" as in Israel (Shalev, Tuval, Frenkiel-Fishman, Hadar, & Eth, 2006). A great many other valuable reports and volumes have been published highlighting not only the impacts of terrorism particularly (e.g., Danieli, Brom, & Sills, 2005) but also war and violence (de Jong, 2002).

2.5. INTERVENTIONS AND EARLY INTERVENTION

Interventions have been a focus of review in terms of current knowledge, effective models, and the need for research and evaluation of interventions that are provided. The chaos and uncertainty of the acute disaster setting means that the ideal of early intervention may be difficult to implement, and there may be serious constraints in terms of testing effectiveness through the standard model of the randomized controlled trial.

While there are significant numbers of more broadly based manuals (Cohen & Ahearn, 1980; Parad et al., 1976), as well as the Australian manual described earlier, there have been very few research studies evaluating these interventions. Some excellent, more recent publications have drawn together research relevant to comprehensive response (Ritchie, Watson, & Friedman, 2006; van Ommeren, Saxena, & Saraceno 2005; WHO, 2003). Several developing themes have progressively informed response in this period.

The debriefing model has tended to dominate early response. However, while the debriefing debate was heralded by strong conviction and extensive uptake of this model, this favor was also balanced by a growing number of studies showing that it was not effective for disaster-affected populations (Raphael & Wilson, 2000; Rose, Bisson, & Wessely, 2002). Indeed, the 2001 consensus conference on mass violence determined that the model was not appropriate for broadly affected disaster populations and that psychological first aid was a more suitable generic approach, meeting the standard of "first do no harm."

The concept of psychological first aid has been critically reviewed, and detailed guidelines have been developed through the National Child Traumatic Stress Network (www.nctsnet.org). These guidelines emphasize goals of engagement, safety and orientation, stabilization and self-regulation, and connectedness. Support empathy, information, comforting, and practical assistance are among such strategies. This emergency response process may lead to triage, processes of registration, follow-up, and linkage to services or outreach as required. Again, this concept needs to be empirically tested, but there are significant challenges for researchers seeking to conduct any randomized controlled trials in the early and acute postincident setting.

Early intervention was strongly recommended and supported both by the consensus process as well as a number of important edited publications presenting the work of experts in this field (Litz, 2004; Ritchie et al., 2006). For the psychological trauma component, the work of Bryant's (2000, 2003) group was significant, demonstrating the benefits in nondisaster settings of cognitive behavioral exposure therapies with those at risk of PTSD because of the presence of acute stress disorder. Phone and Internet or web-based approaches have extended this type of therapeutic intervention. Brief models have been used in postdisaster settings, such as that following the Turkish earthquake (Basoglu, Livanou, Salcioglu, & Kalender, 2003). There have also been clinical studies for pharmacotherapies as a model for early intervention, although effectiveness of these has not been established (Shalev & Ursano, 1998). An interesting development in early intervention is screening/Cognitive behavioral therapy (CBT) and exposure-based techniques using book formats for children to work through in school-based programs with response to natural disaster settings (McDermott, 2007; McDermott & Palmer, 2007) and others dealing with preparedness (Ronan & Johnston, 2005).

Long-term interventions have been chiefly focused on treatments for PTSD, often utilizing evidence-based guidelines such as those of the International Society for Traumatic Stress Studies (United States) (www.istss.org) and the National Institute for Health and Clinical Excellence (NICE) in the United Kingdom (http://www.nice.org.uk). There is a growing recognition of the difficulty of follow-up and outreach over time, the multiple social variables relevant to the recovery process, and the need to address these as well as the emerging mental health problems (Raphael & Wooding, 2006).

Despite these developments, there are many challenges for intervention only now being considered, as for instance with treating those injured as suggested and progressed in a stepped care model (Zatzick, 2003; Zatzick et al., 2004) linked to general hospital or medical care settings. Another challenge is that of medically unexplained physical symptoms (MUPS) that occur after threats such as CBRN and require triage, follow-up, and ongoing monitoring (Engel & Katon, 1999; Engel et al., 2003). Shalev (2007) has demonstrated the difficulties of delivering evidence-based early interventions aimed at those presenting with PTSD. As with the traumatized or bereaved in such devastating settings, establishing the evidence base is very difficult, as is the necessary translational research testing strategies established in nondisaster settings.

2.6. MASSIVE NATURAL DISASTERS

A number of overwhelming natural disasters have reinforced how extensive their impact may be on health, mental health, and survival. The South East Asian Tsunami of December 26, 2004, caused perhaps a quarter of a million deaths; the Kashmir/Pakistan earthquake of 2005 killed an estimated 54,000 people, and the death toll from Hurricane Katrina in 2005 was 1,464 (Louisiana Department of Health and Hospitals, 2006). All of these events had profound and prolonged effects, testing both response systems and the potential for recovery. The impacts in culturally diverse, conflict-affected (e.g., Sri Lanka, Aceh), and already vulnerable communities led to enormous human and economic costs. Mental health consequences from these disasters have been measured to some extent (Kessler, Galea, Jones, & Parker, 2006; Thienkrua et al., 2006), and it is clear that communities will be affected in ongoing ways. These major catastrophes drew a huge response from sources including nongovernment and international agencies and numerous diverse volunteers (both individuals and groups). These converging forces as well as internationally deployed medical and mental health resources that were provided in collaboration with affected regions highlight further logistics and systems issues. For instance, questions and disputes arise in terms of what training should be provided, what requirements have priority, what skills and resources should those offering assistance bring, and how may the responders engage effectively with the resources of the affected areas. The WHO Sphere Standards (WHO, 2007) have attempted to address these broad issues and have within them a mental health and psychosocial guideline component. Nevertheless, little is known about the effectiveness of such standards or how they may be evaluated. They have, however, been widely used as a basis for care, facilitating consistent response strategies.

2.7. THE RISE OF RESILIENCE

Resilience has long been recognized by trauma experts, though they acknowledge it may coexist with painful emotional scars. Resilience was present in survivors following tragedies such as Hiroshima and the Holocaust, and there has been a great renewal of interest in this phenomenon in terms of posttrauma outcomes, perhaps fueled by a number of findings, including the role of hope in positive outcomes (Carr et al., 1997; Henderson & Bostock, 1977) and the concept of posttraumatic growth (Tedeschi, Park, & Calhoun, 1998), recently demonstrated to co-occur with severe trauma experience in Hurricane Katrina (Kessler et al., 2006).

Also important are Bonanno's concepts of resilience involving those affected by loss or catastrophic events; he suggests that resilience means "to maintain relatively stable, healthy levels of psychological and physiological functioning" (Bonanno, 2004). He differentiates this concept from recovery, which occurs where there first was symptomatic response, describing trajectories for the patterns of response over time after September 11th (Bonanno, Galea, Bucciarelli, & Vlahov, 2006). In contrast, others working in this sphere consider resilience to be the tendency to bounce back (Connor, 2006).

While there have been attempts to operationalize and measure resilience, for instance, one or no symptoms of PTSD as suggested by Bonanno and colleagues (2006) or specific scales, such as Resilience Scale (Connor & Davidson, 2003), there remains a need to extend the concepts to domains beyond PTSD symptoms. Further aspects include the significant developmental issues relevant for children and adults (Luthar & Cicchetti, 2000), the time dimension, the possible biological correlates, and the differentiation of risk and resilience (Yehuda & Flory, 2007), as well as considerations of whether resilience in the individual is a state developed in response to a trauma stimulus or a "trait" that protects against trauma impacts.

Furthermore, there is an increasing recognition of societal resilience. Beyond the individual experience of trauma or risk of PTSD, mass events such as disasters and terrorism impact the society and the social fabric. Social support; the perceptions and delivery of social support; and the loss or preservation of social, physical, or institutional resources may impact societal resilience. Social connectedness is another variable of interest, as is social cohesion, which may be increased by the attachments and affiliative behaviors mobilized by the acute incident (Mawson, 2005). These positive acute societal responses – rather than the myth of panic – and the altruism, courage, leadership, and mobilization of community all suggest resilience. In addition, there is the growing awareness of the resilience associated with social capital (Kawachi & Berkman, 2001) and its influence in disaster (Nakagawa & Shaw, 2004). Societal resilience and its mobilization through universal interventions that promote the social institutions, safety, connectedness, and well-being of the community and individuals is an area of increasing interest as it is seen as important for community preparation to deal with terrorism or other mass catastrophe (Reissman et al., 2003).

Norris and colleagues (2008) have provided a very important analysis of community resilience in terms of "metaphor, theory, set of capacities and strategy for disaster readiness." From an extensive evaluation of the existing literature and from their own conceptualization, they set forth a model that identifies (1) economic development in terms of resource volume and diversity and resource equity and social vulnerability; (2) social capital in terms of network structures and linkages, social support, community bonds, roots, and commitments; (3) information and communication in terms of systems and infrastructure for informing the public, as well as communication and narrative; and (4) community competence in terms of collective action and decision making and the network of adaptive capacities. Drawing from their extensive research and experience with both disaster and terrorism, they identify the aspects of stress and stress resistance, resilience and adaption, and wellness as a manifestation of adaptation and psychological and population wellness. They highlight the dynamic aspects of resilience/resources, resource mobilization, and deterioration, and also discuss how the set of capacities identified may be further researched.

Resilience, as a strategy for disaster readiness, could be developed in terms of resource base and equity, engagement of local communities to access and build social capital, the organizational networks that can be mobilized for both surge and sustainability of systems, and the interventions that may help to boost and support social networks. Further, the critical role of flexibility, adaptative capacities, and leadership to deal with the diversity of potential threats are important considerations. It is clear that theory, conceptualization, and research are required to develop this field and its complex interfaces with disaster and terrorism response.

2.8. SYSTEMS FOR RESPONSE: LOCAL, NATIONAL, AND INTERNATIONAL

Effective, flexible systems of response to disaster are critical at all levels. However, there is increasing need for the development of principles for response and the provision of standards for education and training (Weine et al., 2002). There is an increasing international focus in this area, and WHO, UNICEF, World Psychiatric Association, and the World Federation for Mental Health are contributing to the effort. Nevertheless, given the diverse sectors and groups, including large numbers of NGOs and other aid agencies that converge on a traumatized locale after a disaster, it is vital that systems are in place to inform response and serve as "rules of engagement." It is also critical that there are systems for interaction and cooperation with affected nations and populations, that these incorporate a respect for the resilience and strengths of most affected populations, and that they ensure support to meet priority needs. The model developed by Norris and colleagues (2008), discussed in Section 2.7, is also helpful in this context.

As is evident in terms of the evolving understanding of disasters, the new threats they encompass, and their levels of complexity, preparation, and planning are essential. Such preparation and planning should be guided by principles that take into account the governance structures, systems, and organizations that would be involved or hold responsibilities in response efforts, as well as the resources, particularly in terms of workforce, that would be required. Systems of governance need to address such issues with their inherent accountabilities. Attendant challenges certainly lie in the unpredictability in the specific threats; however, risk appraisal processes, such as the monitoring of natural hazard vulnerabilities, are rapidly improving, as with the World Bank (2005) report, *Natural disaster hot spots: a global risk analysis*.

Systems for disaster planning and management traditionally deal with prevention, preparation and planning, response and recovery. They are focused on local, regional, and national needs, supported by formal plans, and frequently exercised to test these plans. They incorporate a legislative infrastructure that delineates command and control and the responsibilities of each agency involved; the plans frequently are implemented through various operating processes during the emergency phase. The WHO has developed a planning template for such emergency responses, known as the WHO AIMS-E (Assessment Instrument for Mental Health Services – Emergency). WHO AIMS-E emphasizes the need for coordination that engages key stakeholders; education and training for persons involved, including those in primary care and nongovernment settings; and systems of communication, information, and documentation. This model also proposes a disaster preparation plan for mental health for implemented in predisaster settings and a disaster response plan formulated and targeted to the specific incident. Mental health response must be situated in such planning processes, whether using the WHO AIMS-E model or another plan determined by the particular country or region (e.g., Flynn, 2007).

While most acute incidents will be chaotic initially – as is the very nature of disasters – structures of response that are flexible and can be adapted to specific need provide the best framework for effective action. The convergence of would-be helpers of every conceivable kind, the control (or lack thereof) of the disaster site, the assessment of impact and ongoing threat, the nature of the incident and any corresponding requirements for criminal and forensic investigation (e.g., as in a terrorist attack), all challenge mental health service provision, such as psychological first aid or early intervention. Similarly, the transition from the emergency state, the identification of those affected and at risk, and the targeting of outreach and follow-up all require formal integration of mental health into these systems (Raphael, 2008). To achieve this, mental health services must be valued as an effective and necessary component of the broader response and recovery.

2.8.1. Challenges for Mental Health Response

Challenges for mental health lie in several aspects of planned response systems. First, a key challenge to be met now and in the future is the active engagement of the mental health field with key responding agencies, from the earliest planning stages and throughout a disaster event. Mental health practitioners may collectively formulate their own plans for action in the face of disaster, but unless they engage with lead agencies during the planning phase as well as throughout the emergency, the role and effectiveness of mental health services will be severely limited. Collaboration may be difficult given that mental health systems are frequently separate and relatively peripheral to other health bodies, including those of emergency response and through to primary care.

A second challenge lies in the development, expertise, and "selling" of the role of mental health in providing effective interventions from the earliest stages. Mental health models have focused on individual or one-on-one care of those with established DSM or ICD disorders. In many settings, funding for services is dependent on such diagnostic precision. Most deal with those clients who have diagnosable psychiatric disorders rather than those who are distressed, vulnerable and at risk. Concepts of screening and the science to support effective early intervention are developing but will need strengthening.

Third, a further aspect of the necessary collaboration lies in building mental health capacity for leadership in developing new roles and managing the evolving complexities. This includes developing collaborations that will enhance the capacity of other diverse agencies to understand the importance of mental health and improve their knowledge and skills in areas such as psychological first aid. Mental health needs to work effectively with other areas of health from emergency services (Ruzek, Cordova, & Flynn, 2004), primary care systems (Engel et al., 2003), and specialty health systems to deal with the complexity of disaster response, including management of inpatient services for the injured (Zatzick, 2007), surge in CBRN incidents (Engel et al., 2007), and the long-term health impacts of MUPS. Such models of interaction need to include not only clinical services but also public health systems, which would be involved in a response to a biological threat such as pandemic influenza. In addition, such engagement needs to recognize the expertise of the collaborating agencies. Thus, mental health must foster creative population and clinical collaborations that will address prevention, early intervention, treatment, and recovery; that will recognize and build resilience; that will extend to all potential morbidity patterns, not just the focus of PTSD; and that will enhance mental health capacity beyond the disaster context.

Fourth, documentation systems, as well as information systems, are critical. All agencies need to provide consistent data on assessment, interventions, and other basic aspects of response. There is a need to link to local and national evaluation frameworks that will contribute to research and development in this field. Standard assessment tools are a critical component of this for mental health, yet there is little agreement or provision for these. Though standardization of measures can be difficult across diverse regions and nations, identification of some common core data requirements is critical. The challenge for mental health lies in effective, brief, critical information, and documentation systems (e.g., hand-held computing devices with relevant programs) to develop the databases essential for effective assessment, care, and evaluation.

A fifth challenge for mental health research is to establish levels of core knowledge, skills, and competencies for basic and advanced levels of response leadership and science and to translate these into effective educational programs. This moves the education and training of personnel well beyond the brief courses so often provided currently. How to build such capacity on top of the existing high demand in mental health services to care for the "seriously mentally ill" – as is usually the priority in the public sector – is a significant consideration. In addition, the cost framework for privately funded providers is another challenge, as indicated above. Programs need to build capacity that will be valuable in everyday work, engage with relevant systems – especially health care – and extend beyond the individual clinical interface to public/population health. In addition, there is the need for modules for specific threats including terrorism (CBRN) settings, just-in-time educational updates and briefings, and continuing professional education. These are very significant yet critical challenges for effective response.

While there are some reports (e.g., Raphael, 2000) addressing training needs, and there is a wide range of available courses, agreement about standards is limited. Weine and colleagues (2002) have developed some educational guidelines to inform international response. There are evidence-based guidelines for PTSD, as noted earlier, but disaster mental health needs extend much more widely. A consensus process in Australia has agreed on a three-level structure for training, the first level dealing with psychological first aid and general support, the second a higher level of competencies, and the third dealing with leadership, management, and other specific skills that might be used by an expert leadership team (Education and Training Consensus Conference, University of Western Sidney; August, 2006). One major contribution just released is the *Textbook of disaster psychiatry*, (Ursano, Fullerton, Weisaeth, & Raphael, 2007), which could provide core material for students in this field. This volume addresses disaster mental health; individual and community responses; epidemiology; impact on children; disaster ecology; neurobiology of disaster experience; clinical care interventions; special topics, including weapons of mass destruction and workplace and health-care system planning; and public health issues.

Finally, there are many emerging systems challenges, for instance, change mechanisms, workplace/workforce occupational mental health, emergency responders' service needs, family issues, and growing, changing systems engaged in disaster management. New technologies and new threats, such as cyber-terrorism, are also part of the picture. Climate change is another evolving factor that is likely to lead to significant system challenges and "tipping points," as well as mental health impacts. Continuous development of response capacity, risk assessment, and flexible, creative, future-focused paradigms are likely to be vital in addressing the potential for expanding, increasingly severe threats. Thus, key challenges for mental health involve engaging the future orientation and new demand contexts of planning and response and contributing to their development in positive ways.

2.9. THE SCIENCE OF DISASTER MENTAL HEALTH

Researchers across the globe have contributed to the expanding science of disaster mental health. There have been multiple studies focused on the stressor components, particularly those related to psychological trauma and PTSD. The epidemiology of "single incident" disasters and terrorism has been explored, and diverse investigations have been conducted across many different disasters and countries. Not only has traumatic stress been a focus of specific journals such as the *Journal of Traumatic Stress Studies*, but mainstream high-quality psychiatric journals, such as *Psychological Medicine*, *British Journal of Psychiatry*, *American Journal of Psychiatry*, and *Archives of General Psychiatry*, have all published research in this field. Physiological and biological issues are an increasing focus, chiefly with respect to PTSD; nevertheless, the science needs are broader than this, particularly given the complex threat and risk analyses associated with potential terrorist attacks. In this context, *Pre-Hospital and Disaster Medicine* is an important journal, particularly in its integration of mental health into the broad health field; for instance, this journal included a paper examining environmental contamination versus mass hysteria (Van de Auwera, Beckers, Devue, Claes, & De Cock, 2007) and a report on the gaps in mental health emergency preparedness (Hawley et al., 2007).

There has now been a number of important specific meta-analyses. Norris and colleagues' (2002) review of disaster mental health research suggests that "research demands that we think ecologically" (p. 240) and goes on to emphasize the need to "design and test societal- and community-level intervention for the population at large" (p. 240). Norris also extended earlier findings on the significance of violent human intent in contributing to more severe mental health impacts and the particular vulnerabilities of some populations, as well as the need to further develop research and methods to fill the gaps in knowledge (Norris, 2005). Norris, Galea, Friedman, and Watson (2006) reviewed the wide variety of research findings and methods; they noted that cross-sectional, postevent research, and small or convenience samples were common to that time, and that the longitudinal design, representative samples were less frequent but provided important data. They emphasized the fundamental value of sound epidemiological research but also noted that latent trajectory modeling and hierarchical linear modeling would be useful in view of the complexity of disasters. The book *Methods of disaster mental health research* (2006) represents an important contribution to this field.

2.9.1. The Challenges and Opportunities Ahead

There remain several important challenges to disaster mental health research. These range from biology to population health and from translational research findings to clinical care. They also encompass the need for research and evaluation systems linked to broader information systems to inform assessments, interventions, and outcomes. The complex domains of chemical, biological, and radiological/nuclear threats and their correspondingly complex biological and psychosocial impacts is emerging as a critical issue. Further, the epidemiology of the culture of fear and the changes this may bring in our society (Furedi, 2002), as well as the nature of risk perception, response to risk, and resilience in all its meanings are areas that need more nuanced understandings and are therefore receiving greater attention in this field.

The biology of postdisaster and posttraumatic morbidity is one area of major focus (Friedman & Pitman, 2007). The possibilities and potential for this field can be noted in advances in neurobiology, explorations of hypothalamic-pituitary-adrenocortical functional systems, technological enablement of brain imaging with fMRI and PET scanning, and greater understandings of early developmental impacts on children with linkages to subsequent disregulation. Vulnerability and resilience, gene–environmental interaction (Kendler & Baker 2007; Kilpatrick et al., 2007), and genetic epidemiology in disaster may also be future themes. The challenge for mental health lies in extending this research to meaningful strategies that might contribute to neuroprotection, neuroplasticity, and resilience (Luthar & Cicchetti, 2000) and that may make for pathways to prevention of PTSD and other posttrauma morbidity.

Measurement strategies are a necessary and increasing research focus in mental health (Sonis, King, King, Lauterbach, & Palmieri, 2007). Stressor components are poorly delineated and rarely consistently measured. The life threat inherent in risk for PTSD, the associated reactive phenomena, and the differing processes of grief have not been adequately investigated for their significance in the disaster setting, although some consistent strategies are evolving. Even though, as Norris (2005) has indicated, malevolent intent is associated with significantly poorer outcomes, there has been no systematic attempt to measure this stressor component and to identify the pathways by which it may make things worse, either psychologically or biologically. While there is emerging data on the negative impacts of complexity, multiple stressors, or the "tipping points" (Lopes et al., 2004; Lopes Cardoza, Vergara, Agani, & Gotway, 2000) of increasing numbers of traumatic events that may overwhelm resilience, frameworks for this are yet to be established. Herein, the field of disaster mental health must promote the development of agreed measures of stressor exposure, including those for life threat, loss, displacement, malevolent intent, as well as the CBRN's threat spectrum of uncertainty, uncontrollability, dread, and health fears.

The science of risk is increasingly relevant; some considerations include actual and perceived risk (Slovic, 1987) and risk as feelings (Lerner, Gonzalez, Small, & Fischhoff, 2003). The mechanisms of risk communication, the human factors influencing response, and short- and long-term risk are all relevant, as are the balancing perceptions of threat and safety. Perceived health risks (Maguire, 2007) are a particular issue with CBRN terrorist threats, as such health fears may have enduring consequences. Disaster mental health researchers must engage in cross-disciplinary risk research, drawing on the expertise of biological, psychological, and social parameters, and investigate the effectiveness of communication strategies in relation to risk.

As described in this chapter, resilience has become a significant issue, yet there is little agreed upon definition and operationalization of this concept at societal levels, although there are several measures of individual "resilience." Norris and colleagues' (2008) review is a major contribution in this context. Consensus on what resilience means is important, and disaster mental health practitioners must clarify whether it is realistic and scientifically sound to characterize it as simply the absence of posttraumatic pathology (Bonanno et al., 2006). While Yehuda and Flory (2007) are examining potential neurobiology of risk and resilience, there are also questions of how to recognize it when it is there, how not to damage it, and how to build/or facilitate it in scientifically sound and effective ways. In addition, it is likely that resilience coexists with problems of living or even with psychiatric disorder (Bleich, Gelkopf, & Solomon, 2003). A further important research theme lies in predisaster conditions and preparing communities and individuals to respond and be resilient in the face of disaster and terrorism (Reissman, Spencer, Tanielan, & Stein, 2003).

An important challenge for disaster mental health is to engage in longitudinal studies that will provide data on the potentially profound impacts of disaster on individual and broader societal development trajectories, especially in terms of how the effects of disasters overlay and interact with existing vulnerabilities and strengths. As commentaries and studies have shown, the challenge of such experiences may lead to personal growth and community renewal; there may be resilience, or there may be more negative effects that alter life opportunities or the potential for the society's development. It is important that researchers examine such changes over time at both individual and societal levels. This is particularly relevant for young children and adolescents, who are at the most vulnerable stage of development, biologically, psychologically, and socially, and for vulnerable populations in transition, including migrants, refugees, and those dealing with massive cultural and social change, such as rapid urbanization.

The field of disaster mental health still has much development to do in the way of a research strategy for both basic and translational research and for research of disaster mental health impacts, interventions, and outcomes. Studies of interventions in disaster contexts remain difficult in part because of the need for before-incident ethically approved study methodologies. Most existing trauma research focuses on PTSD, for instance, psychotherapy outcome research (Schnurr, 2007), but how effectively these modalities can be translated into disaster settings has not been established. Treatment integrity is a further issue in such translational studies, with emphasis on adherence, competence, therapeutic alliance, and outcomes (Barber, Triffelman, & Marmar, 2007). Issues include the systematic assessment of risk and protective factors and diverse impacts, also related is the need to estimate the capacity requirements for mental health services (Siegel, Wanderling, & Laska, 2004). Similarly, triage after terrorism, trauma, and mass casualty events needs further research and evaluation (Engel et al., 2007; Wessely, 2007). Large-scale studies are needed in the field of psychosocial aspects of CBRN threat to address risk, communication strategies, community engagement, and resilience and to gather good baseline data against which to measure program effectiveness (Gibson, Lemyre, Clement, Markon, & Lee, 2007). Shalev's (2006) comprehensive study of outcomes and the whole spectrum of need, treatment, and so forth as related to disaster and terrorism provides an important model that could be adapted to future research and evaluation in this field.

Indeed, the research opportunities in this field are enormous. Important contributions may involve new methodologies to deal with large data sets, innovations linking diverse as well as related research fields, and the utilization of emerging technologies to support research endeavors. Such options can be employed at molecular and nano-levels as well as at the population level and even on a global scale. Increasing urbanization, the growth of mega-cities, and increasing reliance on mass transport may mean greater devastation from disasters and terrorism. The evolution of communication and information technologies means that risk communication and risk amplification will require more comprehensive mental health engagement with such systems. In this regard, collective trauma (Somasundaram, 2005) is an important theme for the field to pursue. Research also has much to offer in terms of furthering understandings of the effects of the multilayering of stressors. Severe natural disasters, possibly caused by or superimposed on global warming should also be a priority area for the field. Understanding economic costs and "benefits" of catastrophes is another important domain (Greenberg, Lahr, & Mantell, 2007). Finally, the need for qualitative, quantitative, longitudinal, context-relevant, family and lifespan, societal, workgroup, and related studies indicate some of the multiplicities that will need to be addressed.

One of the most exciting examples of rising to such challenges is exemplified in Sheri Fink's (2007) "The science of doing good," in which she describes how information technology, satellite imaging, and research in disaster relief areas have contributed to improving the delivery and effectiveness of humanitarian aid, and within that, medical services. If such tools and technologies can make such a difference in the regions of developing environments affected by catastrophe and can also contribute to promote social justice and human rights, then there are important opportunities for mental health to utilize such models. These could include rapid response epidemiology, surveillance of mental heath risk, protective, and impact variables, as well as the use of social resource surveys and many other technologically supported initiatives. The challenge for the field going forward is to encourage enthusiasm, hope, and optimism to utilize new methods and new technologies in creative, innovative, and flexible ways to address the scientific and human challenges of disaster mental health.

REFERENCES

Abrahams, N. J., Price, J., Whitlock, F. A., & Williams, G. (1976). The Brisbane Floods, January 1974: Their impact on health. *Medical Journal of Australia, 2,* 936–939.

Adler, A. (1943). Neuropsychiatric complications in Victims of Boston's Coconut Grove Disaster. *Journal of the American Medical Association, 123,* 1098–1101.

Baker, G., & Chapman, D. (Eds.). (1962). *Man and society in disaster*. New York: Basic Books.

Barber, J., Triffelman, E., & Marmar, C. (2007). Considerations in treatment integrity: Implications and recommendations. *Journal of Traumatic Stress, 20*(5), 793–805.

Barton, A.H. (1969). *Communities in disaster: A sociological analysis of collective stress situations.* Garden City, New York: Doubleday.

Basoglu, M., Livanou, M., Salcioglu, E., & Kalender, D. (2003). A brief behavioural treatment of chronic post-traumatic stress disorder in earthquake survivors: Results from an open clinical trial. *Psychological Medicine, 33*(4), 647–654.

Bleich, A., Gelkopf, M., & Solomon, Z. (2003). Exposure to terrorism, stress-related mental health symptoms, and coping behaviors among a nationally representative sample in Israel. *Journal of the American Medical Association, 290*, 612–620.

Bonanno, G.A. (2004). Loss, trauma, and human resilience. *American Psychologist, 59*(1), 20–28.

Bonanno, G.A., Galea, S., Bucciarelli, A., & Vlahov, D. (2006). Psychological resilience after disaster: New York City in the aftermath of the September 11th terrorist attack. *Psychological Science: A Journal of the American Psychological Society, 17*(3), 181–186.

Bromet, E.J., Parkinson, D.K., Shulberg, H.C., Dunn, L.O., & Gondek, P.C. (1982). Mental health of residents near the Three Mile Island nuclear reactor: A comparative study of selected groups. *Journal of Preventive Psychiatry, 1*, 225–276.

Bryant, R.A., & Harvey, A.G. (2000). *Acute stress disorder: A handbook of theory, assessment and treatment.* Washington DC: American Psychological Association.

Bryant, R.A., Moulds, M.A., & Nixon, R. (2003). Cognitive behaviour therapy of acute stress disorder: A four-year follow-up. *Behaviour Research and Therapy, 41*, 489–494.

Carr, V.J., Lewin, T.J., Kenardy, J.A., Webster, R.A., Hazell, P.L., Carter, G.L., et al. (1997). Psychosocial sequelae of the 1989 Newcastle earthquake: III. Role of vulnerability factors in post-disaster morbidity. *Psychological Medicine, 27*, 179–190.

Carr, V.J., Lewin T.J., Webster, R.A., Hazell, P.L., Kenardy, J.A., & Carter, G.L. (1995). Psychosocial sequelae of the 1989 Newcastle earthquake. I. Community disaster experiences and psychological morbidity 6 months post-disaster. *Psychological Medicine, 25*, 539–555.

Cohen, R.E., & Ahearn, F.L. (1980). *Handbook of mental health care for disaster victims.* Baltimore, MD: John Hopkins University Press.

Connor, K.M. (2006). Assessment of resilience in the aftermath of trauma. *Journal of Clinical Psychiatry, 67*(Suppl. 2), 46–49.

Connor, K.M., & Davidson, J.R. (2003). Development of a new resilience scale: The Connor Davidson Resilience Scale (CD-RISC). *Depression and Anxiety, 18*, 76–82.

Danieli, Y., Brom, D., & Sills, J.B. (Eds.). (2005). *The trauma of terrorism: Sharing knowledge and shared care. An international handbook.* Binghamton, NY: The Haworth Press Inc.

de Jong, J. (2002). *Trauma, war and violence: Public mental health in sociocultural context.* New York: Klewer Academic/ Plenum Publishers.

Difede, J., Roberts, J., Jayasinghe, N., & Leck, P. (2006). Evaluation and treatment of firefighters and utility workers following the World Trade Center attacks. In Y. Neria, R. Gross, R. Marshall, & E. Susser (Eds.), *9/11 mental health in the wake of terrorist attacks.* New York: Cambridge University Press.

DiGiovanni, C. (1999). Domestic terrorism with chemical or biological agents: Psychiatric aspects. *American Journal of Psychiatry, 156*(10), 1500–1505.

Dynes, R.R. (1970). *Organized behavior in disaster.* Lexington, MA: Heath Lexington Books.

Eitinger, L. (1969). Psychosomatic problems in concentration camp survivors. *Journal of Psychosomatic Research, 13*, 183–189.

Engel, C.C., Jaffer, A., Adkins, J., Sheliga, V., Cowan, D., & Katon, W.J. (2003). Population-based health care: A model for restoring community health and productivity following terrorist attack. In R.J. Ursano, C.S. Fullerton, & A.E. Norwood (Eds.), *Terrorism and disaster: Individual and community mental health interventions.* New York: Cambridge University Press.

Engel, C. Jr., & Katon, W. (1999). Population and need-based prevention of unexplained physical symptoms in the community. In L.M. Joellenbeck, P.K. Russell, & S.B. Guze (Eds.). *Strategies to protect the health of deployed Us forces: medical surveilance, record keeping, and risk reduction* (pp. 173–212). Washington D.C.: National Academy Pr.

Engel, C.C., Locke, S., Reissman, D.B., DeMartino, R., Kutz, I., McDonald, M., et al. (2007). Terrorism, trauma, and mass casualty triage: How might we solve the latest mind-body problem? *Biosecurity and Bioterrorism: Biodefense Strategy, Practice, and Science, 5*(2), 155–163.

Erikson, K.T. (1976). Disaster at Buffalo Creek. Loss of communality at Buffalo Creek. *American Journal of Psychiatry, 133*(3), 302–305.

Fink, S. (2007). The science of doing good. *Scientific American Magazine, 29*(5), 98–106.

Flynn, B.W. (2007). Healthcare systems planning. In R.J. Ursano, C.S. Fullerton, L. Weisaeth, & B. Raphael (Eds.), *Textbook of disaster psychiatry.* Cambridge, UK: Cambridge University Press.

Frankl, V. (1984). *Man's search for meaning.* New York: Washington Square Books.

Friedman, M.J.J., & Pitman, R.K. (2007). New findings on the neurobiology of posttraumatic stress disorder. *Journal of Traumatic Stress, 20*(5), 653–655.

Furedi, F. (2002). *Culture of fear: Risk taking and the morality of low expectation*. London: Cassell.

Galea, S., Ahern, J., Resnick, H., Kilpatrick, D., Bucuvalas, M., Gold, J., et al. (2002). Psychological sequelae of the September 11 terrorist attacks in New York City. *New England Journal of Medicine, 346*, 982–987.

Galea, S., Nandi, A., & Vlahov, D. (2005). The epidemiology of post-traumatic stress disorder after disasters. *Epidemiologic Reviews, 27*, 78–91.

Gibson S., Lemyre, L., Clement, M., Markon, M. P. L., & Lee, J. E. C. (2007). Terrorism threats and Preparedness in Canada: The perspective of the Canadian public. *Biosecurity and Bioterrorism: Biodefense, Practice, and Science, 5*(2),134–144.

Gleser G. C., Green, B. L., & Winget, C. N. (1978). Quantifying interview data on psychic impairment of disaster survivors. *Journal of Nervous and Mental Disease, 166*, 209–216.

Green, B. L., Lindy, J. D., Grace, M. C., Gleser, G. C., Leonard, A. C., Korol, M., et al. (1990). Buffalo Creek survivors in the second decade: Stability of stress symptoms. *American Journal of Orthopsychiatry, 60*, 43–54.

Greenberg, M. R., Lahr, M., & Mantell, N. (2007). Understanding the economic costs and benefits of catastrophes and their aftermath: A review and suggestions for the U.S. federal government. *Risk Analysis, 27*(1), 83–96.

Hawley, S. R., Hawley, G. C., Ablah, E., St Romain, T., Molgaard, C. A., & Orr, S. A. (2007). Mental health emergency preparedness: The need for training and coordination at the state level. *Prehospital and Disaster Medicine, 22*(3), 199–204.

Henderson, S., & Bostock, T. (1977). Coping behaviour after shipwreck. *British Journal of Psychiatry, 131*, 15–20.

Hobfoll, S. E. (1989). Conservation of resources. A new attempt at conceptualizing stress. *American Psychologist, 44*, 513–524.

Holloway, H. C., Norwood, A. E., Fullerton, C. S., Engel, C. C., & Ursano, R. J. (1997). The threat of biological weapons: Prophylaxis and mitigation of psychological and social consequences. *Journal of the American Medical Association, 278*(5), 425–427.

Horowitz, M. J. (1976). *Stress response syndromes*. New York: Jason Aronson.

Hoven, C. W., Duarte, C. S., Lucas, C. P., Wu, P., Mandell, D. J., Renee D., et al. (2005). Psychopathology among New York City public school children 6 months. *Archive of General Psychiatry, 62*, 545–551.

Jones, D. R. (1985). Secondary disaster victims: Emotional effects of recovering and identifying human remains. *American Journal of Psychiatry, 142*(3), 303–307.

Kawachi, I., & Berkman, L. F. (2001). Social ties and mental health. *Journal of Urban Health, 78*(3), 458–467.

Kendler, K. S., & Baker, J. H. (2007). Genetic influences on measures of the environment: A systematic review. *Psychological Medicine, 37*(5), 615–626.

Kessler, R. C., Galea, S., Jones, R. T. & Parker, H. A. (2006). Mental illness and suicidality after Hurricane Katrina. *Bulletin of the World Health Organization, 84*(12), 930–931.

Kilpatrick, D. G., Koenen, C. K., Ruggiero, K. J., Acierno, R., Galea, S., Resnick, H. S., et al. (2007). The serotonin transporter genotype and social support and moderation of post-traumatic stress disorder and depression in hurricane-exposed adults. *American Journal of Psychiatry, 164*, 1693–1699.

Kingston, W., & Rosser, R. (1974). Disaster: Effects on mental health and physical state. *Journal of Psychosomatic Research, 18*, 437–456.

Krystal, H., & Niederland, W. (1968). Clinical observations on the survivor syndrome. In H. Krystal (Ed.), *Massive psychic trauma*. New York: International Universities Press.

La Greca, A. M., Silverman, W. S., Vernberg, E. M., & Roberts, M. C. (Eds.) (2002). *Helping children cope with disasters and terrorism*. Washington, DC: American Psychological Association.

Lerner, J. S., Gonzalez, R. M., Small, D. A., & Fischhoff, B. (2003). Effects of fear and anger on perceived risks of terrorism: A national field experiment. *Psychological Science, 14*, 144–150.

Lifton, R. (1967). *Death in life, survivors of Hiroshima*. New York: Random House.

Lindemann, F. (1944). Symptomatology and management of acute grief. *American Journal of Psychiatry, 101*, 141–148.

Lindy, J. D, Green, B. L., Grace, M., & Titchener, J. (1983). Psychotherapy with survivors of the Beverly Hills Supper Club fire. *American Journal of Psychotherapy, 37*, 593–610.

Litz, B. T. (Ed.) (2004). *Early intervention for trauma and traumatic loss*. New York: The Guilford Press.

Logue, J. N., Hansen, H., & Struening, E. (1979). Emotional and physical distress following Hurricane Agnes in Wyoming Valley of Pennsylvania. *Public Health Reports, 94*, 495–502.

Lopes Cardoza, B., Bilukha, O., Gotway Crawford, C., Shaikh, I., Wolfe, M., Gerber, M., et al. (2004). Mental health, social functioning, and disability in postwar Afghanistan. *Journal of American Medical Association (Reprinted), 292*(5), 575–584.

Lopes Cardoza, B., Vergara, A., Agani, F., & Gotway, C. (2000). Mental health, social functioning, and attitudes of Kosovar Albanians following the war in Kosovo. *Journal of American Medical Association (Reprinted), 284*(5), 569–577.

Louisiana Department of Health, and Hospitals. (2006). *Reports of Missing and Deceased.*

Luthar, S., & Cicchetti, D. (2000). The construct of resilience: Implications for interventions and social policies. *Development and Psychopathology, 12,* 857–885.

McDermott, B.M. (2007). *Screening and intervention following cyclone Larry.* Paper presented at the Psychosocial Response and Recovery Conference, Brisbane, Queensland, November 3, 2007.

McDermott, B.M., & Palmer, L. J (2002). Post disaster emotional distress, depression and event-related variables: Findings across child and adolescent developmental stages. *Australian and New Zealand Journal of Psychiatry, 36*(6), 754–761.

McFarlane, A. (1988). The longitudinal course of posttraumatic morbidity. The range of outcomes and their predictors. *The Journal of Nervous and Mental Disease, 176*(1), 30–39.

Maguire, P. (2007). PhD research program, Australian National University.

Mawson, A.R. (2005). Understanding mass panic and other collective responses to threat and disaster. *Psychiatry, 68*(2), 95–113.

Milne, G. (1977). Cyclone Tracy: The effects on Darwin children. *Australian Psychologist, 12,* 55–62.

Mitchell, J.T. (1983). When disaster strikes.... The critical incident stress debriefing process. *Journal of Emergency Medical Services, 8*(1), 36–39.

Nakagawa, Y., & Shaw, R (2004). Social capital: a missing link to disaster recovery. *International Journal of Mass Emergencies and Disasters, 22*(1), 5–34.

Neria, Y., Gross, R., Marshall, R.D., & Susser, E.S. (Eds.). (2006). *9/11: Mental health in the wake of terrorist attacks.* New York: Cambridge University Press

Neria, Y., Gross, R., Litz, B., Maguen, S., & Insel, B. (2007). Prevalence and psychological correlates of complicated grief among bereaved adults 2.5–3.5 years after September 11th attacks. *Journal of Traumatic Stress, 20*(3), 251–262.

Neria, Y., Nandi, Arijit, N., & Galea, S. (2008). Posttraumatic stress disorder after disasters: A systematic review. *Psychological Medicine, 38*(4), 1–14.

Norris, F.H. (2005). *Range, magnitude, and duration of the effects of disasters on mental health: Review update 2005.* Dartmouth: Dartmouth Medical School and National Center for Posttraumatic Stress Disorder.

Norris, F., & Kaniasty, K. (1996). Received and perceived social support in times of stress: A test of the social support deterioration deterrence model. *Journal of Personality and Social Psychology, 71,* 498–511.

Norris, F., Galea, S., Friedman, M.J., & Watson, P.J. (Eds.). (2006). *Methods of disaster mental health research.* New York: The Guilford Press.

Norris, F., Perilla, J., Riad, J., Kaniasty, K., & Lavizzo, E. (1999). Stability and change in stress, resources, and psychological distress following natural disaster: Findings from Hurricane Andrew. *Anxiety, Stress and Coping, 12,* 363–396.

Norris, F., Friedman, M., & Watson, P. (2002). 60,000 disaster victims speak, Part II: Summary and implications of the disaster mental health research. *Psychiatry, 65,* 240–260.

Norris, F.H., Friedman, M.J., Watson, P.J., Byrne, C., & Kaniasty, K. (2002). 60,000 disaster victims speak, Part I. An empirical review of the empirical literature: 1981–2001. *Psychiatry, 65,* 207–239.

Norris, F.H., Stevens, B., Pfefferbaum, Wyche, R. & Pfefferbaum, B. (2008). Community resilience as a metaphor, theory, set of capacities, and strategy for disaster readiness. *American Journal of Community Psychology, 41,* 127–150.

North, C.S., Nixon, S.J., Shariat, S., Mallonee, S., McMillen, J.C., Spitznagel, E.L., et al. (1999). Psychiatric disorders among survivors of the Oklahoma City Bombing. *Journal of the American Medical Association, 282*(8), 755–762.

North, C.S., Tivis, L., McMillen, J.C., Pfefferbaum, B., Cox, J., Spitznagel, E.L., et al. (2002). Coping, functioning and adjustment of rescue workers after the Oklahoma City bombing. *Journal of Traumatic Stress, 15*(3), 755–762.

North, C.S., Tivis, L., McMillen, J.C., Pfefferbaum, B., Spitznagel, E.L., Cox, E.L., et al. (2002). Psychiatric disorders in rescue workers after the Oklahoma City bombing. *American Journal of Psychiatry, 159*(5), 857–859.

Ohbu, S., Yamashina, A., Takasu, N., & Yamaguchi, T. Sarin poisoning on Tokyo subway. *Southern Medical Journal, 90*(6), 587–593.

Ochberg, F.M., & Soskis, D.A. (1982). *Victims of Terrorism.* Boulder, CO: Westview

Parad, H.J., Resnick, H.L.P., & Parad, L.G. (Eds.). (1976). *Emergency and disaster management: A mental health sourcebook.* Bowie, MD: Charles Press.

Pfefferbaum, B., Nixon, S., Tucker, P., Tivis, R., Moore, V., Gurwitch, R.H., et al. (1999). Posttraumatic stress responses in bereaved children after the Oklahoma City bombing. *Journal of the American Academy of Child and Adolescent Psychiatry, 38,* 1372–1379.

Pynoos, R. S., Frederick, C., & Nader, K. (1987). Life threat and posttraumatic stress in school-age children. *Archives of General Psychiatry, 44*, 1057–1063.

Quarantelli, E. (1954). The nature and conditions of panic. *American Journal of Sociology, 60*, 267–275.

Raphael, B. (1977). The Granville train disaster: Psychological needs and their management. *Medical Journal Australia, 1*, 303–305.

(1986). *When disaster strikes: how individuals and communities cope with catastrophe.* New York: Basic Books.

(2000). *NSW mental health disaster manual.* Sydney: Institute of Psychiatry.

Raphael, B., Lundin, T., & Weisaeth, L. (1989). A research method for the study of psychological and psychiatric aspects of disaster. *Acta Psychiatrica Scandinavia 80*(Suppl. 353), 1–75.

Raphael, B., Dunsmore, J., & Wooding, S. (2004). Terror and trauma in Bali: Australia's mental health response. *Journal of Aggression, Maltreatment and Trauma, 9*(2), 245–256.

Raphael, B., & Wilson, J. (Eds.). (2000). *Psychological Debriefing: Theory, Practice and Evidence.* London: Cambridge University Press

Raphael, B., & Wooding, S. (2004). Early mental health interventions for traumatic loss in adults. In B. Litz, (Ed.). *Early intervention for trauma and traumatic loss.* New York: Guilford Press.

(2006). Longer term interventions. In E. Ritchie, T. Watson, & M. Friedman (Eds.), *Interventions following mass violence and disasters.* New York: Guilford Press.

Raphael, B. (2008). Systems, science and populations effective early mental health intervention following mass trauma: the roles of government, clinicians & communities. In M. Blumenfield & R. Ursano (Eds.), *Intervention and resilience after mass trauma.* Cambridge UK: Cambridge University Press.

Reissman, D., Spencer, S., Tanielan, T., & Stein, B. (2003). Integrating behavioral aspects into community preparedness and response systems. In Y. Danieli, D. Brom, & J. B. Sills (Eds.), *The trauma of terror: sharing knowledge and shared care.* Binghamton, NY: The Howarth Press.

Ritchie, E., Watson, T., & Friedman, M. (2006). *Interventions following mass violence and disasters.* New York: Guilford Press.

Ronan, K., & Johnston, D. (2005). *Promoting community resilience in disasters: the role for schools, youth, and families.* New York. Springer

Rose, S., Bisson, J., & Wessely, S. (2002). Psychological debriefing for preventing posttraumatic stress disorder (PTSD). *The Cochrane Database of Systematic Review, 3*, CD000560.

Rubin, G. J. (2007). Enduring consequences of terrorism: 7-month follow-up survey of reactions to the bombings in London on 7 July 2005. *The British Journal of Psychiatry, 190*, 350–356.

Ruzek, J. I. J., Cordova, M. J., & Flynn, B. W. (2004). Integration of disaster mental health services with emergency medicine (Review). *Prehospital & Disaster Medicine, 19*(1), 46–53.

Rynearson, E. K., (Ed.). (2006). *Violent death: resilience and intervention beyond crisis.* New York: Routledge, Taylor & Francis Group.

Schlenger, W. E., Caddell, J. M., Ebert, L., Jordan, B. K. M., Wilson, D., Thalji, L., et al. (2002). Psychological reactions to terrorist attacks: Findings of the National Study of Americans' Reactions to September 11. *Journal of the American Medical Association, 288*, 1235–1244.

Schnurr, P. (2007). The rocks and hard places in psychotherapy outcome research. *Journal of Traumatic Stress, 20*(5), 779–792.

Schuster, M. A., Stein, B. D., Jaycox, L. H., Collins, R. L., Marshall, G. N., Elliott, M. N., et al. (2001). A national survey of stress reactions after the September 11, 2001, terrorist attacks. *The New England Journal of Medicine, 345*(20), 1507–1512.

Shahani, P. J., & Trish, H. M. (2006). Healing after September 11: Short-term group intervention with 9/11 families. In E. K. Rynearson, (Ed.), *Violent death: resilience and intervention beyond the crisis.* New York: Routledge, Francis Taylor Group.

Shalev, A. (2006). Lessons learned from 9/11: The boundaries of a mental health approach to mass casualty events. In Y. Neria, R. Gross, R. D. Marshall, & E. Susser (Eds.), *9/11 mental health in the wake of terrorist attacks.* Cambridge, UK: Cambridge University Press.

Shalev, A., & Ursano, R. (1998). Mapping the multidimensional picture of acute responses to traumatic stress. In U. Schneider, (Ed.), *Early intervention for psychological trauma.* Oxford: Oxford University Press.

Shalev, A., Tuval, R., Frenkiel-Fishman, S., Hadar, H., & Eth, S. (2006). Psychological responses to continuous terror: A study of two communities in Israel. *American Journal of Psychiatry, 163*, 667–673.

Shalev, A. (2007). Terrorism and Its Mental Health Impacts; Impacts and Management; Resilience, Trauma and Long Term: *Presentation at Terrorism: Human Factors and Response Workshop.* 26 November, 2007, Sydney, Australia.

Shear, K., Jackson, C. T., Essock, S. M., Donahue, S. A., & Felton, C. J. (2006). Screening for complicated grief among Project Liberty service recipients 18 months after September 11, 2001. *Psychiatric Services, 57*, 1291–1297.

Shore, J., Tatum, E., & Vollmer, W.M. (1985). Psychiatric findings of Mount St. Helen's disaster. Paper presented at 138th Annual Meeting of the American Psychiatric Association, Dallas, Texas, May 18–24, 1985.

Siegel, C., Wanderling, J., & Laska, E. (2004). Coping with disasters: Estimation of additional capacity of the mental health sector to meet extended service demands. *Journal of Mental Health Policy and Economics*, *7*(1), 29–35.

Silver, R.C., Holman, A., McIntosh, D.N., Poulin, M., & Gil-Rivas, V. (2002). Nationwide longitudinal study of psychological responses to September 11. *JAMA*, *288*, 1235–1244.

Singh, B., & Raphael, B. (1981). Post disaster morbidity of the bereaved. A possible role for preventive psychiatry. *Journal of Nervous and Mental Disease*, *169*(4), 203–212.

Slovic, P. (1987). Perception of risk. *Science*, *236*(4799), 280–285.

Somasundaram D. (2005). Short and long term effects on the victims of terror in Sri-Lanka. In Y. Danieli, D. Brom, J. Sills (Eds.), *The trauma of terrorism*. Binghampton, NY: The Haworth Maltreatment and Trauma Press.

Sonis, J., King, D.W., King, L.A., Lauterbach, D., & Palmieri, P. (2007). Innovations in trauma research methods. *Journal of Traumatic Stress*, *20*(5), 775–777.

Taylor, A.J., & Frazer, G. (1982). The stress of post-disaster body handling and victim identification work. *Journal Human Stress*, *8*(4), 4–12.

Tedeschi, R.G., Park, C.L., & Calhoun, L.G. (1998). Posttraumatic growth: conceptual issues. In R.G. Tedeschi, C.L. Park, & L.G. Calhoun (Eds.), *Posttraumatic growth. Positive changes in the aftermath of crisis*. Mahwah. NJ: Erlbaum.

Thienkrua, W., Lopes Cardozo, B., Chakkraband, M.L.S., Guadamuz, T., Pengjuntr, W., Tantipiwatanaskul, P., et al. (2006). Symptoms of posttraumitc stress disorder and depression among children in tsunami-affected areas in Southern Thailand. *JAMA*, *296*(5), 549–559.

Titchener, J.L., Kapp, F.T., & Winget, C. (1976). The Buffalo Creek Syndrome symptoms and character change after a major disaster. In J.H. Parad, H.L.P. Resnick, & L.P. Parad (Eds.), *Emergency and disaster management: a mental health sourcebook*. Bowie Maryland: Charles Press.

Tyhurst, J.S. (1951). Individual reactions to community disaster: The natural history of psychiatric phenomena. *American Journal of Psychiatry*, *107*(10), 764–769.

Ursano, R.J., Fullerton, C.S., & Norwood, A.F. (Eds.). (2003). *Terrorism and disaster: Individual and community mental health interventions*. Cambridge, UK: Cambridge University Press.

Ursano, R.J., Fullerton, C.S., Weisaeth, L., & Raphael, B. (Eds.). (2007). *Textbook of disaster psychiatry*. Cambridge UK: Cambridge University Press.

Ursano, R.J., McCaughey, B.G., Fullerton, C.S. (1994). *Individual and community responses to trauma and disaster: The structure of human chaos*. Cambridge UK: Cambridge University Press.

Ursano, R.J., Norwood, A.E., & Fullerton, C.S. (Eds.). (2004). *Bioterrorism: Psychological and public health interventions*. Cambridge UK: Cambridge University Press.

Van der Auwera, M., Beckers, R., Devue, K., Claes, P., & Der Cock, A. (2007). Presumed mass illness following a pyridine fumes incident: Environmental contamination versus mass hysteria. *Prehospital Disaster Medicine*, *22*(2), 140–143.

van Ommeren, M., Saxena, S., & Saraceno, B. (2005). Mental and social health during and after acute emergencies: Emerging consensus? *Bulletin of the World Health Organisation*, *83*, 71–75.

Weine, S., Danieli, Y., Silove, D., Van Ommeren, M., Fairbank, J.A., & Saul, J. (2002). Guidelines for international training in mental health and psychosocial interventions for trauma exposed populations in clinical and community settings. For the Task Force on International Trauma Training of the International Society For Traumatic Stress Studies. *Psychiatry*, *65*(2), 156–163.

Weisaeth, L. (1989). A study of behavioural responses to an industrial disaster. *Acta Psychiatrica Scandinavia*, *355*, 13–24.

Wessely, S. (2007). Commentary on "Terrorism, trauma, and mass casualty triage". *Biosecurity and Bioterrorism: Biodefense Strategy, Practice, and Science*, *5*(2), 164–167.

Wilson, J., & Raphael, B. (1993). *Handbook of traumatic stress studies*. New York: Plenum.

Wolfenstein, M. (1957). *Disaster: A psychological essay*. Glencoe, Il: Free Press.

World Bank. (2005). *Natural disaster hotspots: A global risk analysis*. Washington, DC: World Bank Group.

World Health Organization. (1991). *Psychosocial guidelines for preparedness and intervention in disaster*. Geneva: World Health Organization.

(2003). *Mental health in emergencies*. Geneva, Switzerland: World Health Organization, department of Mental Health and Substance Dependence.

(2007). *Benchmarks, standards and indicators for emergency preparedness response*. New Delhi, India: World Health Organization, Regional Office for South-East Asia.

Yehuda, R., & Flory, J.D. (2007). Differentiating biological correlates of risk, Posttraumatic Stress Disorder, and resilience following trauma exposure. *Journal of Trauma Stress*, *20*(4), 435–447.

Yule, W., & Williams, R. (1990). Post-traumatic stress reactions in children. *Journal of Traumatic Stress*, *3*(2), 279–295.

Zatzick, D. (2003). Posttraumatic stress, functional impairment, and service utilization after injury: A public health approach. *Seminars in Clinical Neuropsychiatry*, *8*, 149–157.

(2007). Intervention for acutely injured survivors of individual and mass trauma. In R. J. Ursano, C. S. Fullerton, L. Weisaeth, & B. Raphael (Eds.), *Textbook of Disaster Psychiatry*. Cambridge, UK: Cambridge University Press.

Zatzick, D., Roy-Byrne, P., Russo, J., Rivara, F., Droesch, R, Wagner, A., et al. (2004). A randomized effectiveness trial of stepped collaborative care for the acutely injured trauma survivors. *Archives of General Psychiatry*, *61*, 498–506.

3 The Experience of Disaster: Trauma, Loss, Adversities, and Community Effects

FRAN H. NORRIS AND LESLIE H. WIND

3.1. INTRODUCTION

Exposure to disaster is an inherently complex, multifaceted phenomenon. In some cases it begins even before the disaster strikes and in most cases concludes months or years later. It encompasses objective, observable stressors and subjective beliefs about cause, effect, and response. Exposure may be direct, entailing personal loss, or indirect because of shared community damage, disruption, or threat. In this chapter, we will consider the various ways in which people experience disasters acutely and persistently, objectively and subjectively, personally and collectively. We have organized these experiences into categories of traumatic stressors, loss, ongoing adversities, and community effects and meanings. We do not attempt to provide a comprehensive review of the literature but rather highlight selected studies that illustrate these aspects of disaster exposure and their consequences.

3.2. TRAUMATIC STRESSORS

Disasters are, by definition, potentially traumatic events that have acute onset and are collectively experienced (McFarlane & Norris, 2006). By classifying these events as potentially traumatic, we acknowledge the potential of disasters to engender situations where people are confronted with threats to life or bodily integrity and are likely to experience intense fear, horror, or helplessness (American Psychiatric Association, 1994). The importance of terror and horror as crucial elements of disaster exposure has been recognized for quite some time. As Bolin (1985) noted, these elements derive from exposure to the raw physical power of the disaster. Major earthquakes, hurricanes, bombings, and many other agents of disaster cause sudden and sometimes unimaginable levels of destruction. In this section, we explore the most acutely severe and personally traumatic aspects of disaster exposure: loss of life and traumatic bereavement; threat to life, injury, and fear; and witnessing of horror.

3.2.1. Loss of Life and Traumatic Bereavement

In the worst disasters, people die. The death tolls of some disasters have been profound: over 1,200 in Hurricane Katrina (2005), over 3,000 in the September 11th terrorist attacks (2001), 18,000 in Hurricane Mitch (1998), 25,000 in the Spitak, Armenia, earthquake (1988), 280,000 in the Southeast Asia tsunami (2004). Widespread bereavement and concomitant grief are perhaps the saddest effects of such catastrophic disasters.

Disasters characterized by high mortality are likely to yield substantial psychological morbidity. In their meta-analysis of 31 controlled disaster studies (part of a larger review of 52 studies), Rubonis and Bickman (1991) found that the number of deaths caused by the disaster was strongly associated with psychopathology, uniquely explaining 20% of the variance in the disaster's effect size across studies, with methodology and other study characteristics controlled in the analysis. They noted that high mortality may increase the prevalence of psychological problems because bereavement is added to other disaster-related stressors and may indicate that more surviving victims were threatened by death themselves.

The direct effects of bereavement have been documented in several specific studies, including Gleser, Green, and Winget's (1981) classic study of the 1972 Buffalo Creek dam collapse. Over the course of a few hours, 125 people in this rural area died, approximately 1,000 persons were injured and 4,000 were left homeless. No participant in this study was untouched by the loss of life; 35% lost close friends and 26% lost family members. Two years after the dam collapse, two-thirds of the 380 adults and one-third of the 273 children were evaluated as moderately or severely impaired, with generalized anxiety disorder (60% among adults, 20% among children) and major depressive disorder (70%, 25%) the most prevalent disorders. Many years later, these data were reanalyzed for probable posttraumatic stress disorder (PTSD), which had not been a Diagnostic and Statistical Manual of Mental Disorders (DSM) diagnosis at the time of the original study (Green et al., 1990). The prevalence of PTSD at 2 years was 44% among adults and 32% among children. Those who lost close friends or family members showed higher levels of psychopathology than did persons who lost acquaintances or possessions only.

Similarly, Murphy (1984) examined the effects of bereavement caused by the Mount St. Helens volcanic eruption. Eleven months after the eruption, bereaved persons scored more highly on measures of depression, somatization, and "hassles" (ongoing minor stressors) than controls or property-loss groups. The 39 persons whose loved ones were presumed dead differed little from the 30 persons whose loved ones were confirmed dead.

There is some evidence that bereavement is more closely linked to postdisaster depression than to PTSD, but other studies provide contradictory results. In a study of 1,027 treatment-seeking disaster survivors assessed, on average, 14 months after the 1999 earthquake in Turkey, loss of a family member was predictive of depression but not PTSD in multivariate models that controlled for other disaster experiences and participant characteristics (Livanou, Basoglu, Salcioglu, & Kalender, 2002). Galea and colleagues (2002) reported similar results from their study of 1,008 Manhattan residents 5 to 8 weeks after the September 11, 2001, terrorist attacks on the World Trade Center. In multivariate analyses, having had a friend or relative killed was associated with depression but not with PTSD. Eighteen percent of the bereaved adults met criteria for probable depression compared with 9% of others. However, Neria and colleagues (2008) presented conflicting results. In a systematic sample of 929 adult primary care patients, over one-fourth reported that they knew someone who died in the September 11th attacks. These persons were twice as likely as others to meet clinical criteria for at least one mental disorder (e.g., major depressive disorder, generalized anxiety disorder, and/or PTSD) and, controlling for trauma prior to the attacks, to report pain that resulted in interference in daily activities, loss of work, and functional impairment related to social and family life. Although the prevalence of major depression (29%) was higher than the prevalence of PTSD (17%) in the bereaved group, bereavement (vs. no bereavement) was more strongly related to PTSD (OR = 2.6) than to depression (OR = 1.8).

Neria and colleagues (2007) theorized that sudden death because of extreme acts of violence, such as terrorism or war, might cause additional strain on the natural course of grief. Using a Web-based survey, they studied long-term grief reactions in a sample of 704 bereaved adults 2.5 to 3.5 years after the September 11th terrorist attacks. Complicated grief was often comorbid with depression and PTSD but formed a distinct syndrome. Nearly all of the participants reported one or more current complicated grief symptoms, and 43% met study criteria for complicated grief. Yearning for the deceased and preoccupation with thoughts about the deceased were especially prevalent. Loss of an adult child was particularly likely to lead to complicated grief.

Studies of youth also report linkages between loss of family and friends and depression and posttraumatic stress. Wickrama and Kaspar

(2007) studied 325 exposed adolescents and their mothers in two villages in Sri Lanka 4 months after the 2004 tsunami. Loss of a family member significantly contributed to depression and PTSD symptoms in adolescents. Pfefferbaum and colleagues (2006) surveyed 156 children who lost a parent (5%), sibling (1%), another relative (37%), friend (32%), or acquaintance (42%) in the 1998 U.S. Embassy bombing in Nairobi, Kenya. Ten months after the terrorist attack, bereavement increased the severity of posttraumatic stress symptoms, with loss of a parent the most significant predictor of distress.

Finally, culture shapes beliefs and expectations about death and bereavement and defines death rituals (Rosenblatt, 1997). Two studies report coping among Asian families who had a family member killed in the September 11th World Trade Center attacks. Consistent with collectivistic cultures in which identity lies within the collective experience, Yeh, Inman, Kim, and Okubo (2006) and Inman, Yeh, Madan-Bahel, and Nath (2007) found a sense of shared collective loss referring to not only the loss of a particular person, but the loss of their role in the family, their sense of self, and their shared identity. These researchers discussed the importance of participation in culturally relevant rituals. For example, Hindu cremation ceremonies immediately following death are perceived as the means to release the soul and enable rebirth. Muslim families maintain vigilance over the body of their loved one between death and burial and pray for a safe, painless transition to the afterlife. Inman and colleagues (2007) suggest that among South Asian families who lost family members in the September 11th terrorist attacks, the inability to perform traditional rituals due to unavailability of their bodies may have complicated their bereavement process.

3.2.2. Threat to Life, Injury, and Fear

Threat to life (feeling that one's life was in danger during the incident) can be highly prevalent even in events that do not cause extensive loss of life. For example, in studies of Hurricane Hugo (Norris & Uhl, 1993; Norris, 1989; Thompson, Norris, & Hanacek, 1993), life threat was reported by 46% of respondents in the two stricken cities (Charleston, South Carolina, and Charlotte, North Carolina) though few people on the U.S. Mainland lost their lives in this storm. Perceptions of life threat were even more prevalent (73%) in a subsequent study of several neighborhoods damaged by Hurricane Andrew (Norris, Perilla, Riad, Kaniasty, & Lavizzo, 1999).

In samples with a range of experiences, life threat and injury are consistent risk factors for psychopathology. Briere and Elliott (2000) studied a general population sample of 935 persons, of whom 22% reported exposure to disaster an average of 13 years previously. Disaster exposure was associated with higher scores on six of ten scales of the Trauma Symptom Inventory. The type of disaster was far less important than the characteristics of exposure, especially whether the participant recalled fear of death or physical injury. In a study of 831 adults interviewed 12, 18, and 24 months after Hurricane Hugo, Thompson and colleagues (1993) documented persistent effects of life threat and injury on a variety of domains of mental health (depression, anxiety, somatic complaints, general stress, traumatic stress). In contrast, effects of financial and personal loss were significant at Wave 1 but largely dissipated thereafter. In the Livanou and colleagues (2002) study described earlier, fear experienced during the earthquake was highly predictive of PTSD at 14 months postevent, although it was less predictive of depression. Maes, Mylle, Delmeire, and Altamura (2000) studied 128 victims of a ballroom fire and 55 victims of a mass traffic accident 7 to 9 months after these disasters in Belgium. Threats to life, injury, or both were prevalent in this sample, of which 46% developed PTSD, 13% major depression, and 18% any anxiety disorder other than PTSD. Life threat was strongly associated with the development of psychopathology.

While self-reported "threat to life" and "fear" involve a certain degree of subjectivity (reflecting a transaction between stressor and person), studies that used relatively objective measures confirm these results. In the subgroup exposed to the fire in the Maes and colleagues (2000) study, the severity of burns (burn stage) was strongly related to depression and anxiety disorders. In the Buffalo Creek study described earlier (Gleser et al., 1981), life threat was carefully and objectively scaled on the basis of the extent of contact with the water, and it was significantly correlated with overall severity of psychopathology 2 years after the dam collapsed. Six months after the bombing of the Murrah Federal Building in Oklahoma City, North and colleagues (1999) studied 182 adults from a health department registry of persons documented to have experienced bombing-related injuries. Most participants (77%) had required medical intervention, including hospitalization (20%) and surgery (15%). One-third (34%) of the sample met criteria for PTSD, and 45% had some postdisaster disorder. Participants with postdisaster PTSD reported an average of six injuries, compared with an average of three injuries among others. Number of injuries was also associated with development of disorders other than PTSD.

Threat to life and injury are also risk factors for children and youth. McDermott, Lee, Judd, and Gibbon (2005) studied 222 children of ages 8 to 18 as part of a schoolwide screen 6 months after the Canberra wildfire in Australia. Eleven percent (16% girls and 5% boys) felt they were in danger of dying during the wildfire, and 29% (35% girls and 21% boys) were concerned about a family member dying. Perception of life threat to either self or family was related to more severe posttraumatic stress symptoms. Thienkrua and colleagues (2006) assessed PTSD and depression in 371 Thai children (167 displaced living in camps, 99 living in affected villages, 105 living in unaffected villages) 2 and 9 months after the devastating 2004 tsunami occurred off the coast of Indonesia. Percentages scoring above cut-points were, respectively, 13%, 11%, and 6% for clinically significant PTSD symptoms and 11%, 5%, and 8% for depression. In multivariate analyses, threat to life and panic/fear were significantly and independently associated with PTSD symptoms; threat to life was also significantly associated with depressive symptoms.

3.2.3. Witnessing and Horror

Exposure to the grotesque and aversive sights of disasters can be difficult to disentangle from threat to life and fear. Therefore this component of disaster exposure has been studied less often and shows independent effects on mental health less consistently. In Maes and colleagues' (2000) multivariate analyses, having seen a friend or family member injured or killed in the fire or crash was a significant predictor of postdisaster psychological disorder over and above the effects of threat or loss. The September 11th terrorist attacks provided an excellent context for studying the effects of horror, because, for many people, witnessing the planes fly into the World Trade Center or the collapse of the buildings was the primary mechanism of exposure. In Galea and colleagues' (2002) study described earlier, participants who directly witnessed the events had a higher prevalence of PTSD and depression (10.4% and 10.8%, respectively) than nonwitnesses (5.5% and 9.2%). This variable, however, was not predictive of either condition in multivariate analyses that controlled for panic and loss. Similarly, in Thienkrua and colleagues' (2006) study of young victims of the 2004 tsunami, seeing the waves, seeing anyone dead or injured, and hearing screams were related to PTSD and depression in univariate analyses but not in multivariate analyses that controlled for the effects of panic and loss. Pfefferbaum and colleagues (2003) surveyed 562 middle school children in 38 schools throughout Nairobi, Kenya, 8 to 14 months after the terrorist attack on the U.S. embassy. They used a physical exposure scale comprised of items such as experiencing personal injury, hearing yelling or screaming, seeing others physically injured, seeing blood from injuries, coming into direct contact with another person's blood, and knowing someone injured or killed in the bombings. Physical exposure explained 3% of the unique variance in posttraumatic stress symptoms, and an eight-point increase in physical exposure increased the odds of functional impairment (e.g., functioning at home and school) by 2.20.

Studies of rescue workers and body handlers are particularly important for understanding horror independently of terror. One good example is Epstein, Fullerton, and Ursano's (1998) study of 355 health-care professionals who were exposed to burn victims (55% of the sample) or dead bodies (24%) after planes collided and crashed during the Ramstein Air Force Base air show in 1988. PTSD was assessed at 6, 12, and 18 months, and 14% of participants met study criteria for PTSD at one of these time points. Exposure to burn victims, especially child victims, exposure to bodies, and initial emotional reactions (anxiety, numbness) were all associated with PTSD; exposure to burn victims and initial numbness were retained in multivariate models, along with education and postdisaster stressful life events.

3.3. LOSS

3.3.1. Property Damage and Financial Loss

Damage to home and property, often accompanied by financial loss, may be the prototypical stressor associated with natural disasters, such as floods, hurricanes, and earthquakes. A common, related stressor is the loss of possessions of personal rather than financial value, such as photographs and keepsakes. Accordingly, the consequences of these losses have been studied extensively. For example, total loss in rubles was among the strongest predictors of PTSD experienced anytime over the first 2 years after the 1988 earthquake in Armenia (Armenian et al., 2000); having one's house destroyed was associated with higher symptom levels 6 months after Hurricane Mitch in Nicaragua (Caldera, Palma, Penayo, & Kullgren, 2001), and property damage in combination with injury formed the strongest set of predictors of psychopathology at 3-month follow-up in a study of 357 persons seeking emergency assistance after the 2003 fire storm in California (Marshall, Schell, Elliott, Rayburn, & Jaycox, 2007). In a study of 325 adolescents and their mothers 4 months after the 2004 tsunami, property destruction predicted greater adolescent depression and posttraumatic stress (Wickrama & Kaspar, 2007).

The relative impact of property loss compared to trauma has varied in past research. McFarlane (1989) studied a sample of firefighters 4, 11, and 29 months after the 1983 bushfires in Australia. The sample was highly exposed to traumatic aspects of the event, with an average of 16 hours spent fighting the fire, 20% reporting near-panic, 27% injured, and 7% knowing someone who died. In addition, 23% experienced property damage from the fire itself. In multivariate analyses, property damage was a significant predictor of distress at Month 4, whereas injury, threat to life, hours in the fire, and bereavement were not. However, the effect of property damage was not present at Month 11. Panic showed both initial and more lasting effects on distress.

Other longitudinal studies also have found the effects of property loss to decrease over time. For example, Thompson and colleagues (1993) found that both financial losses and personal losses were significantly correlated with depression, anxiety, somatic complaints, general stress, and traumatic stress 1 year after Hurricane Hugo, but most of these effects dissipated over the next few months, whereas those of life threat and injury did not.

On the other hand, some evidence indicates that disaster-related losses may interfere with recovery from PTSD. Losing a job was the only factor the predicted PTSD at 6 months among persons who met criteria for probable PTSD 1 month after the September 11th terrorist attacks on the World Trade Center (Galea et al., 2003).

3.3.2. Resource Loss

The concept of resource loss has become central in stress theory, primarily because of the influence of Hobfoll's (1988) theory of conservation of resources (CORs). The basic tenet of COR theory is that individuals strive to obtain, retain, protect, and foster those things that they value, which are termed *resources*. In Hobfoll's theory, stress occurs when resources are threatened, when resources are lost, or when individuals fail to gain resources following a significant investment of other resources. Introduced to the disaster field by Freedy, Shaw, Jarrell, and Masters (1992), COR theory has become highly influential in disaster research because disasters and terrorism threaten a host of *object resources* (e.g., housing), *personal resources* (e.g., optimism, safety), *conditions* (e.g., employment, social relationships), and *energies* (e.g., money, free time). Whether scored simply as a count of losses tallied from an inventory or as multiple measures of specific losses, resource loss has correlated highly with symptom severity in several disaster studies that have spanned disaster type, location, and phase of recovery in adults (e.g., Arata, Picou, Johnson, & McNally, 2000; Freedy, Saladin, Kilpatrick, Resnick, & Saunders, 1994; Hobfoll, Tracy, & Galea, 2006; Sattler et al., 2002) and in youth (Dirkzwager, Kerssens, & Yzermans, 2006; Wickrama & Kaspar, 2007). In studies that distinguished between resource domains, loss of conditions (Arata et al., 2000) and loss of personal resources (Sattler et al., 2002; Wickrama & Kaspar, 2007) have emerged as especially predictive of postdisaster symptoms.

Kaniasty and Norris (Kaniasty & Norris, 1993; Norris & Kaniasty, 1996) suggested that loss of social resources is an especially important aspect of disaster exposure. Their "social support deterioration model" – and subsequent "deterioration deterrence model" – built on Erikson's (1976) earlier proposition that the trauma experienced by disaster survivors has two facets: *individual trauma*, the personal psychic impact of the disaster, and *collective trauma*, the impairment of the prevailing sense of community. Many things can lead to postdisaster declines in social support, including violations of expectations, relocation, job loss, disruption of routine social activities, fatigue, and emotional irritability. Scarcity of resources increases the potential for interpersonal conflicts and social withdrawal. The relationship between declines in social support and PTSD is bidirectional, with social support exerting the greater influence in the first few months postdisaster, and PTSD exerting the greater influence as it grows more chronic (Kaniasty & Norris, 2008).

3.4. ONGOING ADVERSITIES

3.4.1. Housing and Rebuilding Issues

The acutely stressful experiences of trauma and loss are soon followed by a host of challenges associated with poor housing conditions, rebuilding, and other stressors in the postdisaster environment. Although subsequently dwarfed by Hurricane Katrina and several catastrophic disasters internationally, Hurricane Andrew remains a good example. Ninety thousand housing units in Southern Dade County (Florida) were completely destroyed (250,000 damaged), and large areas awaited reconstruction 16 months after the hurricane struck (McDonnell et al., 1995). Recognizing the extensiveness of the housing issues, Burnett and colleagues (1997) explored how best to capture perceived disruption during rebuilding after Hurricane Andrew. Their focus on the stress of settling insurance claims, getting repairs done, poor quality of repairs, taking time away from work, and the like, certainly – if anecdotally – rings true. In this study, the frequency and intensity of rebuilding problems explained significant and unique variance in posttraumatic stress and global distress 9 to 12 months postdisaster. Having made similar observations, Norris and colleagues (1999) studied the influence of "ecological stress" (an 11-item scale of living standards that assesses shortages, problems with heat, insects, and sanitation, and perceptions of crowding, isolation, and fear of crime) on depressive symptoms and posttraumatic stress 6 and 30 months after Hurricane Andrew. In multivariate models that controlled for pre-, within-, and other postdisaster factors, postdisaster ecological stress was a significant predictor of both depression and posttraumatic stress at Wave 1, and the extent of improvement in ecological stress between Waves 1 and 2 was significantly predictive of psychological recovery.

3.4.2. Postdisaster Life Events and Chronic Stress

Postdisaster stressors are typically captured in disaster research by measures of stressful life events or chronic stress. Life events refer to discrete changes, usually measured by checklists, whereas hassles, strains, and chronic stress refer to ongoing stressful life circumstances. Life events experienced after the disaster have been studied repeatedly and are consistently among the strongest predictors of postdisaster symptoms over time (e.g., Carr et al., 1997; Creamer, Burgess, Buckingham, & Pattison, 1993; Epstein et al., 1998; Freedy et al., 1994; McFarlane, 1989; Norris et al., 1999). This effect should not be interpreted as a competing cause of postdisaster distress but rather as a mediator or perpetuator of disaster-related effects. A number of studies, dating back to as long as 30 years ago, have shown disaster victims to be at higher risk than general populations for experiencing life events over the ensuing months. Janney, Minoru, and Holmes (1977) studied life change after an earthquake in Peru; they contrasted Huarez, the largest city struck by the quake, and Arequipa, a city untouched but otherwise comparable. During the year of the earthquake, life change units rose in Arequipa but not nearly so much as they did in Huarez.

There is an important limitation of studies that operationalize secondary stress solely in terms of life events or discrete changes: Life events do not measure experienced stress very completely. The stressfulness of any given interval is influenced both by life events and by less dramatic hassles, pressures, and strains. Norris and Uhl (1993) addressed this issue by studying the mediating role of chronic stress, experienced across seven domains of life, in a sample of 930 adults assessed 1 year after Hurricane Hugo. The effects of financial and personal loss on psychological symptoms were completely explained by victims' higher financial, marital, filial, and physical stress over the ensuing months. These same domains largely mediated the effects of injury and, with the addition of neighborhood stress (e.g., concerns about crime, drugs, noise), the effects of life threat. Norris and Uhl concluded that relief efforts directed at restoring housing and basic services only skim the surface of the needs of disaster victims. For quite some time following a major disaster, victims confront a myriad of adaptational requirements in the form of marital strain, filial burden, financial problems, and neighborhood concerns.

Several studies have linked parent functioning with child functioning after disasters. Overall, children of parents who are distressed following a disaster tend to exhibit greater emotional and behavioral problems than those whose parents are having less difficulty. For example, in a study of parent–child dyads in New York City at the time of the September 11th World Trade Center attacks, Fairbrother, Stuber, Galea, Fleischman, and Pfefferbaum (2003) found that children who saw their parents crying were three times more likely to have severe to very severe posttraumatic reactions. Children with parents demonstrating symptoms consistent with PTSD were four times more likely to have severe to very severe posttraumatic reactions. Parental depression was also predictive of children's posttraumatic stress reactions. Endo, Shioiri, Someya, Toyabe, and Akazawa (2007) assessed 756 children preschool age and older 5 months after the Niigata-Chuetsu earthquake using parent survey and clinical assessment. Higher parent scores on the GHQ-12 were related to more persistent behavioral changes in their children. Among older children, poor parent mental health status 1 month postearthquake was significantly associated with posttraumatic stress symptoms. Similar findings have been found following the Bolu earthquake (Kilic, Ozguven, & Sayil, 2003), Hurricane Hugo (Swenson et al., 1996), Hurricane Andrew (Wasserstein & LaGreca, 1998), and an industrial disaster in France (Vila et al., 2001). Children, then, utilize respected adults as sources of information in social referencing processes. Parents (and other significant people in a child's life) serve as models that may either exacerbate or buffer the impact of disaster on the children (Wasserstein & LaGreca, 1998).

3.4.3. Displacement and Relocation

Of all the ongoing adversities experienced by disaster victims, displacement (forced relocation) is among the most disruptive. Relocation should not be confused with evacuation. Evacuation refers to the temporary withdrawal of persons from a potential impact area. Sometimes evacuation turns into relocation when damage to homes is so severe that temporary, or occasionally permanent, alternate housing must be found. Relocation is not necessarily a negative event, but forced (unwanted) relocation due to politics, war, urban renewal, contamination, or disaster is believed to be quite disruptive and stressful (e.g., Steinglass, De-nour, & Shye, 1985; Steinglass & Gerrity, 1990). Quarantelli (1985) argued that the severe psychological consequences of the 1972 Buffalo Creek dam collapse resulted more from the poor sheltering provided to the survivors than from the direct impact of the flood. Little effort was made to relocate the survivors in a way that revived former community and family ties. Gleser and colleagues (1981) found that the extent of displacement (measured in distance) correlated with depression in women and belligerence in children but had minimal effect on men. The investigators believed this happened because men were able to return to their old jobs, whereas children had to change schools and women largely remained at home in the unfamiliar trailer parks. Norris, Baker, Murphy, and Kaniasty (2005) corroborated these interpretations in their longitudinal study of the 1999 floods and mudslides in Villahermosa and Teziutlán, Mexico (four waves; $N=561$). All participants in Teziutlán were relocated to a new settlement far outside of the original city. Comparisons between sample data and population norms suggested substantial deterioration of perceived support and social embeddedness, especially in Teziutlán and especially among women in Teziutlán. Social support disparities according to gender and context grew larger as time passed. Prevalences of postdisaster PTSD and major depression were also significantly greater and more enduring in Teziutlán (46% and 15% at 6 months) than in Villahermosa (14%, 7%) (Norris, Murphy, Baker, & Perilla, 2004). Providing yet another example, Najarian, Goenjian, Pelcovitz, Mandel, and Najarian (2001) compared 25 women who stayed in Gumri, a stricken city, after the 1988 Armenian earthquake to 25 women who relocated to Yerevan. Rates of PTSD were extremely high in both groups (89%–92%), but the relocated women showed higher severity in symptoms.

The mass displacement of survivors of Hurricane Katrina was unprecedented in the United States. Estimates of the number of displaced persons reached 2.5 million at one point (FEMA, 2006, cited in Larrance, Anastario, & Lawry, 2007). Larrance and colleagues (2007) surveyed 366 residents of FEMA group and commercial trailer parks to assess needs as of April to May 2006, approximately 8 to 9 months after the hurricane struck the Gulf Coast and the levees in New Orleans were breeched. Participants had been displaced an average of 246 days. Sixty-eight percent did not feel safe in their new community, especially at night. During the 2 months before the survey, over half of all households had one or more members with a chronic or acute illness. Fifty percent met criteria for major depressive disorder, 20% had suicidal ideation, and 14% had increased substance use since displacement.

Kessler and colleagues (2008) interviewed 815 prehurricane residents of the areas affected by Hurricane Katrina approximately 6 and 18 months postdisaster. In contrast to the norm in disaster studies (Norris et al., 2002), the investigators found psychopathology to increase over time, with rates of PTSD of 21% at Wave 2 (vs. 15% at Wave 1) and rates of other serious mental illness of 14% at Wave 2 (vs. 11% at Wave 1). Unresolved hurricane-related stresses accounted for much of the increase. Interestingly, family living situation (relocation to a different town) was significantly, but not that strongly, related to increases in serious mental illness, explaining approximately 3% of variance in outcomes.

3.5. COMMUNITY EFFECTS AND MEANINGS

3.5.1. Indirect Effects of Disasters

Over 20 years ago, Bolin (1985) observed that there are two broad categories of disaster victims: Whereas *primary victims* are those who directly experience physical, material, or personal losses, *secondary victims* are others who live in the affected area. Although they sustain no personal injuries or property damage, secondary victims do experience a variety of inconveniences and the potential for economic, environmental, governmental, social, and cultural disruptions ranging from mild to severe. Primary and secondary victims alike may experience declines in opportunities for companionship and leisure, and both may be party to community conflicts about the causes of the disaster and appropriate responses. From this conceptualization, it can be inferred that a disaster is more than an individual-level event but is also a community-level event with potential psychological consequences even for those persons who experience no trauma or loss (Norris, 2006).

These consequences are sometimes characterized as direct and indirect effects. In an early study of indirect effects, Smith and colleagues (1986) studied residents of areas in and around Times Beach, Missouri, that had been flooded or exposed to toxic contaminations or both. They categorized study participants as direct victims ($N = 139$), indirect victims ($N = 215$, persons who were exposed via experiences of relatives and close friends), or nonvictims ($N = 189$). The investigators found little evidence of indirect effects in their study, as generally the direct victims differed from both the indirect victims and nonvictims, who did not differ significantly from one another.

On the other hand, Norris and colleagues (1994) did find evidence of indirect effects in their study of the 1981 floods in eastern Kentucky (Appalachia). The 220 respondents in this study were all participating in a larger panel study of older adult mental health and had been interviewed 3 months before as well as four times after the floods. The study spanned ten flooded and five adjacent nonflooded counties and archival data were used to capture county-level damages independently of the self-report measures of personal loss. This measure of "community destruction" explained significant variance in psychological well-being (Phifer & Norris, 1989), physical health (Phifer, Kaniasty, & Norris, 1988), and social functioning (Kaniasty & Norris, 1993) over and above that explained by personal loss. The pattern of findings was instructive. Only primary victims (those with personal loss relative to secondary and nonvictims) showed increases in negative affect from before to after the flood, but both primary and secondary victims (relative to nonvictims) showed decreases in positive affect. Only primary victims showed increases in medical conditions and symptoms, but both showed increases in fatigue. Only primary victims showed declines in perceptions of kin support, but both primary and secondary victims showed declines in nonkin support. Together, the various findings appeared to reflect community-wide tendencies to feel less positive about their surroundings, less enthusiastic, less energetic, and less able to enjoy life in the aftermath of the disaster. No one would suggest that such consequences constitute psychopathology, but they do indicate that disasters may impair the quality of life in the community for quite some time.

The potential of disasters to have indirect effects on mental health is particularly salient in the context of terrorism. This question has intrigued a number of researchers in the aftermath of terrorist attacks (e.g., Bleich, Gelkopf, & Solomon, 2003; Gabriel et al., 2007; Galea et al., 2002; Pfefferbaum et al., 2000; Schuster et al., 2001; Silver, Holman, McIntosh, Poulin, & Gil-Rivas, 2002). With particular emphasis on research following the September 11, 2001, attacks on the World Trade Center in New York City, Galea and Resnick (2005) provided a thoughtful discussion of why psychopathology may emerge in some portion of the general population in the case of terrorism. In the New York example, the prevalence of PTSD was far lower among persons exposed only indirectly, but because they composed a large proportion of the population, there were almost as many indirect cases as direct cases. As the authors noted, the findings from New York raised questions about "what constitutes exposure for PTSD, and by extension, what constitutes PTSD itself" (p. 113). Throughout the New York metropolitan area, people felt terror, helplessness, or horror (PTSD Criterion A2), even if they were not directly affected (witnessing, bereavement, job loss, etc.) by the September 11th attacks.

However, there are concerns that indirect effects may be spurious due to confounds with other variables such as previous trauma and psychiatric family history. In Neria and colleagues' (2006) primary care study, a predisaster history of trauma and having a family psychiatric history increased the likelihood of PTSD among patients exposed only indirectly to the terrorist attacks. In Aber and colleagues' (2004) study of 768 adolescents in New York City, adolescents who had witnessed community violence prior to September 11th were more likely to react to media exposure and report a greater number of posttraumatic stress symptoms.

3.5.2. The Media Controversy

One mechanism of indirect exposure that has been explored in the literature, usually with some controversy, is the media. There is ample evidence (e.g., Ahern et al., 2002; Lau, Lau, Kim, & Tsui, 2006; Pfefferbaum et al., 2001) that PTSD symptoms are positively correlated with exposure to extreme media images (e.g., people jumping from the towers on September 11th; dead bodies in the aftermath of the 2004 tsunami; the iconic dead child in footage of the Oklahoma City bombing). Although Ahern and colleagues (2002) found that frequency of television viewing was related to PTSD and depression only among direct victims of the September 11th attacks, other investigators have found correlations in samples far distant from attacks, none of whom were directly affected (Pfefferbaum et al., 2000; Silver et al., 2002). In the first prospective study of the relationship, Bernstein and colleagues (2007) showed that the number of hours of exposure to coverage of the anniversary of September 11th was significantly associated with new onset PTSD in New York City. The relationship was strongest among persons who evidenced some symptoms of PTSD at baseline although they had not met study criteria for the diagnosis.

What these relations mean is not yet clear, and investigators generally caution against attributing causality. If television viewing is in fact another vehicle of exposure, it may function differently for primary victims and others. For the former, repeated television images may trigger traumatic memories in persons predisposed to PTSD. For example, in the national sample of bereaved adults studied by Neria and colleagues (2007), watching the attacks on television increased the likelihood of reporting complicated grief. The researchers suggested two possible reasons for this finding: (1) Individuals who screened positive for complicated grief may have watched more television reporting of the attacks as a means to obtain more information about loved ones; or (2) as indicated by Ahern and colleagues (2002), exposure to live television coverage of mass violence creates haunting memories that contribute to postdisaster mental health problems. For indirect or secondary victims, media images may convey information that heightens perceptions of threat. Thus the issue may not be the horror of the images per se but the information they convey. Marshall and colleagues (2007) proposed that media effects are explained by "relative risk appraisals" that mediate the relation between an event and its meaning, as influenced by emotional responses and a host of other factors. Typically, media exposure does not result in PTSD because the viewer does not perceive a personal threat. However, in the case of terrorism, and quite possibly in the case of certain other catastrophes, it is quite plausible that the viewer does.

3.5.3. Meanings

One of the most intriguing aspects of Marshall and colleagues' (2007) analysis of relative risk appraisal is that it challenges prevailing notions of exposure. At least in the case of terrorism, the objective, observable experience of an event is de-emphasized relative to the subjective, psychological experience of what that event implies for the future, as evidenced in perceptions of threat. This reframing of the nature of disaster exposure has serious implications, as it virtually abandons the traditional emphasis, reflected by this very chapter, on the immediate trauma, tangible losses, and ensuing adversities experienced by people within more or less geographically defined communities. More important is what the event means to the individual.

This is actually not the first time that the disaster field has struggled with exposure definitions and determined that psychological meanings cannot be ignored. For example, the nuclear accident at Three Mile Island in 1979 posed similar dilemmas. Although there was an extensive and frightening emergency evacuation, residents experienced no property damages, no injuries, and minimal exposure to radiation. How could this event then be a disaster? What accounted for the chronic stress and moderate psychological distress evident in Three Mile Island (e.g., Baum, Gatchel, & Schaeffer, 1983; Cleary & Houts, 1984)? Discussions of these consequences often emphasized the long-term uncertainties regarding the nature of the impact, fears that there might be unseen or delayed consequences, and anxieties regarding threat of recurrence (see, for example, Bolin, 1985).

The adverse meanings of disasters are not limited to threat and uncertainty regarding future harm. The long-standing concern about the heightened potential of human-caused disasters (including various failures of technology) to affect mental health arises essentially because of what these events mean to people about the larger society. As Bolin (1985) noted, human-caused disasters "represent in the eyes of victims a callousness, carelessness, intentionality, or insensitivity on the part of others" (p. 24) and make the sense of victimization intense. Residents of areas afflicted by technological accidents often bitterly debate the severity of the threat, and antagonisms may yield high levels of anger, alienation, and mistrust (Kaniasty & Norris, 1999). In a study of a railroad chemical spill (Bowler, Mergler, Huel, & Cone, 1994), for example, 69% of respondents believed that their community was divided between persons who felt they suffered from the accident and others who claimed there were no adverse consequences, and 36% believed they personally suffered because their own sense of victimization was minimized by friends and neighbors. The divisiveness has numerous implications, not yet fully understood, for what a disaster means for one's sense of community. As the world witnessed the events following Hurricane Katrina, survivors may legitimately perceive neglect and injustices in disaster response that can fundamentally undermine the relationship between citizen and state.

The experience of disaster can also vary by cultural lens. That is, the cultural shaping of values, expectations, and worldview influences the meanings individuals attach to traumatic experiences (Draguns, 1996; Marsella & Christopher, 2004). For example, Palinkas and colleagues (1993) studied 600 residents from different ethnocultural groups who were exposed to the Exxon Valdez oil spill in Alaska. They found Alaskan Natives to be at least twice more likely to develop PTSD and generalized anxiety disorder than non-natives. They suggested that the greater vulnerability of the Alaskan Natives was based not only on the loss of subsistence activities but also on the salience of the destroyed natural resources. The natural resources destroyed by the oil spill were central to the intergenerational sharing of cultural values, which lie at the core of Native identity, ideology, and social organization (Green, 1996).

Among collectivistic cultures such as Arab, Israeli, Chinese, Japanese, Thai, Vietnamese, and other Asian groups, *fatalism* strongly influences the meaning of disaster. Fatalism refers to a collectivistic worldview that control lies within contextual or external forces rather than the individual. In contrast, individuals from individualistic cultures strive for autonomy and control of their environment, placing a value on separateness, internal or personal qualities, and uniqueness (Yeh, Arora, & Wu, 2006). Yeh, Inman, and colleagues (2006) studied collectivistic coping and found that Asian American families who lost a family member in the September 11th World Trade Center attacks utilized fatalistic beliefs to both understand and accept the loss of family members, indicating that the attacks "happened for a reason," were "part of a natural order," and were "part of a larger will" (p. 142).

3.6. IMPLICATIONS FOR FUTURE RESEARCH

In this chapter we have attempted to summarize the complex ways in which people experience disasters. We organized these experiences into categories of traumatic stressors, loss, ongoing adversities, and community effects and meanings. These are not truly discrete categories but rather our effort to present a snapshot of what we know about the multitude of factors affecting psychosocial outcomes of adults and youth in the aftermath of disaster. Understanding the multifaceted nature of disaster exposure should increase our capacity to understand the mental health consequences of disasters.

It should be clear from this chapter, however, that characterizing disaster exposure is no simple matter. Classifications of exposure severity based only on proximity to the "epicenter" are far from adequate to capture the various ways disasters are experienced. We know little about the relative impact of various potential stressors and even less about how they may interact to influence mental health. There is unlikely to be one answer to these questions, as the relative importance of different aspects of exposure is likely to vary across outcomes, events, places, time, culture, and developmental stage.

This review has implications for sampling strategies for epidemiologic disaster research. While this will not always be possible or warranted, in many disasters it appears advisable to sample from populations in ways that ensure that persons affected directly, indirectly, and not at all are represented. This three-tiered approach may be necessary to tease out the nature of direct and indirect effects on the community at large. Where possible, sampling that includes sufficient numbers of diverse groups would support examination of possible developmental, gender, and cultural differences in the experience of disaster.

This review has clearer implications for assessment. Investigators should aim to capture each of the major elements of disaster exposure that make sense for their context, including extent of bereavement; life threat and injury; peri-event panic and fear; witnessing and horror; property and financial loss; other resource loss; housing, rebuilding, and neighborhood stress; other secondary and chronic stressors; evacuation and relocation; and media exposure. Given the absence of a uniform hierarchy of effects (e.g., trauma > loss > rebuilding stress) and the likelihood of substantial correlations among exposure elements, investigators may need to create sample-specific indices that best capture severity of exposure in their context. In addition, examination of the direct and indirect influence of prior traumatic exposure will contribute to a better understanding of the complex dynamics of exposure and psychosocial outcomes postdisaster.

Work on developing quantitative measures of potential adverse meanings (threat, uncertainty, alienation, neglect, injustice), distinct from objective impacts, could be key to answering emerging questions regarding the relative merit of environmental and psychological conceptions of exposure. Such questions may be especially salient in the case of terrorist attacks but not necessarily unique to them. In addition, development and validation of quantitative measures that encompass both universal and culture-specific responses to trauma could help address current cross-cultural and transnational assessment challenges.

ACKNOWLEDGMENTS

Preparation of this chapter was supported by the National Institute of Mental Health through the National Center for Disaster Mental Health Research, P60 MH082598–01 and R25 MH068298 and by the Department of Homeland Security through the National Consortium for the Study of Terrorism and Responses to Terrorism (START), grant number N00140510629. Any opinions, findings, and conclusions or recommendations in this document are those of the authors and do not necessarily reflect views of the Department of Homeland Security or the National Institute of Mental Health.

REFERENCES

Aber, J., Gershoff, E., Ware, A., & Kotler, J. (2004). Estimating the effects of September 11th and other forms of violence on the mental health and social development of New York City's youth: A matter of context. *Applied Developmental Science, 8*(3), 111–129.

Ahern, J., Galea, S., Resnick, H.S., Kilpatrick, D.G., Bucuvalas, M., Gold, J., et al. (2002). Television images and psychological symptoms after the September 11 terrorist attacks. *Psychiatry, 65*(4), 289–300.

American Psychiatric Association. (1994). *Diagnostic and statistical manual of mental disorders (4th ed.)*. Washington, DC: American Psychiatric Association.

Arata, C., Picou, J., Johnson, G., & McNally, T. (2000). Coping with technological disaster: An application of the conservation of resources model to Exxon Valdez oil spill. *Journal of Traumatic Stress, 11*, 23–39.

Armenian, H., Morikawa, M., Melkonian, A., Hovanesian, A., Haroutunian, N., Saigh, P., et al. (2000). Loss as a determinant of PTSD in a cohort of adult survivors of the 1988 earthquake in Armenia: Implications for policy. *Acta Psychiatrica Scandinavica, 102*, 58–64.

Baum, A., Gatchel, R., & Schaeffer, M. (1983). Emotional, behavioral and physiological effects at Three Mile Island. *Journal of Consulting and Clinical Psychology, 51*, 565–572.

Bernstein, K.T., Ahern, J., Tracy, M., Boscarino, J.A., Vlahov, D., & Galea, S. (2007). Television watching and the risk of incident probably posttraumatic stress disorder: A prospective evaluation. *Journal of Nervous and Mental Disease, 195*(1), 41–47.

Bleich, A., Gelkopf, M., & Solomon, Z. (2003). Exposure to terrorism, stress-related mental health symptoms, and coping behaviors among a nationally representative sample in Israel. *Journal of the American Medical Association, 290*(5), 612–620.

Bolin, R. (1985). Disaster characteristics and psychosocial impacts. In B. Sowder (Ed.), *Disasters and mental health: Selected contemporary perspectives* (pp. 3–28). Rockville, MD: NIMH.

Bowler, R., Mergler, D., Huel, G., & Cone, J.E. (1994). Psychological, psychosocial and psychophysiological sequelae in a community affected by a railroad chemical disaster. *Journal of Traumatic Stress, 7*, 601–624.

Briere, J.N., & Elliott, D.M. (2000). Prevalence, characteristics, and long-term sequelae of natural disaster exposure in the general population. *Journal of Traumatic Stress, 13*(4), 661–679.

Burnett, K., Ironson, G., Benight, C.G., Wynings, C.G., Greenwood, D., Carver, C.S., et al. (1997). Measurement of perceived disruption during rebuilding following Hurricane Andrew. *Journal of Traumatic Stress, 10*(4), 673–681.

Caldera, T., Palma, L., Penayo, U., & Kullgren, G. (2001). Psychological impact of the hurricane Mitch in Nicaragua in a one-year perspective. *Social Psychiatry and Psychiatric Epidemiology, 36*(3), 108–114.

Carr, V., Lewin, T., Kenardy, J., Webster, R., Hazell, P., Carter, G., et al. (1997). Psychosocial sequelae of the 1989 Newcastle earthquake: III. Role of vulnerability factors in the post-disaster morbidity. *Psychological Medicine, 27*, 179–190.

Cleary, P., & Houts, P. (1984). The psychological impact of the Three Mile Island incident. *Journal of Human Stress, 10*(1), 28–34.

Creamer, M., Burgess, P., Buckingham, W., & Pattison, P. (1993). Posttrauma reactions following a multiple shooting: A retrospective study and methodological inquiry. In J. Wilson & B. Raphael (Eds.), *International handbook of traumatic stress syndromes* (pp. 201–212). New York: Plenum.

Dirkzwager, A.J.E., Kerssens, J.J., & Yzermans, C.J. (2006). Health problems in children and adolescents before and after a man-made disaster. *Journal of the American Academy Child and Adolescent Psychiatry, 45*(1), 94–103.

Draguns, J.G. (1996). Ethnocultural considerations in the treatment of PTSD: Therapy and service delivery. In A. J. Marsella, M. J. Friedman, E. T. Gerrity, & R. M. Scurfield (Eds.), *Ethnocultural aspects of posttraumatic stress disorder: Issues, research, and clinical applications* (pp. 459–482). Washington, DC: American Psychological Association.

Endo, T., Shioiri, T., Someya, T., Toyabe, S., & Akazawa, K. (2007). Parental mental health affects behavioral changes in children following a devastating disaster: A community survey after the 2004 Niigata-Chuetsu earthquake. *General Hospital Psychiatry, 29*, 175–176.

Epstein, R.S., Fullerton, C.S., & Ursano, R.J. (1998). Posttraumatic stress disorder following an air disaster: A prospective study. *American Journal of Psychiatry, 155*(7), 934–938.

Erikson, K. (1976). Loss of communality at Buffalo Creek. *American Journal of Psychiatry, 133*, 302–305.

Fairbrother, G., Stuber, J., Galea, S., Fleischman, A.R., & Pfefferbaum, B. (2003). Posttraumatic stress reactions in New York City children after the September 11, 2001, terrorist attacks. *Ambulatory Pediatrics, 3*(6), 304–311.

Freedy, J., Saladin, M., Kilpatrick, D., Resnick, H., & Saunders, B. (1994). Understanding acute psychological distress following natural disaster. *Journal of Traumatic Stress, 7*, 257–273.

Freedy, J., Shaw, D., Jarrell, M., & Masters, C. (1992). Towards an understanding of the psychological impact of natural disasters: An application of the conservation resources stress model. *Journal of Traumatic Stress, 5*, 441–454.

Gabriel, R., Ferrando, L., Sainz Corton, E., Mingote, C., Garcia-Camba, E., Fernandez Liria, A., et al. (2007). Psychopathological consequences after a disaster: An epidemiological study among victims, the general population, and police officers. *European Psychiatry, 22*, 339–346.

Galea, S., Ahern, J., Resnick, H., Kilpatrick, D., Bucuvalas, M., Gold, J., et al. (2002). Psychological sequelae of the September 11 terrorist attacks in New York City. *The New England Journal of Medicine, 346*, 982–987.

Galea, S., & Resnick, H. (2005). Posttraumatic stress disorder in the general population after mass terrorist incidents: Considerations about the nature of exposure. *CNS Spectrums, 10*(2), 107–115.

Galea, S., Vlahov, D., Resnick, H. S., Ahern, J., Susser, E. S., Gold, J., et al. (2003). Trends of probably post-traumatic stress disorder in New York City after the September 11 terrorist attacks. *American Journal of Epidemiology, 158*(6), 514–524.

Gleser, G., Green, B., & Winget, C. (1981). *Prolonged psychological effects of disaster: A study of Buffalo Creek*. New York: Academic Press.

Green, B. L. (1996). Cross-national and ethnocultural issues in disaster research. In A. J. Marsella, M. J. Friedman, E. T. Gerrity, & R. M. Scurfield (Eds.), *Ethnocultural aspects of posttraumatic stress disorder: Issues, research, and clinical applications* (pp. 341–361). Washington, DC: American Psychological Association.

Green, B., Lindy, J., Grace, M., Gleser, G., Leonard, A., Korol, M., et al. (1990). Buffalo Creek Survivors in the second decade: Stability of stress symptoms. *American Journal of Orthopsychiatry, 60*, 43–54.

Hobfoll, S. E. (1988) *The ecology of stress*. New York: Hemisphere.

Hobfoll, S. E., Tracy, M., & Galea, S. (2006). The impact of resource loss and traumatic growth on probably PTSD and depression following terrorist attacks. *Journal of Traumatic Stress, 19*(6), 867–878.

Inman, A. G., Yeh, C. J., Madan-Bahel, A., & Nath, S. (2007). Bereavement and coping of South Asian families post 9/11. *Journal of Multicultural Counseling and Development, 35*, 101–115.

Janney, J. G., Minoru, M., & Holmes, T. H. (1977). Impact of a natural catastrophe on life events. *Journal of Human Stress, 3*(2), 22–23.

Kaniasty, K., & Norris, F. (1993). A test of the support deterioration model in the context of natural disaster. *Journal of Personality and Social Psychology, 64*, 395–408.

(1999). Individuals and communities sharing trauma: Unpacking the experience of disaster. In R. Gist & B. Lubin (Eds.), *Psychosocial, ecological, and community approaches to understanding disaster* (pp. 25–62). London: Bruner/Mazel.

(2008). Longitudinal linkages between perceived social support and psychological distress: A test of sequential model of social causation and social selection. *Journal of Traumatic Stress, 21*, 274–281.

Kessler, R. C., Galea, S., Gruber, M. J., Sampson, N. A., Ursano, R. J., & Wessely, S. (2008). Trends in mental illness and suicidality after Hurricane Katrina. *Molecular Psychiatry, 13*, 374–384.

Kilic, E. Z., Ozguven, H. D., & Sayil, I. (2003). The psychological effects of parental mental health on children experiencing disaster: The experience of Bolu Earthquake in Turkey. *Family Process, 42*(4), 485–495.

Larrance, R., Anastario, M., & Lawry, L. (2007). Health status among internally displaced persons in Louisiana and Mississippi travel trailer parks. *Annals of Emergency Medicine, 49*(5), 590–601.

Lau, J. T. F., Lau, M., Kim, J. H., & Tsui, H. Y. (2006). Impacts of media coverage on the community stress level in Hong Kong after the tsunami on 26 December 2004. *Journal of Epidemiology and Community Health, 60*(8), 675–682.

Livanou, M., Basoglu, M., Salcioglu, E., & Kalender, D. (2002). Traumatic stress responses in treatment-seeking earthquake survivors in Turkey. *Journal of Nervous and Mental Disease, 190*(12), 816–823.

Maes, M., Mylle, J., Delmeire, L., & Altamura, C. (2000). Psychiatric morbidity and comorbidity following accidental man-made traumatic events: Incidence and risk factors. *European Archives of Psychiatry and Clinical Neuroscience, 250*(3), 156–162.

Marsella, A. J., & Christopher, M. A. (2004). Ethnocultural considerations in disasters: An overview of research, issues, and directions. *Psychiatric Clinics of North America, 27*, 521–539.

Marshall, G. N., Schell, T. L., Elliott, M. N., Rayburn, N. R., & Jaycox, L. H. (2007). Psychiatric disorders among adults seeking emergency disaster assistance after a wildland-urban interface fire. *Psychiatric Services, 58*(4), 509–514.

Marshall, R. D., Bryant, R. A., Amsel, L. V., Suh, E. J., Cook, J. M., & Neria, Y. (2007). The psychology of ongoing threat: Relative risk appraisal, the September 11 attacks, and terrorism-related fears. *American Psychologist*, *62*(4), 304–316.

McDermott, B. M., Lee, E. M., Judd, M., & Gibbon, P. (2005). Posttraumatic stress disorder and general psychopathology in children and adolescents following a wildfire disaster. *Canadian Journal of Psychiatry*, *50*(3), 173–143.

McDonnell, S., Troiano, R. P., Barker, N., Noji, E., Hlady, W. G., & Hopkins, R. (1995). Long-term effects of Hurricane Andrew: Revisiting mental health indicators. *Disasters*, *19*(3), 235–246.

McFarlane, A. (1989). The aetiology of post-traumatic morbidity: Predisposing, precipitating and perpetuating factors. *British Journal of Psychiatry*, *154*, 221–228.

McFarlane, A. C., & Norris, F. (2006). Definitions and concepts in disaster research. In F. Norris, S. Galea, M. Friedman, & P. Watson (Eds.), *Methods for disaster mental health research* (pp. 3–19). New York: Guilford Press.

Murphy, S. (1984). Stress levels and health status of victims of a natural disaster. *Research in Nursing and Health*, *7*, 205–215.

Najarian, B., Goenjian, A. K., Pelcovitz, D., Mandel, F. S., & Najarian, B. (2001). The effect of relocation after a natural disaster. *Journal of Traumatic Stress*, *14*(3), 511–526.

Neria, Y., Gross, R., Litz, B., Maguen, S., Insel, B., Seirmarco, G., et al. (2007). Prevalence and psychological correlates of complicated grief among bereaved adults 2.5–3.5 years after September 11th attacks. *Journal of Traumatic Stress*, *20*(3), 251–262.

Neria, Y., Gross, R., Olfson, M., Gameroff, M. J., Wickramaratne, P., Das, A., et al. (2006). Posttraumatic stress disorder in primary care one year after the 9/11 attacks. *General Hospital Psychiatry*, *28*, 213–222.

Neria, Y., Olfson, M., Gameroff, M. J., Wickramaratne, P., Gross, R., Pilowsky, D. J., et al. (2008). The mental health consequences of disaster-related loss: Findings from primary care one year after the 9/11 terrorist attacks. *Psychiatry*, *71*, 339–348

Norris, F. (2006). Community and ecological approaches to understanding and alleviating postdisaster distress. In Y. Neria, R. Gross, R. Marshall, & E. Susser (Eds.), *September 11, 2001: Treatment, research, and public mental health in the wake of a terrorist attack*. New York: Cambridge University Press.

Norris, F., Baker, C., Murphy, A., & Kaniasty, K. (2005). Social support deterioration after Mexico's 1999 flood: Effects of disaster severity, gender, and time. *American Journal of Community Psychology*, *36*, 15–28.

Norris, F., Friedman, M., Watson, P., Byrne, C., Diaz, E., & Kaniasty, K. (2002). 60,000 disaster victims speak, Part I: An empirical review of the empirical literature, 1981–2001. *Psychiatry*, *65*, 207–239.

Norris, F., & Kaniasty, K. (1996). Received and perceived social support in times of stress: A test of the social support deterioration deterrence model. *Journal of Personality and Social Psychology*, *71*, 498–511.

Norris, F., Murphy, A., Baker, C., & Perilla, J. (2004). Postdisaster PTSD over four waves of a panel study of Mexico's 1999 flood. *Journal of Traumatic Stress*, *17*, 283–292.

Norris, F., Perilla, J., Riad, J., Kaniasty, K., & Lavizzo, E. (1999). Stability and change in stress, resources, and psychological distress following natural disaster: Findings from Hurricane Andrew. *Anxiety, Stress, and Coping*, *12*, 363–396.

Norris, F., Phifer, J., & Kaniasty, K. (1994). Individual and community reactions to the Kentucky floods: Findings from a longitudinal study of older adults. In R. Ursano, B. McCaughey, & C. Fullerton (Eds.), *Individual and community responses to trauma and disaster*. Cambridge: Cambridge University Press.

Norris, F., & Uhl, G. (1993). Chronic stress as a mediator of acute stress: The case of Hurricane Hugo. *Journal of Applied Social Psychology*, *23*, 1263–1284.

North, C., Nixon, S., Shariat, S., Mallonee, S., McMillen, J., Spitznagel, E., et al. (1999). Psychiatric disorders among survivors of the Oklahoma City bombing. *Journal of the American Medical Association*, *282*, 755–762.

Palinkas, L. A., Downs, M. A., Petterson, J. S., & Russell, J. C. (1993). Social, cultural, and psychological impacts of the Exxon Valdez oil spill. *Human Organization*, *52*(1), 1–13.

Pfefferbaum, B., North, C. S., Doughty, D. E., Gurwitch, R. H., Fullerton, C. S., & Kyula, J. (2003). Posttraumatic stress and functional impairment in Kenyan children following the 1998 American Embassy bombing. *American Journal of Orthopsychiatry*, *73*(2), 133–149.

Pfefferbaum, B., North, C. S., Doughty, D. E., Pfefferbaum, R. L., Dumont, C. E., & Pynoos, R. S. (2006). Trauma, grief, and depression in Nairobi children after the 1998 bombing of the American Embassy. *Death Studies*, *30*, 561–577.

Pfefferbaum, B., Nixon, S. J., Tivis, R. D., Doughty, D. E., Pynoos, R. S., Gurwitch, R. H., et al. (2001). Television exposure in children after a terrorist incident. *Psychiatry*, *64*(3), 202–211.

Pfefferbaum, B., Seale, T., McDonald, N., Brandt, E., Rainwater, S., Maynard, B., et al. (2000). Posttraumatic stress two years after the Oklahoma City bombing in youths geographically distant from the explosion. *Psychiatry*, *63*, 358–370.

Phifer, J., Kaniasty, K., & Norris, F. (1988). The impact of natural disaster on the health of older adults: A multiwave prospective study. *Journal of Health and Social Behavior, 29*, 65–78.

Phifer, J., & Norris, F. (1989). Psychological symptoms in older adults following natural disaster: Nature, timing, duration, and course. *Journal of Gerontology, 44*, 207–217.

Quarantelli, E. L. (1985). An assessment of conflicting views on mental health: The consequences of traumatic events. In C. R. Figley (Ed.), *Trauma and its wake. Vol. I: The study and treatment of posttraumatic stress disorder* (pp. 173–215). New York: Brunner/Mazel.

Rosenblatt, P. C. (1997). Grief in small-scale societies. In C. M. Parkes, P. Laungani, & B. Young (Eds.), *Death and bereavement across cultures* (pp. 27–51). New York: Routledge.

Rubonis, A., & Bickman, L. (1991). Psychological impairment in the wake of disaster: The disaster-psychopathology relationship. *Psychological Bulletin, 109*, 384–399.

Sattler, D. N., Preston, A. J., Kaiser, C. F., Olivera, V. E., Valdez, J., & Schlueter, S. (2002). Hurricane Georges: A cross-national study examining preparedness, resource loss, and psychological distress in the U.S. Virgin Islands, Puerto Rico, Dominican Republic, and the United States. *Journal of Traumatic Stress, 15*(5), 339–350.

Schuster, M. A., Stein, B. D., Jaycox, L. H., Collins, R. L., Marshall, G. N., Elliott, M. N., et al. (2001). A national survey of stress reactions after the September 11, 2001, terrorist attacks. *New England Journal of Medicine, 345*(20), 1507–1512.

Silver, R. C., Holman, E. A., McIntosh, D. N., Poulin, M., & Gil-Rivas, V. (2002). Nationwide longitudinal study of psychological responses to September 11. *Journal of the American Medical Association, 288*(10), 1235–1244.

Smith, E. M., Robins, L. N., Przybeck, T. R., Goldring, E., & Solomon, S. D. (1986). Psychosocial consequences of a disaster. In J. H. Shore (Ed.), *Disaster stress studies: New methods and findings* (pp. 49–76). Washington, DC: American Psychiatric Press.

Steinglass, P., De-nour, A., & Shye, S. (1985). Factors influencing psychosocial adjustment to forced geographical relocation: The Israeli withdrawal from the Sinai. *American Journal of Orthopsychiatry, 55*, 513–529.

Steinglass, P., & Gerrity, E. (1990). Natural disaster and post-traumatic stress disorder: Short-term versus long-term recovery in two disaster-affected communities. *Journal of Applied Social Psychology, 20*, 1746–1765.

Swenson, C. C., Saylor, C. F., Powell, M. P., Stokes, S. J., Foster, K. Y., & Belter, R. W. (1996). Impact of a natural disaster on preschool children: Adjustment 14 months after a hurricane. *American Journal of Orthopsychiatry, 66*, 122–130.

Thienkrua, W., Cardozo, B. L., Chakkraband, M. L. S., Guadamuz, T. E., Pengjuntr, W., Tantipiwatanaskul, P., et al. (2006). Symptoms of posttraumatic stress disorder and depression among children in tsunami-affected areas of southern Thailand. *Journal of the American Medical Association, 296*(5), 549–559.

Thompson, M., Norris, F., & Hanacek, B. (1993). Age differences in the psychological consequences of Hurricane Hugo. *Psychology and Aging, 8*, 606–616.

Vila, G., Witkowski, P., Tondini, M. C., Perez-Diaz, F., Mouren-Simeoni, M. C., & Jouvent, R. (2001). A study of posttraumatic disorders in children who experienced an industrial disaster in the Briey region. *European Child and Adolescent Psychiatry, 10*(1), 10–18.

Wasserstein, S. B., & LaGreca, A. M. (1998). Hurricane Andrew: Parent conflict as a moderator of children's adjustment. *Hispanic Journal of Behavioral Sciences, 20*(2), 212–224.

Wickrama, K. A. S., & Kaspar, V. (2007). Family context of mental health risk in Tsunami-exposed adolescents: Findings from a pilot study in Sri Lanka. *Social Science and Medicine, 64*, 713–723.

Yeh, C. J., Arora, A. K., & Wu, K. A. (2006). A new theoretical model of collectivistic coping. In P. T. P. Wong & L. C. J. Wong (Eds.), *Handbook of multicultural perspectives on stress and coping* (pp. 55–72). New York: Springer.

Yeh, C. J., Inman, A., Kim, A. B., & Okubo, Y. (2006). Asian American families' collectivistic coping strategies in response to 9/11. *Cultural Diversity and Ethnic Minority Psychology, 12*, 134–148.

PART TWO

Psychopathology after Disasters

4 Anxiety Disorders and PTSD

ALEXANDER C. MCFARLANE, MIRANDA VAN HOOFF, AND FREYA GOODHEW

4.1. INTRODUCTION

This chapter reviews the literature on the prevalence and etiology of anxiety disorders, including posttraumatic stress disorder (PTSD), following disasters. We highlight that there is relatively little information about anxiety disorders other than PTSD; the paucity of data is due to the challenge of the shared phenomenology of these disorders and the difficulty of defining their boundaries. A further challenge is explored, namely, how disasters interact with background morbidity in a community. In considering the etiology of anxiety disorders, the differential role of threat is hypothesized to be differentiated from the more enduring effect of the losses sustained in disasters. Anxiety disorders have an enduring effect in the aftermath of disasters, and many issues remain to be examined in future research, especially in expanding beyond PTSD. To begin, however, it is important to understand the settings in which disasters occur and the anticipations that abound following these events, as these have the potential to bias a rational appraisal of the challenges that will impact the affected community.

Managing the psychological impact of disasters is a critical public-health challenge in the aftermath of these events. Informed prevalence and incidence estimates are critical to effective service planning. Unfortunately, there is often dramatization of disaster impact immediately afterward, with fears expressed about the capacity of the population to function and manage effectively (de Ville de Goyet, 2007). Such exaggerated predictions often arise from the media's reporting of these events, with the paradoxical consequence of later disinterest, which, in turn, leads to an underestimation of the long-term impact. Three decades of research has done much to better quantify the effects of these events, particularly those studies that have taken a longitudinal perspective (Norris, 2006).

The psychological impact of disasters can be compared to the impact of war and terrorism on civilian populations. During the early days of World War II, the anticipation of the bombing of London led to predictions of panic and the expectation that overwhelming numbers of individuals would psychologically decompensate (Jones, Woolven, Durodie, & Wessely, 2004). These dire consequences failed to emerge despite the very substantial civilian toll, leading to a counterbelief that these events did not create major mental health consequences. In some regards, the attitude of toughness being the norm is a background issue in some of the U.K. literature surrounding the effects of traumatic stress. A similar literature examining the impact of the Irish Republican Army troubles, during which there were multiple civilian terrorist attacks in Northern Ireland, also took the perspective that this wave of threat had little impact on the psychological adjustment of the targeted population (Curran, 1988).

In the 1970s, Quarantelli and Dynes (1977) also expressed concern about the tendency of mental health professionals to overemphasize the behavioral disorganization of people facing the threat and aftermath of disaster. Their sociological work emphasized the remarkable capacity of communities to remain relatively calm and organized in the aftermath of gross disruption. However, such an approach did not address the fact that overt behavioral disorganization is a very different question from changes in individuals' psychological health, particularly in the longer term. In some regards, the debriefing movement, which emerged in the 1980s, served to similarly maintain the focus on intervention in the immediate days and weeks following disasters. Debriefing was a strategy aimed at preventing the emergence of psychological morbidity (Mitchell, 1983). This movement led to the clarion call for counselors to assist victims in the aftermath of traumatic events, so much so, that in the latter part of the 1990s disaster managers were often overwhelmed by offers for help from "disaster counselors," and their culling and management became a major challenge. Again, the popular perception and media interest focused on the provision of such support. The problem for the field of disaster management is that this approach has tended to distract from the potential for disasters to have a long-term impact on the psychological health and adjustment of communities (McFarlane, 2005).

Psychiatry has long struggled to conceptually understand how individuals can apparently appear to manage and cope effectively at the time of exposure to major and catastrophic stressful situations but still develop consequent psychological morbidity in the longer term (Layton & Krikorian, 2002). The implicit logic that is often applied is that psychological disorders will only arise in those who have high levels of distress and disorganization at the time of the event. This perspective presumes that the critical element in the individual's later adjustment is the failure of their acute distress to mitigate with the passage of time and the emergence of a sense of personal safety and the reestablishment of their life in the aftermath of the event.

4.1.1. The Nature of Posttraumatic Psychological Morbidity

While the primary focus of this chapter is on anxiety disorders and posttraumatic stress disorders after disaster (see Tables 4.1 and Table 4.2), much of the research that has informed our understanding of these conditions comes from the study of other populations, such as individuals after motor vehicle accidents (O'Donnell, Creamer, Bryant, Schnyder, & Shalev, 2003). Looking to these other domains is informative because disasters are unpredictable events, and as a consequence, research that begins in the immediate aftermath of these events and systematically follows individuals is extremely difficult to implement, given the typical funding cycles, the demands of ethical clearance, and the development of research teams. A common presumption is the universality of human distress in response to the loss and threat that characterizes disasters. However, systematic examination of motor vehicle accidents demonstrates that there is a significant percentage of people who have minimal symptoms despite being involved in life threatening events that have substantial consequences for those individuals (Bryant, Creamer, O'Donnell, Silove, in press). The prevalence of the low distress group is underestimated and it is easy for public-health messages to exaggerate the nature and the prevalence of individuals' acute distress. In the aftermath of these events, the public health message often aims to normalize symptoms of anxiety and emotional liability. However, the desire not to stigmatize highly distressed individuals can lead to an underestimation of the significance of the presence of symptoms.

In broad terms, there appear to be three pathways for the emergence of a psychological disorder such as PTSD. A small minority of individuals, generally less than 5%, will become acutely disorganized following a traumatic exposure and will satisfy the diagnosis of acute stress disorder in the immediate aftermath of such an event (Peleg & Shalev, 2006). These are individuals with dissociative anxiety symptoms and intense intrusive preoccupation with the trauma; approximately 80% develop a chronic pattern of psychiatric morbidity, particularly PTSD (Bryant, 2005). Members of this group are the most visible in the aftermath of traumatic events and thus have tended to influence views about the nature of posttraumatic psychopathology.

Table 4.1. PTSD Sequelae in adults after disasters

Author (Year)	Disaster	Sample	Participants	Time after Disaster	Measure	Results
McMillen, North, & Smith (2000)	Northridge earthquake	Adults from area with highest damage	130	3 months	DSM-III-R DIS/DS Clinician interviewed	13% met full criteria 48% met some criteria
Ironson et al. (1997)	Hurricane Andrew	Adults in effected area (advertised study)	180	1 and 4 months	DSM-III-R PTSD criteria & IES	33% met criteria 76% with at least one symptom cluster
Garrison et al. (1995)	Hurricane Andrew	Random-digit dialing sample of 158 Hispanic, 116 black, and 104 white adolescent-parent pairs	378 pairs	6 months	DSM-III-R DIS	3% males 9% females 8.3% blacks 6.1% Hispanics met full criteria
Norris, Murphy, Baker, & Perilla (2004)	Mexico's 1999 Flood	Adults from Tezuitlan and Villahermosa	561	6, 12, 18, and 24 months	CIDI for DSM-IV	MDD and PTSD prevalent but declined over period PTSD = 24% at 6 months
de Bocanegra, Moskalenko, & Kramer (2006)	World Trade Center attack 9/11/2001	Chinese workers in lower Manhattan	148	18 months	PCL-C and CAPS	19% met full criteria
Neria et al. (2006)	World Trade Center attack 9/11/2001	Systematic sample of adult primary care patients	930	7–16 months	PTSD (PCL-C)	4.7% (based on PCL-C score over 50) 10.2% (based on DSM-IV criteria)
North, Pfefferbaum et al. (2004)	World Trade Center attack 9/11/2001	Survivors in direct path of the explosion	137	6 and 17 months	PTSD DIS	32% at 6 months 31% at 17 months
Centers for Disease Control and Prevention (CDC) (2004)	World Trade Center attack 9/11/2001	Rescue and recovery workers and volunteers	1138	9–15 months	PTSD (PCL)	13% met full PTSD criteria 20% met at least one symptom cluster

(continued)

Table 4.1 *(continued)*

Author (Year)	Disaster	Sample	Participants	Time after Disaster	Measure	Results
Stuber, Resnick, & Galea (2006)	World Trade Center attack 9/11/2001	Adults living in New York City metropolitan area (random-digit dialing)	2752	6–9 months	National Women's Study PTSD module-nonclinician administered	Probable event related PTSD = 6.5% females 5.4% males
Tang (2007)	2004 Southeast Asian earthquake-tsunami	Adult Thai survivors	265	2 weeks and 6 months	Traumatic stress symptoms	22% at 2 weeks 30% at 6 months
Kumar et al. (2007)	2004 Southeast Asian earthquake-tsunami	Adults in a severely affected coastal village in India	314	2 months	PTSD (Harvard Trauma Questionnaire)	12.7% met criteria
Armagan, Engindeniz, Devay, Erdur, & Ozcakir (2006)	2004 Southeast Asian earthquake-tsunami	Participants of the Turkish Red Crescent Disaster Relief Team	33 (of 36 member team)	1 month	PTSD (CAPS-1)	24.2% met criteria
Chou et al. (2007)	Chi-Chi earthquake, Taiwan	Cohort population	216	6 months, 2 years, and 3 years	PTSD (MINI & DRPST)	8.3% at 6 months 4.2% at 3 years
Marshall, Schell, Elliott, Rayburn, & Jaycox (2007)	October 2003 California firestorm	Persons in relief centers	357	A few days and 3 months	PTSD (self report)	24% probable PTSD at 3 months
Kuo, Wu, Ma, Chiu, & Chou (2007)	Chi-Chi earthquake, Taiwan	Victims in temporary housing units	272	1 year	PTSD (Davidson Trauma Scale)	16.5% met PTSD criterion 22.2% females 9.2% males
DeSalvo et al. (2007)	Hurricane Katrina August 29, 2005	Web-based survey of employees in New Orleans	1542	6 months	PCL-17 DSM-IV criteria	19.2% met criteria

van Griensven et al. (2006)	2004 Southeast Asian earthquake-tsunami	Displaced/nondisplaced in Phang Nga and nondisplaced in Krabi and Phuket	1061 at 3 months 520 at 9 months	3 and 9 months	Clinician administered Harvard Trauma Questionnaire & Hopkins Checklist-25	PTSD at 3 months 12% of displaced persons (fell to 7% at 9 months) 7% of nondisplaced persons in Phang Nga (fell to 2.3% at 9 months) 3% of nondisplaced persons in Krabi and Phuket
Soldatos, Paparrigopoulos, Pappa, & Christodoulou (2006)	Earthquake	Help seekers	102	0–3 weeks	PTSD (ICD-10)	43% fulfilled PTSD criteria
Onder, Tural, Aker, Kilic, & Erdogan (2006)	1999 Marmara earthquake, Turkey	Random individuals from epicentre	683	3 years	PTSD (CIDI, TSSC)	19.2% met PTSD criteria at some time after event 10.5% current diagnosis at 3 years
Dirkzwager, van der Velden, Grievink, & Yzermans (2007)	Fireworks depot explosion, Netherlands, 2000	Adult survivors who were effected	898	3 weeks and 18 months	PTSD (SRS PTSD)	18% met PTSD criteria
Green, Lindy, Grace, & Leonard (1992)	Buffalo Creek dam collapse 1972	Exposed adults	193	14 years	Clinical Interview for DSM-III PTSD criteria	60% at some time after the flood 25% currently met PTSD criteria
North, Kawasaki, Spitznagel, & Hong (2004)	Great Midwestern Floods, 1993	St Louis area survivors	162	4 and 16 months	PTSD (DIS-III-R)	22% met criteria at 4 months 16% met criteria at 16 months

Notes: CAPS, clinician administered PTSD scale; CIDI, composite international diagnostic interview; DIS, diagnostic interview schedule; DIS/DS, diagnostic interview schedule/disaster supplement; DRPST, disaster related psychological screening test; DSM, Diagnostic and Statistical Manual; IES, impact of events scale; MDD, major depressive disorder; PTSD, posttraumatic stress disorder; MINI, mini international neuropsychiatric interview; PCL-C, PTSD checklist-civilian; SRS PTSD, self-rating scale for PTSD; TSSC, traumatic stress symptom checklist.

Table 4.2. PTSD sequelae in children after disasters

Author (Year)	Disaster	Age/Grade at Time of Diaster	Participants (At Follow-up)	Time after Disaster	PTSD Measure	Prevalence of PTSD
Pynoos et al. (1987)	Sniper attack in schoolyard Feb 24, 1984	5–13 years	159	1 month	PTSD RI	At follow-up: 38.4%: moderate or severe PTSD symptoms 22%: mild symptoms of PTSD
Goenjian et al. (1995)	Earthquake Spitak Armenia 1988		218	1.5 years	CPTSD-RI (cut off score of 40 indicates PTSD)	At follow up: 95% Spitak, 71% Gumri, 26% Yereven
Yule et al. (2000)	Sinking of the cruise ship "Jupiter" 21 Oct, 1988	11–17 years (Mean: 14.7 years)	217 + 29 did part	17–25 years (Mean: 21.3 years)	CAPS	At follow-up: 17.5% Any time since disaster: 51.5%
Goenjian et al. (2001)	Hurricane Mitch Oct–Nov 1998	Approximately 13 years	158	6 months	Child PTSD reaction checklist	At follow-up: 90% most devastated region 55% 2nd most devastated region 14% least devastated region
Hsu, Chong, Yang, & Yen (2002)	Taiwan Earthquake September 21, 1999,	12–14 years	323	6 weeks	SCL-90-R ChIPS earthquake exposure inventory	At follow-up: 21.7%
Green et al. (1991)	Buffalo Creek dam collapse	2–15 years	179	2 years	Psychiatric reports	At follow-up: 37% probable PTSD
Green et al. (1990)	Buffalo Creek dam collapse	2–15 years	135	14 years	SCID	At follow-up: 23% Since disaster: 63%
Kar et al. (2007)	Cyclone Orissa India, Oct, 1999	7–17 years	447	1 year	Clinical examination	At follow-up: 30.6% exposed children had PTSD 13.6% had subsyndromal PTSD 43.7% in HE group had PTSD 11.2% in LE group had PTSD
John, Russell, & Russell (2007)	Tsunami Dec 2004, Tamil Nadu	5–18 years	502	2 months 6 months	IES-8 (cutoff of 17)	At initial assessment: 70.7% At follow-up: 81.6%

Neuner, Schauer, Catani, Ruf, & Elbert (2006)	Tsunami Dec, 2004 Sri Lanka	8–14 years	264	3 to 4 weeks	UCLA PTSD-RI	At follow-up: 4.6% to 8.5% Non-Tsunami PTSD 13.9% to 38.8% Tsunami related PTSD
Thienkrua et al. (2006)	Tsunami Dec, 2004 Thailand	7–14 years	371	2 months 9 months	UCLA PTSD-RI	At 2 months follow-up: 6 to 13% At 9 months follow-up: 10% among children in camps
Garrison et al. (1995)	Hurricane Hugo	11–17 years	1264	1 year	DSM-III-R	At follow-up: 5%
La Greca, Silverman, Vernberg, & Prinstein (1996)	Hurricane Andrew	Grades 3–5	442	3 months 7 months 10 months	PTSD-RI	At 3 months follow-up: 26.7% Moderate 25.3% Severe 3.8% Very severe 39.1% met crit all 3 symptom clusters At 7 months follow-up: 23.3% Moderate 15.2% Severe 3.2% Very severe 24% met crit all 3 symptom clusters At 10 months follow-up: 20.8% Moderate 11.1% Severe 1.6% Very severe 18.1% met crit all 3 symptom clusters
Shannon, Lonigan, Finch, & Taylor (1994)	Hurricane Hugo, Sep 21, 1989	9–19 years	5687	3 months	CPTS-RI	At follow-up: 5.42%
Giannopoulou et al. (2006)	Earthquake Athens, Greece, Sep 7, 1999	9–17 years	2037	6–7 months	CRIES-13 (cutoff of 17)	At follow-up: 35.7% of directly exposed group 20.1% of indirectly exposed group
Hoven et al. (2005)	WTC Bombing, Sep 11, 1001	Grades 4–12	8236	6 months	DISC	At follow-up: 10.6%

Notes: CAPS, clinician administered PTSD scale; ChIPS, child's interview for psychiatric symptoms; CPTSD-RI, child posttraumatic stress disorder-reaction index; CRIES, children's revised impact of event scale; DISC, diagnostic interview schedule for children; IES, impact of events scale; PTSD, posttraumatic stress disorder; SCL-90-R, symptom checklist-90-revised; UCLA PTSD-RI, Unversity of California Los Angeles PTSD reaction index.

For example, in the context of war, many believed that individuals with acute combat stress disorders would often have long-term adverse psychological outcomes arising from their exposure (Shephard, 2001). Concepts such as the role of suggestion, iatrogenesis through pension systems, and long-standing personality and character weaknesses have been evoked to explain these other disorders.

Longitudinal research, however, documents that the majority of people who develop PTSD have some symptoms in the aftermath of the disaster or accident but that these symptoms seem to escalate with the passage of time (Orcutt, Erickson, & Wolfe, 2004). The underlying mechanism is postulated to be sensitization and kindling (Post, Weiss, Li, Leverich, & Pert, 1999). The trauma exposure leads to a conditioned learned response to threat for a number of associated features or stimuli from the environment experienced at the time of the disaster (Shalev, 2000). Subsequent exposure to those reminders evokes fear and anxiety. The link between the trigger and the individual's reactivity grows in amplitude with the passage of time. As a consequence, a series of secondary avoidance behaviors begin to emerge to avert distress arising from this reactivity. Individuals' symptoms will often fluctuate with time. A recent follow up study of Israeli war veterans demonstrates a continuing escalation of symptoms over a 20-year follow-up period (Solomon & Mikulincer, 2006), and there is evidence of the same pattern in disaster victims (Morgan, Scourfield, Williams, Jasper, & Lewis, 2003).

A third pattern of adjustment relates to a group that has fairly continuous and high levels of symptoms that emerge in the first month after an event and then remain for some time (McFarlane, 1988), though a significant proportion of these individuals' symptoms will lessen with the passage of time. One of the difficulties in predicting the patterns of symptoms in the longer term is that much of the data is derived retrospectively from populations (Norris, Friedman, & Watson, 2002). While the burden of symptomatic distress at a population level may remain relatively constant, there is often a significant fluctuation within individuals – at one point an individual may satisfy the diagnostic criteria for an anxiety disorder and PTSD, but months later will not. Thus, a longitudinal perspective is central in understanding the psychiatric morbidity of disasters and how they may be modified with the passage of time. It is also critical to understand the environmental factors that can contribute to the exacerbation of symptoms (Goenjian et al., 2005; McFarlane, 1989).

4.2. THE NATURE OF STRESS IN DISASTER

An earlier section of this book discusses the nature of disasters and their associated threats, but it suffices to state that it is easy to conceptualize a disaster as the period during which a catastrophic event impacts directly upon the population. The point at which control is reestablished and the destruction being wreaked ceases represents the end of the event. Whilst this perspective is appropriate at a population level, the end of a disaster from the perspective of individuals directly affected is very different; a period of considerable stress characterized by major adaptive demands will only be commencing, particularly if relatives have been killed or the individual severely injured. These impacts can be further compounded if the individual's home has been destroyed or their surrounding community severely disrupted, which may also include the loss of the normal place of employment or business from which they derive their income. For these individuals, the disaster has an ongoing impact on their lives, which reverberates in many domains. The stresses and the strains put on the individual are likely to further lead to other life events, such as disruption of marital relationships and the challenges of repeated relocations to temporary housing. The disaster after the disaster is a concept that is often spoken about in relief circles, and these ongoing life events following disasters play a central role in determining the patterns and longitudinal course of the emerging morbidity.

4.2.1. The Nature of Stresses

From the early literature came the hypothesis that anxiety disorders arise from situations associated with threat, whereas depressive disorders result from exposure to loss events (Brown, 1993). However, epidemiological observations suggested that life events also have a nonspecific effect as a risk factor for all disorders (Faravelli, Catena, Scarpato, & Ricca, 2007). Still, what environmental factors predict anxiety disorders versus affective disorders in the aftermath of disasters remains of considerable interest. Furthermore, the specific role of disaster exposure and its immediate impact as compared to its longer-term consequences is a matter that has been inadequately studied as a determinant of the different range of psychiatric disorders that arise in disaster-affected communities. While this chapter will focus specifically on anxiety disorders and PTSD, it should be acknowledged that there is an extensive literature demonstrating the comorbidity of PTSD with not only anxiety disorders but also major depressive disorder. When continuous measures of anxiety and depression are used, these are generally found to be highly correlated phenomena.

Furthermore, it is relatively uncommon, particularly in treatment seeking samples, that individuals only meet one diagnosis. In a significant majority of studies, more than 50% of individuals with PTSD also satisfy the diagnostic criteria for major depressive disorder (Kessler, Sonnega, Bromet, Hughes, & Nelson, 1995). Epidemiological samples similarly find high rates of alcohol abuse in individuals with PTSD (McFarlane, 1998). This high degree of comorbidity implies that the separation of psychopathology into general categories, such as anxiety disorders, depressive disorders, and substance abuse, is an artificial distinction driven by current systems of classification and presumes high degrees of specificity. Hyman (2007) has proposed that the future systems of diagnosis should also include categorical dimensions. Indeed, the early hypothesis that the anxiety disorders arise from a particular type of environmental stressor, in contrast to depressive disorders, is unlikely.

4.3. BACKGROUND PREVALENCE OF DISORDER

There have now been a number of large national mental health surveys that have estimated the prevalence of psychiatric disorders. In the United States, the Epidemiological Catchment Area Survey (Helzer, Robins, & McEvoy, 1987) and the National Comorbidity Study and its replication (Kessler, Chiu, Demler, Merikangas, & Walters, 2005; Kessler et al., 1995) have examined both the lifetime and 12-month prevalence of the more common Axis 1 disorders. Similar surveys have been conducted in Australia, the United Kingdom, and, more recently, in a range of other countries (Wang et al., 2007). In general, these indicate that the lifetime prevalence of PTSD is at approximately 6% to 9%, with the 12-month prevalence of approximately 3%. Similar prevalence estimates exist for panic disorder, generalized anxiety disorder, and agoraphobia (Kessler et al., 2005). Any study of a disaster needs to take into consideration these prevalence estimates.

Disasters are events that impact upon communities, which at the time of the disaster already will have a proportion of people suffering from psychiatric disorders. The general prevalence estimates indicate that at any particular point in time approximately 25% of the population will be suffering from a psychiatric disorder (Kessler et al., 2005). While the prevalence estimates of the community affected by the disaster may vary according to its demographics and risk factors, little is known about the relationship between the preexisting psychiatric morbidity at the time of the event and the disorders that emerge in the aftermath.

A series of possible interactions exist. First, an individual may not develop a new disorder, but rather there may be the worsening of a condition, such as panic disorder, in the aftermath of a disaster. Second, an existing condition such as simple phobia may represent a risk factor for the development of further anxiety disorders after disaster exposure. Finally, the individual may develop a new comorbid disorder above and beyond the condition that they were already experiencing at the time of the traumatic event.

The fact that few studies consider this possibility means that it is often difficult to make precise statements about the incidence of new disorders following a disaster in contrast to the prevalence estimates. Furthermore, prevalence estimates are often based around relatively few diagnoses, such as PTSD, which make it difficult to reflect on the more general pool of psychiatric morbidity within a disaster-affected community. Thus understanding of the prevalence of disorders in disaster-affected communities and the optimal design of treatment services is limited. However, there is little doubt that these events represent major opportunities to improve the quality of care for a range of psychiatric disorders because of the increased concern about the psychological well-being of the community.

A further important issue highlighted by community epidemiological studies is the prevalence of traumatic events. The definition in the DSM-III-R considers traumatic events outside the range of normal human experience. However, as methodological sophistication for documenting trauma exposure has increased, the evidence suggests that at a minimum, approximately 50% of women and 60% of men have had traumatic exposures (Creamer, Burgess, & McFarlane, 2001; Kessler et al., 1995), and more detailed questioning demonstrates even higher prevalence estimates (Breslau, Peterson, Poisson, Schultz, & Lucia, 2004). Disasters are dramatic and critical events in the life of communities, and it should be recognized that many of the exposed individuals also have experienced other major traumatic events that are likely to interact with the effect of the disaster. In a recent longitudinal study of children exposed to a major bushfire in Australia, prior exposure to other traumatic events was more substantial than the disaster in terms of resultant psychiatric morbidity (McFarlane & Van Hooff, 2005). Consequently, there was little difference between the exposed and comparison samples. Furthermore, the data suggested that the increasing number of exposures to traumatic events increased the probability of adverse mental health outcomes. For these reasons, it is critical that the impact of any disaster and its role in determining anxiety disorders, particularly PTSD, be considered against the background prevalence of other trauma exposures within the community.

4.4. RANGE OF DISORDERS

The disaster literature has been dominated by the prevalence of PTSD (see Tables 4.1 and 4.2). This tradition goes back to the work of the Swiss psychiatrist, Stierlin, who carried out the first systematic examination of disaster victims following the 1907 earthquake in Messina, which killed over 70,000 people. He found that 25% of the survivors suffered from sleep disturbances with nightmares and images of extraordinary intensity. Their symptoms were not well predicted by predisposition. He also studied a 1906 mine disaster in Courrieres. He concluded that neurosis was not a good general descriptor and took issue with Krapelin, a highly influential German psychiatrist, over these issues (as cited in Weisaeth & Van der Kolk, 1996).

In both adults and children, questionnaires and interviews have been used for making PTSD prevalence estimates, which range from less than 10% to 70%. The studies listed in Tables 4.1 and 4.2 are not exhaustive but do highlight the challenges in interpreting the findings and developing generalizations from these studies. Challenges revolve around different time periods having elapsed after the disaster, the identification and recruitment of representative samples in the disrupted environment following disaster, and the use of different measures where the cut-offs are not cross-validated. Furthermore, the nature of individual disasters can mean these events have very different exposures and losses – for instance, consider the September 11th terrorist attacks in the United States versus the Indian Ocean tsunami of 2004 – making comparisons relatively meaningless.

The anxiety disorders that have been associated with disasters are generalized anxiety disorder, panic disorder, obsessive-compulsive disorder (OCD), social phobia, and specific phobia. In discussing their relationships, it is important to separate the probability of true independence of symptoms of these disorders from the occurrence of varying patterns of comorbidity with the passage of time. The discussion of these matters is further influenced by the fact that the conventions for recording patterns of comorbidity have changed between DSM-III (American Psychiatric Association, 1980) and DSM-IV (American Psychiatric Association, 1994). Previously it was considered that there were primary disorders and that these conditions existed in a system of hierarchical diagnosis where depressive disorders took precedence over the presence of an anxiety disorder. It was only with the development of highly standardized structured diagnostic interviews that these conventions were challenged, and hence, the true prevalence of some of these disorders has only been examined in the last 15 years. The problem remains, however, that the rates of comorbidity from structured diagnostic interviews are significantly higher than those obtained in most clinical settings, implying that clinicians still impose some degree of disorder hierarchy in clinical practice.

From a phenomenological perspective, a central issue is that there is a very substantial overlay of symptoms between these disorders, and the application of the exclusion criteria is not done in a systematic way. For example, Criterion D for generalized anxiety disorders states

> the focus of the anxiety and worry is not confined to features of an Axis 1 disorder, e.g., the anxiety, worry is not about having a panic attack (as in panic disorder), being embarrassed in public (as in social phobia), being contaminated (as in obsessive compulsive disorder)...and the anxiety and worry do not occur exclusively during posttraumatic stress disorder. (American Psychiatric Association, 1994, p. 436)

In PTSD, one of the symptoms is hypervigilance, which implies a general watchfulness for danger. Determining whether the patient's anxiety about perceived threat and dangerousness in their environment is directly related to the PTSD often involves clinical judgment of considerable subtlety that is unlikely to have interrater reliability. Similarly, in social phobia the exclusion criteria states, "the fear or avoidance is not due to the direct physiological effects of a substance (e.g., drug abuse or medication), or a general medical condition and is not better accounted for by another mental disorder" (American Psychiatric Association, 1994, p. 417). The differentiation of social withdrawal and avoidance of PTSD from the avoidance in phobic disorders can be a challenging clinical question. Further, if the disaster exposure occurred in a public place, such as a shooting in shopping mall, it can be difficult to separate avoidance of open public spaces, typical of agoraphobia, from avoidance of traumatic reminders. Also, in individuals who have been disfigured by injury, being in crowds represents a major challenge if they sense people are looking at their injuries. While the secondary avoidance of these situations is directly related to the traumatic memory, such shame and avoidance can be difficult to separate from social phobia.

In relation to OCD, Criterion D states, "if another Axis 1 disorder is present, the content of the obsessions or the compulsions is not restricted to it" (American Psychiatric Association, 1994, p. 423). Again, the interpretation of these phenomena in PTSD is challenging. There are many similarities between the intrusive and distressing thoughts in PTSD and the associated avoidance and nature of obsessional thoughts. Given that obsessional thoughts often involve intrusive preoccupations about the potential of harm coming to others and that these may directly result from external sources of danger similar to those experienced in disaster, careful dissection of these phenomena is required to determine whether the criteria for obsessions are met. A further complicating factor is the active attempt by individuals with PTSD to avoid their thoughts and feelings associated with the event, similar to the dysphoria that individuals with OCD have for their obsessive thinking. The similarity between the involuntary and unwanted nature of the intrusive thoughts in PTSD and the unbidden nature of obsessional thoughts has received little comment in the scientific literature, despite the obvious diagnostic relevance of the question. In structured diagnostic interviews, which do not allow for a fine-grained analysis of these differences, there is a potential for risk of misclassification of these phenomena.

The relationship between panic disorder and PTSD raises a series of similar questions. In particular, the B4 and 5 diagnostic criteria, namely psychological distress and physiological distress on exposure to traumatic reminders, have few characteristics that differentiate the acute pattern of distress from a panic disorder. Many patients with PTSD do not recognize the symbolic nature of subtle triggers, but structured diagnostic interviews depend upon the individual reporting the link between the reminder and the pattern of distress. Other than the frequency of the episodes, there is no other specific differentiating symptom, leaving substantial error for misclassification. Similarly, an individual may report a simple phobia, such as a fear of wind in extreme weather conditions, without making the link between this fear and a prior exposure to a major bushfire disaster. Thus, it is important to consider the interrelationship between the various anxiety disorders and PTSD in the aftermath of a disaster. On the one hand, individuals with PTSD may be given a range of comorbid anxiety diagnoses arising from the failure of the individual to recognize the link between their symptoms and symbolic reminders. On the other hand, epidemiological studies identify a group of individuals who do not satisfy the diagnostic criteria for PTSD, but are found to have another anxiety disorder. With this group, the possibility exists that some of these individuals may in fact have an "occult" PTSD, where the individual does not make the appropriate links between the provocation stimuli of their symptoms and the disaster. Therefore, the interpretation of the epidemiological data derived from structured diagnostic interviews has a series of limitations that should be taken into account in their interpretation.

4.5. THE IMPACT OF EXISTING ANXIETY DISORDERS ON PERI-DISASTER BEHAVIOR

It commonly has been presumed that individuals with existing psychiatric disorders will behave in excessively fearful and erratic ways at the time of a major disaster. One study specifically examined this question in a cohort of anxiety disorder patients who were being treated at the time of Californian earthquake (Bystritsky, Vapnik, Maidment, Pynoos, & Steinberg, 2000). There was no evidence supporting the hypothesis that these individuals would behave in a maladaptive manner. However, there is a case report (McFarlane, 1986) of a woman with agoraphobia who died as a consequence of her fear of leaving her house though it ignited during a bushfire disaster.

4.6. POSTTRAUMATIC STRESS DISORDER

Posttraumatic stress disorder is the most frequently studied condition in modern disaster literature. From a psychopathological point of view, it is of particular interest because the core of the disorder is the intrusive and distressing recollections of the disaster. From an etiological point of view, these memories drive the hyperarousal and the avoidance and disengagement that emerge in the months and years following the event. The condition has a holistic value because of the immediacy of the link to the disaster as the cause of the disorder. As was the case with veteran populations, this condition is less stigmatized in some regards than other psychiatric disorders because of the obvious critical role of the disaster in its etiology.

It is beyond the scope of this chapter to conduct a complete review of the studies that have estimated the prevalence of PTSD, though this literature has been extensively reviewed elsewhere (Norris et al., 2002; Norris, Friedman, Watson, et al., 2002). Furthermore, the prevalence estimates are very difficult to generalize from because of a number of factors that modify the data. Another review outlined the different approaches that have been used to study disaster-affected populations (McFarlane, 2004). Estimates are significantly influenced by the method used to assess PTSD. For example, ICD-10 criteria generate higher prevalence rates than DSM-IV criteria (Peters, Slade, & Andrews, 1999). In some disasters, such as a wild fire, everyone within the disaster zone has a direct exposure, whereas with an earthquake there is a much larger gradient of exposure from the epicenter to the periphery of the event. Ultimately, the intensity of the exposure is a central factor to the prevalence of the disorder; however, the findings of a particular study are as much likely to be a consequence of the sampling strategy used as an interpretable measure of prevalence. Many of the published studies also do not use representative samples, which creates difficulty in defining hierarchies of effect.

The studies of greatest interest are those that have followed populations longitudinally and have monitored the course of PTSD and the impact of the recovery environment (Neria, Nandi, & Galea, 2007; Norris, 2006). These studies highlight how a matrix of factors affect individuals in the aftermath of these events above and beyond the magnitude of the initial exposure and the losses endured by the individual and the community. Another body of literature of particular relevance is studies that have examined the uptake of services by disaster-affected communities. A striking observation is that there is a substantial delay in treatment seeking, and only a minority will seek formal psychiatric treatment. These findings are similar to the recent replication of the National Comorbidity Study, which showed that the mean duration between the onset of PTSD and seeking treatment was 12 years; only 7% of individuals sought treatment within the initial year following the trauma exposure (Wang et al., 2005). These data combined with other observations, particularly following September 11th, highlight the need to take a very long-term perspective on service provision following disasters (Stuber, Galea, Boscarino, & Schlesinger, 2006). The longest follow-ups that have been conducted, namely those of the Piper Alpha oil field disaster (Hull, Alexander, & Klein, 2002) and the Aberfan disaster (Morgan et al., 2003), highlight the continuing and chronic nature of PTSD.

Subsyndromal PTSD also has attracted considerable interest in epidemiological studies but has only recently attracted the same degree of attention in research on disaster-affected populations (see Table 4.1). The evidence on subsyndromal PTSD indicates that the degree of disability is not dissimilar to the full blown syndrome (Stein, Walker, Hazen, & Forde, 1997). Hence, in dealing with disaster-affected communities, the prevalence of those who potentially may require assistance needs to take into account these broader definitions of morbidity. Recent studies of returning veterans highlight that many seeking treatment from mental health services do not have the full-blown syndrome of PTSD (Milliken, Auchterlonie, & Hoge, 2007).

The relationship between PTSD and the associated comorbidities with other anxiety and depressive disorders is important in determining the chronicity of morbidity following disasters. In general, the findings in disaster-affected populations are that those with comorbid disorders have a greater probability of chronic disorder (McFarlane & Papay, 1992; Onder, Tural, Aker, Kilic, & Erdogan, 2006). In addition, it appears that panic at the time of an event is a risk factor for poorer outcomes (Person, Tracy, & Galea, 2006); this prognostic relationship is particularly apparent with major depressive disorder. Again, this argues for the consideration of a range of dimensions of response following disasters, rather than focusing on individual disorders.

4.7. OTHER ANXIETY DISORDERS

There is little epidemiological research focusing in detail on other anxiety disorders such as OCD, generalized anxiety disorder, specific phobia, and social phobia following disasters. Several studies, such as those of Onder and colleagues (2006), have identified increased rates of these conditions compared with National Mental Health samples up to 3 years following the trauma exposure. One study examined the generalized anxiety disorders in adolescents following a super cyclone found a 12% prevalence of generalized anxiety disorder in a setting where the prevalence of PTSD was 26.9% (Kar & Bastia, 2006). In children there is evidence for prevalence of anxiety disorders after a disaster ranging from 9.9% to 61% (excluding PTSD) depending on the sample and trauma experienced (Bolton, O'Ryan,

Udwin, Boyle, & Yule, 2000; Green et al., 1990; Hoven et al., 2005; Morgan et al., 2003). The lack of research into the prevalence of specific phobia after major disasters, especially weather phobias, is surprising given the theoretical relevance of such events in leading to phobic anxiety (Magee, 1999). Findings derived from the U.S. National Comorbidity Study found a unique relationship between 12 negative types of life events and chronic childhood adversities (Kessler et al., 1995). In particular, specific phobia was associated with chronic childhood trauma, whereas the onset of social phobia was associated with sexual assault. Agoraphobia, however, had a stronger association with life threatening accidents and other natural disasters.

Given the burden of anxiety disorders in community epidemiological studies (Smit et al., 2006), more attention should be focused upon these conditions in disaster-affected populations. It is unlikely that there will be simple relationships between these disorders and disasters, and researchers must consider disasters in the context of the range of other stressors that individuals have experienced in their lives. Patterns of learned fear responses that manifest as anxiety disorders are likely to be a consequence of the interactions between the more recent disaster experience and these prior negative life events. In terms of learning theory, the ability of disasters to reinforce previously conditioned patterns of fear and the link between these two precise elements of the recent disaster exposure are important matters that have received surprisingly scant attention. For example, Conejo-Galindo and colleagues (2007) found in a hospital treatment sample after the terrorist attacks in Madrid increased rates of generalized anxiety disorder, agoraphobia, and panic disorder, and these rates remained similar 1 month after the disaster and 1 year later.

While it is beyond the scope of this chapter, there is another large body of evidence that has looked at the relationship between anxiety disorders and other types of life events. Embedded within this literature is the importance of recent adversity in the onset of these conditions (Hobfoll et al., 2007). However, the specific role of disasters has generally not been explored. Researchers in the field should recognize that important differences are likely to exist between cultures and that the challenge remains to develop instruments that have similar sensitivity and specificity between cultures. For example, a population prevalence study in Nigeria found virtually no generalized anxiety disorder or PTSD, despite the obvious stresses that exist within this community (Gureje, Lasebikan, Kola, & Makanjuola, 2006).

Anxiety disorders other than PTSD have been looked at in more detail in children, in part because of the potential developmental impact of disorders such as separation anxiety. However, the problem remains that the overlap of these conditions suggests a general diathesis of distress, and its severity is marked by the number of disorders.

4.8. CORRELATES OF ANXIETY DISORDERS

The etiology of psychiatric disorders is a scientific question that has been approached using a variety of methodologies, including epidemiology, case control studies, and neurobiological investigations in clinical and population cohorts. There is a vast body of literature examining the role of life events as causative factors in psychological disorders as well as a generation of more recent studies that have examined the interaction of environmental and genetic factors (Cooper, 2001). These studies have often been conducted in the context of a complex matrix of interrelated variables, such as personality, social support, and sociodemographic characteristics of individuals (Kendler, Prescott, Myers, & Neale, 2003). This general literature should be considered in any discussion of PTSD and anxiety disorders following disasters because studies of different populations using the range of methodologies outlined above all make their particular contributions to understanding the multifactorial interaction of predisposing, precipitating, and perpetuating factors for psychiatric disorders.

There is also a specialized literature that has examined the etiology of PTSD and anxiety disorders in the setting of a range of stressors other than disasters. This literature has been summarized in two meta-analyses (Brewin, Andrews, & Valentine, 2000; Ozer, Best, Lipsey, & Weiss, 2003) that have brought together a number of studies of different traumatic events that allow the development of causal modeling. The relevance to disaster-affected populations is based upon the presumption that the causal factors in PTSD are relatively independent of the nature of the stressor. In essence, the substantial difference between disasters and other forms of trauma is the loss of communal resources and the shared traumatization of the broader social network in which the individual lives. However, this is not universally true of disasters involving travel accidents or terrorist incidents because the victim is defined by their chance happening at a particular point in time, such as on a commuter train or on an aircraft. The issues for such an individual are very similar to a person involved in a fatal accident that involved fewer casualties. The main difference with these events is the degree of media interest, and as a consequence, such events have the capacity at times to elicit greater understanding and concern than the victims of individual traumatic events. The etiological variables of particular importance in terms of causal variance explained are the intensity or gradient of trauma exposure and social support in the aftermath of the traumatic experience.

The lack of research into the other anxiety disorders makes it difficult to make any conclusive comments about the precise etiological factors at work. The issue is further complicated by the degree of comorbidity and the lack of longitudinal observations. Hence, this is fertile area for further research.

4.9. FUTURE RESEARCH ISSUES

Norris (2006), in a review of 225 disaster studies, highlighted a number of deficiencies in the literature, such as cross-sectional design, convenience sampling, and small samples. Many of the studies failed to take account of the broader context of the disaster and, in particular, the prevalence of psychiatric morbidity in the affected communities before the event. Of critical interest is the relationship between the existing morbidity within the community and the emerging PTSD and anxiety disorders that follow from the disaster exposure. Furthermore, the intersection with traumatic events in these communities that occur before and after the disaster is critical in better understanding the course and risk of developing PTSD. Too often, disasters are studied in isolation from the other traumatic exposures that individuals have had to contend with before the disaster. A number of studies have particularly identified the role of childhood exposures as risk factors for PTSD, but it is probable that traumatic exposures in adulthood carry with them a cumulative consequence of similar significance.

The importance of other life stresses before and following disasters is a causal matrix of particular importance to PTSD and anxiety disorders. Hobfoll's (1989) conservation of resources theory highlights how individuals' resilience will be significantly affected by the range of choices that they have as determined by their interpersonal and material resources. The impact of social disadvantage is an issue that particularly requires further investigation in terms of the onset and etiology of anxiety disorders and PTSD. Social class is a very blunt measure of individual resources that can protect or aggravate the effects of stress.

Resilience is a challenging concept that attracts considerable interest but has proved somewhat illusive in terms of actual objective findings following disasters. One of the important issues is to ensure uniform definitions are used in future research. An individual who experiences a disastrous event without any substantial distress is different from an individual who becomes symptomatic following some grievous loss but quickly recovers, and both differ still from a person who has been symptomatic following a previous traumatic event and remains symptomatic in the face of a further major threat. These scenarios all represent different forms of positive adaptation and are yet to be adequately captured in quantitative studies that characterize the differentiating features of the individuals. Clearly, temperament and hardiness are critical concepts that deserve careful exploration.

Norris (2006) further highlighted in her review that more recent studies have tended to less frequently use longitudinal designs of representative samples. It is therefore critical that future research does not simply examine a new disaster imposing the same limitations of previous research. Ultimately, it is critical that research on each future disaster aims to elucidate a further scientific question, rather than simply being descriptive of the event at hand. Extending the research beyond PTSD and looking at the other anxiety disorders is an important priority. Benight, McFarlane, and Norris (2006) have highlighted some of the challenges for further investigation of the impact of disasters on the etiology and course of PTSD and the anxiety disorders.

Intervention studies, such as those of Duffy and colleagues (2007), which quantify the benefits or otherwise of evidence-based treatments for PTSD and anxiety disorders should also be an important priority. Ultimately, the purpose of gaining understanding of PTSD and anxiety disorders following disasters is to better identify and treat affected individuals.

4.10. CONCLUSION

The disorder that has attracted greatest interest in the aftermath of disasters is PTSD, and the available data indicate the substantial prevalence and associated burden of morbidity. The variability of the sampling methods and the timing of studies make it difficult to make precise generalizations, and the relative paucity of data about other anxiety disorders means that it is more difficult to make informed incidence and prevalence estimates. However, the critical lesson is that disasters take a substantial toll in psychiatric morbidity that intersects with the existing disadvantage and morbidity in the affected populations.

The attention and concern that is focused on the early days following the disaster needs to be converted into a sustained effort to address the long-term burden arising from PTSD and the other anxiety disorders. Indeed, these events can provide an opportunity for a more general improvement in the mental health of the affected community. Future studies should attempt to better characterize the nature of the comorbidity between PTSD and the other anxiety disorders. Of particular interest are the subsyndromal and more minor anxiety disorder, such as simple phobia, as they may represent the lasting vulnerability within the affected population that could place them at risk of further traumatic stress.

REFERENCES

American Psychiatric Association. (1980). *Diagnostic and statistical manual of mental disorders,* 3rd ed. Washington, DC: Author.

(1994). *Diagnostic and statistical manual of mental disorders,* 4th ed. Washington, DC: Author.

Armagan, E., Engindeniz, Z., Devay, A. O., Erdur, B., & Ozcakir, A. (2006). Frequency of post-traumatic stress disorder among relief force workers after the tsunami in Asia: Do rescuers become victims? *Prehospital and Disaster Medicine, 21*(3), 168–172.

Benight, C. C., McFarlane, A. C., & Norris, F. H. (2006). Formulating questions about post-disaster mental health. In F. Norris, S. Galea, M. Friedman & P. Watson (Eds.), *Methods for disasters mental health research.* New York: The Guilford Press

Bolton, D., O'Ryan, D., Udwin, O., Boyle, S., & Yule, W. (2000). The long-term psychological effects of a disaster experienced in adolescence: II: General psychopathology. *Journal of Child Psychology and Psychiatry, 41*(4), 513–523.

Breslau, N., Peterson, E. L., Poisson, L. M., Schultz, L. R., & Lucia, V. C. (2004). Estimating post-traumatic stress disorder in the community: Lifetime perspective and the impact of typical traumatic events. *Psychological Medicine, 34*(5), 889–898.

Brewin, C. R., Andrews, B., & Valentine, J. D. (2000). Meta-analysis of risk factors for posttraumatic stress disorder in trauma-exposed adults. *Journal of Consulting and Clinical Psychology, 68*(5), 748–766.

Brown, G. W. (1993). Life events and affective disorder: Replications and limitations. *Psychosomatic Medicine, 55*(3), 248–259.

Bryant, R., Creamer, M., O'Donnell, M., Silove, D., & McFarlane, A. C. (2008). A multi-site study of the capacity of acute stress disorder diagnosis to predict posttraumatic stress disorder. *Journal of Clinical Psychiatry, 69*(11), 1694–1701.

Bryant, R.A. (2005). Predicting posttraumatic stress disorder from acute reactions. *Journal of Trauma and Dissociation*, *6*(2), 5–15.

Bystritsky, A., Vapnik, T., Maidment, K., Pynoos, R.S., & Steinberg, A.M. (2000). Acute responses of anxiety disorder patients after a natural disaster. *Depression and Anxiety*, *11*(1), 43–44.

Centers for Disease Control, and Prevention (CDC). (2004). Mental health status of World Trade Center rescue and recovery workers and volunteers – New York City, July 2002–August 2004. *MMWR Morbidity and Mortality Weekly Report*, *53*(35), 812–815.

Chou, F.H., Wu, H.C., Chou, P., Su, C.Y., Tsai, K.Y., Chao, S.S., et al. (2007). Epidemiologic psychiatric studies on post-disaster impact among Chi-Chi earthquake survivors in Yu-Chi, Taiwan. *Psychiatry and Clinical Neuroscience*, *61*(4), 370–378.

Conejo-Galindo, J., Medina, O., Fraguas, D., Teran, S., Sainz-Corton, E., & Arango, C. (2007). Psychopathological sequelae of the 11 March terrorist attacks in Madrid: An epidemiological study of victims treated in a hospital. *European Archives of Psychiatry and Clinical Neuroscience*, *258*(1), 28–34.

Cooper, B. (2001). Nature, nurture and mental disorder: Old concepts in the new millennium. *British Journal of Psychiatry*, *178*(Suppl. 40), s91–101.

Creamer, M., Burgess, P., & McFarlane, A.C. (2001). Post-traumatic stress disorder: Findings from the Australian National Survey of Mental Health and Well-being. *Psychological Medicine*, *31*(7), 1237–1247.

Curran, P.S. (1988). Psychiatric aspects of terrorist violence: Northern Ireland 1969–1987. *British Journal of Psychiatry*, *153*, 470–475.

de Bocanegra, H.T., Moskalenko, S., & Kramer, E.J. (2006). PTSD, depression, prescription drug use, and health care utilization of Chinese workers affected by the WTC attacks. *Journal of Immigration and Minority Health*, *8*(3), 203–210.

de Ville de Goyet, C. (2007). Health lessons learned from the recent earthquakes and Tsunami in Asia. *Prehospital and Disaster Medicine*, *22*(1), 15–21.

DeSalvo, K.B., Hyre, A.D., Ompad, D.C., Menke, A., Tynes, L.L., & Muntner, P. (2007). Symptoms of posttraumatic stress disorder in a New Orleans workforce following Hurricane Katrina. *Journal of Urban Health*, *84*(2), 142–152.

Dirkzwager, A.J., van der Velden, P.G., Grievink, L., & Yzermans, C.J. (2007). Disaster-related posttraumatic stress disorder and physical health. *Psychosomatic Medicine*, *69*(5), 435–440.

Duffy, M., Gillespie, K., & Clark, D.M. (2007). Posttraumatic stress disorder in the context of terrorism and other civil conflict in Northern Ireland: Randomised controlled trial. *BMJ*, *334*(7604), 1147.

Faravelli, C., Catena, M., Scarpato, A., & Ricca, V. (2007). Epidemiology of life events: Life events and psychiatric disorders in the Sesto Fiorentino study. *Psychotherapy and Psychosomatics*, *76*(6), 361–368.

Garrison, C.Z., Bryant, E.S., Addy, C.L., Spurrier, P.G., Freedy, J.R., & Kilpatrick, D.G. (1995). Posttraumatic stress disorder in adolescents after Hurricane Andrew. *Journal of the American Academy of Child and Adolescent Psychiatry*, *34*(9), 1193–1201.

Giannopoulou, I., Strouthos, M., Smith, P., Dikaiakou, A., Galanopoulou, V., & Yule, W. (2006). Posttraumatic stress reactions of children and adolescents exposed to the Athens 1999 earthquake. *Euopean Psychiatry*, *21*(3), 160–166.

Goenjian, A.K., Molina, L., Steinberg, A.M., Fairbanks, L.A., Alvarez, M.L., Goenjian, H.A., et al. (2001). Posttraumatic stress and depressive reactions among Nicaraguan adolescents after hurricane Mitch. *American Journal of Psychiatry*, *158*(5), 788–794.

Goenjian, A.K., Pynoos, R.S., Steinberg, A.M., Najarian, L.M., Asarnow, J.R., Karayan, I., et al. (1995). Psychiatric comorbidity in children after the 1988 earthquake in Armenia. *Journal of the American Academy of Child Adolescent Psychiatry*, *34*(9), 1174–1184.

Goenjian, A.K., Walling, D., Steinberg, A.M., Karayan, I., Najarian, L.M., & Pynoos, R. (2005). A prospective study of posttraumatic stress and depressive reactions among treated and untreated adolescents 5 years after a catastrophic disaster. *American Journal of Psychiatry*, *162*(12), 2302–2308.

Green, B.L., Korol, M., Grace, M.C., Vary, M.G., Leonard, A.C., Gleser, G.C., et al. (1991). Children and disaster: Age, gender, and parental effects on PTSD symptoms. *Journal of the American Academy of Child and Adolescent Psychiatry*, *30*(6), 945–951.

Green, B.L., Lindy, J.D., Grace, M.C., Gleser, G.C., Leonard, A.C., Korol, M., et al. (1990). Buffalo Creek survivors in the second decade: Stability of stress symptoms. *American Journal of Orthopsychiatry*, *60*(1), 43–54.

Green, B.L., Lindy, J.D., Grace, M.C., & Leonard, A.C. (1992). Chronic posttraumatic stress disorder and diagnostic comorbidity in a disaster sample. *Journal of Nervous and Mental Diseases*, *180*(12), 760–766.

Gureje, O., Lasebikan, V.O., Kola, L., & Makanjuola, V.A. (2006). Lifetime and 12-month prevalence of mental disorders in the Nigerian Survey of Mental Health and Well-Being. *British Journal of Psychiatry, 188*, 465–471.

Helzer, J.E., Robins, L.N., & McEvoy, L. (1987). Post-traumatic stress disorder in the general population. Findings of the epidemiologic catchment area survey. *New England Journal of Medicine, 317*(26), 1630–1634.

Hobfoll, S.E. (1989). Conservation of resources. A new attempt at conceptualizing stress. *American Psychology, 44*(3), 513–524.

Hobfoll, S.E., Watson, P., Bell, C.C., Bryant, R.A., Brymer, M.J., Friedman, M.J., et al. (2007). Five essential elements of immediate and mid-term mass trauma intervention: Empirical evidence. *Psychiatry, 70*(4), 283–315.

Hoven, C.W., Duarte, C.S., Lucas, C.P., Wu, P., Mandell, D.J., Goodwin, R.D., et al. (2005). Psychopathology among New York city public school children 6 months after September 11. *Archives of General Psychiatry, 62*(5), 545–552.

Hsu, C.C., Chong, M.Y., Yang, P., & Yen, C.F. (2002). Posttraumatic stress disorder among adolescent earthquake victims in Taiwan. *Journal of American Academy of Child and Adolescent Psychiatry, 41*(7), 875–881.

Hull, A.M., Alexander, D.A., & Klein, S. (2002). Survivors of the Piper Alpha oil platform disaster: Long-term follow-up study. *British Journal of Psychiatry, 181*, 433–438.

Hyman, S.E. (2007). Can neuroscience be integrated into the DSM-V? *National Review of Neuroscience, 8*(9), 725–732.

Ironson, G., Wynings, C., Schneiderman, N., Baum, A., Rodriguez, M., Greenwood, D., et al. (1997). Posttraumatic stress symptoms, intrusive thoughts, loss, and immune function after Hurricane Andrew. *Psychosomatic Medicine, 59*(2), 128–141.

John, P.B., Russell, S., & Russell, P.S. (2007). The prevalence of posttraumatic stress disorder among children and adolescents affected by tsunami disaster in Tamil Nadu. *Disaster Management and Response, 5*(1), 3–7.

Jones, E., Woolven, R., Durodie, B., & Wessely, S. (2004). Civilian morale during the Second World War: Responses to air raids re-examined. *Social History of Medicine, 17*, 463–479.

Kar, N., & Bastia, B.K. (2006). Post-traumatic stress disorder, depression and generalised anxiety disorder in adolescents after a natural disaster: A study of comorbidity. *Clinical Practice and Epidemiology in Mental Health, 2*, 17.

Kar, N., Mohapatra, P.K., Nayak, K.C., Pattanaik, P., Swain, S.P., & Kar, H.C. (2007). Post-traumatic stress disorder in children and adolescents one year after a super-cyclone in Orissa, India: Exploring cross-cultural validity and vulnerability factors. *BMC Psychiatry, 7*, 8.

Kendler, K.S., Prescott, C.A., Myers, J., & Neale, M.C. (2003). The structure of genetic and environmental risk factors for common psychiatric and substance use disorders in men and women. *Archives of General Psychiatry, 60*(9), 929–937.

Kessler, R.C., Chiu, W.T., Demler, O., Merikangas, K.R., & Walters, E.E. (2005). Prevalence, severity, and comorbidity of 12-month DSM-IV disorders in the National Comorbidity Survey Replication. *Archives of General Psychiatry, 62*(6), 617–627.

Kessler, R.C., Demler, O., Frank, R.G., Olfson, M., Pincus, H.A., Walters, E.E., et al. (2005). Prevalence and treatment of mental disorders, 1990 to 2003. *New England Journal of Medicine, 352*(24), 2515–2523.

Kessler, R.C., Sonnega, A., Bromet, E., Hughes, M., & Nelson, C.B. (1995). Posttraumatic stress disorder in the National Comorbidity Survey. *Archives of General Psychiatry, 52*(12), 1048–1060.

Kumar, M.S., Murhekar, M.V., Hutin, Y., Subramanian, T., Ramachandran, V., & Gupte, M.D. (2007). Prevalence of posttraumatic stress disorder in a coastal fishing village in Tamil Nadu, India, after the December 2004 tsunami. *American Journal of Public Health, 97*(1), 99–101.

Kuo, H.W., Wu, S.J., Ma, T.C., Chiu, M.C., & Chou, S.Y. (2007). Posttraumatic symptoms were worst among quake victims with injuries following the Chi-chi quake in Taiwan. *Journal of Psychosomatic Research, 62*(4), 495–500.

La Greca, A., Silverman, W.K., Vernberg, E.M., & Prinstein, M.J. (1996). Symptoms of posttraumatic stress in children after Hurricane Andrew: A prospective study. *Journal of Consulting and Clinical Psychology, 64*(4), 712–723.

Layton, B., & Krikorian, R. (2002). Memory mechanisms in posttraumatic stress disorder. *Journal of Neuropsychiatry and Clinical Neuroscience, 14*(3), 254–261.

Magee, W.J. (1999). Effects of negative life experiences on phobia onset. *Social Psychiatry and Psychiatric Epidemiology, 34*(7), 343–351.

Marshall, G.N., Schell, T.L., Elliott, M.N., Rayburn, N.R., & Jaycox, L.H. (2007). Psychiatric disorders among adults seeking emergency disaster assistance after a wildland-urban interface fire. *Psychiatric Services, 58*(4), 509–514.

McFarlane, A. (1988). The longitudinal course of post-traumatic morbidity: The range of outcomes and their predictors. *Journal of Nervous and Mental Disease, 176*(1), 30–39.

(2004). The contribution of epidemiology to the study of traumatic stress. *Social Psychiatry and Psychiatric Epidemiology, 39*(11), 874–882.

McFarlane, A. (2005). Psychiatric morbidity following disasters: Epidemiology, risk and protective factors. In J. J. López-Ibor, G. Christodoulou, M. Maj, N. Sartorius & A. Okasha (Eds.), *Disasters and mental health.* Chichester, West Sussex, England: John Wiley & Sons.

McFarlane, A., & Van Hooff, M. (2005, November) Adult psychological adjustment following childhood exposure to a disaster: A 20 year longitudinal follow-up of children exposed to the Ash Wednesday Bushfires. Paper presented at ISTSS Conference, Toronto (Currently under second review in *Journal of Abnormal Psychology).*

McFarlane, A. C. (1986). Posttraumatic morbidity of a disaster. A study of cases presenting for psychiatric treatment. *Journal of Nervous and Mental Diseases, 174*(1), 4–14.

(1989). The aetiology of post-traumatic morbidity: Predisposing, precipitating and perpetuating fac tors. *British Journal of Psychiatry, 154*, 221–228.

(1998). Epidemiological evidence about the relationship between PTSD and alcohol abuse: The nature of the association. *Addictive Behaviors, 23*(6), 813–825.

McFarlane, A. C., & Papay, P. (1992). Multiple diagnoses in posttraumatic stress disorder in the victims of a natural disaster. *Journal of Nervous and Mental Diseases, 180*(8), 498–504.

McMillen, J. C., North, C. S., & Smith, E. M. (2000). What parts of PTSD are normal: Intrusion, avoidance, or arousal? Data from the Northridge, California, earthquake. *Journal of Traumatic Stress, 13*(1), 57–75.

Milliken, C. S., Auchterlonie, J. L., & Hoge, C. W. (2007). Longitudinal assessment of mental health problems among active and reserve component soldiers returning from the Iraq war. *JAMA, 298*(18), 2141–2148.

Mitchell, J. T. (1983). When disaster strikes…the critical incident stress debriefing process. *Journal of Emergency Medical Services, 8*(1), 36–39.

Morgan, L., Scourfield, J., Williams, D., Jasper, A., & Lewis, G. (2003). The Aberfan disaster: 33-year follow-up of survivors. *British Journal of Psychiatry, 182*, 532–536.

Neria, Y., Gross, R., Olfson, M., Gameroff, M. J., Wickramaratne, P., Das, A., et al. (2006). Posttraumatic stress disorder in primary care one year after the 9/11 attacks. *General Hospital Psychiatry, 28*(3), 213–222.

Neria, Y., Nandi, A., & Galea, S. (2007). Posttraumatic stress disorder following disasters: A systematic review. *Psychology and Medicine, 38*(4), 467–480.

Neuner, F., Schauer, E., Catani, C., Ruf, M., & Elbert, T. (2006). Post-tsunami stress: A study of posttraumatic stress disorder in children living in three severely affected regions in Sri Lanka. *Journal of Traumatic Stress, 19*(3), 339–347.

Norris, F. H. (2006). Disaster research methods: Past progress and future directions. *Journal of Traumatic Stress, 19*(2), 173–184.

Norris, F. H., Friedman, M. J., & Watson, P. J. (2002). 60,000 disaster victims speak: Part II. Summary and implications of the disaster mental health research. *Psychiatry, 65*(3), 240–260.

Norris, F. H., Friedman, M. J., Watson, P. J., Byrne, C. M., Diaz, E., & Kaniasty, K. (2002). 60,000 disaster victims speak: Part I. An empirical review of the empirical literature, 1981–2001. *Psychiatry, 65*(3), 207–239.

Norris, F. H., Murphy, A. D., Baker, C. K., & Perilla, J. L. (2004). Post-disaster PTSD over four waves of a panel study of Mexico's 1999 flood. *Journal of Traumatic Stress, 17*(4), 283–292.

North, C. S., Kawasaki, A., Spitznagel, E. L., & Hong, B. A. (2004). The course of PTSD, major depression, substance abuse, and somatization after a natural disaster. *Journal of Nervous and Mental Diseases, 192*(12), 823–829.

North, C. S., Pfefferbaum, B., Tivis, L., Kawasaki, A., Reddy, C., & Spitznagel, E. L. (2004). The course of posttraumatic stress disorder in a follow-up study of survivors of the Oklahoma City bombing. *Annals of Clinical Psychiatry, 16*(4), 209–215.

O'Donnell, M. L., Creamer, M., Bryant, R. A., Schnyder, U., & Shalev, A. (2003). Posttraumatic disorders following injury: An empirical and methodological review. *Clinical Psychology Reviews, 23*(4), 587-603.

Onder, E., Tural, U., Aker, T., Kilic, C., & Erdogan, S. (2006). Prevalence of psychiatric disorders three years after the 1999 earthquake in Turkey: Marmara Earthquake Survey (MES). *Social Psychiatry and Psychiatric Epidemiology, 41*(11), 868–874.

Orcutt, H. K., Erickson, D. J., & Wolfe, J. (2004). The course of PTSD symptoms among Gulf War veterans: A growth mixture modeling approach. *Journal of Traumatic Stress, 17*(3), 195–202.

Ozer, E. J., Best, S. R., Lipsey, T. L., & Weiss, D. S. (2003). Predictors of posttraumatic stress disorder and symptoms in adults: A meta-analysis. *Psychological Bulletin, 129*(1), 52–73.

Peleg, T., & Shalev, A. Y. (2006). Longitudinal studies of PTSD: Overview of findings and methods. *CNS Spectrums, 11*(8), 589–602.

Person, C., Tracy, M., & Galea, S. (2006). Risk factors for depression after a disaster. *Journal of Nervous and Mental Disease, 194*(9), 659–666.

Peters, L., Slade, T., & Andrews, G. (1999). A comparison of ICD10 and DSM-IV criteria for posttraumatic stress disorder. *Journal of Traumatic Stress, 12*(2), 335–343.

Post, R. M., Weiss, S. R., Li, H., Leverich, G. S., & Pert, A. (1999). Sensitization components of posttraumatic stress disorder: Implications for therapeutics. *Seminars in Clinical Neuropsychiatry, 4*(4), 282–294.

Pynoos, R. S., Frederick, C., Nader, K., Arroyo, W., Steinberg, A., Eth, S., et al. (1987). Life threat and posttraumatic stress in school-age children. *Archives of General Psychiatry, 44*(12), 1057–1063.

Quarantelli, L. E., & Dynes, R. R. (1977). Response to social crisis and disaster. *Annual Review in Sociology, 3*, 23–49.

Shalev, A. Y. (2000). Biological responses to disasters. *Psychiatry Quarterly, 71*(3), 277–288.

Shannon, M. P., Lonigan, C. J., Finch, A. J., Jr., & Taylor, C. M. (1994). Children exposed to disaster: I. Epidemiology of post-traumatic symptoms and symptom profiles. *Journal of the American Academy of Child and Adolescent Psychiatry, 33*(1), 80–93.

Shephard, B. (2001). *A war of nerves*. Cambridge, MA: Harvard University Press.

Smit, F., Cuijpers, P., Oostenbrink, J., Batelaan, N., de Graaf, R., & Beekman, A. (2006). Costs of nine common mental disorders: Implications for curative and preventive psychiatry. *Journal of Mental Health Policy and Economics, 9*(4), 193–200.

Soldatos, C. R., Paparrigopoulos, T. J., Pappa, D. A., & Christodoulou, G. N. (2006). Early post-traumatic stress disorder in relation to acute stress reaction: An ICD-10 study among help seekers following an earthquake. *Psychiatry Research, 143*(2–3), 245–253.

Solomon, Z., & Mikulincer, M. (2006). Trajectories of PTSD: A 20-year longitudinal study. *American Journal of Psychiatry, 163*(4), 659–666.

Stein, M. B., Walker, J. R., Hazen, A. L., & Forde, D. R. (1997). Full and partial posttraumatic stress disorder: Findings from a community survey. *American Journal of Psychiatry, 154*(8), 1114–1119.

Stuber, J., Galea, S., Boscarino, J. A., & Schlesinger, M. (2006). Was there unmet mental health need after the September 11, 2001 terrorist attacks? *Social Psychiatry and Psychiatric Epidemiology, 41*(3), 230–240.

Stuber, J., Resnick, H., & Galea, S. (2006). Gender disparities in posttraumatic stress disorder after mass trauma. *Gender and Medicine, 3*(1), 54–67.

Tang, C. S. (2007). Trajectory of traumatic stress symptoms in the aftermath of extreme natural disaster: A study of adult Thai survivors of the 2004 Southeast Asian earthquake and tsunami. *Journal of Nervous and Mental Disease, 195*(1), 54–59.

Thienkrua, W., Cardozo, B. L., Chakkraband, M. L., Guadamuz, T. E., Pengjuntr, W., Tantipiwatanaskul, P., et al. (2006). Symptoms of posttraumatic stress disorder and depression among children in tsunami-affected areas in southern Thailand. *JAMA, 296*(5), 549–559.

van Griensven, F., Chakkraband, M. L., Thienkrua, W., Pengjuntr, W., Lopes Cardozo, B., Tantipiwatanaskul, P., et al. (2006). Mental health problems among adults in tsunami-affected areas in southern Thailand. *JAMA, 296*(5), 537–548.

Wang, P. S., Aguilar-Gaxiola, S., Alonso, J., Angermeyer, M. C., Borges, G., Bromet, E. J., et al. (2007). Use of mental health services for anxiety, mood, and substance disorders in 17 countries in the WHO world mental health surveys. *Lancet, 370*(9590), 841–850.

Wang, P. S., Lane, M., Olfson, M., Pincus, H. A., Wells, K. B., & Kessler, R. C. (2005). Twelve-month use of mental health services in the United States: Results from the National Comorbidity Survey Replication. *Archives of General Psychiatry, 62*(6), 629–640.

Weisaeth, L., & Van der Kolk, B. (1996). History. In A. McFarlane, B. V. D. Kolk & L. Weisaeth (Eds.), *Traumatic stress – the effects of overwhelming experience on mind, body and society*. New York: The Guilford Press.

Yule, W., Bolton, D., Udwin, O., Boyle, S., O'Ryan, D., & Nurrish, J. (2000). The long-term psychological effects of a disaster experienced in adolescence: I: The incidence and course of PTSD. *Journal of Child Psychology and Psychiatry, 41*(4), 503–511.

5 Physical Health Problems after Disasters

C. JORIS YZERMANS, BELLIS VAN DEN BERG, AND
ANJA J. E. DIRKZWAGER

5.1. INTRODUCTION

> The term *mental disorder* unfortunately implies a distinction between *mental* disorders and *physical* disorders that is a reductionistic anachronism of mind–body dualism. A compelling literature documents that there is much *physical* in *mental* disorders and much *mental* in *physical* disorders.

This passage from the introduction of the current edition of the *Diagnostic and statistical manual of mental disorders* (DSM-IV-TR) (American Psychiatric Association, 1994) reflects how we still struggle with the Cartesian heritage of the end of the eighteenth century. The linguistic (and the emotional) distinction between mental and physical illness, and the Cartesian mind–body dualism from which this was originally derived, still encourage lay people – and some physicians – to assume that the two are fundamentally different (Kendell, 2001). It often may lead to poor communication between doctors and their patients about the causality and the interpretation of (physical) symptoms and (psychological) problems. Suggesting that symptoms are "between the ears" or "in the mind" is often synonymous to not taking the patient seriously.

In the past decades, the distinction between soma and psyche also played an important role in the research on health problems after disasters. Following military research, especially after the war in Vietnam, approximately 90% of all disaster studies focus on posttraumatic stress disorder (PTSD) and the individual symptoms constituting this disorder. This substantial attention led to the official recognition of this disorder in the 1980s and the successful efforts to include the disorder in the DSM-III. Encouraged by military research after the Gulf War, increased attention was turned to physical symptoms of veterans, especially medically unexplained symptoms (MUS) (Engel, 2001). However, as a consequence of Cartesian dualism mindsets, less research focused on the mutual, causal influence of physical and mental illnesses, and disorders on each other. Likewise, it is not well known that physical symptoms may have a longer duration after disasters than psychological problems and disorders (Galea, 2007; Morren, Dirkzwager, Kessels, & Yzermans, 2007). In general, clinical research is primarily targeted on specific diseases, and symptoms-based research is still an emerging field of scientific inquiry (Kroenke, 2001).

In this chapter we first present a brief introduction to physical issues following disasters as well as disaster studies. In the second section, we present an update of a systematic review on symptoms after disasters, which originally was published in 2005 (van den Berg, Grievink, Yzermans, & Lebret, 2005). Next, we briefly discuss somatic diseases and disorders in disaster survivors, which are not often studied. Moreover, the relation between symptoms and diseases will be described, including attention to the question of what percentage of symptoms presented to the family physician is unexplained and whether relations occur between the two. Subsequently, we will focus on risk factors for physical health outcomes and the relationship between psychological problems and disorders and physical symptoms and diseases. We will discuss which mediating factors are of importance, especially the concurrence of mental and physical health problems. Finally, we will point out gaps in our knowledge and formulate some recommendations for further research.

5.1.1. The Course of Physical Health Problems over Time

Physical health problems that relate to disasters may be distinguished at different points in time.

A. Health problems existing before the disaster. Preexisting health conditions, especially chronic diseases, may be exacerbated during and after the disaster due to stress and excessive attention to bodily symptoms (Norris, Friedman, Watson, Byrne, Diaz, & Kaniasty, 2002). However, a recent study found that disaster survivors who were chronically ill before disaster exposure did not consistently have a different course of general health, physical role limitations, or mental health problems after the disaster than survivors without a preexisting chronic disease (van den Berg, van der Velden, Yzermans, Stellato, & Grievink, 2006).

B. Immediate health problems because of the disaster. Many health problems that may have lasting consequences originate in the acute phase: injuries, burns, fractures, cuts and lacerations, and specific disaster-related symptoms, such as crush syndrome and acute renal failure during and immediately after earthquakes (Pocan, Ozkan, Us, & Cakir, 2002; Vanholder et al., 2007), eye-problems during and after the sarin attack in Tokyo (Kawana, Ishimatsu, Kanda, 2001), hearing-problems directly after the explosion in Toulouse (Lang et al., 2007), burns after a discotheque fire in Volendam (Dorn, Yzermans, Guijt, & van der Zee, 2007), and a cough during and after the World Trade Center attacks in New York (Chen & Thurston, 2002).

C. Health problems in the first weeks after disaster. Apart from injuries, it is expected that in the first days and weeks after a disaster psychological problems and physical symptoms (but not disorders, nor diseases) will be present in many survivors. Uncertainty and fear – and stress in general – after disasters commonly generate symptoms (Bartholomew & Wessely, 2002) and induce anxiety and depression, along with their own somatic and autonomic concomitants (Barsky & Borus, 1999). Psychological problems and physical symptoms are often closely interwoven: Survivors try to regain control over their lives, and at that time, it may be less important whether a doctor diagnoses their problem to be mental (anxiousness, depressed feeling) or physical (neck pain, fatigue). These symptoms and problems are often typified as normal reactions to an abnormal event.

D. Health problems in the first year after disaster. Compared to the first weeks postdisaster, in the first year following the event, physical symptoms with a more chronic nature appear (Norris et al., 2002). After several months the situation may be more or less normalized for many survivors; for others, PTSD, major depression, or a generalized anxiety disorder may appear, often accompanied by physical symptoms. The comorbidity between physical symptoms and PTSD is especially well documented (Andreski, Chilcoat, & Breslau 1998; Dirkzwager, van der Velden, Grievink, & Yzermans, 2007; Engel, 2003; McFarlane, Atchinson, Rafalowicz, & Papay, 1994; Schnurr & Jankowski, 1999). Symptoms experienced by survivors at this stage may be attributed to disaster exposure, and it is difficult to disabuse the individual of this notion.

Notwithstanding the broad range of health problems associated with trauma, survivors are generally highly resilient, and the majority recovers with time. In a study among survivors of the September 11th World Trade Center attacks, within 1 year symptoms resolved in more than half (57%) of the participants (Foa, Stein, & McFarlane, 2006). Evidence suggests that normalcy returns after all significant days of a year (e.g., birthdays, Christmas and commemorations) have passed one time. However, an important factor in postdisaster well-being is the acceptability of living conditions; for example, living in a refugee camp may make it more difficult to return to a normal life. Other factors that play a key role include whether compensation was received in a timely manner (Brooks & McKinlay, 1992), information about any release of chemical substances and their possible health effects is available and well communicated (Yzermans & Gersons, 2002), and actions taken by authorities were transparent and no suspicions or accusations of any concealment arose either in the survivors or the media (Page, Petrie, & Wessely, 2006; Yzermans & Gersons, 2002).

E. Long-term health problems. The majority of disaster survivors do not have long-term health problems. However, a minority of survivors develop chronic symptoms (e.g., fatigue, back pain) and diseases (e.g., hypertension, diabetes mellitus); often they attribute their deteriorated health to disaster exposure.

5.1.2. Medically Unexplained Symptoms

In the aftermath of disasters, survivors experience physical symptoms, whether related or unrelated to distress and/or psychological problems. Some of these symptoms may be presented to a physician, who decides whether the symptom experienced is "medically explained" or "medically unexplained." To understand the concept of medically unexplained symptoms (MUS), it is important to make a distinction between illnesses and diseases. The following definitions were formulated by an international expert consensus group, with the more informal definitions as offered by Wessely provided in parentheses (Clauw et al., 2003; Wessely, 2004; Wessely & Freedman, 2006; Wessely, Nimnuan, & Sharpe, 1999). The term *medically unexplained symptoms* describe physical symptoms that provoke care-seeking but have no clinically determined pathogenesis after an appropriately thorough diagnostic evaluation (unexplained means that no consensual scientific explanation has been advanced that meets with universal acceptance; unexplained is not a code for psychiatric, still less for all in the mind). *Illness* is a subjective lack of wellness that is inferred through words and behavior (in illness a person reports symptomatic distress and suffering, but no pathological condition can be found to explain this as yet), while *disease* is a clinically identified pathophysiological process (in disease there is pathological evidence of dysfunction). Richardson and Engel (2004) add that MUS are *perceptual* (a person feels a symptom), *cognitive* (the person experiencing symptoms decides they are ominous) and *behavioral* (the person with symptoms seeks health care for them).

It is difficult to measure MUS; only examination by a physician can rule out an underlying medical explanation for reported symptoms, making it difficult to assess MUS through self-report questionnaires (van den Berg, Grievink, Stellato, Yzermans, & Lebret, 2005). Another potential problem is that research suggests that at least one-third of all symptoms in both clinical and population-based studies are medically unexplained (Kroenke, 2001), which means that MUS are omnipresent, with or without a disaster. Thus, it is difficult to reach conclusions about the increases in prevalences of symptoms after disaster.

MUS are also present in the general population and intertwine with psychological problems and quality of life. Moreover, MUS are related to functional impairment, increased illness behavior, and comorbid psychological problems. Survivors with more symptoms report significantly lower mean scores on all scales of the RAND-36 questionnaire. The literature suggests depression and anxiety are associated with a number of symptoms; for instance, in one study more than 60% of survivors who reported ten or more symptoms also reported depression and anxiety, compared to 2.4% of survivors with one or no symptoms (van den Berg, Grievink, Stellato, et al., 2005). However, another study found that the psychiatric morbidity in the general population was similar in both medically explained and medically unexplained categories (Kisely & Simon, 2006; Nimnuan, Hotopf, & Wessely, 2001).

In some cases, physicians will have to tell a survivor that current knowledge cannot explain their symptoms, which can negatively affect the doctor–patient relationship. One of the problems of MUS is that physicians tend to consider them the domain of mental health care (somatization, somatoform disorder, or hypochondrias as described in the DSM-IV), while patients perceive them to fall in the domain of somatic health care. However, it is possible that doctors underestimate patients' flexibility: Simon, Gater, Kisely, and Piccinelli (1996) suggest that "frequent somatic presentations of distress to primary care physicians may not reflect patients' inability or unwillingness to reveal emotional problems. Instead such presentations reflect patients' actual experience: Somatic and psychological distress are almost invariably intertwined."

Sometimes a group of MUS is believed to be a syndrome, the so-called functional somatic syndrome, such as fibromyalgia, multiple chemical sensitivity, and the Gulf War syndrome. These syndromes share similar phenomenologies, high rates of co-occurrence, similar epidemiological characteristics, and higher than expected prevalences of psychiatric comorbidity. They are more characterized by comparable, nonspecific, diffuse symptoms than by disease-specific demonstrable abnormalities of structure or function (Barsky & Borus, 1999; Mayou & Farmer, 2002; Wessely et al., 1999). Especially in the aftermath of disasters with intense and perhaps inflammatory media coverage, poor or nontransparent communication by the authorities, and/or perceived exposure to toxic substances, survivors are more likely to report symptoms and construct symptom patterns that take on the name of the disaster. Some examples of this include Bijlmer syndrome, Gulf War syndromes, Balkan war syndrome, and World Trade Center cough (Chen & Thurston, 2002; Rogers, 2000; Wessely, 2001; Yzermans & Gersons, 2002).

MUS are often similar between traumatic events. Military researchers Hyams, Wignall, and Roswell (1996) studied all symptoms presented by veterans of wars in which the United States participated; they concluded that from the Da Costa syndrome (American Civil War) to the Gulf War syndrome, the most common feature has been the similarity of reported symptoms: fatigue, shortness of breath, headache, sleep disturbances, impaired concentration, and forgetfulness. With the exception of the latter two, these symptoms are often found after disasters and in the general population. Additional symptoms may include neck and back pain, stomachache or other abdominal symptoms, cough, and palpitations of the heart.

5.1.3. Methodological Problems in Disaster Studies

When interpreting the results of disaster studies it is important to understand the limitations of the research. Many studies examine only the first months postdisaster or are cross-sectional, often with one or two measurements. Methodological weaknesses may include no baseline data, no denominator of the epidemiological fraction, absence of a proper control group, or a variety of different instruments utilized at different points in time. Studies are often based on self-report, causing issues in terms of nonresponse or recall bias. Moreover, in most circumstances an instrument that is not validated is used to measure physical health problems. In their systematic review, van den Berg, Grievink, Yzermans, and Lebret (2005) found that 21 different questionnaires were used to measure MUS in 57 included studies. It makes a difference whether a survey participant has to select from a list of symptoms (i.e., the somatization domain of the Symptom Checklist 90) or may enumerate all symptoms experienced.

Recently, researchers have begun to use the electronic medical records of family physicians. The strength of this data source is that it utilizes a standard classification system (the International Classification of Primary Care) and that in addition to disorders and diseases, the reason for encounter of the patient is recorded, as much as possible in the words of the patient (Dirkzwager, Grievink, van der Velden, & Yzermans, 2006; Yzermans, Donker, Kerssens, Dirkzwager, & Soeteman ten Veen, 2005; van den Berg et al., 2009). In countries such as Denmark, the Netherlands, and Great Britain, patients are on the list of just one family physician, which provides the opportunity to extract predisaster baseline data, to create reference groups of patients not exposed to the disaster, and to perform longitudinal surveillance. Moreover, the denominator is known and recall bias does not occur. A disadvantage might be that the registration of a contact is always a reduction of reality, especially when a patient presents more than one reason for the encounter. However, one study found the correspondence rate of family physician-registered persistent psychological problems with those self-reported by survivors of a disaster was 73% in a period of 1 to 5 years postdisaster (Drogendijk et al., 2007).

Table 5.1. Key Search Terms

Symptoms	Medically unexplained symptom[a] (MUS), Medically unexplained physical symptom[a] (MUPS), Somatic disorder[a], Psychosomatic symptom[a], Psychosomatic complaint[a], Somatic symptom[a], Somatic complaint[a], Physical symptom[a], Physical complaint[a], Somatization, Functional somatic symptom[a], Stress disorder[a], Posttraumatic stress disorder[a], Signs and symptoms, Distress, Morbidity, Health, Stress
	And
Disaster	Disaster[a], Life event[a], Traumatic event[a], environmental exposure, NOT Disaster planning
	And
Design	Cross-sectional, Prospective, Case-control, Cohort, Causality, Risk, Determinant[a], Predict[a]

Note: [a] Truncation.

5.2. SYMPTOMS IN THE AFTERMATH OF DISASTERS

5.2.1. Systematic Review on Physical Symptoms

The majority of studies after traumatic events such as disasters have focused on psychological problems, such as depression, anxiety, and PTSD, and they have shown a positive relation between exposure to traumatic stress and psychopathology. In the last decade, there has been increased awareness that traumatic events are also related to elevated levels of physical symptoms, such as fatigue, headache, stomachache, and pain in joints and muscles (Clauw et al., 2003; Engel, 2003). For example, a large number of epidemiological studies among military personnel deployed in the Gulf War have confirmed an increase in physical symptoms that could not be explained by a medical disorder, a phenomenon that has come to be known as the "Gulf War syndrome" (Thomas, Stimpson, Weightman, Dunstan, & Lewis, 2006).

Along with war zone exposure, disasters also have been described as precipitating factors for a higher level of physical symptoms. In 2005, two of the authors of this chapter published a systematic review of the literature published between January 1983 and December 2003 on physical symptoms among survivors of disasters; the intent was to provide insight into the prevalence and course of physical symptoms after disasters (van den Berg et al., 2005). Studies were selected in which physical symptoms (but not diagnoses) were measured among survivors of disasters. The keywords that were used to search the literature are shown in Table 5.1. Studies among rescue workers such as police officers and firefighters were excluded from the original review, since these are mostly healthy young men who cannot be easily compared with the survivors of disasters. However, for this chapter we will also describe studies that have examined physical symptoms among rescue workers.

In the original systematic review, 57 studies were selected. For this chapter, 13 additional studies that were published between January 2004 and July 2007 were included. The number of studies published since the original review indicates that in recent years there is an increasing interest in examining physical symptoms among survivors of disasters.

5.2.2. Prevalence of Physical Symptoms among Survivors of Disasters

Several studies have examined the prevalence of specific symptoms among survivors of disasters, and the results are shown in Table 5.2. From this table it becomes clear that the prevalences of the different symptoms vary considerably between studies. For example, shortly after an earthquake in Japan, 78% of survivors reported palpitations (Tainaka et al., 1998), while only 39% did so after an earthquake in the United States (Cardena & Spiegel, 1993). The variation might be due to the type of disaster, the composition of the study population, or the different instruments that are used to measure the symptoms

Table 5.2. Prevalences of self-reported physical symptoms measured in studies after disaster

First Author and Year of Publication	Disaster and Country	Population	Prevalence 0 to 3 Months Postdisaster (%)	Prevalence 3 to 12 Months Postdisaster (%)	Prevalence 1 to 2 Years Postdisaster (%)	Prevalence >2 Years Postdisaster % (No. of Years)
Fatigue						
Lima et al., 1989	Earthquake, Ecuador	A	33			
Tainaka et al., 1998	Earthquake, Japan	A	48	40	23	
Lima et al., 1993	Volcanic eruption, Colombia	A		20		13 (5)
Weisaeth, 1989	Industrial disaster, Norway	A		33		
Donker et al., 2002	Airplane disaster, the Netherlands	A				45 (6)
van den Berg et al., 2005	Fireworks disaster, the Netherlands	A			70	61 (4)
Kar et al., 2007	Cyclone, India	C			27	
Renck et al., 2002	Discotheque fire, Sweden	R	63			
Bartone et al., 1989	Airplane crash, USA	R	20	50		
Huizink et al, 2006	Airplane crash, the Netherlands	R				12–19 (9)
Morren et al., 2005	Fireworks disaster, the Netherlands	R				13 (3)
Headache						
Lima et al., 1989	Earthquake, Ecuador	A	36			
Chen et al., 2001	Earthquake, Taiwan	A	53			
Chen et al., 2007	Earthquake, Taiwan	A				30 (2)
Lima et al., 1993	Volcanic eruption, Colombia	A		60		36 (5)
Guill et al., 2001	Hurricane, Honduras	A		58		
Chae et al., 2005	Typhoon, South Korea	A		34		
Shariat et al., 1999	Terrorist attack, USA	A				30 (2)
Trout et al., 2002	Terrorist attack, USA	A	38			
Brackbill et al., 2006	Terrorist attack, USA	A				21 (2.5)
Donker et al., 2002	Airplane crash, the Netherlands	A				18 (6)
Van den Berg, 2005	Fireworks disaster, the Netherlands	A			47	39 (4)
Dollinger, 1986	Lightning strike, USA	C	31			
Kar, 2007	Cyclone, India	C			24	

Renck, 2002	Discotheque fire, Sweden	R	17			
Bartone, 1989	Airplane crash, USA	R	40	63		
Morren, 2005	Fireworks disaster, the Netherlands	R				21 (3)
Dyspnea						
Escobar, 1992	Flood, Puerto Rico	A			28	
Shariat, 1999	Terrorist attack, USA	A				22 (2)
Trout, 2002	Terrorist attack, USA	A	28			
van den Berg, 2005	Fireworks disaster, the Netherlands	A			33	25 (4)
Bartone, 1989	Airplane crash, USA	R	7	17		
Huizink, 2006	Airplane crash, the Netherlands	R				30 (9)
Morren, 2005	Fireworks disaster, the Netherlands	R				9 (3)
Skin problems						
Donker, 2002	Airplane crash, the Netherlands	A				13 (6)
Trout, 2002	Terrorist attack, USA	A	14			
Brackbill, 2006	Terrorist attack, USA	A				11 (2.5)
Bartone, 1989	Airplane crash, USA	R	9	18		
Huizink, 2006	Airplane crash, the Netherlands	R				52–55 (9)
Morren, 2005	Fireworks disaster, the Netherlands	R				13 (3)
Back pain						
Donker, 2002	Airplane crash, the Netherlands	A				9 (6)
van den Berg, 2005	Fireworks disaster, the Netherlands	A			49	46 (4)
Morren, 2005	Fireworks disaster, the Netherlands	R				17 (3)
Pain in muscles						
Weisaeth, 1989	Industrial disaster, Norway	A		35		
van den Berg, 2005	Fireworks disaster, the Netherlands	A			53	44 (4y)
Dollinger, 1986	Lightning strike, USA	C	31			
Huizink, 2006	Airplane crash, the Netherlands	R				42–54 (9)
Gastrointestinal symptoms						
Lima, 1989	Earthquake, Ecuador	A	29			
Tainaka, 1998	Earthquake, Japan	A	30	23	13	
Lima, 1993	Volcanic eruption, Colombia	A		21		14 (5)
Escobar, 1992	Flood, Puerto Rico	A			22	

(continued)

Table 5.2. *(continued)*

First Author and Year of Publication	Disaster and Country	Population	Prevalence 0 to 3 Months Postdisaster (%)	Prevalence 3 to 12 Months Postdisaster (%)	Prevalence 1 to 2 Years Postdisaster (%)	Prevalence >2 Years Postdisaster % (No. of Years)
Brackbill, 2006	Terrorist attack, USA	A				24 (2.5)
van den Berg, 2005	Fireworks disaster, the Netherlands	A			46	36 (4)
Bartone, 1989	Airplane crash, USA	R	19	45		
Huizink, 2006	Airplane crash, the Netherlands	R				21 (9)
Morren, 2005	Fireworks disaster, the Netherlands	R				18 (3)
Palpitations						
Cardena, 1993	Earthquake, USA	A	39	13		
Tainaka, 1998	Earthquake, Japan	A	78	64	32	
Chen, 2007	Earthquake, Taiwan	A				30 (2)
Chae, 2005	Typhoon, South Korea	A		34		
Clayer et al., 1985	Bushfires, Australia	A		7		
Bartone, 1989	Airplane crash, USA	R	6	12		
Huizink, 2006	Airplane crash, the Netherlands	R				26–29 (9)
Poor digestion						
Lima, 1989	Earthquake, Ecuador	A	17			
Lima, 1993	Volcanic eruption, Colombia	A		24		16 (5)
Chae, 2005	Typhoon, South Korea	A		25		
Trout, 2002	Terrorist attack, USA	A	11			
Kitayama et al., 2000	Earthquake, Japan	C		18	24	
Dollinger, 1986	Lightning strike, USA	C	3			
Poor appetite						
Lima, 1989	Earthquake, Ecuador	A	34			
Tainaka, 1998	Earthquake, Japan	A	33	21	9	
Lima, 1993	Volcanic eruption, Colombia	A		39		17 (5)
Maida et al., 1989	Bushfires, USA	A	20			
Kitayama, 2000	Earthquake, USA	C		30	18	
Kar, 2007	Cyclone, India	C			21	
Dollinger, 1986	Lightning strike, USA	C	3			

Bartone, 1989	Airplane crash, USA	R	7	18		
Dizziness						
Chen, 2001	Earthquake, Taiwan	A	53			
Chen, 2007	Earthquake, Taiwan	A				30 (2)
Shariat, 1999	Terrorist attack, USA	A			34	
van den Berg, 2005	Fireworks disaster, the Netherlands	A			28	23 (4)
Dollinger, 1986	Lightning strike, USA	C	3			
Bartone, 1989	Airplane crash, USA	R	5	15		
Chest symptoms						
Tainaka, 1998	Earthquake, Japan	A	29	19	8	
Chen, 2001	Earthquake, Taiwan	A	53			
Chen, 2007	Earthquake, Taiwan	A				29 (2)
Trout, 2002	Terrorist attack, USA	A	27			
van den Berg, 2005	Fireworks disaster, The Netherlands	A			26	19 (4)
Huizink, 2006	Airplane crash, The Netherlands	R				26–29 (9)
Morren, 2005	Fireworks disaster, The Netherlands					4 (3)
Sleeping problems						
Chae, 2005	Typhoon, South Korea	A		27		
van Griensven et al., 2006	Tsunami, Thailand	A	58			
Donker, 2002	Airplane crash, the Netherlands	A				16 (6)
Kar, 2007	Cyclone, India	C			8	
Renck, 2002	Discotheque fire, Sweden	R	27			
Bartone, 1989	Airplane crash, USA	R	31	45		
Huizink, 2006	Airplane crash, the Netherlands	R				32–48 (9)
Morren, 2005	Fireworks disaster, the Netherlands	R				9 (3)

Notes: A, adult survivors; C, children; R, rescue and relief workers.

(see Section 5.1.3). For example, in some studies, instruments were used that ask about symptoms during the last week, while other instruments ask for symptoms in the last month, resulting in different prevalences. In a study after a fireworks disaster in the Netherlands, survivors were asked whether they regularly suffer from different symptoms, without defining a time frame (van den Berg, Grievink, Stellato, et al., 2005). As a result, the prevalences of the symptoms reported in that study are considerably higher than those found in other studies.

Owing to the large variation between the different studies, it is difficult to draw conclusions about the prevalence of physical symptoms among survivors of disaster. Despite this, some general comments can be made. Overall, the prevalences of physical symptoms vary between 3% and 78% depending on the type of study and the time frame measured. Some symptoms such as headache (ranging from 18% to 58%) and fatigue (13% to 70%) seem to have a higher prevalence that other symptoms such as dyspnea (22% to 33%) and skin problems (11% to 14%). Longitudinal studies indicate that the prevalence of symptoms decreases in the years after the disaster. For example, in a study among survivors of a volcanic eruption in Colombia, Lima and colleagues (1993) found that 60% of the survivors reported headache 1 year postdisaster, and 5 years postdisaster this decreased to 36%. Also, a three-wave longitudinal study after an earthquake in Japan showed significant decreasing prevalences of symptoms; immediately after, 3 months after and 18 months after the earthquake, respectively 48%, 40%, and 23% of survivors reported fatigue (Tainaka et al., 1998).

Although the prevalence of physical symptoms seems to decrease in the years after the disaster, physical symptoms might persist for a long time. For example, 4 years after the fireworks disaster in the Netherlands, 12 of 21 physical symptoms were significantly more prevalent among survivors compared to nonexposed controls (van den Berg et al., 2005a).

Also, in a study 11 years after the Chernobyl accidents, women survivors reported still significantly more symptoms than was reported by a national reference sample (Bromet, Gluzman, Schwartz, Goldgaber, 2002).

Since disasters are unexpected events, predisaster data are seldom available. Only a few studies have examined physical symptoms before and after a disaster. In one study, Escobar and colleagues (1992) evaluated physical symptoms 1 year before and 2 years after a flood in Puerto Rico. Two years after the flood a higher proportion of exposed residents than unexposed residents reported new or persistent physical symptoms (data not shown in Table 5.2). Predisaster data were available in two recent studies after the fireworks disaster in the Netherlands that examined prevalences of physical symptoms presented to the family physician (Table 5.3). One of these studies focused on child survivors (Dirkzwager et al., 2006). This study showed that postdisaster increases were significantly larger in survivors aged 4 to 12 years than in controls for gastrointestinal and musculoskeletal symptoms. For adolescent survivors (13–18 years old), significantly larger postdisaster increases were found for musculoskeletal symptoms (first year postdisaster) and skin problems (second year postdisaster). When compared with self-reported symptoms, the prevalences of symptoms presented to the family physician are considerably lower. Indeed, general population studies indicate that individuals seek medical care for only a small proportion of their symptoms (Green, Fryer, Yawn, Lanier, & Dovey, 2001).

5.2.3. Mean Number of Physical Symptoms among Survivors and Controls

In several studies, the mean number of physical symptoms was compared between survivors of a disaster and a control group. In the majority of these studies, survivors reported a significantly higher mean score than control subjects (Bromet, Havenaar, Gluzman, & Tintle, 2005; Chung, Dennis, Easthope, Farmer, & Werrett, 2005; van den Berg, Grievink, Stellato, et al., 2005; van Kamp et al., 2006). For example, office workers who were exposed to September 11th terrorist attacks on the World Trade Center reported 10.5 times more physical symptoms, such as

Table 5.3. Prevalences of symptoms presented to the general practitioner after the Enschede fireworks disaster

First Author and Year of Publication	Population	Prevalence 0 to 12 Months Predisaster (%)	Prevalence 0 to 12 Months Postdisaster (%)	Prevalence 1 to 2 Years Postdisaster (%)	Prevalence 2 to 3 Years Postdisaster (%)
Gastrointestinal symptoms					
Dirkzwager, 2006	C1	10.0	11.2	10.8	
	C2	10.1	9.9	10	
Morren, 2007	R	1.7	3.7–5.1	4.1–5.7	2.7–0.9
Respiratory symptoms					
Dirkzwager, 2006	C1	22.9	15.8	16.2	
	C2	15.9	16.1	17.8	
Morren, 2007	R	5.4	9.8–14.9	8.7–14.6	4.2–1.5
Musculoskeletal symptoms					
Dirkzwager, 2006	C1	7.1	11.0	10.7	
	C2	21.0	26.6	21.5	
Morren, 2007	R	4.7	8.2–8.0	9.7–9.2	8.5–4.1
Neurological symptoms					
Morren, 2007	R	0.6	2.1–1.9	2.0–1.8	1.5–0.7
Skin problems					
Dirkzwager, 2006	C1	17.5	17.8	17.7	
	C2	20.0	19.8	25.1	

Notes: C1, children aged 4 to 12 years; C2 children aged 13 to 18 years; R, rescue workers (firefighters, police officers, and emergency health personnel). Prevalences for rescue workers in 6-month periods (0–6, 7–12, and 13–18, 19–24, and 25–30, 31–36).

shortness of breath, nausea, and severe headache, 3 months after the attacks than a comparison group of employees in Dallas (Trout et al., 2002). In addition, in a study among 1,526 residents affected by an Australian bushfire, affected residents reported two times more symptoms than nonexposed residents 12 months postdisaster (McFarlane, Clayer, & Bookless, 1997).

5.2.4. Physical Symptoms among Rescue Workers

Table 5.2 also shows the prevalences of symptoms reported by rescue workers, such as police officers and firefighters, who were involved in a disaster. In the study by Morren and colleagues (2005) among volunteer firefighters involved in the Netherlands fireworks disaster, relatively low prevalences were found 3 years after the disaster (ranging between 4% and 21%). Indeed, rescue workers seem to report lower prevalences of symptoms compared with survivors. This may be because of the fact that rescue workers are mostly healthy young men, the so-called healthy worker effect.

Despite this, the prevalences of symptoms among firefighters and police officers responding to an airplane crash in Amsterdam were remarkably high 9 years after the crash. For example, 29% of firefighters reported chest problems 9 years after the airplane crash compared to 4% of firefighters 3 years after the fireworks disaster (Huizink et al., 2006; Morren et al., 2005). The airplane crash was

Table 5.4. Percent of reviewed studies looking at particular postdisaster prevalences of mental and physical outcomes ($N = 139$).

Disaster Type	Distress	PTSD	Depression	Anxiety	Physical	Physical[a]
Natural	52	56	38	18	23	7
Human-made	40	65	26	22	28	8

Note: [a] Percent of studies that looked exclusively at physical symptoms and disease.

followed by a long aftermath of confusing information about the contents of the cargo and possible exposure to toxic substances such as depleted uranium. Also, the media strongly reinforced the idea that health problems were the result of exposure to toxic substances that were released by the cargo of the airplane (Yzermans & Gersons, 2002). Exposed rescue workers were more likely to interpret physical sensations as symptoms of poor health and attributed them to the disaster. Additionally, the media reports might have increased the fears about health effects and may have increased the attribution of symptoms to the disaster (Huizink et al., 2006).

In contrast with the longitudinal studies among affected residents, a study performed among health assistance workers by Bartone and colleagues (1989) showed increased prevalences of symptoms at follow-up. After the airplane crash in Newfoundland, health assistance workers were appointed to help surviving family members for an unusually long period (average 5.5 months). Six months postcrash, the results showed some early effects of exposure to traumatic stress, and 1 year after the crash, the prevalence of health problems increased. For example, 6 months after the crash 19% of assistance workers reported gastrointestinal symptoms, and this prevalence increased to 45% 1 year postdisaster. This study suggests a delayed expression of health effects among rescue workers who had been exposed to traumatic stress for a sustained period.

5.3. DISEASES IN THE AFTERMATH OF DISASTERS

As previously mentioned, the literature demonstrates less attention to "explained" symptoms and diseases. In 2005 two authors of this chapter contributed to the creation of a bibliography for the long-term health consequences of disasters (Yzermans, Dirkzwager, & Breuning, 2005). Using methods for systematic review, 139 studies were selected for the period between 1990 and 2003: 61 concerning natural disasters and 78 human-made. The health outcomes of all studies are presented in Table 5.4. Health outcomes of distress and depression were more often studied after natural disasters and PTSD, anxiety, and physical health more often after human-made disasters. Within the category of physical health outcomes, studies looked at effects on the respiratory tract (after bushfires, floods, hurricanes, volcanic gas and ash exposures, chemical disasters, explosions, and terrorism), the musculoskeletal tract (after earthquakes and terrorism), cancers (chemical and nuclear disasters), fatigue (almost all studies, especially after human-made disasters), eye problems (bushfires, chemical disasters, and terrorism), gastrointestinal tract (earthquakes, bushfires, hurricanes, and floods), and skin (bushfires and chemical disasters). Survivors' general physical condition was measured after earthquakes, floods, transport disasters, nuclear and chemical disasters, and terrorism.

Most physical health outcomes studied are directly related to the disaster, and they may have an immediate or long-term effect. After dioxin exposure in Seveso, Italy, in 1976, people who were in the cloud presented with nausea, headache, and eye irritation. After a few days, exposed persons developed skin lesions and chloracne. In a 15-year follow-up study, increased mortality from chronic ischemic heart disease was found in exposed men and from hypertension and chronic rheumatic heart disease in exposed women. Excess mortality was observed on chronic obstructive pulmonary disease, diabetes mellitus, and dioxin-related cancers for both men and women. For these long-term results a lot of possible confounders may apply (Bertazzi, Bernucci, Brambilla, Consonni, & Pesatori, 1998). With the exception of an increase of thyroid cancer in children, no major physical health effects were substantiated through ionizing radiation on the general health of the population after the Chernobyl disaster (Havenaar et al., 1997). Another well-known chemical disaster is the Union Carbide disaster in Bhopal, India, where on December 2 and 3, 1984, methyl isocyanate, an element of pesticides, leaked from the plant. In the acute phase persistent irritation of the eyes (including ocular lesions), cough, and respiratory impairment were found. Within 1 week 2,500 people died, and by 15 years after the event, between 15,000 and 20,000 had died from effects caused by the exposure. Significant neurological, reproductive, neurobehavioral, and psychological health effects were observed in the long term. Like Bertazzi and colleagues (1998) after the Seveso incident, the authors of a review on the health effects of the Bhopal disaster recommended long-term monitoring of the affected community, including well-designed cohort studies (Dhara & Dhara, 2002).

Dutch authorities implemented such action after the Enschede fireworks disaster (see Chapter 28 in this text), as a reaction on the troublesome aftermath of the Bijlmermeer plane crash (Page et al., 2006; Yzermans & Gersons, 2002). Using data from the electronic medical records of family physicians, statistically significant differences were found for hypertension (Figure 5.1) and diabetes mellitus (Figure 5.2), both chronic diseases, almost immediately post-disaster for survivors of the Enschede fireworks disaster compared with their nonexposed fellow townsmen. The prevalences for the survivors increased at an earlier stage and stayed higher until the end of the study period (Yzermans, Dirkzwager, Kerssens, Cohen-Bendahan, & ten Veen, 2006).

More generally, there appeared to be a strong relation between experiencing a disaster and cardiovascular symptoms and diseases. This relationship was already firmly established in military research, and recently seen again in

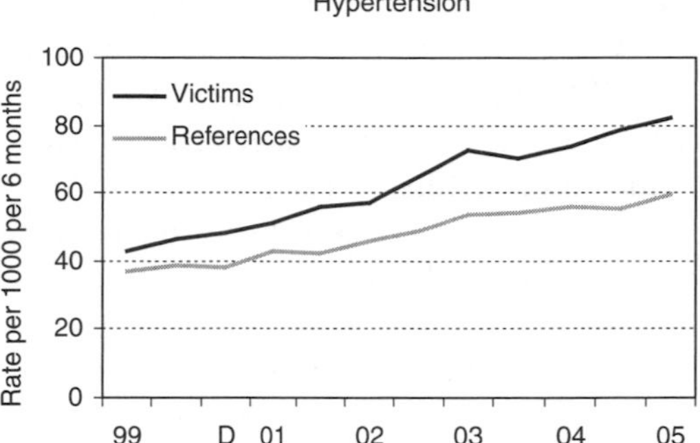

Figure 5.1. Time course for hypertension prevalence rates per 1,000 per 6 months from 16 months before the disaster (D) to 60 months after.

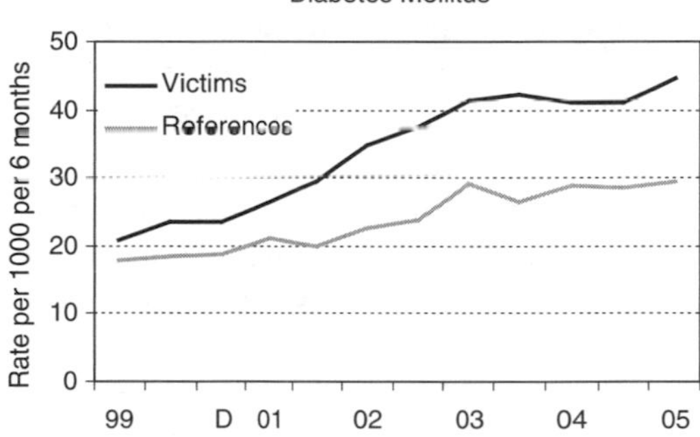

Figure 5.2. Time course for diabetes mellitus prevalence rates per 1,000 per 6 months from 16 months before the disaster (D) to 60 months after.

American veterans from the war in Iraq. One year after their homecoming 16.6% (N=2,815) suffered from self-reported PTSD and odds ratios were high for "chest pain" (OR = 4.98) and pounding or racing heart" (OR = 7.93) (Hoge, Terhakopian, Castro, Messer, & Engel, 2007). Comparison between disaster-exposed civilians and veterans is problematic because the latter are healthy young people, exposed to stress related to jobs that they have voluntarily chosen. However, the relationship between disaster exposure and cardiovascular problems and diseases was confirmed for civilian survivors of a disaster in a longitudinal study including predisaster data. In a study on the health effects of the New Year's Eve discotheque fire in Volendam, the Netherlands, researchers concluded that the risk of becoming hypertensive was 1.48 times higher for parents of adolescent survivors of a discotheque fire. In this study, bereaved parents had the highest risk of becoming hypertensive (OR = 2.42) (Dorn et al., 2007). While these figures describe hypertension as measured in family practice (diagnosed after three independent measurements), in a study with measurements 2 months before and 2 months after the September 11th attacks, systolic blood pressure was measured over 2 months using home telemonitoring. A substantial and sustained increase in blood pressure was found in four sites in the United States, both cross-sectionally and prospectively (Gerin et al., 2005).

Several studies after disasters found musculoskeletal and gastrointestinal diseases and in some cases respiratory and skin diseases (Dirkzwager, Kerssens, & Yzermans, 2006; Dirkzwager, Yzermans, Kessels, 2004; Escobar et al., 1992; McFarlane et al., 1994; Morren et al., 2007). However, the results of these studies are often not unequivocal. Results for occurrence of musculoskeletal diseases were presented after disasters, such as the September 11th attacks in New York City (Berrios-Torres et al., 2003).

One of the problems in measuring MUS after disasters, besides the lack of an appropriate instrument, is that the symptoms are self-reported. How can we be sure that the symptom is unexplained, especially when a survivor is questioned once? We need the clinical judgment of a doctor, especially one who is familiar with the medical history of the patient. This doctor can oversee the episode of care, defined as "a health problem from the first encounter with a health care provider through the completion of the last encounter related to that particular problem" (Hornbrook, Hurtado, & Johnson, 1985). Family physicians often assign a symptom diagnosis early in an episode of care, but this diagnosis may change over time: A cough may develop to bronchitis, and – on the longer run – fatigue to major depression. Okkes and colleagues (2002) analyzed episodes of care in a 10-year study in general practice. The reason for encounter "fatigue," for instance, was associated with several common diseases, such as viral diseases, upper respiratory tract infection, iron deficiency anemia, bronchitis, and major depression.

In one disaster study, symptoms were analyzed using episodes of care (van den Berg, Yzermans 2009) while in another study family physicians were asked whether the symptoms self-reported by their patients belonged to an episode of care (Donker, Yzermans, Spreeuwenberg, & van der Zee, 2002). It appeared that in most cases the diagnosis could not be specified (see Figures 5.3 (a) to (f)). However, remarkable differences appeared between the two studies. Six years after the Bijlmermeer plane crash near Amsterdam, a larger part of self-reported fatigue could be explained ("Fatigue B," Figure 5.3(a)) than one to 18 months after the fireworks disaster in Enschede ("Fatigue E," Figure 5.3(b)). These differences apply also for headache and, especially, shortness of breath/dyspnea.

5.4. CORRELATES/RISK GROUPS

5.4.1. Risk Factors

Since many, but not all, survivors of disasters develop physical symptoms, the question arises as to which factors predict who will and will not develop these symptoms. Although risk factors for psychological problems after exposure to traumatic stress have been investigated in many studies after disasters, only a few risk factors for physical symptoms have been examined after several disasters, which makes drawing conclusions difficult (van den Berg et al., 2005b). Nevertheless, risk factors for physical symptoms after disasters can be divided into predisaster factors (e.g., demographic characteristics, personality traits), disaster-related factors (e.g., injury, relocation, loss of property, and personal belongings) and postdisaster factors (e.g., psychological problems)

5.4.2. Predisaster Risk Factors

Gender has been studied most often as a risk factor for physical symptoms in studies after disasters. Researchers have found that female survivors report significantly more physical symptoms than male survivors after different types of disasters (Bravo, Rubio-Stipec, Canino,

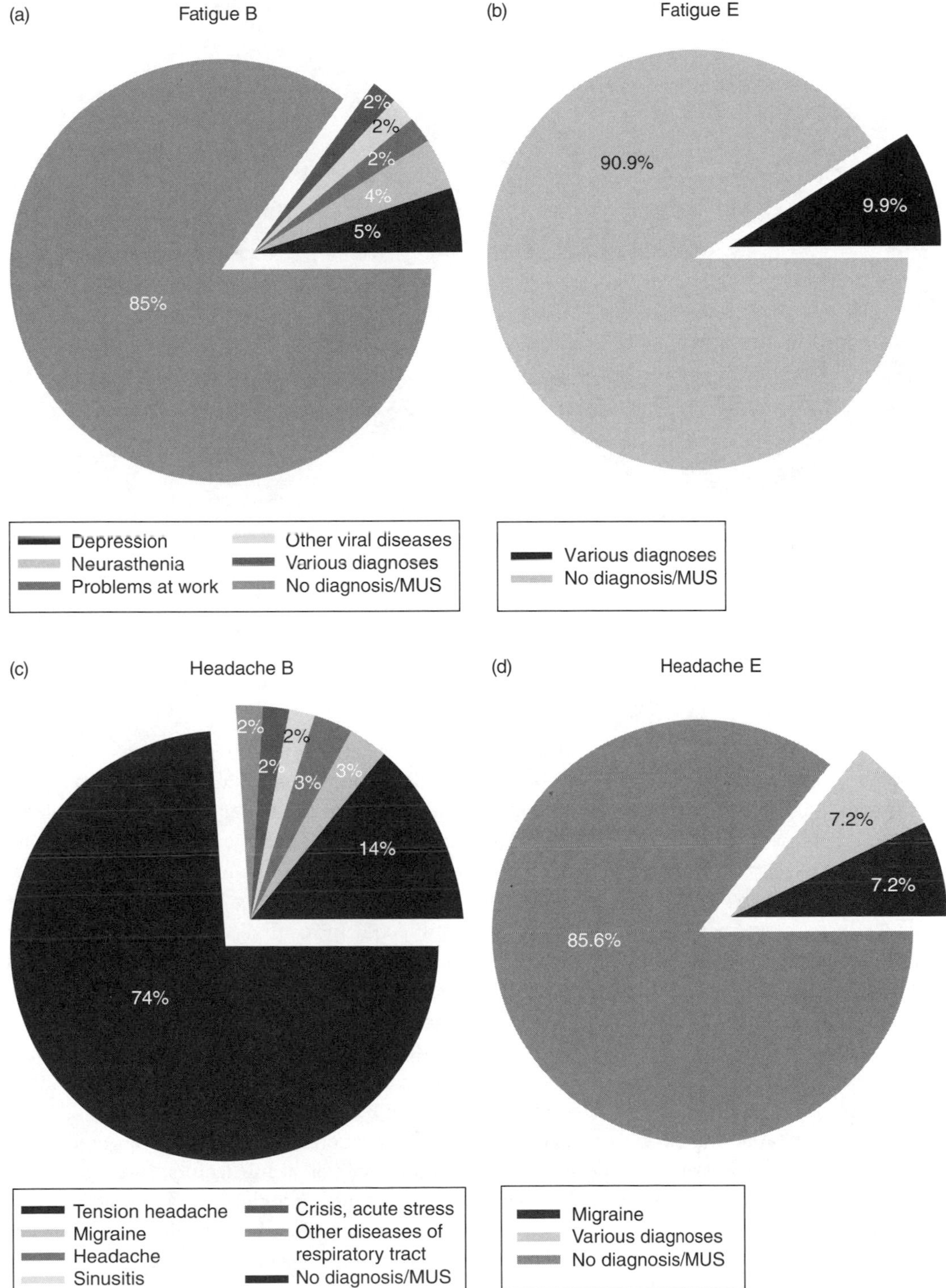

Figure 5.3. Final diagnoses for episodes of care by presenting symptoms such as (a, b) fatigue, (c, d) headache, and (e, f) shortness of breath/Dyspnea after two disasters, the Bijlmermeer plane crash ("B") and the fireworks disaster in Enschede ("E").

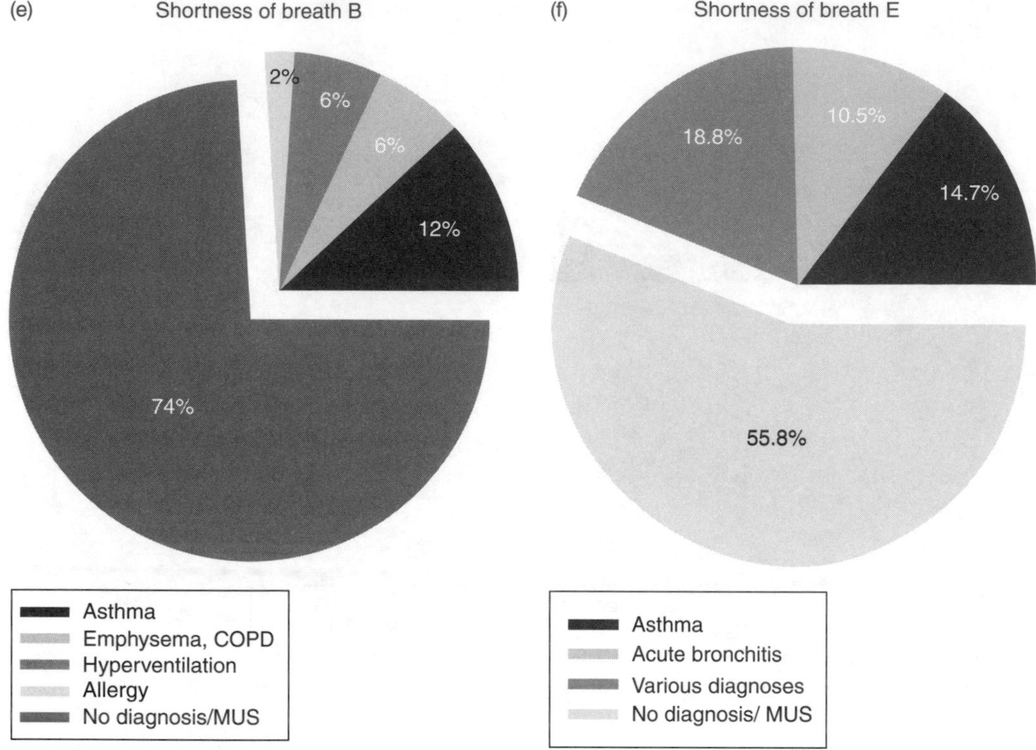

Figure 5.3. (continued)

Woobury, & Ribera, 1990; Karanci & Rustemli, 1995; McFarlane et al., 1997; Norris, Slone, Baker, & Murphy, 2006). Also, several studies have indicated that low socioeconomic status is a risk factor for physical symptoms among survivors. For example, after an earthquake in Turkey the level of education was negatively associated with physical symptoms, indicating that survivors with a higher educational level experienced less physical symptoms (Karanci & Rustemli, 1995). Additionally, in a study among survivors after a fireworks disaster in the Netherlands, public health insurance, which is an indicator of low socioeconomic status, was strongly related to a higher level of physical symptoms presented to the family physician in the years after the disaster (van den Berg, Yzermans, 2009).

These predisaster risk factors are similar to risk factors for physical symptoms in the general population. For example, females and individuals with a low socioeconomic status are at increased risk for physical symptoms in general population studies (Dirkzwager & Verhaak, 2007; Feder et al., 2001; Kroenke & Spitzer, 1998). Although some studies in family practice suggest that older patients report more physical symptoms, the relationship between age and physical symptoms among survivors of disasters is less clear (Dirkzwager & Verhaak, 2007; Feder et al., 2001). In postdisaster settings, some studies showed that older survivors were at an increased risk for physical symptoms (Norris et al., 2006; Karanci & Rustemli, 1995), whereas other studies did not find a relationship between age and symptoms (Bravo et al., 1990; Chung et al., 2005; van den Berg et al., 2008).

The relationship between other predisaster demographic or health factors, such as marital status, religion, ethnicity, and physical symptoms, has not often been studied after disaster (van den Berg, Yzermans, et al., 2005). Although the relation between physical symptoms and marital status and religion is not very clear, ethnicity appears to be a strong predictor of physical symptoms among survivors of the fireworks disaster in the Netherlands. When controlling

Table 5.5. Prevalence rates of all psychological problems of survivors of Turkish and Dutch origin, 1 year predisaster until 4 years postdisaster

Country of Origin	1 Year Predisaster	1 Year Postdisaster	2 Years Postdisaster	3 Years Postdisaster	4 Years Postdisaster
Turkey	22	57	40	48	39
The Netherlands	13	41	26	27	21

for other demographic variables, disaster-related factors, and psychological problems, immigrant survivors were two times more likely to report five or more physical symptoms to the family physician compared with native Dutch survivors (van den Berg, Yzermans, et al., 2009).

Gender, low socioeconomic status, and immigrant status are also important risk factors for physical symptoms in the general population and for that reason are not very specific for physical symptoms after disasters. Indeed, in the population that was affected by the fireworks disaster in the Netherlands, female survivors and immigrant survivors already had more physical symptoms before the disaster took place. As is shown in Table 5.5, medical treatment-seeking and/or morbidity were not influenced by immigration status (Yzermans, Donker, et al., 2005). Moreover, this table illustrates the value of predisaster data for the interpretation of results of disaster studies.

Although predisaster data are seldom available, some studies have indicated that predisaster psychological problems are related to a higher level of physical symptoms after the disaster (North, Kawasaki, Spitznagel, & Hong, 2004; van den Berg, Grievink, et al., 2008;). Norris and colleagues (2006) showed in their study after a flood and mudslides in Mexico that predisaster PTSD and predisaster depressive disorder were significant predictors of postdisaster physical symptoms, even after controlling for postdisaster PTSD and depression. In addition, in a pre–poststudy that examined a community sample before and after an air show disaster in Ukraine, predisaster mental health problems and substance abuse were related to postdisaster physical symptoms (Bromet et al., 2005).

In addition to predisaster psychological problems, predisaster physical symptoms have also been identified as a risk factor for postdisaster symptoms. In a study among 200 older survivors of a severe flood in Kentucky, having any self-reported predisaster physical symptoms was the strongest predictor of postflood physical symptoms (Phifer, 1990). In the studies of the fireworks disaster in the Netherlands, predisaster physical symptoms were the strongest predictor of postdisaster symptoms as well. Since physical symptoms are related to a higher level of health care utilization, a high level of predisaster family physician visits was related to a high level of postdisaster symptoms (Soeteman et al., 2006; van den Berg, Yzermans, et al., 2009).

5.4.3. Disaster-Related Risk Factors

During disaster, survivors might have experiences such as intense fear, injury, and peritraumatic dissociation. Several disaster-related factors, such as the loss of one's house and properties and the loss of a loved one, were risk factors for postdisaster physical symptoms in several disaster studies (van den Berg et al., 2005). For example, in the study among survivors of a flood in Kentucky, a high level of flood exposure was associated with reports of increased physical symptoms 18 months postflood (Phifer, 1990). Also, 7 years after a bus–train collision, those survivors who were in the bus reported the highest level of physical symptoms (Tyano et al., 1996). In addition, Bland and colleagues (2005) studied somatic symptoms among working Italian males 14 years after the 1980 earthquake. Findings showed that, even 14 years postdisaster, those men who experienced damage to their house and those who had financial loss as a result of the earthquake reported higher levels of symptoms than those without damage and financial loss.

The relationship between relocation after a disaster and health problems is less clear. It has been suggested that remaining in the disaster area, which provides the opportunity to maintain cohesion in the family and to contribute to reconstruction, is protective. On the other hand, the constant reminder of the disaster when remaining in the disaster area might be a risk factor for psychological problems (Najarian, Goenjian, Pelcovitz, Mandel, & Najarian, 2001). In a study after a devastating earthquake in Armenia, health problems, including physical symptoms, of women who remained in the earthquake area did not differ from women who were relocated (Najarian et al., 2001). In the study by Bland and colleagues (2005) after an earthquake in Italy, relocation was also not associated with a higher level of physical symptoms among male factory workers.

5.4.4. Postdisaster Risk Factors

Most disaster studies that showed a relationship between disaster exposure and physical symptoms did not control for psychological problems such as depression, anxiety, and PTSD. Several studies have shown that the effect of disaster exposure diminishes or even disappears when controlling for psychological problems. For example, in a study after a severe flood in Mexico, the effect of severity of exposure to the floods and mudslides disappeared when postdisaster PTSD was taken into account (Norris et al., 2006). Also, in a study after the fireworks disaster, the association between disaster-related factors, such as a destroyed house, and physical symptoms diminished considerably after account for PTSD, depression, and anxiety in the regression model (van den Berg, Grievink, et al., 2008). To date, depression and anxiety have seldom been studied as risk factors for postdisaster physical symptoms. The relationship between psychological and physical problems is discussed more explicitly in section 5.5.

Despite the overlap between psychological problems and physical symptoms, not all survivors with a high level of symptoms report a high level of psychological distress. This indicates that physical symptoms can also develop in the absence of psychological problems. In addition, not all survivors of disasters report an elevated level of physical symptoms, while almost all survivors experience psychological distress after the disaster to some degree. It is important to note that the interpretation and amplification of physical symptoms may play an important role in the development and aggravation of the symptoms. Causal attribution of physical symptoms to possible exposure to toxic substances might play a crucial role. Besides cognitions, specific personality traits have also been related to elevated levels of distress and physical symptoms. Higher levels of physical symptoms have been related to high levels of neuroticism and negative affectivity; individuals with these personality factors are more likely to experience distress and a negative mood and self-concept (Watson & Pennebaker, 1989). While these factors might provide more insight into the relationship between traumatic exposure and physical symptoms, relatively little is known about how these cognitions, attributions, and personality traits are related to a higher level of physical symptoms and associated health care utilization.

5.5. RELATIONSHIPS BETWEEN PSYCHOLOGICAL AND PHYSICAL HEALTH PROBLEMS

As described in the previous paragraphs, disaster survivors can report declines in their physical health, and physical and psychological health problems have a tendency to occur together. For instance, studies on medically unexplained physical symptoms in the general population have demonstrated that these symptoms are associated with impaired quality of life and increased psychopathology, such as anxiety and depression (Dirkzwager & Verhaak, 2007; Henningsen, Zimmermann, & Satell, 2003; Hotopf, Mayou, Wadsworth, & Wessely, 1998; Katon, Sullivan, & Walker, 2001; Kroenke & Price, 1993). Significant relationships have also been found between mental disorders and physical diseases. The majority of these studies were focused on depression, and these studies have consistently shown that persons with depression are at an increased risk of cardiovascular disease and cardiac death. Depression has been related to other diseases as well, for instance, multiple sclerosis, Parkinson's disease, migraine, and gastrointestinal disease (Ford, 2004; Glassman, 2007; Nuyen et al., 2006; Siegert & Abernethy, 2005).

With respect to the relationship between psychological and physical health, causality can go both ways; that is, depression can result in a physical disease, and having a chronic disease can result in depression. The impact of depression on subsequent cardiovascular disease has been well described (Ford, 2004). An increased prevalence of depression as a result of medical diseases also has been suggested (Nuyen et al., 2006; van Ede, Yzermans, & Brouwer, 1999). Longitudinal studies are needed to disentangle the temporal association between psychological disorders and physical health problems.

5.5.1. Relationships between Psychological and Self-Reported Physical Health after Disaster

Within the area of traumatic events like disasters, similar results have been found. Most research in this context has focused on PTSD, and it has been argued that PTSD is an important mediator through which trauma can be related to poor physical health outcomes (Schnurr & Green 2003). Studies among combat veterans (e.g., Engel, Liu, McCarthy, Miller, & Ursano, 2000; Litz, Keane, Fisher, Marx, & Monaco, 1992; Norris, Maguen, Litz, Adler, & Britt, 2005; Schnurr & Spiro, 1999; Wolfe, Schnurr, Brown, & Furey, 1994; Zatzick et al., 1997), sexual assault victims (Kimmerling & Calhoun, 1994; Zoellner, Goodwin, & Foa, 2000), and firefighters (McFarlane et al., 1994; Wagner, Heinrichs, & Ehlert, 1998) have shown that exposure to traumatic events and subsequent PTSD is related to increased self-reported physical health problems and a poorer functional status. When we look more closely at the disaster literature, a link between PTSD and physical health problems has been observed for rescue workers involved in the aftermath of disasters. McFarlane and colleagues (1994) investigated firefighters involved in the aftermath of a bushfire disaster, and firefighters with PTSD endorsed a greater number of total physical symptoms, as well as more cardiovascular, musculoskeletal, and neurological symptoms, as compared with those without PTSD. More recently, firefighters with skin rash or lower respiratory symptoms after hurricane Katrina were nearly twice as likely to report depressive symptoms (Tak, Driscoll, Bernard, & West, 2007).

Studies among primary survivors of disasters also suggest significant relationships between psychological and physical health problems. A study on the health problems among children and adolescents who experienced a cyclone in India showed that youngsters with PTSD were more likely to report symptoms such as fatigue, headache, and a decreased appetite (Kar, Mohapatra, Nayak, Pattanaik, Swain, & Kar, 2007). Among a sample of adults who survived the 1999 floods and mudslides in Mexico, postdisaster PTSD symptoms were significantly related to more cardiopulmonary, musculoskeletal, nose–throat, and gastrointestinal/urinary symptoms (Norris et al., 2006).

As already mentioned, most research on the relationship between disaster-related psychological problems and physical health has focused on PTSD; however, some evidence has been provided for a relationship between depression or anxiety and poor physical health outcomes. A study among Israeli immigrants originating from areas exposed to the Chernobyl disaster investigated the relationships between psychological measures and a number of chronic conditions. The chronic conditions most strongly associated with depression and anxiety were heart problems, migraine, problems with the lymphatic system, and musculoskeletal conditions (Cwikel, Abdelgani, Goldsmith, Quastel, & Yevelson, 1997). Survivors of the firework disaster in the Netherlands who reported more physical symptoms after the disaster reported more depressive and anxious feelings as well (van den Berg, Grievink, Stellato, et al.,

2005). Furthermore, a study on the quality of life among Taiwanese earthquake survivors found that compared with a group of mentally healthy persons, survivors with PTSD or major depression reported worse scores on the quality of life subscales relating to physical health (e.g., physical functioning, bodily pain, vitality) (Wu et al., 2006). In a recent review on the prevalence and risk factors of medically unexplained physical symptoms in the aftermath of disasters, it was concluded that psychological distress and posttraumatic stress symptoms were positively associated with MUS in a number of studies of adult survivors (van den Berg et al., 2005).

5.5.2. Relationships between Psychological Problems and Physical Morbidity after Disaster

Although most research on the link between psychological stress and physical health is based on self-reported physical health outcomes, some evidence has shown that traumatic exposure may also be associated with physician-diagnosed morbidity (Schnurr & Green, 2004). The majority of this research was based on male combat veterans, such as Vietnam veterans and veterans of World War II or the Korean War. These studies showed that PTSD was associated with more physician-diagnosed medical disorders (Beckham et al., 1998) and with an increased risk of physician-diagnosed arterial, circulatory, gastrointestinal, dermatological, and musculoskeletal disorders (Ouimette et al., 2004; Schnurr, Spiro, & Paris, 2000). Several other studies, which used objective health measures such as medical examinations or laboratory test results, also observed increased cardiovascular problems among veterans with PTSD (Boscarino, 2004; Boscarino & Chang, 1999; Falger et al., 1992, Shalev, Bleich, & Ursano, 1990). Thus, evidence for a relationship between PTSD and cardiovascular disease is mounting.

Research on the relationship between PTSD and physician-diagnosed physical health problems in the context of disasters is scarce. However, a recent prospective study on the relationship between disaster-related PTSD and physical health found similar results to studies of combat veterans. Survivors of the Enschede firework disaster who had PTSD at 18 months after the disaster were at increased risk of physician-rated vascular, musculoskeletal, and dermatological health problems in the subsequent 2 years (Dirkzwager et al., 2007). Prospectively, PTSD signaled an increased risk of new vascular problems in the subsequent 2 years. (See Table 5.6.)

Table 5.6. Relationship between disaster-related PTSD and new physician-rated physical health problems

New Physical Health Problems[b]	PTSD (%)	No PTSD (%)	OR[c]
Vascular	12.5	6.2	1.92[a]
Gastrointestinal	18.1	16.8	0.96
Respiratory	21.9	17.5	1.09
Dermatological	24.4	20.4	1.15
Musculoskeletal	16.9	17.4	0.94

Notes:

[a] $p < 0.05$.

[b] Health problems present in the 2 years after the PTSD assessment and not present before.

[c] Adjusted for age, gender, insurance type, immigrant status, smoking behavior, and predisaster physical health problems.

Survivors of the Hanshin-Awaji earthquake who experienced acute myocardial infarction during the first 4 weeks after the earthquake reported severe posttraumatic stress levels as well (Suzuki et al., 1997).

5.5.3. Mechanisms Explaining Relationships between Psychological and Physical Health

An important question is how psychological problems, such as PTSD and depression, may influence physical health. One possible explanation for a relationship between disaster-related psychological and physical problems may lie in the fact that disaster survivors are more likely to consult a doctor or another health care provider (Dorn, Yzermans, Kerssens, Spreeuwenberg, & van der Zee, 2006); therefore, psychological as well as physical health problems are more likely to be detected among disaster survivors. It is also possible that survivors with PTSD are more closely monitored by their family physician and, for instance, have their blood pressure measured more frequently. In this case, new physical problems may be discovered earlier among survivors with PTSD than among those without PTSD.

Different mechanisms have been proposed to explain the association between PTSD and physical health. Pathways may include direct effects, such as through PTSD's associated neurobiology (e.g., a decreased immune function, alterations in hormone systems), as well as more indirect effects through cognitive and behavioral mechanisms, such as coping, increased health risk behaviors (e.g., increased smoking or alcohol use), and a heightened symptom perception among people with psychological problems (Boscarino, 2004; Schnurr & Janowski, 1999; Schnurr, Green, 2004). For depression, similar biological, psychosocial, and behavioral processes have been proposed to explain the relationship with adverse physical outcomes. Additionally, medications used to treat depression as well as nonadherence to treatment may also be important factors that can affect physical health (Ford, 2004).

Allostatic load is another concept that may be useful to increase our understanding of how stress can result in poor physical health (McEwen, 1998; McEwen & Stellar, 1993). Allostatic load refers to the cumulative physiological cost of efforts to adapt to prolonged stress, which over time causes wear and tear of bodily systems, and subsequently may increase the likelihood of disease (McEwen, 1998). Central to this approach is the emphasis on the cumulative effects of different factors, which on their own or in the short term would not be sufficient to cause disease. Allostatic load has rarely been examined in samples with traumatic stress exposure or PTSD; an exception is a recent study among mothers of pediatric cancer survivors, which confirmed a relationship between PTSD and an elevated allostatic load (Glover, 2006).

Currently, the question of how exactly psychological disorders may affect physical health remains unanswered, though it is likely that multiple mechanisms contribute in a complex and interactive way. To increase our knowledge and understanding of the relationship between disaster-related psychological disorders and poor physical health, more longitudinal and controlled studies are needed, particularly, those that focus on the possible explanatory mechanisms.

5.6. RECOMMENDATIONS AND GAPS

The central message of this chapter may be abundantly clear: In disaster research, there is a need to realize that psychological problems and disorders on the one side, and physical symptoms and diseases on the other, are strongly intertwined. Dividing soma and psyche is not beneficial to survivors of disasters. Nowadays, there is enough evidence showing that psychological distress is related to symptom reporting but in most cases not directly to organic diseases (i.e., Barsky & Borus, 1999; Dirkzwager et al., 2006; Hotopf et al., 1998; Kroenke & Price, 1993; Page et al., 2006; Schnurr & Jankowski, 1999; van den Berg et al., 2005; Wessely et al., 1999).

We highlight six recommendations for the field, originating from as many gaps in disaster literature. First, there is a need for more longitudinal studies that examine the relationship between mental and physical health (symptoms as well as diseases) in the aftermath of disasters, and information on the health status before the trauma should be used as much as possible. Only in this way we can identify the temporal association between psychological and physical health problems. Second, researchers examining physical health consequences after disasters should improve the methodological quality of their future studies, using methodologically sound instruments and self-reported physical health outcomes as well as clinical judgments. Future studies also should use objective physical health indicators. Third, as thus far most studies have focused on the role of PTSD in the development of physical health problems, more research should focus on the relationship between depression and physical health in the context of disasters. Additionally, since PTSD and depression are highly comorbid, it is important to increase our knowledge on the unique contribution of these specific disorders. It is, for instance, unclear if these psychological disorders coincide with the same physical symptoms and diseases. We may hypothesize that a stronger relationship with physical symptoms and diseases will exist for those survivors who suffer from both PTSD and major depression, whether at the same time or alternately. Fourth, more attention should be given to specific patterns in which mental and physical health problems are (subjectively) intertwined. For example, there are indications that depression and low back pain are comorbid in the intermediate-term after disasters. We even wonder whether there is any difference between the two. Fifth, little is known about the possible mechanisms that may explain the relationships between disasters and their psychological and physical health problems; future studies should consider such issues. Finally, in disaster research there is an ongoing need for knowledge about the attribution process and about cognitions of MUS (e.g., causal illness perceptions).

REFERENCES

American Psychiatric Association. (1994). *Diagnostic and statistical manual of mental disorders, 4th ed.* Washington, DC: American Psychiatric Association.

Andreski, P., Chilcoat, H., & Breslau, N. (1998). Posttraumatic stress disorder and somatisation symptoms: A prospective study. *Psychiatry Research, 79*, 131–138.

Barsky, A. J., & Borus, J. F. (1999). Functional somatic syndromes. *Annals Internal Medicine, 130*, 910–921.

Bartholomew, R. E., & Wessely, S. (2002). Protean nature of mass sociogenic illness. *British Journal of Psychiatry, 180*, 300–306.

Bartone, P. T., Ursano, R. J., Wright, K. M., & Ingraham, L. H. (1989). The impact of a military air disaster on the health of assistance workers. A prospective study. *Journal of Nervous and Mental Disease, 177*(6), 317–328.

Beckham, J. C., Moore, S. D., Feldman, M. E., Hertzberg, M. A., Kirby, A. C., & Fairbank, J. A. (1998). Health status, somatization, and severity of posttraumatic stress disorder in Vietnam combat veterans with posttraumatic stress disorder. *American Journal of Psychiatry, 155*, 1565–1569.

Berrios-Torres, S. I., Greenko, J. A., Phillips, M., Miller, J. R., Treadwell, T. & Ikeda, R. M. (2003). World Trade Center rescue worker injury and illness surveillance, New York, 2001. *American Journal of Preventive Medicine, 25*(2), 79–87.

Bertazzi, P. A., Bernucci, I., Brambilla, G., Consonni, D. & Pesatori, A. C. (1998). The Seveso studies on early and long-term effects of dioxin exposure: A review. *Environmental Health Perspectives, 106*, 625–633.

Bland, S. H., Valoroso, L., Stranges, S., Strazzullo, P., Farinaro, E. & Trevisan, M. (2005). Long-term follow-up of psychological distress following earthquake experiences among working Italian males: A cross-sectional analysis. *Journal of Nervous and Mental Disease, 193*(6), 420–423.

Boscarino, J. A. (2004). Posttraumatic stress disorder and physical illness. Results from clinical and epidemiology studies. *Annals of the New York Academy of Sciences, 1032*, 141–153.

Boscarino, J. A., & Chang, M. P. H. (1999). Electrocardiogram abnormalities among men with stress-related psychiatric disorders: Implications for coronary heart disease and clinical research. *Annals of Behavioral Medicine, 21*(3), 227–234.

Brackbill, R. M., Thorpe, L. E., DiGrande, L., Perrin, M., Sapp, J. H. 2nd, Wu, D., et al. (2006). Surveillance for World Trade Center disaster health effects among survivors of collapsed and damaged buildings. *Morbidity and Mortality Weekly Report Surveillance, 55*(2), 1–18.

Bravo, M., Rubio-Stipec, M., Canino, G. J., Woodbury, M. A., & Ribera, J. C. (1990). The psychological sequelae of disaster stress prospectively and retrospectively evaluated. *American Journal of Community Psychology, 18*(5), 661–680.

Bromet, E. J., Gluzman, S., Schwartz, J. E., & Goldgaber, D. (2002). Somatic symptoms in women 11 years after the Chornobyl accident: Prevalence and risk factors. *Environmental Health Perspectives, 110*(Suppl. 4), 625–629.

Bromet, E. J., Havenaar, J. M., Gluzman, S. F., & Tintle, N. L. (2005). Psychological aftermath of the Lviv air show disaster: A prospective controlled study. *Acta Psychiatrica Scandinavica, 112*, 194–200.

Brooks, N., & McKinlay, W. (1992). Mental health consequences of the Lockerbie disaster. *Journal of Traumatic Stress, 5*(4), 527–543.

Cardena, E., & Spiegel, D. (1993). Dissociative reactions to the San Francisco Bay area earthquake of 1989. *American Journal of Psychiatry, 150*, 474–478.

Chae, E. H., Tong Won, K., Rhee, S. J., & Henderson, T. D. (2005). The impact of flooding on the mental health of affected people in South Korea. *Community Mental Health Journal, 41*(6), 633–645.

Chen, C. C., Yeh, T. L., Yang, Y. K., Chen, S. J., Lee, I. H., Fu, L. S., et al. (2001). Psychiatric morbidity and post-traumatic symptoms among survivors in the early stage following the 1999 earthquake in Taiwan. *Psychiatry Research, 105*(1–2), 13–22.

Chen, C.H., Tan, H.K., Liao, L.R., Chen, H.H., Chan, C.C., Cheng, J.J., et al. (2007). Long-term psychological outcome of 1999 Taiwan earthquake survivors: A survey of a high-risk sample with property damage. *Comprehensive Psychiatry*, *48*(3), 269–275.

Chen, L.C., & Thurston, G. (2002). World Trade Center cough. *The Lancet*, *360*, s37–s38

Chung, M.C., Dennis, I., Easthope, Y., Farmer, S., & Werrett, J. (2005). Differentiating posttraumatic stress between elderly and younger residents. *Psychiatry*, *68*(2), 164–173.

Clauw, D.J., Engel C.C., Aronowitz, R., Jones, E., Kipen, H.M., Kroenke, K., et al. (2003). Unexplained symptoms after terrorism and war: An expert consensus statement. *Journal of Occupational and Environmental Medicine*, *45*(10), 1040–1048.

Clayer, J.R., Bookless-Pratz, C., & Harris, R.L. (1985). Some health consequences of a natural disaster. *The Medical Journal of Australia*, *143*, 182–184.

Cwikel, J., Abdelgani, A., Goldsmith, J.R., Quastel, M., & Yevelson, I.I. (1997). Two-year follow-up study of stress-related disorders among immigrants to Israel from the Chernobyl area. *Environmental Health Perspectives*, *105*(Suppl. 6), 1545–1550.

Dhara, V.R., & Dhara, R. (2002). The Union Carbide disaster in Bhopal: A review of health effects. *Archives of Environmental Health*, *57*(5), 391–404.

Dirkzwager, A.J., & Verhaak, P.F. (2007). Patients with persistent medically unexplained symptoms in general practice: Characteristics and quality of care. *BMC Family Practice*, *8*, 33.

Dirkzwager A.J., Yzermans C.J., & Kessels F.J. (2004). Psychological, musculoskeletal, and respiratory problems and sickness absence before and after involvement in a disaster: A longitudinal study among rescue workers. *Occupational and Environmental Medicine*, *61*(10), 870–872.

Dirkzwager, A.J.E., Grievink, L., van der Velden, P.G., & Yzermans, C.J. (2006). Risk factors for psychological and physical health problems after a man-made disaster. *British Journal of Psychiatry*, *189*, 144–149.

Dirkzwager, A.J.E., Kerssens, J.J., & Yzermans, C.J. (2006). Health problems in children and adolescents before and after a man-made disaster. *Journal of the American Academy of Child and Adolescent Psychiatry*, *45*(1), 94–103.

Dirkzwager, A.J.E., van der Velden, P.G., Grievink, L., & Yzermans, C.J. (2007). Disaster-related posttraumatic stress disorder and physical health. *Psychosomatic Medicine*, *69*, 435–440.

Dollinger, S.J. (1986). The measurement of children's sleep disturbances and somatic complaints following a disaster. *Child Psychiatry and Human Development*, *16*, 148–153.

Donker, G.A., Yzermans, C.J., Spreeuwenberg, P., & van der Zee, J. (2002). Symptom attribution after a plane crash: comparison between self-reported symptoms and GP records. *British Journal of General Practice*, *52*, 917–922.

Dorn, T., Yzermans, C.J., Guijt, H., & van der Zee, J. (2007). Disaster-related stress as a prospective risk factor for hypertension in parents of adolescent fire victims. *American Journal of Epidemiology*, *165*, 410–417.

Dorn, T., Yzermans, C.J., Kerssens, J.J., Spreeuwenberg, P.M., & vn der Zee, J. (2006). Disaster and subsequent health care utilization: A longitudinal study among victims, their family members and control subjects. *Medical Care*, *44*(6), 581–589.

Drogendijk, A.N., Dirkzwager, A.J.E., Grievink, L., van der Velden, P.G., Marcelissen, F.G.H., et al. (2007). The correspondence between persistent self-reported post-traumatic problems and general practitioners' reports after a major disaster. *Psychological Medicine*, *37*, 193–202.

Engel, C.C. (2001). Outbreak of medically unexplained physical symptoms after military action, terrorist threat, or technological disaster. *Military Medicine*, *166*, 47–48.

(2003). Somatization and multiple idiopathic physical symptoms: Relationship to traumatic events and post-traumatic stress disorder. In P.P. Schnurr & B.L. Green (Eds.), *Trauma and health. Physical consequences of exposure to extreme stress*. Washington DC: American Psychological Association.

Engel, C.C., Liu, X., McCarthy, B.D., Miller, R.F., & Ursano, R. (2000). Relationship of physical symptoms to posttraumatic stress disorder among veterans seeking care for Gulf War-related health concerns. *Psychosomatic Medicine*, *62*, 739–745.

Escobar, J.I., Canino, G., Rubio-Stipec, M., & Bravo, M. (1992). Somatic symptoms after a natural disaster: A prospective study. *American Journal of Psychiatry*, *149*, 965–967.

Falger, P.R.J., Op den Velde, W., Hovens, J.E., Schouten, E.G., de Groen, J.H., & van Duijn, H. (1992). Current posttraumatic stress disorder and cardiovascular disease risk factors in Dutch resistance veterans from World War II. *Psychotherapy and Psychosomatics*, *57*, 164–171.

Feder, A., Olfson, M., Gameroff, M., Fuentes, M., Shea, S., Lantigua, R.A., et al. (2001). Medically unexplained symptoms in an urban general medicine practice. *Psychosomatics*, *42*, 261–268.

Foa, E.B., Stein, D.J., & McFarlane, A.C. (2006). Symptomatology and psychopathology of mental health problems after disaster. *Journal of Clinical Psychiatry*, *67*(Suppl. 2), 15–25.

Ford, D.E. (2004). Depression, trauma, and cardiovascular health. In P.P. Schnurr, & B.L. Green (Eds.), *Trauma and health: Physical health consequences of extreme stress*. Washington, DC: American Psychological Association.

Galea, S. (2007). The long-term health consequences of disasters and mass traumas. *Canadian Medical Association Journal, 176*(9), 1293–1294.

Gerin, W., Chaplin, W., Schwartz, J.E., Holland, J., Alter, R., Wheeler, R., et al. (2005). Sustained blood pressure increase after an acute stressor: The effects of the 11 September 2001 attack on the New York City World Trade Center. *Journal of Hypertension, 23*, 279–284.

Glassman, A.H. (2007). Depression and the cardiovascular comorbidity. *Dialogues in Clinical Neurosciences, 9*(1), 9–17.

Glover, D.A. (2006). Allostatic load in women with and without PTSD symptoms. *Annals of the New York Academy of Sciences, 1071*, 442–447.

Green, L.A., Fryer, G.E., Yawn, B.P., Lanier, D., & Dovey, S.M. (2001). The ecology of medical care revisited. *New England Journal of Medicine, 344*(26), 2021–2025.

Guill, C.K., & Shandera, W.X. (2001). The effects of hurricane Mitch on a community in northern Honduras. *Prehospital Disaster Medicine, 16*, 124–129.

Havenaar J., Rumyantzeva, G., Kasyanenko, A., Kaasjager, K., Westermann, A., Van den Brink, W., et al. (1997). Health effects of the Chernobyl disaster: Illness or illness behavior? A comparative general health survey in two former Soviet regions. *Environmental Health Perspectives, 105*(Suppl. 6), 1533–1537.

Henningsen, P., Zimmermann, T., & Sattel, H. (2003). Medically unexplained physical symptoms, anxiety, and depression: A meta-analytic review. *Psychosomatic Medicine, 65*(4), 528–533.

Hoge, C.W., Terhakopian, A., Castro, C.A., Messer, S.C., & Engel, C.C. (2007). Association of Posttraumatic Stress Disorder with somatic symptoms, health care visits, and absenteeism among Iraq war veterans. *American Journal of Psychiatry, 164*(1), 150–153.

Hornbrook, M.C., Hurtado, R.V., & Johnson, R.E. (1985). Health care episodes: Definition, measurement and use. *Medical Care Review, 42*, 163–218.

Hotopf, M., Mayou, R., Wadsworth, M., & Wessely, S. (1998). Temporal relationships between physical symptoms and psychiatric disorder; results from a national birth cohort. *British Journal of Psychiatry, 173*, 255–261.

Huizink, A.C., Slottje, P., Witteveen, A.B., Bijlsma, J.A., Twisk, J.W., Smidt, N., et al. (2006). Long term health complaints following the Amsterdam Air Disaster in police officers and fire-fighters. *Occupational and Environmental Medicine, 63*(10), 657–662.

Hyams, K.C., Wignal, F.S., & Roswell, R. (1996). War syndromes and their evaluation: From the U.S. civil war to the Persian Gulf war. *Annals of Internal Medicine, 125*(5), 398–405.

Kar, N., Mohapatra, K.P., Nayak, K.C., Pattanaik, P., Swain, S.P., & Kar, H.C. (2007). Post-traumatic stress disorder in children and adolescents one year after a super-cyclone in Orissa, India: Exploring cross-cultural validity and vulnerability factors. *BMC Psychiatry, 7*, 8.

Karanci, A., & Rustemli, A. (1995). Psychological consequences of the 1992 Erzincan (Turkey) earthquake. *Disasters, 19*(1), 8–18.

Katon, W., Sullivan, M., & Walker, E. (2001). Medical symptoms without identified pathology: Relationship to psychiatric disorders, childhood and adult trauma, and personality traits. *Annals of Internal Medicine, 134*, 917–925.

Kawana, N., Ishimatsu, S., & Kanda, K. (2001). Psychophysiological effects of the terrorist sarin attack on the Tokyo subway system. *Military Medicine, 166*(12), 23–26.

Kendell, R.E. (2001). The distinction between mental and physical illness. *British Journal of Psychiatry, 178*, 490–493.

Kimmerling, R., & Calhoun, K. (1994). Somatic symptoms, social support, and treatment seeking among sexual assault victims. *Journal of Consulting and Clinical Psychology, 62*, 333–340.

Kisely, S., & Simon, G. (2006). An international study comparing the effect of medically explained and unexplained somatic symptoms on psychosocial outcome. *Journal of Psychosomatic Research, 60*, 125–130.

Kitayama, S., Okada, Y., Takumi, T., Takada, S., Inagaki, Y., & Nakamura, H. (2000). Psychological and physical reactions on children after the Hanshin-Awaji earthquake disaster. *Kobe Journal of Medical Science, 46*, 189–200.

Kroenke, K. (2001). Studying symptoms: Sampling and measurement issues. *Annals of Internal Medicine, 134*, 844–853.

Kroenke, K., & Price, R.K. (1993). Symptoms in the community; prevalence, classification and psychiatric comorbidity. *Archives of Internal Medicine, 153*, 2474–2480.

Kroenke, K., & Spitzer, R.L. (1998). Gender differences in the reporting of physical and somatoform symptoms. *Psychosomatic Medicine, 60*, 150–155.

Lang, T., Schwoebel, V., Diene, E., Bauvin, E., Garrigue, E., Lapierre-Duval, K., et al. (2007). Assessing post-disaster consequences for health at the population level: Experience from the AZF factory explosion in Toulouse. *Journal of Epidemiology and Community Health, 61*, 103–107.

Lima, B.R., Chavez, H., Samaniego, N., Pompei, M.S., Pai, S., Santacruz, H., et al. (1989). Disaster severity and emotional disturbance: Implications for primary mental health care in developing countries. *Acta Psychiatrica Scandinavia, 79*, 74–82.

Lima, B.R., Pai, S., Toledo, V., Caris, L., Haro, J.M., Lozano, J., et al. (1993). Emotional distress in disaster victims: A follow-up study. *Journal of Nervous and Mental Disease, 181*, 388–393.

Litz, B.T., Keane, T.M., Fisher, L., Marx, B., & Monaco, V. (1992). Physical health complaints in combat related post-traumatic stress disorder: A preliminary report. *Journal of Traumatic Stress, 5*(1), 131–141.

Maida, C.A., Gordon, N.S., Steinberg, A., Carl, A., & Gordon, G. (1989). Psychosocial impact of disasters: Victims of the Baldwin hills fire. *Journal of Traumatic Stress, 2*, 37–48.

Mayou, R., & Farmer, A. (2002). Functional somatic symptoms and syndromes. *British Medical Journal, 325*, 265–268.

McEwen, B.S. (1998). Protective and damaging effects of stress mediators. *Seminars in Medicine of the Beth Israel Deaconess Medical Center, 338*(3), 171–179.

McEwen, B.S., & Stellar, E. (1993). Stress and the individual; mechanisms leading to disease. *Archives of Internal Medicine, 153*, 2093–2101

McFarlane, A.C., Atchinson, M., Rafalowicz, E., & Papay, P. (1994). Physical symptoms in post-traumatic stress disorder. *Journal of Psychosomatic Research, 38*(7), 715–726.

McFarlane, A.C., Clayer, J.R., & Bookless, C.L. (1997). Psychiatric morbidity following a natural disaster: An Australian bushfire. *Social Psychiatry Psychiatric Epidemiology, 32*, 261–268.

Morren, M., Dirkzwager, A.J.E., Kessels, F.J.M., & Yzermans, C.J. (2007). The influence of a disaster on the health of rescue workers: A longitudinal study. *Canadian Medical Association Journal, 176*(9), 1279–1283.

Morren, M., Yzermans, C.J., van Nispen, R.M., & Wevers, S.J. (2005). The health of volunteer firefighters three years after a technological disaster. *Journal of Occupational Health, 47*(6), 523–532.

Najarian, L.M., Goenjian, A.K., Pelcovitz, D., Mandel, F., & Najarian, B. (2001). The effect of relocation after a natural disaster. *Journal of Traumatic Stress, 14*(3), 511–526.

Nimnuan, C., Hotopf, M., & Wessely, S. (2001). Medically unexplained symptoms; an epidemiological study in seven specialties. *Journal of Psychosomatic Research, 51*, 361–367.

Norris, F.H., Friedman, M.J., Watson, P.J., Byrne, C.M., Diaz, E., & Kaniasty, K. (2002). 60,000 disaster victims speak: Part 1. An empirical review of the empirical literature, 1981–2001. *Psychiatry, 65*(3), 207–239.

Norris, F.H., Slone, L.B., Baker, C.K., & Murphy, A.D. (2006). Early physical consequences of disaster exposure and acute disaster-related PTSD. *Anxiety, Stress, and Coping, 19*(2), 95–110.

Norris, R.L., Maguen, S., Litz, B.T., Adler, A.B., & Britt, T.W. (2005). Physical health symptoms in peacekeepers: Has the role of deployment stress been overrated? *Stress, Trauma, and Crisis, 8*(4), 251–265.

North, C.S., Kawasaki, A., Spitznagel, E.L., & Hong, B.A. (2004). The course of PTSD, major depression, substance abuse, and somatisation after a natural disaster. *Journal of Nervous and Mental Disease, 192*(12), 823–829.

Nuyen, J., Schellevis, F.G., Satariano, W.A., Spreeuwenberg, P.M., Birkner, M.D., van den Bos, G.A.M., et al. (2006). Comorbidity was associated with neurologic and psychiatric diseases: A general practice-based controlled study. *Journal of Clinical Epidemiology, 59*, 1274–1284.

Ouimette, P., Cronkite, R., Henson, B.R., Prins, A., Gima, K., & Moos, R.H. (2004). Posttraumatic stress disorder and health status among female and male medical patients. *Journal of Traumatic Stress, 17*(1), 1–9.

Okkes, I.M., Oskam, S.K., & Lamberts, H. (2002). The probability of specific diagnoses for patients presenting with common symptoms to Dutch family physicians. *The Journal of Family Practice, 51*(1), 31–36.

Page, L.A., Petrie, K.J., & Wessely, S. (2006). Psychosocial responses to environmental incidents: A review and a proposed typology. *Journal of Psychosomatic Research, 60*, 413–422.

Phifer, J.F. (1990). Psychological distress and somatic symptoms after natural disaster: Differential vulnerability among older adults. *Psychology and Aging, 5*(3), 412–420.

Pocan, S., Ozkan, S., Hulusi, M., & Cakir, O. (2002). Crush syndrome and acute renal failure in the Marmara earthquake. *Military Medicine, 167*(6), 516–518.

Renck, B., Weisaeth, L., & Skarbö, S. (2002). Stress reactions in police officers after a disaster rescue operation. *Nordic Journal of Psychiatry, 56*(1), 7–14.

Richardson, R.D., & Engel, C.C. (2004). Evaluation and management of medically unexplained physical symptoms. *The Neurologist, 10*(1), 18–30.

Rogers, L. (April 16, 2000). Ailing troops sue over Balkan War syndrome. *The Sunday Times of London News*.

Schnurr, P.P., & Green, B.L. (2003). Understanding relationships among trauma, posttraumatic stress disorder, and health outcomes. In P.P. Schnurr & B.L. Green (Eds.), *Trauma and health. Physical Consequences of Exposure to Extreme Stress*. Washington DC: American Psychological Association.

Schnurr, P.P., & Jankowski, M.K. (1999). Physical health and post-traumatic stress disorder: Review and synthesis. *Seminars in Clinical Neuropsychiatry*, *4*(4), 295–304.

Schnurr, P.P., & Spiro, A. (1999). Combat exposure, posttraumatic stress disorder symptoms, and health behaviors as predictors of self-reported physical health in older veterans. *Journal of Nervous and Mental Disease*, *187*(6), 353–359.

Schnurr, P.P., Spiro, A., & Paris, A.H. (2000). Physician-diagnosed medical disorders in relation to PTSD symptoms in older male military veterans. *Health Psychology*, *19*(1), 91–97.

Shalev, A., Bleich, A., & Ursano, R.J. (1990). Posttraumatic stress disorder: Somatic comorbidity and effort tolerance. *Psychosomatics*, *31*(2), 197–203.

Shariat, S., Mallonee, S., Kruger, E., Farmer, K., & North, C. (1999). A prospective study of long-term health outcomes among Oklahoma City bombing survivors. *Journal of Oklahoma State Medical Association*, *92*, 178–186.

Siegert, R.J., & Abernethy, D.A. (2005). Depression in multiple sclerosis: A review. *Journal of Neurology, Neurosurgery, and Psychiatry*, *76*, 469–475.

Simon, G., Gater, R., Kisely, S., & Piccinelli, M. (1996). Somatic symptoms of distress: An international primary care study. *Psychosomatic Medicine*, *58*, 481–488.

Soeteman, R.J.H, Yzermans, C.J., Kerssens, J.J., Dirkzwager, A.J.E., Donker, G.A., van den Bosch, W.J.H.M., et al. (2006). The course of post-disaster health problems of victims with pre-disaster psychological problems as presented in general practice. *Family Practice*, *23*(3), 378–384.

Suzuki, S., Sakamoto, S., Koide, M., Fujita, H., Sakuramoto, H., Kuroda, T., et al. (1997). Hanshin-Awaji earthquake as a trigger for acute myocardial infarction. *American Heart Journal*, *134*, 974–977.

Tainaka, H., Oda, H., Nakamura, S., Tabuchi, T., Noda, T., & Mito, H. (1998). Workers' stress after Hanshin-Awaji earthquake in 1995 – symptoms related to stress after 18 months [In Japanese]. *Sangyo Eiseigaku Zasshi*, *40*, 241–249.

Tak S., Driscoll, R., Bernard, B., & West C. (2007). Depressive symptoms among firefighters and related factors after the response to hurricane Katrina. *Journal of Urban Health*, *84*(2), 153–161.

Thomas, H.V., Stimpson, N.J., Weightman, A., Dunstan, F., & Lewis, G. (2006). Pain in veterans of the Gulf War of 1991: A systematic review. *BMC Musculoskeletal Disorders*, *7*, 74.

Trout, D., Nimgade, A., Mueller, C., Hall, R., & Scott Earnest, G. (2002). Health effects and occupational exposures among office workers near the World Trade Center disaster site. *Journal of Occupational and Environmental Medicine*, *44*(7), 601–605.

Tyano, S., Iancu, I., Solomon, Z., Sever, J., Goldstein, I., Touviana, Y., & Bleich, A. (1996). Seven-year follow-up of child survivors of a bus-train collision. *Journal of the American Academy of Child & Adolescent Psychiatry*, *35*(3), 365–373.

van den Berg, B., Grievink, L., Stellato, R.K., Yzermans, C.J., & Lebret, E. (2005). Symptoms and related functioning in a traumatized community. *Archives of Internal Medicine*, *165*(20), 2402–2407.

van den Berg, B., Grievink, L., van der Velden, P.G., Yzermans, C.J., Stellato, R.K., Lebret, E., et al. (2008) Risk factors for physical symptoms after a disaster: a longitudinal study. *Psychological Medicine*, *38*, 499–510.

van den Berg, B., Grievink, L., Yzermans, C.J., & Lebret, E. (2005). Medically unexplained physical symptoms in the aftermath of disasters. *Epidemiologic Reviews*, *27*, 92–106.

van den Berg, B., van der Velden, P.G., Yzermans, C.J., Stellato, R.K., & Grievink, L. (2006). Health-related quality of life and mental health problems after a disaster: Are chronically ill survivors more vulnerable to health problems? *Quality of Life Research*, *15*, 1571–1576.

van den Berg, B., Yzermans, C.J., Grievink, L., Stellato, R.K., van der Velden, P.G., Brunekreef, B., et al. (2009). Risk factors for unexplained symptoms after a disaster: A 5-year longitudinal study in general practice. *Psychosomatics*, *50*, 69–77.

van Ede, L., Yzermans, C.J., & Brouwer, H.J. (1999). Prevalence of depression in patients with chronic obstructive pulmonary disease: A systematic review. *Thorax*, *54*, 688–692.

van Griensven, F., Chakkraband, M.L., Thienkrua, W., Pengjuntr, W., Lopes Cardozo, B., Tantipiwatanaskul, P., et al. (2006). Thailand Post-Tsunami Mental Health Study Group. Mental health problems among adults in tsunami-affected areas in southern Thailand. *Journal of the American Medical Association*, *296*(5), 537–548.

Vanholder, R., van der Tol, A., de Smet, M., Hoste, E., Koc, M., Hussain, A., et al. (2007). Earthquakes and crush syndrome casualties: Lessons learned from the Kashmir disaster. *Kidney International*, *71*, 17–23.

Van Kamp, I., Van der Velden, P.G., Stellato, R.K., Roorda, J., Van Loon, J., Kleber, R.J., et al. (2006). Physical and mental health shortly after a disaster: first results from the Enschede fireworks disaster study. *European Journal of Public Health*, *16*(3), 253–259.

Wagner, D., Heinrichs, M., & Ehlert, U. (1998). Prevalence of symptoms of posttraumatic stress disorder in German professional firefighters. *American Journal of Psychiatry*, *155*, 1727–1732.

Watson, D., & Pennebaker, J. W. (1989). Health complaints, stress and distress: Exploring the central role of negative affectivity. *Psychological Review*, *96*(2), 234–254.

Weisaeth, L. (1989). The stressors and the post-traumatic stress syndrome after an industrial disaster. *Acta Psychiatrica Scandinavica*, *80*, (Suppl. 355) 25–37.

Wessely, S. (2001). Ten years on: What do we know about the Gulf War syndrome? *Clinical Medicine*, *1*(1), 28–37.

Wessely, S. (2004). There is only one functional somatic syndrome. *British Journal of Psychiatry*, *185*, 95–96.

Wessely, S., & Freedman, L. (2006). Reflections on Gulf War illness. *Philosophical Transactions of the Royal Society*, *361*, 721–730.

Wessely, S., Nimnuan, C., & Sharpe, M. (1999). Functional somatic syndromes: One or many? *The Lancet*, *354*, 936–939.

Wolfe, J., Schnurr, P. P., Brown, P. J., & Furey, J. (1994). Posttraumatic stress disorder and war-zone exposure as correlates of perceived health in female Vietnam war veterans. *Journal of Consulting and Clinical Psychology*, *62*(6), 1235–1240.

Wu, H., Chou, P., Chou, F., Su, C., Tsai, K., Ou-Yang, W., et al. (2006). Survey of quality of life and related risk factors for a Taiwanese village population three years post-earthquake. *Australian and New Zealand Journal of Psychiatry*, *40*(4), 355–361.

Yzermans, C. J., & Gersons, B. P. R. (2002). The chaotic aftermath of an airplane crash in Amsterdam: A second disaster. In J. Havenaar, J. Cwikel, & E. J. Bromet (Eds.), *Toxic turmoil: Psychological and societal consequences of ecological disasters*. New York: Plaenum/Kluwer.

Yzermans, C. J., Donker, G. A., Kerssens, J. J., Dirkzwager, A. J. E., Soeteman, J. H., & ten Veen, P. M. H. (2005). Health problems of victims before and after disaster: A longitudinal study in general practice. *International Journal of Epidemiology*, *34*, 820–826.

Yzermans, C. J., Dirkzwager, A. J. E., & Breuning, E. (2005). *Long-term health consequences of disaster: A bibliography*. Utrecht Netherlands Institute for Health Services Research.

Yzermans, C. J., Dirkzwager, A. J. E., Kerssens, J. J., Cohen-Bendahan, C. C. C., & ten Veen, P. M. H. (2006). *Gevolgen van de vuurwerkramp in Enschede voor de gezondheid [Health effects of the Enschede fireworks disaster]*. Utrecht: Netherlands Institute for Health Services Research.

Zatzick, D. F., Marmar, C. R., Weiss, D. S., Browner, W. S., Metzler, T. J., Golding, J. M., et al. (1997). Posttraumatic stress disorder and functioning and quality of life outcomes in a nationally representative sample of male Vietnam veterans. *American Journal of Psychiatry*, *154*, 1690–1695.

Zoellner, L., Goodwin, M., & Foa, E. (2000). PTSD severity and health perceptions in female victims of sexual assault. *Journal of Traumatic Stress*, *13*, 635–649.

6 Substance Use and Misuse after Disasters: Prevalences and Correlates

PETER G. VAN DER VELDEN AND ROLF J. KLEBER

6.1. INTRODUCTION

Exposure to various traumatic events, as well as resulting disturbances such as posttraumatic stress disorder (PTSD), is associated with increased substance use (Breslau, Davis, & Schultz, 2003; Feldner, Babson, & Zvolensky, 2007; McFarlane, 1998; Morissette, Tull, Gulliver, Kamholz, & Zimering, 2007; Stewart, 1996). In particular, studies have shown that alcohol and tobacco consumption increase through both initiation of and increasing use of these substances. It is, however, unclear whether this is also true in the aftermath of large-scale catastrophes or disasters. The distinction between individual traumatic experiences and collective experiences (e.g., disasters) may be sometimes unclear (Galea, Nandi, & Vlahov, 2005). Moreover, comorbidity profiles of PTSD and substance use and misuse, as well as the population under study, may differ between types of trauma (Deering, Glover, Ready, Eddleman, & Alarcon, 1996).

Insight into substance use and misuse after disaster is important for several reasons. First, similar to PTSD and other mental health disturbances, understanding the prevalence of substance use and misuse after disasters is necessary in estimating the need for mental health services (see Cao, McFarlane, & Klimidis, 2003) and in organizing programs to prevent prolonged and increased use to minimize adverse affects on health and functioning. Second, information on comorbidity (e.g., PTSD, depression), correlates, and predictors of substance use may help to identify victims who are at risk for substance disorders and increased substance use in the short, medium and/or long term.

In this chapter, we provide a detailed overview of the current literature on substance use after disasters in affected populations. Studies examining effects in rescue workers or any individuals or populations that were not more or less direct victims of the disaster were beyond the scope of this chapter (see Melnik et al., 2002; Richman, Wislar, Flaherty, Fendrich, & Rospenda, 2004); however, results of some nationwide studies are included. In addition, we do not focus on clinical samples, help-seeking people, or patient samples (see Deren, Shedlin, Hamilton, & Hagan, 2002; Pfefferbaum & Doughty, 2001; Weissman et al., 2005).

In line with the literature, we have made a distinction between the three types of disasters: natural disasters, technological disasters (man-made, nonintentional disasters), and mass violence and terrorism (man-made, intentional disasters). Intentional events generally lead to poorer levels of health than nonintentional events (e.g., Kessler, Sonnega, Hughes, & Nelson, 1995). We first focus on prevalences and comorbidity of substance use (including changes in substance use). Next, we present correlates of substance use, that is, predictors of substance use as well as substance use as a predictor for mental health disturbances.

It should be noted that researchers have used a variety of categories (definitions and measures) to examine substance use or misuse. The criteria for substance dependency-abuse in the *Diagnostic and statistical manual of mental disorders* (DSM) (American Psychiatric Association

[APA], 1980, 1987, 1994, 2000) and substance use patterns (e.g., binge drinking; daily substance consumption; increased substance use, with and without clear cut offs) have been varied. Furthermore, studies have differed on time intervals for questions on substance (e.g., past weeks, past months, past 6 months, past year). With respect to correlates and predictors, the same diversity in assessment emerges. In addition, studies have been conducted from approximately 1 month to 14 years postevent in relatively small ($N < 20$) and large samples ($N > 1000$). Since these details are crucial in comparing and interpreting findings, for each study we describe relevant characteristics.

Several studies examined different aspects of substance use, such as prevalence, comorbidity, correlates and/or predictors of alcohol, tobacco and drugs use. They are cited more than once and should not be interpreted as different studies with independent results. The specific characteristics are only described when a study is mentioned for the first time.

6.2. PREVALENCES AND COMORBIDITY

This section outlines the prevalence of substance dependency-abuse, changes in substance use (other than changes in substance dependency-abuse), and associations between substance use and PTSD or other mental health problems after different categories of disasters.

6.2.1. Natural Disasters

6.2.1.1. Prevalences of Substance Dependency-Abuse

To what extent do increased substance use disorders accompany natural disasters in the short, intermediate, and long term? One month following a 1988 tornado in northern Florida, North and her colleagues (North, Smith, McCool, & Lightcap, 1989) examined alcohol dependency-abuse (DSM-III) in affected citizens ($N = 42$). No (new) cases of alcohol dependency-abuse were reported, and none of the respondents reported using alcohol to help them deal with their feelings. Comparable results were found 6 to 12 months after Hurricane Andrew struck South Florida in 1992. Among people living in the most severely affected areas ($N = 61$), there were no mental disorders (DSM-III-R) in the 6 months preceding the disaster, and only 2% developed alcohol dependency (David et al., 1996).

In the long term, similar results were found among displaced tribal and nontribal victims ($N = 351$) 6 years after a 1991 volcanic eruption of Mount Pinatubon in the Philippines. Prevalences of alcohol abuse (DSM-IV) were 5.6% and 10.3% in nontribal and tribal people, respectively (Howard et al., 1999). The study found no significant differences in the prevalence of alcohol abuse between disaster victims and the unaffected U.S. population (Spitzer et al., 1994), or between nontribal and tribal people.

Along with the absence of a large increase of substance use disorders in the short term, the absence of a strong increase was also clearly demonstrated in three longitudinal studies up to 3 years postevent. Researchers assessed victims of the great Midwestern floods in the St. Louis area in 1993 approximately 4 months ($N = 162$) and 16 months ($N = 142$) postevent (North, Kawasaki, Spitznagel, & Hong, 2004). In the 4 months postdisaster, prevalence of alcohol and drug use disorders (DSM-III-R) was 9.0% and 1.2%, respectively, with only one respondent (0.7%) developing a new alcohol disorder and no respondents (0.0%) developing drug use disorder. Current substance use disorders at follow-up were 5.9% and 0.7%, respectively, with three new cases of alcohol disorder not identified at the first wave (see also McMillen, North, Mosley, & Smith, 2002).

After the 1999 Chi-Chi disaster in Taiwan, alcohol and drug abuse-dependency (DSM-IV) were examined at 6 months, 2 years, and 3 years postevent ($N = 216$) (Chou et al., 2007). Alcohol abuse-dependency at 6 months, 2 years, and 3 years was relatively stable (4.2%, 5.1%, and 4.6%, respectively), as were all other assessed disorders. Drug abuse-dependency gradually increased (2.3%, 2.35%, and 5.1%). In addition, Wu and colleagues (2006) found that prevalences of alcohol and drug abuse-dependency in respondents who participated in the third survey (3 years postevent, $N = 405$) were 5.4% and 6.4%, respectively.

A study after a flooding disaster in the Caribbean Island of Puerto Rico in 1985 found similar results. This study used a rigorous longitudinal study design, with pre-event assessments and control subjects (Bravo, Rubio, Canino, Woodbury, & Ribera, 1990). Two groups were assessed: the first sample of persons were interviewed after the disaster (retrospective group, $N = 537$) and the second sample of persons were interviewed 1 year predisaster ($N = 375$). In the prospective sample, predisaster alcohol dependency (DSM-III) differed between nonexposed and the near-exposed ($M = 1.03$ vs. $M = 1.73$). In the retrospective group, severe-exposed people differed from the nonexposed ($M = 0.94$ vs. $M = 0.45$). Level of lifetime alcohol dependency at follow-up (1987) in the retrospective group differed between severe exposed and nonexposed ($M = 1.11$ vs. $M = 0.58$); however, differences between non-, near-, moderate-, and severe-exposed did not reach statistical significance in the prospective group.

Finally, one alternative way to assess the association between disaster and the consumption of substances on a population level is to prospectively examine objective sales statistics. Using this method, researchers analyzed quarterly (from 1990 to 1996) sales statistics of alcohol consumption before and after the Great Hanshin Earthquake (Japan, 1995), (Shimizu et al., 2000). Sales of alcoholic liquids in the affected areas decreased in 1995 and 1996. However, a decline of alcohol consumption (sales) on a population level does not necessarily indicate that all victims decreased their alcohol consumption. For example, Shinfuku (1999) reported – on the basis of his own experiences as a medical doctor and as a victim of the disaster – that 1 month postdisaster the consumption of alcohol increased and led to an epidemic of alcohol-related problems in some shelters. In addition, he observed that after 3 years alcohol problems were increasingly reported among those living in temporary housing.

6.2.1.2. Changes in Substance Use

Does the relative absence of an increase in substance use disorders imply that there are no changes in substance use? Larrance, Anastario, and Lawry (2007) conducted interviews among internally displaced people in Louisiana and Mississippi travel trailer camps ($N = 366$) approximately 9 months after Hurricanes Katrina and Rita in 2005. In this study, 14% reported an increase in alcohol or drug use, 12% a decrease, and 74% reported stable substance use since displacement.

Further evidence for possible increased substance use stems from the prospective study of Parslow and Jorm (2006). In young adults ($N = 2063$) affected by a major bush fire in Australia in 2003, 29% smoked at the first predisaster wave (1999–2000), and 28.1% reported increased cigarette consumption at 3 months postevent. Of past smokers at the first wave, 36.8% resumed smoking in the 3 months postevent in contrast to the 1.5% of the nonsmokers.

6.2.1.3. Comorbidity and Using Substances as a Way of Coping

Low comorbidity was found 10 months after the Chi-Chi earthquake in a study of two rural communities (18 years or older, $N = 252$) near the epicenter of the earthquake (Lai, Chang, Connor, Lee, & Davidson, 2004). Current alcohol abuse-dependency (DSM-IV) was reported in 3.8% of the PTSD cases, in 8.3% of the respondents with posttraumatic stress symptoms, and interestingly, in 7.3% of the non-PTSD cases. Four to six months after the disaster, no significant association was found ($N = 442$) between PTSD and alcohol and drug dependency-abuse (Chou et al., 2005). Furthermore, among the survivors of this Chi-Chi disaster, drug dependency-abuse was significantly associated with a higher risk for suicidality (Chou et al., 2007).

Researchers found a higher comorbidity rate 1 year after the 1980 volcanic eruption of Mount Saint Helens. Current alcohol use and drug use disorder (DSM-III) was examined in two rural communities ($N = 548$; Shore, Vollmer, & Tatum, 1989). Of the 37 respondents with current PTSD, 27% had alcohol disorder, and 8.1% had drug use disorder. After Hurricanes Katrina and Rita, increased substance use since displacement was associated with a 3.3-fold risk for major depressive disorder after adjusting for age, ethnicity, gender, and income (Larrance, Anastario, & Lawry, 2007).

An older retrospective comparative study 5 years (n = 562) after *Hurricane Agnes* (US, 1972), reported that among drinkers, victims (n = 169, 41.5%) more often obtained relief using alcohol compared to residents (n = 49, 31.6%) in the control group (Logue, Hansen, & Stuening, 1979). Following the great Midwestern floods (North et al., 2004), postdisaster alcohol use disorder was diagnosed in 42% of those who acknowledged drinking alcohol to cope with the flood but only in 2% of others. Of those with a postdisaster alcohol use disorder, 77% reported coping with the flood by drinking alcohol in contrast to 7% of others. However, in the prospective study assessing the impact of a major bush fire, current PTSD symptoms (hyperarousal and reexperiencing at the second wave) and neuroticism (wave 1) were not independently associated with increased cigarette smoking (started or increased frequency of smoking), uptake of smoking (nonsmoker in 12 months before first wave but had smoked in the 12 months preceding the second wave), or increased level of smoking (smoked less than one cigarette per day in first wave, and smoked one or more cigarettes at second wave or increased consumption) (Parslow & Jorm, 2006).

6.2.2. Technological Disasters

6.2.2.1. Prevalences of Substance Dependency-Abuse

Three studies provide insight in substance use disorders after technological disasters. The first study was conducted 4 to 6 weeks after a plane crashed into a hotel in 1987 (Smith, North, McCool, & Shea, 1990). In total, 12% of the hotel employees ($N = 46$) reported alcohol abuse-dependency (DSM-III). Approximately half of the cases met the criteria before disaster (lifetime 4 out of 6), indicating that 4% ($N = 2$) were new onset cases. No significant differences were found in alcohol abuse-dependency between onsite and offsite employees.

The second study was longitudinal, conducted 2 and 14 years after the Buffalo Creek Dam Collapse of 1972. Of the 143 responding families, 44% reported increased smoking levels immediately after the flood to 2 years after the flood (cited in Feldner et al., 2007), and 30% reported increased alcohol consumption in this period (cited in Stewart, 1996). Follow-up surveys 2 and 14 years postevent ($N = 120$) reported that alcohol abuse (DSM-III) was low at 2 years postevent ($M_{males} = 1.26$ and $M_{females} = 1.07$, where 1.0 means no impairment) and at 14 years postevent ($M_{males} = 1.09$ and $M_{females} = 1.01$) (Green et al., 1990).

Finally, Dooley and Gunn (1995) described the results of an assessment of psychological injury in a selective group of 75 survivors of 1987's *Herald of Free Enterprise* shipping disaster in Belgium, as well as relatives of victims who were referred by their solicitors to the authors (mid-1987 to early 1989). Of the 10 bereaved survivors, 6 (60%) met the criteria for alcohol abuse (DSM-III-R) at any time since the disaster. In other survivors ($N = 37$) and bereaved relatives ($N = 28$), 49% and 29%, respectively, met these criteria.

6.2.2.2. Changes in Substance Use

Are technological disasters accompanied by change in substance use in the short, intermediate, and long term, as was partly demonstrated in studies after natural disasters? Two months after the Three Miles Island (TMI) disaster in 1979, 13.3% of the regular alcohol drinkers living in the 5-mile ring of TMI reported increased use ($N_{total} = 691$) (Hu & Slaysman, 1984). During follow-up in January 1980 (9 months postevent), 2% reported increased drinking in relation to the event. Within the 5-mile exposure ring, 43% of the responders were regular smokers, consuming approximately one pack (20 cigarettes) a day. In total, 32% increased smoking during the first

2 weeks (additional 10 cigarettes). At follow-up, 8% reported an increase in smoking related to the disaster.

Six months after the *Herald of Free Enterprise* shipping disaster a study found high rates of increased substance use. Of the survivors ($N = 73$), 73% reported that their alcohol consumption and 44% reported that their cigarette consumption had increased in the preceding 6 months (increased a lot or a little more than usual) (Joseph, Yule, Williams, & Hodgekinson, 1993). In the 6 months preceding the second survey (30 months postdisaster), these percentages were 58% and 39%, respectively. Differences in mean scores of substance use at both surveys indicated a significant decrease in consumption.

After the *Exxon Valdez* oil tanker ran aground in Alaska in 1989, spilling 11 million gallons of crude oil, a somewhat different research methodology was used (Palinkas, Downs, Petterson, & Russel, 1993). The study was conducted 1 year postevent. Because of cultural sensitivity in the affected rural Alaskan communities over the issues of alcohol and drug use, people ($N = 594$) were asked if they thought friends/family and their particular community were using alcohol and drugs (more than before, or about the same or less than that before the spill). In addition, researchers asked respondents if the amount of substance use was leading to problems that did not exist before the spill. Of the high, low, and not exposed Native respondents, 47.3%, 37.1%, and 2.1%, respectively, reported increased alcohol use in family or friends. In addition, 46.9%, 25.8%, and 6.0%, respectively, reported more drinking problems. With respect to drug use and problems with drug use, percentages of high, low, and not exposed Native respondents were 42.1%, 42.5%, and 24.4%, and 14.9%, 5.3%, and 4.8%, respectively. The same pattern in non-Natives was demonstrated, although lower percentages in the three exposure groups were found. With respect to observed substance use and substance problems in the communities, Natives and non-Natives reported more and comparable increased substance use and substance use problems.

Another longitudinal comparative study suggests that in the intermediate and long term, increase of substance use may also be restricted to pre-event users, as relatively few nonsmokers begin to smoke after a disaster (see Parslow & Jorm, 2006). Eighteen months and almost 4 years after a 2000 fireworks disaster in the Netherlands, no differences were found between affected native citizens ($N = 662$) and a control group in the proportion of nonsmokers, past smokers, and current smokers ($N = 526$) (Van der Velden, Grievink, Olff, Gersons, & Kleber, 2007).

6.2.2.3. Comorbidity and Using Substances as a Way of Coping

A few studies have examined comorbidity after technological disasters. Survivors of the Kegworth air disaster in the United Kingdom in 1989 were interviewed in the period 6 to 12 months postdisaster ($N = 68$) (Gregg et al., 1995). Of the PTSD cases (39.7%, DSM-III-R), 33% increased alcohol consumption (slightly or heavily) in contrast to 12% of the non-PTSD cases, although change in alcohol use was unknown in 29.3% of the non-PTSD cases. Ten years after the *Piper Alpha* oil platform disaster in 1988, survivors with current psychiatric problems (GHQ caseness) were significantly more likely to have developed alcohol problems after the disaster (Hull, Alexander, & Klein, 2002).

In a study after the Buffalo Creek disaster ($N = 193$), Green and colleagues (1992) reported a lifetime postflood (14 years) prevalence of substance abuse of 10.4%. Among respondents with lifetime-disaster-related PTSD (59.4%), 10.5% met the criteria for substance abuse (substance disorder was almost entirely accounted for by alcohol diagnoses). Approximately 6% had lifetime-disaster-related PTSD and substance abuse disorder. Current prevalence of substance abuse 14 years postevent was 3.6%, and of the respondents with current PTSD (14 years postevent), 8.3% met the criteria for substance abuse.

Finally, a study among a small group of volunteers ($N = 13$) who responded to the Swissair

Flight 111 disaster in 1998 assessed the association between PTSD symptomatology and using alcohol or drugs to think less about the event and drinking to decrease or avoid negative internal states. The study was conducted over a period of 9 months between July 2001 and April 2002 (Stewart, Mitchell, Wright, & Loba, 2004). Results showed that PTSD symptom severity and frequency were strongly correlated with this coping strategy.

6.2.3. Mass Shooting and Terrorism

6.2.3.1. Prevalences of Substance Dependency-Abuse

North and colleagues (1994, 1997, 2001) examined substance use in the short and intermediate term after a 1991 mass shooting in Killeen. First, they examined drug use disorder (DSM-III-R) after 6 to 8 weeks (*N* = 136) (North et al., 1994, 1997). Current alcohol and drug use disorder at 4 to 6 weeks postevent was 7.5% and 0.0%, respectively. No new postdisaster drug use disorders were found 4 to 6 weeks postevent. Researchers then reassessed 124 survivors at 1 year (North et al., 1997), and 113 at 3 years (North et al., 2001). At 1-year follow-up, 5.7% and 0.8% had current alcohol and drug use disorder, respectively. Of 11 cases of postdisaster alcohol use disorder identified at the first or second wave, five were diagnosed 4 to 6 weeks postevent and all 11 at follow-up, indicating a small increase in alcohol use disorder.

Four to eight months after the Oklahoma City bombing in 1995, North and colleagues (1999) demonstrated that postdisaster alcohol and drug use disorder in survivors (*N* = 182) was 9.4% and 2.2%, respectively (DSM-III-R). They found no new postdisaster substance disorders. Furthermore, North and colleagues (2005) compared substance use after the terrorist bombings in Oklahoma City and Nairobi (*N* = 227) at 8 to 10 months postevent (North et al., 2005). Among men and women, more survivors of the Oklahoma City bombing than survivors of the Nairobi bombing showed predisaster alcohol disorder. After the bombings, only differences between the women in the two samples remained (8.7% vs. 0.0%; among men, 10.2% and 11.1%, respectively). As after the Oklahoma bombing, no new postdisaster alcohol disorders were identified after the Nairobi terrorist attacks.

After the September 11th terrorist attacks in the United States, substance use was systematically and extensively examined in a series of epidemiological studies among citizens of Manhattan. In these studies, approximately one-third were directly affected by the disaster (i.e., were injured in the attacks, had a friend or relative killed, had lost or damaged possessions, lost a job, or were involved in rescue effort) (see Nandi, Galea, Ahern, & Vlahov, 2005; Vlahov et al., 2006).

Vlahov and colleagues (2006) compared alcohol use in the 6 months before the event with consumption in the 6 months after the event (*N* = 1570). The prevalence of drinking problems (indicative for alcohol use disorder, CAGE criteria) was 3.7% before and 4.2% after the event. In total, 2.1% were new cases (*N* = 46) of drinking problems, double that of those who resolved problem drinking (*N* = 22).

Somewhat lower prevalences of alcohol problems (using the same CAGE criteria) were reported in a longitudinal study (*N* = 1,681) 1 and 2 years postevent (Boscarino, Adams, & Galea, 2006). Of the respondents, 1.6% reported alcohol dependency in the year before September 11th, 2.8% reported alcohol dependency in the first year postevent and 2.7% in the year before the second wave (no significant changes in dependency). In addition, 15.9% reported binge drinking (six or more drinks on one occasion) during the first year postevent and 14.9% in the year before the second wave (14.4% in the year before September 11th).

One study examined nicotine dependency (Nandi et al., 2005). Four months after September 11th, 24.9% (*N* = 2001) of the citizens smoked. Approximately one-tenth (10.1%) reported three or more symptoms of nicotine dependency (DSM-IV).

6.2.3.2. Change in Substance Use

In the study among victims of the Nairobi bombing, 5.1% reported increased alcohol and 4.1% increased tobacco consumption (North et al., 2005). Almost all other studies on changes in substance use after mass violence and terrorism are of the September 11th terrorist attacks.

A study 5 to 8 weeks after September 11th showed that in the week before the event, 22.6%, 59.1%, and 4.4% used cigarettes, alcohol, and marijuana, respectively (*N* = 988) (Vlahov et al., 2002). In the week before the survey 23.4%, 64%, and 5.7% respectively used these substances. Compared to the week before September 11th, 9.7% reported an increase in cigarette consumption (increased frequency in the week before the survey but not the week before September 11th). With respect to alcohol and marijuana, increases of 24.6% and 3.2% were reported. A survey 4 months postevent found that 69.4% of the nicotine dependent respondents increased smoking, in contrast to 2.2% of the noncases (Nandi et al., 2005).

Similar results with respect to cigarettes and marijuana were found 6 to 9 months postevent (*N* = 1,570) (Vlahov et al., 2004). In total, 9.9% reported any increase in cigarette consumption, 17.5% in alcohol, and 2.7% in marijuana consumption. Researchers also found that 22.9% of participants reported use of cigarettes, 34.1% of alcohol, and 4.8% of marijuana, in the 30 days before the attacks. A very small group used substances in the month before the survey, but not in the 30 days before the attacks (1.9%, 5.3%, and 0.4%, respectively).

In another study, two samples of citizens who lived south of 110th street in Manhattan were examined approximately 1 month (*N* = 988) and 6 months (*N* = 854) postevent (Vlahov, Galea, Ahern, Resnick, & Kilpatrick, 2004). Comparison of the two samples showed that percentages of increased use of alcohol, cigarettes or marijuana were 30.8% and 27.3%, respectively. Results suggested a modest decline in alcohol and cigarette consumption and a modest increase in marijuana use. There were no significant differences in patterns between directly affected and not directly affected citizens.

In a longitudinal study 1 and 2 years postevent, at the 2 years postevent time point, 10% reported an increase of 4 or more days of drinking per month as compared to 1 year postevent, and 9.3% reported an increase of two or more drinks per day (Adams, Boscarino, & Galea, 2006a). Drinking two or more drinks per day increased from 6.3% at the first wave to 14.3% at second wave, but the percentages of respondents with alcohol dependency and of binge drinking did not increase (Boscarino et al., 2006). In another study among adult Manhattan residents 3 to 6 months after September 11th, Delisi and colleagues (2003) found only 6.8% of participants increased alcohol use. Of those interviewed (*N* = 1,009), 4.8% and 4.0% reported the use of any "street drugs" before or after September 11th, respectively.

In addition, a study among military and civilian staff of the Pentagon 6 months after the attacks found that 13% staff of the Pentagon (*N* = 77) reported that they used more alcohol since the attack than they meant to (Grieger, Fullerton, & Ursano, 2003). Ford and colleagues (2006) assessed a sample of Connecticut citizens (*N* = 2,741), of whom a substantial number worked in, regularly traveled to, or had family or close friends living in New York City. Five to fifteen months after the attacks, 19.6% were current smokers and 67.3% were current drinkers; 2.1% reported an increase of smoking and 6.4% reported an increase in alcohol consumption.

6.2.3.4. Comorbidity and Using Substances as a Way of Coping

Six to eight weeks after the mass shooting in Killeen, among men with postdisaster PTSD, almost none had comorbid substance use disorder, and among females with PTSD-only a few had alcohol use disorder. Drinking alcohol did not differentiate respondents with postdisaster PTSD from those without PTSD (North et al., 1994). The study 6 months after the Oklahoma City bombing (North et al., 1999) partly confirms these findings. Those with PTSD and comorbid diagnosis or with non-PTSD-diagnosis only more often reported drinking alcohol as a way of coping with the event compared with survivors without postdisaster diagnoses (32.4%, 40.0%, and 5.6% respectively). However, PTSD-only cases and no-diagnoses cases did not differ significantly (13.0% vs. 5.6%). After the mass shooting in Killeen, 15% coped with the event by drinking alcohol (North et al., 1994). The same pattern (15.9%) was found among the survivors of the Oklahoma City bombing (North et al., 1999). However, more Oklahoma victims (15.4%) than victims of the Nairobi bombings (8.5%) used alcohol to cope with the event.

The frequency of direct and indirect exposure to terrorists attacks may influence substance use because a somewhat lower rate of this coping strategy was found in populations exposed to the terrorist attacks on Israeli society since 2000 (Bleich, Gelkopf, & Solomon, 2003). In total, 5.3% reported ever using alcohol or cigarettes as a way to cope with the event(s), and 0.7% reported always using these substances as a way to cope with the attacks. However, the researchers interviewed a nationally representative population sample ($N = 512$), which included citizens who were not directly or indirectly affected (55.6%). As was shown in other studies, more respondents using than not using this coping style reported posttraumatic stress symptoms (controlling for gender, low sense of safety, use of tranquilizers, avoidance of television/radio, and faith in God); in addition, they were more likely to report PTSD symptoms (controlling for associations with gender, low sense of safety, and use of tranquilizers).

Five to eight weeks after September 11th, current disaster-related PTSD and depression were more frequent in those reporting increased cigarette consumption than those who did not report such increase (24.2% vs. 5.6% and 22.1% vs. 8.2%, respectively) and more frequent in those reporting increased marijuana use as compared with those who did not report such increase (36.0% vs. 6.6% and 22.3% vs. 9.4%, respectively) (Vlahov et al., 2002). In contrast to PTSD, depression was more prevalent in victims who have increased alcohol consumption as compared with those who did not report such increase (15.5% vs. 8.3%).

Four months postevent, nicotine dependent citizens more than nonnicotine dependent citizens had disaster-related PTSD (18.1% vs. 5.7%) and depression (23.6% vs. 6.0%) after the attacks (Nandi et al., 2005). Increased consumption was associated with PTSD among nicotine dependent cases (23.4% vs.6.4%) and noncases (15.1% vs. 5.5%), but with respect to depression only among cases of nicotine dependency (28.3% vs. 13.3%). Among non-cigarette-dependent cases those who increased cigarette consumption were not significantly more likely to be depressed than those who did not increase consumption (8.5% vs. 5.9%).

Six to nine months postevent, more respondents reporting increased smoking than respondents without increased use had PTSD (4.3% vs. 1.2%) and depression (14.6% vs. 5.2%) in the past month (Vlahov, Galea, Ahern, Resnick, Boscarino, et al., 2004). In addition, increases in alcohol and, especially, marijuana consumption were associated with depression compared with respondent without increased use (11.8% vs. and 34.1 vs. 5.3%, respectively). The percentages of depression were higher in those reporting an increase in two to three substances compared with respondents reporting an increase in one substance (data not presented).

Vlahov and colleagues (2006) also assessed prevalence of PTSD in the 6 months after September 11th in respondents with drinking problems in the 6 months before and/or after the event (PTSD any time since September 11th). In total, 2% reported drinking problems before and after (PTSD = 34.2%), 2.2% after but not before (PTSD = 28.4%), and 1.7% before but not after September 11th (PTSD = 15.4%); 40.5% were consistently drinking without drinking problems (PTSD = 5.1%), and 53.6% were nondrinkers in both time intervals (PTSD = 7.0%). Similar patterns were found for depression and subsyndromal PTSD at any time since September 11th. Current (past 30 days) PTSD in the five drinking groups was 9.5%, 17.1%, 1.1%, 0.4%, and 1.4%. Higher prevalences of depression were found in citizens who either changed from nonproblem to problem or from problem to nonproblem drinking (23.5% and 28.3%, respectively).

Of the Pentagon staff, people with PTSD were 5.6 times more likely to report an increase in alcohol consumption than those without PTSD (Grieger et al., 2003). In another study, Pentagon personnel ($N = 4{,}739$) were assessed in the period October 2001 to January 2002 (Jordan et al., 2004). In total, 2.5% were considered to be at high risk for alcohol abuse, of whom 52.6% reported functional impairment. Functional impairment was independently associated with alcohol abuse, after controlling for postevent mental health problems (PTSD, depression, panic attacks, and generalized anxiety). In the Ford and colleagues (2006) study, however, measures of substance use were not significantly associated with reported disaster-related psychological problems in Connecticut citizens. Approximately 9 months after September 11th, Lating and colleagues (2004) assessed substance use in American airline attendants ($N = 2050$). Those with PTSD had significantly lower scores in substance use (not specified) as part of functioning than those without PTSD, but their mean scores indicated healthy functioning in this domain.

One prospective study after September 11th had baseline measures in 1991 and 1992 and 1- and 10-year follow-ups of an adult community sample of drinkers (i.e., had consumed five or more drinks at one occasion during the 12 months before baseline) living approximately 12 miles from the World Trade Center ($N = 791$) (Hasin, Keyes, Hatzenbuehler, Aharonovich, & Alderson, 2007). Ten percent were 0 to 5 miles from the World Trade Center at the time of the attacks, and 32.1% knew someone who was lost or killed. Approximately 11% reported drinking to cope with feelings about September 11th.

6.2.4. Conclusions

A comprehensive overview of the main conclusions on prevalence and comorbidity with regard to substance use and abuse is presented in Table 6.1.

Empirical studies are characterized by great variation in measures for substance use and misuse (see Stewart, 1996), types of disaster, the use of prospectively and retrospectively collected data (e.g., lifetime prevalences), study designs (e.g., cross-section, longitudinal), time-frames, postdisaster mental health problems, and geographical area (most studies have been conducted in Western countries, especially those after technological disasters, mass violence, and terrorism). Compared to PTSD symptomatology (see Galea et al., 2005; Norris, Watson, Byrne, Diaz, & Kaniasty, 2002), substance use after disasters is far less often examined.

The large diversity in study designs and methodology makes it very difficult to draw firm conclusions, especially because many of the studies were not primarily focused on substance abuse after disasters and calamities. In addition, it is unclear to what extent differences in reported increase use of substance can be, among other factors, attributed to the use and effects of mental health-care utilization at earlier stages after the disaster.

Nevertheless, we can draw one general conclusion: disasters are *not* accompanied by a large increase of substance use disorders in affected citizens. New onset cases of substance use disorders in the first years after disasters, particularly alcohol and drug use disorders, tend to be the exception rather than the rule; new postdisaster cases are zero to a few percent. Thus, empirical results suggest that prevalence and incidence of substance dependency-abuse after disasters and prevalences in comparable nonaffected populations are more or less equivalent. Although it is plausible that these findings are applicable to nicotine dependency as well, further longitudinal research on the development of nicotine dependency is warranted.

However, after disasters, a variable group has been found to report an increase of substance use or problematic use of cigarettes, marijuana, and, especially, alcohol (when available). In other words, when substance use after disasters increases, it does not appear to translate into *new* abuse-dependence cases (see North et al., 2004). Nevertheless, the observed increase and the well-known negative effects of high levels of tobacco, alcohol, and drug consumption on health (e.g., liver disease, heart disease, and

Table 6.1. Main conclusion on prevalences and comorbidity

- Compared to PTSD and other mental health disturbances, substance use in the short, intermediate, and long term has received less attention in empirical studies after technological disasters, natural disasters, and disasters caused by mass violence and terrorism
- There is a large variety in study designs and research methods of studies on substance abuse-dependency, increased use, and comorbidity. Assessments of use other than by self-reports are almost absent. More uniform prospective study designs and methods with multiple follow-ups in future research would facilitate lucid conclusions about the course of substance use
- Since most studies after technological disasters and disasters caused by mass violence and terrorism were conducted in western countries, their findings may not be applicable to the disasters in non-Western countries
- Relatively few studies examined substance use and comorbidity prospectively in the long term (>5–10 years postevent). Since studies with multiple follow-ups are almost absent and existing studies differ as described earlier, it is difficult to draw firm conclusions about the course of substance use or pattern of use over the years after the three types of disasters
- Nevertheless, there are no indications that disasters are accompanied by a (strong) increase of substance use disorders in the short, intermediate, or in the long term, and thus, postdisaster prevalences appear more or less equal to prevalences in comparable nonaffected residents
- The available empirical evidence indicates that increases in substances such as tobacco, alcohol, and drugs are almost restricted to predisaster users, and that a very small proportion of the nonusers will start using substances after the disaster
- In most cases, a minority will show an increase in substance use, although increases of alcohol consumption have been reported up to 73%. In general, increases in substance use decline when time passes by as posttraumatic stress reactions do (although, a further increase in alcohol consumption was reported in some studies)
- Reported increases in alcohol consumption tend to be higher than reported increases in cigarettes and drug consumption. However, compared to alcohol use, cigarette use and drug consumption were less often examined
- Substance use disorder or increased use and postdisaster mental disturbances are mostly, thus not always, positively – although on the whole weakly to modestly – associated, that is, comorbidity in general is lower than approximately 30%–40%. Thus, comorbidity of substance use disorder and, for example, PTSD or depression is not high but may be a noteworthy problem
- The interassociations between alcohol, cigarette, and drug use is a relatively neglected topic in disaster research, as well as mental health disturbances among affected residents who are multiusers (or increased consumption of alcohol, cigarettes, and drugs)
- Other studies have shown that a part of the disaster victims seek treatment or receives some kind of mental health care. It is unclear to what extent differences in reported (increased) use of substances can be, among other factors, attributed to differences in mental health-care utilization and its effects

Note: PTSD, posttraumatic stress disorder.

cancer) necessitate special attention in mental health programs after disasters. Results suggest that only a very small group *began* to use substances after the disaster. Increased use in the aftermath of a catastrophic event can continue for years, as posttraumatic symptoms do, though a (slow) decline can be observed.

Interestingly, findings also suggest that a very small group of victims *decrease* substance use. However, in general, the majority of disaster-affected people demonstrate rather stable substance use in the intermediate and long term. In addition, (increased) substance use after a disaster and postdisaster mental health disturbances such as PTSD and depression are mostly positively – although in general modestly – associated, although results are mixed. Findings suggest that after disasters a minority of (increased) substance users or substance dependent-abuse victims suffer from these disturbances or vice versa. However, there are indications that mental health disturbances are more prevalent in substance-dependent victims who increase substance use than in nondependent victims who increase substance use.

At last, interassociations between alcohol, cigarettes, and drug use has received relatively little attention in disaster research to date. Mental health disturbances in multiusers, or increased consumption of alcohol, cigarettes, *and* drugs, have rarely been examined in postdisaster research.

6.3. PREDICTORS

In the preceding paragraphs, we described the associations between substance use and mental health disturbances (comorbidity) after several types of disasters. In the following section, we present correlates of (increased) substance use or misuse in detail, that is, (independent) predictors of substance use, as well as substance use as a (independent) predictor for PTSD and other postdisaster mental health disturbances.

6.3.1. Natural Disasters

6.3.1.1. Predictors of Substance Use

There is little consensus across studies on natural disasters that substance is significantly associated with exposure level and disaster experiences (including being displaced). In the study of Bravo and colleagues (1990), after the flooding in the Caribbean island of Puerto Rico postevent lifetime alcohol dependency-abuse was not independently predicted by exposure level. Similar results were found approximately 2 months after the Tsunami disaster (Asia, 2005) in displaced ($N = 371$) and nondisplaced victims ($N = 322$) in the Phang Nga province ($N = 322$), and nondisplaced people in the provinces of Krabi and Phuket in Thailand ($N = 368$) (Van Griensven et al., 2006). No significant differences were found in reported use of illicit drugs in displaced (4.9%) and nondisplaced people (3.7%) in the Phang Nga province, and nondisplaced people in the provinces of Krabi and Phuket (4.9%). In addition, the three groups also did not differ in alcohol consumption (daily three glasses or more).

Solomon and colleagues (1993) compared relationships between alcohol abuse symptoms (DSM-III) on the one hand and levels of disaster exposure, emotional support, and support burden on the other hand, in victims of the flooding in Puerto Rico and victims of the flooding in St. Louis (United States, 1982; 1 year [$N = 543$, SL] and 2 years [$N = 912$, PR]) after the flooding. In the St. Louis sample, only those reporting heavy support burdens showed more alcohol abuse than those reporting low or moderate support burden (after controlling for lifetime alcohol abuse before the disaster and family role). Furthermore, no significant differences were found in alcohol abuse symptoms between exposed and nonexposed people. Interestingly, in the Puerto Rico sample exposed people and those with heavy support burden reported more alcohol abuse than nonexposed and low/moderate support burden respectively (see results in Bravo et al., 1990). In addition, those reporting high emotional support showed less alcohol abuse than those reporting low/moderate emotional support.

After a major bush fire (Parslow & Jorm, 2006) the number of firework-related experiences independently predicted increased smoking and uptake smoking.

Age also yielded the same mixed results, in contrast to gender. In the just mentioned study by Parslow and Jorm (2006), females were less likely to increase level of smoking, and those with more years of education were less likely to increase cigarette consumption and uptake smoking.

After Hurricane Mitch in Honduras (1998) alcohol misuse was examined in three age groups, that is, 15 to 24 year olds, 25 to 59 year olds, and 60 years or older ($N = 800$; Kohn et al., 2005). Approximately 1 to 2 months postevent, 5.5%, 5.0%, and 3.9% respectively reported alcohol misuse and no statistical differences were found between the three groups. Additional regression analyses controlling for demographics, "prior" nerves, high-low impact neighborhood, exposure (and several interaction affects) did not alter these findings. In contrast, lifetime alcohol dependency-abuse after the flooding in the Caribbean island of Puerto Rico (Bravo et al., 1990) in the prospective group was independently predicted by younger age.

In the already mentioned studies on the bush fire (Parlow & Jorm, 2006) and the flooding (Bravo et al., 1990) females were less likely to increase the level of smoking. Lifetime alcohol dependency-abuse after the flooding was more prevalent in males than females. Four to six months after the Chi-Chi disaster, significantly lower prevalences were found in females than in males for drug and alcohol dependence-abuse (DSM-IV) that is, 0.8% versus 4.7%, and 0.0% versus 11.7% (Chou et al., 2005).

Finally, the study of McMillen and colleagues (2002), focusing on the first wave of studies after the Great Midwestern flood (see previous text), showed that those with a prior psychiatric history were also more likely to drink alcohol to cope with the flood (24% vs. 8%).

6.3.1.2. Substance Use as Predictor of Postdisaster Mental Health Problems

Associations reported in empirical studies between substance use and later postdisaster mental health problems (including substance use) are confusing: they were found to be nonsignificant, positive, and negative.

Six months after the Marmara, Turkey, earthquake in 1999, employees of a factory in the affected area, their spouses, and their adult children affected by the disaster ($N = 1{,}288$) were examined (Çorapçlolu, Tural, Yargiç, & Kocabaolu, 2004). In the group of respondents with PTSD (DSM-IV), with subthreshold PTSD and without (subthreshold) PTSD, respectively 3.4%, 2.2%, and 0.8% reported alcohol abuse before the disaster. Alcohol abusers were more likely to be PTSD cases and subthreshold PTSD cases compared to noncases, when controlling for demographics, experienced events during the disaster (e.g., horror and loss of lost ones), and a history of psychiatric disorder and previous trauma. PTSD cases and subthreshold PTSD cases did not differ from each other.

Results of a longitudinal study ($N = 640$) after the Newcastle, Australia, earthquake (1989) showed that regular tobacco and alcohol use before the disaster (yes or no; assessed 6 months postdisaster) did not independently predict general distress and intrusions and avoidance reactions 2 years postevent, after controlling for 20 other variables assessed at the first wave (e.g., demographics, neuroticism, lifestyles, and history of emotional problems) (Carr et al., 1997).

Similar results were found in another prospective study after the Chi-Chi disaster. In total, 268 people aged 65 and older were interviewed 3 to 8 days before and 1 year after the disaster (Lin, Huang, Huang, Tsai, & Chiu, 2002). No differences were found between predisaster smokers and nonsmokers as well as pre-event alcohol users and nonalcohol users with regard to changes in physical capacity, psychological well-being, and social relationships from baseline to 12 months after the earthquake.

However, one study found that alcohol use after the disaster was negatively associated with later postdisaster depression but not associated with cigarette consumption (Armenian et al., 2002). This study was conducted after the earthquake in Armenia (1988) among employees of the Ministry of Health (between 16 and 70-years old) living in the earthquake region. It used longitudinal designs starting in 1989, with a second survey in the period of June 1991 to June 1992 ($N = 1{,}785$). Those without PTSD, major depression, panic disorder, general anxiety disorder, and phobia (controls), were compared with respondents (cases) with major depression but without comorbidity (DSM-III-R). At follow-up, nondrinkers at baseline (summer 1989) were more likely to be cases (25.8%) than drinkers (14.8%). No significant differences were found between nonsmokers and smokers at baseline (25.1% vs. 18.6%). After adjusting for gender, postdisaster support, company during earthquake, change in postdisaster space, and cumulative loss, drinkers were still less likely to be depressive than nondrinkers were.

In contrast, in the longitudinal study of Van Griensven and colleagues (2006), after the Tsunami disaster, users of illicit drug were more likely to suffer from anxiety symptoms at follow-up 9 months postevent, but not from PTSD or depression (when controlling for displacement status, demographics, several disaster experiences, and prior diagnoses or mental illness; Phang Nga group, $N = 270$ and $N = 250$ respectively, see preceding text). In the study of Bravo et al. (1990), predisaster alcohol dependency symptoms independently predicted post-event lifetime alcohol dependency-abuse after the flooding in the Caribbean island of Puerto Rico.

Approximately 3 years after an extended period of gradual upward or downward shifting of the land (so-called bradyseism; Italy, 1983–1984), which resulted in the evacuation of approximately 25,000 (of the 70,000) inhabitants of Pozzuoli, Bland and her colleagues (2000) examined male factory workers ($N = 693$). Results showed that daily consumption of cigarettes did not differ between evacuated and nonevacuated workers, between workers with and without financial loss due to the disaster, between those who did not and did return to their houses, between those who now lived at increased distance of family/friends and those who did not, and between those who decreased contacts with family/friends and those who had the same number of contacts.

6.3.2. Technological Disasters

6.3.2.1. Predictors of Substance Use

Two studies investigated correlates of substance and again showed partly inconsistent results. The study after the TMI disaster (Hu & Slaysman, 1984) showed that cigarette consumption during March 1979 was independently and negatively associated with age. Furthermore, consumption was negatively associated with being pregnant, and positively associated with psychosomatic symptoms such as headache and pain, and behavioral symptoms in this period such as insomnia irritability, in contrast to gender, income, marital status, family size, and work status. Alcohol consumption in this period was only independently associated with age (negative) and behavioral symptoms (positive). At follow-up (January 1980), cigarette consumption was associated with the aforementioned variables, and with income (positive) and education (negative). Alcohol consumption was not significantly and independently associated with these variables.

However, among the survivors of the *Herald of Free Enterprise* disaster, gender and age were not associated with increased alcohol and cigarette consumption at 6 and 30 months postevent (Joseph et al., 1993). Consumption assessed at the first wave was strongly related to consumption assessed at the second wave.

6.3.2.2. Substance Use as Predictor of Postdisaster Mental Health Problems

Among the survivors of the *Herald of Free Enterprise* disaster, those reporting higher alcohol and cigarette consumption in the 6 months before the second wave reported significantly less well-being and more intrusions and more intrusions and avoidance reactions respectively.

Comparable results were found in the longitudinal study after the Enschede fireworks disaster (The Netherlands, 2000) (Van der Velden et al., 2007). Findings showed that current smoking 18 months postdisaster was independently associated with a two- to three-fold risk for disaster-related PTSD, severe anxiety, and hostility symptoms among affected citizens 4 years postdisaster, compared with nonsmoking respondents (after controlling for demographic characteristics, severe depression, anxiety symptoms, and hostility symptoms at 18 months postdisaster and life events in the period 2 to 5 years before the last survey). No differences were found between nonsmokers and past smokers, and smoking did not predict depression symptoms 4 years postevent. In the control group, smoking did not independently predict anxiety and hostility symptoms.

The only study examining the predictive value of alcohol consumption at the time of the traumatic event was conducted after a fire at New Years Eve in a hotel (Belgium, 1994). Maes and colleagues (2001) assessed the association between alcohol consumption (more or less

100 ml pure alcohol) and (perceived) intoxication until the event (at midnight when the fire started) and PTSD at 7 to 9 months postevent ($N = 127$). Results showed that both consumption and intoxication independently predicted PTSD (DSM-III-R), when controlling for previous trauma, sense of control, and loss of control during the disaster and simple phobia before the disaster, that is, decreased the odds of PTSD.

6.3.3. Mass Violence and Terrorism

6.3.3.1. Predictors of Substance Use

With regard to age, Bleich and colleagues (2005) found that older people (in the categories 65 to 74 years and 75 years or older) used cigarettes/alcohol and tranquilizers *more* often to cope with the situation than younger people (18 to 64 years old; 19.5%, 39.6% vs. 9.6% respectively).

North and colleagues (1999) examined the relationship between predisaster mental health disorders and postdisaster substance use disorders after the Oklahoma City bombings in detail. Prevalences of postdisaster alcohol and drug use disorders in respondents with (no) predisaster lifetime disorders were as follows: in PTSD cases ($N = 27$), 14.8% and 3.7%; in major depression cases ($N = 23$), 17.4% and 4.3%; in panic disorder cases ($N = 5$), 20.0% and 20.0%; in generalized anxiety cases ($N = 5$), 20.0% and 20.0%; in alcohol disorder cases ($N = 48$), 35.4% and 4.2%; in drug disorder cases ($N = 17$), 23.5% and 23.5%; and no-disorder cases ($N = 103$), 0.0% and 0.0% respectively. In addition, those with predisaster alcohol disorder were more likely to have postdisaster alcohol disorder and only those with predisaster drug disorder were more likely to have postdisaster drug disorder. However, the majority of predisaster alcohol and drug disorders were reported as inactive after the disaster.

Studies among New York citizens after the September 11th attacks assessed a variety of correlates of substance use, such as demographics (e.g., age, gender, marital status, education, income, location of residence before September 11th; ethnic background), life stressors in 12 months before September 11th, fear of personal injury or death, panic attacks during first hours, loss of job due to September 11th, (media) exposure, PTSD and depression after the attacks, social support, self-esteem, and poor health. Subsequently, we focus on independent predictors. Since these studies differ (slightly) in assessed correlates, for reasons of parsimony we refer to these studies to obtain a complete list of covariates assessed.

Five to eight weeks postevent (Vlahov et al., 2002), more citizens in the age of 35 to 44 years than citizens in the age of 18 to 24 years increased cigarette and marijuana consumption. Compared with citizens with high income ($\geq 100{,}000$ U.S. dollars), citizens with low income ($< 20{,}000$ U.S. dollars) were less likely to increase cigarettes and marijuana consumption. Those who were not married (either divorced or separated or never married) more often had increased marijuana consumption than married citizens. Citizens reporting attacks, more often increased cigarettes and marijuana consumption. Compared with citizens not reporting life stress stressors, citizens reporting one or more life stressors more often increased cigarette consumption. Increased alcohol consumption was only independently predicted by media exposure: those reporting high media exposure were more likely to increase alcohol consumption than those reporting low exposure.

Four months after September 11th (Nandi et al., 2005) more citizens with a college degree than citizens with only high school degree reported cigarette dependency. Those reporting four or more life stressors, high media exposure, depression after September 11th, and those directly affected were more likely to be dependent compared with reference categories (not, lowest score). PTSD since September 11th was not an independent predictor.

Six to nine months postevent (Vlahov, Galea, Ahern, Resnick, Boscarino, et al., 2004), those who were receiving high social support and did not lose their job were less likely to increase smoking. Compared with citizens in the age of 18 to 24 years, citizens of 25 to 34 years and 55 years and older less often increased alcohol consumption. In addition, females compared to males, Asian citizens compared to White citizens, and separated people compared to those married were less likely to increase alcohol consumption. However, widows and citizens having experience of more than three lifetime stressors before September 11th and panic attacks during the attacks were more likely to increase alcohol consumption. Compared with citizens of 18 to 24 years old, citizens of 35 years and older were less likely to increase marijuana smoking. Concerning race/ethnicity, Asians and Hispanics were less likely to increase marijuana smoking. A marital status of never being married and being involved in rescue work was independently associated with increased marijuana smoking.

Boscarino et al. (2006) examined predictors of binge drinking in the first year, binge drinking in the second year, alcohol dependency in the past 2 years, and increased drinking between first and second wave (in total four drinking categories). Results showed that younger citizens (18–44 years) were more likely to report the four drinking categories than older citizens (65 years or older), except alcohol dependency. Males more often reported the four drinking categories than females and Latinos more often than Whites, except binge drinking in the first year postevent. Those who experienced high to very high disaster exposure were more likely to report binge drinking in the first year and alcohol dependency in the 2 years postevent, than citizens reporting low exposure. Antisocial behavior was associated with binge drinking in the first and second year. Interestingly, those reporting high social support were more likely to be alcohol dependent than those reporting low support. Citizens with and without PTSD in the first year did not differ in the four drinking categories.

In addition, Vlahov et al. (2006) examined predictors of incident drinking in the 6 months after September 11th among those without drinking problems in the 6 months before September 11th. Compared with citizens 18 to 24 years old, citizens of 65 or older reported less problem drinking. Likewise, unmarried couples and those with panic attacks were more likely to report problem drinking than married couples and citizens without panic attacks, respectively.

Another study focused on military and civilian staff of the Pentagon. Results showed that in comparison with men, females were 6.8 times more likely to report more alcohol consumption than they meant to (Grieger et al., 2003), but females were also 5.4 times more likely to have PTSD than males. Peritraumatic dissociation during the attacks and lower current perceived safety (work, home, travel, daily activities) after the attacks were, on a bivariate level, associated with increased consumption. No relationships with age, previous trauma, degree of exposure, or initial emotional response to the attack were found.

In the only prospective study on the effects of terrorism, Hasin and her colleagues (2007) showed that a personal history of alcohol dependence (DSM-IV), and especially physical proximity (within 5 miles of WTC), independently predicted the number of drinks per day in the 7 days after September 11th. Knowing someone who was lost or killed, having a family history and personal history of major depression, and a family history of alcoholism were not independently associated. Physical proximity was the only independent predictor for the number of drinks per day in the 16 weeks after September 11th. Other control variables included were age, gender, race, and the time between September 11th and follow-up (mean 381 days).

6.3.3.2 Substance Use as Predictor of Postdisaster Mental Health Problems

The longitudinal study of Adams et al. (2006a) after the September 11th terrorist attacks found that alcohol dependency in the 2 years postevent, when controlling for demographics, stress (exposure, negative life events, lifetime traumatic events), and resources (social support and self-esteem) predicted subsyndromal PTSD, PTSD symptom severity, depression in the period one to two postevent, and psychiatric symptoms. Similar analyses showed that binge drinking in the first year postevent independently predicted PTSD symptom severity, and that increased drinking (4 or more months and 2 or more days) independently predicted subsyndromal PTSD and poor physical health. In another study, Adams and colleagues (2006b) showed that alcohol dependency in the 1 to 2 years postevent, independently predicted (poor) mental health.

Using a nationwide probability sample Silver and colleagues (2002) assessed predictors of September 11th-related posttraumatic stress symptoms (DSM-IV) during 6 months postevent (with surveys 9–23 days, 2 months, and 6 months postevent) (Silver, Holman, McIntosh, Poulin, & Gil-Rivas, 2002). Findings showed that using substances (alcohol or drugs) as a way of coping with terrorist attacks during the first 9 to 23 days was not independently associated with posttraumatic stress symptoms and global distress at 6 months, after adjusting for demographics, predisaster physician diagnosed mental disorder and physical illness, other early coping strategies (such as denial and acceptance), and exposure (including TV-watching).

Hasin and colleagues (2007) found that a personal and family history of alcohol dependence did not independently predict posttraumatic stress symptoms following September 11th, and found no significant interaction effects between physical proximity and previous alcohol dependence, major depression, and gender in predicting drinking in the 7 days and 16 weeks after September 11th.

6.3.4. Conclusions

A comprehensive overview of the main conclusions with respect to correlates and predictors of substance dependency-abuse and increased substance use after disasters is presented in Table 6.2. Results of empirical studies are varied and sometimes contradictory. This is an indication that the relationships are complex. However, it should be emphasized that in addition to differences between studies as described earlier (see 2.4), studies vary extensively in assessed covariates, which seriously complicate comparisons of results. It is unclear whether different outcomes can be attributed to, for example, differences between categories of disasters, provided health care, and local circumstances and habits. Insight in predictors of substance use after mass violence and terrorism, for example, is largely based on the September 11th studies. Possible predictors related to work (workload, job satisfaction, etc.) and related to significant others, for instance those who survived the disaster, such as spouse, family, and friends (their personal disaster experiences, substance use, and mental health disturbances) have hardly been investigated (see Richman et al., 2004).

What can we conclude about predictors of substance abuse? Concerning the level of exposure, there are indications that high levels of disaster exposure and predisaster life-vents are independently associated with (increased) substance use, but this pattern has not been consistently found. Furthermore, findings suggest that social support or being married may protect against (increased) substance use, although one study found that those reporting high social support were more likely to be alcohol dependent. Similarly, a higher education level is negatively associated with (increased) substance use. The factor of age produced mixed results, whereby younger age was associated with more substance use in several studies, but not always. With regard to gender, results suggest that males are more at risk for increased substance use or abuse than females, although, one study (Grieger et al., 2003) found that females more often than males reported that they used more substances than they meant to. However, they were more likely than males to suffer from PTSD. Using substances (especially alcohol) as a way to cope with the impact of the event, which may be considered as a method of self-medication (McFarlane, 1998), is associated with (increased) substance use or misuse in most studies. Nevertheless, possible attempts to quit use, duration of these attempts and withdrawal symptoms after quitting substance use, have not been systematically examined yet.

North and colleagues (1999) systematically examined the association between (retrospectively) lifetime pre-event substance

Table 6.2. Main conclusion on predictors

- Disaster studies on risk factors for substance use vary extensively in assessed covariates and study designs, which complicate comparisons of results. Prospective studies using more uniform measures of smoking are warranted to determine whether different factors predict substance use in the short, intermediate, and long term
- Although studies examined a variety of predictors of substance use, there are no studies available that systematically examined factors related to the work situation, such as workload, relationships, social support at work; job satisfaction; conflicts; and work autonomy
- Little is known about the influence of factors related to significant others who were also affected by the disaster, such as their personal disaster experiences, substance use, and mental health disturbances. Factors related to work and significant others need to be examined in future research
- Predictors such as gender (males), age (younger), direct or media exposure, education level (low), social support (low) were negatively associated with (increased) substance use in several studies, but did not consistently predict use in other studies
- In general, results with respect to predictors of substance use are mixed. However, studies differ in measure of substance use (dependency, abuse, global increase, qualified increase), which partly may explain these different outcomes
- There are clear indications that victims with predisaster mental disorders are more at risk for substance use disorder than noncases. Pre-event nonusers hardly develop substance use after the disaster
- There is emerging evidence that smoking predicts later posttraumatic stress symptoms. Pre-event alcohol use and postevent use are negatively, nonsignificant, and positively associated with later symptoms. One study remarkably found that being drunk when the disaster occurred protected against the development of PTSD
- Using substances, especially alcohol, as a coping strategy was associated with mental health problems in several studies. However, attempts to quit in the aftermath of the disaster, duration of quit attempts, and withdrawal symptoms experienced during these attempts, and relationships with mental health disturbances have not been examined

Note: PTSD, posttraumatic stress disorder.

dependency-abuse and several other mental disorders, and postdisaster alcohol and drug use disorders. Results clearly indicate that victims with pre-event lifetime mental disorders more than victims without pre-event mental disorders are at risk for alcohol and drug use disorders. However, Hasin and colleagues (2007) found no indication in their prospective study that a history of major depression (examined approximately 10 years before September 11th), independently predicted alcohol use after September 11th, in contrast to history of alcohol dependence that predicted (only) drinking in the 7 days after September 11th.

With respect to reverse relationships between substance abuse and mental health disturbances, there is emerging evidence that those who smoke or report increased smoking are more at risk for later PTSD and other mental health disturbances than those who do not (Van der Velden, Kleber, & Koenen, 2008). However, a few studies using other research methods found no indications that smoking and drinking were independent risk factors. In addition, results indicate that postdisaster substance disorders are more prevalent among those with predisaster substance use disorders (and other predisaster mental disorders). Interestingly, alcohol use is found to be negatively, nonsignificantly, and also positively associated with later posttraumatic stress symptoms.

6.4. EPILOGUE

This chapter focused on residents affected by natural and technological disasters as well as disasters caused by mass violence and terrorism. Our main conclusion is that there are no indications for a (strong) increase of substance dependency-abuse (alcohol, nicotine, or other substances). In most cases, only a minority of the victims will show increased substance use, while substance use has been partly associated with postevent mental health disturbances. Several factors have been associated with substance use, but the results of empirical studies are mixed. There is no evidence that is replicated in several studies following other disasters for one or two clear risk factors other than being a pre-event user. Although some studies examined predictors or alcohol and cigarette use and found that some factors were related to alcohol and not to cigarette use (or vice versa), more research is needed to further examine possible differences.

Remarkably, of the 55 empirical studies after disasters on substance use in this chapter, 91% ($N = 50$) examined alcohol use, whereas only 27% ($N = 15$) assessed cigarette use and 35% ($N = 19$) drug use (4% substance in general, $N = 2$). Since part of the users will be multiusers, only alcohol, and only cigarette users, these subgroups need to be distinguished in future research (see Vlahov, Galea, Ahern, Resnick, & Kilpatrick, 2004) to examine possible predictors.

Nevertheless, prevalences of increased substance use indicate that mental health interventions after disasters should at least include questions about alcohol abuse of directly affected disaster victims. One should definitely screen and monitor disaster-affected people with regard to substance use.

Unfortunately, most research has been conducted among adults. There are only a few studies on children and adolescents, but the results of these studies are mostly not different from those with adults. In the prospective comparative study of Reijneveld and colleagues (2003, 2005) with pre-event measures, on the effects of a fire disaster in the Netherlands (2001), it was found that exposed adolescents underwent a significant increase in self-reported use of alcohol, but not with respect to smoking or use of marijuana and ecstasy in the 12 months postevent (Reijneveld, Crone, Schuller, Verhulst, & Verloove-Vanhorick, 2005; Reijneveld, Crone, Verhulst, & Verloove-Vanhorick, 2003). Thirty-three years after the Aberfan disaster (U.K., 1996), Morgan and colleagues (2003) found that (child) survivors were not more likely than control subjects to show increased risk of anxiety-related substance misuse. Schroeder and Polusny (2004) reported that higher levels of binge drinking were associated with age (older), prior drinking involvement, prior trauma history 6 months after a series of tornados (U.S., 1998). Prior trauma history and current levels of disaster-related PTSD symptomatology were significantly related with adolescents' report of increased alcohol consumption.

Finally, empirical studies reviewed in this chapter suggest that the type of disaster is not highly relevant with regard to substance use and abuse. We have made a distinction between three types of disasters, but the results did not provide a clear picture or a noteworthy trend of differences in (increased) substance use, substance dependency-abuse and correlates, or predictors of use between these types of disasters. Furthermore, it became clear that compared to alcohol consumption, cigarette use and nicotine dependency after disasters are a relatively neglected topic and need further attention. Future research is needed to investigate whether increased substance use in the intermediate and long term sustain in the presence of resolving mental health problems with possible adverse effects on health (see Vlahov et al., 2004).

ACKNOWLEDGMENTS

We gratefully thank Peter Hoonakker (Center for Quality and Productivity Improvement, University of Wisconsin, Madison, U.S.), Henk Koenen (Schouten & Nelissen, Zaltbommel, The Netherlands), and Annelieke Drogendijk (Institute for Psychotrauma, Zaltbommel, The Netherlands) for their help and assistance.

REFERENCES

American Psychiatric Association. (1980). *Diagnostic and statistical manual of mental disorders, 3rd ed. (DSM-III)*. Washington, DC: American Psychiatric Association.

(1987). *Diagnostic and statistical manual of mental disorders, 3rd ed. Revised (DSM-III-R)*.

Washington, DC: American Psychiatric Association.

(1994). *Diagnostic and statistical manual of mental disorders, 4th ed. (DSM-IV).* Washington, DC: American Psychiatric Association.

(2000). *Diagnostic and statistical manual of mental disorders, 4th ed. Text Revision (DSM-IV-TR).* Washington, DC: American Psychiatric Association.

Adams, R. E., Boscarino, J. A., & Galea, S. (2006a). Alcohol use, mental health status and psychological well-being 2 years after the World Trade Center attacks in New York City. *The American Journal of Drug and Alcohol Dependency, 32,* 203–224.

(2006b). Social and psychological resources and health outcomes after the World Trade Center disaster. *Social Science & Medicine, 62,* 76–188.

Armenian, H. K., Morikawa, M., Melkonian, A. K., Hovanesian, A., Akiskal, K., & Akiskal, H. S. (2002). Risk factors for depression in the survivors of the 1988 earthquake in Armenia. *Journal of Urban Health, 82,* 370–377.

Bland, S. H., Farinaro, E., Krogh, V., Jossa, F., Scottoni, A., & Trevisan, M. (2000). Long term relations between earthquake experiences and coronary heart disease risk factors. *American Journal of Epidemiology, 151,* 1086–1090.

Bleich, A., Gelkopf, M., & Solomon, Z. (2003). Exposure to terrorism, stress-related mental health symptoms, and coping behaviors among a nationally representative sample in Israel. *JAMA, 290,* 612–620.

Bleich, A., Gelkopf, M., Melamed, Y., & Solomon, Z. (2005). Emotional impact of exposure to terrorism among young-old and old-old Israeli citizens. *American Journal of Geriatric Psychiatry, 13,* 705–712.

Boscarino, J. A., Adams, R. E., & Galea, S. (2006). Alcohol use in New York after the terrorist attacks: A study of the effects of psychological trauma on drinking behavior. *Addictive Behaviors, 31,* 606–621.

Bravo, M., Rubio-Stipec, M., Canino, G. J., Woodbury, M. A., & Ribera, J. C. (1990). The psychological sequelae of disaster stress prospectively and retrospectively evaluated. *American Journal of Community Psychology, 18,* 661–680.

Breslau, N., Davis, G. C., & Schultz, L. R. (2003). Posttraumatic stress disorder and the incidence of nicotine, alcohol, and other drug disorders in persons who have experienced trauma. *Archives of General Psychiatry, 60,* 289–294.

Cao, H., McFarlane, A. C., & Klimidis, S. (2003). Prevalence of psychiatric disorder following the 1988 Yun Nan (China) earthquake. The first 5-month period. *Social Psychiatry and Psychiatric Epidemiology, 38,* 204–212.

Carr, V. J., Lewin, T. J., Kenardy, J. A., Webster, R. A., Hazell, P. L., Carter, G. L., et al. (1997) Psychosocial sequelae of the 1989 Newcastle earthquake: III. Role of vulnerability factors in postdisaster morbidity. *Psychological Medicine, 27,* 179–190.

Chou, F. H., Su, T. T., Chou, P., Ou-Yang, W. C., Lu, M. K., & Chien, I. C. (2005). Survey of psychiatric disorders in a Taiwanese village population six months after a major earthquake. *Journal of Formosa Medical Association, 104,* 308–317.

Chou, F. H., Wu, H. C., Chou, P., Su, C. Y., Tsai, K. Y., Chao, S. S., et al. (2007). Epidemiologic psychiatric studies on post-disaster impact among Chi-Chi earthquake survivors in Yu-Chi, Taiwan. *Psychiatry and Clinical Neuroscience, 61,* 370–378.

Çorapçlolu, A., Tural, Ü., Yargiç, I., & Kocabaolu, N. (2004). Subthreshold post traumatic stress disorder in the survivors of Marmara earthquake. *Primary Care Psychiatry, 9,* 137–143.

David, D., Mellman, T. A., Mendoza, L. M., Kulick-Bell, R., Ironson, G., & Schneiderman, N. (1996). Psychiatric morbidity following Hurricane Andrew. *Journal of Traumatic Stress, 9,* 607–612.

Deering, C. G., Glover, S. G., Ready, D., Eddleman, H. C., & Alarcon, R. D. (1996). Unique patterns of comorbidity in posttraumatic stress disorder from different sources of trauma. *Comprehensive Psychiatry, 37,* 336–346.

DeLisi, L. E., Maurizio, A., Yost, M., Papparozzi, C. F., Fulchino, C., Katz, C. L., et al. (2003). A survey of New Yorkers after the Sept. 11, 2001, terrorist attacks. *American Journal of Psychiatry, 160,* 780–783.

Deren, S., Shedlin, M., Hamilton, T., & Hagan, H. (2002) Impact of the September 11th attacks in New York city on drug users: A preliminary assessment. *Journal of Urban Health, 79,* 409–412.

Dooley, E., & Gunn, J. (1995). The psychological effects of disaster at sea. *British Journal of Psychiatry, 167,* 233–237.

Feldner, M. T., Babson, K. A., & Zvolensky, M. J. (2007). Smoking, traumatic event exposure, and post-traumatic stress: A critical review of the empirical literature. *Clinical Psychological Review, 27,* 4–45.

Ford, J. D., Adams, M. L., & Dailey, W. F. (2006). Factors associated with receiving help and risk factors for disaster-related distress among Connecticut adults 5–15 months after the September 11th terrorist incidents. *Social Psychiatry and Psychiatric Epidemiology, 41,* 261–270.

Galea, S., Nandi, A., & Vlahov, D. (2005). The epidemiology of posttraumatic stress disorder after disasters. *Epidemiologic Reviews, 27,* 78–91.

Green, B. L., Lindy, J. D., Grace, M. C., Gleser, G. C., Leonard, A. C., Korol, M., et al. (1990). Buffalo Creek survivors in the second decade: Stability of stress symptoms. *American Journal of Orthopsychiatry*, *60*, 43–54.

Green, B. L., Lindy, J. D., Grace, M. C. & Leonard, A. C. (1992). Chronic posttraumatic stress disorder and diagnostic comorbidity in a disaster sample. *Journal of Nervous and Mental Disease*, *180*, 760–766.

Gregg, W., Medley, I., Fowler-Dixon, R., Curran, P., Loughrey, G., Bell, P., et al. (1995). Psychological consequences of the Kegworth air disaster. *British Journal of Psychiatry*, *167*, 812–817.

Grieger, T. A., Fullerton, C. S., & Ursano, R. J. (2003). Posttraumatic stress disorder, alcohol use, and perceived safety after the terrorist attack on the Pentagon. *Psychiatric Services*, *54*, 1380–1382.

Hasin, D. S., Keyes, K. M., Hatzenbuehler, M. L., Aharonovich, E. A., Alderson, D. (2007). Alcohol consumption and posttraumatic stress after exposure to terrorism: Effects of proximity, loss, and psychiatric history. *American Journal of Public Health*, *97*, 2268–2275.

Howard, W. T., Loberiza, F. R., Pfohl, B. M., Thorne, P. S., Magpantay, R. L., & Woolson, R. F. (1999). Initial results, reliability, and validity of a mental health survey of Mount Pinatubo disaster victims. *Journal of Nervous and Mental Disease*, *187*, 661–672.

Hu, T. W., & Slaysman, K. S. (1984). Health-related economic costs of the Three-Mile Island accident. *Socio-economic Planning Sciences*, *18*, 183–193.

Hull, A. M., Alexander, D. A., & Klein, S. (2002). Survivors of the Piper Alpha oil platform disaster: Long-term follow-up study. *British Journal of Psychiatry*, *181*, 433–438.

Jordan, N. N., Hoge, C. W., Tobler, S. K., Wells, J., Dydek, G. J., & Egerton, W. E. (2004). Mental health impact of 9/11 Pentagon attack: Validation of a rapid assessment tool. *American Journal of Preventive Medicine*, *26*, 284–293.

Kessler, R. C, Sonnega, A., Hughes, M., & Nelsson, C. B. (1995). Posttraumatic stress disorder in the national comorbidity survey. *Archives of General Psychiatry*, *52*, 1048–1060.

Kohn, R., Levav, I., Donaire, I., Donnaire Machuca, M. E., & Tamashiro, R. (2005). Psychological and psychopathological reactions in Honduras following Hurricane Mitch: Implications for service planning. *International Journal of Geriatric Psychiatry*, *20*, 835–841.

Lai, T. J., Chang, C. M., Connor, M. M., Lee, L. C., & Davidson, J. R. T. (2004). Full and partial PTSD among earthquake survivors in rural Taiwan. *Journal of Psychiatric Research*, *38*, 313–322.

Larrance, R., Anastario, M., & Lawry, L. (2007). Health status among internally displaced persons in Louisiana and Mississippi travel trailer parks. *Annals of Emergency Medicine*, *49*, 590–601.

Lating, J. M., Sherman, M. F., Everly, G. S. Jr., Lowry, J. L., & Peragine, T. F. (2004). PTSD reactions and functioning of American airlines flight attendants in the wake of September 11. *Journal of Nervous and Mental Disease*, *192*, 435–441.

Lin, M. R., Huang, W., Huang, C., Hwang, H. F., Tsai, L. W., & Chiu, Y. N. (2002). The impact of the Chi-Chi earthquake on quality of life among elderly survivors in Taiwan: A before and after study. *Quality of Life Research*, *11*, 379–388.

Logue, J. N., Hansen H., & Struening E. (1979). Emotional and physical distress following Hurricane Agnes in Wyoming Valley of Pennsylvania. *Public Health Reports*, *94*, 495–502.

Maes, M., Delmeire, L., Mylle, J., & Altamura, C. (2001). Risk and preventive factors of post-traumatic stress disorder (PTSD): Alcohol consumption and intoxication prior to a traumatic event diminishes the relative risk to develop PTSD in response to that trauma. *Journal of Affective Disorders*, *63*, 113–121.

McFarlane, A. C. (1998). Epidemiological evidence about the relationship between PTSD and alcohol abuse: The nature of the association. *Addictive Behaviors*, *23*, 813–825.

McMillen, C., North, C., Mosley, M., & Smith, E. (2002). Untangling the psychiatric comorbidity of posttraumatic stress disorder in a sample of flood survivors. *Comprehensive Psychiatry*, *43*, 478–485.

Melnik, T. A, Baker, C. T., Adams, M. K., Mokdad, A. H., Brown, D. W., Murphy, W., et al. (2002). Psychological and emotional effects of the September 11 attacks on the World Trade Center-Connecticut, New Jersey, and New York, 2001. *JAMA*, *288*, 1467–1468.

Morissette, S. B., Tull, M. T., Gulliver, S. B., Kamholz, B. W., & Zimering, R. T. (2007). Anxiety, anxiety disorders, tobacco use, and nicotine: A critical review of interrelationships. *Psychological Bulletin*, *133*, 245–272.

Morgan, L., Scourfield, J., Williams, D., Jasper, A., & Lewis, G. (2003). The Aberfan disaster: 33-year follow-up of survivors. *British Journal of Psychiatry*, *182*, 532–536.

Nandi, A., Galea, S., Ahern, J., & Vlahov, D. (2005). Probable cigarette dependence, PTSD, and depression after an urban disaster: Results from a population survey of New York City residents 4 months after September 11, 2001. *Psychiatry*, *68*, 299–310.

Norris, F. H., Friedman, M., Watson, P. J., Byrne, C. M., Diaz, E., & Kaniasty, K. (2002). 60,000 disaster victims speak: Part I. An empirical review of the empirical literature, 1981–2001. *Psychiatry: Interpersonal and Biological Processes*, *65*, 207–239.

North, C. S., Kawasaki, A., Spitznagel, E. L., & Hong, B. A. (2004). The course of PTSD, major depression, substance abuse, and somatization after a natural disaster. *Journal of Nervous and Mental Disease*, *192*, 823–829.

North, C. S., Nixon, S. J., Shariat, S., Mallonee, S., McMillen, J. C., Spitznagel, E. L., et al. (1999). Psychiatric disorders among survivors of the Oklahoma City bombing. *JAMA*, *282*, 755–762.

North, C. S., Pfefferbaum, B., Narayanan, P., Thielman, S., McCoy, G., Dumont, C., et al. (2005). Comparison of post-disaster psychiatric disorders terrorist bombings in Nairobi and Oklahoma City. *British Journal of Psychiatry*, *186*, 487–493.

North, C. S., Smith, E. M., & Spitznagel, E. L. (1994). Posttraumatic stress disorder in survivors of a mass shooting. *American Journal of Psychiatry*, *151*, 82–88.

(1997). One-year follow-up of survivors of a mass shooting. *American Journal of Psychiatry*, *154*, 1696–1702.

North, C. S., Smith, E. M., McCool, R. E., & Lightcap, P. E. (1989). Acute postdisaster coping and adjustment. *Journal of Traumatic Stress*, *2*, 353–360.

North, C. S., Spitznagel, E. L, & Smith, E. M. (2001). A prospective study of coping after exposure to a mass murder episode. *Annals of Clinical Psychiatry*, *13*, 81–87.

Palinkas, L. A., Downs, M. A., Petterson, J. S., & Russell, J. (1993). Social, cultural, and psychological impacts of the Exxon Valdez oil spill. *Human Organization*, *52*, 1–13.

Parslow, R. A., & Jorm, A. F. (2006). Tobacco use after experiencing a major natural disaster: Analysis of a longitudinal study of 2063 young adults. *Addiction*, *101*, 1044–1050.

Pfefferbaum, B., & Doughty, D. E. (2001) Increased alcohol use in a treatment sample of Oklahoma City bombing victims. *Psychiatry*, *64*, 296–303.

Reijneveld, S. A., Crone, M. R., Schuller, A. A., Verhulst, F. C., & Verloove-Vanhorick, S. P. (2005). The changing impact of a severe disaster on the mental health and substance misuse of adolescents: Follow-up of a controlled study. *Psychological Medicine*, *35*, 367–376.

Reijneveld, S. A., Crone, M. R., Verhulst, F. C., & Verloove-Vanhorick, P. (2003). The effect of a severe disaster on the mental health of adolescents: A controlled study. *The Lancet*, *362*, 691–696.

Richman, J. A., Wislar, J. S., Flaherty, J. A., Fendrich, M., & Rospenda, K. M. (2004). Effects on alcohol use and anxiety of the September 11, 2001, attacks and chronic work stressors: A longitudinal cohort study. *American Journal of Public Health*, *94*, 2010–2015.

Schroeder, J. M., & Polusny, M. A. (2004). Risk factors for adolescent alcohol use following a natural disaster. *Prehospital Disaster Medicine*, *19*, 122–127.

Silver, R. C., Holman, E. A., McIntosh, D. N., Poulin, M., & Gil-Rivas, V. (2002). Nationwide longitudinal study of psychological responses to September 11. *JAMA*, *288*, 1235–1244.

Shimizu, S., Aso, K., Noda, T., Ryukei, S., Kochi, Y., & Yamamoto, N. (2000). Natural disasters and alcohol consumption in a cultural context: The Great Hanshin Earthquake in Japan. *Addiction*, *95*, 529–536.

Shinfuku, N. (1999). To be a victim and a survivor of the Great Hanshin Awaji earthquake. *Journal of Psychosomatic Research*, *46*, 541–548.

Shore, J. H., Vollmer, W. M., & Tatum, E. L. (1989). Community patterns of posttraumatic stress disorders. *Journal of Mental and Nervous Disease*, *177*, 681–685.

Smith, E. M., North, C. S., McCool, R. E., & Shea, J. M. (1990). Acute postdisaster psychiatric disorders: Identification of persons at risk. *American Journal of Psychiatry*, *147*, 202–206.

Joseph, S., Yule, W., Williams, R., & Hodgekinson, P. (1993). Increased substance use in survivors of the Herald of Free Enterprise Disaster. *British Journal of Medical Psychology*, *66*, 185–191.

Stewart, S. H. (1996). Alcohol abuse in individuals exposed to trauma: A critical review. *Psychological Bulletin*, *120*, 83–112.

Stewart, S. H., Mitchell, T. L., Wright, K. D., & Loba, P. (2004). The relations of PTSD symptoms to alcohol use and coping drinking in volunteers who responded to the Swissair Flight 111 airline disaster. *Journal of Anxiety Disorders*, *18*, 51–68.

Solomon, S. D., Bravo, M., Rubio-Stipec, M., & Canino, G. (1993). Effects of family role on response to disaster. *Journal of Traumatic Stress*, *6*, 255–269.

Spitzer, R. L., Williams, J. B., Kroenke, K., Linzer, M., deGruy III, F. V., Hahn, S. R., et al. (1994). Utility of a new procedure for diagnosing mental disorders in primary care. The PRIME-MD 1000 study. *JAMA*, *272*, 1749–1756.

Velden, P. G., Van der, Grievink, L., Olff, M., Gersons, B. P. R., & Kleber, R. J. (2007). Smoking as a risk factor for mental health disturbances after a disaster: A prospective comparative study. *Journal of Clinical Psychiatry*, *69*, 87–92.

Velden, P. G., van der, Kleber, R. J., & Koenen, K. C. (2008). Smoking predicts posttraumatic stress symptoms among rescue workers: A prospective study of ambulance personnel involved in the Enschede Fireworks Disaster. *Drugs and Alcohol Dependence*, *94*, 267–271.

Van Griensven, F., Chakkraband, M. L. S., Thienkrua, W., Pengjuntr, W., Lopes Cardozo, B., Tantipiwatanaskul, P., et al. (2006). Mental health problems among adults in Tsunami-affected areas in southern Tailand. *JAMA, 296*, 537–548.

Vlahov, D., Galea, S., Ahern, J., Resnick, H., Boscarino, J. A., Gold, J., et al. (2004). Consumption of cigarettes, alcohol, and marijuana among New York City residents six months after the September 11 terrorist attacks. *American Journal of Drug and Alcohol Abuse, 30*, 385–407.

Vlahov, D., Galea, S., Ahern, J., Resnick, H., & Kilpatrick., D. (2004). Sustained increased consumption of cigarettes, alcohol, and marijuana among Manhattan residents after September 11, 2001. *American Journal of Public Health, 94*, 253–254.

Vlahov, D., Galea, S, Ahern, J, Rudenstine, S., Resnick, H, Kilpatrick, D., et al. (2006). Alcohol drinking problems among New York residents after the September 11 terrorist attacks. *Substance Use and Misuse, 41*, 1295–1311.

Vlahov, D., Galea, S., Resnick, H., Ahern, J., Boscarino, J. A., Bucuvalas, M., et al. (2002). Increased use of cigarettes, alcohol, and marijuana among Manhattan, New York, residents after the September 11th terrorist attacks. *American Journal of Epidemiology, 155*, 988–996.

Weissman, M. M., Neria, Y., Das, A., Feder, A., Blanco, C., Lantigua, R., et al. (2005). Gender differences in posttraumatic stress disorder among primary care patients after the World Trade Center attack of September 11, 2001. *Gender Medicine, 2*, 76–87.

Wu, H. C., Chou, P., Chou, F. H., Su, C. Y., Tsai, K. Y., Ou-Yang, W. C., et al. (2006). Survey of quality of life and related risk factors for a Taiwanese village population 3 years post-earthquake. *Australian and New Zealand Journal of Psychiatry, 40*, 355–361.

7 Depression and Prolonged Grief in the Wake of Disasters

SHIRA MAGUEN, YUVAL NERIA, LAUREN M. CONOSCENTI, AND BRETT T. LITZ

7.1. INTRODUCTION

In the days, weeks, and months following a disaster, survivors struggle to regain a sense of who they were before the event as they try to adapt to various resource losses and to the emotional residue of their traumatic experiences. Intense and function-impairing sadness is commonplace in survivors as they try to make sense of the event and piece their lives back together, especially those who were directly impacted. While most individuals recover and return to baseline, others may continue to be affected after the initial shock of the disaster has passed. A variety of pre-, peri-, and post disaster factors interact to create risk for the development of mental health problems, and it is not surprising that in addition to posttraumatic stress disorder (PTSD), a spectrum of affective disorders may emerge, especially in those with a prior mental health history.

At one end of the continuum are those who may experience fleeting or periodic dysphoria and other symptoms of major depression (e.g., anhedonia), but these experiences are bearable (and understandable), and functioning is not compromised. At the opposite end of the spectrum are those with major depressive disorder (MDD) and/or prolonged grief disorder (PGD). MDD is the most likely affective disorder to surface post disaster and is one of the most widely studied to date. PGD, formerly referred to as either complicated grief (Prigerson et al., 1995, 1996) or traumatic grief (Prigerson, 1999, 2001; Prigerson, Bierhals, Kasl, et al., 1997) is another affective disorder that may arise when a disaster causes loss of intimates. PGD is not a current nosological classification, but it is under consideration, and a wealth of research has shown its incremental diagnostic validity and clinical significance (e.g., Bonanno et al., 2007). MDD and PGD should only be diagnosed after intense symptoms linger and impair multiple domains of functioning. Individuals with these diagnoses may or may not have had an affective disorder before the disaster.

This chapter explores both MDD and PGD as responses to disasters and terrorist events. In particular, we discuss the differences between the two disorders, how they relate to PTSD, and the prevalence of each. We also relay findings on correlates of post disaster MDD and PGD. Finally, we describe interventions for each disorder, with an emphasis on empirically-supported treatments.

7.2. MAJOR DEPRESSION

Major depressive disorder (MDD) should be diagnosed in individuals for whom intense dysphoria and feelings of sadness persist and who experience related depressive symptoms, such as anhedonia (i.e. loss of interest in activities they used to enjoy), low self-worth, guilt, changes in sleep, changes in appetite, and corresponding functional impairment related to these problems. Although feelings of dysphoria and other symptoms of MDD are common postdisaster, they typically remit as individuals regain lost resources, including sources of support and connectedness, reclaim various habits and repertoires, and generate positive expectations for a good future life. There is virtually no research on the trajectory of mood problems over time post-disaster. Conceptually, the rate at which mood symptoms diminish will depend on the magnitude of the event, the degree to which resources and supports are lost, and various individual differences. Difficulty meeting basic needs, such as obtaining clean water, loss of personal effects, and problems contacting loved ones because of disruptions in communications systems, are all stressors that can leave individuals feeling helpless, hopeless, and without a sense of control over their lives (Stimpson, 2006). All of these circumstances are high-probability precipitators of MDD.

Disasters that result in the loss of significant others create a serious risk for mood disorders and functional disturbances. Low-income primary care patients who experienced the loss of a loved one in the September 11, 2001 terrorist attacks in the United States were twice as likely to screen positive for MDD as compared with patients who did not experience loss on September 11th. Loss on September 11th also was significantly associated with extreme pain, interference in daily activities, work loss and functional impairment (Neria et al., 2008). Individuals who have survived a terrorist attack may also have the additional burden of trying to make sense of the political and social implications of human maliciousness, which can be particularly toxic. Because symptoms of MDD thwart instrumentality and action that would otherwise promote recovery, it is important to identify individuals who are having a depressive episode and need more help to heal.

7.3. PROLONGED GRIEF DISORDER

Prolonged grief disorder is a relatively new mental health diagnosis (Lichtenthal et al., 2004; Prigerson & Jacobs, 2001; Prigerson, Vanderwerker, & Maciejewski, 2007), but psychiatrists (Freud, 1917; Lindemann, 1944), psychologists (Marwit, 1991), oncologists (Penson, Green, Chabner, & Lynch, 2002), social workers (Lacey, 2005), geriatricians (Berezin, 1970), nurses (Dunne & Dunne-Maxim, 2004), family members and friends (Swarte, van der Lee, van der Bom, van den Bout, & Heintz, 2003) of bereaved individuals have all recognized that grief may, in certain instances, be acutely distressing, unremitting, and functionally impairing. Indeed, PGD is more severe and unremitting than normal grief. Distinguishable from depression or PTSD, it is marked by chronic mourning, prolonged intense yearning for and rumination about the deceased, loneliness, bitterness, emptiness, interpersonal disengagement, a sense of meaninglessness, and difficulty coping with day-to-day demands. PGD is associated with considerable functional impairment, physical and mental health morbidity, lost productivity, suicide, and fewer quality adjusted life years (see Lichtenthal, Cruess, & Prigerson, 2004 for review). The specific symptoms of PGD are (1) constant longing, yearning or pining for the lost person; (2) feeling on edge or jumpy; (3) having trouble accepting the loss; (4) finding it hard to trust others; (5) feeling angry or bitter about the loss; (6) feeling uneasy about moving on with life; (7) feeling emotionally numb; (8) having trouble feeling connected to others; and (9) feeling like there is no future or that the future holds no meaning without the lost person.

Studies have shown that PGD symptoms form a coherent cluster distinct from bereavement-related depressive and anxiety symptom clusters (Boelen & van den Bout, in press; Boelen, van den Bout, & de Keijser, 2003; Chen et al., 1999; Ogrodniczuk, Piper, & Joyce, 2003; Prigerson et al., 1995, 1996, 1997; Prigerson, Frank, Kasl, et al., 1995) and that PGD has a different array of risk factors, course, and outcomes (see Prigerson et al., 2007). Symptoms of sadness, impassivity, and psychomotor retardation are all depressive symptoms, whereas, separation distress (symptoms of yearning for the deceased and trouble "moving on" without the deceased), an inability to accept the death and the reality that the deceased is truly gone, feeling detached from significant others since the death, and feeling bitter and agitated about the death are all specific indicators of PGD (Prigerson et al., 1996, Prigerson, Frank, Kasl, et al., 1995).

Prolonged grief disorder is a widespread condition associated with considerable suffering, functional impairment, and morbidity (Melhem, Day, & Shear, 2004; Neria et al., 2007; Ott, Lueger, Kelber, & Prigerson, 2007 Prigerson, 1999; Prigerson, Bierhals, Kasl, & Reynolds, 1997; Prigerson, Frank, Kasl, et al., 1995), with indications that once individuals develop PGD they are at substantial risk for chronic problems that may be unresponsive to current treatment interventions (Reynolds et al., 1999). While research has demonstrated the efficacy of treatment such as interpersonal psychotherapy (IPT) and nortriptyline for the reduction of bereavement-related depression, these have not proven effective for the reduction of grief-related symptoms (Pasternak, Reynolds, & Schlernitzauer, 1991; Reynolds et al., 1999).

Symptoms of PGD and PTSD may co-occur in the event of traumatic loss (Neria & Litz, 2004), but avoidance of fear-inducing stimuli associated with psychic trauma does not occur with PGD following a natural death. Rather, there is a hyperfocus on the loss and reminders of the deceased, a desire for reconnection with the deceased, and in most cases, comfort and/or longing (not aversive physiological reactivity) when exposed to symbolic cues that conjure thoughts of the deceased. Generally speaking, fears of violent – especially physical – harm to self or significant others and the hypervigilance triggered by a sense of impending attack play a more significant role for trauma victims than they do for people with PGD (Boelen et al., 2003; Prigerson et al., 2000). Additionally, not included among criteria for PTSD are the unique separation distress symptoms of PGD, such as longing and pining for the deceased and interpersonal attachment problems of mistrust of others and difficulty forming new relationships arising from concerns about interpersonal abandonment (Prigerson et al., 2000).

Prolonged grief disorder is particularly important to study in the context of disasters because oftentimes individuals are lost suddenly, horrifically, and unexpectedly. Interestingly, we know least about traumatic loss because the majority of studies of PGD have focused on conjugal bereavement. Sudden and horrific loss is especially complex in instances where it occurs as a result of human maliciousness, which is known to be a risk factor for PTSD (Norris et al., 2002). In the aftermath of disasters, loss might be difficult to integrate and accept, and avoidance of the loss may be prevalent because of the horrific nature of the disaster, which may serve as an additional trigger in the context of a particular loss.

7.4. PREVALENCES OF DEPRESSION AND PGD POSTDISASTER

Postdisaster prevalence of depression varies considerably across disasters and estimates can be misleading without additional information. To best understand depression estimates, it is important to take into account a variety of factors, including the prevalence of depression in the general population, the nature of the disaster, distance from the epicenter, long-term symptom trajectory, and the method used to measure depression. First, it is important to place estimates of postdisaster depression in the context of prevalence of depression in the general population in any given year. Kessler, Chiu, Demler, Merikangas, and Walters (2005) found that the 1-year prevalence of depression was 6.7% as compared to the prevalence of PTSD (3.5%) and general anxiety (3.1%). We would expect these estimates to rise following a disaster; however, to accurately measure postdisaster prevalence, it is necessary to know predisaster prevalence. Ideally, the prevalence of postdisaster depression would be measured prospectively, controlling for predisaster depression. Most often, studies have to utilize retrospective lifetime assessments, which is a limitation. For example, current mood or litigation can bias reports of past depression difficulties.

The nature and magnitude of the event is the single most important variable to consider. Although the magnitude of disasters can be quantified in terms of the monetary value of the damage or the number of lives lost, subtle differences in the types of events may lead to greater or smaller estimates of postevent symptomatology.

For example, Maes, Mylle, Delmeire, and Altamura (2000) found that 7 to 9 months after exposure to fire and/or motor vehicle accidents, the prevalence of depression was 13.4% (using a DSM-III-R structured interview). Acierno and colleagues (2007) found the prevalence of depression following a series of hurricanes to be somewhat lower, with 6.1% meeting criteria for depression postdisaster (using the Structured Clinical Interview for DSM-IV). The prevalence of depression in hurricane victims is no higher than would be found in the general population at any given time. Do those who experience hurricanes recover more quickly than those involved in a motor vehicle accident or a fire? Or is it possible that natural disasters, compared to man-made events such as car accidents, do not engender high rates of depression because of causality attributions? Or perhaps a third variable, such as community support, accounts for these differences?

For some events, it is necessary to take into account physical distance from the disaster. Following an earthquake in Turkey, 16% of those in the epicenter met criteria for depression 14 months later (as measured by the Traumatic Stress Symptom Checklist, which contains six depression symptoms and has been validated using the depression module of the SCID), with 8% of those a short distance away also meeting criteria (Başoğlu, Salcioğlu, & Livanou, 2004). There may also be an interaction between distance from the disaster and community cohesion and support in the aftermath in predicting mental health response (e.g., Somer, Maguen, Moin, Boehm, Metzler, & Litz, 2008). Consequently, those who are displaced may exhibit greater depression prevalence in the immediate aftermath if removed from sources of community support. Following the 2004 tsunami in Southeast Asia, symptoms of depression were assessed in displaced and nondisplaced individuals in Thailand at two time periods. Two months after the tsunami, 30% of displaced and 21% of nondisplaced individuals reported depression symptoms (as measured by the Birleson Depression Self-Rating Scale), and at 9 months these rates decreased to 17% and 14% respectively (van Griensven et al., 2006).

Another important factor to consider when examining prevalence estimates is the limitation of cross-sectional data and the trajectory of symptom change. Although we know that in the aftermath of a disaster symptoms may be higher and likely will improve over time, it is unclear how long symptoms generally last, and norms for improvement are ambiguous at best. In a prospective study of Hurricane Katrina survivors attending an outpatient clinic who were surveyed 1 month before and 1 month after Katrina, depression symptoms (as measured by Center for Epidemiologic Studies–Depressed Mood Scale [CES-D]) increased while PTSD symptoms did not (McLeish & Del Ben, 2008). In a study that tracked symptoms in a community following an earthquake, individuals' PTSD symptoms improved significantly when measured at 1 month and at 13 months following the disaster; however, there was no significant improvement in depression symptoms (as measured by the Beck Depression Inventory [BDI]) (Altindag, Ozen, & Sir, 2005). Similarly, Norris, Perilla, Riad, Kaniasty, and Lavizzo (1999) found that in the aftermath of a hurricane, measurement at 6 and 30 months postdisaster indicated a significant improvement in PTSD symptoms but not in depression symptoms (as measured by CES-D). Interestingly, Chou, and colleagues (2007) found that among earthquake survivors in Taiwan who were surveyed at 6 months, 2 years and 3 years, PTSD and depression symptoms seem to decline at the 2 year mark (as measured by the Mini-International Neuropsychiatric Interview). Survivors of the Oklahoma City bombing were interviewed 6.5 to 7 years after the terror event, and those interviewed were matched with controls. Depression symptoms (as measured by the BDI) were not significantly different in survivors and controls; however, differences were found in relation to PTSD symptoms, especially with respect to autonomic reactivity (Tucker et al., 2007). Collectively, these studies suggest that while depression symptoms may linger in the first few years postdisaster, they eventually dissipate with time in most people. However, more research is needed to better understand these trajectories, with attention to the differential impacts of disaster type, extent of damage, and cultural factors.

In deciphering varying estimates of depression, it is important to account for how depression is measured, the time period over which it is evaluated, and whether figures refer to assessments of current as opposed to past depression. Some measurement instruments may have greater validity; furthermore, cut points may be different depending on the measure employed. Some instruments may focus only on symptoms; others may consider both symptoms and functional impairment. Some studies utilize self-report instruments, while others employ structured clinical interviews. Related, some studies report symptom prevalence as the main outcome variable, while others employ diagnostic rates of a particular disorder. There are drawbacks to each approach. Many studies examining prevalence use clinical diagnostic instruments; however, these studies exclude those individuals with subthreshold mental health problems. Additionally, it is necessary to consider whether individuals are asked to report about their symptoms within the prior month, or over a 6-month period, as the latter may be a greater source of measurement error.

Sampling issues are also important. Some studies employ telephone interviews, while others utilize field interviews at or near individuals' homes. If the particular disaster has caused displacement, sampling issues become even more complex, and researchers must struggle with how to create the most representative sample. Sampling decisions must also be made about the circumference of inclusion and proximity from the disaster. Refusal rates are also important to consider, as it is possible that those that are most severely impacted cannot participate because of issues of emotional distress. Issues of generalizability are always at the forefront; decisions must be made about how to collect data that are most representative of those impacted.

An excellent example of the measurement and sampling issues is reflected in studies attempting to understand rates of depression following terrorism. After September 11th, Ahern and Galea (2006) found that the prevalence of depression at 6 months was 12.4% in a representative sample of those residing in New York City. Person, Tracy, and Galea (2006) found somewhat lower rates following the attacks on the World Trade Center; they reported a 9.4% prevalence of probable depression over the 6 month period that followed. Current rates were much lower, with 3.9% of individuals meeting criteria for probable current depression (Person et al., 2006). Following the Madrid train bombings, the prevalence of depression was 8% in a period 1 to 3 months after the event (Miguel-Tobal et al., 2006). These three studies demonstrate the varying prevalence of postdisaster depression. While all three studies utilized random digit dialing and employed the same depression measure (MDD module of the SCID), each looked at a particular time frame following terrorism (e.g., 3 months vs. 6 months). Two of the aforementioned samples were drawn from the same larger random digit dialing study of individuals residing in New York City following the terrorist attacks of September 11th; Ahern and Galea (2006) used a smaller sample than Persons and colleagues (2006) and utilized only those who reported specific information about their neighborhood of residence.

Overall, what is clear is that depression estimates vary, and it is challenging to make sense of the various findings because of procedural variability. Clearly more uniform and longitudinal epidemiological research is needed to better understand the mental health impact of disasters. In the next section, we will look to specific correlates of depression that may help account for some of the variability in mental health response to disasters.

The prevalence of PGD is somewhat more challenging to quantify because few disaster studies have measured the disorder. Nonetheless, some research exists. Following the terrorist attacks of September 11th Neria and colleagues (2007) found that 43% of a sample of over 700 individuals who lost a loved one screened positive for PGD several years after the terrorist event. Similarly, in a smaller sample of those who lost loved ones on September 11th, Shear, Jackson, Essock, Donahue, and Felton (2006) found that 44% screened positive for complicated grief 1.5

years afterward. Owing to the lack of knowledge on prevalence of PGD in the general population, it is somewhat difficult to make sense of these findings. However, the findings underscore the painful, often debilitating and enduring consequences of traumatic loss in the context of mass violence events. Despite limitations, the two studies examining prevalence of PGD seem to be consistent, highlighting a potential post-disaster public health concern requiring greater attention.

In addition to a dearth of information on prevalence of prolonged grief, we know very little about the trajectory of recovery in the context of disasters. We can glean important information from trajectory studies on conjugally bereaved individuals; however, these studies should be interpreted with caution since it is unclear how they generalize to those who have lost a loved one as a consequence of disaster. One study of PGD in conjugally bereaved older adults demonstrated that following a loss, individuals can be categorized into three trajectories: common, resilient, and chronic grief (Ott, Lueger, Kelber, & Prigerson, 2007). About half of all individuals followed the common grief trajectory, with elevated grief and depression symptoms postloss decreasing over time. Approximately one-third of the sample was resilient, demonstrating low rates of grief and depression, and a higher quality of life. Finally, 17% experienced chronic grief, demonstrating the highest levels of grief and depression. This chronic grief group also reported more sudden deaths of their loved ones, and most of the individuals in this group also met criteria for a diagnosis of complicated grief. One conclusion we can draw from this research is the possibility that those who suffer from sudden losses in the context of disasters are at greater risk of PGD. This would help explain the elevated rates in the studies described earlier. Future research should continue to explore this important question.

Another study found five trajectories of bereavement, quite similar to the ones outlined earlier, with the addition of two depression trajectories: common grief, chronic grief, chronic depression, depression followed by improvement, and resilience (Bonanno, Wortmann, & Nesse, 2004). Individuals were surveyed before their loss, 6 months postloss and 18 months postloss. Bonanno and colleagues (2007) found that the chronic grief group was different than the others in their continued search for meaning concerning the loss, higher yearning for the lost loved one, greater emotional pangs, and talking and thinking about the lost person more at 6 months postloss. The chronic depression group reported the highest perceived difficulties after the loss (e.g., financial). The authors conclude that providers should help those in the chronic grief group in the construction of a new meaning of the loss and help those with chronic depression with self-esteem, and the daily strains resulting from their loss. These findings suggest that those who suffer from chronic grief in the context of disasters are at greater risk of a range of psychological sequelae that deserve grief-focused treatment postdisaster.

For both postdisaster depression and prolonged grief, comorbidity issues should be explored. For example, of those with probable depression during some period in the 6 months following September 11th, 24.2% of those individuals also had probable PTSD (Person et al., 2006). However, for those with current probable depression, only 8.3% also met criteria for current probable PTSD (Person et al., 2006). With these comorbidity rates in mind, the next important question to ask is whether comorbidity is associated with differential recovery trajectories. Indeed, following an earthquake, those with comorbid depression and PTSD were slower to recover; furthermore, 37.5% of those with a PTSD diagnosis still met criteria for depression 36 months later (Onder, Tural, Aker, Kilic, & Erdogan, 2006). In those screening positive for PGD following loss of a loved one on September 11th, 43% also had probable PTSD and 36% probable depression (Maguen, Litz, Neria, Marshall, & Gross, 2004; Neria et al., 2007).

Although prior theoretical formulations questioned whether PGD was a distinct entity and comorbidity certainly has been found to be common, there has been a great deal of support for PGD as a stand-alone diagnosis. In their study of September 11th bereaved individuals, Neria and colleagues (2007) found that complicated grief was associated with functional impairment, independent of depression, and PTSD symptoms. In fact, criteria for depression or PTSD were not met in 32% of those screening positive for complicated grief. Similarly, Simon and colleagues 2007 found that 25% of those who met criteria for PGD did not evidence a DSM-IV diagnosis. When individuals did meet criteria for another disorder, grief severity was greater than for those without a comorbid disorder. Even when controlling for comorbidity, PGD was associated with impairments in employment and social functioning. Moreover, in a study of two samples of bereaved individuals, including one in which several different measures of functioning (i.e., interviewer ratings, friend ratings, self-report, and autonomic arousal) were used, PGD emerged as a unique predictor of functioning both at a single time point and longitudinally (Bonanno et al., 2007).

7.5. CORRELATES OF DEPRESSION AND PROLONGED GRIEF

Risk and resilience factors can be temporally categorized into three categories: preevent predictors, perievent predictors, and postevent predictors. Prior mental health problems are preevent predictors of postevent depression. Among those who were injured in the March 11, 2004, terrorist attacks in Madrid, prior psychotropic medication was the main predictor of both depression and PTSD following the event (Gabriel et al., 2007). Following the Oklahoma City bombing, 26% of individuals reported preexisting depression that had worsened since the bombing (Shariat, Mallonee, Kruger, Farmer, & North, 1999). When examining depression rates more closely, North and colleagues (1999) found that 13% of individuals met criteria for predisaster major depression disorder, evaluated retrospectively, and 23% met criteria postdisaster. Seventy-eight percent of individuals who reported predisaster depression reported a persistence or reoccurrence of the disorder following the bombing. Similarly, Norris and colleagues (2004) examined depression rates in individuals in two cities impacted by floods in Mexico, assessing lifetime predisaster MDD (13%, 16%), postdisaster MDD (7%, 15%), and first onset MDD (2%, 5%). They found that postdisaster rates differed among individuals in the two cities; however, first onset MDD rates did not, suggesting that postdisaster differences resulted from reoccurrence rates in those with prior MDD. This highlights the possibility that a significant percentage of the variance in mental health symptoms postdisaster may be accounted for by predisaster symptoms.

Prior trauma is another important preevent predictor of depression. History of exposure to a traumatic event was found to be a predictor of depression following September 11th (Person et al., 2006), with those who reported experiencing four or more traumatic events before the attacks demonstrating a greater likelihood of depression. Similarly, past exposure to a traumatic event was a predictor of depression following hurricane exposure (Acierno et al., 2007) and earthquake exposure (Sattler et al., 2006). Preevent stressors, such as having a close friend die, being seriously injured or ill, getting married or divorced, having family problems, and/or having low levels of social support, can also be significant preevent predictors. Level of stress before September 11th was found to predict depression in the aftermath, with those experiencing two or more life stressors in the year before attacks demonstrating a higher likelihood of depression (Person et al., 2006). Low social support in the 6 months before hurricane exposure also significantly predicted depression (Acierno et al., 2007).

There are also several demographic factors that have been shown to be predictors of depression. Younger age was a risk factor for depression following exposure to hurricanes (Acierno et al., 2007). Similarly, older age (being 65 or older) was a protective factor against depression following September 11th. Additionally, being single and having low income were also found to be risk factors for depression after September 11th (Ahern & Galea., 2006). Low socioeconomic status was associated with depression following other disasters, such as earthquakes (e.g., Seplaki, Goldman, Weinstein, & Lin, 2006). Finally, female gender was found to be a risk factor for depression in several different disaster contexts (e.g., Armenian et al., 2002; Kuo et al., 2003; Somer, Maguen, Or-Chen, Litz, 2009).

In terms of perievent factors, Person et al. (2006) found that having a panic attack within close proximity of the time of a terror event was a predictor of depression symptoms 6 months later. While this variable also has been found to predict PTSD, which is conceptualized along the anxiety continuum, it is informative that it is also a predictor of subsequent depression, suggesting a possible common pathway. Among earthquake survivors, being with someone at the time of the disaster was a protective factor against depression (Armenian et al., 2002). Furthermore, the severity and intensity of exposure (e.g., Kohn, Levav, Garcia, Machuca, & Tamashiro, 2005) and proximity of exposure (e.g., Armenian et al., 2002; Başoğlu et al., 2004) are important disaster-related predictors of depression.

A host of postevent variables influence adaptation to disasters. For example, resource loss (e.g., loss of home, income, social supports) following disaster has been shown to be an important predictor of mental health in several studies. Hobfoll's conservation of resources (COR) theory is particularly germane to disasters. COR posits that individuals strive to maintain precious resources, including internal and external resources and physical and psychological resources, and that by doing so, psychosocial welfare is maintained. In the context of terrorism, Hobfoll, Tracy, and Galea (2006) found that resource loss was a significant predictor of probable depression. Similarly, property damage after wildfires (Marshall, Schell, Elliott, Rayburn, & Jaycox, 2007) and following earthquakes (Seplaki et al., 2006) is a strong predictor of depression. Following earthquakes in El Salvador, Sattler and colleagues (2006) found that damage to the home and loss of object resources were important predictors of depression almost 2 months later. Among tsunami survivors, loss of livelihood was the strongest predictor of depression in the aftermath of the disaster (van Griensven et al., 2006). Displacement and relocation can also be important measures of well-being following disaster. Among earthquake and tsunami survivors, those that were forced to relocate demonstrated more severe depression (Kilic et al., 2006; van Griensven et al., 2006). Relocation may also be a proxy for decreased social support, as individuals are forced to leave core communities that may offer emotional and physical support.

Social support is a resource that promotes well-being and quality of life, and social support losses or deficits in the aftermath of disasters are important predictors of mental health outcome. Social support can come in many forms, manifesting at the individual level, the family unit level, the community level, the national level, and several levels in between. Firefighters assisting with Hurricane Katrina were less likely to report depression symptoms if they were living with their families, as opposed to living alone during the disaster (Tak, Driscoll, Bernard, & West, 2007). Conversely, social isolation is found to be associated with greater depressive symptoms (Seplaki et al., 2006). One important finding over a series of studies is that although social support may be readily available in the immediate aftermath of a disaster, the sources, quantity, and quality of social support deteriorates over time. In one study looking at depression as the outcome following floods, deterioration of social support mediated the immediate and delayed impact of disaster stress (Kaniasty & Norris, 1993). Future studies should continue to explore the relationship between social supports at all levels and its association with depression following disasters.

Resource loss can also be conceptualized in terms of physical health capacities. For example, physical injury is a strong predictor of depression in the context of fires (e.g., Maes et al., 2000; Marshall et al., 2007). There is also evidence that physical symptoms are associated with depression; in a survey of firefighters 13 weeks after Hurricane Katrina, those who developed skin rashes or lower respiratory symptoms were twice as likely to report symptoms of depression (Tak et al., 2007). At present, we do not know the direction of the causal relationship between physical injury and depression; it is more likely than not that the relationship is reciprocal.

Life stressors in the aftermath of a disaster have also been shown to have a profound impact on subsequent healing. Norris and Uhl (1993) found that following Hurricane Hugo, chronic stress (e.g., financial, marital, physical stress) mediated the long-term effects of acute disaster stress on psychological distress, such as depression.

When examining relationships between pre-, peri-, and post-event predictors after Hurricane Andrew, Norris and colleagues (1999) found that for PTSD symptoms, pre- (e.g., demographics) and peri-event predictors were most significant, while for depression, postevent predictors (i.e., stress and resources) carried the most weight. Future studies should continue to explore how pre-, peri-, and postevent predictors are associated with symptoms and recovery.

Only one known study directly examined correlates of PGD postdisaster. Following September 11th, Neria and colleagues (2007) found that PGD was more prevalent in the older age group, in individuals with lower educational attainment, and in those not gainfully employed. Likelihood for PGD was highest among participants who had lost a son or daughter, as compared to those who lost a spouse or a sibling. People who were at the World Trade Center site during the attacks were over two times more likely to have PGD than those who were at other locations.

7.6. INTERVENTIONS FOR PROLONGED GRIEF AND DEPRESSION POSTDISASTER: CURRENT STATUS AND FUTURE DIRECTIONS

Grief and depression-focused treatments are rarely implemented systematically in the wake of disasters. Yet treatment research for both conditions exists, suggesting that a number of treatment modalities may be appropriate after disasters.

7.6.1. Treatment for Postdisaster Depression

A large number of clinical trials suggest that IPT is efficacious as acute and maintenance treatment for depression across age, gender, and culture (de Mello, de Jesus Mari, Bacaltchuk, Verdeli, & Neugebauer, 2005; Klerman, Chevron, Weissman, & Rounsaville, 1984; Klerman & Weissman, 1993; Weissman & Markowitz, 2007; Weissman, Markowitz, & Klerman, 2000). IPT can be delivered in a flexible format (e.g., over the phone; Donnelly et al., 2000; Miller & Weissman, 2002; Neugebauer et al., 2007) and may be especially attractive to people who have many logistic barriers to coming in for treatment. It addresses a range of conditions that are known to be prevalent among disaster-exposed populations, such as increased exposure to stressful life events associated with the depressive symptoms (Weissman & Markowitz, 1994). IPT is based on the premise that depression, regardless of biological vulnerability or personality, occurs in a psychosocial and interpersonal context. Exploration of the context associated with the onset of depression and examination of the possibility of renegotiating difficulties in current psychosocial/interpersonal domains are viewed as central to recovery from a depressive episode. IPT is focused on exploring coping strategies for social and interpersonal problems associated with the onset and maintenance of depressive symptoms. This goal includes dealing with one or more problem areas that may have triggered the patient's index episode. The problems are highly prevalent in traumatized populations: grief, interpersonal disputes, role transitions, and interpersonal deficits. The therapist works with the patient to resolve difficulties experienced in the most prominent problem area. IPT can be easily translated to a range of cultures and contexts, including non-Western societies. When IPT has been applied following disaster in Africa in the context of the HIV/AIDS epidemic (Bolton et al., 2003; Verdeli et al., 2003) and among internally displaced people in northern Uganda (Bolton et al., 2007), IPT was highly efficacious in reducing depression and dysfunction.

Interestingly, although cognitive-behavioral therapy (CBT) has been shown to be an effective treatment for depression in multiple randomized controlled trials (RCTs), no known study specifically tests its efficacy in reducing depression symptoms in the context of disasters. While some studies examine the efficacy of CBT with respect to PTSD symptoms postdisaster, depression is often examined as a comorbid complication, rather than an outcome in its own right. This is surprising given the plethora of evidence demonstrating CBT's efficacy for depression. In a flexible manualized CBT treatment for PTSD following terrorism on September 11th, one study demonstrated that after 12 to 25 sessions, depression (and PTSD) symptoms decreased significantly, with moderate to large effect sizes, similar in those found in RCTs (Levitt, Malta, Martin, Davis, & Cloitre, 2007). The lack of studies employing CBT for disaster-related depression represents an important gap in our understanding of how to provide evidence-based care in the aftermath of disasters. Without explicit studies testing CBT within the context of disasters, we cannot conclude that it is efficacious in reduction of postdisaster depression.

7.6.2. Treatment for Postdisaster Grief

Bereavement interventions have been classified as primary, secondary, and tertiary (Schut, 2001). Primary interventions are broad-based interventions for all individuals who recently experienced loss with the goal of facilitating the grieving process. Secondary interventions seek to prevent PGD in those most at risk for PGD. Tertiary interventions are for those already experiencing PGD. Several meta-analyses have examined the efficacy of these types of interventions (e.g., Center for the Advancement of Health, 2004). While broadly focused primary interventions do not appear to be helpful and may in fact exacerbate grief symptoms (Schut, 2001), some tertiary interventions for PGD have been shown to reduce PGD symptoms and related dysfunction (Boelen, de Keijser, van den Hout, & van den Bout, 2007; Shear, Frank, Houck, & Reynolds, 2005). Almost all of these studies use a modified exposure therapy approach in which painful memories of the deceased are reviewed and the negative aspects are challenged with cognitive therapy techniques. In one of the most comprehensive interventions to date, Shear and colleagues (2005) conducted a randomized controlled clinical trial of a tertiary intervention for PGD in 95 participants with PGD approximately 2 years after their loss. The treatment package combined exposure therapy (e.g., imaginal and in vivo exposure to the memory of the death and avoided people and places), cognitive restructuring techniques, IPT techniques (e.g., focusing on illness role and interpersonal role transitions and disputes), and techniques focused on reviewing positive memories of the deceased to help promote accommodation to the loss (PGD-specific techniques). This trial demonstrated that the specified treatment led to significantly greater improvements in PGD symptoms and general functioning than IPT alone (51% vs. 28% were treatment responders, respectively). However, it is important to note that even in the PGD enhanced treatment condition approximately half of participants were not identified as treatment responders, highlighting the need for more efficacious treatments.

In another study using CBT models in the conceptualization and treatment of PGD, Boelen and colleagues (2007) assigned 54 participants who demonstrated high levels of prolonged grief symptoms because of both traumatic and non-traumatic losses to: (1) exposure therapy focused on avoidance symptoms followed by cognitive restructuring, (2) cognitive restructuring followed by exposure therapy, or (3) supportive counseling. Results suggest that CBT-based interventions were more effective than supportive counseling, and that the exposure therapy was more effective than cognitive restructuring as a stand-alone treatment. Furthermore, exposure therapy followed by cognitive restructuring was most effective in reducing PGD symptoms at the 6-month follow-up.

IPT also has been considered as an intervention for PGD; however, there is little empirical research on IPT targeting PGD symptoms, and it appears that IPT is not a particularly effective treatment for PGD. As noted previously, Shear and colleagues (2005) found that CBT treatment augmented with some IPT techniques was superior to IPT alone. In another study, Reynolds and colleagues (1999) compared the effects of nortriptyline and IPT alone and in combination against a placebo for bereavement-related depression and grief symptoms. Results indicated that IPT alone evidenced the lowest level of remission in bereavement-related depression (29%), scoring much lower than the placebo alone (45%), nortriptyline (56%), or nortriptyline, and IPT together (69%). No treatment condition resulted in decreases in grief symptoms.

These studies suggest that future treatments for disaster-related grief should include exposure techniques, yet studies have shown that this component may not be sufficient to address core symptoms of PGD. Previous studies that have examined the daily diaries of people with pathological grief reactions found that they showed significantly less contact with others, missed more meals, started work later, and were involved in fewer outdoor activities than healthy controls (Jacobs & Prigerson, 2000; Monk, Houck, & Shear, 2006). This underscores the necessity of fostering reengagement and reattachment to facilitate recovery from loss. Exposure-based treatments arguably do not address the entire picture of attachment-related core symptoms of PGD and may not represent the ideal treatment paradigm for PGD. We therefore believe that it is important to generate and test a more focused and parsimonious approach to PGD treatment by adapting a technique that (1) focuses on core symptoms of functional and emotional disengagement, (2) targets ruminative and avoidant behaviors that disconnect individuals from sources of positive reinforcement and psychosocial resources, (3) promotes stable, active self-care routines, and (4) encourages reengagement with pleasurable activities and social resources postdisaster.

7.7. SUMMARY AND CONCLUSIONS

Depression and PGD are important to examine following disasters of all magnitudes, and each of these affective disorders should be conceptualized along a continuum. Most individuals heal with time, with a minority exhibiting long-term mental health symptoms; those displaying exacerbated symptoms and unremitting functional impairment are at the far end of the continuum.

The prevalence of postdisaster depression and PGD varies tremendously, and predisaster estimates among the general population, the nature of the disaster, distance from the disaster, social support in the aftermath, long-term symptom trajectories, sampling strategies, and methods used to measure depression and grief outcomes are each crucial to consider when trying to decipher varying estimates of prevalence. Predictors of depression and PGD explain some additional variance in measured outcomes and can be parsed into preevent predictors, perievent predictors and postevent predictors, with preevent prior mental health diagnoses often explaining a large proportion of the variance in postdisaster mental health outcomes. Future research in this area should particularly examine how prevalence and predictors vary over time. While several studies exist in the immediate aftermath, the long-term trajectory of recovery from depression and PGD seems ambiguous at best for those who exhibit more severe symptoms.

Research specifically concerning treatment of depression and PGD in a postdisaster environment is in its infancy, and although some studies exist, few examine these outcomes as distinct entities. Future studies should examine evidence-based treatments for MDD and PGD longitudinally rather than making assumptions about their efficacy as generalized from studies of individuals in different contexts.

REFERENCES

Acierno, R., Ruggiero, K. J., Galea, S., Resnick, H. S., Koenen, K., Roitzsch, J., et al. (2007). Psychological sequelae resulting from the 2004 Florida hurricanes: Implications for postdisaster intervention. *American Journal of Public Health, 97*, S103–S108.

Ahern J., & Galea, S. (2006). Social context and depression after a disaster: The role of income inequality. *Journal of Epidemiology and Community Health, 60*, 766–770.

Altindag, A., Ozen, S., & Sir, A. (2005). One-year follow-up study of posttraumatic stress disorder among earthquake survivors in Turkey. *Comprehensive Psychiatry, 46*, 328–333.

Armenian, H. K., Morikawa, M., Melkonian, A. K., Hovanesian, A., Akiskal, K., & Akiskal, H. S. (2002). Risk factors for depression in the survivors of the 1988 earthquake in Armenia. *Journal of Urban Health, 79*, 373–382.

Başoğlu, M., Kiliç, C., Salcioğlu, E., & Livanou, M. (2004). Prevalence of posttraumatic stress disorder and comorbid depression in earthquake survivors in Turkey: An epidemiological study. *Journal of Traumatic Stress, 17*, 133–141.

Berezin, M. A. (1970). The psychiatrist and the geriatric patient: Partial grief in family members and others who care for the elderly patient. *Journal of Geriatric Psychiatry, 4*, 53–70.

Boelen, P. A., & van den Bout, J. (2008). Complicated grief and uncomplicated grief are distinguishable constructs. *Psychiatry Research, 157*, 311–314.

Boelen, P. A., van den Bout, J., & de Keijser, J. (2003). Reliability and validity of the Dutch version of the Inventory of Traumatic Grief (ITG). *Death Studies, 27*, 227–247.

Boelen, P. A., de Keijser, J., van den Hout, M. A., & van den Bout, J. (2007). Treatment of complicated grief: A comparison between cognitive-behavioral therapy and supportive counseling. *Journal of Consulting and Clinical Psychology, 75*, 277–284.

Bolton, P., Bass, J., Betancourt, T., Speelman, L., Onyango, G., & Clougherty, K. F. (2007). Interventions for depression symptoms among adolescent survivors of war and displacement in northern Uganda: A randomized controlled trial. *Journal of the American Medical Association, 298*, 519–527.

Bolton, P., Bass, J., Neugebauer, R., Verdeli, H., Clougherty, K. F., & Wickramaratne, P. (2003). Group interpersonal psychotherapy for depression in rural Uganda: A randomized controlled trial. *Journal of the American Medical Association, 289*, 3117–3124.

Bonanno, G. A., Neria, Y., Mancini, A., Coifman, K. G., Litz, B., & Insel, B. (2007). Is there more to complicated grief than depression and posttraumatic stress disorder? A test of incremental validity. *Journal of Abnormal Psychology, 116*, 342–351.

Bonanno, G. A., Wortman, C. B., & Nesse, R. M. (2004). Prospective patterns of resilience and maladjustment during widowhood. *Psychology of Aging, 19*, 260–271.

Center for the Advancement of Health (CAH). (2004). Report on bereavement and grief research. *Death Studies, 28*, 491–575.

Chen, J. H., Bierhals, A. J., Prigerson, H. G., Kasl, S. V., Mazure, C. M., & Jacobs, S. (1999). Gender differences in the effects of bereavement-related psychological distress in health outcomes. *Psychological Medicine, 29*, 367–380.

Chou, F. H., Wu, H. C., Chou, P., Su, C. Y., Tsai, K. Y., Chao, S. S., et al. (2007). Epidemiologic psychiatric studies on post-disaster impact among Chi-Chi earthquake survivors in Yu-Chi, Taiwan. *Psychiatry and Clinical Neurosciences, 61*, 370–378.

De Mello, M. F., de Jesus Mari, J., Bacaltchuk, J., Verdeli, H., & Neugebauer, R. (2005). A systematic review of research findings on the efficacy of interpersonal therapy for depressive disorders. *European Archives of Psychiatry and Clinical Neuroscience, 255*, 75–82.

Donnelly, J. M., Kornblith, A. B., Fleishman, S., Zuckerman, E., Raptis, G., & Hudis, C. A. (2000). A pilot study of interpersonal psychotherapy by telephone with cancer patients and their partners. *Psychooncology, 9*, 44–56.

Dunne, E. J., & Dunne-Maxim, K. (2004). Working with families in the aftermath of suicide. In F. Walsh & M. McGoldrick (Eds.), *Living beyond loss: Death in the family 2nd ed.* New York: W. W. Norton & Co.

Freud, S. (1917). *The history of the psychoanalytic movement.* Washington, DC: Nervous and Mental Disease Publishing Company.

Gabriel, R., Ferrando, L., Cortón, E. S., Mingote, C., García-Camba, E., Liria, A. F., et al. (2007). Psychopathological consequences after a terrorist attack: An epidemiological study among victims, the general population, and police officers. *European Psychiatry, 22*, 339–346.

Hobfoll, S. E., Tracy, M., & Galea, S. (2006). The impact of resource loss and traumatic growth on probable PTSD and depression following terrorist attacks. *Journal of Traumatic Stress, 19*, 867–878.

Jacobs, S., & Prigerson, H. (2000). Psychotherapy of traumatic grief: A review of evidence for psychotherapeutic treatments. *Death Studies, 24*, 479–495.

Kaniasty, K., & Norris, F. H. (1993). A test of the social support deterioration model in the context of natural disaster. *Journal of Personality and Social Psychology, 64*, 395–408.

Kessler, R. C., Chiu, W. T., Demler, O., Merikangas, K. R., & Walters, E. E. (2005). Prevalence, severity, and comorbidity of 12-month DSM-IV disorders in the National Comorbidity Survey Replication. *Archives of General Psychiatry, 62*, 617–627.

Kilic, C., Aydin, I., Taskintuna, N., Ozcurumez, G., Kurt, G., Eren, E., et al. (2006). Predictors of psychological distress in survivors of the 1999 earthquakes in Turkey: Effects of relocation after the disaster. *Acta Psychiatrica Scandinavica, 114*, 194–202.

Klerman, G.L., Chevron, E.S., Weissman, M.M., & Rounsaville, B. (1984). *Interpersonal psychotherapy of depression* New York: Basic Books.

Klerman, G.L., & Weissman, M.M. (1993). *New applications of interpersonal psychotherapy*. Washington, DC: American Psychiatric Press.

Kohn, R., Levav, I., Garcia, I.D., Machuca, M.E., & Tamashiro, R. (2005). Prevalence, risk factors and aging vulnerability for psychopathology following a natural disaster in a developing country. *International Journal of Geriatric Psychiatry, 20*, 835–841.

Kuo, C.J., Tang, H.S., Tsay, C.J., Lin, S.K., Hu, W.H., & Chen, C.C. (2003). Prevalence of psychiatric disorders among bereaved survivors of a disastrous earthquake in Taiwan. *Psychiatric Services, 54*, 249–251.

Lacey, D. (2005). Nursing home social worker skills and end-of-life planning. *Social Work in Health Care, 40*, 19–40.

Levitt, J.T., Malta, L.S., Martin, A., Davis, L., & Cloitre, M. (2007). The flexible application of a manualized treatment for PTSD symptoms and functional impairment related to the 9/11 World Trade Center attack. *Behaviour Research and Therapy, 45*, 1419–1433.

Lichtenthal, W.G., Cruess, D.G., & Prigerson, H.G. (2004). A case for establishing complicated grief as a distinct mental disorder in DSM-V. *Clinical Psychology Review, 24*, 637–662.

Lindemann, E. (1944). Symptomatology and management of acute grief. *American Journal of Psychiatry, 101*, 141–148.

Maes, M., Mylle, J., Delmeire, L., & Altamura, C. (2000). Psychiatric morbidity and comorbidity following accidental man-made traumatic events: Incidence and risk factors. *European Archives of Psychiatry and Clinical Neurosciences, 250*, 156–162.

Maguen, S., Litz, B.T., Neria, Y., Marshall, R., & Gross, R. (2004). Predictors of traumatic grief resulting from loss on 9-11-01. Paper presented at The International Society for Traumatic Stress 20th Annual Meeting, New Orleans, LA.

Marshall, G.N., Schell, T.L., Elliott, M.N., Rayburn, N.R., & Jaycox, L.H. (2007). Psychiatric disorders among adults seeking emergency disaster assistance after a wildland-urban interface fire. *Psychiatric Services, 58*, 509–514.

Marwit, S.J. (1991). DSM-III-R, grief reactions, and a call for revision. *Professional psychology: Research and practice, 22*, 75–79.

McLeish, A.C., & Del Ben, K.S. (2008). Symptoms of depression and posttraumatic stress disorder in an outpatient population before and after Hurricane Katrina. *Depression and Anxiety, 25*, 416–421.

Melhem, N.M., Day, N., & Shear, M.K. (2004). Traumatic grief among adolescents exposed to a peer's suicide. *American Journal of Psychiatry, 161*, 1411–1416.

Miguel-Tobal, J.J., Cano-Vindel, A., Gonzalez-Ordi, H., Iruarrizaga, I., Rudenstine, S., Vlahov, D., et al. (2006). PTSD and depression after the Madrid March 11 train bombings. *Journal of Traumatic Stress, 19*, 69–80.

Miller, L., & Weissman, M. (2002). Interpersonal psychotherapy delivered over the telephone to recurrent depressives: A pilot study. *Depression and Anxiety, 16*, 114–117.

Monk, T.H., Houck, P.R., & Shear, M.K. (2006). The daily life of complicated grief patients – what gets missed, what gets added? *Death Studies, 30*, 77–85.

Neria, Y., & Litz, B.T. (2004). Bereavement by traumatic means: The complex synergy of trauma and grief. *Journal of Loss and Trauma, 9*, 73–87.

Neria, Y., Gross, R., Litz, B., Maguen, S., Insel, B., Seirmarco, G., et al. (2007). Prevalence and psychological correlates of traumatic grief among bereaved adults 2.5–3.5 years after September 11th attacks. *Journal of Traumatic Stress, 20*, 251–262.

Neria, M., Olfson, M., Gameroff, R., Gross, D., Pilowsky, P.C., Blanco, J. et al. (2008). The Mental Health Sequelae of Loss: Findings from a New York City Primary Care Practice One Year after the 9/11 Attacks. *Psychiatry, 71*, 339–348.

Neugebauer, R., Kline, J., Bleiberg, K., Baxi, L., Markowitz, J.C., Rosing, M., et al. (2007). Preliminary open trial of interpersonal counseling for subsyndromal depression following miscarriage. *Depression and Anxiety, 24*, 219–222.

Norris, F., Friedman, M.J., Watson, P.J., Byrne, C.M., Diaz, E., & Kaniasty, K. (2002). 60,000 disaster victims speak: Part I. An empirical review of the empirical literature, 1981–2001. *Psychiatry: Interpersonal and Biological Processes, 65*, 207–239.

Norris, F.H., & Uhl, G.A. (1993). Chronic stress as a mediator of acute stress: The case of Hurricane Hugo. *Journal of Applied Social Psychology, 23*, 1263–1284.

Norris, F.H., Murphy, A.D., Baker, C.K., Perilla, J. L. (2004). Postdisaster PTSD over four waves of a panel study of Mexico's 1999 flood. *Journal of Traumatic Stress, 17*, 283–292.

Norris, F.H, Perilla, J.L., Riad, J.K., Kaniasty, K.Z., & Lavizzo, E.A. (1999). Stability and change in stress, resources, and psychological distress following natural disaster: Findings from Hurricane Andrew. *Anxiety, Stress, and Coping, 12*, 363–396.

North, C.S., Nixon, S.J., Shariat, S., Mallonee, S., McMillen, J.C., Spitznagel, E.L., et al. (1999). Psychiatric disorders among survivors of the Oklahoma City bombing. *JAMA, 282*, 755–762.

Ogrodniczuk, J. S., Piper, W. E., & Joyce, A. S. (2003). Differentiating symptoms of complicated grief and depression among psychiatric outpatients. *The Canadian Journal of Psychiatry*, *48*, 87–93.

Onder, E., Tural, U., Aker, T., Kilic, C., & Erdogan, S. (2006). Prevalence of psychiatric disorders three years after the 1999 earthquake in Turkey: Marmara Earthquake Survey (MES). *Social Psychiatry and Psychiatric Epidemiology*, *41*, 868–874.

Ott, C. H., Lueger, R. J., Kelber, S. T., & Prigerson, H. G. (2007). Spousal bereavement in older adults: Common, resilient, and chronic grief with defining characteristics. *Journal of Nervous and Mental Disease*, *195*, 332–341.

Pasternak, R. E., Reynolds, C. F., & Schlernitzauer, M. (1991). Acute open-trial nortriptyline therapy of bereavement-related depression in late life. *Journal of Clinical Psychiatry*, *52*, 307–310.

Penson, R. T., Green, K. M., Chabner, B. A., & Lynch, T. J. (2002). When does the responsibility of our care end: Bereavement. *Oncologist*, *7*, 251–258.

Person, C., Tracy, M., & Galea, S. (2006). Risk factors for depression after a disaster. *Journal of Nervous and Mental Disease*, *194*, 659–666.

Prigerson, H. (1999). Traumatic grief as a risk factor for suicidal ideation among young adults. *American Journal of Psychiatry*, *156*, 1994–1995.

(2001). *Diagnostic criteria for traumatic grief: A rationale, consensus criteria, and preliminary empirical test. part II. Theory, methodology, and ethical issues*. Washington, DC: American Psychological Association Press.

Prigerson, H. G., & Jacobs, S. C. (2001). Caring for bereaved patients: 'All the doctors just suddenly go.' *Journal of the American Medical Association*, *286*, 1369–1375.

Prigerson, H. G., Bierhals, A. J., Kasl, S. V., Reynolds, C. F. III, Shear, M. K., & Day, N. (1997). Traumatic grief as a risk factor for mental and physical morbidity. *American Journal of Psychiatry*, *154*, 616–623.

Prigerson, H. G., Bierhals, A. J., Kasl, S. V., Reynolds, C. F. III, Shear, M. K., Newsom, J. T. (1996). Complicated grief as a disorder distinct from bereavement-related depression and anxiety: A replication study. *American Journal of Psychiatry*, *153*, 1484–1486.

Prigerson, H. G., Bierhals, A. J., Kasl, S. V., & Reynolds, C. F. III. (1997). Traumatic grief as a risk factor for mental and physical morbidity. *American Journal of Psychiatry*, *154*, 616–623.

Prigerson, H. G., Frank, E., Kasl, S. V., Reynolds, C. F. III, Anderson, B., Zubenko, G. S., et al. (1995). Complicated grief and bereavement-related depression as distinct disorders: Preliminary empirical validation in elderly bereaved spouses. *American Journal of Psychiatry*, *152*, 22–30.

Prigerson, H. G., Maciejewski, P. K., Newsom, J., Reynolds, C. F. III, Frank, E., Bierhals, E. J., et al. (1995). The Inventory of Complicated Grief: A scale to measure maladaptive symptoms of loss. *Psychiatry Research*, *59*, 65–79.

Prigerson, H. G., Monk, T. H., Reynolds, C. F. III, Kupfer, D. J., Begley, A., Houck, P. R., et al. (1995). Lifestyle regularity and activity levels as protective factors against bereavement-related depression. *Depression*, *3*, 297–302.

Prigerson, H. G., Shear, M. K., Jacobs, S. C., Kasl, S. V., Maciejewski, P. K., Silverman, G. K., et al. (2000). Grief and its relationship to PTSD. In D. Nutt, & J. R. T. Davidson (Eds.), *Post traumatic stress disorders: Diagnosis, management and treatment*. NY: Martin Dunitz.

Prigerson, H. G., Vanderwerker, L. C., & Maciejewski, P. K. (2007). Complicated grief as a mental disorder: Inclusion in DSM. In M. Stroebe, R. Hansson, H. Schut, & W. Stroebe (Eds.), *Handbook of bereavement research and practice: 21st century perspectives*. Washington, DC: American Psychological Association Press.

Reynolds, C. F. III, Miller, M. D., Pasternak, R. E., Frank, E., Perel, J. M., Cornes, C. (1999). Treatment of bereavement-related major depressive episodes in later life: A controlled study of acute and continuation treatment with nortriptyline and interpersonal psychotherapy. *American Journal of Psychiatry*, *156*, 202–208.

Sattler, D. N., de Alvarado A. M., de Castro, N. B., Male, R. V., Zetino, A. M., & Vega, R. (2006). El Salvador earthquakes: Relationships among acute stress disorder symptoms, depression, traumatic event exposure, and resource loss. *Journal of Traumatic Stress*, *19*, 879–893.

Schut, H. (2001). *The efficacy of bereavement interventions: Determining who benefits*. Washington, D. C.: American Psychological Association.

Seplaki, C. L., Goldman, N., Weinstein, M., & Lin, Y. H. (2006). Before and after the 1999 Chi-Chi earthquake: Traumatic events and depressive symptoms in an older population. *Social Science and Medicine*, *62*, 3121–3132.

Shariat, S., Mallonee, S., Kruger, E., Farmer, K., & North, C. (1999). A prospective study of long-term health outcomes among Oklahoma City bombing survivors. *Journal of the Oklahoma State Medical Association*, *92*, 178–186.

Shear, K., Frank, E., Houck, P. R., & Reynolds, C. F. III. (2005). Treatment of complicated grief: A randomized controlled trial. *Journal of the American Medical Association*, *293*, 2601–2608.

Shear, K. M., Jackson, C. T., Essock, S. M., Donahue, S. A., & Felton, C. J. (2006). Screening for complicated grief among Project Liberty service recipients 18 months after September 11, 2001. *Psychiatric Services, 57*, 1291–1297.

Simon, N. M., Shear, K. M., Thompson, E. H., Zalta, A. K., Perlman, C., Reynolds, C. F., et al. (2007). The prevalence and correlates of psychiatric comorbidity in individuals with complicated grief. *Comprehensive Psychiatry, 48*, 395–399.

Somer, E., Maguen, S., Moin, V., Boehm, A., Metzler, T., & Litz, B. T. (2008). The effects of perceived in community cohesion on stress symptoms following a terrorist attack. *Journal of Psychological Trauma*, 7, 73–90.

Somer, E., Maguen, S., Or-Chen, K., & Litz., B. T. (2009). Managing terror: Differences between Jews and Arabs in Israel. *International Journal of Psychology 44*(2), 138–146.

Stimpson, J. P. (2006). Short communication: Prospective evidence for a reciprocal relationship between sense of control and depressive symptoms following a flood. *Stress and Health, 22*, 161–166.

Swarte, N. B., van der Lee, M. L., van der Bom, J. G., van den Bout, J., & Heintz, A. P. M. (2003). Effects of euthanasia on the bereaved family and friends: A cross sectional study. *British Medical Journal, 327*, 189–192.

Tak, S., Driscoll, R., Bernard, B., & West, C. (2007). Depressive symptoms among firefighters and related factors after the response to Hurricane Katrina. *Journal of Urban Health, 84*, 153–161.

Tucker, P. M., Pfefferbaum, B., North, C. S., Kent, A., Burgin, C. E., Parker, D. E., et al. (2007). Physiologic reactivity despite emotional resilience several years after direct exposure to terrorism. *American Journal of Psychiatry, 164*, 230–235.

van Griensven, F., Chakkraband, M. L., Thienkrua, W., Pengjuntr, W., Lopes Cardozo, B., Tantipiwatanaskul, P., et al. (2006). Thailand Post-Tsunami Mental Health Study Group: Mental health problems among adults in tsunami-affected areas in southern Thailand. *Journal of the American Medical Association, 296*, 537–548.

Verdeli, H., Clougherty, K., Bolton, P., Speelman, L., Lincoln, N., & Bass, J. (2003). Adapting group interpersonal psychotherapy for a developing country: Experience in rural Uganda. *World Psychiatry, 2*, 114–120.

Weissman, M. M., & Markowitz, J. C. (1994). Interpersonal psychotherapy: Current status. *Archives of General Psychiatry, 51*, 599–606.

(2007). *Clinician's quick guide to interpersonal psychotherapy*. USA: Oxford University Press.

Weissman, M. M., Markowitz, J. C., & Klerman, G. L. (2000). *Comprehensive guide to interpersonal psychotherapy*. New York, NY: Basic Books.

8 What is Psychopathology after Disasters? Considerations about the Nature of the Psychological and Behavioral Consequences of Disasters

ROBERT J. URSANO, CAROL S. FULLERTON, AND DAVID M. BENEDEK

8.1. INTRODUCTION

Disasters are an unexpected but not uncommon aspect of our lives. In 2005, an estimated 162 million people worldwide were affected by disasters (i.e., natural disasters, industrial and other accidents, and epidemics). Over 105,000 people died, and damages totaled over $176 million (World Health Organization, 2006). Earthquakes illustrate the burden of natural disasters. Globally, there are over 20,000 earthquakes a year, and over half are magnitude five or greater. Earthquakes can result in significant loss of human life; an earthquake in Iran in 1990 killed 50,000 people. In the Armenian earthquake of 1988 over 25,000 died, and the 1976 earthquake in Tangshan, China, resulted in at least 255,000 deaths and perhaps as many as 655,000 (U.S. Geological Survey, 2007). Human-made disasters include war and terrorism. Over 29 armed conflicts are occurring now around the globe involving 25 countries (Project Plowshares, 2007). Over two million children have been killed in war in the last decade and six million permanently disabled or injured (Project Plowshares, 2005; Ursano & Shaw, 2007). One and a half million people are displaced because of war and conflict in Uganda alone (Bolton et al., 2007).

Apart from causing death and dislocation, disasters exert a substantial psychological burden on affected populations (Neria, Nandi, & Galea, 2008). The nature of this burden varies from one disaster to another and, within a given disaster, from one individual to another. We begin this chapter by describing the interface of mental health and disaster generally. We then describe the range of psychological and behavioral responses to disaster, from subsyndromal symptoms of distress, to alterations in behavior, to the development of specific psychiatric disorders. We then focus on one specific disaster-related psychiatric disorder – posttraumatic stress disorder (PTSD). After a brief description of conceptual models of PTSD, we explore the challenges associated with understanding the range of pathology associated with this disease and identify key issues that may be better clarified through investigations in the context of conceptual models.

8.2. MENTAL HEALTH AND DISASTERS

Mental illness affects behavior, cognition, and function, and sadly, carries a greater burden of stigma than most – but not all – other medical disorders. The burden of mental illness for families, communities, and nations is substantial (World Health Organization, 2003, 2005), and the mental illness that follows extreme traumatic events, including disasters, is part of this global burden (Kessler, 2000). In general, human-made disasters have been shown to cause more frequent and more persistent psychiatric symptoms and distress. A review of the empiric literature describing multiple disaster types from 160 disaster samples involving over 60,000 victims noted that 67% of the samples who experienced mass violence were severely impaired, compared with 39% of the samples exposed to technological disasters and 34% of samples exposed to natural disasters (Norris et al., 2002). However, the distinction between natural and human-made disasters is increasingly difficult to make. The etiology and consequences of natural disasters often are the result of human beings.

Over time, the resilience of individuals and communities is the expected response to a disaster, but for some, the effects can be severe and lasting. Experiencing an altered sense of safety, increased fear and arousal, and concern for the future affects not only those who may develop mental health problems but also those who continue to work and care for their families and loved ones.

The public-health response to large-scale emergencies and catastrophes requires consideration of the disorders (e.g., PTSD, depression), distress (e.g., sleep disturbance, fear, changes in economic behaviors such as purchasing a house), and health risk behaviors (e.g., increased alcohol and tobacco use, evacuation behaviors) of those exposed (Institute of Medicine, 2003; Ursano, Fullerton, Weisaeth, & Raphael, 2007). Displaced disaster populations, from natural as well as human-made disasters of war and terrorism, also carry with them the endemic risks of disease that were present before the disaster. Disasters require that we respond not only to those who need direct care but also populations that may need support, assistance, guidance, and psychological and health-related information. Emergency-care providers must identify physical and anxiety symptoms to assure the integrity of the medical system (Ursano, Fullerton, Weisaeth, & Raphael, 2007a), and mental health providers must respond to a range of emotional and behavioral consequences, such as anger, fear, depression, and increased substance use. In some disasters, such as epidemics or bioterrorism, there are the additional special stresses related to quarantine and shelter in place directives, including altered travel behaviors and movement restrictions that affect the economic stability of a nation. Mental health and behavior are critically important elements of our health-care system for responses to disasters. Mental health and behavioral preparedness are one step in the process.

Accurate and real-time health surveillance information on the population rates of mental health and illness and the barriers to care are needed to address the mental and behavioral health-care needs of disaster populations. Health surveillance can inform disaster care and provide the basis for disaster mental health research to address the effectiveness of new care models that include psychological first aid (Benedek & Fullerton, 2007; Center for the Study of Traumatic Stress [CSTS], 2005; Flynn, 2007; Hobfoll et al., 2007; Watson, 2007; Watson & Shalev, 2005), resource restoration, primary care models of mental health care, Internet-based interventions, and the role of public education and messaging. The National Comorbidity Replication Study surveyed the mental health of the Katrina disaster region before the hurricane; thus, we know that the rates of mental disorder had doubled 6 months after Katrina, going from approximately 15% to 30%. (Galea et al., 2007; Kessler et al., 2006; Ursano, 2006). The mental health costs of this disaster still continue over 2 years after the disaster. Such disasters, as well as those caused by terrorism and war, remind us that recovery of populations is a long and arduous task. Optimizing management of this task requires planning and must encompass the pathology of disasters across the domains of suffering, impairment, altered functional capacity, and disability.

8.3. PSYCHOLOGICAL AND BEHAVIORAL RESPONSES TO DISASTER

8.3.1. Initial Behaviors

Disaster behavior, how one acts at the time of impact of a disaster, affects morbidity and, at times, mortality. Studies of evacuation from the World Trade Center towers in 1993 after a terrorist truck bombing showed that those evacuating in groups greater than 20 took over 6 minutes longer to decide to evacuate (Aguirre, Wenger, & Vigo, 1998). In addition, the more people knew each other in the group, the longer the group took to initiate evacuation. After the September 11th attacks, rather than leave the disaster area, victims from the twin towers tended to congregate at the site (Gershon, Hogan, Qureshi,

& Doll, 2004). Overdedication to one's group can also lead firefighters, police, and other first responders to needlessly risk their lives. In pandemics or after a bioterrorism attack, adherence to medical recommendations is a lifesaving behavior. Interventions at the public health level must attempt to minimize certain behaviors (e.g., delay in evacuation) and encourage others (e.g., compliance with shelter in place or social distancing recommendations).

8.3.2. Distress and Health Risk Behaviors

Distress and health risk behaviors related to disaster include nonspecific distress (for review, see Norris et al., 2002); stress-related psychological and psychosomatic symptoms (Ford, 1997; McCarroll, Ursano, Fullerton, Liu, & Lundy, 2002); sleep disturbance; increased alcohol, caffeine, and cigarette use (Shalev, Bleich, & Ursano, 1990; Vlahov et al., 2002). Following the July 7, 2005 bombings in London, 31% of Londoners reported substantial distress, and 32% of Londoners reported behavioral changes, such as the intent to travel less (Rubin, Brewin, Greenberg, Simpson, & Wessely, 2005). Anger, disbelief, sadness, anxiety, fear, and irritability are the expected responses following trauma, and there also may be an increase in family conflict and family violence. Anxiety and family conflict can accompany the distress and fear of recurrence of a traumatic event, the ongoing threat of terrorism, and the economic impact of lost jobs and companies closed or moving as a result of a disaster. After the September 11th terrorist attacks in the United States, substantial numbers of people wished to stay home and might well have met a modified version of the diagnosis of separation anxiety.

Somatization is common after a disaster and must be managed both in the community at large and in individual patients (Engel & Katon, 1999; Rundell & Ursano, 1996). Somatic symptoms can also be an indicator of disaster-related distress and may persist long after a disaster has passed. Disaster and rescue workers also report increased somatic symptoms after disaster exposure (McCarroll et al., 2002). Somatization is a frequent presentation of anxiety and depression in patients seeking care in medical clinics. Though after a disaster, overburdened primary care physicians may overlook the assessment of exposure to disaster events in patients with chronic somatic symptoms; recognizing these symptoms as an indicator of distress is important as it can help in the appropriate diagnosis and treatment and minimize inappropriate medical treatments. Medical evaluation, which includes inquiring about family conflict, can provide reassurance, initiate a discussion for referral, and be a primary preventive intervention for children whose first experience of a disaster or terrorist attack is mediated through their parents.

Sleep disturbances following trauma are common clinical problems that present to clinicians for treatment. Sleep difficulties can be due to grief, anxiety related to recurrent disaster events (e.g., aftershocks), the ongoing threat of terrorist attacks, or an underlying psychiatric disease such as depression or PTSD (Mellman, Kulick-Bell, Ashlock, & Nolan, 1995). Posttraumatic distress must be considered in the differential diagnosis and appropriate treatments initiated. Hostility, with its accompanying features of social disruption, feelings of frustration, and perception of chaos, is also common following disaster (Forster, 1992; Ursano, Fullerton, Bhartiya, & Kao, 1995). Although, in some cases it is helpful for individuals to recognize that the return of anger can be a sign of a return to normal (i.e., it is again safe to be angry and express one's losses, disappointments, and needs), in others, hostility should remind the care provider to assess the risk of family violence and substance abuse.

8.3.3. Disorders

The constellation of psychiatric symptoms most often associated with disaster is PTSD (Galea et al., 2003; Neria et al., 2007), and we deal with this disorder in greater detail in Section 4.0. However, PTSD is neither the only trauma-related disorder nor, perhaps, the most common (Fullerton & Ursano, 1997; Norris et al., 2002; North et al., 1999). People exposed to disaster are at increased risk for depression (e.g., Miguel-Tobal et al., 2006), generalized anxiety disorder, panic disorder, and increased substance use (Breslau, Davis, Andreski, & Peterson, 1991; Kessler, Sonnega, Bromet, Hughes, & Nelson, 1995; North et al., 1999, 2002; Vlahov et al., 2002). Nearly 40% of disaster workers following a plane crash met the criteria for at least one diagnosis (i.e., acute stress disorder, PTSD, or depression) in a 13-month longitudinal study (Fullerton, Ursano, & Wang, 2004). Exposed disaster workers with acute stress disorder (ASD) were over seven times more likely to meet PTSD criteria at 13 months. Forty-five percent of survivors of the Oklahoma City bombing had a postdisaster psychiatric disorder. Of these, 34.3% had PTSD, and 22.5% had major depression; nearly 40% of those with PTSD or depression had no previous history of psychiatric illness (North et al., 1999).

Acute stress disorder was introduced into the diagnostic nomenclature in DSM-IV (American Psychiatric Association, 1994). ASD is a constellation of symptoms very similar to PTSD but persists for a minimum of 2 days to a maximum of 4 weeks and occurs within 4 weeks of the trauma (Bryant & Harvey, 2000). The only difference in symptom requirements between the two diagnoses is that dissociative symptoms must be present to diagnose ASD. The dissociative symptoms can occur during the traumatic event or after it. A common early response to traumatic exposure is disturbance in an individual's internal time clock, resulting in time distortion where time feels sped up or slowed down (Ursano & Fullerton, 2000). Along with other dissociative symptoms, time distortion indicates over four times greater risk for chronic PTSD and may also be an accompaniment of depressive symptoms. ASD is diagnosed in 15% to 20% of survivors of civilian trauma (Brewin, Andrews, Rose, & Kirk, 1999); as many as 80% of persons with ASD will develop PTSD at 6 months. However, not everyone who develops PTSD had ASD in the first month. A recent review suggests that although acute dissociation is an important factor in early response to trauma, many people develop PTSD in the absence of dissociative symptoms (Bryant, 2005).

Major depression, generalized anxiety disorder, substance abuse, and adjustment disorders in disaster victims have been less often studied than ASD and PTSD, but available data suggest that these disorders also occur at higher than average rates (Galea et al., 2002; Kessler et al., 1999; Miguel-Tobal et al., 2006). Major depression, substance abuse, and adjustment disorders (anxiety and depression) may be relatively common in the 6 to 12 months after a disaster and may reflect survivors' reactions to their injuries, to feelings stimulated by the disaster, and/or to their attributions of symptoms to the disaster. Secondary stressors mediate the occurrence of these psychiatric disorders following a disaster (Epstein, Fullerton, & Ursano, 1998; Vlahov et al., 2002); these include the problems of disaster recovery, such as negotiations with insurance companies for reimbursement, or unemployment secondary to destroyed businesses. Major depression and substance abuse (drugs, alcohol, and tobacco) are frequently comorbid with PTSD and warrant further study (Davidson & Fairbank, 1992; Rundell, Ursano, Holloway, & Silberman, 1989; Shalev et al., 1990). Increased substance use (without abuse) is also seen and effects morbidity and mortality through potential risk behaviors such as motor vehicle accidents, risky sexual behaviors, and family violence (Galea et al., 2002; Fullerton et al., 2004).

Grief reactions are common after all disasters, and increasingly, traumatic loss and the bereavement and grief associated with the traumatic loss are recognized as posing special challenges to survivors of disasters and other traumatic events (Fullerton, Ursano, Kao, & Bharitya, 1999; Prigerson et al., 1999, 2000; Neria, Nandi, & Galea, 2008; Raphael, Martinek, & Wooding, 2004; Raphael & Minkov, 1999; Raphael & Wooding, 2004; Shear et al., 2001; Shear, Frank, Houck, & Reynolds, 2005). While the death of loved ones is always painful, an unexpected and violent death is most difficult. Even when not directly witnessing the death, family members may develop intrusive images on the basis of the information gleaned from authorities or the media. In children, traumatic play, a phenomenon similar to intrusive symptoms in adults, is both a sign of distress and an effort at mastery

(Terr, 1981). However, little is known about complex grief as a disaster-specific outcome. Available studies of grief reactions following trauma do not greatly aid our understanding of who is at risk for persistent depression, although risk factors for complicated grief have been identified (Neria et al, 2007b). Single parents may be at high risk for developing psychiatric disorders since they often have fewer resources to begin with, and they loose some of their social support after a disaster (Solomon & Smith, 1994). At the individual level, cognitive-behavioral psychotherapeutic interventions for children and adults with complex grief are under investigation (Shear, 2005). At the population level, effective leadership after disasters includes "grief leadership," an important aspect of giving permission for and teaching and showing people how to grieve (Ursano & Fullerton, 1990).

After a disaster or terrorist event, the contribution of the psychological factors to medical illness can also be pervasive and range from heart disease (Leor, Poole, & Kloner, 1996) to diabetes (Jacobson, 1996). Injured survivors often have psychological factors affecting their physical condition (Benedek, Holloway, & Becker, 2002; Kulka et al., 1990; North et al., 1999; Shore, Vollmer, & Tatum, 1989; Smith, North, McCool, & Shea, 1990; Zatzick et al., 2001).

8.4. THE COMPLEXITY OF MODELING PSYCHOPATHOLOGY AFTER DISASTER: UNDERSTANDING PTSD

Posttraumatic stress disorder (PTSD) has been widely studied following both natural and human-made disasters (for review, see, Breslau, Reboussin, Anthony, & Storr, 2005; Saigh & Bremner, 1999). The National Comorbidity Survey (NCS) found rates of PTSD to be 7.8%, while the National Women's Study (NWS) found rates of PTSD to be 12.3%. In an epidemiological study of people belonging to an urban health-maintenance organization in the United States, Breslau, Davis, Andreski, and Peterson (1991) found the lifetime prevalence of PTSD to be 9.2% for adults. PTSD symptoms can be debilitating and require psychotherapeutic and/or pharmacological intervention. The illness of PTSD – illness meaning the interaction of the disorder with an individual in a particular social context – is classically a waxing and waning illness that results in suffering, altered functional capacity, impairment, and disability across the domains of cognitive, emotional, social, and occupational function. These characteristics highlight various models of how PTSD becomes a disease and an illness. Such models for PTSD are more conceptually developed than for other trauma-related disorders and are necessary to direct future research and understanding for care provision.

PTSD can be considered the result of "resetting" our behavioral and physiologic response point. For example, the equations that describe the response of steel at room temperature are not the same as the equations that describe the response at zero degrees Kelvin. The actual system has changed because of exposure to an extreme environment. Might our brain and psychological system respond similarly to disasters? Or is PTSD actually the glue that holds the three primary symptom clusters – intrusion, avoidance, and arousal – together? For large segments of a disaster-exposed population, the transient occurrence of some symptoms of PTSD is not uncommon following traumatic events, ranging from terrorism to motor vehicle accidents or industrial explosions (Breslau et al., 1991, 2005). In this acute form, posttraumatic symptoms may be more like the common cold, experienced at some time in one's life by nearly all. Some colds of course progress to pneumonia and may create substantial illness, involve impairment of function, and be debilitating. Like the common cold, the symptoms that define PTSD may represent more serious illness if they persist and progress. For example, while we most often think of identification as a normally growth-promoting, health protective, and adaptive cognitive mechanism, the contribution of overidentification with the dead ("It could have been me. It could have been my child.") as a cognitive risk factor for development of PTSD (Ursano, Fullerton, Vance, & Kao, 1999; Ursano, Kao, & Fullerton, 1992) indicates excessive operation of this mechanism. Identification with the aggressor and the Stockholm syndrome are additional examples of identification gone awry.

PTSD can also be considered a "breakdown" of our usual neural functions. Engineering models are often built around the concept of "failure mode analysis," that is, "How can we break the machine? How does it breakdown?" Breakdown is not the same as function. It draws our attention to the neurobiology that may be least redundant, most subject to interference or disruption. PTSD perhaps is most basically a disorder of forgetting even more than of remembering; it is the inability to forget that leads to the pathology and suffering in PTSD. Forgetting is often overlooked or even avoided in clinical practice, yet it is a critical component of recovery. Of course if we could not "forget," our brains would rapidly be cluttered with information and observations and perhaps be more limited in cognitive control functions for other activities (Kuhl, Dudukovic, Kahn, & Wagner, 2007). Recent studies have demonstrated that forgetting is itself an active process accomplished through new learning. Thus, failure of the active extinction learning (failure to forget) exemplifies PTSD as modeled through failure mode analysis. How our "forgetting system" may break down is intrinsically a different question from how does it function. If PTSD is the failure to recover (rather than the onset of disease), what is the breakdown that has occurred?

8.4.1. Key Challenges in Understanding PTSD after Disaster

In the context of these overarching questions of disease modeling, considerations related to the observed variations in the clinical presentation of PTSD in terms of the nature and intensity of symptoms, time course and progression of symptoms, and relationship to putative biological markers for disease come to the fore. Models that contribute to an understanding of the illness for PTSD must account for phenomena such as delayed onset of symptoms and variability in the degree of disability resulting from traumatic exposure. Emerging understanding of the molecular pathophysiology of stress response, if not consistent with well-designed and replicated studies, will necessitate a reconsideration of the validity of the models themselves.

8.4.1.1. Delayed Onset

Delayed PTSD is likely a reflection of persistent low-level symptoms that only later manifest as symptoms meeting full diagnostic criteria. However, true delayed disorder (i.e., absence of symptoms for months to years following exposure, with subsequent full symptom presentation) is also well documented. The NCS reported 12% delayed onset for combat-related PTSD, which was four and a half times more likely than any other trauma (Kessler et al., 1995). Approximately 40% of those diagnosed with PTSD in the first 7 months after combat did not have the diagnosis until 7 months after combat injury (Grieger et al., 2006). Although longer-term data for the vast majority of natural disasters is lacking, well-designed longitudinal studies of war veterans provide additional evidence of the phenomenon of delayed onset PTSD. Of Israeli veterans of the 1982 Lebanon War followed for 20 years after the war, about 5% of those who had a combat stress reaction but *no PTSD* in the first 3 years postcombat met PTSD criteria at 20 years postcombat. Of those who had no combat stress reaction and no diagnosis of PTSD by 3 years postcombat, approximately 9% had PTSD 20 years postcombat. This study also demonstrated the waxing and waning of PTSD symptoms over time with significant changes in the persons meeting diagnostic criteria at the 1-, 2-, 3-, and 20-year time points in the study (Solomon & Mikulinver, 2006).

8.4.1.2. Disability and Impaired Function

In its acute form, such as after a motor vehicle accident, recovery from PTSD may occur in 6 to 12 months. Most studies suggest that PTSD is chronic (i.e., lasting greater than 6 months) and enduring (Institute of Medicine, Committee on

Veterans Compensation for PTSD, 2007; Institute of Medicine, Subcommittee on Posttraumatic Stress Disorder of the Committee on Gulf War and Health, 2007; Kessler et al., 1995). The symptoms and impaired function may be continuous or sporadic and are often aggravated by present adversity or new life stressors. Stressors associated with aging and accompanying changes in family, job, and health can contribute to exacerbations or new degrees of impairment. Some data indicate that aging and its accompanying loss of cognitive executive function may increase PTSD symptom severity and frequency in later life. Impaired sleep, jumpiness, startle, and intrusive thoughts or flashbacks can be greatly impairing or "under control," depending on the day and additional stress load. The frequency of symptoms, especially symptoms of arousal and numbing, can be particularly impairing. The severity of these symptoms can also vary greatly. Knowing the range of severity can provide some estimate of possible near-term disability. Comorbidity can substantially increase disability. In particular, the co-occurrence of depression (major depression, dysthymic disorder) and/or substance abuse is both common and generally increases functional impairment across all domains. The individual with PTSD may have high levels of symptoms with little evident impairment of social or vocational function. However, even without evidence of gross occupational or social dysfunction, substantial loss of the quality of life may result from having to avoid situations, having to delay or avoid being in certain environments with friends or family, or having to pick and choose when to be in situations which may be stressful.

Treatment intensity reflects the level of intervention necessary to effectively resolve the impairment caused by initial symptoms but also encompasses possible interaction with treatment for other comorbid disorders, the goal of relapse prevention, and the trajectory (to health or chronicity) of the psychopathology and required treatment interventions. One can make the case that the true target of treatment or intervention is never a disorder (i.e., merely the symptoms that define the disorder) but rather the impairment that it causes, from pain to loss of function. Understanding and quantifying impaired function after trauma exposure is essential for informing treatment, but the process inherently involves a great deal of complexity. A recent and thorough consideration of functional impairment in PTSD has been presented by a National Academies Institute of Medicine panel. This document identifies five areas of assessment for functional impairment: (1) degree of symptoms, (2) occupational impairment, (3) psychosocial impairment, (4) treatment intensity, complexity, and response, and (5) health-related quality of life. This comprehensive model of disability that has been proposed for PTSD is applicable to other mental illnesses and provides a roadmap to consider treatment of pathology across its five domains. Thus, quantifying the pathology of PTSD amounts to more than describing the frequency and intensity of operational criteria for reexperience, hyperarousal, and avoidance on an analog scale. Measures of pathology must account for the degree to which these symptoms result in loss of the ability to work, to form and sustain meaningful relationships, and to enjoy or find meaning in one's life.

8.4.2. Neuroscience, Genetics and the Psychopathology of Traumatic Exposure

Over the past few years we have seen the first studies of postmortem PTSD human brain tissue. The power of translating knowledge across human tissues, animal models, and biomarker studies is remarkable and offers opportunities to identify treatment targets not previously known (Ursano et al., 2008). These exciting and groundbreaking studies (Duric, Kang, Newton, Duman, and the PTSD Brain Bank Consortium, 2007; Zhang, Li, Li, & Ursano, 2007) have shown the possibility of identifying critical gene activity in PTSD related to various brain regions. In the prefrontal cortex and the amygdale, for instance, the studies have suggested unique genes in PTSD, some of which (i.e., *p11* gene) have also been shown in animal models of PTSD and initial biomarker studies. Recent studies of hurricane victims have shown that those with short/short genotype of the serotonin transporter gene (*5-HTTLPR*) and lower social supports were 20 times more likely to develop PTSD (Kilpatrick et al., 2007). The science of PTSD now requires a well-developed brain bank (Osuch et al., 2004) as exists for other psychiatric (e.g., schizophrenia, depression/mania) and neurological (e.g., amyotrophic lateral sclerosis, Alzheimer's) disorders.

Historically, adequate animal models have been central to developing effective therapeutic treatments, and the development of animal models is critical for the study of therapeutic and prophylactic treatments of stress-associated psychiatric disorders like PTSD. Our increased ability to identify end phenotypes – specific genetically linked behavioral characteristics/phenotypes (Gottesman & Gould, 2003) – that relate to PTSD will greatly enhance our neurobiological understanding of the disorder. Our present animal models of PTSD include models of predator stress, social defeat, shock, restraint and shock, and serial prolonged stress. None is complete, but each models different symptoms of the trauma response. Different strains as well as knock out and knock in strains offer additional sources of study. As yet, animal models have rarely addressed the observation that even in animals, not all animals (as in humans) develop PTSD-like symptoms in the particular model; this is an important area of additional future study for identifying resilience and risk gene targets.

8.5. CONCLUSION

Psychological responses to the traumatic events of disaster are diverse, and understanding their psychological, interpersonal, community, and neurobiological onset, as well as the factors sustaining responses, is only beginning. We have a good taxonomy describing the types of responses to expect, and we have a reasonable and evolving epidemiology quantifying the prevalence and time course of pathological responses. However, we are only now developing models for understanding the complexity of the unfolding disorder, distress, changed behavior, or, more importantly, the impairments that may occur and that may be assisted by intervention. Intervention studies of other psychiatric disorders such as depression, schizophrenia, and substance abuse now focus not only on the resolution of disease-specific symptoms, but also on measures such as frequency of clinic visits or hospitalization, employability, and changes in quality of life. Our conceptualization of postdisaster pathology and of PTSD certainly requires a broader view across the domains of suffering, altered functional capacity, and disability. Better understanding of the traumatic stress response that results in PTSD (whether acute and transient, protracted and severe, or delayed) may also shed light on the treatment of illnesses such as depression, substance use disorders, or other forms of anxiety when they emerge in the aftermath of disaster.

REFERENCES

Aguirre, B. E., Wenger, D., & Vigo, G. (1998). A test of the emergent norm theory of collective behavior. *Sociological Forum*, *13*, 301–320.

American Psychiatric Association (1994). *Diagnostic and statistical manual of mental disorders, 4th ed.* Washington, DC: American Psychiatric Press.

Benedek, D. M., & Fullerton, C. S. (2007). Translating five essential elements into programs and practice. *Psychiatry, 70*(4), 345–349.

Benedek, D. M., Holloway, H. C., & Becker, S. M. (2002). Emergency mental health management in bioterrorism events. *Emergency Medicine Clinics of North America*, *20*, 393–407.

Bolton, P., Bass, J., Betancourt, T., Speelman, L., Onyango, G., Clougherty, K. F., et al. (2007). Interventions for depression symptomatology among war-affected adolescents in Northern Uganda: A randomized controlled trial. *Journal of the American Medical Association*, *298*, 519–527.

Breslau, N., Davis, G. C., Andreski, P., & Peterson E. (1991). Traumatic events and posttraumatic stress disorder in an urban population of young adults. *Archives of General Psychiatry*, *48*, 216–222.

Breslau, N., Reboussin, B. A., Anthony, J. C., & Storr, C. L. (2005). The structure of posttraumatic stress disorder. Latent class analysis in 2 community samples. *Archives of General Psychiatry*, *62*, 1343–1351.

Brewin, C. R., Andrews, B., Rose, S., & Kirk, M. (1999). Acute stress disorder and posttraumatic stress disorder in victims of violent crime. *American Journal of Psychiatry, 156*, 360–366.

Bryant, R. A. (2005). Predicting posttraumatic stress disorder from acute reactions. *Journal of Trauma Dissociation, 6*(2), 5–15.

Bryant, R. A., & Harvey, A. G. (2000). *Acute stress disorder: A handbook of theory, assessment, and treatment.* Washington, DC: American Psychological Association.

Center for the Study of Traumatic Stress. (2005). *Courage to care. Psychological first aid: Helping victims in the immediate aftermath of disaster.* Bethesda, MD (February 2007); http://www.centerforthestudyoftraumaticstress.org/downloads/CTCPsychological FirstAid.pdf

Davidson, J. R. T., & Fairbank, J. A. (1992). The epidemiology of posttraumatic stress disorder. In J. R. T. Davidson, & E. B. Foa (Eds.), *Posttraumatic stress disorder: DSM-IV and beyond.* Washington, DC: American Psychiatric Press.

Duric, V., Kang, H. J., Newton, S. S., Duman, R. S., & the PTSD Brain Bank Consortium. (2007). Microarray-based analysis of gene expression in postmortem brains from patients diagnosed with PTSD. Neuroscience Society Annual Meeting, San Diego, CA.

Engel, C. C., & Katon, W. J. (1999). Population and need-based prevention of unexplained physical symptoms in the community (Appendix A). In L. M. Jollenbeck, P. K. Russell, & S. B. Guze (Eds.), *Strategies to protect the health of deployed US forces.* Washington, DC: National Academy Press.

Epstein, R. S., Fullerton, C. S., & Ursano, R. J. (1998). Posttraumatic stress disorder following an air disaster: A prospective study. *American Journal Psychiatry, 155*, 934–938.

Flynn, B. W. (2007). A sound blueprint for building a stronger home. *Psychiatry, 70*(4), 366–369.

Ford, C. V. (1997). Somatic symptoms, somatization, and traumatic stress: An overview. *Nordic Journal of Psychiatry, 51*, 5–13.

Forster, P. (1992). Nature and treatment of acute stress reactions. In L. S. Austin (Ed.), *Responding to disaster: A guide for mental health professionals.* Washington, DC: American Psychiatric Press.

Fullerton, C. S., & Ursano, R. J. (Eds.). (1997). *Posttraumatic stress disorder: Acute and long term responses to trauma and disaster.* Washington DC: American Psychiatric Press.

Fullerton, C. S., Ursano, R. J., & Wang, L. (2004). Acute stress disorder, posttraumatic stress disorder, and depression in disaster or rescue workers. *The American Journal of Psychiatry, 161*, 1370–1376.

Fullerton, C. S., Ursano, R. J., Kao, T. C., & Bharitya, V. R. (1999). Disaster-related bereavement: Acute symptoms and subsequent depression. *Aviation, Space, and Environmental Medicine, 70*, 902–909.

Galea, S., Ahern, J., Resnick, H., Kilpartick, D., Bucuvalas, M., Gold, J., et al. (2002). Psychological sequelae of the September 11 terrorist attacks in New York City. *The New England Journal of Medicine, 346*, 982–987.

Galea, S., Brewin, C. R., Jones, R. T., King, D. W., King, L. A., McNally, R. J., et al. (2007). Exposure to hurricane related stressors and mental illness after Katrina. *Archives of General Psychiatry, 64*(12), 1427–1434.

Galea, S., Vlahov, D., Resnick, H., Ahern, J., Susser, E., Gold, J., et al. (2003). Trends of probable posttraumatic stress disorder in New York City after the September 11 terrorist Attacks. *American Journal of Epidemiology, 158*(6), 514–524.

Gershon, R., Hogan, E., Qureshi, K. A., & Doll, L. (2004). Preliminary results from the world trade center evacuation study – New York City. *MMWR: Morbidity and Mortality Weekly Reports, 53*, 815–817.

Gottesman, I. I., & Gould, T. D. (2003). The endophenotype concept in psychiatry: Etymology and strategic intentions. *American Journal of Psychiatry, 160*, 636–645.

Grieger, T. A., Cozza, S. J., Ursano, R. J., Hoge, C., Martinez, P. E., Engel, C. C., et al. (2006). Posttraumatic stress disorder and depression in battle-injured soldiers. *American Journal of Psychiatry, 163*(10), 1777–1783.

Hobfoll, S. E., Watson, P., Bell, C. C., Bryant, R. A., Brymer, M. J., Friedman, M. J., et al. (2007). Five essential elements of immediate and mid-term mass trauma intervention: Empirical evidence. *Psychiatry, 70*(4), 283–315

Institute of Medicine. (2003). *Preparing for the psychological consequences of terrorism: A public health strategy.* Washington, DC: National Academies of Science, National Academies Press.

Institute of Medicine, Committee on Veterans Compensation for PTSD. (2007). *Posttraumatic stress disorder compensation and military service.* Washington, DC: National Academies of Science, National Academies Press.

Institute of Medicine, Subcommittee on Posttraumatic Stress Disorder of the Committee on Gulf War and Health. (2007). *Posttraumatic stress disorder: Diagnosis and assessment.* Washington, DC: National Academies of Science, National Academies Press.

Jacobson, A. M. (1996). The psychological care of patients with insulin-dependent diabetes mellitus. *New England Journal of Medicine, 334*, 1249–1253.

Kessler, R. C. (2000). Posttraumatic stress disorder: The burden to the individual and to society. *Journal of Clinical Psychiatry, 61*(5), 4–14.

Kessler, R., Brewin, C., Galea, S., Jones, R. T., Kendrick, D., King, D., et al. (2006). *Overview of baseline survey results: Hurricane Katrina community advisory group*. (February 2008); http://hurricanekatrina.med.harvard.edu/pdf/baseline_report%208-25-06.pdf.

Kessler, R. C., Barber, C., Birnbaum, H. G., Frank, R. G., Greenberg, P. E., Rose, R. M., et al. (1999). Depression in the workplace: Effects of short-term disability. *Health Affairs, 18*, 163–171.

Kessler, R. C., Sonnega, A., Bromet, E., Hughes, M., Nelson, C. B. (1995). Posttraumatic stress disorder in the National Comorbidity Survey. *Archives of General Psychiatry, 52*, 1048–1060.

Kilpatrick, D. G., Koenen, K. C., Ruggiero, K. J., Acierno, R., Galea, S., Resnick, H. S., et al. (2007). The serotonin transporter genotype and social support and moderation of post-traumatic stress disorder and depression in hurricane-exposed adults. *American Journal of Psychiatry, 64*, 1693–1699.

Kuhl, K. A., Dudukovic, N. M., Kahn, I., & Wagner, A. D. (2007). Decreased demands on cognitive control reveal the neural processing benefits of forgetting. *Nature Neuroscience, 10*(7), 908–914.

Kulka, R. A., Schlenger, W. E., Fairbank, J. A., Jordan, B. K., Hough, R. L., Marmar, C. R., et al. (1990). *Trauma and the Vietnam war generation*. New York: Brunner/ Mazel.

Leor, J., Poole, W. K., & Kloner, R. A. (1996). Sudden cardiac death triggered by an earthquake. *New England Journal of Medicine, 334*, 413–419.

McCarroll, J. E., Ursano, R. J., Fullerton, C. S., Liu, X., & Lundy, A. (2002). Somatic symptoms in Gulf War mortuary workers. *Psychosomatic Medicine, 64*, 29–33.

Mellman, T. A., Kulick-Bell, R., Ashlock, L. E., & Nolan, B. (1995). Sleep events among veterans with combat-related posttraumatic stress disorder. *American Journal of Psychiatry, 52*, 110–115.

Miguel-Tobal, J. J., Cano-Vindel, A., Gonzalez-Ordi, H., Iruarrizaga, I., Rudenstine, S., Vlahov, D., et al. (2006). PTSD and depression after the Madrid March 11 train bombings. *Journal of Traumatic Stress, 19*, 69–80.

Neria, Y., Gross, R., Litz, B., Maguen, S., Insel, B., Seirmarco, G., et al. (2007). Prevalence and psychological correlates of complicated grief among bereaved adults after September 11th attacks. *Journal of Traumatic Stress, 20*(3), 251–262.

Neria, Y., Nandi, A., & Galea, S. (2008). Post-traumatic stress disorder following disasters: A systematic review. *Psychological Medicine, 38*(4), 467–480.

Norris, F. H., Friedman, M. J., Watson, P. J., Byrne, C. M., Diaz, E., & Kaniasty, K. (2002). 60,000 disaster victims speak, Part I. An empirical review of the empirical literature: 1981–2001. *Psychiatry, 65*, 207–239.

North, C. S., Nixon, S. J., Shariat, S., Mallonee, S., McMillen, J. C., Spitznagel, E. L., et al. (1999). Psychiatric disorders among survivors of the Oklahoma City bombing. *Journal of the American Medical Association, 282*, 755–762.

North, C. S., Tivis, L., McMillen, J. C., Pfefferbaum, B., Spitznagel, E. L., Cox, J., et al. (2002). Psychiatric disorders in rescue workers after the Oklahoma City bombing. *American Journal of Psychiatry, 159*, 857–859.

Osuch, E., Ursano, R., Li, H., Webster, M., Hough, C., Fullerton, C., et al. (2004). Brain environment interactions: Stress, posttraumatic stress disorder, and the need for a postmortem brain collection. *Psychiatry, 67*, 353–383.

Prigerson, H. G., Shear, M. K., Jacobs, S., Kasl, S. V., Maciejewski, P. K., Silverman, G. K., et al. (2000). Grief and its relationship to posttraumatic stress disorder. In D. Nutt, J. R. Davidson, & J. Zohar (Eds.), *Posttraumatic stress disorders: Diagnosis, management and treatment*. New York, NY: Martin Dunitz Publishers.

Prigerson, H. G., Shear, M. K., Jacobs, S. C., Reynolds, C. F., Maciejewski, P. K., Davidson, J. R., et al. (1999). Consensus criteria for traumatic grief: A preliminary empirical test. *British Journal of Psychiatry, 174*, 67–73.

Raphael, B., Martinek, N., & Wooding, S. (2004). Assessing traumatic bereavement. In J. P. Wilson & T. M. Keane (Eds.), *Assessing psychological trauma and PTSD, 2nd ed*. New York: Guilford Press.

Raphael, B., & Minkov, C. (1999). Abnormal grief. *Current Opinion in Psychiatry, 12*, 99–102.

Raphael, B., & Wooding, S. (2004). Early mental health interventions for traumatic loss in adults. In B. T. Litz (Ed.), *Early intervention for trauma and traumatic loss*. New York: Guilford Press.

Rubin, G. J., Brewin, C. R., Greenberg, N., Simpson, J., & Wessely, S. (2005). Psychological and behavioural reactions to the bombings in London on 7 July 2005: Cross sectional survey of a representative sample of Londoners. *British Medical Journal, 331*, 606.

Rundell, J. R., & Ursano, R. J. (1996). Psychiatric responses to trauma. In R. J. Ursano & A. E. Norwood (Eds.), *Emotional aftermath of the persian gulf war: Veterans, communities, and nations*. Washington, DC: American Psychiatric Press.

Rundell, J.R., Ursano, R.J., Holloway, H.C., & Silberman, E.K. (1989). Psychiatric responses to trauma. *Hospital and Community Psychiatry, 40*, 68–74.

Saigh, P. A., & Bremner, J. D. (Eds.). (1999). *Posttraumatic stress disorder: A comprehensive text*. Boston, MA: Allyn & Bacon.

Shalev, A., Bleich, A., & Ursano, R.J. (1990). Posttraumatic stress disorder: Somatic comorbidity and effort tolerance. *Psychosomatics, 31*, 197–203.

Shear, K., Frank, E., Houck, P.R., & Reynolds, C.F. III (2005). Treatment of Complicated Grief: a Randomized Controlled Trial *JAMA, 293*, 2601–2608

Shear, M.K., Frank, E., Foa, E., Cherry, C., Reynolds, C.F., Vander Bilt, J., et al. (2001). Traumatic grief treatment: A pilot study. *The American Journal of Psychiatry, 158*, 1506–1508.

Shear, M.K., Frank, E., Houck, P.R., & Reynolds, C.F. (2005). Treatment of complicated grief. A randomized controlled trial. *Journal of the American Medical Association, 293*(21), 2601–2608.

Shore, J.H., Vollmer, W.M., & Tatum, E.L. (1989). Community patterns of posttraumatic stress disorders. *Journal of Nervous and Mental Disease, 177*, 681–685.

Smith, E.M., North, C.S., McCool, R.E., & Shea, J.M. (1990). Acute postdisaster psychiatric disorders: Identification of those at risk. *American Journal of Psychiatry, 147*, 202–206.

Solomon, S., & Mikulinver, M. (2006). Trajectories of PTSD: A 20 year longitudinal study. *American Journal of Psychiatry, 163*(4), 659–666.

Solomon, S.D., & Smith, E.M. (1994). Social support and perceived control as moderators of responses to dioxin and flood exposure. In R.J. Ursano, B.G. McCaughey, & C. S. Fullerton (Eds.), *Individual and community responses to trauma and disaster*. Cambridge: Cambridge University Press.

Terr, L.C. (1981). "Forbidden games": Post-traumatic child's play. *Journal of the American Academy of Child Psychiatry, 20*, 741–760.

Project Plowshares. (2005). *Armed conflicts report*. (July 2007); http://www.ploughshares.ca/libraries/monitor/monj05f.htm

(2007). *Armed conflicts report*. (August 2007); http://www.ploughshares.ca/libraries/ACRText/Summary2006.pdf

U.S. Geological Survey. (2007). *National earthquake information center*. (February, 2008); http://earthquake.usgs.gov/eqcenter/

Ursano, R.J. (2006). Hurricane Katrina: Science and research. Presented at the 22nd Annual Rosalynn Carter Symposium on Mental Health Policy. U.S. Psychology Congress: Mental health in the wake of hurricane Katrina. The Carter Center: Atlanta, Georgia.

Ursano, R.J., & Fullerton, C.S. (1990). Cognitive and behavioral responses to trauma. *The Journal of Applied Psychology, 20*, 1766–1775.

(2000). Posttraumatic stress disorder: Cerebellar regulation of psychological, interpersonal and biological responses to trauma. *Psychiatry, 62*, 325–328.

Ursano, R.J., Fullerton, C.S., Bhartiya, V., & Kao, T.C. (1995). Longitudinal assessment of posttraumatic stress disorder and depression after exposure to traumatic death. *The Journal of Nervous and Mental disease, 183*, 36–42.

Ursano, R.J., Fullerton, C.S., Vance, K., & Kao, T.C. (1999). Posttraumatic stress disorder and identification in disaster workers. *The American Journal of Psychiatry, 156*, 353–359.

Ursano, R.J., Fullerton, C.S., Weisaeth, L., & Raphael, B. (2007). Individual and community responses to disasters. In R. J. Ursano, C. S. Fullerton, L. Weisaeth, & B. Raphael (Eds.), *Textbook of disaster psychiatry*. Cambridge: Cambridge University Press.

(2007a). Public health and disaster mental health: Preparing, responding and recovering. In R. J. Ursano, C. S. Fullerton, L. Weisaeth, & B. Raphael (Eds.), *Textbook of disaster psychiatry*. Cambridge: Cambridge University Press.

(2007b). Individual and community responses to disasters. In R. J. Ursano, C. S. Fullerton, L. Weisaeth, & B. Raphael (Eds.), *Textbook of disaster psychiatry*. Cambridge: Cambridge University Press.

Ursano, R.J., Kao, T.C., & Fullerton C.S. (1992). Posttraumatic stress disorder and meaning: Structuring human chaos. *The Journal of Nervous and Mental Disease, 180*, 756–759.

Ursano, R.J., Li, H., Zhang, L., Hough, C.J., Fullerton, C.S., Benedek, D.M., et al. (2008). Models of PTSD and traumatic stress: The importance of research "from bedside to bench to bedside" in neuroscience of PTSD. In R. de Kloet & E. Vermetten (Eds.), *Progress in brain research*. Amsterdam: Elsevier Press.

Ursano, R.J. & Shaw, J.A. (2007). Children of war and opportunities for peace. *Journal of the American Medical Association, 298*, 567–568.

Vlahov, D., Galea, S., Resnick, H., Boscarino, J.A., Bucuvalas, M., Gold, J., et al. (2002). Increased use of cigarettes, alcohol, and marijuana among Manhattan, New York, residents after the September 11th terrorist attacks. *American Journal of Epidemiology, 155*, 988–996.

Watson P.J. (2007). Early intervention for trauma-related problems following mass trauma. In R.J. Ursano, C. S. Fullerton, L. Weisaeth, & B. Raphael (Eds.), *Textbook of disaster psychiatry*. Cambridge: Cambridge University Press.

Watson, P.J., & Shalev, A.Y. (2005). Assessment and treatment of adult acute responses to traumatic stress following mass traumatic events. *CNS Spectrums*, *10*(2), 123–131.

World Health Organization. (2006). *Mental health atlas: Implications for policy development*. Geneva, Switzerland: Department of Mental Health and Substance Dependence.

(2003). *Mental health in emergencies: Mental and social aspects of health of populations exposed to extreme stressors*. Geneva, Switzerland: Department of Mental Health and Substance Dependence.

World Health Organization, Collaborating Centre for Research on the Epidemiology of Disasters. (2006). *EM-DAT: The OFDA/CRED International Disaster Database*. (February 2008); http://www.em-dat.net/

Zatzick, D.F., Kang, S.M., Hinton, L., Kelly, R.H., Hilty, D.M., Franz, C.E., et al. (2001). Posttraumatic concerns: A patient-centered approach to outcome assessment after traumatic physical injury. *Medical Care*, *39*, 327–339.

Zhang, L., Li, H., Li, X.X., & Ursano, R.J. (2007). *P11 a potential biomarker for PTSD. Poster. Presented at Society of Neuroscience*. San Diego, California.

PART THREE

Vulnerability and Resilience

9 Resilience after Disaster

GEORGE A. BONANNO AND SUMATI GUPTA

9.1. INTRODUCTION

Although, we may wish otherwise, disasters do happen. In any given year, human beings can be subject to severe flooding, devastating hurricanes, war, and, especially in recent years, the threat and sometimes horror of a large-scale terrorist attack. When imagining what the dread victims must face after unexpected and catastrophic events, people often assume that they will suffer lasting emotional damage. However, this is usually not the case. Research on potentially traumatic events (PTEs) has consistently revealed a wide range of reactions; apart from a limited subset of people who suffer extreme distress, most people cope with such events extremely well (Bonanno, 2004, 2005). In this chapter, we use the phrase "potentially traumatic" to underscore that there are measurable and important individual differences in how people respond to such events (Bonanno, 2005). Simply put, highly aversive events that fall outside the range of normal experience are "potentially" traumatic because not everyone experiences them as traumatic.

We begin by briefly reviewing the historical background on the construct of psychological trauma, and then consider recent empirical studies on individual differences in response to PTEs. We consider common outcomes people exhibit after exposure to PTEs, including both chronic and pathological reactions as well as relatively healthy reactions. We focus, in particular, on the growing evidence for the human capacity to thrive even after the most difficult of experiences and on the emergent concept of psychological resilience. Finally, we review the available evidence on factors that predict who will and who will not cope well with such events and suggest ways in which these data might inform a more empirically sound public health conception of traumatic events.

9.2. A BRIEF HISTORY OF THE CONCEPT OF PSYCHOLOGICAL TRAUMA

Almost since the beginning of psychology and psychiatry as formal disciplines, researchers, theorists, and practitioners have looked at violent or life-threatening events as antecedents to psychological and physiological dysfunction (Ellenberger, 1970; Lamprecht & Sack, 2002). In one of the first theoretical accounts of psychological trauma, Erichsen (1866) proposed a hypothetical link between psychological dysfunction and microtraumas of the spinal cord caused by railway accidents or "railroad spine syndrome." Later, Oppenheim (1889) inaugurated the use of a medical term, "trauma," to describe psychological reactions to acute stressors. Around this same time, Charcot (1887) and Janet (1889) published highly influential accounts of the links between traumatic experiences and dissociative symptoms.

Over the next several decades, war and an unprecedented military technology brought increasing attention to combat-related traumata. During the U.S. Civil War, the terms "soldier's heart" or "Da Costa's Syndrome" were used to describe the emotional and physical symptoms experienced by severely distressed veterans (Da Costa, 1871; Myers, 1870). Later, Myers (1915) coined the term "shell shock" to describe the psychological devastation wrought by trench warfare in World War I. Although, in the years that followed, there was considerable confusion and controversy over the nature of traumatic events and whether to consider psychological reactions as malingering, weakness, or genuine dysfunction worthy of compassion and treatment (Lamprecht & Sack, 2002; McFarlane & Yehuda, 1996), the lucid accounts of genuine combat trauma reactions during World War II (Keegan, 1976) again shifted debate in the direction of our current conceptions of posttraumatic stress disorder (PTSD). These accounts were captured in Kardiner's (1941) pioneering description of the "*Traumatic neuroses of war*." Kardiner's formulation still tended to place responsibility for traumatic events, primarily within the individual, as for example, in his retention of the term "neurosis." However, as traumatic reactions were gradually formalized and objectified, first as "gross stress reactions" in the *Diagnostic and statistical manual of mental disorders* (DSM)-I (APA, 1952), then as "transient situational disturbance" in the DSM-II (APA, 1968), and finally as PTSD in DSM-III (APA, 1980), the emphasis continued to shift toward an understanding of these symptoms as natural human reactions to unnatural or highly aversive situations.

Since its emergence as a legitimate diagnostic category, PTSD has dominated both scholarly and lay conceptions of psychological trauma (McNally, 2003). An obvious reason for the focus on PTSD is its crucial implications for public health. PTSD is a debilitating condition, and given the prevalence with which people are exposed to PTEs during a lifetime, even at low frequencies, it presents a potentially serious public health burden. A second reason why the field has focused on PTSD has to do with lingering controversies about its definition and use. For example, as several studies have now shown (Browman-Fulks et al., 2006; Ruscio, Ruscio, & Keane, 2002) PTSD symptoms do not tend to behave like a taxon or categorical variable, but rather as a continuous marker of dysfunction. Such an analysis suggests the sobering conclusion that however PTSD is defined, it will always be to some extent an arbitrary categorization.

Of even greater relevance to the concerns of this article, however, is the sometimes elusive distinction between genuine psychological trauma and malingering. This distinction has played an important role in the experiences of recent U.S. soldiers fighting in Iraq and Afghanistan. Media accounts have dramatized their reports of fears about stigmatization or even retribution for mental duress (Zwerdling, 2006). Moreover, an encompassing research study found that while many Army and Marine Corps returning from Iraq and Afghanistan were at significant risk of mental health problems, they desired but did not seek treatment because of prevailing stigmas about perceptions of weakness (Hoge et al., 2004).

The same historical patterns are evident in the literature on bereavement. The first systematic empirical study of the grieving processes was not conducted until near the midpoint of the twentieth century (Lindemann, 1944). Several decades passed before further bereavement studies would appear (e.g., Marris, 1958; Parkes 1964; Parkes & Brown, 1972). Because these earlier studies were cross-sectional and retrospective, however, they tended to overrepresent acute and chronic grief reactions and offered little insight about the possibility of resilience in the face of loss. In a report summarizing current knowledge about bereavement at the time of its writing, Osterweis, Soloman, and Green (1984) concluded that it was commonly assumed, particularly by clinicians "that the absence of grieving phenomena following bereavement represents some form of personality pathology" (p. 18). Bowlby (1980) considered the "prolonged absence of conscious grieving" (p. 138) as a type of disordered mourning. Similarly, according to Rando (1993), bereaved individuals who do not experience intense distress following a loss are in a state of denial and have "a powerful ability to block out reality" (p. 158). In 1993, Middleton, Moylan, and their colleagues surveyed self-identified bereavement experts and reported that a majority (65%) endorsed beliefs that "absent grief" exists, that it usually stems from denial or inhibition, and that it is generally maladaptive in the long run.

9.3. INDIVIDUAL DIFFERENCES

In stark contrast to the binary view of traumatic stress, empirical studies reveal a number of unique and variable patterns amongst individual responses to PTEs. Most of the variability can be captured by four prototypical trajectories: chronic dysfunction, delayed reactions, resilience, and recovery (Bonanno, 2004). We present these trajectories graphically in Figure 9.1 and elaborate on each trajectory briefly in the subsequent text.

9.3.1. Chronic Dysfunction

Despite the highly aversive nature of PTEs, it is now well established that only a relatively small subset of those exposed to such events will typically exhibit chronic pathological reactions. Although there is considerable variability in the type, severity, and duration of PTEs, PTSD is typically observed in 5% to 10% of exposed individuals (Kessler, Sonnega, Bromet, Hughes, & Nelson, 1995). In cases when exposure is exceptionally prolonged or aversive, the proportion for PTSD or other types of psychopathology may reach higher levels, sometimes as high as one-third of the sample. For example, a population-based survey conducted 1 month after the September 11th terrorist attack in New York City estimated that PTSD among Manhattan residents was 7.5% and that 17.4% would meet criteria for subsyndromal PTSD (high symptom levels that do not meet full diagnostic criteria) (Galea et al., 2002). PTSD was more likely if traumatic exposure was high. Among those physically injured in the attack, for example, PTSD prevalence rose to 26% (Bonanno, Galea, Bucciarelli, & Vlahov, 2006). Similarly, in a careful reanalysis of the National Vietnam Veterans Readjustment data, a representative sample of 1,200 veterans, chronic PTSD was estimated at 9% but rose to 28% among veterans with the highest levels of combat exposure (Dohrenwend et al., 2006).

Studies of psychopathology during bereavement also suggest similar proportions. Typically only approximately 10% of bereaved people will exhibit chronically elevated grief reactions (Bonanno &

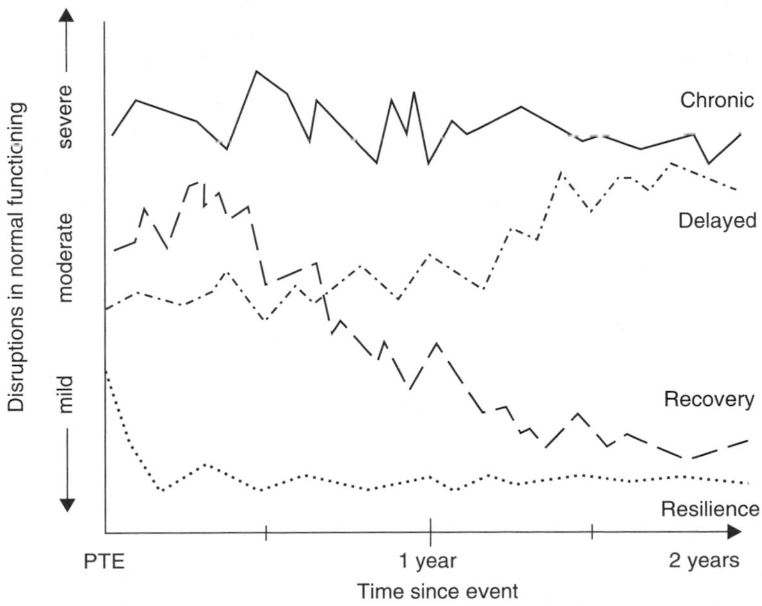

Figure 9.1. Prototypical patterns of disruption in normal functioning across time following interpersonal loss and potentially traumatic events. Figure adapted from Bonanno (2004).

Kaltman, 2001). However, as was the case for PTEs in general, chronic grief reactions tend to be more prevalent following more extreme losses, such as when the death-event involves violence (Kaltman & Bonanno, 1999, 2003; Zisook, Chentsova-Dutton, & Shuchter, 1998) or when the lost loved one is a child (Bonanno, Papa, Lalande, Zhang, & Noll, 2005).

Somewhat surprising, there is relatively little data on traumatic events and grief reactions among children. Systematic studies of children's bereavement reactions report similar levels of complicated grief as in adult studies (e.g., Christ, 2000). The data that are available on PTSD, however, suggest that the disorder may be less frequent among children and young adults (Copeland, Keeler, Angold, & Costello, 2007). However, as we discuss later, it is important to keep in mind that the question of adjustment is in many ways more complex among children, and therefore these proportions should be considered with caution. For example, children exposed to aversive events may fail to evidence PTSD or complicated grief but show increased externalizing symptoms, substance use, academic problems, or peer conflict.

9.3.2. Delayed Reactions

It has been widely assumed in the bereavement literature that the absence of overt signs of grieving, by virtue of its assumed link with denial, will eventually manifest in delayed grief reactions (e.g., Bowlby, 1980; Deutsch, 1937; Osterweis et al., 1984; Parkes & Weiss, 1983; Rando, 1993; Sanders, 1993). Although this assumption has been widely endorsed by self-identified grief experts (Middleton et al., 1993), reliable empirical evidence for delayed grief has never been reported (Bonanno & Kaltman, 1999; Wortman & Silver, 1989), even in longitudinal studies explicitly designed to measure the phenomenon (e.g., Bonanno & Field, 2001; Middleton, Burnett, Raphael, & Martinek, 1996). There is some evidence for delayed PTSD reactions following potentially traumatic events, occurring in approximately 5% to 10% of exposed individuals (Bonanno et al., 2005; Buckley, Blanchard, & Hickling, 1996). However, this pattern does not tend to conform to the traditional idea of denial manifesting in delayed reactions. Rather, exposed individuals who eventually manifest delayed PTSD tend to have had relatively high levels of symptoms in the aftermath of the stressor event (e.g., Bonanno et al., 2005; Buckley et al., 1996). Thus, the delayed pattern is more appropriately conceptualized as subthreshold psychopathology that gradually grew worse over time (Bonanno, 2006; Buckley et al., 1996).

9.3.3. Resilience and Recovery

Until recently, it was widely assumed that the enduring absence of trauma symptoms following exposure to a PTE was rare and would occur only in people with exceptional emotional strength (Casella & Motta, 1990; McFarlane & Yehuda, 1996; Tucker et al., 2002). Additionally, as noted earlier, bereavement theorists have persistently regarded the relative absence of grief as a form of denial or hidden psychopathology (Middleton et al., 1993). There is compelling evidence, however, that the ability to continue functioning after exposure to PTE is not rare and neither a sign of exceptional strength nor of psychopathology. Rather, this kind of resilience is common and appears to be a fundamental feature of normal coping skills (Bonanno, 2004). Moreover, as a growing number of studies have shown, resilience and recovery can be mapped as discrete and empirically separable outcome trajectories. Distinctions between resilience and recovery have been identified following loss (e.g., Bonanno et al., 2002), major illness (e.g., Deshields, Tibbs, Fan, Taylor, 2006), and close exposure to large-scale terrorist attack (e.g., Bonanno et al., 2005).

9.4. RESILIENCE TO TRAUMATIC EVENTS

Major advances in theory and research on resilience to adversity came from developmental psychologists and psychiatrists during the 1970s. These pioneering researchers documented the large number of children who, despite growing up in harsh socioeconomic circumstances, nonetheless evidenced healthy developmental trajectories (e.g., Garmezy, 1991; Murphy & Moriarty, 1976; Rutter, 1979; Werner & Smith, 1982). A surprising feature of this work was that resilience in children at risk turned out to be surprisingly common, a kind of "ordinary magic" (Masten, 2001). Whereas traditional deficit-focused models of development had assumed that only children with remarkable coping ability could thrive in such adverse contexts, a growing body of evidence began to suggest that resilience is a result of normal human adaptational mechanisms (Masten, 2001).

Trauma theorists also offered early theoretical accounts of widespread resilience (Janis, 1951; Rachman, 1978). However, much of this work was based on anecdotal and unsystematic accounts. It is only more recently that the resilience construct has gained currency among trauma researchers and the differences between resilience in response to chronic and acute stressors have become apparent (Bonanno, 2004, 2005). One of the key differences appears to be in the way different types of stressors influence outcome. While the definition of healthy adaptation is a complex issue in developing children (Luthar, Cicchetti, & Becker, 2000; Masten, 2001), this situation is arguably more straightforward for adults exposed to PTEs (Bonanno, 2004; 2005). For example, children at risk may evidence competence in one domain but fail to meet long-term developmental challenges in other domains (e.g., Luthar, Doernberger, & Zigler, 1993). For adults, most – but certainly not all – of the PTEs they might be confronted with can be classified as isolated stressor events (e.g., an automobile accident) that occur in a broader context of otherwise normative (i.e., low stress) circumstances. Of course, adults may also be exposed to concomitant stressors accompanying or extending the PTE (e.g., enduring health problems or change in financial situation). However, this level of variability is usually straightforward and can be measured with a reasonable degree of reliability (Bonanno, Moskowitz, Papa, & Folkman, 2005). Finally, because developmental considerations are less pronounced in adults, responses to PTEs can usually be assessed in terms of deviation from or return to normative (baseline) functioning (Carver, 1998) rather than in terms of long-term changes in developmental trajectory.

On the basis of the aforementioned considerations, Bonanno (2004) extended previous definitions of resilience developed in response to chronic adversity by proposing a definition of "resilience" in specific reference to isolated PTEs. Accordingly, "resilience to traumatic events" was defined as

> the ability of adults in otherwise normal circumstances who are exposed to an isolated and potentially highly disruptive event such as the death of a close relation or a violent or life-threatening situation to maintain relatively stable, healthy levels of psychological and physical functioning...as well as the capacity for generative experiences and positive emotions (p. 20–21).

This definition contrasts resilience with a more traditional *recovery* from trauma pathway, which is characterized by readily observable elevations in psychological symptoms that endure for at least several months before gradually returning to baseline, pretrauma levels. It is important to note that although some resilient individuals manage to endure PTEs without any signs of distress or any disruptions in functioning, the complete absence of any trauma response appears to be a relatively rare phenomenon (Bonanno et al., 2002). Most of the people who ultimately show a resilient profile do tend to experience at least some form of temporary stress reaction. However, these reactions are typically only mild in degree, transient, and do not significantly interfere with the ability to continue functioning (Bonanno et al., 2002, 2005; Bisconti, Bergman, & Boker, 2006; Ong, Bergman, Bisconti, & Wallance, 2006). For example, resilient individuals may have difficulty sleeping or experience intrusive thoughts or memories of the event for several days or even weeks, but most can still manage to adequately perform the tasks of their daily life, career, or care for others. This is not to say, of course, that people showing resilient outcomes were not upset, disturbed, or unhappy about the occurrence of the event. Our point is merely that as undesirable as PTEs might be, resilient individuals manage to cope with such events reasonably well and are able to continue meeting the daily demands of their normal lives.

Some of the first direct evidence for widespread adult resilience in the face of an isolated but potentially devastating stressor event came from studies of how people cope with the death of a loved one (Bonanno et al., 2002, 2005). Across these studies, the proportions of bereaved people exhibiting resilient outcomes consistently hovered near half of the sample. It was also noteworthy that the prevalence remained relatively consistent across studies using both longitudinal and prospective designs (Bonanno et al., 2002) and across a variety of measures of adaptation, including low levels of psychopathological symptoms, but also measures of positive adjustment, such as anonymous ratings of different types of adjustment obtained from close friends and measures of positive emotional experiences (Bonanno et al., 2005). One possible criticism of the evidence from bereavement studies, however, is that the death of a spouse does not capture the same potential for severe trauma inherent in more violent or life-threatening events (Litz, 2005; Roisman, 2005).

A study of resilience among high-exposure survivors of the 2001 terrorist attack on the World Trade Center (WTC) in New York City partially addressed this concern (Bonanno et al., 2005). The sample was comprised of individuals either in or near the WTC towers at the time of the attack. Resilient individuals were defined as having little or no symptoms of PTSD or depression across the first 18 months following exposure. Resilient individuals in this study were also defined as having high levels of positive adjustment on the basis of anonymous ratings obtained from their close friends and relatives, and again, they had higher levels of positive effect compared with other participants. An important limitation of this study, however, was the relatively small size of the sample, which raises questions about generalizability and possible selection biases.

The issue of trauma exposure was examined more directly and more broadly in another study of resilience after September 11th. Bonanno, Galea, Bucciarelli, and Vlahov (2006) examined the prevalence of resilient outcomes in New York City and the contiguous geographic area during the first 6 months following the attack using data from a large probability sample ($N = 2{,}752$). The sample closely matched the most recent New York census data (Galea, Ahern, et al., 2002; Galea et al., 2002, 2003). What is more, measurements of PTSD symptoms in this sample were shown to be highly reliable at 1, 4, and 6 months post–September 11th (Resnick, Galea, Kilpatrick, & Vlahov, 2004). Of particular importance, as the sample varied in both geographic location and experiences during and after the attacks, it was possible to directly compare the prevalence of resilient outcomes across different levels of potential traumatic event exposure. Owing to the large-scale nature of the study, it was not possible to use the same multifaceted measures of resilience employed in other trauma studies. For this reason, these researchers adopted the relatively conservative approach used in studies of the absence of depression (e.g., Judd, Akiskal, & Paulus, 1997) and defined a resilient outcome as either one or zero PTSD symptoms during the first 6 months after the attack. Despite this conservative definition, widespread resilience was again observed. Across most exposure groups, the proportion with resilient outcomes was at or above 50% of the sample. Even among the groups with the most pernicious levels of exposure and highest probable PTSD, the proportion that was resilient never dropped below one-third of the sample.

Although the virtual absence of PTSD symptoms among these participants suggests that the study participants had coped well after the disaster, it is possible that the potential distress of the attack may have manifested in other domains of adjustment (Bonanno et al., 2005; Luthar et al., 1993). Specifically, high-exposure participants may have become more depressed or increase their substance use (e.g., alcohol or cigarettes). This was not the case; however, as resilient individuals in the study had extremely low levels of depression (1.3%), reported significantly lower use of cigarettes (19.9%) and marijuana (3.8%) compared with other participants, and showed no differences from other participants in alcohol consumption. Together, these findings argue that participants with a resilient outcome had indeed experienced a healthy course of adjustment.

Similar findings on resilience have also begun to emerge following potentially traumatic (i.e., life-threatening) medical stressors. Deshields and colleagues (2006) mapped the same outcome trajectories depicted in Figure 9.1 using depression scores obtained from women immediately following radiation treatment for breast cancer and again 3 and 6 months after treatment. Although 21% of the sample evidenced clinically significant levels of depression at 6 months, the majority (61%) had extremely low levels of depression throughout the study.

Evidence for widespread resilience among survivors of the severe acute respiratory syndrome (SARS) epidemic has also recently been reported (Bonanno et al., in press). SARS is a highly contagious respiratory illness first reported in Guangdong Province, People's Republic of China, toward the end of 2002. Unknown before its first appearance, it spread rapidly and broadly, and by the spring of 2003 over 8,000 individuals were infected in over 30 different countries, which led to the perception of this event as a prototype for a global biological pandemic. Moreover, SARS was potentially lethal. When it was finally contained in the summer of 2003, through a combination of stringent hygiene precautions and quarantine measures, SARS had already claimed 800 lives (Ho, 2003; Ho, Kwong-Lo, Mak, & Wong, 2005; Peiris et al., 2003).

The sample used in the Bonanno and colleagues (in press) study comprised the majority of hospitalized survivors of the 2003 epidemic in Hong Kong. The data from Hong Kong was particularly well suited for examination of individual differences. Due to its function as major port city and locus of international travel contiguous with the Chinese mainland, Hong Kong was hard hit by the epidemic. Although comparatively small in size and population, Hong Kong was, nonetheless, second only to mainland China in total number of infected individuals (N = 1,755) and total number of SARS-related deaths (N = 299) (World Health Organization, 2003). Moreover, because a central public institution, the Hospital Authority, manages most hospital care in Hong Kong, it was possible to follow the majority of the hospitalized survivors over time and to examine factors that most clearly predicted long-term psychological outcome.

Measures of psychological functioning in this sample indicated that on an average the survivors were functioning well below normal levels at each assessment point during the first 18 months after hospitalization. Such a low level of psychological functioning clearly demonstrated the potentially devastating impact of a biological epidemic. However, a different story, one consistent with other disaster and traumatic event studies, emerged when we examined long-term adjustment from an individual differences perspective. Using latent class growth curve modeling, we found ample evidence for the psychological cost of SARS. Forty-two percent of the sample had chronically low levels of psychological functioning across the first 18 months after hospitalization. However, we also found ample evidence for resilience. Thirty-five percent of the sample had high levels of psychological functioning at each assessment point through 18 months, a proportion comparable to that observed in other disaster and traumatic event studies.

9.5. A HETEROGENEOUS ARRAY OF RISK AND PROTECTIVE FACTORS

If we assume, as traditional theorists have, that resilience is rare, then it would make sense to look for a single dominant resilience factor, most likely the one located within the individual (i.e., a resilient personality characteristic). However, since resilience is not rare, then it follows that there must be multiple protective factors that might buffer against adversity, including person-centered variables (e.g., coping skills, personality) (Bonanno, 2005) and sociocontextual factors (e.g., supportive relations, community resources) (Hobfoll, 2002).

A particularly compelling aspect of this story is that resilience does not result even from any one dominant set of factors. Rather, there appears to be multiple independent risk and protective factors, each contributing to or subtracting from the overall likelihood of a resilient outcome. Consider, for example, the idea of a resilient personality. There is undoubtedly some role for personality in resilience to traumatic events. However, as Mischel (1969) famously observed, personality rarely explains more than 10% of the actual variance in people's behavior across situations. It is more appropriate and more accurate, therefore, to conceive of personality as one of many potential sources of resilient outcomes.

9.5.1. Demographic Variables

Previous studies have documented the link between trauma-related psychopathology and a number of demographic variables (Brewin, Andrews, & Valentine, 2000). For example, a study of survivors of the 2005 Hurricane Katrina found that those who suffered from any DSM-IV anxiety or mood disorders tended to be less than 60 years old, female, unemployed, unmarried, and had not completed an undergraduate education (Galea et al., 2007). In contrast, resilience to trauma following disaster has been associated with male gender, older age, and greater education (Bonanno, Galea, Bucciarelli, Vlahov, 2007; Bonanno et al., in press). Racial/ethnic minority status is often identified as a risk factor for the development of PTSD (e.g., Breslau, Peterson, Poisson, Schultz, & Lucia, 2004). The risk for PTSD appears to be greatest for Hispanics (e.g., Kulka et al., 1990; Perilla, Norris, & Lavizzo, 2002), whereas, the findings are somewhat more equivocal for African Americans (Mainous, Smith, Acierno, & Geesey, 2005; Perilla et al., 2002). However, in Western industrialized cultures, race, and ethnicity often are often confounded with low socioeconomic status, and studies reporting racial/ethnic differences in PTSD often fail to account for this overlap (McGruder-Johnson et al., 2000). Consequently, when socioeconomic status is statistically controlled, racial/ethnic effects in response to PTEs tend to disappear (e.g., Adams & Boscarino, 2005). A recent exception, however, was a finding that among New Yorkers, ethnic Chinese were considerably more likely to be resilient following the September 11th attack (Bonanno et al., 2007).

9.5.2. Personal and Social Resources

A number of theorists have argued for the crucial role played by social and personal resources in successful coping with stress (Hobfoll, 2002; Holahan & Moos, 1991; Lazarus & Folkman, 1984; Murrell & Norris, 1983). There is also considerable research linking resources or change in resources with adjustment following PTEs (Freedy, Shaw, Jarrel, & Master, 1992; Ironson et al., 1997; Kaniasty & Norris, 1993; Norris & Kaniasty, 1996). One of the most influential theories in this area, Hobfoll's (1989; 2002) conservation of resources (CORs) theory, allots a central role for resource change (i.e., resource loss or gain) and its influence on the generation or amelioration of stress.

Social resources are one of the most consistently identified predictors of adjustment following PTEs. For example, Hobfoll, Freedy, and colleagues (1990) argued that people strive to maintain and protect their resources in times of stress and that social resources (e.g., social support) act as a major vehicle for resources that are beyond one's personal resources. Across several studies investigating PTSD in, both, civilian and combat-exposed populations, lower levels of social support during and after PTE exposure were associated with increased symptoms (Brewin et al., 2000). Furthermore, following the September 11th terrorist attacks, lower levels of social support among New Yorkers in the months before the attacks were associated with increased PTSD symptoms (Galea, Ahern, et al., 2002; Galea, Resnick, et al., 2002) and decreased probability of resilience (Bonanno, Galea, et al., 2006). Similarly, a loss in resources after the attacks was associated with probable depression and PTSD in the year following the attacks (Hobfoll, Tracy, & Galea, 2006). In addition to war and terrorism, natural disasters are also events for which social support is likely to minimize distress (Norris & Kaniasty, 1996). Specifically, following hurricanes Hugo and Andrew, perceived social support mediated the relationship between disaster exposure and long-term distress and the relationship between received support and long-term distress (Norris & Kaniasty, 1996). Supportive resources have also been found to predict resilience following biodisaster, such as SARS (Bonanno et al., in press).

Some theorists believe that personality characteristics of survivors of PTEs influence the extent to which they seek social support and perceive their social support networks (e.g., Hobfoll & Freedy, 1990; Sarason et al., 1991). One such characteristic includes a ruminative coping style in which survivors repeatedly and passively think about their reactions to a traumatic event (Nolen-Hoeksema, 1991). Ironically, bereaved people with a ruminative coping style have been found to seek out more social support, probably as a result of their excessive worry about the loss, and to benefit more from the support they received (Nolen-Hoeksema & Davis, 1999). This effect is moderated, however, by the availability and quality of support. Bereaved ruminators who felt their family or friends were critical and unsupportive tended to experience greater levels of distress. A related factor, cognitive ability, has also been widely observed as a protective resource against PTSD in both children (Breslau, Lucia, & Alvarado, 2006) and adults (Brewin et al., 2000). Although there is not yet data linking cognitive resources to resilience in adults exposed to PTEs, such a link is highly probable.

9.5.3. Additional Life Stress

There is solid evidence linking PTSD with increased life stress before and following the traumatic event (Brewin et al., 2000; Kubiak, 2005; Shalev, Bonne, & Eth, 1996). For example, a study of the March 2004 terrorist bombing of the railways in Madrid, Spain found that life stressors in the year before the attack – such as recent loss of relatives, loss of work, and accidents – were strongly associated with depressive and anxiety disorders after the attack (Gabriel et al., 2007). Recent evidence suggests an even stronger relationship between the relative absence of current and prior life stress and resilience to traumatic events (Bonanno et al., 2007). An important qualifier of these findings, however, is how the previous stressors were experienced. One of the few prospective studies to examine this issue suggests that only those prior stressors that result in PTSD (i.e., that cause serious trauma reactions) will put people at risk for PTSD at subsequent exposures (Breslau, 2002). It may also be that resilience to past stressors will predict subsequent resilience.

9.5.4. Flexible Adaptation and Pragmatic Coping

Although, as we noted previously, personality factors most likely play a smaller role in coping with traumatic events than is usually assumed, they still do play a role. The available research suggests that the role of personality in coping with PTEs can be grouped into two broad categories: pragmatic coping and flexible adaptation (Bonanno, 2005; Mancini & Bonanno, 2006, in press). By definition, a PTE is an extreme event that occurs outside the range of normal human experience. As a consequence, PTEs often pose unique and highly specific coping demands. Successfully meeting these demands suggests the need for a highly *pragmatic* or "whatever it takes" approach that is single-minded and goal-directed. Sometimes pragmatic coping involves behaviors that under normal circumstances may be less effective or even maladaptive. This type of coping has also been referred to as "coping ugly" (Bonnano, 2006; Bonanno & Mancini, 2008) to emphasize the pragmatic nature of coping in highly adverse situations; it does not necessarily need to be a thing of beauty but rather just needs to get the job done.

Pragmatic coping can also be observed as a consequence of relatively rigid personality characteristics. For example, the construct of *trait self-enhancement* describes people who are narcissistic and habitually utilize self-serving biases. Trait self-enhancers tend to suffer social liabilities as they often receive negative evaluations from peers and observers (Colvin, Block, & Funder, 1995; Paulhus, 1998). However, they also enjoy high self-esteem and cope extremely well with isolated PTEs, such as war (Bonanno, Field, Kovacevic, & Kaltman, 2002), terrorist attack (Bonanno, Rennicke, & Dekel, 2005), and various PTEs experienced in young adulthood (Gupta & Bonanno, under review). Another group of individuals, known as repressive copers, tend to avoid unpleasant emotional experiences and are possibly susceptible to health deficits. Yet, repressive copers have also been found to cope extremely well with adversity (Bonanno, Keltner, Holen, & Horowitz, 1995; Coifman, Bonanno, Ray, & Gross, 2007). The confluence of costs and benefits associated with these personality types suggests that they may be something of a "mixed blessing" (Paulhus, 1998).

A more genuinely health personality dimension is suggested by the concept of *adaptive flexibility*. A core aspect of flexibility is the capacity to shape and modify one's behavior to meet the demands of a given stressor event. This capacity for flexibility has been observed very early in development, yet it can change over time as a result of the dynamic interplay of personality and social interactions with key attachment figures (Block & Block, 2006). Practically speaking, then, flexibility is a personality resource that helps bolster resilience to aversive events, such as childhood maltreatment (Flores, Cicchetti, & Rogosch, 2005), but may also be enhanced or reduced by developmental experiences (Shonk & Cicchetti, 2001). Preliminary research on flexibility in adults suggests that the construct does eventually become stable and can effectively predict resilience to PTEs (Bonanno, Papa, Lalande, Westphal, & Coifman, 2004; Fredrickson, Tugade, Waugh, & Larkin, 2003).

9.6. IMPLICATIONS FOR INTERVENTION

Our understanding of how people react to and cope with traumatic events and disaster has come a long way since the initial theorizing in the mid to late nineteenth century. Widespread acceptance of the reality of severe psychological trauma was excruciatingly slow in coming. It was not until the late twentieth century that pathological reactions to psychological trauma were formally ensconced in the diagnostic nomenclature in the form of PTSD. With that development, however, the pendulum swung so far in the opposite direction that the literature became dominated by an almost exclusive focus on extreme trauma reactions. By the end of the twentieth century, ideas about resilience to traumatic events seemed to have all but disappeared. However, once again, as we move into the twenty-first century, the pendulum has begun to swing back toward the middle. Recent empirical studies have focused on individual differences in response to PTEs and have begun to move beyond the simple binary distinction of PTSD versus the absence of PTSD. These studies have begun to map a number of prototypical and readily observable outcome trajectories, including a pattern characterized by the relative absence of trauma response and by a stable trajectory of health functioning across time. Once thought to be the province of only a small handful of exceptionally healthy individuals, it is now clear that many and sometimes the majority of exposed individuals will exhibit this kind of psychological resilience.

Moving beyond the documentation of resilience to traumatic events and disaster, researchers have also begun to identify the factors that predict resilient outcomes. It seems clear at this point that there are many independent and additive risk and protective factors that might inform adjustment. That most of these factors appear to explain only a small portion of the variance in postevent outcome suggests that they may exert an additive influence on resilience. Developmental theorists have for years argued that resilience to aversive childhood contexts results from a cumulative mix of person-centered variables (e.g., disposition, personality) and sociocontextual (e.g., family interaction, community support systems) risk and protective factors (Garmezy, 1991; Rutter, 1979; Werner, 1995). The recent work on adults exposed to disaster suggests a similar conclusion.

These findings offer some compelling implications for prophylactic intervention in the aftermath of disaster (Bonanno et al., 2007; Litz, Gray, Bryant, & Adler, 2002; Shalev, 2004). Conceptualizations of mental health response to disaster have been dominated by the focus on early interventions, such as critical incident stress debriefing (Mitchell, 1983; Everly, Flannery, & Mitchell, 2000). A growing body of evidence has indicated, however, that such brief (typically one session) interventions are often ineffective (Rose, Brewin, Andres, & Kirk, 1999) and possibly even harmful (Bisson, Jenkins, Alexander, & Bannister, 1997; Mayou, Ehlers, & Hobbs, 2000; for a review see McNally, Bryant, & Ehlers, 2003). In response to this sobering news, some investigators have argued that early psychological interventions could be improved by targeting only those most at risk (e.g., Litz et al., 2002). One obvious category for this type of targeted intervention would be people who show early signs of elevated distress or PTSD symptoms. However, several studies have now shown that survivors with the highest initial symptom levels are actually more likely to experience the negative effects of early intervention (Mayou, 2000; Sijbrandij, Olff, Reitsma, Carlier, & Gersons, 2006).

A more promising conclusion, and one more compatible with the existing evidence, was suggested by Shalev (2004), who argued that "early interventions in communities suffering mass traumatic events should consist of general support and bolstering of the recovery environment rather than psychological treatment." In this context, candidates for early risk assessment might include people with relatively low social support or limited economic resources. It seems feasible that such individuals could be identified and offered assistance relatively soon after the event. It might also be possible to assess other longer-term risk factors, such as marked loss of income or additional life stressors after the PTE, which would become apparent only after a greater interval of time. Eventually, these factors, too, might be targeted for intervention. These considerations also suggest that early psychological interventions might yet be effective, provided they are enacted as part of a broader ecological approach that includes the assessment of and intervention on a range of sociocontextual factors (Sandler et al., 2003).

Finally, it will also be important to consider how the literature on resilience may inform broader social and governmental interventions. One possible avenue for consideration at this level is the way a disaster is framed in the media and in communications from government agencies and whether and how such communications might be modified so as to reduce fear and promote calm in the public (Menon & Goh, 2005; Wallis & Nerlich, 2005). Event-related worries and fears have been associated with poorer adjustment in the aftermath of natural disasters, such as earthquakes (e.g., Livanou et al., 2005). Studies of the psychological reactions to the SARS epidemic of 2003, in many ways a prototype for large-scale biological disaster, have also consistently pointed to the harmful role of SARS-related fears and worries (Bonanno, Ho, et al., in press; Ho et al., 2005; Yu, Ho, So, & Lo, 2005). Preliminary reports from Southeast Asian countries in the aftermath of SARS, however, affirm that thoughtful governmental communications can be effective. On basis of an analysis of 17 cities in China, Shi and colleagues (2003) concluded that providing the public with realistic information about risk and recovery did appear to help assuage SARS-related worry. Similarly, Ng and colleagues (2006) reported promising data on a brief group intervention for at-risk populations during the SARS epidemic that included among its aims "help participants cope with fear" (p. 56). It is our hope that continued research on the factors that promote resilience following disaster will provide still further insights into effective individual, community, and societal interventions.

REFERENCES

Adams, R. E., & Boscarino, J. A. (2005). Differences in mental health outcomes among Whites, African Americans, and Hispanics following a community disaster. *Psychiatry*, *68*(3), 250–265.

American Psychiatric Association. (1952). *Diagnostic and statistical manual of mental disorders* 1st ed. Washington, DC: Author.

(1968). *Diagnostic and statistical manual of mental disorders* 2nd ed. Washington, DC: Author.

(1980). *Diagnostic and statistical manual of mental disorders* 3rd ed. Washington, DC: Author.

Bisconti, T.L., Bergeman, C.S., & Boker, S.M. (2006). Social support as a predictor of variability: An examination of the adjustment trajectories of recent widows. *Psychology and Aging, 21*(3), 590–599.

Bisson, J.I., Jenkins, P.L., Alexander, J., & Bannister, C. (1997). Randomized controlled trial of psychological debriefing for victims of acute burn trauma. *British Journal of Psychiatry, 171*, 78–81.

Block, J., & Block, J.H. (2006). Venturing a 30-year longitudinal study. *American Psychologist, 61*, 315–327.

Bonanno, G.A. (2004). Loss, trauma, and human resilience: Have we underestimated the human capacity to thrive after extremely aversive events? *American Psychologist, 59*(1), 20–28.

(2005). Resilience in the face of potential trauma. *Current Directions in Psychological Science, 14*, 135–138.

(2006). Grief, trauma, and resilience. In E. K. Rynearson (Ed.), *Violent death: Resilience and intervention beyond the crisis* (pp. 31–46). New York: Routledge.

Bonanno, G.A., & Field, N.P. (2001). Evaluating the delayed grief hypothesis across 5 years of bereavement. *American Behavioral Scientist, 44*, 798–816.

Bonanno, G.A., & Kaltman, S. (1999). Toward an integrative perspective on bereavement. *Psychological Bulletin, 125*, 705–734.

(2001). The varieties of grief experience. *Clinical Psychology Review, 21*(5), 705–734.

Bonanno, G.A., & Mancini, A.D. (2008). The human capacity to thrive in the face of extreme adversity. *Pediatrics, 121*(2), 369–375.

Bonanno, G.A., Field, N.P., Kovacevic, A., & Kaltman, S. (2002). Self-enhancement as a buffer against extreme adversity: Civil war in Bosnia and traumatic loss in the United States. *Personality and Social Psychology Bulletin, 28*(2), 184–196.

Bonanno, G.A., Galea, S., Bucciarelli, A., & Vlahov, D. (2006). Psychological resilience after disaster: New York City in the aftermath of the September 11th Terrorist Attack. *Psychological Science, 17*, 181–186.

(2007). What predicts psychological resilience after disaster? The role of demographics, resources, and life stress. *Journal of Consulting and Clinical Psychology, 75*(5) 671–682.

Bonanno, G.A., Ho, S.M.Y., Chan, J.C.K., Kwong, R.S.Y., Cheung, C.K.Y., & Wong, C.P.Y. (2008). Psychological resilience and dysfunction among hospitalized survivors of the SARS epidemic in Hong Kong: A latent class approach. *Health Psychology, 27*(5), 659–667.

Bonanno, G.A., Keltner, D., Holen, A., & Horowitz, M.J. (1995). When avoiding unpleasant emotions might not be such a bad thing: Verbal-autonomic response dissociation and midlife conjugal bereavement. *Journal of Personality and Social Psychology, 69*, 975–989.

Bonanno, G.A., Moskowitz, J.T., Papa, A., & Folkman, S. (2005). Resilience to loss in bereaved spouses, bereaved parents, and bereaved gay men. *Journal of Personality and Social Psychology, 88*(5), 827–843.

Bonanno, G.A., Papa A., Lalande K., Zhang N., & Noll J.G. (1995). Grief processing and deliberate grief avoidance: A prospective comparison of bereaved spouses and parents in the United States and the People's Republic of China. *Journal of Consulting and Clinical Psychology, 73*(1), 86–98.

Bonanno, G.A, Papa, A., Lalande, K., Westphal, M., & Coifman, K. (2004). The importance of being flexible: The ability to both enhance and suppress emotional expression predicts long-term adjustment. *Psychological Science, 15*(7), 482–487.

Bonanno, G.A., Rennicke, C., & Dekel, S. (2005). Self-enhancement among high-exposure survivors of the September 11th terrorist attack: Resilience or social maladjustment? *Journal of Personality and Social Psychology, 88*(6), 984–998.

Bonanno, G.A., Wortman, C.B., Lehman, D.R., Tweed, R.G., Haring, M., Sonnega, J., et al. (2002). Resilience to loss and chronic grief: A prospective study from preloss to 18-months postloss. *Journal of Personality & Social Psychology, 83*(5), 1150–1164.

Bowlby, J. (1980). *Loss: Sadness and depression (Attachment and loss, Vol. 3)*. New York: Basic Books.

Breslau, N. (2002). Epidemiologic studies of trauma, posttraumatic stress disorder, and other psychiatric disorders. *Canadian Journal of Psychiatry, 47*(10), 923–929.

Breslau, N., Lucia, V.C., & Alvarado, G.F. (2006). Intelligence and other predisposing factors in exposure to trauma and posttraumatic stress disorder. *Archives of General Psychiatry, 63*(11), 1238–1245.

Breslau, N., Peterson, E.L., Poisson, L.M., Schultz, L.R., & Lucia, V.C. (2004). Estimating post-traumatic stress disorder in the community: Lifetime perspective and the impact of typical traumatic events. *Psychological Medicine, 34*, 889–898.

Brewin, C.R., Andrews, B., & Valentine, J.D. (2000). Meta-analysis of risk factors for posttraumatic stress disorder in trauma-exposed adults. *Journal of Consulting and Clinical Psychology, 68*, 748–766.

Browman-Fulks, J. J., Ruggiero, K. J., Green, B. A., Kilpatrick, D. G., Danielson, C. K., Resnick, H. S., et al. (2006). Taxometric investigation of PTSD: Data from two nationally representative samples. *Behavior Therapy*, *37*, 364–380.

Buckley, T. C., Blanchard, E. B., & Hickling, E. J. (1996). A prospective examination of delayed onset PTSD secondary to motor vehicle accidents. *Journal of Abnormal Psychology*, *105*(4), 617–625.

Carver, C. S. (1998). Resilience and thriving: Issues, models, and linkages. *Journal of Social Issues*, *54*(2), 245–266.

Casella, L., & Motta, R. W. (1990). Comparison of characteristics of Vietnam veterans with and without posttraumatic stress disorder. *Psychological Reports*, *67*, 595–605.

Charcot, J. M. (1887). *Lecons Sur les Maladies du Système Nervuex Faites à la Salpêtrière*. Paris: Progrès Médicial en A. Delahaye & E. Lecrosnie.

Christ, G. H. (2000). *Healing children's grief*. New York: Oxford.

Coifman, K. G., Bonanno, G. A., Ray, R. D., & Gross, J. J. (2007). Does repressive coping promote resilience? Affective-autonomic response discrepancy during bereavement. *Journal of Personality and Social Psychology*, *92*(4), 745–758.

Colvin, C. R., Block, J., & Funder, D. C. (1995). Overly positive self-evaluations and personality: Negative implications for mental health. *Journal of Personality and Social Psychology*, *68*, 1152–1162.

Copeland, W. E., Keeler, G., Angold, A., & Costello, E. J. (2007). Traumatic events and posttraumatic stress in childhood. *Archives of General Psychiatry*, *62*, 577–584.

Da Costa, J. M. (1871). On irritable heart; a clinical study of a form of functional cardiac disorder and its consequences. *American Journal of the Medical Sciences*, *61*, 17–52.

Deshields, T., Tibbs, T., Fan, M. Y., & Taylor, M. (2006). Differences in patterns of depression after treatment for breast cancer. *Psycho-Oncology*, *15*, 398–406.

Deutsch, H. (1937). Absence of grief. *Psychoanalytic Quarterly*, *6*, 12–22.

Dohrenwend, B. P., Turner, J. B., Turse, N. A., Adams, B. G., Koenen, K. C., & Marshall, R. (2006). The psychological risks of Vietnam for U.S. veterans: A revisit with new data and methods. *Science*, *313*, 979–982.

Ellenberger, H. F. (1970). *The discovery of the unconscious: History and evolution of dynamic psychiatry*. New York: Basic Cooks.

Erichsen, J. E. (1866). *On railway and other injuries of the nervous system*. London: Walton & Maberly.

Everly, G. S., Flannery, R. B., & Mitchell, J. T. (2000). Critical incident stress management (CISM): A review of the literature. *Aggression and Violent Behavior*, *5*(1), 23–40.

Flores, E., Cicchetti, D., & Rogosch, F. A. (2005). Predictors of resilience in maltreated and non-maltreated Latino children. *Developmental Psychology*, *41*, 338–351.

Fredrickson, B. L., Tugade, M. M., Waugh, C. E., & Larkin, G. R. (2003). What good are positive emotions in crises? A prospective study of resilience and emotions following the terrorist attacks on the United States on September 11th, 2001. *Journal of Personality & Social Psychology*, *84*, 365–376.

Freedy, J. R., Shaw, D. L., Jarrell, M. P., & Masters, C. R. (1992). Towards an understanding of the psychological impact of natural disasters: An application of the conservation resources stress model. *Journal of Traumatic Stress*, *5*(3), 441–454.

Gabriel, R., Ferrando, L., Cortón, E. S., Mingote, C., García-Camba, E., Liria, A. F., et al. (2007). Psychopathological consequences after a terrorist attack: An epidemiological study among victims, the general population, and police officers. *European Psychiatry*, *22*, 339–346.

Galea, S., Ahern, J., Resnick, H., Kilpatrick, D., Bucuvalas, M., Gold, J., et al. (2002). Psychological sequelae of the September 11 terrorist attacks in New York City. *The New England Journal of Medicine*, *346*(13), 982–987.

Galea, S., Resnick, H., Ahern, J., Gold, J., Bucuvalas, M., Kilpatrick, D., et al. (2002). Posttraumatic stress disorder in Manhattan, New York City, after the September 11th terrorist attacks. *Journal of Urban Health*, *79*, 340–353.

Galea, S., Vlahov, D., Resnick, H., Ahern, J., Susser, E., Gold, J., et al. (2003). Trends of probably posttraumatic stress disorder in New York City after the September 11 terrorist attacks. *American Journal of Epidemiology*, *158*(6), 514–524.

Garmezy, N. (1991). Resilience and vulnerability to adverse developmental outcomes associated with poverty. *American Behavioral Scientist*, *34*(4), 416–430.

Gupta, S., & Bonanno, G. A. (Submitted). Trait self-enhancement as a buffer against potentially traumatic events: A prospective study.

Ho, W. (2003). Guidelines on management of severe acute respiratory syndrome (SARS). *Lancet*, *316*, 1319–1325.

Ho, S. M. Y., Kwong-Lo, R. S. Y., Mak, C. W. Y., & Wong, J. S. (2005). Fear of severe acute respiratory syndrome (SARS) among health care workers. *Journal of Consulting and Clinical Psychology*, *75*, 344–349.

Hobfoll, S. E. (1989). Conservation of resources: A new attempt at conceptualizing stress. *American Psychologist, 44*, 513–524.

(2002). Social and psychological resources and adaptation. *Review of General Psychology, 6*(4), 307–324.

Hobfoll, S. E., & Freedy, J. R. (1990). The availability and effective use of social support. *Journal of Social and Clinical Psychology, 9*, 91–103.

Hobfoll, S. E., Freedy, J. R., Lane, C., & Geller, P. (1990). Conservation of social resources: Social support resource theory. *Journal of Social and Personal Relationships, 7*, 465–478.

Hobfoll, S. E., Tracy, M., & Galea, S. (2006). The impact of resource loss and traumatic growth on probably PTSD and depression following terrorist attacks. *Journal of Traumatic Stress, 19*(6), 867–878.

Hoge, C. W., Castro, C. A., Messer, S. C., McGurk, D., Cotting, D. I., & Koffman, R. L. (2004). Combat duty in Iraq and Afghanistan, mental health problems, and barriers to care. *New England Journal of Medicine, 351*(1), 13–22.

Holahan, C. J., & Moos, R. H. (1991). Life stressors, personal and social resources, and depression: A 4-year structural model. *Journal of Abnormal Psychology, 100*(1), 31–38.

Ironson, G., Wynings, C., Schneiderman, N., Baum, A. Rodriguez, M., Greenwood, D., et al. (1997). Posttraumatic stress symptoms, intrusive thoughts, loss, and immune function after Hurricane Andrew. *Psychosomatic Medicine, 59*(2), 128–141.

Janet, P. (1889). *L'Automatisme psychologique*. Paris: Alcan.

Janis, I. L. (1951). *Air war and emotional stress*. New York: McGraw Hills.

Judd, L. L., Akiskal, H. S., & Paulus, M. P. (1997). The role and clinical significance of subsyndromal depressive symptoms (SSD) in unipolar major depressive disorder. *Journal of Affective Disorders, 45*, 5–17.

Kaltman, S., & Bonanno, G. A. (2003). Examining the impact of sudden and violent deaths. *Journal of Anxiety Disorders, 17*(2), 131–147.

Kaniasty, K., & Norris, F. H. (1993). A test of the social support deterioration model in the context of natural disaster. *Journal of Personality and Social Psychology, 64*(3), 395–408.

Kardiner, A. (1941). *The traumatic neuroses of war*. New York: Jason Aaronson.

Keegan, J. (1976). *The face of battle*. New York: Viking Press.

Kessler, R. C., Sonnega, A., Bromet, E., Hughes, M., & Nelson, C. B. (1995). Posttraumatic stress disorder in the National Comorbidity Survey. *Archives of General Psychiatry, 52*(12), 1048–1060.

Kubiak, S. P. (2005). Trauma and cumulative adversity in women of a disadvantaged social location. *American Journal of Orthopsychiatry, 75*(4), 451–465.

Kulka, R. A., Schlenger, W. E., Fairbank, J. A., Hough, R. L., Jordan, B. K., Marmar, C. R. (1990). *Trauma and the Vietnam War generation: Report of findings from the National Vietnam Veterans Readjustment Study*. New York, NY: Brunner\Mazel.

Lamprecht, F., & Sack, M. (2002). Posttraumatic stress disorder revisited. *Psychosomatic Medicine, 64*(2), 222–237.

Lazarus, R. S., & Folkman, S. (1984). *Stress, appraisal, and coping*. New York: Springer.

Lindemann, E. (1944). Symptomatology and management of acute grief. *American Journal of Psychiatry, 101*, 141–148.

Litz, B. T. (2005). Has resilience to severe trauma been underestimated? *American Psychologist, 60*(3), 265–267.

Litz, B. T., Gray, M. J., Bryant, R. A., & Adler, A. B. (2002). Early intervention for trauma: Current status and future directions. *Clinical Psychology: Science and Practice, 9*(2), 112–134.

Livanou, M., Kasvikis, Y., Basoglu, M., Mytskidou, P., Sotiropoulou, V., Spanea, E., et al. (2005). Earthquake-related psychological distress and associated factors 4 years after the Parnitha earthquake in Greece. *European Psychiatry, 20*, 137–144.

Luthar, S. S., Cicchetti, D., & Becker, B. (2000). The construct of resilience: A critical evaluation and guidelines for future work. *Child Development, 71*(3), 543–562.

Luthar, S. S., Doernberger, C. H., & Zigler, E. (1993). Resilience is not a unidimensional construct: Insights from a prospective study of inner-city adolescents. *Development & Psychopathology, 5*(4), 703–717.

Mainous, A. G., Smith, D. W., Acierno, R., & Geesey, M. E. (2005). Differences in posttraumatic stress disorder symptoms between elderly non-Hispanic Whites and African Americans. *Journal of the National Medical Association, 97*, 546–549.

Mancini, A. D., & Bonanno, G. A. (2006). Resilience in the face of crisis: Clinical practices and interventions. *Journal of Clinical Psychology: In Session, 62*(8), 971–985.

Marris, P. (1958). *Widows and their families*. London: Routledge & Kegan Paul.

Masten, A. S. (2001). Ordinary magic: Resilience processes in development. *American Psychologist, 56*(3), 227–238.

Mayou, R. A., Ehlers, A., & Hobbs, M. (2000). Psychological debriefing for road traffic accident victims: Three-year follow up of a randomized controlled trial. *Journal of Clinical and Consulting Psychology, 176,* 589–593.

McFarlane, A. C., & Yehuda, R. (1996). Resilience, vulnerability, and the course of posttraumatic reactions. In B. A. van der Kolk, A. C. McFarlane, & L. Weisaeth (Ed.), *Traumatic stress (pp.* 155–181). New York: Guilford.

McGruder-Johnson, A. K., Davidson, E. S., Gleaves, D. H., Stock, W., & Finch, J. F. (2000). Interpersonal violence and posttraumatic symptomatology: The role of ethnicity, gender, and exposure to violent events. *Journal of Interpersonal Violence, 15*(2), 205–221.

McNally, R. J. (2003). Progress and controversy in the study of posttraumatic stress disorder. *Annual Review of Psychology, 54,* 229–252.

McNally, R. J., Bryant, R. A., & Ehlers, A. (2003). Does early psychological intervention promote recovery from posttraumatic stress? *Psychological Science in the Public Interest, 4*(2), 45–79.

Menon, K. U., & Goh, K. T. (2005). Transparancy and trust: Risk communications and the Singapore experience in managing SARS. *Journal of Communication Management, 9,* 375–383.

Middleton, W., Burnett, P., Raphael, B., & Martinek, N. (1996). The bereavement response: A cluster analysis. *British Journal of Psychiatry, 169,* 167–171.

Middleton, W., Moylan, A., Raphael, B., Burnett, P., & Martinek, N. (1993). An international perspective on bereavement related concepts. *Australian and New Zealand Journal of Psychiatry, 27,* 457–463.

Mischel, W. (1969). Continuity and change in personality. *American Psychologist, 24*(11), 1012–1018.

Mitchell, J. T. (1983). When disaster strikes…the critical incident stress debriefing process. *Journal of Emergency Medical Services, 8*(1), 36–39.

Murphy, L. B., & Moriarty A. E. (1976). *Vulnerability, coping, and growth.* New Haven, CT: Yale University Press.

Murrell, S. A., & Norris, F. H. (1983). Resources, life events, and changes in psychological states: A prospective framework. *American Journal of Community Psychology, 11*(5), 473–491.

Myers, A. R. (1870). *On the etiology and prevalence of diseases of the heart among soldiers.* London: J. Churchill.

Myers, C. S. (1915). A contribution to the study of shell shock. *Lancet, 1,* 316–320.

Ng, S. M., Chan, T. H. Y., Chan, C. L. W., Lee, A. M., Yau, J. K. Y., Chan, C. H. Y., et al. (2006). Group debriefing for people with chronic diseases during the SARS pandemic: Strength-focused and Meaning-oriented Approach for Resilience and Transformation (SMART). *Community Mental Health Journal, 42,* 53–63.

Nolen-Hoeksema, S. (1991). Response to depression and their effects on the duration of depressive episodes. *Journal of Abnormal Psychology, 100,* 569–582.

Nolen-Hoeksema, S., & Davis, C. G. (1999). "Thanks for sharing that": Ruminators and their social support networks. *Journal of Personality and Social Psychology, 77*(4), 801–814.

Norris, F. H., & Kaniasty, K. (1996). Received and perceived social support in times of stress: A test of the social support deterioration deterrence model. *Journal of Personality and Social Psychology, 71*(3), 498–511.

Ong, A. D., Bergeman, C. S., Bisconti, T. L., & Wallace, K. A. (2006). Psychological resilience, positive emotions, and successful adaptation to stress in later life. *Journal of Personality and Social Psychology, 91*(4), 730–749.

Oppenheim, H. (1889). *Die traumatische neurosen.* Berlin: Hirschwald.

Osterweis, M., Solomon, F., & Green, M. (1984). *Bereavement: Reactions, consequences and care.* Washington, DC: National Academy Press.

Parkes, C. M. (1964). The effects of bereavement on physical and mental health: A study of the case records of widows. *British Medical Journal, 2,* 274–279.

Parkes, C. M., & Brown R. J. (1972). Health after bereavement. A controlled study of young Boston widows and widowers. *Psychosomatic Medicine, 34*(5), 449–461.

Parkes, C. M., & Weiss, R. S. (1983). *Recovery from bereavement.* New York: Basic Books.

Paulhus, D. L. (1998). Interpersonal and intrapsychic adaptiveness of trait self-enhancement: A mixed blessing? *Journal of Personality and Social Psychology, 74,* 1197–1208.

Peiris, J. S. M., Lai, S. T., Poon, L. L. M., Guan, Y., Yam, L. Y. C., Lim, W., et al. (2003). Coronavirus as a possible cause of severe acute respiratory syndrome. *Lancet, 361,* 1319–1325.

Perilla, J. L., Norris, F. H., & Lavizzo, E. A. (2002). Ethnicity, culture, and disaster response: Identifying and explaining ethnic differences in PTSD six months after Hurricane Andrew. *Journal of Social and Clinical Psychology, 21,* 20–45.

Rachman S. J. (1978). *Fear and courage.* New York: Freeman.

Rando, T. A. (1993). *Treatment of complicated mourning.* Champaign, IL: Research Press.

Resnick, H., Galea, S., Kilpatrick, D., & Vlahov, D. (2004). Research on trauma and PTSD in the aftermath of 9/11. *PTSD Research Quarterly, 15*(1), 1–3.

Roisman, G. I. (2005). Conceptual clarifications in the study of resilience. *American Psychologist, 60,* 264–265.

Rose, S., Brewin, C.R., Andrews, B. & Kirk, M. (1999). A randomised controlled trial of psychological debriefing for victims of violent crime. *Psychological Medicine, 29*, 793–799.

Ruscio, A.M., Ruscio, J., & Keane, T.M. (2006). The latent structure of posttraumatic stress disorder: A taxonomic investigation of reactions to extreme stress. *Journal of Abnormal Psychology, 111*, 290–301.

Rutter, M. (1979). Protective factors in children's responses to stress and disadvantage. In M. W. Kent, J. E. Rolf (Eds.), *Primary prevention of psychopathology: Social competence in children Vol. 3*. New Hampshire: University Press of New England.

Sanders, C.M. (1993). Risk factors in bereavement outcome. In M. S. Stroebe, W. Stroebe, & R. O. Hansson (Eds.), *Handbook of bereavement: Theory, research, and intervention*. Cambridge, England: Cambridge University Press.

Sandler, I.N., Ayers, T.S., Wolchik, S.A., Tein, J.Y., Kwok, O.M., Haine, R.A., et al. (2003). The Family Bereavement Program: efficacy evaluation of a theory-based prevention program for parentally-bereaved children and adolescents. *Journal of Consulting and Clinical Psychology, 71*, 587–600.

Sarason, B.R., Pierce, G.R., Shearin, E.N., Sarason, I.G., Waltz, J.A., & Poppe, L. (1991). Perceived social support and working models of self and actual others. *Journal of Personality and Social Psychology, 60*, 273–287.

Shalev, A.Y. (2004). Further lessons on 9/11: Does stress equal trauma. *Psychiatry, 67*, 174.

Shalev, A.Y., Bonne, O., & Eth, S. (1996). Treatment of posttraumatic stress disorder: A review. *Psychosomatic Medicine, 58*, 165–182.

Shi, K., Fan, H., Jia, J., Li, W., Song, Z., Gao, J., et al. (2003). The risk perception of SARS and socio-psychological behaviors of urban people in China. *Acta Psychologia Sinica, 35*, 546–554.

Shonk, S.M., & Cicchetti, D. (2001). Maltreatment, competency deficits, and risk for academic and behavioral maladjustment. *Developmental Psychology, 37*, 3–17.

Sijbrandij, M., Olff, M., Reitsma, J.B., Carlier, I.V.E., & Gersons, B.P.R. (2006). Emotional or educational debriefing after psychological trauma. *British Journal of Psychiatry, 189*, 150–155.

Tucker, P., Pfefferbaum, B., Doughty, D.E., Jones, D. E, Jordan, F.B., & Nixon, S.J. (2002). Body handlers after terrorism in Oklahoma City: Predictors of posttraumatic stress and other symptoms. *American Journal of Orthopsychiatry, 72*(4), 469–475.

Wallis, P., & Nerlich, B. (2005). Disease metaphors in new epidemics: The UK media framing of the 2003 SARS epidemic. *Social Science and Medicine, 60*, 2629–2649.

Werner, E.S., & Smith, R.S. (1982). *Vulnerable but invincible: A longitudinal study of resilient children and youth*. New York: Adams, Bannister, & Cox.

Werner, E.E. (1995). Resilience in development. *Current Directions in Psychological Science, 4*, 81–85.

World Health Organization. (2003). Summary of probable SARS cases with onset of illness from 1 November 2002 to 31 July 2003. From http://www.who.int/csr/sars/country/table2004_04_21/en/index.html

Wortman, C.B., & Silver, R.C. (1989). The myths of coping with loss. *Journal of Consulting and Clinical Psychology, 57*, 349–357.

Yu, Y.R.H., Ho, S.C., So, K.F.E., & Lo, Y.L. (2005). The psychological burden experienced by Hong Kong midlife women during the SARS epidemic. *Stress and Health, 21*, 177–184.

Zisook, S., Chentsova-Dutton, Y., & Shuchter, S.R. (1998). PTSD following bereavement. *Annals of Clinical Psychiatry, 10*(4), 157–163.

Zwerdling, D. (December 4, 2006). Investigative report on soldiers with PTSD. *All things considered*. National Public Radio Network.

10 Social and Cognitive Frameworks for Understanding the Mental Health Consequences of Disasters

CHARLES C. BENIGHT, ROMAN CIESLAK, AND EDWARD WALDREP

10.1. INTRODUCTION

Research on disaster mental health has made significant gains over the past 25 years; yet, it has also shown significant theoretical and methodological limitations (Norris et al., 2002; Norris, Friedman, & Watson, 2002). An old adage shared by Leonardo da Vinci captures this issue nicely: "One who loves practice without theory is like the sailor who boards a ship without a rudder and compass and never knows where he or she may be cast." In this chapter we hope to provide a bit of a compass for disaster mental health research by presenting the guiding theories proposed to explain disaster mental health and the primary constructs within those theories.

This chapter focuses exclusively on social and cognitive theories that have gained significant empirical support in predicting mental health consequences of disaster. Although other theoretical approaches, such as stress diathesis models testing the interaction between disaster exposure and gene susceptibility, are obviously important, we have chosen to limit our focus. It is our view that the field has had difficulty developing testable theory-based models, and, as such, our targeted view provides an opportunity to integrate critical, social, and cognitive variables that have been previously tested.

The theories that we do target range from very broad explanations for human behavior (i.e., social cognitive theory – SCT) to very specific trauma-based theories (i.e., dual processing theory). We will review the more broad theoretical frameworks first, then move progressively to the more specific theories. In each section we offer some critique of the different approaches and the empirical evidence available within the disaster context. This, we believe, should provide the disaster mental health researcher with not only an overview but also a more rich appreciation for the pros and cons of different theoretical approaches. At the end of the chapter we provide a cross-theoretical model that depicts the interactions among the major constructs presented. Figure 10.1 depicts the theories we discuss, and in it the theories are stacked relative to their breadth, with SCT at the top and trauma-specific theories in the center. Table 10.1 outlines the major constructs, theories, and primary publications for quick reference.

10.2. SOCIAL COGNITIVE THEORY

Social cognitive theory is a comprehensive theory of human behavior (Bandura, 1997). SCT outlines the importance of bidirectional interactions between the environment, the person, and behavior (see Figure 10.2). Called *triadic reciprocal determinism*, this framework demonstrates the dynamic nature of human adaptation where human beings self-regulate behavior through feedback systems both internally (cognitive appraisal processes) and externally (changes in environmental conditions). The self-regulation process is primarily driven through self-evaluation of successful or unsuccessful achievement of desired goals. Through forethought and strategic planning, humans are able to be shapers of their environments compared to reactive organisms responding to changes in external contexts.

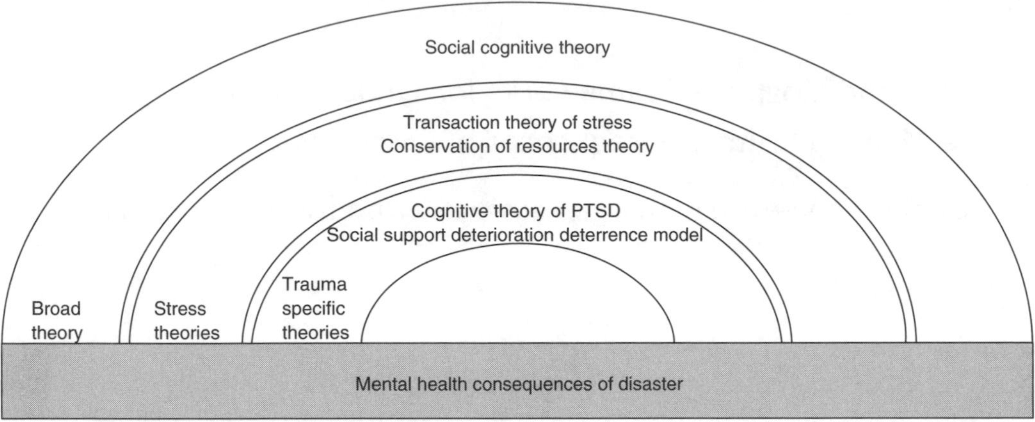

Figure 10.1. Theories utilized for understanding disaster mental health recovery.

Table 10.1. Theory and key constructs in order of presentation for disaster or trauma mental health research

Theory	Key Constructs	Reference
Social cognitive theory	Coping self-efficacy	Bandura, 1997; Benight & Bandura, 2004
	Mastery	Murphy, 1988; Kaniasty, 2006
	Collective efficacy	Benight, 2004
Stress and coping theory	Primary appraisal, secondary appraisal, problem-focused; emotion-focused coping	Lazarus & Folkman, 1984
Conservation of resources theory	Loss of resources, resource gains, loss spirals	Hobfoll, 2001
Social support deterioration deterrence model	Received social support, perceived social support	Norris & Kaniasty, 1996
Theory of shattered assumptions	Shattered assumptions	Janoff-Bulman, 1992
Emotional processing theory	Self and world schemas Negative cognitions about self and the world	Foa & Rothbaum, 1998; Foa, Ehlers, Clark, Tolin, & Orsillo, 1999; Ehlers & Clark, 2000
Dual processing theory	Verbal accessible memory (VAM), Situational accessible memory (SAM)	Brewin, Dalgleish, & Joseph, 1996

A key construct within SCT is self-efficacy. Self-efficacy is defined as the perception of capability to enact a certain behavior. Self-efficacy perceptions have been found to be highly predictive of behavior across multiple domains of human functioning (e.g., athletics, education, health, stress) (see Bandura, 1997). Self-efficacy perceptions are developed through interactive feedback with success or failure as one strives toward valued goals. For example, school children develop specific self-efficacy perceptions for different subjects, such as math or English, as they progress through the primary grades. If one has repeated difficulty mastering a subject,

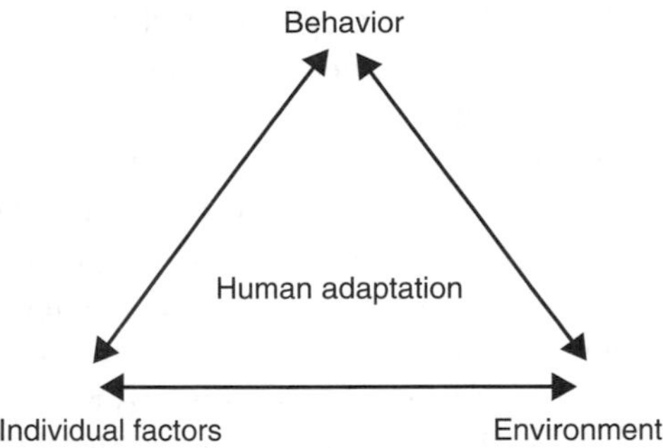

Figure 10.2. According to SCT, triadic bidirectional determinism among individual, environmental, and behavioral factors regulates human adaptation.

the self-efficacy perception will be predictably low, whereas, if someone is consistently successful, self-efficacy perceptions will be high. These perceptions are important in that they are highly predictive of motivational behaviors, such as goal setting, perseverance, or giving up.

Self-efficacy perceptions also have been investigated within the context of disaster trauma. Benight and Bandura (2004) demonstrated the importance of coping self-efficacy (i.e., the perceived capability to manage postdisaster or posttrauma recovery demands) in predicting psychological recovery in a variety of disaster settings. Disaster recovery requires extensive coping efforts across multiple domains that are consistently changing (e.g., securing funding for rebuilding one's home, dealing with changes in employment, managing emotional reactions resulting from the disaster itself along with the aftermath). These recovery demands tax individuals in ways they have often never encountered, necessitating extensive adaptation. Benight and Bandura argued that the interactive aspect of self-evaluation within this "pressure cooker" environment is critical to understanding the unfolding dynamic process of trauma (disaster) recovery and that successful or maladaptive outcomes are strongly influenced by coping self-efficacy.

Research on disaster specific coping self-efficacy perceptions, has found these perceptions to be predictive of psychological adjustment within multiple disaster settings (e.g., hurricanes, fires, floods, and earthquakes) (Benight, Antoni, Kilbourn, & Ironson, 1997; Benight et al., 1999; Benight & Harper, 2002; Benight, Swift, Sanger, Smith, & Zeppelin, 1999; Sumer, Karanci, Berument, & Gunes, 2005). These effects were seen after taking into account a number of control variables, including loss of resources, age, damage, threat of death, gender, income, and education. Coping self-efficacy was also predictive of posttraumatic distress following a terrorist attack (Benight et al., 2000). Although some of these studies were cross-sectional, limiting the interpretation of causation, many were longitudinal, suggesting coping self-efficacy may serve as a causal agent.

Studies have investigated a related construct to self-efficacy called *mastery*, which is a more general form of self-efficacy integrating efficacy perceptions across multiple domains. These studies found mastery or general efficacy to be predictive of psychological outcomes following disaster (Kaniasty, 2006; Murphy, 1988). Bandura (1997), however, argues that such global assessments weaken the predictive capacity of these perceptions within different contexts and suggests the strongest explanatory power will be within domain-specific measures of efficacy (i.e., posttraumatic coping self-efficacy).

Collectively, these studies demonstrate the importance of self-perceptions of coping capability following a disaster. Higher levels of coping self-efficacy to manage postdisaster recovery demands provides an internal sense of control (Baum, Cohen, & Hall, 1993) that supports positive cognitions about the self, increases motivation to respond to ongoing demands, assists in self-management of emotions, and promotes effective decision making (Bandura, 1997). Alternatively, lower levels of coping self-efficacy beliefs contribute to an increasing sense of despair in survivors as recovery demands accumulate, leading to uncontrolled emotions, significant negative self-scrutiny, avoidance, and eventual capitulation.

In addition to the general predictive power of coping self-efficacy, disaster studies have demonstrated that these beliefs may play a mediational role in translating the effects of other important environmental (e.g., loss of resources, social support) and individual (e.g., optimism) factors on adjustment outcomes (Benight & Harper, 2002; Benight, Ironson, Klebe, et al., 1999; Benight, Swift, et al., 1999; Sumer et al., 2005). For example, Benight and Harper (2002) demonstrated that coping self-efficacy perceptions mediated the longitudinal effect of peritraumatic distress on psychological outcomes a year later.

Social cognitive theory also offers a construct for community response to natural disasters. Collective efficacy is the perceived ability for a group to organize and perform actions that produce desired results (Bandura, 1997). Individual self-efficacy beliefs do play a role in collective efficacy, but the latter is not a simple summation of individual beliefs. Rather, the collective efficacy of a group can be attributed to the group as a whole. In a disaster setting, collective efficacy is the perceived capability for a group, or community, to organize, set goals, and perform the necessary courses of action to respond to a future disaster. Within a given community there may be a wide range of individuals who possess complementary skills or knowledge that may contribute to a high perceived ability to react to disaster events. Such a group may consist of members with emergency medical training, paramedics, and former military or firefighters, for example. Benight (2004) investigated the role of collective efficacy on psychological distress outcomes within a community that had suffered extensive damage from both a severe wildfire and subsequent flash flooding. Collective efficacy was found to function as a buffer under conditions of high loss, where higher collective efficacy resulted in lower reported distress. A similar finding was reported for social support.

The challenge of operationalizing SCT within the disaster recovery environment is finding ways to measure the bidirectional relationships between environmental conditions, self-evaluative appraisals, and behavior across time. Current approaches to measuring environmental influences rely on event characteristic checklists (i.e., extent of exposure) that are usually assessed at one point in time. Behavioral assessments of coping rely on noncontextualized assessments of coping strategies that are thought to cut across stress domains (e.g., the COPE or the Ways of Coping Checklist). Coping self-efficacy measurements should be situationally specific (Bandura, 1997; see for example, the Hurricane Coping Self-Efficacy measure, Benight, Ironson, & Durham, 1999). However, coping demands are dynamic, changing as disaster recovery unfolds. Thus, coping self-efficacy measurement should change as well to capture the most pressing demands survivors are facing. Having psychometrically sound measures of coping self-efficacy perceptions that relate to changing disaster recovery demands available for diverse and dynamic disaster environments is unrealistic. Thus, this vein of research struggles with significant measurement issues that must be addressed to fully test theoretical predictions. Although many of the studies testing the predictive power of coping self-efficacy were longitudinal in nature, more sophisticated designs and analyses are necessary to truly model the complex dynamics of disaster recovery. Advanced dynamic modeling techniques, such as structural equation modeling or latent growth curve modeling, provide more options and should be utilized (see Benight, Ironson, Klebe, et al., 1999).

10.3. STRESS AND COPING PERSPECTIVE

In contrast to the more comprehensive SCT, the transactional theory of stress is a theory directly addressing the interactive process between environmental stress demands and the individual (Lazarus, 1966; Lazarus & Folkman, 1984). Lazarus and Folkman (1984) emphasize the role of cognitive appraisals within the dynamic relationship (i.e., transactions) between environmental demands and the person specific to understanding stress. This theory of stress distinguishes between two fundamental, intraindividual constructs: primary appraisal and secondary appraisal. In primary appraisal, individuals evaluate how important a specific person × environment interaction is for their own well-being, judging it to be irrelevant, positive, (i.e., the transaction may lead to positive consequences without taxing or exceeding recourses), or stressful (i.e., the transaction may lead to positive or negative consequences, but resources need to be engaged). For situations that are deemed relevant and stressful, appraisals of harm/loss, threat, and challenge are made. Only challenge is related to a perception that the consequences of a specific stress transaction may be positive, despite the amount of resources invested, whereas, harm/loss or threat appraisals are made under situations where stress demands exceed available resources, leading to negative outcomes.

Lazarus and Folkman (1984) described secondary appraisal as the perception of available resources. These appraisals relate to an evaluation of available physical, social, psychological, and material resources, as well as the ability to use them in dealing with environmental demands (Folkman, 1984). Through the process of primary and secondary appraisal, specific coping strategies are initiated. Lazarus and Folkman (1984) defined coping as "constantly changing cognitive and behavioral efforts to manage specific external and/or internal demands that are appraised as taxing or exceeding the resources of the person" (p. 141). Thus, similar to SCT, this theory emphasizes cognitive appraisal processes.

Applications of this comprehensive stress theory to studying disasters have usually focused on coping behaviors and their effectiveness with little attention to the cognitive appraisal aspect of the theory. The theory suggests that coping behaviors can be broken into two broad categories of problem-focused or emotion-focused coping. Problem-focused coping constitutes the cognitive and behavioral coping strategies designed to modify the existing environmental conditions that are creating the stress. An example from disaster recovery might be calling the insurance company to initiate a claim on a destroyed or damaged house. Emotion-focused coping relates to efforts both internal and external to manage emotional reactions to the stress, such as calling a friend to vent about the difficulties of getting an insurance agent on the phone. Researchers have also dichotomized coping actions into active and avoidant categories.

Folkman and Moskowitz (2004) argued that researchers should consider that coping is a process and should be analyzed dynamically; for example, a specific coping strategy used in the early stage of dealing with stress may be ineffective when used at a later stage. In addition, the outcomes used to evaluate the effectiveness of coping should be carefully selected because a specific coping behavior may be beneficial in the case of one outcome and, at the same time, detrimental if other outcomes are considered. Overall, the interactional stress theory suggests a complex assessment of coping effectiveness. While this has not been done in most disaster studies that have focused on assessing coping, there are, however, some studies that assessed coping with disaster trauma in a more comprehensive way.

In a series of studies with adolescents following a disaster, a group of researchers proposed a conceptual model based on the interactional theory of stress for predicting traumatic distress in children following a natural disaster (La Greca, Silverman, Vernberg, & Prinstein, 1996; Vernberg, La Greca, Silverman, & Prinstein, 1996). This model assumes that the effect of disaster exposure on traumatic distress is mediated by specific efforts to cope. These coping efforts are affected by properties of the postdisaster environment (e.g., life events and social support) and preexisting individual characteristics of the child. Although the model has not been fully tested, Vernberg and colleagues (1996) showed that the direct effects of all factors included in the model (i.e., disaster exposure, coping efforts, postdisaster environment, and individual characteristics) on posttraumatic stress disorder (PTSD) symptoms explained up to 62% of the variance. Dynamics and complexity of coping processes are well illustrated by the differential effects of coping strategies on PTSD symptoms measured at 7-month and at 10-month follow-up assessments. Positive strategies, blame–anger, and social withdrawal at 3 months after disaster predicted higher traumatic distress at 7-month follow-up. Using blame–anger strategy at the 3-month follow-up also predicted higher 10-month traumatic distress. Traumatic distress declined over time, and we may conclude that the reduction of symptoms was at least partially influenced by coping strategies used after the hurricane (La Greca et al., 1996).

Coping studies with adult disaster survivors have also been conducted, yet typically in a more simplified manner. The longitudinal analyses of data gathered among adult survivors of the 1993 Midwest Flood focused on the effects of active coping versus avoidant coping (Smith, 1996). The study showed that active coping measured at 6 weeks after the flood predicted low general distress and high positive effect 5 months later, whereas, 6-week avoidant coping predicted high general distress measured 5 months later. However, longitudinal data analyses indicated that neither active coping nor avoidant coping predicted physical symptoms. The effects of demographic variables and flood exposure were controlled in all analyses. This study suggests that active coping may be associated with more positive outcomes measured at short-term follow-ups. The strength of this study was its longitudinal design and multiple outcomes.

In a more typical coping disaster study, problem- and emotion-focused coping were evaluated cross-sectionally for individuals exposed to either an aircraft or train crash. Results suggested that both forms of coping were positively related to traumatic distress and negative health outcomes (Chung, Dennis, Easthope, Werrett, & Farmer, 2005). This result should be read with caution because of the cross-sectional nature of the study. The dynamic relationships between coping and mental/physical health post disaster may differ as longer time gaps between measurements of coping and outcomes are considered. In addition, more attention to other critical factors should be integrated into future studies (e.g., cognitive appraisal processes, social support deterioration, preexisting psychiatric problems).

Coping self-efficacy may be a pivotal mediating resource factor that is influential for understanding the relationship between coping behaviors after trauma and important health outcomes. For example, one study suggested that the effect of exposure to a hurricane and resulting loss of resources on avoidant coping behaviors may be mediated by coping self-efficacy, as those adult survivors who had higher level of trauma exposure and lost more resources had lower coping self-efficacy (Benight, Ironson, Klebe, et al., 1999). Beliefs about one's ability to manage trauma demands, in turn, were negatively related to using avoidant coping strategies. Yet surprisingly, coping self-efficacy remained unrelated to active coping behaviors. This study showed that coping self-efficacy as a cognitive variable is involved in the process of coping with trauma. However, we need more research to understand how coping self-efficacy is related to using adaptive and nonadaptive strategies of coping with trauma and how these mechanisms influence health outcomes.

In summary, coping strategies are primary constructs of Lazarus and Folkman's transactional theory of stress that have been addressed in disaster research. Little attention has been paid to the cognitive appraisal factors (e.g., primary and secondary appraisals) and the dynamic of coping. The studies that do exist, typically suffer from limited research design (largely cross-sectional in nature) and poor assessments. The effects of changes in postdisaster coping processes and adaptive value of coping strategies over shorter and longer time periods still remain unclear and need further investigation.

10.4. CONSERVATION OF RESOURCES THEORY

Conservation of resources (COR) theory emphasizes that both individual and environmental factors are predictive of stress. The primary tenet of the theory is that people act to obtain, retain, and protect their resources (Hobfoll, 1989; 2001). Stress occurs when at least one of the three conditions is met (1) resources are threatened with a loss, (2) resources are actually lost, or (3) there is no sufficient gain of resources after investing them. Resources are defined in COR theory as "objects, personal characteristics, conditions, or energies that are valued in their own right, or that are valued because they act as conduits to the achievement or protection of valued resources"

(Hobfoll, 2001, p. 339). Hobfoll (2001) listed 74 such resources and categorized them as objects (e.g., a house), conditions (e.g., marriage), personal characteristics (e.g., social skillfulness), and energies (e.g., credits).

Hobfoll (1991) applied COR theory to traumatic stress suggesting that trauma is the sudden, unexpected, rapid loss of resources; a description quite appropriate to the disaster context. COR theory was first tested in disaster research by Freedy, Shaw, Jarrell, and Masters (1992) with positive findings for the importance of lost resources in the aftermath of a major hurricane. Several other studies support aspects of COR theory in a context of disaster (Freedy, Saladin, Kilpatrick, Resnick, & Saunders, 1994; Kaiser, Sattler, Bellack, & Dersin, 1996; Norris, Perilla, Riad, Kaniasty, & Lavizzo, 1999; Sattler et al., 2002, 2006; Smith & Freedy, 2000). Collectively, these studies suggest that lost resources, broadly defined, are important predictors of psychological outcomes following a disaster.

Norris and colleagues (1999), for example, analyzed data collected among 241 victims of Hurricane Andrew. This longitudinal study, in a time interval of 24 months, tested if predisaster, within-disaster, and postdisaster factors predicted depression and PTSD symptoms measured at 30 months after the hurricane. This study exemplifies high-quality research methodology unique in the disaster field, with predata on participants and a long-term follow-up. Personal resources (i.e., self-esteem and perceived control), social resources (i.e., social embeddedness), and stress-related variables (i.e., life events, acculturative stress) constituted the postdisaster factors. After controlling for the effects of predisaster, within-disaster, and postdisaster factors measured at Time 1, low self-esteem at Time 2 was predictive of high levels of depression ($\beta = -0.41$, $p < 0.001$), avoidance ($\beta = -0.28$, $p < 0.001$), intrusion ($\beta = -0.30$, $p < 0.001$), and arousal ($\beta = -0.26$, $p < 0.001$), all measured at Time 2. The initial levels of these outcome variables were controlled. Low levels of social embeddedness at Time 2 was also predictive of high depression at Time 2 ($\beta = -0.26$, $p < 0.001$) and high avoidance at Time 2 ($\beta = -0.26$, $p < 0.001$) when respective Time 1 outcomes and disaster factors were controlled.

Although this study demonstrated that personal and social resources are important in predicting mental health after a disaster, the analyses did not directly test loss of resources in predicting psychological outcomes postdisaster. Other studies have shown support for level of resource loss as a predictor of psychological outcomes across a variety of disasters (see Freedy et al., 1994; Kaiser et al., 1996; Langley & Russell, 2005; Sattler et al., 2006). What has been disappointing in this line of research has been the lack of advancement in understanding the dynamics of resource loss or gains *across time* and the effects of these "cycles" in predicting community level or individual level recovery. However, this area of research is not alone in its lack of forward development. Indeed, disaster mental health research more broadly has become less sophisticated over the last 25 years (Norris, 2005).

Besides predicting trauma effects directly, loss of resources may play a mediating role in the relation between disaster exposure and health outcomes. A longitudinal study conducted among flood-affected communities located along the Missouri and Mississippi rivers indicated that loss of resources mediated the effects of flood exposure on general distress and physical symptoms (Smith & Freedy, 2000).

What remains unclear from COR theory is how psychosocial resources (e.g., coping self-efficacy, mastery, social support) interact with material losses other than to compound them if both are compromised. One hypothesis is that specific psychological resources, such as coping self-efficacy, mediate material losses. In a study conducted among Hurricane Opal survivors, Benight, Swift, and colleagues (1999) investigated the effects of the loss of resources in predicting general and trauma-related distress. They predicted that the effect of loss of resources on these outcomes would be mediated by coping self-efficacy. Coping self-efficacy was a more powerful predictor of general and trauma-related distress than loss of resources, and as expected, the effect of a loss of resources on general and traumatic distress was mediated through coping self-efficacy appraisals. Although the study was cross-sectional and involved a relatively small sample, it showed the possible avenue for a development of COR theory or perhaps a combination theory linking COR and SCT together.

Applying SCT to COR theory seems to be justified, particularly, in a context of traumatic stress and overcoming its after-effects. In another study drawing from both COR and SCT, the crucial role of coping self-efficacy and loss of resources was confirmed. In a longitudinal study of Hurricane Andrew survivors, coping self-efficacy mediated the effect of resource loss on general distress following the disaster (Benight, Ironson, Klebe, et al., 1999).

Since it was introduced to disaster mental health research, COR theory has been one of the most utilized theoretical frameworks in the field (Freedy et al., 1992). However, many untested aspects of the theory await further investigation. Future studies that look at the effects of interactive elements of the theory (e.g., loss spirals) across time and how these influence mental health outcomes would be invaluable.

10.5. SOCIAL SUPPORT DETERIORATION DETERRENCE MODEL

Social support is a unique environmental resource that has received more comprehensive evaluation within the context of disaster recovery. The Social Support Deterioration Deterrence (SSDD) model was formulated and tested by Norris and Kaniasty (1996). It is an extension of the previous Social Support Deterioration (SSD) model (Kaniasty & Norris, 1993). The SSDD model was developed to explain the role of two primary constructs (i.e., received and perceived social support) in the context of the relationships between the scope of disaster and subsequent distress. Other social support models (see House, 1981; Karasek & Theorell, 1990) do not consider different facets of social support (e.g., received vs. perceived social support). The SSDD model is a dynamic picture of the interplay between social resources that flow into disaster affected communities and the availability of social support perceived by the individual. The hypothesis tested by Norris and Kaniasty (1996) implied that received social support following a disaster serves as a mediator between the effect of disaster scope on perceived social support and subsequent distress.

The two fundamental mechanisms that explain the influence of disaster on received and perceived social support are the postdisaster mobilization of support and the postdisaster deterioration of perceived social support. The deterioration of perceived support after a disaster is because of the devastation of the community social fabric as a result of the disaster (obviously variable based on the type and scope of the disaster). The SSDD model suggests that this effect is reduced by the postdisaster mobilization of support. Therefore, regardless of the disaster damage and disruption of social relationships, beliefs about the receipt of assistance provide a protective role against psychological distress (Norris & Kaniasty, 1996).

Evidence for the SSDD model is strong. It was tested across a variety of natural disasters. For example, in two independent studies conducted among survivors of Hurricane Hugo ($N = 498$) and Hurricane Andrew ($N = 404$), received social support mediated the effects of disaster scope on perceived social support. This mediating effect counteracted a deterioration of social support availability (i.e., perceived social support) after the disaster (Norris & Kaniasty, 1996). The longitudinal analyses demonstrated that although the direct impact of disaster scope (measured early after a disaster) on distress level at follow-up was nonsignificant, this relationship was mediated by received and perceived social support (Norris & Kaniasty, 1996). However, the positive effect of postdisaster mobilization of support has not always been observed (e.g., among adults affected by the 1999 flood and mudslides in Mexico) (Norris, Baker, Murphy, & Kaniasty, 2005).

In addition, individual and contextual variables explained differences in the processes of mobilization and deterioration of social support. For example, Tyler (2006) indicated that women received more support after the flood and perceived higher social support than men. By contrast, Norris and colleagues (2005) showed that men may receive and perceive more support than women. These contradictory results suggest that, potentially, other factors (e.g., cultural differences) have to be controlled for in further investigation of the processes suggested in the SSDD model.

In line with previous studies utilizing SCT and COR theory, it has been shown that relations between social support and posttraumatic distress may be accounted for by cognitive self-regulatory factors (e.g., coping self-efficacy). For example, the effect of perceived social support on general and traumatic distress was mediated by coping self-efficacy for Hurricane Opal survivors (Benight, Swift, et al., 1999). Although these conclusions are based on cross-sectional data, the results suggest that further developments of the SSDD model might include cognitive self-regulatory factors, such as coping self-efficacy, as key mechanisms through which social resources influence psychological outcomes. Although one of the important advantages of the SSDD model is its parsimony, the model does not explain why perceived social support should be the most proximal determinant of posttraumatic distress. As Benight, Swift, and colleagues (1999) demonstrated, it is possible that these pathways are rather indirect and that perceptions of social support operate via perceptions of self-competence. Perceived social support may contribute to self-evaluative capability to manage the disaster-related demands (i.e., coping self-efficacy), and when this self-evaluation of one's own capabilities is positive, distress symptoms may be perceived as less threatening to the individual.

The quality of the research on the SSDD model is exemplary and should serve as a guide to future disaster mental health studies. The studies had excellent sample sizes and measurement of main constructs and were longitudinal in nature. Improvements in this research might be to include more individual appraisal-based factors (e.g., coping self-efficacy) that seem to be important in other disaster recovery studies.

10.6. INFORMATION PROCESSING THEORIES OF TRAUMA PSYCHOPATHOLOGY

Consistent with a focus on cognition as an important factor to consider in disaster mental health, several trauma-specific theories have been developed that highlight the importance of information processing in understanding trauma recovery. One of the pioneers in this area was Horowitz (1976), who outlined a theory of human adaptation to trauma that had cognition as a central factor. Horowitz argued that individuals vacillate between avoidance and assimilation of traumatic material in an attempt to process what has just happened. This "natural" process allows for the traumatic experience to be integrated into the life experience of the person. However, for a subset of people, this integration process fails and the intensity of the intrusions of traumatic material remains elevated in combination with an increase in avoidance of thoughts related to the trauma. Thus, the normal processing does not take place and the hallmark symptoms of PTSD (i.e., intrusions and avoidance) worsen. Multiple disaster studies have utilized the PTSD symptom measures of intrusions and avoidance developed by Horowitz, yet none have attempted to capture the dynamic processing outlined in his theory.

A key component of Horowitz theory is the struggle to come to terms with the traumatic event, and Janoff-Bulman's (1992 theory of shattered assumptions also emphasizes this challenge. In her work, Janoff-Bulmann suggests that the key to what makes an event traumatic is the confrontation of cherished beliefs about the world (e.g., the world is a safe place, the world is just, etc.) and the self (e.g., I'm a competent person) through a crisis experience. Within the disaster context, for example, one could only imagine the cognitive cataclysm resulting from the horrific experiences in the aftermath of Katrina as individuals struggled for survival and saw loved ones perish. In this environment, the world was definitely not safe and, one could argue, not just.

Emotional processing theory (Foa & Rothbaum, 1998) is quite similar to these other theories in that it emphasizes the importance of cognitively working through a traumatic experience to get past it. Foa and colleagues emphasize the disturbance of this process as critical to the development of PTSD, particularly focusing on distorted cognitions relative to the trauma itself, current perceptions of personal safety, and self-assessments of competence. This theory has been extremely influential in shaping current cognitive trauma interventions for those suffering from PTSD. Specifically, emotional processing theory as applied to trauma research posits that there are three kinds of cognitions responsible for the development and maintenance of PTSD symptoms: negative beliefs about self, negative beliefs about the world, and self-blame schemas (Foa, Ehlers, Clark, Tolin, & Orsillo, 1999). The model describes complex factors involved in the formation of negative cognitions: pretrauma schemas, the trauma memory, and posttraumatic experiences, which all interrelate in the posttrauma recovery. However, it assumes a simple, direct link between negative cognitions and recovery or development of posttraumatic distress. Results of our studies provide evidence that the relationship between negative cognitions and traumatic distress is more complex, with coping self-efficacy mediating this effect. Negative cognitions about the world and self render an individual less capable to manage trauma-related demands. The perceived incapability to manage trauma-related demands contributes to development and maintenance of traumatic symptoms (Cieslak, Benight, & Lehman, 2008).

Ehlers and Clark (2000) developed a cognitive theory of PTSD that emphasizes the role of cognitive appraisals during the trauma and in the aftermath of the experience. The authors propose that many of the problems faced by individuals with PTSD relate to the lack of autobiographical integration of the trauma memory (i.e., memory fragmentation) combined with ongoing, negative self-appraisals relating to the event or subsequent coping attempts. These problems are then compounded by behavioral and cognitive strategies, such as alcohol and drug use, avoidance behaviors, cognitive distractions, and thought suppression, which keep the individual from integrating the trauma into their autobiographical memory.

Brewin and colleagues have also focused on memory processing in trauma (Brewin, Dalgleish, & Joseph, 1996). They proposed dual representation theory to help explain memory function, cognitive appraisals, and emotional responses following trauma. This theory builds upon advances in neuroscience and observations from SCT and differentiates between immediate trauma memory consolidation and subsequent self-appraisals. The primary constructs proposed are *verbally accessible memory* (VAM) and *situational accessible memory* (SAM). These two memory systems operate in parallel, although one or the other might dominate at any given moment. The VAM system is an autobiographical verbal representation of the trauma, linking the event to the person's individual life history (past, present, and future). The SAM, in contrast, is a nonverbal memory system that is based at a more primal or lower perceptual level where processing of the trauma experience is linked to information that has not been verbally processed (e.g., sights, sounds, smells, and raw emotions) during the trauma. It is through integration of the SAM memories into the more contemporary VAM (i.e., verbal integration of peritraumatic sensory memories) that enables the individual to not react with the intensity of the original trauma when reminded of the event. This theory has important implications for disaster mental health research: Traumatized survivors often are faced with living conditions that serve as constant reminders of the trauma, leading to specific testable hypotheses relative to the interplay between the SAM and the VAM as disaster survivors attempt to cope with the ongoing stress demands of rebuilding their lives.

Collectively, the cognitive theories of trauma adaptation provide a series of similar assumptions concerning trauma recovery. They all emphasize the dynamic cognitive processing of a traumatic experience as central to healthy adaptation. Most were designed primarily to help understand the symptoms that emerge with PTSD and to assist in treatment development. Their application to disaster recovery has been extremely limited.

We identified only one study, on Three-Mile Island survivors, that tested aspects of Janoff-Bulman's theory; its findings around loss of faith in experts supported the shattered assumptions hypothesis (Prince-Embury & Rooney, 1995).

Going forward, an area for further expansion in disaster mental health research is targeting these theories and beginning to test specific hypotheses emanating from them. For example, through the use of digital diary systems, studies could test the hypothesis that individuals shift back and forth between cognitive avoidance and intrusions of traumatic material. More studies could also assess the impact of disasters on world beliefs as suggested by Janoff-Bulmann. Critical elements for such studies will be clearly outlined in theoretical hypotheses that are dynamic in nature and are tested utilizing advanced longitudinal modeling techniques to help us understand adaptation across time. Moreover, future research should determine how these more trauma-specific informational processing theories relate to the broader theories already outlined. The next section provides some suggestions for how the different theories interact and ends with a theoretical model that is inclusive of the major constructs outlined in the chapter.

10.7. THEORETICAL INTEGRATION AND EVALUATION

Social cognitive theory (SCT), COR theory and the transactional theory of stress all feature an interaction between environmental conditions and individual variables as central to the prediction of behavior. The key differences appear to be one of emphasis. In SCT and the transactional theory of stress, cognitive appraisals (e.g., appraisal of environmental threat or perceptions of self-competence) serve as critical determinants of behavior. COR theory, in contrast, emphasizes social and environmental resources, although personal resources are also included. The more trauma-specific theories (SSDD, informational processing theories) also emphasize either more social or environmental processes (e.g., SSDD) or internal cognitive interpretative mechanisms that influence trauma outcomes. All of these theories also emphasize to some degree the importance of preexisting psychosocial factors (e.g., personality, socioeconomic status).

It is clear that a useful theoretical approach to disaster mental health research must take into account environmental conditions and internal cognitive processes related to the disaster and recovery. The theory should be dynamic, thereby capturing the evolving conditions that are a critical part of the recovery experience. It is our belief that the self-regulatory process outlined by SCT is extremely useful for understanding how these variables interact across time. Coping with the trauma of a major disaster thrusts the individual into a novel environment where self-regulation will rely heavily on self-evaluative mechanisms (e.g., coping self-efficacy). Thus, Figure 10.3 is an attempt to depict a comprehensive theoretical model of coping with disaster stress as it unfolds across time with an emphasis on the self-evaluative process as a collection point for the impact of other factors (e.g., external resources, memory consolidation).

The value of this model is that it captures critical biopsychosocial factors that are interacting at different points of the recovery trajectory (e.g., sympathetic arousal, social support, and cognitive appraisal processes). The model provides testable relationships among these variables that will move the field beyond the current exposure/outcome approach. For example, researchers can utilize this model to test whether different aspects of memory consolidation directly influence perceptions of coping self-efficacy in the acute phase of recovery and how this translates into better or worse psychological recovery. One could hypothesize that more fragmented verbal memory of the trauma would predict lower coping self-efficacy perceptions on the basis of the premise that initial cognitive processing of the trauma is stalled, making coping more difficult. Studies could also investigate the hypothesis that social support resources (social support received and perceived) influence critical psychological recovery factors either directly or through the mediation of cognitive self-appraisals. Such findings would provide knowledge needed to assist in the development of postdisaster interventions

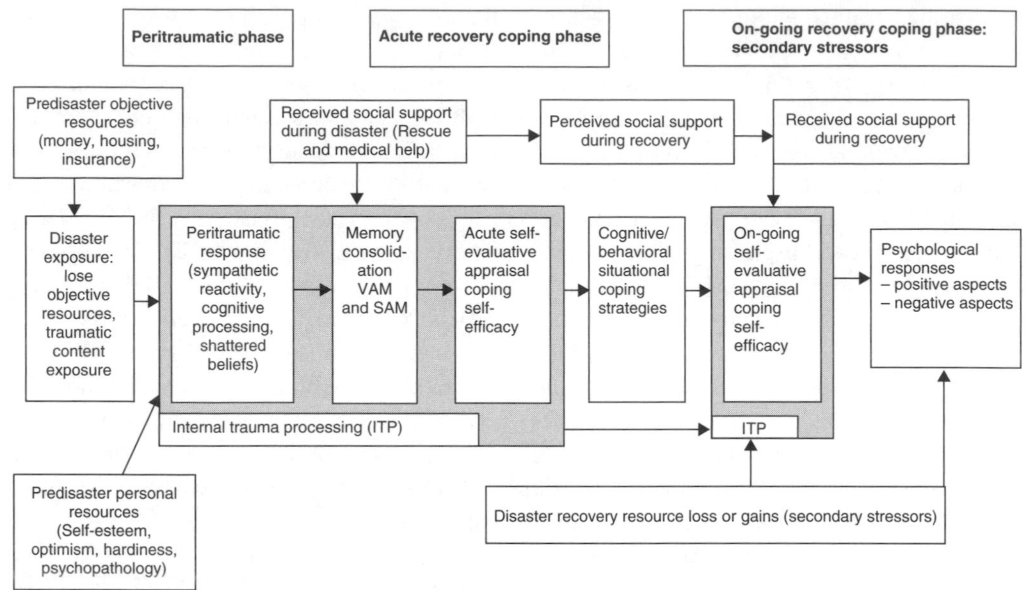

Figure 10.3. Transtheoretical model for investigating dynamic processes that lead to positive and negative responses to disaster exposure.
Note: SAM, Situational accessible memory; VAM, Verbal accessible memory.

that target the most influential variables for recovery at critical points in time.

Perhaps even more valuable would be the utilization of structural modeling techniques to test possible bidirectional relationships. For example, infusing a community with external resources will most likely have effects on social support perceptions, and greater beliefs in social support availability could enhance the attainment of more critical resources (i.e., enhanced collective efficacy). One could also test the bidirectional relationship between resource gains or losses and coping self-efficacy appraisals. The key here would be to determine the relative strengths of the different pathways at different points in recovery to determine the most important areas for intervention. It is conceivable that early after a major catastrophe, infusion of resources might be more helpful than focusing on enhancing individual perceptions of mastery. However, these hypotheses need to be tested, and this transtheoretical model provides the framework to begin these types of studies.

The final important aspect of this model is that it depicts a dynamic recovery process. Changes in crucial factors (e.g., resources lost, memory consolidation, social support disruption, or coping self-efficacy) may be more important than changes in static levels from one point in time to the next. These change variables represent an evolving biopsychosocial process (e.g., gaining a sense of mastery or seeing a community recover as resources are gained). Evaluation of the significance of these dynamic change processes awaits further testing.

In conclusion, the field of disaster mental health is starving for research studies that test theoretically based models with testable hypotheses. Studies should be designed to disprove theoretical predictions, if possible, or test competing hypotheses on the basis of different theoretical propositions (Popper, 1957). One might test for differential psychological outcomes between a subpopulation targeted to enhance individual perceptions of coping efficacy versus another subgroup that receives information on utilizing social support most effectively. Studies are needed that assess critical constructs and determine which variables are most important at which points in time. These studies will enable us to refine our theoretical frameworks and inform the development of more targeted interventions that promote resilience and growth as well as reduce pathological outcomes.

REFERENCES

Bandura, A. (1997). *Self-efficacy. The exercise of control.* New York: W.H. Freeman and Company.

Baum, A., Cohen, L., & Hall, M. (1993). Control and intrusive memories as possible determinants of chronic stress. *Psychosomatic Medicine, 55,* 274–286.

Benight, C.C. (2004). Collective efficacy following a series of natural disasters. *Anxiety, Stress, and Coping, 17,* 401–420.

Benight, C.C., Antoni, M.H., Kilbourn, K., & Ironson, G. (1997). Coping self-efficacy buffers psychological and physiological disturbances in HIV-infected men following a natural disaster. *Health Psychology, 16,* 248–255.

Benight, C.C., & Bandura, A. (2004). Social cognitive theory of posttraumatic recovery: The role of perceived self-efficacy. *Behaviour Research and Therapy, 42,* 1129–1148.

Benight, C.C., Freyaldenhoven, R.W., Hughes, J., Ruiz, J.M., Zoschke, T.A., & Lovallo, W.R. (2000). Coping self-efficacy and psychological distress following the Oklahoma City bombing. *Journal of Applied Social Psychology, 30,* 1331–1344.

Benight, C.C., & Harper, M.L. (2002). Coping self-efficacy perceptions as a mediator between acute stress response and long-term distress following natural disasters. *Journal of Traumatic Stress, 15,* 177–186.

Benight, C.C., Ironson, G., & Durham, R.L. (1999). Psychometric properties of a hurricane coping self-efficacy measure. *Journal of Traumatic Stress, 12,* 379–386.

Benight, C.C., Ironson, G., Klebe, K., Carver, C., Wynings, C., Greenwood, D., et al. (1999). Conservation of resources and coping self-efficacy predicting distress following a natural disaster: A causal model analysis where the environment meets the mind. *Anxiety, Stress, and Coping, 12,* 107–126.

Benight, C.C., Swift, E., Sanger, J., Smith, A., & Zeppelin, D. (1999). Coping self-efficacy as a prime mediator of distress following a natural disaster. *Journal of Applied Social Psychology, 29,* 2443–2464.

Brewin, C.R., Dalgleish, T., & Joseph, S. (1996). A dual representation theory of post traumatic stress disorder. *Psychological Review, 103,* 670–686.

Cieslak, R., Benight, C.C., & Lehman, V.C. (2008). Coping self-efficacy mediates the effects of negative cognitions on traumatic distress. *Behaviour, Research, and Therapy, 46*(7), 788–798.

Chung, M.C., Dennis, I., Easthope, Y., Werrett, J., & Farmer, S. (2005). A multiple-indicator multiple-cause model for posttraumatic stress reactions: Personality, coping, maladjustment. *Psychosomatic Medicine, 67,* 251–259.

Ehlers, A., & Clark, D.M. (2000). A cognitive model of posttraumatic stress disorder. *Behaviour Research and Therapy, 38,* 319–345.

Foa, E.B., Ehlers, A., Clark, D.M., Tolin, D.F., & Orsillo, S.M. (1999). The Posttraumatic Cognitions Inventory (PTCI): Development and validation. *Psychological Assessment, 11,* 303–314.

Foa, E.B., & Rothbaum, B.O. (1998). *Treating the trauma of rape. Cognitive-behavioral therapy for PTSD.* New York: Guilford Press.

Folkman, S. (1984). Personal control and stress and coping processes: A theoretical analysis. *Journal of Personality and Social Psychology, 46* (4), 839–852.

Folkman S., & Moskowitz, J.T. (2004). Coping: Pitfalls and promise. *Annual Review of Psychology, 55,* 745–774.

Freedy, J.R., Saladin, M.E., Kilpatrick, D.G., Resnick, H.S., & Saunders, B.E. (1994). Understanding acute psychological distress following natural disaster. *Journal of Traumatic Stress, 7,* 257–273.

Freedy, J.R., Shaw, D.L., Jarrell, M.P., & Masters, C.R. (1992). Towards an understanding of the psychological impact of natural disasters: An application of the conservation of resources stress model. *Journal of Traumatic Stress, 5,* 441–454.

Hobfoll, S.E. (1989). Conservation of resources: A new attempt at conceptualizing stress. *American Psychologist, 44,* 513–524.

(1991). Traumatic stress: A theory based on rapid loss of resources. *Anxiety Research, 4,* 187–197.

(2001). The influence of culture, community, and the nested-self in the process: Advancing conservation of resources theory. *Applied Psychology: An International Review, 50,* 337–421.

Horowitz, M.J. (1976). *Stress response syndromes.* New York: Aronson.

House, J.S. (1981). *Work stress and social support.* Reading, MA: Addison-Wesley.

Janoff-Bulman, R. (1992). *Shattered assumptions: Towards a new psychology of trauma.* New York: Free Press.

Kaiser, C.F., Sattler, D.N., Bellack, D.R., & Dersin, J. (1996). A conservation of resources approach to a natural disaster: Sense of coherence and psychological distress. *Journal of Social Behavior and Personality, 11,* 459–476.

Kaniasty, K. (2006). Sense of mastery as a moderator of long-term effects of disaster impact on psychological distress. In J. Strelau & T. Klonowicz (Eds.), *People under extreme stress.* Hauppauge, NY: Nova Science Publishers.

Kaniasty, K., & Norris, F. (1993). A test of the support deterioration model in the context of natural disaster. *Journal of Personality and Social Psychology, 64,* 395–408.

Karasek, R., & Theorell, T. (1990). *Healthy work.* New York: Basic Books.

La Greca, A.M., Silverman, W.K., Vernberg, E.M., & Prinstein, M.J. (1996). Symptoms of posttraumatic stress in children after Hurricane Andrew: A prospective study. *Journal of Consulting and Clinical Psychology, 64,* 712–723.

Langley, A.K., & Russell, T.J. (2005). Coping efforts and efficacy, acculturation, and post-traumatic symptomatology in adolescents following wildfire. *Fire Technology, 41,* 125–143.

Lazarus, R.S. (1966). *Psychological stress and the coping process.* New York: McGraw–Hill.

Lazarus, R.S., & Folkman, S. (1984). *Stress, appraisal, and coping.* New York: Springer.

Murphy, S. (1988). Mediating effects of intrapersonal and social support on mental health 1 and 3 years after natural disaster. *Journal of Traumatic Stress, 1,* 155–172.

Norris, F. (2005). *Disaster research methodology: Past progress and future directions.* (May 2005); http://www.redmh.org/research/general/methods.html

Norris, F.H., Baker, C.K., Murphy, A.D., & Kaniasty, K. (2005). Social support mobilization and deterioration after Mexico's 1999 flood: Effects of context, gender, and time. *American Journal of Community Psychology, 36,* 15–28.

Norris, F.H., Friedman, M.J., & Watson, P.J. (2002). 60,000 disaster victims speak: Part II. Summary and implications of the disaster mental health research. *Psychiatry, 65,* 240–260.

Norris, F.H., Friedman, M.J., Watson, P.J., Byrne, C.M., Diaz, E., & Kaniasty, K. (2002). 60,000 disaster victims speak: Part I. An empirical review of the empirical literature, 1981-2001. *Psychiatry, 65,* 207–239.

Norris, F.H., & Kaniasty, K. (1996). Received and perceived social support in times of stress: A test of the social support deterioration deterrence model. *Journal of Personality and Social Psychology, 71,* 498–511.

Norris, F.H., Perilla, J.L., Riad, J.K., Kaniasty, K., & Lavizzo, E.A. (1999). Stability and change in stress, resources, and psychological distress following natural disaster: Findings from Hurricane Andrew. *Anxiety, Stress, and Coping, 12,* 363–396.

Popper, K. (1957). Science: Conjectures and refutations. (2008); http://poars1982.files.wordpress.com/2008/03/science-conjectures-and-refutations.pdf

Prince-Embury, S., & Rooney, J.F. (1995). Psychological adaptation among residents following restart of Three Mile Island. *Journal of Traumatic Stress, 8,* 47–89.

Sattler, D.N., Glower de Alvarado, A.M., de Castro N.B., van Male, R., Zetino, A.M., & Vega R. (2006). El Salvador earthquakes: Relationships among Acute Stress Disorder symptoms, depression, traumatic event exposure, and resource loss. *Journal of Traumatic Stress, 19,* 879–893.

Sattler, D.N., Preston, A., Kaiser, C.F., Olivera, V.E., Valdez, J., & Schlueter, S. (2002). Hurricane Georges: A cross-national study examining preparedness, resource loss, and psychological distress in the U.S. Virgin Islands, Puerto Rico, Dominican Republic, and the United States. *Journal of Traumatic Stress, 15,* 339–350.

Smith, B.W. (1996). Coping as a predictor of outcomes following the 1993 Midwest flood. *Journal of Social Behavior and Personality, 11,* 225–239.

Smith, B.W., & Freedy, J.R. (2000). Psychosocial resource loss as a mediator of the effects of flood exposure on psychological distress and physical symptoms. *Journal of Traumatic Stress, 13,* 349–357.

Sumer, N., Karanci, A.N., Berument, S.K., & Gunes, H. (2005). Personal resources, coping self-efficacy, and quake exposure as predictors of psychological distress following the 1999 earthquake in Turkey. *Journal of Traumatic Stress, 18,* 331–342.

Tyler, K.A. (2006). The impact of support received and support provision on changes in perceived social support among older adults. *International Journal of Aging and Human Development, 62,* 21–38.

Vernberg, E.M., La Greca A.M., Silverman, W.K., & Prinstein, M.J. (1996). Prediction of posttraumatic stress symptoms in children after Hurricane Andrew. *Journal of Abnormal Psychology, 105,* 237–248.

11 Distinctions that Matter: Received Social Support, Perceived Social Support, and Social Embeddedness after Disasters

KRZYSZTOF KANIASTY AND FRAN H. NORRIS

11.1. INTRODUCTION

Disasters elicit strong and quick physiological, emotional, and social reactions. Even in the most dramatic circumstances, survivors seldom become psychologically paralyzed. Instead, they burst into action, doing what they can to rescue and help others. A century ago, after his stay at Leland (Stanford) University during the 1906 San Francisco earthquake, William James (1912) coined the term "universal equanimity" to describe how "the steadfastness of tone was universal" among survivors in the midst of their suffering (p. 225). He concluded his essay, "On some mental effects of the earthquake," with these words:

> At San Francisco the need will continue to be awful, and there will doubtless be a crop of nervous wrecks before the weeks and months are over, but meanwhile the commonest men, simply because they *are* men, will go on, singly and collectively, showing this admirable fortitude of temper. (p. 226)

These insightful words serve to remind us that individual and community resilience to disasters rests on ongoing cooperative action.

Other writers have since echoed James' observations in describing high levels of mutual helping engrossing whole communities in the aftermath of disaster. This phenomenon has been referred to in the disaster literature with a variety of terms: "democracy of distress" (Kutak, 1938), "post-disaster utopia" (Wolfenstein, 1957), "stage of euphoria" (Wallace, 1957), "altruistic community" (Barton, 1969), and "heroic and honeymoon phases" (Frederick, 1980). The most distinguishing features of such collectives are heightened internal solidarity, sense of unity, disappearance of community conflicts, utopian mood, overall sense of altruism, and heroic action. Newly emerging social entities begin to govern themselves spontaneously, discovering unconventional ways for communication and collective action. Previous class, race, ethnic, and social barriers may crumble, at least temporarily (Bolin, 1989; Eränen & Liebkind, 1993). In his essay about the 1937 Louisville flood, Kutak (1938) observed White and Black survivors, people whose life paths would have never crossed in the segregated south of the 1930s, cooking and praying together. He noted that "a pleasant and cordial atmosphere prevailed in the church, and the transition to a communal manner of living was made easily and happily" (p. 60). As a result of these early writings, it became widely believed that enhanced social cohesion creates "therapeutic communities" that can mitigate the adverse psychological consequences of disasters (Fritz, 1961; see also Quarantelli, 1985).

In our age of global communication, we are exposed to continuous transmissions unveiling horror, grief, and heroism displayed by survivors of major disasters. Such ubiquitous reporting provides numerous illustrations of spontaneously occurring support and concern in the aftermath of hurricanes, floods, earthquakes, or other (mainly natural) disasters. Although a sense of solidarity and heightened levels of help are evidently abundant immediately after many catastrophic events, we must be careful not to romanticize suffering with heartwarming expressions such as "democracy of common disaster," or "altruistic community." These comforting metaphors may inadvertently create a false image that all victims are equally enveloped by these supporting efforts. Altruistic or therapeutic communities do develop, but they are not all-inclusive. Likewise, these instances of post-crisis benevolence may create false images that these collectives inevitably perpetuate. Answers to some key questions are thus essential. What are the rules governing the development of altruistic communities? Do they develop in all contexts of collective disasters? How long do they last?

In this chapter, we will consider various post-disaster social dynamics in considerable depth, with particular focus on social support. After defining the various facets of social support, we summarize existing empirical research on the "mobilization of support"; this is the research that descends most directly from the early observations of Kutak, Fritz, Barton, and other disaster sociologists. We then summarize research on "deterioration of support," an observation that emerged later in disaster studies, but just as prominently, that sense of community was sometimes destroyed by catastrophic events. We then summarize research that has attempted to integrate these seemingly paradoxical perspectives.

11.2. SOCIAL SUPPORT DEFINED

Social support is most often referred to as social interactions that provide individuals with actual assistance and embed them into a web of social relationships perceived to be loving, caring, and readily available in times of need. This definition points to the three prominent facets of social support. The first, "received support," is probably the most prominent facet of social support for the majority of people. Most of us think of support as being actually helped by others in times of need. Instruments measuring received support are concerned with (1) assessments of specific behaviors that are involved in the expression of support ("[How often someone] provided you with some transportation?") (see Barrera, Sandler, & Ramsay, 1981) or (2) estimation of "natural helping behaviors," that is, actions that others perform when they render assistance to a person ("Whenever you wanted to talk how often was there someone willing to listen to you after the disaster?") (see Joseph, 1999).

The second facet of social support is "perceived support." This is probably the most prominent facet for the majority of researchers because it is most often assessed in stress and coping studies. Perceived social support is defined as the cognitive appraisal of being reliably connected to others. Measures of perceived support attempt to (1) assess an individual's confidence that adequate support would be available if needed ("If I were sick and needed someone to take me to the doctor, I would have trouble finding someone") (see Cohen, Mermelstein, Kamarck, & Hoberman, 1985) or (2) characterize the primary social environment as helpful or cohesive ("Who accepts you totally, including both your worst and your best points?") (see Sarason, Sarason, Shearin, & Pierce, 1987).

Both perceived and received social support may take on different kinds or types. Various types of social support are cataloged in the literature, but most frequently investigated are emotional support, informational support, and tangible support. Each kind of these supportive resources may be linked to specific sources such as kin relations (those connected by blood or marriage), nonkin informal networks (friends, neighbors, coworkers, and others known from religious or social settings), and people outside immediate support circles (people not known personally, such as community leaders, charitable organizations, professional service providers).

The third facet of social support, "social embeddedness," represents more structural aspects of social networks. It refers to the number of connections individuals have with significant others in their social environments ("How many of your neighbors do you visit or talk to at least once every 2 weeks?") (see Cohen, Doyle, Skoner, Rabin, & Gwaltney, 1997). The existence of social ties based on marital status, numbers of friends and neighbors, or frequency of participation in community activities are broad indicators of embeddedness. In a nutshell, perceived support is helping behavior that might happen, received support is helping behavior that did happen, and social embeddedness represents the network of people who might provide or did provide these supportive acts.

11.3. MOBILIZATION OF SOCIAL SUPPORT IN THE AFTERMATH OF DISASTERS

11.3.1. The Rule of Relative Needs

The mobilization of support refers to the power of a disaster to generate help for its victims. The rules that govern the receipt of support have been of interest to us (the authors) for many years, beginning with our study of Hurricane Hugo. In the fall of 1990, 1 year after Hurricane Hugo devastated large areas of North and South Carolina, we interviewed a total of 1,000 persons – 500 survivors (i.e., respondents residing in two stricken cities, Charleston, SC, and Charlotte, NC) and 500 nonvictims (i.e., respondents residing in two "control" sites, Greenville, SC, and Savannah, GA). We asked all the respondents 16 questions about the frequency with which they received tangible (e.g., money, a place to stay, help with improving property), informational (e.g., information about how to do something, how to understand a situation, suggestion on what action to take) and emotional (e.g., expressions of interest/concerns, reassurance, comfort with physical affection) help in the first 2 months following the hurricane. Because we asked about any support received regardless of the reason (therefore not necessarily linked to the disaster experience) we were able to compare disaster victims to nonvictims on the amounts of support received in that time frame (e.g., "In the time period between Hugo and Thanksgiving, did anyone loan you or give you tools, appliances, or equipment that you needed? Regardless of the reasons, did this happen: never [1], once or twice [2], a few times [3], many times [4]").

Disaster exposure, operationalized as loss (of property and belongings) and trauma (injury or threat to life), was strongly associated with the amount of help received (Kaniasty & Norris, 1995). Between-group differences were pervasive: Respondents who experienced Hugo received much more help than nonvictims, and high-impact survivors generally received more support than low-impact survivors. Appropriately, priority was given to those affected by the hurricane that experienced the greatest exposure to the disaster's destructive powers; this is the "rule of relative need."

Such a norm of relative need has governed social support and aid distribution in many other disasters (Bolin, 1982; Carr, Lewin, Carter, & Webster, 1992; Drabek & Key, 1984). Our subsequent studies of Hurricane Andrew (Kaniasty & Norris, 2000), Hurricane Paulina (Norris, Murphy, Kaniasty, Perilla, & Ortis, 2001), and the 1997 flood in Poland (Kaniasty, 2003) similarly showed that the extent of disaster losses and exposure to trauma are typically predictive of the level of help received (see also Beggs, Haines, & Hurlbert, 1996; Pickens, Field, Prodromidis, Pelaez-Nogueras, & Hossain, 1995; Tyler, 2006).

11.3.2. Matching Help with Needs

What types of social support are received most frequently after disasters? The efficacy of social support is determined by the extent to which it functions to promote preservation or recovery of important physical and psychological resources necessary for successful adaptation (Hobfoll, 1998; Lazarus & Folkman, 1984). To be useful in aiding recovery, informal support networks must provide those resources that are the most challenged by the stressful event and most needed for coping (Cutrona & Russell, 1990). Many disasters entail destruction of the physical environment and loss of possessions. Consequently, the rule of relative needs should be expected to govern distribution of tangible aid. Indeed, in our studies of hurricanes and floods, differences between groups with low, moderate, and high losses have been greatest for tangible support. Twelve months after the 1999 Marmara earthquake, Kasapoĝlu, Ecevit, and Ecevit (2004) asked 210 survivors about their social support needs. Finances were the utmost concern, followed by needs for education of children and protection of life and property. These needs were associated quite predictably with survivors' sociodemographic characteristics. For example, people with lower education reported the highest needs for financial support. Childcare and education needs were clearly important for the younger portion of the sample. Although they are not surprising, such findings should be nevertheless instructive for researchers. Assessments of tangible support are infrequent in disaster studies, which tend to rely on global measures of social support that emphasize emotional support.

Support in the form of information and guidance is also a valuable resource for disaster victims whose success in recovery often depends on finding quick and practical solutions to many exacting predicaments. Survivors must efficiently organize their clean-up efforts and protect what is left of their property and belongings. Navigating through a maze of local, governmental, or insurance agencies to obtain formal assistance can be a lonely and daunting task. For these reasons, we hypothesized and documented that informational support was also predicted by severity of disaster impact following Hurricanes Hugo, Andrew, and flooding in Poland.

Although the extent of disaster losses best determines the amount of tangible and informational support received by survivors, in absolute terms it is the emotional social support that seems to be exchanged most frequently and in greatest amounts after disasters and other stressful events (see Joseph, 1999; Wills & Shinar, 2000). Being surrounded by those loving and understanding maintains sense of safety, concern, love, and hope in times when the world appears brutal, dangerous, and unjust (Lindy & Grace, 1986). "The best help was from those who could *listen* and just *spend* time," a survivor reflected in the aftermath of the 1980 volcanic eruption of Mount St. Helens (Murphy, 1986, p. 71). While emotional support is reliably the most frequent form of support, highly exposed survivors are not as different from less severely exposed survivors and nonvictims in receiving emotional support as they are in receiving tangible and informational support (Kaniasty, 2003; Kaniasty & Norris, 1995). Furthermore, emotional support was determined less by disaster impact measures and more by measures standing for person characteristics than were tangible and emotional support.

The need for concrete forms of social support in terms of instrumental aid and advice are generally determined by demands of the stressors, whereas people may desire emotional support all the time. Moreover, emotional support seems to be ubiquitous in daily interpersonal contacts, regardless of need (Kaniasty & Norris, 1997; Leatham & Duck, 1990). Its emergence could be assumed even if it has not actually materialized. This speculation implies that reports about emotional support receipt, especially on the part of low-impact victims and nonvictims, may be vulnerable to psychological and psychometric distortions. On the one hand, the belief that one experienced many signs of love and concern from others may be just another positive illusion in the service of generally inflated self-presentations (see Paulhus, 1991; Taylor & Brown, 1988). On the other hand, it could be that measures of emotional support suffer from "ceiling effects" and are not sensitive enough to variations in receiving this type of support.

The findings regarding types of support received after disasters have both theoretical and practical importance. We will argue that because emotional support seems to be a resource readily available to most people, disaster researchers might benefit from extending their attention to careful assessments of tangible and informational support because this could be where differences between less exposed and more exposed victims lie. Likewise, intervention efforts and psychological help should be built around providing tangible and informational help. Expressions of love and words of encouragement can be effectively communicated when passing a survivor a bottle of water, handing him a blanket, or assisting her in filling out an insurance form.

11.3.3. The Pyramid of Postdisaster Support

Who provides help to disaster survivors? Literature on help-seeking behavior and help utilization in all contexts of needs often evokes an image of a "pyramid" to describe the sequence of people's reliance on different sources of help (e.g., Wills & DePaulo, 1991). The broad base of the pyramid is the family and other primary support groups. Its narrow top, the apex not always readily available or recognized is the aid provided by formal agencies. The pyramid analogy implies that the closer the source of support is to the victim, the greater the amounts of social support he or she provides. Allen Barton (1969) in the now-classic monograph, *Communities in disasters,* termed this immediate reliance on assistance within primary groups as an "informal mass assault." In other words, survivors rely mainly on their families, relatives, friends, and neighbors. They may be more reticent in utilizing assistance or less aware of availability of aid from sources outside their immediate networks. Of course, this statement must be qualified by the fact that in many instances the (mainly tangible) aid from governments and other formalized support organizations should and must predominate, yet the primary reliance on informal support networks is rather all-pervading (see Golec, 1983; Hill & Hansen, 1962; Ibañez et al., 2003; Kasapoĝlu et al., 2003; Quarantelli, 1960). Disaster survivors turn to formal aid agencies when their needs exceed available resources and if the types of needed provisions depart from routinely offered kinds of social support (Beggs et al., 1996; Solomon, 1986).

In a study of Hurricane Andrew, we asked about help received from different sources (Kaniasty & Norris, 2000). Specifically, we assessed the support respondents received from their family, friends (including neighbors and coworkers), and people outside their immediate circle. In general, survivors reported receiving substantial amounts of help from all three sources, in the rank order of greatest reliance on family, followed by friends, followed by outsiders. Moreover, this hierarchy emerged with each of the three ethnic groups studied (European Americans, African Americans, and Latinos). A similar "pyramid" in reliance on support from different sources has been reported by many studies investigating disasters in different countries and cultures, including the United States, Australia, Poland, and Mexico (e.g., Bolin, 1982; Carr et al., 1992; Kaniasty, 2003; Norris et al., 2001).

However, other patterns of help utilization by source have been observed. Caldera, Palma, Penayo, and Kullgren's (2001) study of Hurricane Mitch (Nicaragua and Honduras, 1998) showed that only 4% of their respondents sought help from families, whereas 29% of them turned to friends, and 29% turned to medical professionals. Our investigation of the 1999 flood and mudslides in Mexico (Norris, Baker, Murphy, & Kaniasty, 2005) presented evidence of very minimal mobilization of support from family and friends in two studied cities, Villahermosa and Teziutlán. The only substantial help came from the outsiders. In a study of an earthquake in Turkey (Kasapoĝlu et al., 2003), 20% of survivors reported receiving help from the government, 14.3% from family, and 10.3% of respondents mentioned received help from other nonkin sources.

These contradictory findings can be considered as surprising given that the locations of examined events are regarded as endorsing collectivistic values emphasizing strong kin relationships (see Triandis, 1995). Although available evidence in disaster research at times allows for making generalizations (e.g., "dependence on family in times of crisis is universal"), we must recognize that economic, societal, and cultural factors of specific disaster locales may produce social support dynamics that contradict these overarching expectations.

11.3.4. The Rule of Relative Advantage and Help-Seeking Comfort

Besides relative need, what other factors affect the distribution of social support in postdisaster communities? Empirical and common observations alike suggest that, irrespective of needs, certain individuals may have a relative advantage in receiving support. Basic person characteristics such as gender, age, ethnicity, and education level (as proxy for income) tend to impart their influence in development and maintenance of social support networks (see House, Umberson, & Landis, 1988;

Vaux, 1988; Wills & Shinar, 2000). Such forces create "the rule of relative advantage," which operates quite apart from need.

Who are the people who have advantage in receiving social support following disasters? People with larger support networks typically receive more social support (Beggs et al., 1996; Drabek & Key, 1984; Kaniasty, 2003; Kaniasty & Norris, 1995). Most studies, as expected, show that women routinely receive more support than men, particularly in the domain of emotional help (Beggs et al., 1996; Kaniasty, 2003; Kaniasty & Norris, 1995; Tyler, 2006). Survivors who are younger, have more years of education, and have higher income are also afforded higher levels of assistance (Kaniasty, 2003; Kaniasty & Norris, 1995; Norris et al., 2005; Tyler, 2006). Marriage has been traditionally regarded as a proxy measure for "having social support"; therefore, it was not surprising to observe that marital status predicted social support receipt after Hurricanes Hugo and Andrew (Kaniasty & Norris, 1995; Norris & Kaniasty, 1996).

Nevertheless, again there are studies that provided evidence contrary to these seemingly established rules of advantage in receiving help in the aftermath of disasters. For example, an investigation of psychometric properties of the Crisis Support Scale, a frequently used instrument assessing received support in trauma studies (see Joseph, 1999), revealed that female gender was associated with lower scores on the majority of items (Elklit, Pedersen, & Jind, 2001). People who were unmarried received more help after the 1993 U.S. Midwest floods (Tyler, 2006) and flooding in Poland (Kaniasty, 2003). The role of ethnicity is not always clear-cut either (see Bolin & Bolton, 1986; Kaniasty & Norris, 1995, 2000).

Of all the relevant person attributes, one variable that seems to most reliably and strongly predict the amount of social support received is the individual's willingness to ask for help. Vaux, Burda, and Steward (1986) state, "Support resources of whatever quality are useless if the individual, for one reason or another, is reluctant to utilize them." People may fail to solicit help because they believe help is not available or because help-seeking engenders feelings of indebtedness and threatens self-esteem (see DePaulo, Nadler, & Fisher, 1983; Nadler, 1997). Notwithstanding the complexity of theses intervening and background factors, the most direct and most proximal predictor of whether or not an individual receives help is that person's willingness to ask for it.

Constructs such as social network orientation (Tolsdorf, 1976; Vaux et al., 1986), discomfort in seeking support (Hobfoll & Lerman, 1989), help-seeking beliefs (Eckenrode, 1983), or active social orientation (Nadler, 1997) capture individuals' preconceptions about, and evaluation of, seeking and receiving help. People with positive network orientations are less reluctant to seek help from a variety of sources. Williams, Hodgkinson, Joseph, and Yule (1995) examined attitudes toward emotional expression and support received in crisis among 73 survivors of a capsized ferry. Four questions assessed respondents' unwillingness to seek help ("I think you should not burden other people with your problems") and formed a reliable scale whose content validity the authors labeled as reflecting a "stiff upper lip" attitude. This negative attitude toward emotional expression was associated with lower levels of received social support and higher levels of symptomatology. In our examinations of social support dynamics after Hurricane Andrew (Kaniasty & Norris, 2000) and the 1997 flood in Poland (Kaniasty, 2003) we also asked respondents about how comfortable they felt when requesting help (tangible, informational, emotional) from different sources (family, friends, outsiders). Predictably, help-seeking comfort affected the amount of received help after both disasters. However, two additional findings were somewhat surprising. Help-seeking comfort was strong or even stronger predictor of support receipt than the extent of disaster losses. In other words, survivors' willingness to ask for help "competed" with relative needs in predicting help received. In the context of disaster, where many people simultaneously require help, readiness to seek support may yield a strong advantage.

The second unexpected finding was the fact that survivors of Hurricane Andrew who experienced greater disaster impact were more uncomfortable seeking help from others. This relation was later replicated with victims of flooding in Poland. Thus, a vicious cycle is closed. Although people in need after disasters do receive help, they receive altogether less help than they might have because of their reticence in asking for support. People get what they ask for, or, more precisely, do not get what they do not ask for. Thus, help-seeking discomfort, or its opposite, help-seeking comfort, as an important psychological asset affecting the efficacy of coping processes could render some individuals more vulnerable to additional loss in crisis situations (see Hobfoll, 1998). Outreach efforts in the wake of community-level events are always essential (Norris, Friedman, & Watson, 2002).

Recent disasters point to a new person characteristic (or attribute) that might serve as an important advantage in mobilizing social support – familiarly with the Internet. Procopio and Procopio (2007) presented relevant data from a sample of New Orleans residents who used the Internet in the first week after Hurricane Katrina. Close to half of the sample reported using the Internet to contact people with whom they had not been in touch for over a year, a trend particularly visible among victims who incurred greater losses. Furthermore, the authors concluded that the Internet should be considered as a viable medium for sustaining geographic community in crisis. It appears that the Internet will become an asset in catalyzing postdisaster support from both strong (proximal) and weak (distal) social ties, and its influence on recovery dynamics must be from now on systematically considered by researchers (e.g., Jones & Rainie, 2002).

11.3.5. Patterns of Neglect and Concern

Investigations of mobilization of postdisaster helping processes generally suggest that people who are poor, older, less educated, or belong to racial or ethnic minorities may be less involved in postdisaster altruistic communities. Disaster survivors with higher socioeconomic status, whether assessed via income or education, routinely receive more social support from their social networks, whereas victims of less prominent socioeconomic status must rely more on formal support agents, which are not always easily accessible (Bolin, 1982; Drabek, 1986, Drabek & Key, 1984). Our first study of helping behavior following disasters is a disheartening illustration of how scarcity of resources weakened mobilization of social support, far below the levels heralded by "altruistic communities" (Kaniasty, Norris, & Murrell, 1990). People affected by the Kentucky floods were disadvantaged in many ways; they were older adults who averaged only 8 years of education and lived in an impoverished rural area characterized by substandard housing and high unemployment (20% at the time the study was conducted). Furthermore, unlike many contemporary disasters, the Kentucky floods attracted little attention from the media and general public. Because the floods occurred in the midst of an ongoing panel study in the area, we were afforded pre- as well as postdisaster measures (see Norris, Phifer, & Kaniasty, 1994). Using a prospective design, we were able to examine how expectations of help ("In an emergency, how much help would your immediate family be able to give you?") in a hypothetical life crisis fared during an actual emergency ("During the flood, how much help did friends give you?"). These elderly survivors generally received little help, and what they received appeared to be far below what they had expected. These results were not congruent with the image of widespread altruism following disasters.

Apparently, older age may be associated with unequal involvement in postdisaster helping communities. Following the Topeka tornado, Drabek and Key (1984) found that families headed by persons over 60 received aids far less frequently from all sources than families headed by persons under 60. The authors concluded that "elderly families simply did not participate as fully in the emergent postdisaster therapeutic community as did the younger victims" (p. 100). In fact, it was this situation that inspired Kilijanek and Drabek (1979) to coin the term "pattern of neglect." Other disaster studies showed that age was inversely related to the amount of received support (e.g., Norris et al., 2005; Tyler, 2006).

However, the idea of "the pattern of neglect" is best demonstrated by a statistical interaction. For instance, in the presence of high material losses due to flooding in Poland, adults older than 64 years of age received considerably less support from outsiders (but not other sources) than their middle-aged and younger counterparts (Kaniasty, 2003). Thus, disaster exposure sharpened their relative disadvantage, resulting in a clear pattern of neglect.

Still, the impact of older age on receiving social support in disasters is even more complicated. We did not find the pattern of neglect in the Hugo study where we also tested an interaction of age and tangible losses and damages (Kaniasty & Norris, 1995). What we found instead were statistically reliable interactions between age and disaster trauma (physical harm and threat to life). The form of these interactions was such that older adults received as much help as equally threatened younger survivors, who routinely receive more support in disasters than elderly victims. Hence, with regard to property damage, older adults may sometimes suffer from a pattern of neglect; however, with regard to physical illness and injury there may actually be a "pattern of concern" that mobilizes support networks to provide more assistance to the elderly. Most reasonably, informal support networks may be especially attentive to health threats experienced by elderly because of their assumed vulnerability in the physical health domain.

Whereas in our studies older people experienced both a pattern of neglect and a pattern of concern, the findings from the same investigations indicated that survivors representing racial/ethnic minorities or lower socioeconomic status tended to experience only a pattern of neglect. Interactions between disaster impact and race or education level were statistically significant. Blacks consistently received less tangible, informational, and emotional help than equally affected victims who were white (Kaniasty & Norris, 1995). This pattern also emerged among Hugo victims who had little education. Likewise, in the first 2 months after a flood in Poland, persons with fewer years of formal schooling (eight or less) consistently received lower levels of support (tangible, informational, emotional, from kin sources, from nonkin sources) than their more educated counterparts (Kaniasty, 2003). In all these cases, the experience of disaster losses augmented the relative disadvantage of minorities and persons with lower socioeconomic status in receiving postdisaster social support.

Some studies document more equitable distributions of social support after disasters (e.g., Kaniasty & Norris, 2000), but disparities in allocation of aid predominate. Although we have not yet seen many published empirical analyses of social support exchanges following Hurricanes Katrina and Rita, and recent scholarly reports dispel many (negative) images that prevailed in the media at that time (e.g., Rodríguez, Trainor, & Quarantelli, 2006; Tierney, Bevc, & Kuligowski, 2006), we would argue that the dynamics resembling pattern of neglect were present in the immediate recovery after these events. In fact, as researchers of disaster social support, we would have predicted just that. Bluntly speaking, the chances for speedy, or at least equitable, recovery of people from economically disadvantaged and politically marginalized societal strata are frequently hampered by their restricted involvement in postdisaster helping communities (see also, Bolin & Bolton, 1986; Norris et al., 2005; Oliver-Smith, 1996).

To summarize thus far, high levels of helping and social support generally emerge after disasters. However, these postdisaster helping communities cannot escape the preexisting societal conditions of inclusion and exclusion. Quite simply, they are not ruled in the most egalitarian way. The often talked about altruism and fellowship that the public marshals in times of crisis should not obscure the fact that not all people fully participate in these emergent altruistic communities.

11.3.6. Qualifications Concerning Mobilization of Postdisaster Social Support

Most of the research reviewed here has concerned helping behavior and received social support following natural disasters. There is simply much more empirical work on receipt of social support in the aftermath of events generally considered as acts of nature or "acts of God." In the context of such events, human activities are by and large, rightly or wrongly, absolved as reasons for their occurrence and consequences. Of course, this overreliance on the investigations of natural disasters is a qualifier to the generality of the metaphor of altruistic community. Hence the question: Do altruistic communities with their defining features of benevolence, altruism, and solidarity develop in the context of human-induced catastrophes?

We attempted to answer this question in an earlier synthesis of postdisaster social support literature (Kaniasty & Norris, 2004). The answer was tentatively "no" for the context of human-induced disasters that are considered acts of omission. Disastrous acts of human omission are generally consequences of errors, negligence, poor planning, ignorance, or motivation to increase revenues and savings often at the expense of safety and preservation. Most environmental disasters, such as contamination of groundwater, leaking toxic waste sites, or chemical spills, are apparent acts of omission. This category also includes large industrial and transportation accidents, as well as nuclear accidents, such as those that occurred at Three Mile Island or in Chernobyl. The impact of technological disasters is quite frequently slowly evolving, uncertain, and not readily perceptible (see Bolin, 1993; Cuthbertson & Nigg, 1987; Erikson, 1994). The aftermath of these human-made catastrophes seems to be packed with interpersonal conflicts and erosion of social cohesion, a point to which we will return later.

In contrast to inadvertent human-made disasters, the answer to the question is tentatively "yes" in the category of events that are caused by humans deliberately and with malice. Such acts of commission generally include premeditated acts of violence and terrorism motivated by an intention to inflict death, injury, fear, and pain for the purpose of economic and political gains. The ultimate goal of acts of terror is to induce a sense of horror, helplessness, and chaos that extends well beyond the targeted individuals and groups. In the short run, this is exactly what happens. However, as the initial waves of terror extend far past "ground zero," more and more people rally against it, and a passionate collective sense of resolve and determination emerges. Just as the survivors of natural disasters have their "heroic" stage, the victims of terrorism may have their "patriotic" stage. Fullilove and Saul (2006, p. 167) described their impression of "altruistic community" in the New York City's neighborhoods after September 11th attacks,

> People felt a common pain and despair and turned to each other for comfort. In this unique hiatus, black people smiled at police, rich people cared about poor people, and Jews were concerned about attacks on Arabs. In Lower Manhattan, people helped each other to find shelter, to search for loved ones, and to endure months of uncertainty and displacement.

Similar accounts of solidarity and resolve transpired following the March 11th Madrid bombings (e.g., Conejero & Etxebarria, 2007; Páez, Basabe, Ubillos, & González-Castro, 2007) and the July 7th London bombings (e.g., Sheppard, Rubin, Wardman, & Wessely, 2006). Furthermore, new research emerging from these tragic events tends to describe patterns of results concerning help-seeking (e.g., Stein et al., 2004) and social support receipt and provision (e.g., Ford, Adams, & Dailey, 2006; Pulcino et al., 2003) similar to those described in the context of natural disasters (see also Kaniasty, 2006a).

Interestingly, there is another similarity pertaining to emergent altruistic communities in the aftermath of both natural disasters and acts of terror: They do not persist for long (see, Conejero & Etxebarria, 2007; Collins, 2004; Penner, Barnnick, Webb, & Connell, 2005; Raphael & Wilson, 1993). The heightened level of helping and concern inevitably must cease "and in no case can it be expected to last the length of the recovery process" (Bolin, 1982, p. 60). Although many disasters occur suddenly, and often quickly move beyond the low point, the challenges and losses they cause are not short term. Like many other major stressful events, disasters evoke an array of secondary stressors that challenge survivors and strain their coping resources at a rate faster than the progress of recovery (Norris, Friedman, Watson, et al., 2002). The salient heroic phase, with its therapeutic features of increased cohesiveness and altruism, a stage somewhat infelicitously labeled as "honeymoon," is soon overtaken by a gradual disillusionment and outright realization of the harsh reality of grief, loss and destruction. President Bill Clinton, during his visit to areas of the Midwestern floods of 1993, appropriately remarked, "Folks are brave and good-humored and courageous. But then, the reality of the losses sinks in and grief takes over" (Adler, 1993). As a "rise and fall of utopia" (see Giel, 1990), disasters and catastrophes are vivid portrayals of how communal upheavals move from an initial abundance of social support to an often inadvertent longer-term deterioration of supportive resources.

11.4. DETERIORATION OF SOCIAL SUPPORT IN THE AFTERMATH OF DISASTERS

11.4.1. Sudden and Slowly Evolving Collective Traumas

A number of forces combine to cause social support deterioration after disasters (Kaniasty & Norris, 1997, 1999, 2004). The foremost and usually the most dramatic factor is that disasters disrupt social networks. Disasters of all kinds remove significant supporters from survivors' networks through death, injury, and relocation. Some people move away and never return, changing the structure social relations permanently (e.g., Hutchins & Norris, 1989; Smith & Belgrave, 1995). Even if relocation is short term, the experience of loss of social support is unavoidable given the intransigent practice of creating temporary housing that seldom reflects predisaster personal relationships and neighborhood patterns (e.g., Bland et al., 1997; Bolin & Stanford, 1990; Golec, 1983; Riad & Norris, 1996).

The interpersonal losses brought on by disasters are unambiguous and undeniable. Hence, severe natural disasters, serious technological accidents, or bloody acts of terror are "a blow to the tissues of social life that damages the bonds linking people together and impairs the prevailing sense of communality" (Erikson, 1976, p. 154). However, beyond these most tragic losses, the progression of declining quality and quantity of personal relationships is more diffused, often delayed, and not easily recognized, at least initially. In his powerful account of the Buffalo Creek dam collapse and flood, Kai Erickson (1976) wrote,

> The collective trauma works its way slowly and even insidiously into the awareness of those who suffer from it, so it does not have the quality of suddenness normally associated with "trauma." But it is a form of shock all the same, a gradual realization that the community no longer exists as effective source of support and that an important part of the self has disappeared. (p. 154)

11.4.2. Erosion of Perceived Social Support

Whereas the instant mobilization of postdisaster helping behavior is a clear manifestation of received social support, the deterioration processes following disasters are more directly pertinent to expectations regarding social support availability and sense of companionship. These are, of course, the other two facets of social support mentioned earlier, perceived support and social embeddedness. The Kentucky flood study provided a clear demonstration of disaster's potential to diminish perceived social support (Kaniasty et al., 1990). Controlling for preflood assessments of perceived availability of social support in time of emergencies, Kaniasty and colleagues (1990) found that the extent of losses incurred in disaster was directly associated with declines in perceived support from both kin and nonkin sources. Similar declines in expectations of social support may be inferred from numerous studies that either showed significant bivariate negative correlations between measures of exposure and the measures of postdisaster perceived support or documented an analogous association in more complex multiple regression or path analyses (e.g., Benight, 2004; Benight, Swift, Sanger, Smith, & Zeppelin, 1999; Bokszczanin, 2004; Kaniasty, 2003; Khoury et al., 1997; Norris & Kaniasty, 1996; Solomon, Bravo, Rubio-Stipec, & Canino, 1993; Tyler, 2006; Warheit, Zimmerman, Khoury, Vega, & Gil, 1996). Norris and colleagues (2005) showed that 6 months after the 1999 Mexican floods and mudslides, survivors scored below norms for Mexico on both perceived support and social embeddedness. This deterioration in perceptions of being reliably connected to others and in sense of companionship was most dramatically salient among women in Teziutlán, where bereavement was common and displacement universal.

In part, these lower levels of perceived support may reflect a sense of disappointment that the help from relatives and friends was not provided as readily as anticipated. "Friends who you have loved and trusted turn out to be selfish and self-serving," said one of the victims of the 1993 Midwestern floods (Harvey et al., 1995, p. 328). People have typically high expectations concerning how much help they should receive, and the amount of support actually received may not meet these expectations (see Kaniasty et al., 1990; Kasapoĝlu et al., 2003). The likelihood is high that potential support providers will themselves be victims, and as a result, the need for support among all affected persons frequently surpasses its availability. Concerns about depleting resources, the resulting sense of competition, and lack of transparency and inadequacies in allocation of aid may add to disappointments with the quantity and the manner in which the help was received. For the Polish flood study, we created an index of "postdisaster bitterness" measuring survivors' unfavorable evaluations and perceptions concerning "altruistic community" (Kaniasty, 2003, 2006b). The items asked about (1) satisfaction with received help and aid from all different sources (e.g., "In general, I believe that I received adequate amount of help and aid"), (2) about evaluation of the process of aid distribution (e.g., "Some victims were omitted or neglected in the process of help distribution and received much less help than others"), and (3) respondents' beliefs in the presence of postdisaster altruistic community at the time of the first interview (12 months after the flood) (e.g., "The sense of solidarity and unity that we experienced immediately after the flood is still present among us today"). Multiple regression analyses that controlled for sociodemographic and flood exposure variables showed the respondents who reported feeling more postdisaster bitterness 12 months after the flood exhibited lower levels of perceived social support 20 and 28 months after the event.

Loss of perceived support is not limited to "primary victims," those survivors who are personally affected by disasters (see Bolin, 1985). In the Kentucky floods study we showed that expectations of support declined also for "secondary victims," those residents who lived in the affected area but sustained no personal injuries or damages. Thus, declines in expectations of support reported by both primary and secondary victims were in large part veridical assessments of their postdisaster reality. All people residing in disaster areas must adjust downward their perceptions of how much social support is available to them at any particular point in time. Although not necessarily uniformly for all victims or all sources or types of support, at some later time when more and more residents of the affected areas become less burdened by their recovery efforts, these social support estimates should recover to their more usual and higher levels (see Kaniasty et al., 1990; Norris et al., 2005).

11.4.3. Declines in Sense of Companionship and Sense of Community

There are many other factors generally responsible for postdisaster social support deterioration (see Kaniasty & Norris, 1997, 1999, 2004). Obviously, disasters interfere with many routine social activities and consequently undermine a sense of companionship. Communal activities may be thwarted for all residents of affected areas simply because physical environments, settings, and places instrumental for maintaining a sense of community and interpersonal contacts are damaged or destroyed. Residents of disaster-stricken areas often report decreased participation in activities with relatives, friends, neighbors, and community organizations (Bolin, 1993; Brown & Perkins, 1992; Golec, 1983; Hutchins & Norris, 1989; Kaniasty, 2003; Norris et al., 2005). Peculiarly, recovery may also be a very lonely and isolating process. Survivors must prioritize the use of their resources and prudently expend their energies, often putting their "social life" on hold. People feel overwhelmed by their responsibilities and are reluctant to "fritter away" their time for social contacts. In the Polish flood study, both measures of disaster exposure (material losses and experience of trauma) correlated negatively with a measure assessing withdrawal from interpersonal relationships 20 months (stronger effect) and 28 months (weaker effect) after the impact (Kaniasty, 2003). According to Rook (1985), the companionship domain of social support embraces taking part in communal activities, sharing with others the moments of leisure, or just simply enjoying being together. It appears that communities affected by disasters may be denied for a long while this particular aspect of social relationships.

Changes in social support occur also due to factors other than physical destruction, relocation, or depletion of resources like money or time. There are, undoubtedly, social and psychological dynamics of the victimization experience that may also contribute to the diminished quality and quantity of interpersonal and communal relations. Coping with community stressors such as disasters creates a shared "energy field" wherein reactions and efforts of so many people inadvertently rub off on each other. People may experience stress contagion wherein psychological difficulties experienced by some may grate on the others, all augmenting the adverse effects of disaster on entire families and other social groups (e.g., Bokszczanin, 2008; Gil-Rivas, Silver, Holman, McIntosh, & Poulin, 2007; Hobfoll & London, 1986; McFarlane, 1987; McFarlane, Policansky, & Irwin, 1987; Rustemli & Karanci, 1996; Swenson et al., 1996). In addition, social networks may become saturated with stories of and feelings about the event. Residents in disaster-stricken communities sometimes begin to downplay or reject the importance of revealed emotions and even escape interacting. Polish flood victims who were exposed to trauma or who felt more disappointed with their community immediately after disaster reported later that their social networks were more constrained, negative, and disinterested in their accounts of experiences and feelings about the event (Kaniasty, 2003). Four weeks after the Loma Prieta earthquake, T-shirts appeared on the streets of San Francisco that read "Thank you for not sharing your earthquake experience" (Pennebaker & Harber, 1993; see also, Smith & Belgrave, 1995). Interactions with people who are insensitive, uninterested, or dismissive impede recovery from all traumas (see Lepore, 2001; Maercker & Müller, 2004; Ullman & Filipas, 2001). Furthermore, physical fatigue, emotional irritability, scarcity of resources, the ongoing social pressures, and the unending chain of continuing burden of recovery enhance the potential for competition and interpersonal conflict (see, Adams & Adams, 1984; Golec, 1983; Ibañez et al., 2003; Norris & Uhl, 1992; Oliver-Smith, 1996; Steinglass & Gerrity, 1990).

11.4.4. Toxic Communities

"When the *Exxon Valdez* ran aground in Prince Sound, it spilled oil into a social as well as a natural environment" (Palinkas, Downs, Petterson, & Russell, 1993).

Victims of technological disasters are often trapped in fuzzy, chaotic, secretive, convoluted, and extended dramas. The social and community consequences of human-caused disasters are determined, in large part, by the slowly evolving, vague, and not readily perceptible nature of the impact. More often than not, the postdisaster reality of persons affected by such events is that of deterioration of social support and erosion of sense of community. In fact, the terms "toxic" or "corrosive" communities can be frequently found in the literature describing social and psychological fallouts of human-caused disasters (Bolin, 1993; Cuthbertson &

Nigg, 1987; Erikson, 1994; Freudenburg & Jones, 1991; Kroll-Smith & Couch, 1990). Kaniasty and Norris (2004) reviewed most rudimentary aspects associated with social support deterioration in these contexts.

The distinction between human-induced disasters and natural disasters is not as clear as the language used to differentiate between them (human vs. natural) would suggest. Less and less frequently are natural disasters perceived as politically neutral acts of nature or acts of God. Both victimized communities and the general public begin to see natural disasters as "unnatural" in origin and, thus, controllable. When inquires into causal factors move away from "natural" toward "human" agents, community divisions are even more likely to surface (Rochford & Blocker, 1991). Advances in technological control over the forces of nature may eventually change the way people assess and react collectively to so-called natural disasters (see Drabek, 1986).

11.4.5. Rhetoric of Disasters: Protecting the Status Quo versus Instigating Social Change

Regardless of their origins, disasters vividly expose and augment preexisting social inequities along the lines of ethnicity, race, and socioeconomic status. Bolin and Stanford (1990) reported that in some communities damaged by the Loma Prieta earthquake, the process of allocation of temporary housing to survivors inspired allegations of racism, political and cultural discrimination, and further marginalization of minorities, the elderly, and the poor. The aftermath of Hurricane Katrina dramatically uncovered the potential of the politics of disaster recovery to demoralize the victimized community's sense of unity and justice in shared struggle. Napier, Mandisodza, Andersen, and Jots (2006) conducted extensive analyses of messages and statements communicated by national and local governments, social elites, and media as the hurricane havoc unfolded. Regrettably, too many of these communications too readily and too eagerly endorsed victim-blaming attributions aimed at deflecting the responsibility for this "disaster in disaster" away from political leaders, administrators, and other mainstream stakeholders. For many Americans as well as the worldwide audience, it seemed unthinkable that residents of New Orleans would suddenly find themselves in conditions of despair, chaos, lawlessness, and neglect. The inadequate disaster response exposed governmental and organizational weaknesses, apathy of leadership, and undeniable racial and economic divisions.

According to Napier and her colleagues, faced with these failures, the political status quo, media, and the general public, as well as many victims themselves, resorted to a range of system-justifying mechanisms to support, defend, and restore perceived legitimacy of existing sociopolitical arrangements. Of course, the problem is that engaging in victim-blaming, stereotyping, and internalization of inequity, all inflict a "second injury" to the survivors, inhibit public empathy, discourage supportive responses, and undermine internal sense of unity among survivors themselves (see also, Golec, 1983; Symonds, 1980). Anecdotal evidence suggests that indeed unfavorable perceptions of refugees from New Orleans might have made their efforts in integrating themselves into hosting communities even more difficult. More to the point are empirical findings of Weems and colleagues (2007) who examined regional differences in the social and psychological impact of Katrina. Two to five months after the hurricane, residents of Orleans Parish were more likely than other regional groups (Greater New Orleans, Mississippi Gulf Coast) to report experiencing discrimination following the storm. Residents of the Mississippi Gulf Coast perceived greater levels of social support than did survivors who lived in metropolitan New Orleans and adjacent areas.

Tierney, Bevc, and Kuligowki's (2006) insightful debunking of the mass media reporting after Katrina steers in a direction of similar reflections. The media's relentless perpetuation of disaster myths (e.g., panic, looting, crime) and adherence to "war zone" metaphors should be held responsible for some immediate negative consequences for the residents of New Orleans. Curfews and military involvement interfered with survivors' abilities to help one another, hindered the emergence of the goodwill and altruistic spirit in the community, and destroyed prospects for collaborative efforts that major disasters necessitate. The researchers wrote,

> This militaristic approach stands in sharp contrast with foundational assumptions concerning how disasters should be managed, which emphasize the need for strengthening community resilience, building public-private partnerships, reaching out to marginalized community residents and their trusted institutions... (p. 76)

11.5. THE IMPACT OF RECEIVED AND PERCEIVED SOCIAL SUPPORT ON THE MENTAL HEALTH OF DISASTER SURVIVORS

11.5.1. Two Dominant Theoretical Models

Altogether, the evidence gathered across a variety of disasters suggests that a short-lived therapeutic phase of increased cohesion and helpfulness is overtaken by a protracted and diffused process of social support erosion. Thus, on the one hand, disasters mobilize social support and on the other hand, disasters deteriorate social support. What seems a paradox can be easily resolved by turning again to defining features of social support mentioned at the beginning of this chapter. The instantaneous mobilization of help following traumatic events occurs in the domain of received support, whereas a lingering sense of deterioration of interpersonal and community relationships occurs in the domains of perceived support and social embeddedness. It should be apparent now that, at the very least, the nature and timing of social support must be considered when trying to understand the impact of this most valuable resource on physical and psychological health of disaster victims.

Most studies that specifically aimed to investigate social support in the context of disasters were based conceptually on two theoretical models that have been dominating social support research for the past three decades: the stress buffer (interactive) model and the main effect (additive) model (see Lakey & Cohen, 2000; Uchino, 2004). The buffering model suggests that social support benefits individuals in crisis through protection from negative consequences of stressful conditions. The most frequent form of this model refers to social support as moderating the effects of stress, which is evidenced by a significant statistical interaction between the exposure to the stressor and social support in predicting outcome variables such as psychical and psychological health. This model implies that in the absence of stress the beneficial effect of social support is not expected (Cassel, 1976; Cobb, 1976).

To our knowledge, the first study in the area of disasters that addressed the buffering function of social support compared a group of people living near the Three Mile Island (TMI) nuclear power plant with a randomly selected group of control respondents residing in demographically similar areas. Fleming, Baum, Gisriel, and Gatchel (1982) showed that the level of perceived social support statistically interacted with accident exposure. TMI residents with lower levels of perceived support exhibited more symptoms of global distress, depression, alienation, and anxiety than did respondents from other groups. Conversely, the victims of this technological disaster who reported higher levels of perceived support were protected by it and experienced the adverse impact of the TMI accident to a lesser extent. There are many different explanations, not necessarily competing, of the stress-buffering mechanism. Social support is credited assisting in appraising the stress encounter as less taxing; sustaining self-efficacy, self-esteem, and optimism; hastening a return to physiological and emotional equilibrium; and of course, providing concrete resources needed for coping (Cohen & Wills, 1985; Cutrona & Russell, 1990; Hobfoll, 1998; Kessler, 1992: Thoits, 1986; Vaux, 1988).

The alternative model, the main or direct effect model, states that social support has an equivalent impact on well-being, regardless of whether the stress is low or high. Accordingly, this model suggests that social support has salutary effects on physical and psychological health independently of the stress process. Findings of studies consistent with this model typically show main effects of social support on the outcome variables that are not qualified by a significant interaction between the stressor and support (i.e., more support, less distress, regardless of whether the stress is low or high). The fundamental assumption of the direct effect model is that humans have basic needs for attachment, affiliation, protection, and social control, and social support provides these needs (Bowlby, 1969; Lakey & Cohen, 2000; Uchino, 2004).

Overall, the literature suggests that main effects and interactive effects of social support both occur, and the presence of either, or both, is determined by the ecological context of stressful encounters and the type of social support assessed (Cohen & Wills, 1985; Cutrona & Russell, 1990). In fact, it is rather unusual not to observe, in one form or another, and at least at a bivariate level, the beneficial effects of social support on symptomatology in the context of any life circumstances (see Kaniasty, 2005; Sarason & Sarason, 2006; Taylor, 2007).

11.5.2. Received Social Support and Postdisaster Distress

Somewhat oddly, there are not that many studies in disaster research that attempted to examine the psychological benefits of received social support. Bolin (1982) and Bolin and Bolton (1986) have observed that primary group aid facilitated emotional recovery from several disasters. Drabek and Key (1984) documented similar effects in their analysis of social functioning 3 years after a Topeka, Kansas, tornado. Controlling for the degree of damage, tornado survivors who received help from friends or relatives, compared with those who did not, reported being less alienated, healthier, happier in their marriages, and more involved in activities with friends, churches, or social organizations. Numerous studies that used the Crisis Support Scale also clearly showed that greater levels of received support both immediately and later after disasters had direct salutary associations with lower posttraumatic distress (e.g., Dalgleish, Joseph, Thrasher, Tranah, & Yule, 1986; Joseph, Andrews, Williams, & Yule, 1992; Udwin, Boyle, Yule, Bolton, & O'Ryan, 2000; see also, Joseph, 1999). The classic studies of receipt of help by survivors did not attempt the tests of stress-buffering properties of received support, but their results are consistent with the main effect model.

Studies that specifically aimed to examine the buffer model of social support received after disasters are even less frequent. Solomon (1985) hypothesized the buffer function of received support in a study of mothers of young children 12 months after the TMI accident. Received social support did not moderate the impact of stress (TMI site vs. control site); nevertheless, received emotional support had direct beneficial effects on occurrence of new episodes of major depression and generalized anxiety. Tangible support was unrelated to any of the outcome measures. In a sample of survivors of Hurricane Andrew, Sanchez, Korbin, and Viscarra (1995) showed some buffering effects of received support (from employers), but these effects were restricted to very specific outcomes (i.e., work tension, not anxiety or physical symptoms). There are also studies that simply did not register any clear influence of social support receipt in the aftermath of disasters (e.g., Murphy, 1988; Morgan, Matthews, & Winton, 1995; see also Pickens, Field, Prodromidis, Pelaez-Nogueraz, & Hossain, 1995).

This apparent neglect of received social support by disaster mental health researchers is not at all unique because the studies of psychological impact of actually receiving help are not common in the general stress and coping literature. The reason for this indifference is most likely the fact that findings of studies assessing social support as actual provisions of help are less consistent than those of the studies that examined perceived social support. In fact, many studies that examined coping with a variety of different stressors revealed no effects, or worse, documented positive associations between receiving help and psychological distress (e.g., Dunkel-Schetter, 1984; Helgeson, 1993; Hobfoll & London, 1986; Husaini, Neff, Newbrough, & Moore, 1982; Riley & Eckenrode, 1986; Sandler & Barrera, 1984; see also, Bödvarsdóttir, Elklit, & Gudmundsdóttir, 2006). Such an association may be artifactual in that the presence of psychological suffering constitutes a clear cue for support networks to mobilize their efforts to provide for those in need.

11.5.3. Perceived Social Support and Postdisaster Distress

Just as it is in the case of stress and coping research, perceived support is the principal facet of social support investigated in studies of natural disasters, technological catastrophes, and acts of terrorism. Some of these investigations sought evidence of the stress-buffering properties of perceived social support. For example, with the data from a small sample of residents of areas affected by fires and floods, Benight (2004) showed a classic pattern of a fan-shaped (synergistic) stress-buffering interaction. Of all the victims, those who incurred high losses and reported low levels of perceived support (or low levels of collective efficacy) exhibited the highest levels of psychological distress a year after the events. However, not many disaster studies found the pristine and unqualified buffering effects as this study or earlier-mentioned investigation of Fleming and his colleagues (1982). When present, stress-buffering properties of perceived social support are likely to be confined to specific subgroups, locales, or contexts of disasters (Palinkas, Russell, Downs, & Petterson, 1992; Solomon, Smith, Robins, & Fishbach, 1987; Tyler & Hoyt, 2000). Very limited buffer effects were reported by other investigations (e.g., Cook & Bickman, 1989), and there are reports that revealed null findings regarding the buffer model (e.g., Bokszczanin, 2008; Kaniasty, 2006b; Murphy, 1988).

The lack of strong empirical evidence for perceived social support as a buffer of disaster stress does not at all mean that having greater levels of perceived support is inconsequential for better psychological outcomes among people subjected to disaster events. In fact, almost all investigations have documented that perceived availability of support is directly related to victims' well-being (e.g., Acierno, Ruggiero, Kilpatrick, Resnick, & Galea, 2006; Bananno, Galea, Bucciarelli, & Vlahov, 2007; Bartone, Ursano, Wright, & Ingraham, 1989; Benight et al., 1999; Bokszczanin, 2008; Bromet, Parkinson, Schulberg, & Gondek, 1982; Carr, Webster, Hazell, Kenardy, & Carter, 1995; Hobfoll, Tracy, & Galea, 2006; Khoury et al., 1997; La Greca, Silverman, Vernberg, & Prinstein, 1996; Lutgendorf et al., 1995; Ullman & Newcomb, 1999; Vernberg, La Greca, Silverman, & Prinstein, 1996; Warheit et al., 1996; Watanabe, Okumura, Chiu, & Wakai, 2004). Likewise, meta-analytical studies place low levels of perceived social support on the top of the lists of risk factors for posttraumatic stress disorder (Brewin, Andrews, & Valentine, 2000; Ozer, Best, Lipsey, & Weiss, 2003).

Whereas both the stress buffer model and the main effects model are viable ways of describing how social support operates, they do not account for all possible relations between stress, social support, and psychological functioning. A major conceptual problem with these two dominant hypotheses is that they consider stress as a static phenomenon. The principal assumption of both theoretical formulations is that stress and social support are unrelated to each other; in fact, the link between stressor and social support has been largely ignored or considered a conceptual or methodological inconvenience (see Barrera, 1986). However, a closer inspection of correlation tables in most disaster and trauma studies reveals that perceived support is frequently negatively correlated with stress exposure measures. Simply, whenever stressful circumstances meaningfully influence social support and personal relationships, buffering and main effects models offer only limited grounds for explaining dynamics of the stress process.

11.5.4. Social Support as a Mediator of Disaster Impact on Distress

The present review of literature provided strong evidence for declines in quality of personal relationships and social support following disasters.

What are the mental health consequences of this disaster-induced erosion of social support for the survivors? Most reasonably, the postevent declines in social support could contribute to the detrimental impact of stress rather than counteract (buffer) it. Consequently, a mediating, not a moderating model (see Baron & Kenny, 1986), may be more appropriate for describing the role of social support in disaster recovery.

The social support deterioration model (see Barrera, 1986; Ensel & Lin, 1991; Wheaton, 1985) describes a mechanism whereby stressful experiences instigate declines in social support that in turn contribute to the detrimental impact of stress on psychological health. We tested this model in the context of the Kentucky floods (Kaniasty & Norris, 1993). Our hypothesis was that declines in social support following disaster would account, to an extent, for the impact of disaster stress on survivors' psychological well-being. Using a methodologically conservative design that controlled for preevent levels of functioning (symptoms and social support), we found that victims experienced the psychological consequences of flooding (i.e., an increased in depressive symptomatology) both directly, through immediate damage and exposure to trauma, and indirectly, through deterioration of perceived support and sense of embeddedness. The loss of social support has also been found to mediate psychological consequences of Hurricanes Hugo and Andrew (Norris & Kaniasty, 1996). In recent years, studies investigating a variety of potentially traumatic events, such as forced relocation, war combat exposure, interpersonal violence, child abuse, or crime, have presented evidence congruent with the social support deterioration model and shown how declines in social support (mainly perceived support), fully or partially explained the translation of trauma exposure into symptoms of enduring distress (e.g., Hwang, Xi, Cao, Feng, & Qiao, 2007; Taft, Stern, King, & King, 1999; Thompson et al., 2000; Vranceanu, Hobfoll, & Johnson, 2007; Yap & Devilly, 2004). In trauma research, the social support deterioration model represents a viable alternative to the stress buffering and the main effect models.

However, the present review of literature also provided enough evidence that people affected by disastrous events, particularly victims of natural disasters, receive substantial amounts of help and often experience heightened levels of postcrisis benevolence and solidarity. Thus, important questions remain. What is the role of received social support when perceived social support deteriorates as a result of disaster experience? Can these two seemingly contradictory facets of social support processes – the instantaneous mobilization of received support and subsequent deterioration of perceived support – be combined into one comprehensive explanatory model?

On the basis of our research with survivors of floods and hurricanes, we developed a conceptual model that attempts to capture many of the complexities of social functioning in the aftermath of disasters and its impact on victims' and community's well-being. The social support deterioration deterrence model (SSDD) (Kaniasty & Norris, 1997, 1999, 2004; Norris & Kaniasty, 1996) is an extension of the social support deterioration hypothesis, and thus it also begins with the proposal that disastrous events exert their adverse impact on psychological health both directly and indirectly, through disruptions of social relationships and loss of perceived social support (Figure 11.1). First of all, disasters have a powerful adverse direct effect on psychological distress (direct impact). Preexisting social and psychological conditions and resources of individuals (i.e., age, gender, social status) influence the extent of exposure to the stressor (differential exposure). At their onset, many catastrophic events mobilize social support networks (support mobilization). Although receipt of help is influenced by the extent of losses incurred in disaster (relative needs), it is not completely equitable (relative advantage), and it is governed by diverse norms and rules of inclusion and exclusion. Most importantly, the initial rush of spontaneous helping inevitably ceases long before the stress of disaster is over, and the survivors eventually face the sad reality of declining social support (support deterioration). The erosion of perceived social support and sense of belonging

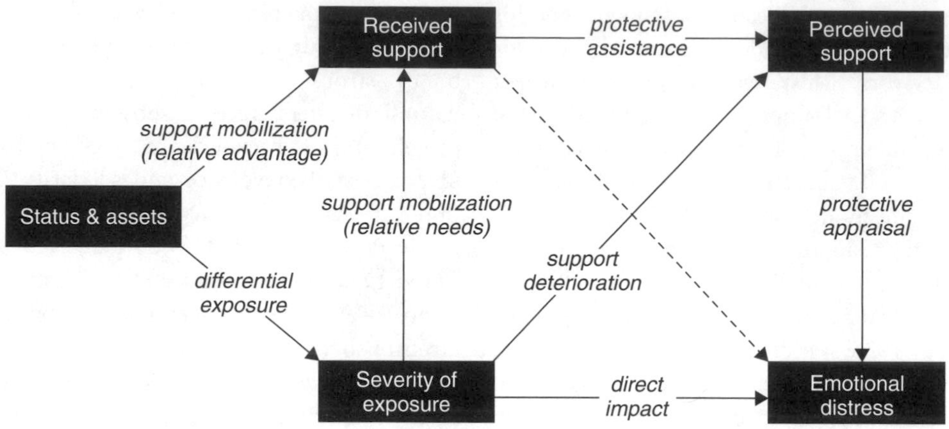

Figure 11.1. Social support deterioration deterrence (SSDD) model.

may inevitably contribute to poorer physical and mental health. To an important but incomplete extent, the initial mobilization of received support counteracts this deterioration and preserves perceptions that supportive networks are still in place (protective assistance). Through the process of deterioration deterrence (paths – support mobilization and protective assistance combined), mobilization of received support indirectly affects mental health by preserving perceptions of social support. Thus, perceived support plays its usual protective role (protective appraisal).

Our analyses (Norris & Kaniasty, 1996) of data collected 12 and 24 months following Hurricane Hugo and 6 and 28 months following Hurricane Andrew provided strong evidence for the hypothesized model. Importantly, perceived support mediated the long-term effects on psychological distress of both disaster stress and postdisaster received support. Although disaster stress led to deterioration of perceived support, the total effects of disaster on perceived support were less severe than they might have been because the stress of disaster was positively associated with received support. Received support was, in turn, positively associated with ensuing beliefs regarding the perceived availability of support (see also, Kaniasty, 2003; Tyler, 2006). Clearly, the deterioration of social support following disasters is not inevitable. When victims receive high levels of help following a disaster, they are protected against salient erosion in their evaluations of support availability. Protecting perceived support may be the most important function of received support. The value of the more comprehensive SSDD model is in that it explicitly connects the processes of mobilization and deterioration in social resources and provides clear predictions regarding how these contrasting paths account for psychological well-being of the people and communities affected by disasters.

11.6. RECOMMENDATIONS FOR RESEARCH

Presently, both researchers and practitioners consider social support as a central construct in exploring and understanding the relations between stressors and health. For many contemporary studies that examine how different stressors impact physical, psychological, and social well-being, it is almost imperative to include some feature of this multifaceted resource. Social support has become an expected companion to standard status variables in stress and coping research, such as gender, age, education, or ethnicity. Consequently, over the years social support has been given a leading role in the complex nets of nearly all theoretical formulations attempting to describe consequences of the stress experience.

For disaster mental health research the importance of social support is paramount because interpersonal and social dynamics play a dominant role in coping with catastrophic events. Understanding postdisaster social support processes augments the comprehensiveness of our theories and precision of our hypotheses. Understanding postdisaster social support processes is also a direct step in translating our sophisticated theoretical and empirical notions into practice. Social support, with its intrapsychic and interpersonal manifestations, is simply a prerequisite matter for the practice of postdisaster mitigation and interventions. Helping disaster survivors inherently involves addressing their social support needs and contexts.

How can our studies assure that social support that is enacted by the survivors themselves as well as provided to them is ultimately what it is intended to be – supportive? We must recognize the distinctions among its different facets because they matter. At the very least, the "method sections" of our manuscripts should clearly declare which facet (e.g., perceived, received, embeddedness) of social support was assessed, hopefully with more than one or two items. Too often, otherwise informative trauma and disaster studies refer to social support generically and seem to assume its commonsense validity just as if the meaning of social support was as apparent as the meaning of status variables such as gender, age, or race.

We believe that the potential for practical usefulness of our research will benefit from more frequent investigations of social support actually received. The types of received social support (e.g., tangible, informational, emotional) and timing of their receipt (e.g., immediately after the impact vs. later in the process of recovery) are also significant. From whom social support is received matters, for both the recipients and the providers, and less traditional sources that capably enter the stage and that activate social support networks should be included in the assessments (e.g., media, Internet). Although this review did not directly address the role of social support provided by victims to other victims, investigations of social support provisions attest to the psychological relevance of this aspect of social support in disaster preparedness and recovery processes.

Besides the most rudimentary distinctions among received social support, perceived social support, and social embeddedness, there are many related constructs that help capture the meaning of postdisaster social support dynamics. Help-seeking comfort, sense of companionship, sense of community, collective efficacy or mastery, or postdisaster growth in social relationships are promising variables that explore tributaries of social support's roles in coping with disasters and catastrophes. However, because within the ecology of collective stress every asset has its liabilities and every benefit has its costs, we must also recognize that postdisaster social support exchanges inadvertently encompass negative social interactions. Inquiries into the origins and consequences of postdisaster social bitterness, negative social reactions to victims, feelings of rejection, neglect, social network constraints, and conflicts are equally instructive.

Finally, the "old and reliable" statement that "nothing is as practical as a good theory" is definitely true for disaster social support research. Our studies must be guided by continuously evolving theoretical frameworks that diversely place social support in the stress process. Whether or not social support moderates the impact of disasters on mental health is an important question, but it is not the only question. Routine subscription to both the main effects and stress buffer models limits our understanding of all possible linkages between the exposure, social support, and recovery. Social support, especially in the context of shared traumas, is a malleable entity; hence, dynamic (e.g., mediating) models should be more useful for delineating its constructive and unconstructive functions. The majority of disaster social support studies are cross-sectional, and even if they follow survivors longitudinally, very few have pre-event measures of psychological and social well-being. Likewise, nearly all these investigations explain the importance of social support for disaster mental health based on the idea that social support resources are antecedents of well-being, and lack of them increases psychological distress ("social causation" hypothesis).

However, a converse view is also viable, which suggests that via "social selection processes" healthy individuals are selected, or welcomed, into thriving social relationships. Therefore, persons with psychological distress (e.g., disaster survivors) may experience a subsequent decline in their social support resources (e.g., postdisaster deterioration of support). The inquiry into the relative importance of these two causal processes, social causation or social section, must continue.

In sum, we must accept that social support is not a generic or a proxy variable standing for "just good social relationships." Social support with its multitude of facets and functions is ridden with complexities. It's often remarkable effects must be rigorously examined to expand the theory and practice beyond the perfunctory statement that social support is a critical resource for people coping with disasters.

REFERENCES

Acierno, R. Ruggiero, K., Kilpatrick, D., Resnick, H., & Galea, S. (2006). Risk and protective factors for psychopathology among older versus younger adults after the 2004 Florida hurricanes. *American Journal of Geriatric Psychiatry, 14*, 1051–1059.

Adams, P., & Adams, G. (1984). Mount St. Helen ashfall: Evidence for a disaster stress reaction. *American Psychologist, 39*, 252–260.

Adler, J. (1993). Troubled waters. *Newsweek, July, 26*, 23.

Baron, R., & Kenny, D.A. (1986). The moderator-mediator variable distinction in social psychological research: Conceptual, strategic, and statistical considerations. *Journal of Personality and Social Psychology, 51*, 1173–1182.

Barrera, M. (1986). Distinctions between social support concepts, measures, and models. *American Journal of Community Psychology, 14*, 413–445.

Barrera, M., Sandler, I.N., & Ramsay, T.B. (1981). Preliminary development of a scale of social support: Studies on college students. *American Journal of Community Psychology, 9*, 435–447.

Barton, A.M. (1969). *Communities in disaster*. Garden City, NJ: Doubleday.

Bartone, P., Ursano, R., Wright, K., & Ingraham, L. (1989). The impact of a military air disaster on the health of assistance workers: A prospective study. *Journal of Nervous and Mental Disease, 177*, 317–328.

Beggs, J.J., Haines, V.A., & Hurlbert, J.S. (1996). Situational contingencies surrounding the receipt of informal support. *Social Forces, 75*, 201–223.

Benight, C. (2004). Collective efficacy following a series of natural disasters. *Anxiety, Stress & Coping: An International Journal, 17*, 401–420

Benight, C.C., Swift, E., Sanger, J., Smith, A., & Zeppelin, D. (1999). Coping self-efficacy as a mediator of distress following a natural disaster. *Journal of Applied Social Psychology, 29*, 2443–2464.

Bödvarsdóttir, Í., Elklit, A., & Gudmundsdóttir, D. (2006). Post-traumatic stress reactions in children after two large Earthquakes in Iceland. *Nordic Psychology, 58*, 91–107.

Bokszczanin, A. (2004). Negatywne efekty powodzi 1997 roku dla dorastających: Deterioracja wsparcia społecznego oraz symptomy stresu pourazowego. [*Negative consequences of 1997 Polish flood on adolescents: Deterioration of social support and posttraumatic distress*]. In J. Strelau, (Ed.), *Osobowość a Ekstremalny Stres*. Gdańsk: Gdańskie Wydawnictwo Psychologiczne.

(2008). Parental support, family conflict, and overprotectiveness: Predicting PTSD symptom levels of adolescents 28 months after a natural disaster. *Anxiety, Stress, & Coping: An International Journal, 21*, 325–335.

Bonanno, G., Galea, S., Bucciarelli, A., & Vlahov, D. (2007). What predicts psychological resilience after disaster? The role of demographics, resources, and life stress. *Journal of Consulting and Clinical Psychology, 75*, 671–682.

Bland, S., O'Leary, E., Farinaro, E., Jossa, F., Krogh, V., Violanti, J., et al. (1997). Social network disturbances and psychological distress following earthquake evacuation. *Journal of Nervous and Mental Disease, 185*, 188–194.

Bolin, R. (1982). *Long-term family recovery from disaster*. Boulder, CO: University of Colorado.

(1985). Disaster characteristics and psychosocial impacts. In B.T. Sowder (Ed.), *Disasters and mental health: Selected contemporary perspectives*. Rockville, MD: National Institute of Mental Health.

(1989). Natural disasters. In R. Gist & B. Lubin (Eds.), *Psychological aspects of disaster*. New York: Wiley.

(1993). Natural and technological disasters: Evidence of psychopathology. In A.-M. Ghadirian & H.E. Lehmann (Eds.), *Environment and Psychopathology*. New York: Springer, New York.

Bolin, R., & Bolton, P. (1986). *Race, religion, and ethnicity in disaster recovery*. Boulder, CO: University of Colorado.

Bolin, R., & Stanford, L. (1990). Shelter and housing issues in Santa Cruz County. In R. Bolin (Ed.),

The Loma Prieta earthquake: Studies of short-term impacts. Bolder, CO: University of Colorado.

Bowlby, J. (1969). *Attachment and loss: Vol. 1. attachment.* New York: Basic Books.

Brown, B.B., & Perkins, D.D. (1992). Disruptions in place attachment. In I. Altman & S. Low (Eds.), *Place attachment.* New York: Plenum Press.

Brewin, C., Andrews, B., & Valentine, J. (2000). Meta-analysis of risk factors for posttraumatic stress disorder in trauma-exposed adults. *Journal of Consulting and Clinical Psychology, 68,* 748–766.

Bromet, E.J., Parkinson, D., Schulberg, H., & Gondek, P. (1982). Mental health of residents near the Three Mile Island reactor: A comparative study of selected groups. *Journal of Preventive Psychiatry, 1,* 225–276.

Caldera, T., Palma, L., Penayo, U., & Kullgren, G. (2001). Psychological impact of the Hurricane Mitch in Nicaragua in a one-year perspective. *Social Psychiatry and Psychiatric Epidemiology, 36,* 108–114.

Carr, V.J., Lewin, T.J., Carter, G., & Webster, R. (1992). Patterns of service utilization following the 1989 Newcastle earthquake: Findings from phase 1 of the Quake Impact study. *Australian Journal of Public Health, 16,* 360–369.

Carr, V.J., Lewin, T., Webster, R., Hazell, P., Kenardy, J., & Carter, G. (1995). Psychological sequelae of the 1989 Newcastle Earthquake: I. Community disaster experiences and psychological morbidity 6 months post-disaster. *Psychological Medicine, 25,* 539–555.

Cassel, J. (1976). The contribution of the social environment to host resistance. *American Journal of Epidemiology, 104,* 107–123.

Cobb, S. (1976). Social support as a moderator of life stress. *Psychosomatic Medicine, 38,* 300–314.

Cohen, S., & Wills, T.A. (1985). Stress, social support, and the buffering hypothesis. *Psychological Bulletin, 98,* 310–357.

Cohen, S., Doyle, W.J., Skoner, D.P., Rabin, B.S., & Gwaltney, J.M., Jr. (1997). Social ties and susceptibility to the common cold. *Journal of the American Medical Association, 277,* 1940–1944.

Cohen, S., Mermelstein, R., Kamarck, T., & Hoberman, H. (1985). Measuring the functional components of social support. In I.G. Sarason & B.R. Sarason (Eds.), *Social support: Theory, research and application.* The Hague, Holland: Martinus Nijhoff.

Collins, R. (2004). Rituals of solidarity and security in the wake of terrorists attack. *Sociological Theory, 22,* 53–87.

Conejero, S., & Etxebarria, I. (2007). The impact of the Madrid bombing on personal emotions, emotional atmosphere and emotional climate. *Journal of Social Issues, 63,* 273–287.

Cook, J., & Bickman, L. (1990). Social support and psychological symptomatology following a natural disaster. *Journal of Traumatic Stress, 3,* 541–556.

Cuthbertson, B., & Nigg, J. (1987). Technological disaster and the nontherapeutic community: A question of true victimization. *Environment and Behavior, 19,* 462–483.

Cutrona, C., & Russell, D. (1990). Type of social support and specific stress: Toward a theory of optimal matching. In B. R. Sarason, I. G. Sarason, & G.R. Pierce (Eds.), *Social support: An interactional view.* New York: Wiley.

Dalgleish, T., Joseph, S., Thrasher, S., Tranah, T., & Yule, W. (1996). Crisis support following the herald of free-enterprise disaster: A longitudinal perspective. *Journal of Traumatic Stress, 9,* 833–845.

DePaulo, B., Nadler, A., & Fisher, J. (Eds.). (1983). *New directions in helping Vol. 2. Help-seeking.* New York: Academic Press.

Drabek, T.E. (1986). *Human system responses to disaster.* New York: Springer-Verlag.

Drabek, T.E., & Key, W.M. (1984). *Conquering disaster: Family recovery and long-term consequences.* New York: Irvington Publishers.

Dunkel-Schetter, C. (1984). Social support and cancer: Findings based on patient interviews and their implications. *Journal of Social Issues, 40,* 77–98.

Eckenrode, J. (1983). The mobilization of social supports: Some individual constraints. *American Journal of Community Psychology, 11,* 509–528.

Elklit, A., Pedersen, S.S., & Jind, L. (2001). The Crisis Support Scale: Psychometric qualities and further validation. *Personality and Individual Differences, 31,* 1291–1302.

Ensel, W., & Lin, N. (1991). The life stress paradigm and psychological distress. *Journal of Health and Social Behavior, 32,* 321–341.

Eranen, L., & Liebkind, K. (1993). Coping with disaster: The helping behavior of communities and individuals. In J.P. Wilson & B. Raphael (Eds.), *International handbook of traumatic stress syndromes.* New York: Plenum Press.

Erikson, K. (1976). *Everything in its path.* New York: Simon & Schuster.

(1994). *A new species of trouble: The human experience of modern disasters.* New York: W.W. Norton & Company.

Fleming, R., Baum, A., Gisriel, M., & Gatchel, R. (1982). Mediating influences of social support on stress at Three Mile Island. *Journal of Human Stress, 8,* 14–22.

Fullilove, M.T., & Saul, J. (2006). Rebuilding communities post-disaster in New York. In Y. Neria,

R. Gross, R. Marshall, & E. Susser (Eds.), *9/11: Mental health in the wake of terrorist attacks.* New York: Cambridge University Press.

Ford, J., Adams, M., & Dailey, W. F. (2006). Factors associated with receiving help and risk factors for disaster-related distress among Connecticut adults 5–15 months after the September 11th terrorist incidents. *Social Psychiatry and Psychiatric Epidemiology, 41,* 261–270.

Frederick, C. (1980). Effects of natural vs. human-induced violence upon victims. *Evaluation and Change, (Special Issue),* 71–75.

Freudenburg, W. R., & Jones, T. R. (1991). Does an unpopular facility cause stress? A test of the Supreme Court Hypothesis. *Social Forces, 69,* 1143–1168.

Fritz, C. E. (1961). Disasters. In R. K. Merton & R. A. Nisbet (Eds.), *Contemporary social problems.* New York: Harcourt.

Giel, R. (1990). Psychosocial process in disasters. *International Journal of Mental Health, 19,* 7–20.

Gil-Rivas, V., Cohen, S. R., Holman, E. A., McIntosh, D., & Polin, M. (2007). Parental response and adolescent adjustment to the September 11, 2001 attacks. *Journal of Traumatic Stress, 20,* 1063–1068

Golec, J. A. (1983). A contextual approach to the social psychological study of disaster recovery. *International Journal of Mass Emergencies and Disaster, 1,* 255–276.

Harvey, J., Stein, S., Olsen, N., Roberts, R., Lutgendorf, S., & Ho, J. (1995). Narratives of loss and recovery from a natural disaster. *Journal of Social Behavior and Personality, 10,* 313–330.

Helgeson, V. (1993). Two important distinctions in social support: Kind of support and perceived versus received. *Journal of Applied Social Psychology, 23,* 825–845.

Hill, R., & Hansen, D. A. (1962). Families in disaster. In G. W. Baker & D. W. Chapman (Eds.), *Man and society in disaster.* New York: Basic Books.

Hobfoll, S. E. (1998). *Stress, culture and community: The psychology and philosophy of stress.* New York: Plenum Press.

Hobfoll, S. E., & Lerman, M. (1989). Predicting receipt of social support: A longitudinal study of parents' reactions to their child's illness. *Health Psychology, 8,* 61–77.

Hobfoll, S. E., & London, P. (1986). The relationship of self-concept and social support to emotional distress among women during war. *Journal of Social and Clinical Psychology, 12,* 87–100.

Hobfoll, S., Tracy, M., & Galea, S. (2006). The impact of resource loss and traumatic growth on probable PTSD and depression following terrorist attacks. *Journal of Traumatic Stress, 19,* 867–878.

House, J., Umberson, D., & Landis, K. (1988). Structures and processes of social support. *Annual Review of Sociology, 14,* 293–318.

Husaini, B., Neff, J., Newbrough, J., & Moore, M. (1982). The stress-buffering role of social support and personal competence among the rural married. *Journal of Community Psychology, 10,* 409–426.

Hutchins, G., & Norris, F. H. (1989). Life change in the disaster recovery period. *Environment and Behavior, 21,* 33–56.

Hwang, S., Xi, J., Cao, Y., Feng, X., & Qiao, X. (2007). Anticipation of migration and psychological stress and the Three Gorges Dam project, China. *Social Science & Medicine, 65,* 1012–1024.

Ibañez, G., Khatchikian, N., Buck, C., Weisshaar, D., Abush-Kirsh, T., Lavizzo, E., et al. (2003). Qualitative analysis of social support and conflict among Mexican and Mexican-American disaster survivors. *Journal of Community Psychology, 31,* 1–23.

James, W. (1912). *Memories and studies (On some mental effects of the earthquake).* New York: Longmans, Green, and Co.

Jones, S., & Rainie, L. (2002). Internet use and the terror attacks. In B. S. Greenberg (Ed.), *Communication and terrorism: Public and media responses to 9/11.* Cresskill, NJ: Hampton Press.

Joseph, S. (1999). Social support and mental health following trauma. In W. Yule (Ed.), *Post-traumatic stress disorders. Concepts and therapy.* Chichester, UK: John Wiley & Sons.

Joseph, S., Andrews, B., Williams, R., & Yule, W. (1992). Crisis support and psychiatric symptomatology in adult survivors of the Jupiter cruise ship disaster. *British Journal of Clinical Psychology, 31,* 63–73.

Kaniasty, K. (2003). *Klęska żywiołowa czy katastrofa społeczna? Psychospołeczne konsekwencje polskiej powodzi 1997 roku.* (Natural disaster or social catastrophe? Psychosocial consequences of the 1997 Polish Flood). Gdańsk, Poland: Gdańskie Wydawnictwo Psychologiczne.

(2005). Social support and traumatic stress. *PTSD Research Quarterly, 16* (2). The National Center for PTSD.

(2006a). Searching for points of convergence: A commentary on prior research on disasters and some community programs initiated in response to September 11, 2001. In Y. Neria, R. Gross, R. Marshall, & E. Susser (Eds.), *9/11: Mental health in the wake of terrorist attacks.* New York: Cambridge University Press.

(2006b). Sense of mastery as a moderator of longer-term effects of disaster impact on psychological distress. In J. Strelau & T. Klonowicz (Eds.), *People under extreme stress.* Hauppauge, NY: Nova Science Publishers.

Kaniasty, K., & Norris, F. H. (1995). In search of altruistic community: Patterns of social support mobilization following Hurricane Hugo. *American Journal of Community Psychology, 23*, 447–477.

(1997). Social support dynamics in adjustment to disasters. In S. Duck (Ed.), *Handbook of personal relationships (2nd ed.)*. London, UK: Wiley.

(1999). The experience of disaster: Individuals and communities sharing trauma. In R. Gist & B. Lubin (Eds.), *Response to disaster: Psychosocial, community, and ecological approaches*. Philadelphia, PA: Brunner/Maze.

(2000). Help-seeking comfort and receiving social support: The role of ethnicity and context of need. *American Journal of Community Psychology, 28*, 545–581.

(2004). Social support in the aftermath of disasters, catastrophes, and acts of terrorism: Altruistic, overwhelmed, uncertain, antagonistic, and patriotic communities. In R. Ursano, A. Norwood, & C. Fullerton (Eds.), *Bioterrorism: Psychological and public health interventions*. Cambridge: Cambridge University Press.

Kaniasty, K., Norris, F. H., & Murrell, S. A. (1990). Received and perceived social support following natural disaster. *Journal of Applied Social Psychology, 20*, 85–114.

Kasapoĝlu, A., Ecevit, Y., & Ecevit, M. (2004). Support needs of the survivors of the August 17, 1999 Earthquake in Turkey. *Social Indicators Research, 66*, 229–248.

Kessler, R. (1992). Perceived support and adjustment to stress: methodological considerations. In H. Veiel & U. Baumann (Eds.), *The meaning and measurement of social support*. New York: Hemisphere.

Khoury, E. L., Warheit, G. J., Hargrove, M. C., Zimmerman, R. S., Vega, W. A., & Gil, A. G. (1997). The impact of Hurricane Andrew on deviant behavior among a multi-racial/ethnic sample of adolescents in Dade County, Florida: A longitudinal analysis. *Journal of Traumatic Stress, 10*, 71–91.

Kilijanek, T., & Drabek, T. E. (1979). Assessing long-term impacts of a natural disaster: A focus on the elderly. *The Gerontologist, 19*, 555–566.

Kroll-Smith, J. S., & Couch, S. (1990). *The real disaster is above ground: A mine fire and social conflict*. Lexington: University Press of Kentucky.

Kutak, R. I. (1938). The sociology of crises: The Louisville flood of 1937. *Social Forces, 16*, 66–72.

La Greca, A., Silverman, W., Vernberg, E., & Prinstein, M. (1996). Symptoms of post-traumatic stress in children after Hurricane Andrew: A prospective study. *Journal of Consulting and Clinical Psychology, 64*, 712–723.

Lakey, B., & Cohen, S. (2000). Social support theory and measurement. In S. Cohen, L. Underwood, & B. Gottlieb (Eds.), *Social support measurement and interventions: A guide for health and social scientists*. New York: Oxford University Press.

Leatham, G., & Duck, S. (1990). Conversations with friends and the dynamic of social support. In S. Duck & R. Silver. (Ed.), *Personal relationships and social support*. London: Sage.

Lazarus, R. S., & Folkman, S. (1984). *Stress, appraisal, and coping*. New York: Springer.

Lepore, S. J. (2001). A social-cognitive processing model of emotional adjustment to cancer. In A. Baum & B. Andersen (Eds.), *Psychosocial interventions for cancer*. Washington, DC: American Psychological Association.

Lindy, J., & Grace, M. (1986). The recovery environment: Continuing stressor versus a healing psychosocial space. In B. Sowder & M. Lystad (Eds.), *Disasters and mental health*. Washington, DC: American Psychiatric Press.

Lutgendorf, S. K., Antoni, M. H., Ironson, G., Fletcher, M. A., Penedo, F., Baum, A., et al. (1995). Physical symptoms of chronic fatigue syndrome are exacerbated by the stress of Hurricane Andrew. *Psychosomatic Medicine, 57*, 310–323.

Maercker, A., & Müller, J. (2004). Social acknowledgment as a victim or survivor: A scale to measure a recovery factor of PTSD. *Journal of Traumatic Stress, 17*, 345–351.

McFarlane, A. C. (1987). Family functioning and overprotection following a natural disaster: The longitudinal effects of post-traumatic morbidity. *Australian and New Zealand Journal of Psychiatry, 21*, 210–218.

McFarlane, A. C., Policansky, S., & Irwin, C. (1987). A longitudinal study of the psychological morbidity in children due to a natural disaster. *Psychological Medicine, 17*, 727–738.

Morgan, I., Matthews, G., & Winton, M. (1995). Coping and personality as predictors of post-traumatic intrusions, numbing, avoidance and general distress: A study of victims of the Perth Flood. *Behavioural and Cognitive Psychotherapy, 23*, 251–264.

Murphy, S. (1986). Perceptions of stress, coping, and recovery one and three years after a natural disaster. *Issues in Mental Health Nursing, 8*, 63–77.

(1988). Mediating effects of intrapersonal and social support on mental health 1 and 3 years after a natural disaster. *Journal of Traumatic Stress, 1*, 155–172.

Nadler, A. (1997). Personality and help seeking: autonomous versus dependent seeking of help. In G. Pierce, B. Lakey, I. Sarason, & B. Sarason (Eds.), *Sourcebook of social support and personality*. New York: Plenum Press.

Napier, J.L., Mandisodza, A., Andersen, S., & Jost, J.T. (2006). System justification in responding to the poor and displaced in the aftermath of Hurricane Katrina. *Analyses of Social Issues and Public Policy*, *6*, 57–73.

Norris, F.H., & Kaniasty, K. (1996). Received and perceived social support in times of stress: A test of the social support deterioration deterrence model. *Journal of Personality and Social Psychology*, *71*, 498–511.

Norris, F.H., & Uhl, G. (1993). Chronic stress as a mediator of acute stress: The case of Hurricane Hugo. *Journal of Applied Social Psychology*, *23*, 1263–1284.

Norris, F.H., Baker, C., Murphy, A., & Kaniasty, K. (2005). Social support mobilization and deterioration after Mexico's 1999 flood: Effects of context, gender, and time. *American Journal of Community Psychology*, *36*, 15–28.

Norris, F.H., Friedman, M., & Watson, P. (2002). 60,000 disaster victims speak: Part II. Summary and implications for the disaster mental health research. *Psychiatry*, *65*, 240–260.

Norris, F.H., Friedman, M., Watson, P., Byrne, C., Diaz, E., & Kaniasty, K. (2002). 60,000 disaster victims speak, Part I: An empirical review of the empirical literature, 1981–2001. *Psychiatry*, *65*, 207–239.

Norris, F.H., Murphy, A. Kaniasty, K., Perilla, J., & Ortis, D.C. (2001). Postdisaster social support in the U.S. and Mexico: Conceptual and contextual considerations. *Hispanic Journal of Behavioral Sciences*, *23*, 469–497.

Norris, F.H., Phifer, J., & Kaniasty, K. (1994). Individual and community reactions to the Kentucky floods: Findings from a longitudinal study of older adults. In R. Ursano, B. McCaughey, & C. Fullerton (Eds.), *Individual and community responses to trauma and disaster: The structure of human chaos*. Cambridge, U.K.: Cambridge University Press.

Oliver-Smith, A. (1996). Anthropological research on hazards and disasters. *Annual Reviews of Anthropology*, *25*, 303–328.

Ozer, E., Best, S., Lipsey, T., & Weiss, D. (2003). Predictors of posttraumatic stress disorder and symptoms in adults: A meta-analysis. *Psychological Bulletin*, *129*, 52–73.

Páez, D., Basabe, N., Ubillos, S., Gonzalez-Castro, J., & Páez, D. (2007). Social sharing, participation in demonstrations, emotional climate, and coping with collective violence after the March 11th Madrid bombings. *Journal of Social Issues*, *63*, 323–337.

Palinkas, L.A., Downs, M.A., Petterson, J.S., & Russell, J. (1993). Social, cultural, and psychological impacts of the *Exxon Valdez* oil spill. *Human Organization*, *51*, 1–13.

Palinkas, L.A., Russell, J., Downs, M.A., & Petterson, J.S. (1992). Ethnic differences in stress, coping, and depressive symptoms after the Exxon Valdez oil spill. *The Journal of Nervous and Mental Disease*, *180*, 287–295.

Paulhus, D.L. (1991). Measurement and control of response bias. In J.P. Robinson, P.R. Shaver, & L.S. Wrightsman (Eds.), *Measures of personality and social psychological attitudes*. San Diego, CA: Academic Press.

Pennebaker, J.W., & Harber, K. (1993). A social stage model of collective coping: The Loma Prieta Earthquake and the Persian Gulf War. *Journal of Social Issues*, *49*, 125–145.

Penner, L. Brannick, M. T., Webb, S., & Connell, P. (2005). Effects on volunteering of the September 11, 2001 attacks: An archival analysis. *Journal of Applied Social Psychology*, *35*, 1333–1360.

Pickens, J., Field, T., Prodromidis, M., Pelaez-Nogueraz, M., Hossain, Z. (1995). Post-traumatic stress, depression and social support among college students after Hurricane Andrew. *Journal of College Student Development*, *36*, 152–161.

Procopio, C.H., & Procopio, S.T. (2007). You know what it means to miss New Orleans? Internet communication, geographic community, and social capital in crisis. *Journal of Applied Communication Research*, *35*, 67–87.

Pulcino, T., Galea, S., Ahern, J., Resnick, H., Foley, M., & Vlahov, D. (2003). Posttraumatic stress in women after the September 11 terrorist attacks in New York City. *Journal of Women's Health*, *12*, 809–820.

Quarantelli, E.L. (1960). A note on the protective function of the family in disasters. *Marriage and Family Living*, *22*, 263–264.

(1985). An assessment of conflicting views on mental health: The consequences of traumatic events. In C. Figley (Ed.), *Trauma and its wake*. New York: Brunner-Mazel.

Raphael, B., & Wilson, J.P. (1993). Theoretical and intervention considerations in working with victims of disasters. In J.P. Wilson & B. Raphael (Eds.), *International handbook of traumatic stress syndromes*. New York: Plenum Press.

Riad, J., & Norris, F. (1996). The influence of relocation on the environmental, social, and psychological stress experienced by disaster victims. *Environment and Behavior*, *28*, 163–182.

Riley, D., & Eckenrode, J. (1986). Social ties: Subgroup differences in costs and benefits. *Journal of Personality and Social Psychology*, *51*, 770–778.

Rochford, B., & Blocker, T. (1991). Coping with "natural" hazards as stressors. *Environment and Behavior, 23*, 171–194.

Rodríguez, H., Trainor, J., & Quarantelli, E. (2006). Rising to the challenges of a catastrophe: The emergent and prosocial behavior following Hurricane Katrina. *Annals of the American Academy of Political and Social Science, 604*, 82–101.

Rook, K.S. (1985). Functions of social bonds: Perspectives from research on social support, loneliness and social isolation. In I.G. Sarason & B.R. Sarason (Eds.), *Social support: Theory, research and application*. Dordrecht, the Netherlands: Martinus Nijhoff.

Rustemli, A., & Karanci, A. (1996). Distress reactions and earthquake-related cognitions of parents and their adolescent children in a victimized population. *Journal of Social Behavior and Personality, 11*, 767–780.

Sanchez, J.I., Korbin, W.P., & Viscarra, D.M. (1995). Corporate support in the aftermath of a natural disaster of natural disaster: Effects on employee strains. *Academy of Management Journal, 38*, 504–521.

Sandler, I., & Barrera, M. (1984). Toward a multimethod approach to assessing the effects of social support. *American Journal of Community Psychology, 12*, 37–52.

Sarason, B., & Sarason, I.G. (2006). Close relationships and social support: Implications for the measurement of social support. In A. Vangelisti & D. Perlman (Eds.), *The Cambridge handbook of personal relationships*. New York: Cambridge University Press.

Sarason, I.G., Sarason, B.R., Shearin, E.N., & Pierce, G.R. (1987). A brief measure of social support: Practical and theoretical implications. *Journal of Social and Personal Relationships, 4*, 497–510.

Sheppard, B., Rubin, G.J., Wardman J., & Wessely, S. (2006). Terrorism and dispelling the myth of a panic prone public. *Journal of Public Heath Policy, 27*, 219–245

Smith, K.J., & Belgrave, L.L. (1995). The reconstruction of everyday life: Experiencing Hurricane Andrew. *Journal of Contemporary Ethnography, 24*, 244–269.

Solomon, S.D. (1986). Mobilizing social support networks in times of disaster. In C.R. Figley (Ed.), *Trauma and its wake: Vol. 2. Traumatic stress theory, research, and intervention*. New York: Brunner/Mazel.

Solomon, S.D., Bravo, M., Rubio-Stipec, M., & Canino, G. (1993). Effect of family role on response to disaster. *Journal of Traumatic Stress, 6*, 255–270.

Solomon, S.D., Smith, E., Robins, L., & Fischbach, R. (1987). Social involvement as a mediator of disaster-induced stress. *Applied Journal of Social Psychology, 17*, 1092–1112.

Solomon, Z. (1985). Stress, social support and affective disorders in mothers of pre-school children: A test of the stress-buffering effect of social support. *Social Psychiatry, 20*, 100–105.

Stein, B., Elliott, M., Jaycox, L., Collins, R., Berry, S., Klein, D., et al. (2004). A national longitudinal study of the psychological consequences of the September 11, 2001 terrorist attacks: Reactions, impairment, and help-seeking. *Psychiatry: Interpersonal and Biological Processes, 67*, 105–117.

Steinglass, P., & Gerrity, E. (1990). Natural disasters and post-traumatic stress disorder: Short-term versus long-term recovery in two disaster-affected communities. *Journal of Applied Social Psychology, 20*, 1746–1765.

Swenson, C.C., Saylor, C.F., Powell, M P., Stokes, S.J., Foster, K.Y., & Belter, R.W. (1996). Impact of a natural disaster on pre-school children: Adjustment 14 months after a hurricane. *American Journal of Orthopsychiatry, 66*, 122–129.

Symonds, M. (1980). The "second injury to victims." In L. Kivens (Ed.), *Evaluation and change: Services for survivors*. Minneapolis: Minneapolis Medical Research Foundation.

Taft, C., Stern, A., King, L., & King, D. (1999). Modeling physical health and functional health status: The role of combat exposure, posttraumatic stress disorder and personal resource attributes. *Journal of Traumatic Stress, 12*, 3–23.

Taylor, S.E. (2007). Social support. In H. Friedman & R. Silver Cohen (Eds.), *Foundations of health psychology*. New York: Oxford University Press.

Taylor, S.E., & Brown, J.D. (1988). Illusion and well-being: A social psychological perspective on mental health. *Psychological Bulletin, 103*, 193–210.

Thoits, P.A. (1986). Social support as coping assistance. *Journal of Consulting and Clinical Psychology, 54*, 416–423.

Thompson, M., Kaslow, N., Kingree, J., Rashid, A., Puett, R., Jacobs, D., et al. (2000). Partner violence, social support, and distress among inner-city African American women. *American Journal of Community Psychology, 28*, 127–143.

Triandis, H. (1995). *Individualism and collectivism*. Boulder, CO: Westview Press.

Tolsdorf, C. (1976). Social networks, support, and coping: An exploratory study. *Family Process, 15*, 407–417.

Tierney, K., Bevc, C., & Kuligowski, E. (2006). Metaphors matter: Disaster myths, media frames, and their consequences in Hurricane Katrina. *Annals of the American Academy of Political and Social Science, 604*, 57–81.

Tyler, K. (2006). The impact of support received and support provision on changes in perceived social support among older adults. *International Journal of Aging & Human Development, 62*, 21–38.

Tyler, K., & Hoyt, D. (2000). The effects of an acute stressor on depressive symptoms among older adults: The moderating effects of social support and age. *Research on Aging, 22*, 143–164.

Uchino, B.N. (2004). *Social support and physical health: understanding the health consequences of our relationships*. New Haven, CT: Yale University Press.

Udwin, O., Boyle, S., Yule, W., Bolton, D., & O'Ryan, D. (2000). Risk factors for long-term psychological effects of a disaster experienced in adolescence: Predictors of PTSD. *Journal of Child Psychology and Psychiatry and Allied Disciplines, 41*, 969–979.

Ullman, J., & Newcomb, M. (1999). I felt the earth move: A prospective study of the 1994 Northridge Earthquake. In P. Cohen, C. Slomkowski, & L. Robins (Eds.), *Historical and geographical influences on psychopathology*. Mahwah: Lawrence Erlbaum.

Ullman, S., & Filipas, H. (2001). Predictors of PTSD symptom severity and social reactions in sexual assault victims. *Journal of Traumatic Stress, 14*, 369–389.

Vaux, A. (1988). *Social support: Theory, research, and intervention*. New York: Praeger.

Vaux, A., Burda, P., & Steward, D. (1986). Orientation toward utilization of support resources. *Journal of Community Psychology, 14*, 159–170.

Vranceanu, A., Hobfoll, S., & Johnson, R. (2007). Child multi-type maltreatment and associated depression and PTSD symptoms: The role of social support and stress. *Child Abuse & Neglect, 31*, 71–84.

Vernberg, E.M., La Greca, A.M., Silverman, W.K., & Prinstein, M.J. (1996). Prediction of post-traumatic stress symptoms in children after Hurricane Andrew. *Journal of Abnormal Psychology, 105*, 237–248.

Wallace, A. (1957). *Tornado in Worcester*. (Disaster Study Number Three). Committee on Disaster Studies, National Academy of Sciences: National Research Council.

Warheit, G.J., Zimmerman, R.S., Khoury, E.L., Vega., W.A., & Gil, A.G. (1996). Disaster related stresses, depressive signs and symptoms, and suicidal ideation among a multi-racial/ethnic sample of adolescents: A longitudinal analysis. *Journal of Child Psychology and Psychiatry, 37*, 435–444.

Watanabe, C., Okumura, J., Chiu, T., & Wakai, S. (2004). Social support and depressive symptoms among displaced older adults following the 1999 Taiwan earthquake. *Journal of Traumatic Stress, 17*, 63–67.

Weems, C., Watts, S., Marsee, M., Taylor, L., Costa, N., Cannon, M., et al. (2007). The psychosocial impact of Hurricane Katrina: Contextual differences in psychological symptoms, social support, and discrimination. *Behaviour Research and Therapy, 45*, 2295–2306.

Wheaton, B. (1985). Models for stress-buffering functions of coping resources. *Journal of Health and Social Behavior, 26*, 352–364.

Williams, R.M., Hodgkinson, P., Joseph, S., & Yule, W. (1995). Attitudes to emotion, crisis support and distress: 30 months after the capsize of a passenger ferry disaster. *Crisis Intervention & Time-Limited Treatment, 1*, 209–214.

Wills, T., & DePaulo, B. (1991). Interpersonal analysis of the help-seeking process. In C.R. Snyder & D. Forsyth (Eds.), *Handbook of social and clinical psychology: The health perspective*. New York: Pergamon Press.

Wills, T., & Shinar, O. (2000). Measuring perceived and received social support. In S. Cohen, L. Underwood, & B. Gottlieb (Eds.), *Social support measurement and interventions: A guide for health and social scientists*. New York: Oxford University Press.

Wolfenstein, M. (1957). *Disaster: A psychological essay*. Glencoe, Ill.: Free Press.

Yap, M., & Devilly, G. (2004). The role of perceived social support in crime victimization. *Clinical Psychology Review, 24*, 1–14.

PART FOUR

Special Groups

12 Women and Disasters

RACHEL KIMERLING, KATELYN P. MACK, AND JENNIFER ALVAREZ

12.1. INTRODUCTION

Specific consideration of gender differences in the prevalence of mental health conditions and their gender-specific risk factors can contribute to a more comprehensive understanding of the disaster mental health literature. Women tend to be diagnosed with markedly higher rates of unipolar depression, anxiety disorders, and somatization disorders, and they tend to have higher rates of comorbidity than do men. Men are reliably diagnosed with higher rates of substance use disorders and neuro-developmental conditions (see Blehar, 2006, for review). A variety of biological and social explanations have been proposed to understand gender differences in psychopathology, but questions remain as to the contexts, cultures, and populations that may increase or decrease gender differences.

These questions are particularly relevant for the disaster literature. For example, women's increased risk for posttraumatic stress disorder (PTSD) following exposure to trauma, relative to that of men, is well documented (for reviews see Kimerling, Ouimette, & Weitlauf, 2005; Tolin & Foa, 2002). The disaster literature reflects a similar trend, where women demonstrate an elevated risk for PTSD postdisaster compared to men (Norris et al., 2002). However, disasters differ from other types of trauma in that they constitute not only an individual experience but also a community-wide event. Thus, studying the impact of disasters on women and their mental health outcomes can provide valuable insight into the role that social context plays in women's responses. In this chapter, we review recent literature on natural disasters and discrete incidences of mass violence in an effort to elucidate the factors that shape women's experiences and outcomes.

Our basic assumption is that gender issues are most meaningful when interpreted within a social context (Yoder & Kahn, 2003). In this chapter, we use the word "sex" to refer to the biological fact of being male or female, whereas we use "gender" to signify the interaction between sex and social context, or the psychological experience of a male or female individual in a given society and culture (Kimerling et al., 2005). This framework allows us to identify a diversity of women's experiences, which are shaped by a variety of factors that play a key role in recovery from disaster. For example, we analyze studies in our review separately for developed and developing nations using the International Monetary Fund definition of "advanced economies" (Central Intelligence Agency, 2007). This distinction takes into account various aspects of culture and socioeconomic differences between countries, and it provides a structured basis for our review.

In prior reviews of the disaster research, Norris and colleagues (Norris, Friedman, & Watson, 2002; Norris, Friedman, Watson, et al., 2002) found that the risk of poor outcomes following disaster was higher among residents of non-Western/developing nations. While the authors caution that this could indicate that only more severe events that occur outside the United States are likely to be studied, it may also be that the relative lack of socioeconomic resources in these communities contributes to poorer outcomes. In addition, disasters in developing countries do tend to be more severe (e.g., greater number of deaths, higher displacement), which may contribute to the higher prevalence of mental health problems in these areas (Dominici, Levy, & Louis, 2005; Shultz, Russell, & Espinel, 2005). Women's experiences are likely to differ in developing nations because their resource context is determined by social, economic, political, or religious factors that likely differ from those experienced by women in the United States and in other developed nations. Indeed, certain gender roles, such as being the primary caregiver, have emerged as gender-specific risk factors for PTSD following trauma; if gender roles are more delineated in developing countries, this may explain gender differences in mental health outcomes.

Women's experiences also may be unique from men's because of both "differential exposure" and "differential vulnerability" (Perilla, 2002). Differential exposure examines the extent to which women's outcomes are a function of higher levels of exposure to the traumatic effects of disaster. Women's social roles or physical characteristics could increase the likelihood of danger, physical injury, or bereavement. Differential vulnerability suggests that women may be more severely impacted by disaster exposure than men because of a greater number of predisaster risk factors for poor outcome, such as predisaster trauma exposure, mental health conditions, or low socioeconomic status. Women might also be more vulnerable to the effects of disaster because of gender-specific risk factors. For example, women may be more affected by displacement and property loss than men, especially in communities where women rely on domestic activities and the informal economy to meet their needs. Whereas men may more easily migrate to find work following disasters, women might be limited because of their traditional gender role and responsibilities and face greater economic insecurity postdisaster (Bradshaw, 2004; Enarson, 2000). Disruption of social support networks following disasters may disproportionately impact women.

In this chapter, we explore these issues by reviewing key studies that report exposure by gender and examining women's reports of both subjective and objective exposure. We also review study samples to highlight potential vulnerability factors that could interact with gender to produce more severe postdisaster mental health outcomes among women.

12.2. WOMEN AND EXPOSURE

Disasters are often assumed to be random "gender-neutral" forms of trauma exposure, but relatively few studies have explored whether the experience of disaster is similar for men and for women. Differential exposure to trauma is, thus, an important hypothesis to explore with respect to disasters. Objective trauma exposure is most often operationalized as threatened or actual injury, near-death experiences, displacement or property loss, and loss of close friends or family members. Peri- or postdisaster activities, such as participation in rescue work or repeated encounters with related media reports, also increase trauma exposure via witnessing of death and destruction. Subjective exposure includes reactions of fear, horror, and helplessness, as defined in DSM-IV criterion A2 for PTSD. While the PTSD literature generally finds that men, relative to women, report more traumatic events in their lifetime, women report more pronounced subjective reactions to these events.

The most informative comparisons of men's and women's experiences of disaster can be drawn from studies of representative samples, which identify participants using methodologies such as random-digit-dial telephone surveys. These types of samples are particularly difficult to obtain in the aftermath of disaster, especially in developing countries where probabilistic sampling techniques are often infeasible. Potential bias in sample selection can be important to bear in mind when interpreting studies that compare men and women. The site of recruitment (i.e., temporary housing), the characteristics of treatment seekers, and the displacement of individuals may affect study findings. To the extent that these similar findings are reported across studies, we can draw more specific conclusions about the different experiences of women and men in these contexts.

12.2.1. Disaster Exposure in Developed Countries

A number of recently published studies of the September 11th World Trade Center (WTC) attacks have provided good data on gender differences in both disaster-related trauma exposure and vulnerability factors associated with PTSD (Agronick, Stueve, Vargo, & O'Donnell, 2007; Pulcino et al., 2003; Stuber, Resnick, & Galea, 2006). Two studies in particular have utilized representative samples of men and women. Pulcino and colleagues (2003) studied 988 randomly selected men ($N=474$) and women ($N=514$), drawn from the Manhattan neighborhoods in proximity to the WTC 6 to 8 weeks following the collapse of the towers. Their data indicated that men were significantly more likely than women to directly witness the event (42.6% vs. 34.1%), and women were more likely to volunteer time at rescue centers (10.5% vs. 6.5%). No gender differences emerged for vicarious exposure or resource loss, such as having friends, relatives, or acquaintances killed; losing possessions; or losing a job. However, women were significantly more likely than men to report peri-event panic (17.4% vs. 7.3%), subjective exposure-related distress consistent with criterion A2 for PTSD. Women also reported higher levels of concern over issues such as the war on terror, the risk of future attacks, and harm from chemical or dust exposures. Pulcino and colleagues (2003) also identified a number of vulnerability factors associated with PTSD that were reported more often by women: Women were significantly more likely than men to be the primary caretaker of children in their home and to report a past history of unwanted sexual contact, mental health problems in the past year, and more life stressors in the past year. Men, as compared to women, reported a greater number of lifetime traumatic events.

A subsequent study using a random sample of 2,752 Manhattan residents (1,273 men and 1,479 women) approximately 6 to 9 months following the September 11th attacks did not find gender differences in direct exposure to the event, such as having been in the WTC, getting injured, participating in rescue efforts, knowing about the death of a close friend or family member, or losing one's job (Stuber et al., 2006). Consistent with the study by Pulcino and colleagues (2003), women were significantly more likely than men to report peri-event panic. Women participating in the study also reported more vulnerability factors for PTSD than did men, including lower socioeconomic status, and were more likely to be divorced, widowed, or separated; to be a parent; and to report prior sexual assault and preexisting mental health problems.

Two other studies of the September 11th attack did not use representative sampling but are important to note for use of low socioeconomic and diverse samples. Weissman and colleagues (2005) used a systematic sample of 688 women and 294 men seeking treatment at a large primary care practice in northern Manhattan. The majority of participants were Hispanic immigrants with low levels of income and education. Women were more likely to be Hispanic (83.6% vs. 77.9%), less likely to be married (25.4% vs. 45.6%), and had lower levels of education as compared to men. The study found no gender differences in the rates or nature of exposure to the September 11th attack, including directly witnessing the attacks, having a loved one at the WTC or Pentagon, knowing some one who was injured or killed, or being exposed to rescue and recovery efforts. Notably, when gender comparisons were adjusted for race/ethnicity, marital status, and education, men were slightly more likely to be exposed (AOR = 1.12, 95% CI = 1.00–1.23), suggesting that these vulnerability factors were associated with greater levels of exposure. Similar to other studies, women were more likely to have a history of sexual assault victimization and to report higher levels of subjective distress related to the attacks, including concerns for the safety of their family and their own safety. Men were more likely to report a history of nonsexual assault. These gender differences were not accounted for by demographic characteristics.

There were no gender differences in the likelihood of prior trauma.

The second analysis capitalized on a longitudinal study of low-income African Americans and Latinos recruited from Brooklyn high schools and followed through young adulthood (Agronick et al., 2007). This study of 542 women and 413 men was conducted approximately 8 months following the September 11th attacks. The researchers found that men were significantly more likely to witness the disaster (38% vs. 28%) but found no other gender differences on objective indicators of exposure. Results for subjective elements of exposure revealed that women were more likely to report hopelessness after the event than were men. Agronick and colleagues (2007) also assessed several gender-linked vulnerability factors for the impact of exposure and found no significant gender differences for income and employment status; however, they found that women were significantly more likely to have the primary responsibility of raising children and to participate in public assistance programs.

12.2.2. Disaster Exposure in Developing Countries

A number of studies of the 1999 earthquake in Turkey have reported the characteristics of exposure separately for men and women. Livanou and colleagues (2002) studied 1,027 adults consecutively self-referred to a community treatment center 4 to 14 months following the earthquake. No gender differences emerged for most objective characteristics of exposure, such as being trapped under rubble or loss of family members or friends. Men reported higher levels of some types of exposure, such as damage to the home and loss of property, and were more likely to have participated in rescue work. Women reported significantly higher levels of fear during the earthquake (Livanou, Başoğlu, Salcioğlu, & Kalendar, 2002). This research team also asked similar questions to 586 adults (337 women, 249 men) living in temporary housing sites approximately 20 months after the same earthquake (Salcioğlu, Başoglu, & Livanou, 2003). Similarly, this study found few gender differences for most objective indicators of exposure, including being trapped under rubble, loss of close family members or friends, or damage to the home. Women were more likely to report loss of second degree relatives, and men were significantly more likely to have participated in rescue work.

Another study of the 1999 earthquake in Turkey (Sumer, Karanci, Berument, & Gunes, 2005) 4 to 6 months following the disaster examined personal resources relevant to coping with trauma exposure. While no gender differences were found for direct exposure to events, women reported more earthquake-related distress. Women also reported significantly lower self-efficacy for coping with the event, perceived control, and optimism. A fourth study investigated residents of supported housing sites approximately 3.3 years following the earthquake (Salcioğlu, Başoglu, & Livanou, 2007); as the sample was comprised of individuals still homeless over 3 years after the earthquake, this could indicate that the sample experienced more severe exposure or had fewer predisaster resources. In this study of 507 women and 262 men, slightly more gender differences emerged in reports of exposure. Men were significantly more likely to report being trapped under rubble, losing property, and participating in rescue work. As with previous studies, women reported more fear during the earthquake.

In three of these studies (Livanou et al., 2002; Salcioğlu et al., 2003, 2007), women reported social contextual vulnerability factors. Women were more likely to be married, had lower levels of education, and had higher rates of personal and family past psychiatric illness. However, each of these studies found men significantly more likely to report past traumatic events.

Several other studies in developing societies have elucidated interesting dimensions of subjective responses to trauma exposure associated with female gender, even in the absence of gender differences in objective measures of exposure. In a study of a random sample of 446 women and 212 men assessed 6 weeks to 2 years following a large-scale flood in Puebla and Tobasco, Mexico, there were no gender differences found for objective indicators such as the loss of friends and family or property damage, but women were more likely than men to report perceptions of threat to life during the flood (63.7% vs. 73.1%) (Norris, Baker, Murphy, & Kaniasty, 2005). Similarly, a study of college students 1 month after an earthquake in El Salvador in 2001 assessed 164 women and 89 men and found no gender differences on objective exposure to events (Sattler et al., 2006); the study did find that men reported higher levels of optimism and sense of purpose in life as compared to women.

12.3. WOMEN AND POSTDISASTER PSYCHOPATHOLOGY

Exposure to disasters may result in a wide range of negative mental health consequences. Of these, PTSD is arguably the most common and debilitating, and certainly the most frequently studied (Galea, Nandi, & Vlahov, 2005; Norris, Friedman, Watson, et al., 2002). Elevated rates of depression are also reliably found among disaster survivors. For example, in a random community sample following the September 11th attacks, 9.4% of the population reported a major depressive episode in the 6 months following the attacks, and nearly one-quarter of these individuals (24.2%) also reported PTSD (Person, Tracy, & Galea, 2006). Disaster exposure, subjective distress (i.e., peri-event panic), and vulnerability factors (i.e., being unmarried, high levels of predisaster trauma exposure, and number of stressful life events) increased risk for depression.

An emerging literature has also documented complicated grief reactions following disaster. Complicated grief is distinct from PTSD and depression and focuses on the specific reactions to traumatic loss of friends and family as a result of disaster. It has been noted (Neria et al., 2007) that grief reactions may not follow the expected dose–response relationship between exposure and outcome because these reactions are specific to the loss experiences of disaster exposure. Gendered roles, such as care-giving responsibilities, may make bereavement reactions an especially salient issue for women.

Most of the postdisaster literature indicates that women are at greater risk for postdisaster distress than men and that these differences may be exacerbated in more traditional societies (Norris, Foster, & Weisshaar, 2002; Norris, Perilla, Ibanez, & Murphy, 2001). Several studies conducted in Mexico and Chile after natural disasters found the rate of PTSD among female survivors to be more than twice the rate among male survivors (de la Fuente, 1990; Durkin, 1993; Norris et al., 2001). Research aimed at identifying factors associated with the development of psychological distress in the aftermath of disasters has not uniformly examined gender as a risk factor. In Norris and colleagues' (2002) review of 49 studies reporting significant gender differences in postdisaster psychopathology, 46 (94%) found women to be at higher risk, particularly for PTSD. The three exceptions had certain important common factors, including chronic rather than sudden onset, low severity of exposure, and adjustment for predisaster mental health. Our review of postdisaster psychopathology considers a wide range of disaster types as is evident in our discussion of gender differences in disaster exposure. We do, however, limit our discussion of mass violence to discrete incidents, rather than events of war or chronic community-based violence.

12.3.1. Methodological Considerations

A specific issue for the interpretation of gender differences in risk for postdisaster psychopathology is the measurement of symptoms or conditions. For example, studies have used a variety of assessment tools and diagnostic criteria to measure PTSD following disasters, which may have affected gender differences. Studies using criteria from the DSM-III were inconsistent: Some found no gender differences (Bravo, Rubio-Stipec, Canino, Woodbury, & Ribera, 1990) or higher rates of psychopathology among men (Smith, Robins, Przybeck, Goldring, & Solomon, 1986), while other studies found higher rates of PTSD among women (Durkin, 1993; Steinglass & Gerrity, 1990). Recent studies, particularly those examining psychopathology after the

September 11th attacks, have begun to examine rates of disaster-specific PTSD, rather than lifetime or postdisaster PTSD, which may be linked to any trauma. This has led to more precise data on the psychological impact of disasters.

The limitations of postdisaster assessment may be more pronounced when evaluating rates of depression and anxiety, since these symptom criteria are less clearly linked to a specific event. The distinction between prevalence and incidence is an important one in this case. Prevalence refers to the proportion of a population who meet criteria for a condition, such as depression, at a given time point, whereas incidence refers to new cases of a condition within a specified period. True incidence can be difficult to assess in disaster studies where investigators are often unable to measure predisaster functioning. Studies of postdisaster psychopathology can look for elevated rates of depression and anxiety compared with what would be expected in the community. Associations of mental health conditions with exposure to the disaster can play an important role in the interpretation of these data, though the reader should bear in mind the possibility that vulnerable populations experience elevated rates of mental health conditions but may also be at risk for greater exposure to effects of disaster.

12.3.2. Studies of Developed Countries

Studies using random or probability samples of New York City residents after the September 11th attacks have found higher rates of both PTSD and depression among women as compared to men (Hobfoll, Tracy, & Galea, 2006; Pulcino et al., 2003). In the previous section, we examined the extent of gender differences in exposure characteristics and vulnerability factors to better understand gender differences in postdisaster psychopathology. Pulcino and colleagues (2003) found that women were twice as likely as men to meet criteria for PTSD 5 to 8 weeks following the attacks (9.9% vs. 4.8%), and in this case, gender differences in exposure and vulnerability factors accounted for women's higher rates of PTSD. Factors explaining women's higher rates included volunteering at a rescue center, experiencing peri-event panic, being the primary caretaker for children at home, and having predisaster mental health problems. The prevalence of lifetime PTSD was significantly higher among women compared to men (17.2% vs. 12.1%) in the study by Stuber and colleagues (2006). PTSD prevalence associated with the September 11th attacks did not significantly differ by gender (6.5% vs. 5.4% in women and men, respectively), though women reported significantly greater reexperiencing and hyperarousal symptoms. While the authors did not include objective indicators of exposure in their statistical models predicting PTSD (because these did not differ between men and women), their results did indicate that subjective exposure and vulnerability factors explained much of the observed differences between men and women. In multivariate models that accounted for all of these factors, peri-event panic, history of interpersonal violence, and preevent mental health problems were associated with women's higher rates of both lifetime and event-specific reports of PTSD symptoms. The authors were able to conclude that the observed gender difference in post-September 11th reexperiencing and arousal symptoms was partially determined by women's greater likelihood of sexual assault history and peri-event panic.

Similarly, in Weissman and colleagues' (2005) primary care study, women had significantly higher rates of PTSD (13.4% vs. 8.4%) and depression (24.3% vs. 8.4%) as compared to men. Gender differences in PTSD were most pronounced among Hispanic patients (15.0% vs. 9.5%) and were no longer significant when adjusted for race/ethnicity, education, and marital status. Gender differences in depression were not accounted for by these factors. The authors did not examine other predictors of depression and PTSD, so it is unclear whether the observed gender differences in depression are consistent with a differential vulnerability to the impact of the attacks, or whether they reflect expected gender differences in rates of depression in primary care. Another study of primary care patients recruited from the same clinics assessed

647 women and 283 men 7 to 16 months following the attacks and showed higher rates of PTSD among women as compared to men (11.6% vs. 7.1%) (Neria et al., 2006). PTSD was significantly associated with knowing someone who was killed in the attacks, and the relationship of this variable to PTSD was not accounted for by gender or other social factors, such as race/ethnicity, nativity, martial status, education, or prior trauma. The effect size for gender in this equation was not displayed, so it is unknown whether gender was still a significant predictor of PTSD when exposure and social factors were taken into account.

In the Agronick sample (2007) of economically disadvantaged African American and Latino young adults, the authors found that women were significantly more likely than men to report PTSD symptoms after the September 11th attacks. In a multivariate model, the authors examined not only the independent contribution of exposure and vulnerability factors but also the interaction between gender and exposure. This is one of the few studies that has statistically tested a differential exposure hypothesis, that is, whether objective characteristics of exposure to disasters differentially affects men's and women's risk for PTSD. Results indicated that objective exposure, history of violent victimization, and prior psychological distress were associated with PTSD. Despite few gender differences in reports of objective exposure, exposure had a more pronounced effect on PTSD symptoms for women than for men. The results of this study suggest that exposure to a disaster may affect women differently, with the same level of exposure leading to more PTSD symptoms for women relative to men. The findings that gender differences in vulnerability factors partially explained women's higher psychological reactions to the September 11th attacks (Pulcino et al., 2003) support the hypothesis that the social context of disaster may have a greater impact on the development of PTSD for women than for men.

More research is needed on disaster-related complicated grief reactions. In a large community convenience sample of 704 largely female (79%), white (93%), and college educated (64%) individuals assessed approximately 2.5 to 3.5 years after the September 11th attacks, Neria and colleagues (2007) found that 43% of the sample reported complicated grief reactions. When analyses were adjusted for age and education differences between men and women, female gender emerged as a significant predictor of grief (AOR = 2.67, 95% CI = 1.42–5.03). In a multivariate model, the strongest predictors of grief were loss of a child and vicarious exposure, but these factors did not account for gender effects.

Studies of Hurricane Katrina and other recent disasters have also found higher rates of postdisaster psychopathology among women, though these studies did not examine gender-specific rates of exposure. Using a community sample of 386 participants from several areas impacted by Hurricane Katrina, Weems and colleagues (2007) found that female gender was a significant predictor of PTSD, depression, and anxiety 2 to 5 months after the disaster. DeSalvo and colleagues (2007) assessed PTSD among a sample of Tulane University employees 6 months after the hurricane; PTSD prevalence was significantly higher among women than men (21.9% vs. 14.7%). While objective characteristics of exposure, such as being evacuated for longer than 1 month, knowing someone who died, and relocating to a new or temporary housing, were associated with PTSD, these factors did not fully account for women's increased risk. Because gender was only examined in the multivariate model, it cannot be determined whether these factors partially contributed to women's increased risk for PTSD relative to men.

Miguel-Tobal and colleagues (2006) conducted a cross-sectional study of Madrid citizens 1 to 3 months after the March 11, 2004, train bombings. Multivariate analyses indicated women were more than twice as likely as men to report both PTSD and depression, even after controlling for objective exposure and potentially gender-linked exposure factors such as peri-event panic, low social support, and pre-event life stressors. Female gender has also been associated with PTSD risk among survivors of the Taiwan Chi-Chi earthquake. One study of community members affected by the Chi-Chi earthquake found a higher prevalence of PTSD symptoms among women compared to men (61.55% vs. 28.5%) (Chen et al., 2007). This gender difference in PTSD was significant both in bivariate and multivariate analyses controlling for age, marital status, education, destruction of property, and current living environment. In a larger sample of survivors of the same earthquake, women were significantly more likely than men to report PTSD symptoms in the bivariate analyses, but this gender difference was no longer significant when variables such as age, education, occupation, and exposure were controlled (Kuo, Wu, Ma, Chiu, & Chou, 2007).

A study examining PTSD among 46 flood survivors in a small Colorado town (Benight & Harper, 2002) indicated that women were more likely to report PTSD symptoms 1 year postdisaster. While objective indicators of exposure were not included in the study, a subjective measure for self-efficacy for coping with the disaster was included and revealed lower scores for women. Poorer self-efficacy for coping with the disaster emerged as a significant mediator for long-term PTSD symptoms.

12.3.3. Studies of Developing Countries

The majority of studies in developing nations find women to have higher rates of postdisaster psychopathology or identify female gender as a significant risk factor. Several studies of communities affected by the 1999 Marmara earthquake in Turkey examined gender-specific risk factors and found that women had greater risk for PTSD and depression than men (Salcioğlu et al., 2003, 2007). In particular, Salcioğlu and colleagues (2007) identified twice the rate of PTSD among women as compared to men (46.4% vs. 27.9%). Gender, as well as both objective (i.e., trapped under rubble, losing friends or neighbors) and subjective (i.e., fear during the earthquake) components of exposure were significantly related to PTSD. Lower education level was the only vulnerability factor that emerged as a significant predictor of PTSD in a rather conservative multivariate model controlling for comorbid depression symptoms. Twenty months following the same earthquake, a study found that women had an elevated risk for greater severity of both PTSD and depression, even after adjusting for demographic characteristics, prior psychiatric illness, earthquake-related loss, and objective and subjective aspects of exposure, though gender-aggregated prevalence estimates for PTSD and depression by gender were not reported (Salcioğlu et al., 2003). Sumer and colleagues (2005) examined gender differences in general distress and symptoms of intrusion and avoidance. They found that women reported more intrusion symptoms and general distress. As noted, women also reported less education, self-efficacy, self-esteem, perceived control, and optimism, and more general distress. Gender differences in self-efficacy, however, did not explain women's increased symptoms. Vulnerability and exposure factors associated with increased distress and intrusion symptoms included lower level of education, greater direct exposure to the disaster, increased perceived threat, and greater general distress.

Two studies of treatment-seeking survivors of this earthquake also found that women had a higher prevalence of PTSD and depression compared to men (Aksaray, Kortan, Erkaya, Yenilmez, & Cem, 2006; Livanou et al., 2002). It should be noted that, consistent with other research, women were more likely than men to seek treatment. Aksaray and colleagues (2006) found that women scored significantly higher than men on PTSD. Female gender, history of past psychiatric illness, and injury to self were associated with posttraumatic stress symptom levels in a multiple regression analysis. Although gender differences in education and financial strain were found, these were not included in the multivariate model. The second study also found higher rates of PTSD among women compared to men (71% vs. 46%) (Livanou et al., 2002). Even when controlling for gender differences in vulnerability factors for PTSD, such as education, marital status, past psychiatric illness, and previous trauma, gender still emerged as a significant predictor of PTSD. The authors noted that greater fear during the earthquake most strongly predicted PTSD outcomes.

Another study assessed 105 treatment-seeking individuals (20 men and 55 women) 1 month following a 1998 earthquake in Turkey and reevaluated them 1 year later; the researchers did not find gender differences in the prevalence of PTSD at either point in time (Altindag, Ozen, & Sir, 2005). Injuries and low social support were associated with PTSD at 1 month, but at 13 months no exposure or vulnerability factors were associated with PTSD. The lack of correspondence of these findings to other studies of this earthquake could be due to its use of a treatment-seeking population and its relatively small sample size.

A few other studies outside of Turkey also lend insight into association between gender and psychopathology after disasters in the developing world. A study conducted with a very large sample of 33,340 Chinese flood survivors of all ages found that female gender was a significant risk factor for PTSD, even after accounting for significant predictors of age and degree of exposure (Liu et al., 2006). The rate of postdisaster PTSD among females was 9.2% compared with 8.1% among males. This study did not assess other vulnerability factors for PTSD. In a representative sample of 211 male and 189 female survivors of the Bam earthquake in Iran, gender emerged as a key risk factor for complicated grief reactions (Ghaffari-Nejad, Ahmadi-Mousavi, Gandomkar, & Reihani-Kermani, 2007). While loss of a first-degree family member was the most potent risk factor, more severe exposure and lower levels of education were also significant risk factors. Even after adjusting for all of these variables, female gender was still a significant risk factor for complicated grief.

12.3.4. Studies Comparing Developed and Developing Countries

It has been hypothesized that the more traditional gender roles common to cultures in developing countries may increase the gender differences in postdisaster PTSD. Gender differences in vulnerability factors, including socioeconomic status, may be greater in developing countries, contributing to more pronounced differences in mental health outcomes. We know of only two studies that have directly compared the effects of a disaster in a developing nation to the effects of a similar disaster in a developed nation. The first study, conducted by Norris and colleagues (2001), identified a gender-by-country interaction predicting PTSD symptoms in the aftermath of Hurricanes Paulina and Andrew. Several vulnerability characteristics and exposure factors differed by gender within cultural groups: In the United States, Black women were more educated than Black men, whereas Mexican women were less educated than Mexican men. There was a higher percentage of household injury among both Black women in the United States and Mexican women as compared to men in the same communities. The prevalence of PTSD differed by gender within the white sample in the United States (19.4% among women, 5.4% among men) and the Mexican sample (43.8% among women, 14.4% among men), but for all three cultural groups, the severity of PTSD symptoms was significantly greater among women than men. After adjusting for age, education, and the severity of exposure, there was a larger gender difference in the severity of PTSD symptoms among Mexican survivors than among survivors in the United States, with Mexican women reporting the highest rates of PTSD symptoms.

The second study compared the rates of PTSD among 182 men and women exposed to terrorist bombings in Oklahoma City and 227 individuals exposed to a terrorist bombing in Nairobi (North et al., 2005). The researchers did not document gender differences in exposure or vulnerability factors, but they did report rates of postdisaster psychopathology by gender and by country. The strength of this study was the assessment of both lifetime and current symptoms, so postdisaster incidence of mental health conditions could be estimated. Nairobi and Oklahoma women had very similar incidence rates of any psychopathology (40.6% in Nairobi; 40.4% in Oklahoma), including PTSD and depression. In both countries, women had higher rates of bombing-related PTSD than did men (35.1% vs. 25.8% in Nairobi; 34.0% vs. 19.5% in Oklahoma), but gender differences in the postbombing incidence of depression were found only among the Oklahoma sample (15.5% vs. 11.6% in Nairobi; 17.0% vs. 8.0% in Oklahoma for men and women, respectively). The authors note that this pattern may mirror the general prevalence of depression, where elevated rates among women are more consistently observed in U.S. populations as compared to African countries.

12.4. DISCUSSION

Consistent with previous literature reviews (Norris, Friedman, Watson, et al., 2002), almost all recent studies reviewed for this chapter suggest that women are at greater risk for postdisaster mental health symptoms when compared to men. However, studies did not consistently report rates of mental health conditions by gender or bivariate associations between gender and symptom severity. Given the consistent findings for women's increased risk, disaster studies should report descriptive statistics that examine key outcome variables separately for men and women more frequently. This information can help determine the extent to which prevalence rates differ after disasters and which specific aspects of men's and women's experiences of disasters contribute to gender disparities in mental health outcomes. Reporting results in this manner could more precisely identify disaster-related risk for poor mental health outcomes for both men and women.

Women's increased risk for PTSD, depression, and grief reactions was found across developed and developing countries, though this finding was slightly more consistent among studies from developing countries. Comparison of the magnitude of gender differences in each group of studies is difficult given varying statistical methods employed across studies and the lack of gender-stratified prevalence data. However, there is some evidence that women's risk for PTSD may be more pronounced among women from developing countries (Norris et al., 2001; Webster, McDonald, Lewin, & Carr, 1995). Interpreting the evidence highlights the complexity of the gender issues in disaster response. Gender may interact not only with culture but also with exposure and with other vulnerability factors to determine women's experiences of disasters.

In this chapter, we explored two themes for these interactions: differential exposure and differential vulnerability. We examined whether women experience more severe exposure, or different types of exposure, than do men, which could explain higher rates of PTSD. We also examined whether women are more vulnerable to PTSD following disaster exposure as compared to men and the extent to which gender specific-risk factors for PTSD, such as parenting roles, contributed to women's increased risk. Investigation of differential exposure requires more research. Relatively few studies reported characteristics of exposure stratified by gender, despite consistent gender differences in postdisaster outcomes. Few gender differences in exposure were found in studies of the September 11th attacks (Pulcino et al., 2003; Stuber et al., 2006) or earthquakes in Turkey (Livanou et al., 2002; Salcioğlu et al., 2003, 2007), but when differences were identified, men seemed to experience more direct exposure than women. More consistent are findings that women experience more subjective elements of exposure than do men, such as more peri-event panic and concern about harm to themselves and others, and lower levels of perceived control. This is a pattern consistent with gender differences in responses to other traumatic events, where men may experience higher levels of exposure, but women are more likely to experience trauma exposure that meets criterion A2 for PTSD, the immediate reactions (fear, horror, and helplessness) to events that characterize them as traumatic, as compared to other types of stressful experiences. These reactions are consistently associated with PTSD in both developed and developing countries.

Furthermore, there is some evidence that even the objective indicators of disaster exposure do not impact men and women in the same way. Agronick and colleagues (2007) included a gender by exposure interaction term in their model predicting PTSD symptoms and found that the same types of exposure had a more severe impact on women as compared to men.

Theoretical work has posited that women would be more affected by disaster-related damage to the home and by community disruption due to their greater involvement with family and local social networks (Morrow & Enarson, 1996). On the most empirical level, the findings by Agronick and colleagues (2007) suggest that we can rule out neither the roles of objective nor subjective characteristics of disaster exposure in explanations for women's increased risk for PTSD. More research is needed to understand how exposure might differentially impact men and women; particularly informative would be large, random samples in developing countries and a larger variety of disaster types in developed countries.

Disaster exposure may also have more pronounced effects for women because of a differential vulnerability for PTSD. Gender-specific risk factors for PTSD, determined by women's social roles, such as wife and mother, are linked to PTSD risk (Norris, Friedman, Watson, et al., 2002). These risk factors should be more consistently included in studies of disaster, as well as other indicators of help-giving roles, as these roles are more common to women and appear to partially account for gender differences in rates of PTSD (Livanou et al., 2002; Pulcino et al., 2003). Care-giving responsibilities may partially explain the differential impact of exposure on women if this increases the stress associated with displacement, property damage, or other aspects of a difficult living environment. Physical injury or psychological consequences of the disaster experienced by children or partners may also cause more severe vicarious trauma to women as a result of their close relationships and care-taking role.

Specific psychological vulnerabilities for PTSD also emerged as more common among women. Women consistently reported higher rates of predisaster mental health conditions and predisaster exposure to sexual or interpersonal violence, which were associated with increased risk for PTSD in both developed and developing countries (Agronick et al., 2007; Aksaray et al., 2006; Livanou et al., 2002; Pulcino et al., 2003; Salcioğlu et al., 2003; Stuber et al., 2006; Sumer et al., 2005). Given the strong association of these factors with postdisaster psychopathology, the role of mental health history and victimization history on postdisaster recovery should be routinely investigated. Interestingly, women's risk for sexual and interpersonal violence, which appears to broadly account for epidemiological observations of women's higher rates of PTSD (Foa, Stein, & McFarlane, 2006), appears to also play a specific role in women's higher rates of postdisaster distress.

While a number of studies have accounted for women's history of sexual assault and other forms of violence against women, few studies have examined the role of postdisaster crime in the development of PTSD. The data on this topic is sparse, as epidemiological studies of crime incidence are especially difficult in the aftermath of disaster. A recent study of New Orleans post-Hurricane Katrina suggests that homicide rates may have increased by as much as 69% in 2006 (Van Landingham, 2007). A study of 124 Katrina evacuees in Houston, Texas, shelters found that witnessing interpersonal violence during the floods or in the immediate aftermath was significantly associated with increased risk for PTSD (Coker et al., 2006). Anecdotal reports of increased rates of intimate partner violence following disasters have also been observed (Enarson, 1999; Fothergill, 1999). A World Bank report on postdisaster recovery and reconstruction in Nicaragua after Hurricane Mitch found that incidents of familial violence decreased in the immediate aftermath of the disaster but then steadily increased during later phases of reconstruction (Delaney & Sharader, 2000) In contrast, a community-based study of women working in eastern North Carolina after Hurricane Floyd did not find a rise in intimate partner violence in the 6 months following the hurricane (Frasier et al., 2004). Other studies have reported a rise in intimate partner violence following disasters, such as in California following the 1989 Loma Prieta Earthquake (Pan American Health Organization, 2002), in Washington after the Mt. St. Helen's eruption (World Health Organization, 2005), in the Philippines after the eruption of Mt. Pinatubo, and in El Salvador after earthquakes in 2001 (World Health Organization,

2005). Unfortunately, these studies lack rigorous comparative data on predisaster incidence of violence.

Theoretical work suggests that the association of disaster-related stress and associated marital strain could result in increased emotional and/or physical violence (Menendez, Molloy, & Magaldi, 2006). The community and individual psychological consequences of disaster may also interfere with women and men's ability to assume their normal cultural, social, and economic roles, which may lead to frustration and aggression toward women. Anecdotal evidence from studies documenting economic well-being and health following Hurricane Mitch in Nicaragua and Guatemala suggests that women tend to be disproportionately affected by displacement and disruption of social networks following disasters (Delaney & Schrader, 2000). For example, the percentage of female-headed households was estimated to have more than doubled after Hurricane Mitch. Therefore, both care giving and provision of resources became the responsibility of many women, increasing stressors, and potentially increasing the psychological impact of the disaster.

Norris and colleagues (2005) found that women's perceptions of social support and embeddedness were lower than men's 6 months following floods and mudslides in Mexico, but there were not significant sex differences in received support. The difference of social support deterioration between men and women was exaggerated in Teziutlán compared with Villahermosa; notably, the community of Teziutlán experienced greater disaster impact resulting in higher rates of displacement and mass causalities. This may indicate that gender differences in social support following disasters may be greatest in communities severely affected by disasters. The disruption of social networks and loss of housing in the aftermath of disasters may also reduce access to battered women's shelters, social support networks, or other strategies women use to maintain safety in relationships where violence was present before the disaster (Enarson, 1999). An increase in intimate partner violence was reported after the 1997 Grand Forks flood, and decreased levels of social support were found to be a determinant of intimate partner violence perpetration (Clemens, Hietala, Rytter, Schmidt, & Reese, 1999). Additional research is needed to assess the extent to which community violence, and specifically family violence, increases among communities impacted by disaster.

12.5. CONCLUSION

In sum, women's elevated risk for PTSD following disaster appears to stem both from differential exposure as well as differential vulnerabilities. While women do not demonstrate higher levels of disaster exposure than do men, disaster exposure appears to have a more pronounced impact on women's risk for PTSD. There are also a number of gender-specific vulnerabilities for PTSD that stem from women's social roles as caregivers and their personal histories of interpersonal violence and mental health conditions. However, the majority of studies found that exposure and vulnerability factors only partially accounted for women's increased risk of postdisaster psychopathology. A number of unexplored factors could also shape women's experiences, such as the differential impact of displacement, disruptions in social embeddedness, or increased incidence of postdisaster violence. It follows that women with multiple risk factors might also face disasters with lower levels of self-efficacy and perceived control. Future research should focus on the mechanisms through which women are impacted by and recover from disasters.

There is sufficient evidence to refute the notion of disasters as "gender-neutral" forms of trauma. Many of the parameters that define women's unique experiences are similar to the gender-specific risks observed for other forms of traumatic exposure. However, there are sufficient hypotheses specific to the experience of disasters that we cannot attribute the whole of women's outcomes to a sex-linked vulnerability for PTSD. More research on the factors that could define the unique experiences of women, especially women in developing countries, is essential to a full understanding of the effects of disaster on our communities.

REFERENCES

Agronick, G., Stueve, A., Vargo, S., & O'Donnell, L. (2007). New York City young adults' psychological reactions to 9/11: Findings from the Reach for Health longitudinal study. *American Journal of Community Psychology, 39*(1–2), 79–90.

Aksaray, G., Kortan, G., Erkaya, H., Yenilmez, C., & Cem, K. (2006). Gender differences in psychological effect of the August 1999 earthquake in Turkey. *Nordic Journal of Psychiatry, 60*(5), 387

Altindag, A., Ozen, S., & Sir, A. (2005). One-year follow-up study of posttraumatic stress disorder among earthquake survivors in Turkey. *Comprehensive Psychiatry, 46*(5), 328.

Benight, C. C., & Harper, M. L. (2002). Coping self-efficacy perceptions as a mediator between acute stress response and long-term distress following natural disasters. *Journal of Traumatic Stress, 15*(3), 177–186.

Blehar, M. C. (2006). Women's mental health research: The emergence of a biomedical field. *Annual Review of Clinical Psychology, 2*, 135–160.

Bradshaw, S. (2004). *Socio-economic impacts of natural disasters: A gender analysis*. Santiago: United Nations, Sustainable Development and Human Settlements Division, Women and Development Unit.

Bravo, M., Rubio-Stipec, M., Canino, G., Woodbury, M., & Ribera, J. (1990). The psychological sequelae of disaster stress prospectively and retrospectively evaluated. *American Journal of Community Psychology, 18*, 661–680.

Central Intelligence Agency. (2007). *The world factbook: Appendix B – international organizations and groups*. (October, 2007); https://www.cia.gov/library/publications/the-world-factbook/appendix/appendix-b.html

Chen, C. H., Tan, H. K. L., Liao, L. R., Chen, H. H., Chan, C. C., Cheng, J. J. S., et al. (2007). Long-term psychological outcome of 1999 Taiwan earthquake survivors: A survey of a high-risk sample with property damage. *Comprehensive Psychiatry, 48*(3), 269–275.

Clemens, P., Hietala, J. R., Rytter, M. J., Schmidt, R. A., & Reese, D. J. (1999). Risk of domestic violence after flood impact: Effects of social support, age, and history of domestic violence. *Applied Behavioral Science Review, 7*(2), 199–206.

Coker, A. L., Hanks, J. S., Eggleston, K. S., Risser, J., Tee, P. G., Chronister, K. J., et al. (2006). Social and mental health needs assessment of Katrina evacuees. *Disaster Management & Response, 4*(3), 88–94.

de la Fuente, R. (1990). The mental health consequences of the 1985 earthquakes in Mexico. *International Journal of Mental Health, 19*, 21–29.

Delaney, P. L., & Sharader, E. (2000). *The case of Hurricane Mitch in Honduras and Nicaragua* (Decision Review Draft). Washington, DC: The World Bank, LCSPG/LAC Gender Team.

DeSalvo, K. B., Hyre, A. D., Ompad, D. C., Menke, A., Tynes, L. L., & Muntner, P. (2007). Symptoms of posttraumatic stress disorder in a New Orleans workforce following Hurricane Katrina. *Journal of Urban Health, 84*(2), 142.

Dominici, F., Levy, J. I., & Louis, T. A. (2005). Methodological challenges and contributions in disaster epidemiology. *Epidemiologic Reviews, 27*, 9–12.

Durkin, M. (1993). *Major depression and post-traumatic stress disorder following the Coalinga and Chile earthquakes*. Corte Madera: Select Press.

Enarson, E. (1999). Violence against women in disasters: A study of domestic violence programs in the United States and Canada. *Violence Against Women, 5*(7), 742–768.

(2000). *Working paper 1. Gender and natural disasters*. Geneva: International Labor Organization, Recovery and Reconstruction Department.

Foa, E. B., Stein, D. J., & McFarlane, A. C. (2006). Symptomatology and psychopathology of mental health problems after disaster. *Journal of Clinical Psychiatry, 67(Suppl. 2)*, 15–25.

Fothergill, A. (1999). An exploratory study of woman battering in the Grand Forks flood disaster: Implications for community responses and policies. *International Journal of Mass Emergencies and Disasters, 17* (1), 79–98.

Frasier, P. Y., Belton, L., Hooten, E., Campbell, M. K., DeVellis, B., Benedict, S., et al. (2004). Disaster down east: Using participatory action research to explore intimate partner violence in Eastern North Carolina. *Health Education & Behavior, 31*(4), 69S–84S.

Galea, S., Nandi, A., & Vlahov, D. (2005). The epidemiology of post-traumatic stress disorder after disasters. *Epidemiologic Reviews, 27*, 78–91.

Ghaffari-Nejad, A., Ahmadi-Mousavi, M., Gandomkar, M., & Reihani-Kermani, H. (2007). The prevalence of complicated grief among Bam earthquake survivors in Iran. *Archives of Iranian Medicine, 10*(4), 525–528.

Hobfoll, S. E., Tracy, M., & Galea, S. (2006). The impact of resource loss and traumatic growth on probable PTSD and depression following terrorist attacks. *Journal of Traumatic Stress, 19*(6), 867–878.

Kimerling, R., Ouimette, P. C., & Weitlauf, J. (2005). Gender Issues in PTSD. In M. J. Friedman, T. M. Keane, & P. A. Resick (Eds.), *PTSD: Science and practice – a comprehensive handbook*. New York: Guilford Press.

Kuo, H. W., Wu, S. J., Ma, T. C., Chiu, M. C., & Chou, S. Y. (2007). Posttraumatic symptoms were worst among quake victims with injuries following the Chi-chi quake in Taiwan. *Journal of Psychosomatic Research, 62*(4), 495–500.

Liu, A., Tan, H., Zhou, J., Li, S., Yang, T., Wang, J., et al. (2006). An epidemiologic study of posttraumatic stress disorder in flood victims in Hunan China. *Canadian Journal of Psychiatry, 51*(6), 350.

Livanou, M., Başoğlu, M., Salcioğlu, E., & Kalendar, D. (2002). Traumatic stress responses in treatment-seeking earthquake survivors in Turkey. *Journal of Nervous and Mental Disease, 190*(12), 816–823.

Menendez, A. M., Molloy, J., & Magaldi, M. C. (2006). Health responses of New York City firefighter spouses and their families post-September 11, 2001 terrorist attacks. *Issues in Mental Health Nursing, 27*(8), 905.

Miguel-Tobal, J. J., Cano-Vindal, A., Gonzalez-Ordi, H., Iruarrizaga, I., Rudenstine, S., Vlahov, D., et al. (2006). PTSD and depression after the Madrid March 11 train bombings. *Journal of Traumatic Stress, 19*(1), 69–80.

Morrow, B. H., & Enarson, E. (1996). Hurricane Andrew through women's eyes: Issues and recommendations. *International Journal of Mass Emergencies and Disasters, 14*(1), 5–22.

Neria, Y., Gross, R., Litz, B., Maguen, S., Insel, B., Seirmarco, G., et al. (2007). Prevalence and psychological correlates of complicated grief among bereaved adults 2.5–3.5 years after September 11th attacks. *Journal of Traumatic Stress, 20*(3), 251–262.

Neria, Y., Gross, R., Olfson, M., Gameroff, M. J., Wickramaratne, P., Das, A., et al. (2006). Posttraumatic stress disorder in primary car one year after the 9/11 attacks. *General Hospital Psychiatry, 28*, 213–222.

Norris, F. H., Baker, C. K., Murphy, A. D., & Kaniasty, K. (2005). Social support mobilization and deterioration after Mexico's 1999 flood: Effects of context, gender, and time. *American Journal of Community Psychology, 36* (1–2), 15.

Norris, F. H., Foster, J. D., & Weisshaar, D. L. (2002). The epidemiology of sex differences in PTSD across developmental, societal, and research contexts. In R. Kimerling, P. Ouimette, & J. Wolfe (Eds.), *Gender and PTSD*. New York: The Guilford Press.

Norris, F. H., Friedman, M. J., & Watson, P. J. (2002). 60,000 disaster victims speak: Part II. Summary and implications of the disaster mental health research. *Psychiatry, 65*(3), 240–260.

Norris, F. H., Friedman, M. J., Watson, P. J., Byrne, C. M., Diaz, E., & Kaniasty, K. (2002). 60,000 disaster victims speak: Part I. An empirical review of the empirical literature, 1981–2001. *Psychiatry, 65*(3), 207–239.

Norris, F. H., Perilla, J. L., Ibanez, G. E., & Murphy, A. E. (2001). Sex differences in symptoms of posttraumatic stress disorder: Does culture play a role? *Journal of Traumatic Stress, 14*(1), 7–28.

North, C. S., Pfefferbaum, B., Narayanan, P., Thielman, S., McCoy, G., Dumont, C., et al. (2005). Comparison of post-disaster psychiatric disorders after terrorist bombings in Nairobi and Oklahoma City. *The British Journal of Psychiatry, 186*, 487–493.

Pan American Health Organization. (2002). *Gender and natural disasters*. Washington, DC: World Health Organization, PAHO, Program on Women, Health, & Development.

Perilla, J. L, Norris, F. H, Lavizzo, E. A. (2002). Ethnicity, culture, and disaster response: identifying and explaining ethnic differences in PTSD six months after Hurricane Andrew. *Journal of Social and Clinical Psychology. 21*(1), 20–45.

Person, C., Tracy, M., & Galea, S. (2006). Risk factors for depression after a disaster. *The Journal of Nervous and Mental Disease, 194*(9), 659–666.

Pulcino, T., Galea, S., Ahern, J., Resnick, H., Foley, M., & Vlahov, D. (2003). Posttraumatic stress in women after the September 11 terrorist attacks in New York City. *Journal of Women's Health, 12*(8), 809–820.

Salcioğlu, E., Başoglu, M., & Livanou, M. (2003). Long-term psychological outcome for non-treatment-seeking earthquake survivors in Turkey. *Journal of Nervous and Mental Disease, 191*(3), 154–160.

(2007). Post-traumatic stress disorder and comorbid depression among survivors of the 1999 earthquake in Turkey. *Disasters, 31*(2), 115–129.

Sattler, D. N., de Alvarado, A. M. G., de Castro, N. B., Male, R. V., Zetino, A. M., & Vega, R. (2006). El Salvador earthquakes: Relationships among acute stress disorder symptoms, depression, traumatic event exposure, and resource loss. *Journal of Traumatic Stress, 19*(6), 879–893.

Shultz, J. M., Russell, J., & Espinel, Z. (2005). Epidemiology of tropical cyclones: The dynamics of disaster, disease, and development. *Epidemiologic Reviews, 27*, 21–35.

Smith, E., Robins, L., Przybeck, T., Goldring, E., & Solomon, S. (1986). *Psychosocial consequences of disaster*. Washington, DC: American Psychiatric Press.

Steinglass, P., & Gerrity, E. (1990). Natural disasters and post-traumatic stress disorder: Short-term versus long-term recovery in two disaster affected communities. *Journal of Applied Social Psychology, 20*, 1746–1765.

Stuber, J., Resnick, H., & Galea, S. (2006). Gender disparities in posttraumatic stress disorder after mass trauma. *Gender Medicine, 3*(1), 54–67.

Sumer, N., Karanci, A. N., Berument, S. K., & Gunes, H. (2005). Personal resources, coping self-efficacy, and quake exposure as predictors of psychological distress following the 1999 earthquake in Turkey. *Journal of Traumatic Stress, 18*(4), 331–342.

Tolin, D. F., & Foa, E. B. (2002). Sex differences in vulnerability for posttraumatic stress disorder: A cognitive model. In R. Kimerling, P. Ouimette, & J. Wolfe (Eds.), *Gender and PTSD*. New York: The Guilford Press.

Van Landingham, M. J. (2007). Murder rates in New Orleans, La, 2004–2006. *American Journal of Public Health, 97*(9), 1614–1616.

Webster, R. A., McDonald, R., Lewin, T. J., & Carr, V. J. (1995). Effects of a natural disaster on immigrants and host population. *Journal of Nervous and Mental Disease, 183*(6), 390–397.

Weems, C. F., Watts, S. E., Marsee, M. A., Taylor, L. K., Costa, N. M., Cannon, M. F., et al. (2007). The psychosocial impact of Hurricane Katrina: Contextual differences in psychological symptoms, social support, and discrimination. *Behaviour Research and Therapy, 45*, 2295–2306.

Weissman, M. M., Neria, Y., Das, A., Feder, A., Blanco, C., Lantigua, R., et al. (2005). Gender differences in posttraumatic stress disorder among primary care patients after the World Trade Center attack of September 11, 2001. *Gender and Medicine, 2*(2), 76–87.

World Health Organization. (2005). *Violence and disasters: Factsheet*. Geneva: World Health Organization, Department of Injuries and Violence Prevention.

Yoder, J. D., & Kahn, A. S. (2003). Making gender comparisons more meaningful: A call for more attention to social context. *Psychology of Women Quarterly, 27*, 281–290.

13 Child Mental Health in the Aftermath of Disaster: A Review of PTSD Studies

CHRISTINA W. HOVEN, CRISTIANE S. DUARTE, J. BLAKE TURNER, AND DONALD J. MANDELL

13.1. INTRODUCTION

Epidemiological investigations provide strong evidence that experiencing disaster-related traumatic events in childhood can have significant adverse psychopathological consequences (Hoven et al., 2005; La Greca, Silverman, Vernberg, & Prinstein, 1996; Lonigan, Shannon, Finch, Jr., Daugherty, & Taylor, 1991). Clearly, understanding how such exposure to disaster affects children's mental health and psychosocial development is important, both for elucidating vulnerabilities specific to children, and for informing and guiding appropriate responses, including treatment, which fosters resilience and speeds recovery. The greatest promise for advancing knowledge on this topic depends upon systematic assessment, using diagnostic-based measures in well-designed, longitudinal investigations of representative samples of children (in sufficient numbers) to allow for meaningful analyses. Unfortunately, to date, no study with children that includes all of these elements could be identified.

As a nascent field of inquiry, disaster mental health research in children is now ideally poised to review its own recent research, including emphasis and approach, so as to determine a future trajectory. In an effort to stimulate and facilitate this process and to identify critical knowledge gaps, this chapter systematically examines the extant literature, focusing on methodological issues. In an effort to identify lacunae in our collective research agenda, we offer a conceptual typology, or classification schema, for reviewing the kinds of disasters that have been studied and the research methods employed. We hope, therefore, that this chapter will stimulate the kind of thinking and dialogue required for the development of rigorous investigations that address the many remaining unanswered questions concerning child mental health in the aftermath of disaster.

13.2. METHODOLOGICAL CONSIDERATIONS

Children present different, and often greater, challenges to epidemiologic research than do adults. These challenges, however, can be viewed positively, because of the requisite ecological, developmental approach. In fact, postdisaster studies of children afford unique opportunities to explicate how the intersecting contexts of childhood experiences meld in a maturing mind. From this perspective, children represent the ideal age group to study in order to gain insight into the etiology of psychopathology in the aftermath of disaster.

As Comer and Kendall (2007) and La Greca (2007) have recently pointed out, we should currently be in a position to systematically address priority areas in child mental health research and to better understand a wider range of postdisaster outcomes, including less commonly studied psychiatric disorders, impairments, and contextual influences. Yet, in spite of such admonitions and evidence from many published postdisaster studies of psychological impact on children, there remains a glaring lack of consensus concerning (1) what constitutes appropriate study design, especially as to sampling frames and study methods; (2) which children (e.g., what ages) should be assessed, in which time frame, and utilizing which measures; and (3) what are the most useful contrasts (relationships between exposures, mediating factors, and outcomes) to examine.

Appropriate assessment requires that the children's developmental stages should first be considered, and recognize that the measurement strategies to be employed must vary accordingly. As a general rule, the younger the children, the more limited the assessment options. Additionally, when the research goal is to learn about children's reactions to a disaster, judiciously selected adult informants may be necessary, and in some cases, more than one may be required (e.g., both a parent and a teacher). The choice of optimal informant(s) depends on several factors: the type of child reaction of interest (e.g., internalizing or externalizing behavior), the age range (e.g., early childhood or adolescence), and interview logistics (e.g., feasibility of interviewing both a child and an adult informant). A further complication, except in certain anonymous studies, is the need to obtain parental approval for children to participate in an interview or other form of assessment. In certain postdisaster settings, the logistics of obtaining such approval may be compromised by the separation of family members, legal questions regarding guardianship, or even parental death.

Generally, in the child trauma literature, very little attention has been devoted to methodological issues involved in the evaluation of children's exposure. Research, to date, has failed to provide a conceptual or empirical rationale for selecting child-specific extreme traumatic events. Problems associated with reliability and validity of widely used checklists, which rely on broad categories describing extreme mass events (Dohrenwend, 2006), may well be exacerbated for children. It is not always clear as to when, and to what extent, both parental and child reports of child exposure are necessary to characterize an exposure.

Any postdisaster child assessment should necessarily involve a two-step process, including a detailed characterization of the child's exposure and the possible related reactions. Reviews of postdisaster child measures are available elsewhere (Balaban, 2006; Duarte Bordin, Green & Hoven, 2009; Ohan, Myers, & Collett, 2002; Strand, Sarmiento, & Pasquale, 2005), so they are not addressed here. Rather, we have focused on reviewing the available literature on child mental health after disasters, which we have classified according to a useful typology.

13.3. DISASTER TYPOLOGY

Disasters can be defined in a variety of ways, depending on one's objectives. To facilitate methodological considerations of postdisaster child mental health assessment strategies, we propose a three-category disaster typology based on the distribution of different types of disaster exposures (see Table 13.1). This typology is not meant to exhaustively characterize all possible dimensions of disaster experiences relevant to children's mental health. Instead, it distinguishes disaster categories according to dimensions which would require specific research design and methods, an approach best suited to inform the effective study of psychological aftermath in children. It is, after all, the type of exposure that is particularly relevant in guiding how to best assess the impact of a specific disaster. Across the three proposed disaster types, the research approach will necessarily be quite different; while within each type the research approach is likely to be similar.

13.3.1. Disaster Type 1: Diffuse, Geographically Spread Exposure

Type I disasters are geographically spread events with a wide range of exposures and threat-to-life-and-physical-integrity, as well as other adverse postdisaster consequences, across differently affected areas or regions. The most common disasters of this type are large-scale weather events (e.g., hurricanes, severe tornadoes) and other natural disasters (e.g., earthquakes).

The signature U.S. example of this type of event was Hurricane Katrina on August 29, 2005, which affected a very large geographic area. Within a wide area, there was substantial variation in both the degree and type of hurricane-related adversity. In the areas most directly affected

Table 13.1. Disaster type

	Type I: Diffuse, Wide Geographic Spread	**Type II: Exposure to Noxious Agent**	**Type III: Intense, Circumscribed Exposure; Clear Demarcation of the Exposed Population**
Defining characteristics	Catastrophic event dispersed over potentially wide geographic area, with considerable variation in level of exposure; secondary effects of mass evacuation, sheltering, and disrupted social systems often compound the initial effect of the triggering event and lengthen exposure phase	Exposure defined by the location, concentration, and path of a noxious agent; in the case of infectious disease, the agent is generally tracked through the identification of new disease cases	Single catastrophic event that affects a geographically circumscribed area, often within a brief time period, with little diffusion of the destructive agent beyond the affected area
Examples	Major weather events (e.g., hurricanes, tornadoes); large geophysical events (e.g., earthquakes, tsunamis); major flooding; large area fires; and so on	Biological or chemical attacks; pandemic flu; water-supply contamination	Bombings, such as World Trade Center attack, London buses or Madrid train attacks; landslides; major building fire, such as Triangle Shirtwaist Factory; other mass murders, such as Virginia Tech shootings
Sampling (1) considerations (2) constraints (3) strategies	(1) Sample frame complicated by multiple exposures (initial event, response to event, subsequent displacement and social disorganization); (2) Although affected geographic areas may be identified, challenge to locate dispersed populations; (3) Cluster sampling strategies could be used given disaster-related groupings, such as FEMA congregate shelter sites, or aggressive tracking efforts. Ideally, researchers would have access to Red Cross or FEMA lists	(1) Agent difficult to track; exposed population often only identifiable via symptoms. Important to identify especially vulnerable populations (elderly, young children) (2) As with Type I, dislocation of segments of the population could cause bias (3) Sampling procedures could combine GIS mapping with cluster strategies	(1) Well-defined exposed population; (2) Need to enumerate the exposed; (3) Ability to use "membership" lists, such as building tenants, employees, or area residents as sampling frame; absent that, potential for posthoc registry based on care-seeking activities

Notes: FEMA, federal emergency management agency; GIS, geographic information system.

by failed levees, there was a substantial amount of immediate, life-threatening danger from drowning. Large numbers of New Orleans' residents were stranded for protracted periods without adequate food and water, not only those housed in the Superdome and Convention Center but also those perched on the roofs of houses and other neighborhood locations. Many people lost their loved ones. In other areas, property damage was responsible for much of the adversity.

While Hurricane Katrina is among the most severe of such examples, Type I disasters do occur quite frequently. A number of weather events, not only hurricanes and tornadoes, but also blizzards, ice storms, and even thunderstorms can, if severe and extensive enough, overwhelm the available resources a community has for dealing with them. Geophysical events, such as earthquakes (e.g., the May 12, 2008, Sichuan, China, earthquake), tsunamis (e.g., the December 26, 2004, Southeast Asia tsunami), and volcanic eruptions are also included in Type 1 disasters. Severe flooding, even if it comes from a slow accumulation of precipitation, can result in dislocation experiences similar to those caused by hurricanes and earthquakes (e.g., the June 2008 Mississippi River floods).

13.3.2. Disaster Type II: Agent-Related Exposure

Type II exposure is defined by the location, concentration, and path of a noxious agent, for instance, a poisonous chemical after a major leak, spill, or malevolent attack; an infectious (biological) agent spreading after a leak, spill, or malevolent attack or because of a natural outbreak, as with a flu epidemic; dangerous radiation level after a nuclear power accident or malevolent attack.

Type II disasters are much rarer than Type I disasters; nevertheless, many have occurred in recent history. The most extreme example occurred in Bhopal, India, in 1984 when approximately 40 tons of methyl isocyanate gas were released from a nearby Union Carbide pesticide plant. Nearly 3,000 people died initially and estimates of the ultimate death toll from related illness vary between 15,000 and 20,000.

Most disasters of this type are not nearly as extensive as Bhopal, but nonetheless, they tend to cause substantial panic. For example, in May of 2000, the water supply for Walkerton, Ontario, Canada, became contaminated with a dangerous strain of *Escherichia coli* bacteria, apparently from farm runoff. Seven people died before the authorities issued an announcement informing citizens not to drink the water. After a widespread outbreak of severe acute respiratory syndrome (SARS) in mainland China, which resulted in the deaths of nearly 800 people, a substantial amount of public anxiety arose in other countries (e.g., Canada) that experienced very small and localized outbreaks (Maunder et al., 2004; Nickell et al., 2004; Reynolds et al., 2007).

13.3.3. Disaster Type III: Circumscribed Exposure

Type III disasters are characterized by intense, circumscribed exposure, with a generally clear demarcation between the exposed and unexposed and between groups with different forms or levels of exposure. Disasters of this type include explosions (whether accidental or intentional), building collapses, school shootings, major building fires, terrorist attacks and landslides.

The signature U.S. example of this type of disaster was the September 11, 2001, terrorist attack on the World Trade Center in New York City and the subsequent collapse of the Twin Towers. Without any extensive postdisaster investigation, exposure groups could be easily demarcated:

- Those definitely exposed – evacuees from the towers, rescue workers in, or immediately proximal to the towers.
- Those with markedly lower exposure – for example, those who came in contact with the spreading dust cloud and smoke after the collapse of the buildings.
- Groups with qualitatively different types of exposure – for example, the bereaved, witnesses of jumpers from the towers, family members of evacuees and rescue workers, and so on.

In Type I and Type II disasters, parents and children are frequently jointly exposed to most of the consequent adversities. In Type III disasters, however, the direct exposure is often limited to one group. This creates the need for considering "indirect exposure" – for example, mental health outcomes in children of parents who were evacuated from a building; mental health outcomes in parents of children who witnessed a mass shooting in their school.

13.4. OVERVIEW OF PUBLISHED STUDIES

Most attempts to summarize existing evidence about the impact of mass disasters on children have focused on the impact of terrorism on child mental health (Fremont, 2004; Hoven, Duarte, & Mandell, 2003; Pfefferbaum et al., 2003; Pine, Costello, & Masten, 2005); others have addressed important conceptual issues in the field (Shalev, Tuval-Mashiach, & Hadar, 2004; Steinberg, Brymer, Steinberg, & Pfefferbaum, 2006). However, we could not identify any review that systematically examined the literature on child mental health across different types of disasters. This is an important omission as the number of published papers in the field has increased substantially, particularly after September 11th, and there is a pressing need to compile what has been learned in response to different types of disaster and to consider which issues should be addressed to move the field forward. We concluded, therefore, that a thorough examination of the contribution and limitations of published studies, to date, across types of disaster would be very useful in advancing the study of postdisaster child mental health.

For clarity, this review focuses exclusively on reports of reactions related to posttraumatic stress disorder (PTSD) in children after mass traumatic events, with studies being reviewed within the context of the proposed typology. Included in this literature review are studies about children and adolescents who were exposed to mass disasters and who were subsequently assessed for the development of posttraumatic stress reactions as a result of such exposure. All articles reviewed here were published between January 1, 1984, and December 31, 2007, inclusively, and indexed in Medline or PsychInfo. Investigations about chronic exposure to specific mass traumatic events (e.g., war or terrorism threat) were included, but studies reporting on posttraumatic reactions in adults, even if the exposure occurred during childhood, were not. Studies about reactions to personal traumatic experiences (e.g., child abuse) which did not occur in the context of a specific mass traumatic event, as well as reports about postdisaster intervention or policy strategies, were excluded. Studies that focused exclusively on psychometric properties of posttraumatic stress assessment measures were not included either.

The systematic literature search focused on child posttraumatic reactions following disasters that occurred throughout the world and fulfilled the criteria described earlier generated 139 reports.

Table 13.2 lists different disasters about which a published report was found, organized according to the typology of disasters previously described. The majority of the articles report on disaster Type I ($N = 87$), followed by Type III ($N = 48$). Only three studies described child PTSD after disaster Type II, and one paper was not classified because it could not be located (only the abstract is available). The number of articles reporting on each specific disaster Type can also be found in Table 13.2. The 87 publications reporting on Type I disasters related to 45 different events, while 21 events were described in the 48 papers reporting on Type III disasters. The Oklahoma City bombing, the September 11th attack, and terrorist acts/threats in Israel are disasters with the largest number of publications (10 each), suggesting that terrorist attacks have provided the strongest motivation for systematic investigation.

The typology of disasters presented here appears to be useful when considering children's exposure to disaster. The paucity of Type II, investigations, while mostly resulting from the lower frequency of these types of disasters, calls for consideration of increasing research effort following such events.

13.4.1. General Characteristics of Studies Reviewed

During the last 12 years there has been a marked increase in the number of papers published on child and adolescent posttraumatic reactions after mass disasters (see Figure 13.1). Over 80% of the studies included here were published during this brief period. The number of papers published per year and the year of occurrence of a specific disaster suggests that there is generally a lag of approximately 4 to 5 years between the occurrence of a major disaster and the publication

Table 13.2. Disasters with published reports on posttraumatic reactions in children and adolescents[a]

Type I (*N* = 87)	Type II (*N* = 3)	Type III (*N* = 48)
Cyclone, India, 1999 (2)	Fire in PCB warehouse, Canada, 1988	Air show disaster, Ukraine, 2002
Earthquake, Colombia, 1999	Nuclear waste disaster, U.S.A, 1984	Automotive collision, Israel, 1985
Earthquake, U.S.A., 1990	Nuclear waste disaster, Chernobyl, Russia, 1986	Boat disaster, Iran, 2002
Earthquake, Taiwan, 1999		Buffalo Creek Dam collapse, U.S.A., 1972
Earthquake, Japan – Nigata, Chuetsu, 2004		Café fire, Korea, 1999
Earthquake, Japan – Hanshin-Awaji, 1995		Café fire, Netherlands, 2001
Earthquake, U.S.A., 1994 (2)		Challenger explosion, U.S.A., 1986
Earthquake, Greece, 1999 (4)		Children taken hostage, Russia, 2004
Earthquake, Armenia, 1988 (6)		Children taken hostage, France, 1995
Earthquake, Turkey, 1999 (6)		Discotheque fire, Sweden, 1998
Flood, Poland, 1997		Embassy bombing, Kenya, 1998 (2)
Flood, U.S.A., 1982 and 1983		Fireworks disaster, Netherlands, 2000
Genocide, Kurdistan, 1986–1989		Gas explosion, Japan, 1998
Genocide, Bosnia, 1992–1995		Industrial fire, U.S.A., 1991
Genocide, Rwanda, 1994 (2)		Jupiter shipping disaster, Greece, 1988 (5)
Hostilities, Tibet		Oklahoma City bombing, U.S.A., 1995 (10)
Hostilities, West Bank		School fatality, U.K, 1991
Hurricane Hugo, U.S.A. , 1989 (4)		School shooting, U.S.A., 1988
Hurricane Andrew, U.S.A., 1992 (8)		School shooting, U.S.A., 1984 (3)
Hurricane Floyd, U.S.A., 1999 (2)		World Trade Center attack, U.S.A., 1993
Hurricane Iniki, U.S.A., 1992		World Trade Center attack, U.S.A., 2001 (10)
Hurricane Katrina, U.S.A., 2005		
Hurricane Mitch, Nicaragua, 1998		
Industrial disaster, Toulouse, France, 2001		
Land movement due to mining, France, 1996		
Missile attack, Israel, 1996		
Missile attack SCUD, Israel, 1991		
Ongoing threats/acts thereof, Israel (10)		
Refugee camp, Cuba		
Refugees, Cambodia		
Refugees, Kurdistan		
Refugees, Bosnian War, Bosnia, 1992–1995 (2)		
Refugees, Sudanese War, Sudan, 1983–2005		
Tornado, U.S.A.		
Tsunami, Thailand, Sri Lanka, India, 2004 (7)		
Typhoon Rusa, South Korea, 2002		
War: Bosnia, Bosnia, 1992–1995 (4)		
War: Cambodia, Cambodia,		
War: Persian Gulf, Iraq, 1991 (3)		
War: Uganda, Uganda		
Wildfire, U.S.A., 1990		
Wildfire, Australia, 1994		
Wildfire, Australia, 2003		
Wildfire Ash Wednesday, Australia, 1983 (2)		
World War II, Germany, 1939–1945		

[a] Year of disaster occurrence, region and number of papers (reporting on each specific disaster are indicated).

of a series of papers, at least about children's reactions. This was the case for several major disasters for example, the Oklahoma City bombing (Pfefferbaum et al., 1999) and the September 11th attack (Hoven et al., 2005; Pfefferbaum, Stuber, Galea, & Fairbrother, 2006).

Sixty-one percent of studies reviewed included children between 6 and 11 years of age.

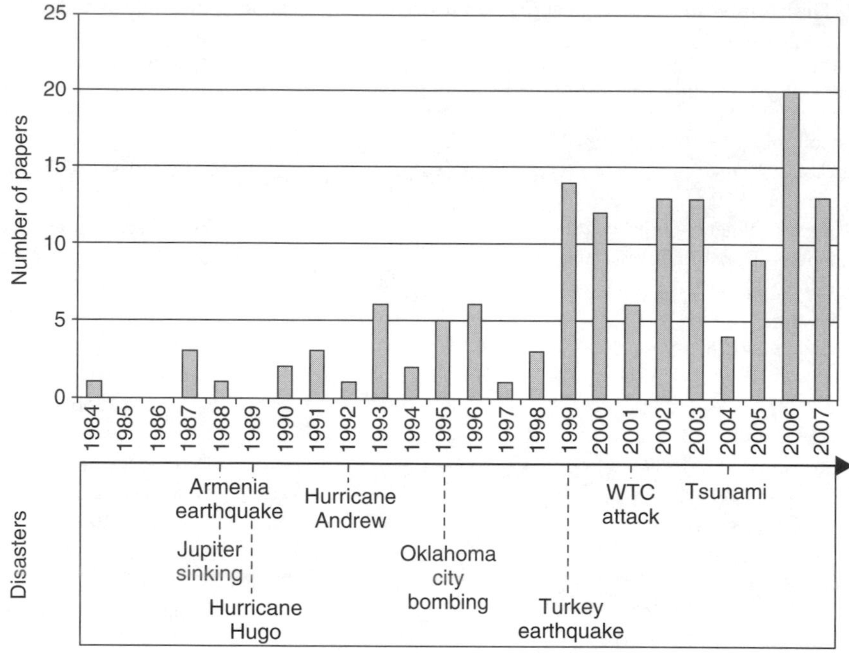

Figure 13.1. Chronology of child PTSD publications and mass disaster events (1984–2007).

Only 18 studies (12.9%) reported on preschool children. Almost 80% of all studies included youth between the ages of 12 and 18 in their samples. Thirty-six (25.9%) of the studies had less than 100 participants, while 29 investigations (20.9%) assessed posttraumatic reactions in more than 1,000 youth. Most studies (N = 81) were conducted less than 1 year after the disaster; however, 17 studies were not classified on this dimension as they involved exposure to continuous threats, such as exposure to war or other ongoing threats. Schools were the preferred setting for recruitment (61.9% of the investigations); in very few instances (seven studies), participants were recruited in a service setting, and the rest (30.2%) were part of a community-based sample. Approximately 65% of the studies used convenience samples, meaning that only immediately available and easily accessible participants were included, without consideration for how representative the sample would be of a specific population. In 27.3% of the studies, some type of randomization was employed to identify the sample, and in the remaining instances, mixed methods were used. The vast majority of the studies (76.3%) had a cross-sectional design, while 31 of them were longitudinal. Posttraumatic reactions were assessed by a range of instruments, mostly self-report scales. The UCLA PTSD-RI (Steinberg, Brymer, Decker, & Pynoos, 2004) was most frequently used. In 92 (62.2%) of the 139 studies, other emotional reactions, in addition to PTSD, were also assessed.

Among the published papers reviewed, 18 studies included more than 100 participants, conducted the first assessment less than 1 year after the disaster, and employed some type of randomization strategy to select the study sample. These 18 studies are displayed in Table 13.3. For each one of them, we indicate when it was conducted, sample size, age range, instrument employed, and prevalence of a posttraumatic reaction.

These 18 publications report on ten different events that correspond to 13 independent studies (Bulut, Bulut, & Tayli, 2005; Fairbrother, Stuber, Galea, Fleischman, & Pfefferbaum, 2003; Garrison et al., 1995; Giannopoulou et al., 2006; Godeau et al., 2005; Hoven et al., 2005; Kiliç, Ozguven, & Sayil, 2003; La Greca et al., 1996; Lonigan et al., 1991; Proctor et al., 2007; Terr et al., 1999;

Table 13.3. Selected studies about posttraumatic stress reactions in children and adolescents after mass disasters

Disaster Type	First Author	Year	Country	Traumatic Event	Time After	*N*	Age	Instruments	PTSD Reaction
I	Kilic EZ	2003	Turkey	Earthquake	6 months	114	7–14 years old	Child PTSD Reaction Index (CPTSD-RI)	Mean PTSD score = 30.3; SD=12.2
I	Bulut S	2005	Turkey	Earthquake	11 months	200	Grades 4–5	The Sefa Bulut Child – PTSD Inventory	High impact = 73.3%; low impact = 73.7%
I	Giannopoulou I	2006	Greece	Earthquake	6–7 months	2037	Grades 4–12	Children's Revised Impact of Event Scale (CRIES-13)	Directly exposed = 35.7%; indirectly exposed = 20.1%
I	Proctor LJ	2007	U.S.A.	Earthquake	8 months	117	4–5 years old	Earthquake impact survey developed for study including PTSD	Distress/PTSD symptoms: 1 month = 90.7%; 8 months later = 71.8%
I	Thabet AA	2000	West Bank	Hostilities – Middle East	1 year apart	234	7–12 years old	CPTSD-RI	Moderate/severe PTSD reactions = T1 40.6% and T2 10.0%.
I	Vernberg EM	1996	U.S.A.	Hurricane Andrew	4 months	568	Grades 3–5	CPTSD-RI	Severe/very severe PTSD symptoms = 30%
I	La Greca AM	1996	U.S.A.	Hurricane Andrew	3, 7, 10 months	442	Grades 3–5	CPTSD-RI	Severe/very severe = T1 29.8%; T2 18.1%; T3 12.5%
I	Garrison CZ	1995	U.S.A.	Hurricane Andrew	6 months	400	12–17 years old	PTSD Module of Diagnostic Interview Schedule (DIS)	Males = 2.9%; females = 9.2%
I	Lonigan CJ	1991	U.S.A.	Hurricane Hugo	3 months	5687	9–19 years old	CPTSD-RI	Severe PTSD symptoms: High exposure ~7%; mild exposure ~<5%

(continued)

Table 13.3 *(continued)*

Disaster Type	First Author	Year	Country	Traumatic Event	Time After	*N*	Age	Instruments	PTSD Reaction
I	Lonigan CJ	1994	U.S.A.	Hurricane Hugo	3 months	5687	9–16+ years old	CPTSD-RI	PTSD: High exposure = 16%; little exposure = 4.1%
I	Godeau E	2005	France	Industrial accident	9 months	1477	11, 13, 15, and 17 years old	Horowitz scale adapted by Dyregrov and Yule, the Revised Impact of Events Scale (R-IES)	Direct exposure = 44.6% (11 and 13 years old); indirect exposure = 22.1%
I	Wickrama KA	2007	Thailand	Tsunami	4 months	325	12–19 years old	17 DSM-IV diagnostic interview items for PTSD	PTSD = 40.9%
III	Terr LC	1999	U.S.A.	Challenger explosion	5–7 weeks /14 months	153	Grades 3 and 10	298-item, 45-minute structured interview of own design	3 children met DSM-III-R for PTSD at T1, none at T2
III	Fairbrother G	2003	U.S.A.	WTC	4–5 months	434	4–17 years old	20-item Posttraumatic Stress Disorder Reaction Index – Child Revision with parents as respondents	Severe/very severe = 18%; moderate = 66%
III	Pfefferbaum B	2006	U.S.A.	WTC	6–9 months	161	12 and 17 years old	DIS for panic attacks, the UCLA PTSD Index for DSM-IV (update of CPTSD-RI)	Probable PTSD = 12.6%; subthreshold PTSD = 26.2%
III	Hoven CW	2005	U.S.A.	WTC	6 months	8236	Grades 4–12	PTSD and other eight disorder modules of DISC Predictive Scales (DPS)	Probable PTSD = 10.6%; severe exposure = 18.4%
III	Duarte CS	2006	U.S.A.	WTC	6 months	8236	Grades 4–12	PTSD module of DISC Predictive Scales (DPS)	Probable PTSD = 18.9% in children with EMTs in their families
III	Wu P	2006	U.S.A.	WTC	6 months	2731	Grades 6–12	DPS	Probable PTSD = 5.7%

Note: Highlighted publications indicate longitudinal analyses.

Thabet & Vostanis, 2000; Wickrama & Kaspar, 2007). Seven countries are represented, although the majority (12) of the studies was conducted in the United States. The earliest of these studies was published in 1991 (Lonigan et al., 1991) and focused on reactions of children following Hurricane Hugo. This was one of three studies conducted most immediately after this event, only 3 months after the hurricane. Another such study was conducted following Hurricane Andrew (La Greca et al., 1996; Vernberg, Silverman, La Greca, & Prinstein, 1996), and another study, which examined reactions to the Challenger explosion (Terr et al., 1999), started 5 weeks after that disaster. Six months was the most frequent interval between the occurrence of a mass disaster and assessment. Within this select group of 18 publications, sample sizes varied considerably, from 114 participants in one of the Turkish earthquake investigations (Kiliç et al., 2003) to 8,236 youth in one of the September 11th studies (Hoven et al., 2005). Variations in the age range of participants are also noteworthy. A population-based assessment of adults in Manhattan, which interviewed parents about their children, was able to include the youngest children (4 years old) of any study, as it relied on parental reporting (Fairbrother et al., 2003). Most investigations, however, began interviewing children when they were between 9 and 10 years of age.

The Child PTSD Reaction Index (CPTSD-RI) (Steinberg et al., 2004; Pynoos, Steinberg, Ornitz, & Goenjian, 1997) was used in five out of the ten studies for which results are presented in Table 13.3 (Kiliç et al., 2003; La Greca et al., 1996; Lonigan et al., 1991; Pfefferbaum et al., 2006; Thabet & Vostanis, 2000), and adaptations of the Impact of Events Scale (Horowitz, Wilner, & Alvarez, 1979) were used in two studies (Giannopoulou et al., 2006; Godeau et al., 2005). It is important to note that *not one* study of child PTSD after a mass disaster used a full structured diagnostic interview. Hoven et al's (2005) World Trade Center Study, however, used the Diagnostic Predictive Scales (Lucas et al., 2001), derived from the DSM-IV Diagnostic Interview Schedule for children (Shaffer, Fisher, Lucas, Dulcan, & Schwab-Stone, 2000).

13.4.2. Findings and Limitations of Recent Studies

Although all of the 18 studies presented here (Table 13.3) examined children's reactions following large-scale traumatic events throughout the world, employed reasonably large sample sizes, assessed individuals within less than 1 year of the event, and adopted some type of randomization to select their samples, using these data to make meaningful comparisons of the reported prevalence rates of posttraumatic reactions remains problematic because of the significant study design differences across investigations. As described earlier, and easily visible in Table 13.3, there are meaningful variations in the PTSD reaction measure, nature of the exposures and age ranges of the populations assessed. The fact that structured diagnostic interviews were never employed most probably afforded another source of significant variation in reported prevalence. In addition, even when random strategies were used to select participants, samples were generally not representative of the larger, potentially affected population, either because of the study design or because of low participation rates. Thus, comparing rates across studies could be misleading, if not impossible. As previously noted (Hoven et al., 2003), after natural disasters, for example, reported rates of PTSD-related syndromes varied substantially, from 3% in children exposed to a tornado (Stoppelbein & Greening, 2000) to 90% in children after exposure to a hurricane (Goenjian et al., 2001). Among the 18 selected publications in Table 13.3, we also see a wide variation in rates of posttraumatic reactions.

Out of the 18 publications in Table 13.3, only four have a longitudinal design (La Greca et al., 1996; Proctor et al., 2007; Terr et al., 1999; Thabet & Vostanis, 2000). However, findings from the few existing longitudinal studies of children's exposure to mass trauma are contradictory regarding posttraumatic stress reactions, with only some studies suggesting that these reactions persist over time (Dyregrov, Gjestad, & Raundalen, 2002; Kitayama et al., 2000; La Greca et al., 1996; Proctor et al., 2007). Interestingly, some studies were able to take advantage of rare opportunities to examine preexisting factors (La Greca, Silverman, & Wasserstein, 1998; Lengua, Long, Smith, & Meltzoff, 2005; Weems et al., 2007). Two studies were able to benefit from ongoing data collection, including one at the time of an earthquake, to show that prior anxiety symptoms was the only factor that significantly predicted subsequent development of PTSD in children (Asarnow et al., 1999), and the other assessed the distal impact of September 11th (Costello, Erkanli, Keeler, & Angold, 2004).

13.4.3. Correlates of Child Stress Reactions after Disasters

The majority of studies examining the effects of exposure to disasters have not included an in-depth investigation of the possible effects of familial exposure on children, or the impact of a multiplicity of exposures within large-scale disasters, including the cumulative effects of numerous exposures. These effects might prove to be particularly relevant for children. Studies have documented that children are highly sensitive to familial conflict and distress after a disaster (La Greca et al., 1998) and that they tend to mirror their parents' distress (Swenson et al., 1996). Conversely, parents' experience of distress after a disaster is influenced not only by the reactions of their children but also by the children's increased dependence on them (La Greca et al., 1998). For example, being a mother has been identified as a risk factor for experiencing greater distress after a traumatic event (Havenaar et al., 1997). Familial transmission, therefore, is one of a number of possible mechanisms that may help to explain the development of posttraumatic stress and other mental health problems in children following indirect exposure to a devastating event (e.g., children of first responder parents).

Media exposure to an event has also been shown to be associated with children's posttraumatic stress reactions (Pfefferbaum et al., 2000; Hoven et al., 2002). For example, media exposure was an important correlate of child PTSD after the Oklahoma terrorist acts (Pfefferbaum et al., 2000); media exposure was also a factor associated with psychopathology after the September 11th attack (Hoven et al., 2002; Saylor, Cowart, Lipovsky, Jackson, & Finch, Jr., 2003). Prior exposure to trauma may also make the development of PTSD more likely (Hoven et al., 2002, 2005). However, prior exposure to interpersonal violence or loss of a family member may be more closely related to the development of PTSD than the type of precipitating traumatic event (Davis & Siegel, 2000).

Psychiatric disorders observed in children after large-scale traumatic events include a range of disorders, with PTSD and depression being the most commonly assessed. Other mental disorders in children are frequently co-morbid with PTSD, particularly other anxiety disorders (Asarnow et al., 1999; Goenjian et al., 2001). PTSD and depression co-occurrence rates as high as 79% have been found in children living in highly exposed areas (Goenjian et al., 2001). The results of a US national survey of adolescents showed that exposure to individual trauma increases the risk of PTSD, major depressive episodes, and substance abuse/dependence in adolescents, with PTSD more likely to present co-morbidly than the latter two (Kilpatrick et al., 2003).

13.5. CONCLUSION

In spite of the fact that funding for disaster research designed to be conducted immediately after mass disaster events is often made available, partially explaining the recent exponential increase in literature on postdisaster childhood psychopathology, information deficits continue. Leaders in the field (Pfefferbaum et al., 2001, 2002; Pynoos et al., 1987; Steinberg et al., 2004) have helped to shape our understanding of children's postdisaster reactions. As a result of their work for example, on the effects of direct versus indirect exposure (Pynoos et al., 1987), media (Pfefferbaum, Nixon, et al., 2001), and distance (Pfefferbaum, Seale, et al., 2000), these topics are now routinely considered by researchers when assessing postdisaster psychological reactions in children. Yet, in spite of their outstanding efforts and the field's current extensive literature, important questions remain unanswered and frequently unaddressed. For example, we still do not know much about some very basic aspects of disaster response, such as which types of disasters are most likely to generate the most intractable forms of child psychopathology or impaired functioning. Further, this chapter illustrates (see Figure 13.1) the heightened interest over the past few decades in studying child mental health sequelae resulting from exposure (both direct and indirect) to disasters (both natural and human-caused), and although a large number of investigators have focused on specific mental health outcomes, most of the research has employed different study designs, diverse sampling strategies and has been conducted at varying time intervals following a disaster.

From a small number of well-designed, child-focused postdisaster studies, we have already learned that many children exhibit short-term, elevated rates of negative psychological reactions to specific disasters (Hoven, 2002; La Greca, 2006; Pfefferbaum, Nixon, et al., 1999; Pynoos et al., 1987), while another meaningful proportion of exposed children will exhibit longer lasting adverse reactions (La Greca et al., 1996; Proctor et al., 2007; Terr et al., 1997; Thabet & Vostanis, 2000). Across studies, age and gender are almost always important determinants of outcome. However, few well-designed, longitudinal, large-scale epidemiological investigations utilizing adequate population-based samples, from which answers to many of the most pressing questions might be gleaned, have been conducted.

Unfortunately, at this time, most studies have not reached their potential to answer some of these important questions. By example, we cite our own study (Hoven, Mandell & Duarte, 2002, 2005; Hoven et al., 2006), which was the first large-scale (*N* = 8,236) epidemiological investigation of a representative sample of children following a major human-made disaster and was carried out among public school children from throughout New York City 6 months after the September 11th terrorist attack on the World Trade Center. This study provided many important insights into the relationship of eight DSM-IV probable disorders (PTSD, major depression, panic disorder, separation anxiety, agoraphobia, generalized anxiety disorder, alcohol abuse/dependence, conduct disorder), as well as functional impairment in relationship to levels and types of personal exposure, age, gender, event proximity, ethnicity, prior exposure, and parental exposure, and so on. However, even this landmark study failed to reach its full scientific potential, primarily by not employing (not permitted) a longitudinal design. As a cross-sectional study, this investigation was therefore unable to explore the long-term psychological consequences of September 11th, including subsequent impairment, resilience, and recovery.

In an attempt to characterize the large body of existing research, we have presented here a typology relevant for considering postdisaster child mental health. We hope this effort is helpful. Yet, without greater agreement concerning the common use of standard measures, appropriate sampling strategies and study designs, the kind of specific detail necessary to draw firm conclusions about the relationships between disaster types and forms of psychopathology evoked remains wanting.

Clearly, the type of disaster, geographic spread, media coverage, affected populations, individual and collective contextual factors, potential ameliorative resources, treatment access and availability – all potentially multifaceted influences on child mental health outcomes – should inform postdisaster study design, choice of study methods and appropriate time frames. Just as predisaster planning has become a ubiquitous requirement for every institutional, federal, state, and city government budget appropriation, particularly after September 11th, it is important to expand this process to developing scientifically sound, child-focused mental health research agendas and methodologies in advance of disasters. It is only by preplanning such research agendas that we will be able to develop the necessary rigorous scientific approaches requisite for improving our understanding of developmental pathways of postdisaster psychopathology and, thus, appropriately design new, targeted interventions.

Finally, a main objective of this chapter has been to offer a call for a general "conversation" among mental health researchers whose work is child focused and related to postdisaster investigation. Agreements resulting from discussions of important research matters, such as those raised here, could influence an opus of work that would then draw on systematic comparisons from future studies. Such focused, collaborative efforts would facilitate major advances for which the field is currently poised to take advantage.

REFERENCES

Asarnow, J., Glynn, S., Pynoos, R.S., Nahum, J., Guthrie, D., Cantwell, D. P., et al. (1999). When the earth stops shaking: Earthquake sequelae among children diagnosed for pre-earthquake psychopathology. *Journal of the American Academy of Child and Adolescent Psychiatry, 38*, 1016–1023.

Balaban, V. (2006). Psychological assessment of children in disasters and emergencies. *Disasters, 30*, 178–198.

Bulut, S., Bulut, S., & Tayli, A. (2005). The dose of exposure and prevalence rates of post traumatic stress disorder in a sample of Turkish children eleven months after the 1909 Marmara earthquakes. *School Psychology International, 26*, 55–70.

Comer, J. S., & Kendall, P. C. (2007). Terrorism: The psychological impact on youth. *Clinical Psychology: Science and Practice, 14*, 179–212.

Costello, E. J., Erkanli, A., Keeler, G., & Angold, A. (2004). Distant trauma: A prospective study of the effects of September 11th on young adults in North Carolina. *Applied Developmental Science, 8*, 211–220.

Davis, L., & Siegel, L. J. (2000). PTSD in children and adolescents: A review and analysis. *Clinical Child and Family Psychology Review, 3*, 135–154.

Dohrenwend, B. P. (2006). Inventorying stressful life events as risk factors for psychopathology: Toward resolution of the problem of intracategory variability. *Psychological Bulletin, 132*, 477–495.

Duarte, C. S., Bordin, I. A. S, Green, R., & Hoven C. W. (2009). Measuring child exposure to violence and mental health reactions in epidemiological studies: challenges and current issues. *Cienc. Saude Coletiva, 13*, 487–496.

Duarte, C.S., Hoven, C.W., Wu, P., Cotel, S., Mandell, D.J., Nagasawa, M., Balaban, V, Wernikoff, L. & Markenson, D., et al. (2006). Posttraumatic stress in children with first responders in their families. *Journal of Traumatic Stress, 19*, 301–306.

Dyregrov, A., Gjestad, R., & Raundalen, M. (2002). Children exposed to warfare: A longitudinal study. *Journal of Traumatic Stress, 15*, 59–68.

Fairbrother, G., Stuber, J., Galea, S., Fleischman, A. R., & Pfefferbaum, B. (2003). Posttraumatic stress reactions in New York City children after the September 11, 2001, terrorist attacks. *Ambulatory Pediatrics, 3*, 304–311.

Fremont, W. P. (2004). Childhood reactions to terrorism-induced trauma: A review of the past 10 years. *Journal of the American Academy of Child and Adolescent Psychiatry, 43*, 381–392.

Garrison, C. Z., Bryant, E. S., Addy, C. L., Spurrier, P. G., Freedy, J. R., & Kilpatrick, D. G. (1995). Posttraumatic stress disorder in adolescents after Hurricane Andrew. *Journal of the American Academy of Child and Adolescent Psychiatry, 34*, 1193–1201.

Giannopoulou, I., Strouthos, M., Smith, P., Dikaiakou, A., Galanopoulou, V., & Yule, W. (2006). Posttraumatic stress reactions of children and adolescents exposed to the Athens 1999 earthquake. *European Psychiatry, 21*, 160–166.

Godeau, E., Vignes, C., Navarro, F., Iachan, R., Ross, J., Pasquier, C., et al. (2005). Effects of a large-scale industrial disaster on rates of symptoms consistent with posttraumatic stress disorders among schoolchildren in Toulouse. *Archives of Pediatric and Adolescent Medicine, 159*, 579–584.

Goenjian, A. K., Molina, L., Steinberg, A. M., Fairbanks, L. A., Alvarez, M. L., Goenjian, H. A., et al. (2001). Posttraumatic stress and depressive reactions among Nicaraguan adolescents after Hurricane Mitch. *American Journal of Psychiatry, 158*, 788–794.

Havenaar, J. M., Rumyantzeva, G. M., Van den Brink, W., Poelijoe, N. W., Van den Bout, J., et al. (1997). Long-term mental health effects of the Chernobyl disaster: An epidemiologic survey in two former Soviet regions. *American Journal of Psychiatry, 154*, 1605–1607.

Horowitz, M., Wilner, N., & Alvarez, W. (1979). Impact of Event Scale – Measure of Subjective Stress. *Psychosomatic Medicine, 41*, 209–218.

Hoven, C. W. (2002). *Testimony: The United States Senate, Hearing Before the Committee on Health, Education, Labor and Pensions, (Chair, Hillary Rodham Clinton), Children of September 11: The Need for Mental Health Services, June 10, 2002. Senate Hearing No. 107-540, Document No. 552-070-29-035-4.* U.S. Government Printing Office.

Hoven, C. W., Duarte, C. S., Lucas, C. P., Mandell, D. J., Cohen, M., Rosen, C., et al. (2002). *Effects of the World Trade Center Attack on NYC public school students: Initial report to the New York City Board of Education.* New York: Columbia University Mailman School of Public Health-New York State Psychiatric Institute and Applied Research and Consulting, LLC, New York City.

Hoven, C. W., Duarte, C. S., Lucas, C. P., Wu, P., Mandell, D. J., Goodwin, R. D., et al. (2005).

Psychopathology among New York City public school children six months after September 11. *Archives of General Psychiatry, 62*, 545–552.

Hoven, C. W., Duarte, C. S., & Mandell, D. J. (2003). Children's mental health after disasters: The impact of the World Trade Center attack. *Current Psychiatry Reports, 5*, 101–107.

Hoven, C. W., Mandell, D. J., & Duarte C. S. (2003). Mental Health in NYC Public School Children Post 9/11: an Epidemiological Investigation. In S. W. Coates, J. L. Rosenthal, & D. S. Schechter (eds.), *September 11: trauma and human bonds*. Analytic Press. Hillsdale, N.J.

Hoven, C. W., Mandell, D. J., Duarte, C. S., Wu, P., & Giordano, V. (2006). An epidemiological response to disaster: the post 9/11 psychological needs assessment of New York City public school students. In Y. Neria, R. Gross, & R. D. Marshall (eds.), *9/11: mental health in the wake of terrorist attacks*. Cambridge University Press,.

Kiliç, E. Z., Ozguven, H. D., & Sayil, I. (2003). The psychological effects of parental mental health on children experiencing disaster: The experience of Bolu earthquake in Turkey. *Family Process, 42*, 485–495.

Kilpatrick, D. G., Ruggiero, K. J., Acierno, R., Saunders, B. E., Resnick, H. S., & Best, C. L. (2003). Violence and risk of PTSD, major depression, substance abuse/dependence, and comorbidity: Results from the National Survey of Adolescents. *Journal of Consulting and Clinical Psychology, 71*, 692–700.

Kitayama, S., Okada, Y., Takumi, T., Takada, S., Inagaki, Y., & Nakamura, H. (2000). Psychological and physical reactions on children after the Hanshin-Awaji earthquake disaster. *The Kobe Journal of Medical Sciences, 46*, 189–200.

La Greca, A. M. (2006). School-based studies of children following disasters. In F. Norris, S. Galea, M. J. Friedman, & P. Watson (Eds.), *Methods for disaster mental health research*. New York: Guilford Press.

(2007). Understanding the psychological impact of terrorism on youth: Moving beyond posttraumatic stress disorder. *Clinical Psychology: Science and Practice, 14*, 219–223.

La Greca, A. M., Silverman, W. K., Vernberg, E. M., & Prinstein, M. J. (1996). Symptoms of posttraumatic stress in children after Hurricane Andrew: A prospective study. *Journal of Consulting and Clinical Psychology, 64*, 712–723.

La Greca, A. M., Silverman, W. K., & Wasserstein, S. B. (1998). Children's predisaster functioning as a predictor of posttraumatic stress following Hurricane Andrew. *Journal of Consulting and Clinical Psychology, 66*, 883–892.

Lengua, L. J., Long, A. C., Smith, K. I., & Meltzoff, A. N. (2005). Pre-attack symptomatology and temperament as predictors of children's responses to the September 11 terrorist attacks. *Journal of Child Psychology and Psychiatry, 46*, 631–645.

Lonigan, C. J., Shannon, M. P., Finch, A. J., Jr., Daugherty, T. K., & Taylor, C. M. (1991). Children's reactions to a natural disaster: Symptom severity and degree of exposure. *Advances in Behaviour Research and Therapy, 13*, 135–154.

Lucas, C. P., Zhang, H. Y., Fisher, P. W., Shaffer, D., Regier, D. A., Narrow, W. E., et al. (2001). The DISC Predictive Scales (DPS): Efficiently screening for diagnoses. *Journal of the American Academy of Child and Adolescent Psychiatry, 40*, 443–449.

Maunder, R. G., Lancee, W. J., Rourke, S., Hunter, J. J., Goldbloom, D., Balderson, K., et al. (2004). Factors associated with the psychological impact of severe acute respiratory syndrome on nurses and other hospital workers in Toronto. *Psychosomatic Medicine, 66*, 938–942.

Nickell, L. A., Crighton, E. J., Tracy, C. S., Al Enazy, H., Bolaji, Y., Hanjrah, S., et al. (2004). Psychosocial effects of SARS on hospital staff: Survey of a large tertiary care institution. *Canadian Medical Association Journal, 170*, 793–798.

Ohan, J. L., Myers, K., & Collett, B. R. (2002). Ten-year review of rating scales. IV: Scales assessing trauma and its effects. *Journal of the American Academy of Child and Adolescent Psychiatry, 41*, 1401–1422.

Pfefferbaum, B., Doughty, D. E., Reddy, C., Patel, N., Gurwitch, R. H., Nixon, S. J., et al. (2002). Exposure and peritraumatic response as predictors of posttraumatic stress in children following the 1995 Oklahoma City bombing. *Journal of Urban Health, 79*, 354–363.

Pfefferbaum, B., Gurwitch, R. H., McDonald, N. B., Leftwich, M. J., Sconzo, G. M., Messenbaugh, A. K., et al. (2000). Posttraumatic stress among young children after the death of a friend or acquaintance in a terrorist bombing. *Psychiatric Services, 51*, 386–388.

Pfefferbaum, B., Nixon, S. J., Krug, R. S., Tivis, R. D., Moore, V. L., Brown, J. M., et al. (1999). Clinical needs assessment of middle and high school students following the 1995 Oklahoma City bombing. *American Journal of Psychiatry, 156*, 1069–1074.

Pfefferbaum, B., Nixon, S. J., Tivis, R. D., Doughty, D. E., Pynoos, R. S., Gurwitch, R. H., et al. (2001). Television exposure in children after a terrorist incident. *Psychiatry, 64*, 202–211.

Pfefferbaum, B., Nixon, S. J., Tucker, P. M., Tivis, R. D., Moore, V. L., Gurwitch, R. H., et al. (1999). Posttraumatic stress responses in bereaved children after the Oklahoma City bombing. *Journal of the American Academy of Child and Adolescent Psychiatry, 38*, 1372–1379.

Pfefferbaum, B., North, C. S., Flynn, B. W., Ursano, R. J., McCoy, G., DeMartino, R., et al. (2001). The emotional impact of injury following an international terrorist incident. *Public Health Reviews, 29*, 271–280.

Pfefferbaum, B., Pfefferbaum, R. L., Gurwitch, R. H., Nagumalli, S., Brandt, E. N., Robertson, M. J., et al. (2003). Children's response to terrorism: A critical review of the literature. *Current Psychiatric Reports, 5*, 95–100.

Pfefferbaum, B., Seale, T. W., McDonald, N. B., Brandt, E. N., Jr., Rainwater, S. M., Maynard, B. T., et al. (2000). Posttraumatic stress two years after the Oklahoma City bombing in youths geographically distant from the explosion. *Psychiatry, 63*, 358–370.

Pfefferbaum, B., Stuber, J., Galea, S., & Fairbrother, G. (2006). Panic reactions to terrorist attacks and probable posttraumatic stress disorder in adolescents. *Journal of Traumatic Stress, 19*, 217–228.

Pine, D. S., Costello, J., & Masten, A. (2005). Trauma, proximity, and developmental psychopathology: The effects of war and terrorism on children. *Neuropsychopharmacology, 30*, 1781–1792.

Proctor, L. J., Fauchier, A., Oliver, P. H., Ramos, M. C., Rios, M. A., & Margolin, G.(2007). Family context and young children's responses to earthquake. *Journal of Child Psychology and Psychiatry, 48*, 941–949.

Pynoos, R. S., Frederick, C., Nader, K., Arroyo, W., Steinberg, A., Eth, S., et al. (1987). Life threat and posttraumatic stress in school-age children. *Archives of General Psychiatry, 44*, 1057–1063.

Pynoos, R. S., Steinberg, A. M., Ornitz, E. M., & Goenjian, A. K. (1997). Issues in the developmental neurobiology of traumatic stress. *Annals of the New York Academy of Sciences, 821*, 176–193.

Reynolds, D. L., Garay, J. R., Deamond, S. L., Moran, M. K., Gold, W., & Styra, R. (2008). Understanding, compliance and psychological impact of the SARS quarantine experience. *Epidemiology and Infection, 136*, 997–1007.

Saylor, C. F., Cowart, B. L., Lipovsky, J. A., Jackson, C., & Finch, A. J., Jr. (2003). Media exposure to September 11: Elementary school students' experiences and posttraumatic symptoms. *American Behavioral Scientist, 46*, 1622–1642.

Shaffer, D., Fisher, P., Lucas, C. P., Dulcan, M. K., & Schwab-Stone, M. E. (2000). NIMH Diagnostic Interview Schedule for Children Version IV (NIMH DISC-IV): Description, differences from previous versions, and reliability of some common diagnoses. *Journal of the American Academy of Child and Adolescent Psychiatry, 39*, 28–38.

Shalev, A. Y., Tuval-Mashiach, R., & Hadar, H. (2004). Posttraumatic stress disorder as a result of mass trauma. *Journal of Clinical Psychiatry, 65*(Suppl. 1), 4–10.

Steinberg, A. M., Brymer, M. J., Decker, K. B., & Pynoos, R. S. (2004). The University of California at Los Angeles Post-traumatic Stress Disorder Reaction Index. *Current Psychiatric Reports, 6*, 96–100.

Steinberg, A. M., Brymer, M. J., Steinberg, J. R., & Pfefferbaum, B. (2006). Conducting research with children and adolescents after disaster. In F. Norris, S. Galea, M. J. Friedman, & P. Watson (Eds.), *Methods for disaster mental health research*. New York: Guilford Press.

Stoppelbein, L., & Greening, L. (2000). Posttraumatic stress symptoms in parentally bereaved children and adolescents. *Journal of the American Academy of Child and Adolescent Psychiatry, 39*, 1112–1119.

Strand, V. C., Sarmiento, T. L., & Pasquale, L. E. (2005). Assessment and screening tools for trauma in children and adolescents: A review. *Trauma, Violence, & Abuse, 6*, 55–78.

Swenson, C. C., Saylor, C. F., Powell, M. P., Stokes, S. J., Foster, K. Y., & Belter, R. W. (1996). Impact of a natural disaster on preschool children: Adjustment 14 months after a hurricane. *American Journal of Orthopsychiatry, 66*, 122–130.

Terr, L. C., Bloch, D. A., Michel, B. A., Shi, H., Reinhardt, J. A., & Metayer, S. A. (1997). Children's thinking in the wake of Challenger. *American Journal of Psychiatry, 154*, 744–751.

Terr, L. C., Bloch, D. A., Michel, B. A., Shi, H., Reinhardt, J. A., & Metayer, S. (1999). Children's symptoms in the wake of Challenger: A field study of distant-traumatic effects and an outline of related conditions. *American Journal of Psychiatry, 156*, 1536–1544.

Thabet, A. A., & Vostanis, P. (2000). Post traumatic stress disorder reactions in children of war: A longitudinal study. *Child Abuse and Neglect, 24*, 291–298.

Vernberg, E. M., Silverman, W. K., La Greca, A. M., & Prinstein, M. J. (1996). Prediction of posttraumatic stress symptoms in children after hurricane Andrew. *Journal of Abnormal Psychology, 105*, 237–248.

Weems, C. F., Pina, A. A., Costa, N. M., Watts, S. E., Taylor, L. K., & Cannon, M. F. (2007). Predisaster trait anxiety and negative affect predict posttraumatic stress in youths after hurricane Katrina. *Journal of Consulting and Clinical Psychology, 75*, 154–159.

Wickrama, K. A., & Kaspar, V. (2007). Family context of mental health risk in Tsunami-exposed adolescents: Findings from a pilot study in Sri Lanka. *Social Science and Medicine, 64*, 713–723.

14 Disaster Mental Health in Older Adults: Symptoms, Policy, and Planning

JOAN M. COOK AND DIANE L. ELMORE

14.1. INTRODUCTION

There is a large body of empirical evidence illustrating that disasters can have considerable mental health effects for a significant proportion of survivors, ranging from temporary stress reactions to more persistent and severe psychopathology (Norris, Friedman, & Watson, 2002). Although there is still some ongoing debate regarding risk and protective factors for mental health vulnerability in the face of disasters, some evidence suggests that those at greater risk are children, women, people of low socioeconomic status, individuals with physical and mental disabilities, ethnic minorities, first responders, the uninsured, residents of rural areas, and subgroups of older adults (Johnson et al., 2006; Johnson & Langlieb, 2005; Mokdad et al., 2005; Norris et al., 2002).

Advances in public health, biomedicine, and socioeconomic and living conditions have all contributed to making older adults one of the fastest growing segments of the population in the United States and other industrialized countries (He, Sengupta, Velkoff, & DeBarros, 2005). Among those 65 years of age and older, women far outnumber men, and there is increasing heterogeneity in race and ethnicity (He et al., 2005). Since female gender and ethnic minority status are two potential risk factors for vulnerability in the event of a disaster, this may compound concern for those among the older adult population.

There are numerous views regarding why older adults are or are not expected to be differentially vulnerable to the effects of disasters. Four explanations of potential differential effects of age are the resource, exposure, inoculation, and burden perspectives (Thompson, Norris, & Hanacek, 1993). Two of these, namely, the resource and the exposure perspectives contend that older adults are more vulnerable to disasters, while the other two, the inoculation and the burden perspectives, posit that older adults are less vulnerable to disaster. More specifically, the resource position suggests that older adults are more vulnerable to disasters because of declining physical health and functional capacity as well as lower socioeconomic resources. The exposure perspective maintains that older adults would be more vulnerable because they are less likely to receive warnings of impending disasters and more likely to be injured and to feel a greater sense of deprivation due to losses. The inoculation perspective proposes that older adults are less vulnerable to disasters because of their past experience and enhanced attitudes of acceptance of loss and suffering. These proposed age-related changes apparently result in increased coping capacity. The burden perspective claims that older adults are less vulnerable than middle-aged individuals, who have more familial and work roles to fill and thus greater responsibilities to shoulder in the recovery period.

The purpose of this chapter is to review the empirical evidence regarding mental health consequences of disasters in older adults. Summary conclusions are made in regards to differential effects, and a tentative new conceptual framework is presented. In addition, important implications for disaster policy and planning for the needs of the aging population are discussed.

In this chapter, the literatures on natural, human-made, and technological disasters are reviewed separately and in chronological order. It is important to note that this review includes only research that has been published in English. Although not directly addressed in this chapter, there are numerous potential physical health consequences of disasters (e.g., infectious disease, food and waterborne illness, electrocution, punctures and wounds, burns) that may bring their own unique problems, exacerbate other chronic physical conditions, and likely negatively impact mental or social functioning in older individuals (Ehrenreich & McQuaide, 2001; Lister, 2005).

14.2. REVIEW OF THE EMPIRICAL LITERATURE

A recent quantitative review of mental health in a broad range of disaster survivors reported differential protective effects associated with older age in only 2 of 17 distinct samples that included older adults (Norris et al., 2002). In contrast, 15 of the 17 samples indicated that the mental health effects of disasters declined with age. The review here provides a critical examination of the 17 distinct samples reported in 16 studies, highlighting some important factors that were previously not emphasized, and presents analysis of additional disaster mental health studies that include older adults. Table 14.1 presents a summary of key variables and findings in quantitative studies of mental health with older adult samples.

14.2.1. Natural Disasters

A natural disaster is the consequence of a potential natural hazard becoming a physical event. This may be geological in nature, such as an avalanche, earthquake, or landslide; hydrological, such as a flood or tsunami; or climatic, such as a drought, hurricane, tornado, or a fire. The majority of scientific investigation on the mental health of older adults and disasters is in the area of natural disasters.

On the basis of his review of hundreds of unstructured interviews with adult survivors of tornados and a hurricane in several states across the United States during the 1950s, Friedsam (1961) formulated a broad hypothesis on differential reactions of younger and older adults to natural disasters. Two themes of relative deprivation were identified in older adults: the loss of symbolic assets, particularly homes, and the preoccupation with time. In the interviews, older adults spoke of having spent a lifetime sacrificing and building their homes, only to have them destroyed by the disaster. Additionally, they expressed concern that not only objects were lost, but time itself was gone. In other words, these older individuals felt they did not have the time to rebuild their lives, including the homes and possessions that they had lost.

Six hundred and seventy-six survivors of the 1966 Topeka Kansas tornado and individuals not affected by the event were compared on the definition and evaluation of losses, the role of external help, economic recovery, and physical and mental health (Kilijanek & Drabek, 1979). As opposed to younger survivors, older adults: (1) reported the loss of material items and house-related damage as being more important, (2) received less community aid (i.e., relatives; friends; American Red Cross, Salvation Army, or other voluntary organizations, strangers; and employers), (3) used less automobile or household item insurance and other economic sources (e.g., savings, credit cards, bank credit) in recovery, and (4) perceived less significant long-term negative physical or mental health consequences. Indeed, in this sample, the tornado did not appear to have any significant long-term negative impact on self-reports of physical or mental health among older individuals.

To ascertain short- and long-term effects of the 1972 floods from Hurricane Agnes in Pennsylvania, 250 older adults (age 60 and older) were interviewed at three different time points over a two and a half year period (Cohen & Poulshock, 1979). The results of the first survey revealed that over 90% of older adults reported immediate and serious housing problems, with most having to move at least three times over the next year (Poulshock & Cohen, 1975). However, over time 38% of older adults

Table 14.1. Summary of key variables and findings in quantitative studies of mental health with older adult samples

	Disaster Type	Where Occurred		Sample Type			
Source	**Type**	**State or Country**	**Population**	**Number**	**Age**	**Gender**	**Ethnicity**
Younger Adults in More Distress							
Acierno et al., 2006	Hurricane	Florida	Households with telephones in Florida counties that were impacted directly by the hurricanes	1,543	Older adult group (aged 50 and older) $M=71.0$, SD = 7.9; Younger adult group $M=42.9$, SD = 10.5	Females ($N=984$); Males ($N=552$); Not Specified ($N=7$)	White ($N=1354$); Black ($N=101$); Asian/Pacific Islander ($N=23$); Native American/ Alaskan ($N=26$); Missing ($N=39$)
Bell, Kara, & Batterson, 1978	Tornado	Nebraska	Victims residing in the urban areas of Omaha, Nebraska	200	18–92 ($M=52.9$); Aged 18–59 ($n=90$), 60 and older ($n=110$) Controls: 18–59 ($n=45$), 60 and older ($n=55$)	Females ($N=110$); Males ($N=90$)	White ($N=198$)
Kato & Kato, 1998[a]; Kato et al., 1996	Earthquake	Japan	Evacuees in shelter	142	12–84 ($M=58.6$); Aged under 60 ($N=67$), 60 and older ($N=75$)	Females ($N=81$); Males ($N=61$)	
Kilijanek & Drabek, 1979	Tornado	Kansas	Communities surrounding the tornados path	665	Aged 39 and younger ($N=170$), Aged 40–59 ($N=247$), Aged 60 and older ($N=248$)		
Norris, Kaniasty, et al., 2002	Hurricane	Mexico	Residents of Acapulco Bay	404	18–81 Young-aged ($N=85$, $M=39.6$); Middle-aged ($N=64$, $M=48.3$); Older-aged ($N=49$, $M=68.6$)	Females ($N=91$); Males ($N=107$) Younger-aged (39 Females, 46 Males) Middle-aged: (29 Females, 35 Males); Older-aged: (23 Females, 26 Males)	Latino ($N=134$); Non-Hispanic Black ($N=135$); Non-Hispanic White ($N=135$)

(*continued*)

Table 14.1 *(continued)*

	Disaster Type	Where Occurred		Sample Type			
Source	**Type**	**State or Country**	**Population**	**Number**	**Age**	**Gender**	**Ethnicity**
Huerta & Horton, 1978	Dam collapse	Idaho	Telephone interview of residents of the damaged area	387	Younger than 65 ($N =^{a}$); Older than 65 ($N =^{a}$)	Females ($N = 259$); Males ($N = 128$)	
Tracy & Galea, 2006	Terrorism	New York City	Telephone survey of NYC metropolitan area residents	2,282	18 and older; 18–34, 35–54, and 55 and older		
Middle-Aged Adults in More Distress							
Gleser, Green, & Winget, 1981	Dam collapse and flood	West Virginia	Buffalo Creek, VA community impacted by the floods	588	281 Adults, 207 Children (Grouped as 16–24; 25–39; 40–54; and 55 and older)	Females ($N = 163$); Males ($N = 131$); Girls ($N = 135$); Boys ($N = 138$)	Sample was made up of both Caucasian Americans and African-Americans, although numbers were not specified
Green et al., (follow-up, 1996)	Dam collapse and flood	West Virginia	Residents who lived in the area surrounding dam	120	16–23 ($N = 27$); 24–38 ($N = 28$); 39–49 ($N = 33$); 53–63 ($N = 32$)	Females ($N = 71$); Males ($N = 49$)	
Logue, Hansen, & Struening, 1981	Flood	Pennsylvania	On the basis of a directory, every fourth household in the towns surrounding the flooded town were used	562	21–88; Aged less than 55; 55 to 64; 64 years and older	Females	

Norris et al., 2002	Hurricane	Florida	Neighborhoods in South Miami	404	18–88 Younger-Aged ($N=89$, $M=30$); Middle-Aged ($N=82$, $M=48$); Older-Aged ($N=96$, $M=70$)	Females ($N=133$); Males ($N=134$)	Latinos ($N=134$); Non-Hispanic Black ($N=135$); Non-Hispanic White ($N=135$) [d]Note: Latinos were excluded because 79% immigrated to the U.S.
Phifer, 1990	Flood	Kentucky	15 counties around Kentucky	222	Working age group: 55–64; Young–old: 65–74; Old: 75+	Females ($N=142$); Males ($N=80$)	
Shore, Tatum, & Vollmer, 1986	Volcanic eruption	Oregon and Washington	Two rural Northwest logging communities	1,025	18–79 ($M=45.7$, SD = 14.7)	Females ($N=512$); Males ($N=513$)	Caucasian
Thompson, Norris, & Hanacek, 1993	Hurricane	Southeastern U. S. (South Carolina, North Carolina, Georgia)	Urban communities	831	18–89; ($M=48$; SD = 18) Young (19–39), Middle-aged (40–59), Older (over 60)	Female ($N=432$); Males ($N=399$)	White ($N=407$); Black ($N=424$)
Lewin, Carr, & Webster, 1998	Earthquake	Australia	New Castle, Australia; local community ($N = 541$), Special interest groups ($N = 304$)	845	17–91 ($M = 43.4$)	Females ($N = 429$), Males ($N = 416$)	
Older Adults in More Distress							
Bolin & Klenow, 1988	Two Tornados	Texas	Local Paris, Texas, community ($N=431$)	431	18–64 ($N=267$); 65 and older ($N=164$)		White ($N=212$); Black ($N=219$)

(*continued*)

Table 14.1 *(continued)*

	Disaster Type	Where Occurred		Sample Type			
Source	Type	State or Country	Population	Number	Age	Gender	Ethnicity
Ticehurst et al., 1996	Earthquake	Australia	Community	3,007	Younger than 65 (N=2371, M=40); Older than 65 (N=636, M=73)	Females (N=1,726) Males (N=1,281)	Non-English Speaking backgrounds (N=250)
Norris, Kaniasty et al., 2002	Flood	Poland	Community in the city of Opole	285	18–87; Young (N = 84, M = 29.1); Middle-Aged (N = 127, M = 48.4); Older (N = 73, M = 67.2)	Females (N = 180); Males (N = 104)	Polish
Ohta et al., 2003[b]	Volcano eruption	Japan	Displaced evacuees	248	19–85 (M = 53.2, SD = 16.9); Younger than 29 (N = 26); 30–39 (N = 40); 40–49 (N = 38); 50–59 (N = 32); 60–69 (N = 65); Older than 70 (N = 47)	Females (N = 124); Males (N = 124)	Japanese
Salcioglu, Basolu, & Livavanou, 2003	Earthquake	Turkey	Samples taken from 3 "tent cities," 7 prefabricated housing sites, two permanent housing sites, and one community center	586	M = 38.1, SD = 14.6	Females (N = 337); Males (N = 249)	
Suar, Misgra, & Khuntia, 2007	Supercyclone	India	Temporary camps	130	18–80 Aged 18–35 (N = 71); 36–55 (N = 46); 56–80 (N = 13)	Females (N = 53); Males (N = 77)	

Trautman et al., 2002	Bombing	Oklahoma City	At-risk minority population provided by Project Heartland	45	19–75 ($M = 43.9$); 19–29 ($N = 8$); 30–39 ($N = 10$); 40–49 ($N = 11$); 50–59 ($N = 10$); Older than 60 ($N = 6$)	Females ($N = 26$); Males ($N = 18$)	Asian and Middle Eastern
Van Griensven et al., 2006[c]	Tsunami	Thailand	Displaced persons	371	Aged 15–90 ($M = 39.5$)	Females ($N = 219$); Males ($N = 152$)	Thai
Yang et al., 2003	Earthquake	Taiwan	Sample was taken from the community of Pu-Li (one of the most severely damaged communities); provided by hospitals and outpatient clinics	663	Younger than 45 years ($N = 227$); 45–64 ($N = 196$); Older than 65 years ($N = 203$)	Females ($N = 387$); Males ($N = 276$)	
Hansson, Noulles, & Bellovich, 1982	Flood	Oklahoma	Random sample of the residents of Tulsa, Oklahoma	176	Median age (46 years)		
Knight et al., 2000	Earthquake	Los Angeles, California	Sample was provided by the Longitudinal Study of Generations (LSOG)	166	Aged 30–102 (Median = 64); 30–54, 31% of sample; 55–75, 45%; 76+, 24%	Females ($N = 106$); Males ($N = 60$)	White, non-Hispanic ($N = 156$); Latino ($N = 7$); African-Americans ($N = 2$); Asian-American ($N = 1$)

(*continued*)

Table 14.1 (*continued*)

	Disaster Type	Where Occurred		Sample Type			
Source	Type	State or Country	Population	Number	Age	Gender	Ethnicity
No Differences Between Younger and Older Adults							
Bleich et al., 2005	Bombing	Israel	Telephone contact from Israeli Dahaf Institute database	444	18–85 (M=43.64); Aged 18–64 (N=385, M=39.5, SD=12.6); 65–74 (N=41, M=67.3, SD=2.8); 74+ (N=18, M=78.2, SD=2.8)	Females (N=221); Males (N=223)	Jewish-Israeli
Chung, Dennis, Easthope, Farmer, & Werrett, 2005	Train collision and aircraft crash	United Kingdom	Community residents	148	45 and younger (N=83); Older than 60 (N=103)	Females (N=97); Males (N=51)	
Chung et al., 2004	Train collision and aircraft crash	United Kingdom	Community residents	148	18+ (M=52.36); 18–39 (N=47); 40–64 (N=48); 65+ (N=53)	Females (N=97); Males (N=51)	Caucasian (N=146); Afro-Caribbean (N=2)
Goenjian et al., 1994	Earthquake	Armenia	Residents of three cities (Spitak, Gumri, and Yerevan) Spitak older adults 59–81 (N=15); Gumri older adults 65–87 (N=39); Gumri younger adults 23–63 (N=66); Yerevan adults 18–53 (N=59)	179	18–87	Females (N=134); Males (N=45)	Armenian

Kohn et al., 2005	Hurricane	Honduras	Sheltered neighborhood	800	15–97; 15–24 ($N=219$, $M=19.5$, SD = 2.6); 25–59 ($N=478$, $M=38.9$, SD = 9.4); 60–97 ($N=103$, $M=69.3$, SD = 7.9)	Females ($N=497$); Males ($N=303$)	
Livingston, Livingston, Brooks, & McKinlay, 1992[d]	Airplane explosion	Scotland	Surrounding neighborhood to explosion	55	18+; 18–65 ($N=24$, $M=39$, SD = 17.5); 65+ ($N=31$, $M=73$, SD = 4.90)	Females ($N=46$); Males ($N=19$)	Scottish
Only Includes Older Adults							
Brenna, Horowitz, & Reinhart, 2003	Terrorism	New York	Sample from Lighthouse International	584	65–98 ($M=81$); Young–Old (65–74); Middle–Old (75–84); Old–Old (85 years +)	Females ($N=327$); Males ($N=257$)	Caucasian ($N=479$); Black ($N=93$); Hispanic ($N=12$)
Phifer, Kaniasty, & Norris, 1988	Floods	Kentucky	Data was provided by two studies previously conducted	222	55–59 ($N=31$); 60–64 ($N=56$); 6–69 ($N=52$); 70–74 ($N=33$); 75–79 ($N=30$); 80–84 ($N=17$); 85 and older ($N=3$)	Females ($N=141$); Males ($N=81$)	
Ferraro, Morton, Knuston, Zink, & Jacobson, 1999	Flood	North Dakota	Recruited from University of North Dakota retired faculty and the local community	68	$M=71$	Females ($N=43$); Males ($N=25$)	
Ferraro, 2003	Flood	North Dakota	Residents of Grand Forks, North Dakota community	37	67–90	Females ($N = 23$); Males ($N = 14$)	

(*continued*)

Table 14.1 *(continued)*

	Disaster Type	Where Occurred		Sample Type			
Source	**Type**	**State or Country**	**Population**	**Number**	**Age**	**Gender**	**Ethnicity**
Krause, 1987	Hurricane	Texas	Community of Galveston, Texas	351	65 years and older M = 73.4, SD = 6.2	Female (N = 232); Male (N = 119)	White (N = 226); Black (N = 96); Hispanic (N = 25); Other races (N = 4)
Melick and Logue, 1985–1986	Flood	Pennsylvania	Residents of designated flooded (N=120) and non-flooded (N=39) areas of Wyoming Valley	167	65–88	Women	
Tyler & Hoyt, 2000	Flood	Iowa	Iowa Health Poll (statewide survey)	651	55–69; 70 and older	Female (N=449); Male (202)	
Watanabe, Okumura, Chiu, & Wakai, 2004	Earthquake	Taiwan	Participants were evacuated and set up in temporary housing	54	M=68.1, SD=9.5		
Cohen & Poulshock, 1979	Hurricane; Flood	Pennsylvania	Sample was taken from Luzerne County where the flood occurred	250	60 years and older (M=71); 87 participants were over the age of 75	Females (N=167); Males (N=83)	Less than 1% of the population was nonwhite
Ollendick & Hoffman, 1982	Flood	Minnesota	Households were provided by the Rochester Area Churches Emergency Response organization	124 adults 54 children	24–59 (M=41.9); 60–93 (M=74.5)	Females (N=90); Males (N=34); Girls (N=23); Boys (N=31)	

Notes:

[a] Older and younger adults equally distressed after 3 weeks, but differences occurred 5 weeks later.

[b] Both middle-aged and older adults had more distress and slower recovery than younger adults.

[c] Old age was not a factor associated with higher prevalence of anxiety but was for depression.

[d] PTSD symptoms were similar, but older adults had a higher incidence of coexisting major depression.

reported that they were better off in regards to housing than before the flood, with most finding shelter with family and friends (Cohen & Poulshock, 1979). The majority of the impact of the flood was within 1 year, and thus the authors suggested that planning for services for older adults in the event of a disaster should be directed at the period between 1 week and 1 year following a disaster, with the most attention paid to the first 100 days.

Although this investigation was before the official entry of posttraumatic stress disorder (PTSD) into the psychiatric nomenclature, approximately 24% said that the most significant result of the flood was experiencing nervousness, fear, nightmares, depression, and isolation (Poulshock & Cohen, 1975). However, only 14 older individuals reported that they thought the flood had directly related to a decline in their physical health (Cohen & Poulshock, 1979). While social services were readily available, most older adults indicated a relatively minor need for counseling.

Logue, Hansen, and Struening (1981) also conducted a study on the long-term health effects of Hurricane Agnes on Pennsylvania residents. The sample consisted of 396 residents of flood areas and 155 controls. Both the older and the younger adults in the flood group consistently had higher scores on depression than the controls, but the differences were not significant. Among the flood groups, on one measure, those 65 and older demonstrated the least mental health problems, while on another measure, those 55 and younger demonstrated the least mental health problems. On both of these mental health indices, those 55 to 64 had the most mental health problems. This middle-aged group also reported the most physical health problems. This study had very low response rates, with many nonrespondents being older individuals with more health problems, perhaps underestimating the effects of the flood.

Five years following Hurricane Agnes and its flood in Pennsylvania, 122 women over the age of 65 and 45 controls were interviewed (Melick & Logue, 1985–1986). Sixty percent of the survivors reported that the length of their recovery period was over 1 year, while 30% reported that their recovery period lasted over 2 years. There were numerous differences in self-perception and somatization between the groups, with survivors reportedly having poorer "state of mind" after the flood, greater distress during recovery, poorer quality of life, greater frequency of thinking about the flood, and more physical health problems. However, there were no differences on anxiety or depressive symptoms. Although differential response rates and self-selected samples may account for some of these nongroup differences in mental health, the authors speculated that the older adult survivors may have taken an active role in personal and community recovery, thus counteracting additional potential mental health consequences.

In structured interviews with 200 Caucasian adult survivors of a 1975 tornado and 100 controls in Nebraska, Bell (1978) found significant differences in disruption and recovery by age. Specifically, mental and physical health was poorer in younger adults (18–59 years) compared with older adults (60 and older). Younger adults rated their 1-week emotional reactions to the tornado in more negative terms (e.g., afraid, fearful, frightened) than older adults. However, there were no differences in ratings of more long-term (30-week) anxiety reactions between the groups. The authors concluded that there may be a tendency for earlier anxiety resolution on the part of older adults. In general, there were no differences in routine community interactions between the younger and older groups. In other words, both groups still continued to frequent the same shops, purchase the same items and seek medical services from the same places as they did before the tornado. However, younger adults reported more disruption and less time spent after the tornado in interpersonal relations with family and friends than older adults.

Additionally, there was no consistent pattern of age-specific perceived needs expressed between younger and older adults (Bell, Kara, & Batterson, 1978). However, interviews and consultation with disaster recovery service providers revealed differential service utilization by age.

Older adults placed fewer demands upon service agencies (i.e., American Red Cross, Salvation Army, Food Stamp Program, Internal Revenue Service, Federal Disaster Assistance Center, police, National Guard) than younger adults. This group of older adults was apparently atypical of national norms in regards to having higher education and income and thus potentially had greater access to resources in coping with a disaster.

Three hundred and two survivors of two 1979 Texas tornados, randomly selected from individuals seeking assistance at disaster service centers, were examined for losses incurred in the storm, utilization of formal and informal aid sources, social and psychological impacts, and economic and emotional recovery (Bolin & Klenow, 1982–1983). There was little difference between older and younger victims in terms of absolute material losses. Compared with younger adults, twice as many older adults reported that their situation post-tornado was worse than those around them. Older adults experienced an injury rate twice that of younger adults. Although they had higher rates of utilization for the Salvation Army and American Red Cross, older adults underutilized other resources such as federal and state agencies for aid in housing, grants and loans. Older adults scored consistently lower than younger adults on several measures of psychosocial impact, such as irritability, fatigue, nightmares, and strains in family relationships. Despite endorsing less distress, between 21% and 80% of older adults continued to report some persistent emotional effects 1 year post-tornado.

A systematic random sample of 300 Oklahoma residents completed questionnaires several months after a major flood season (year not provided) (Hansson, Noulles, & Bellovich, 1982). While unrelated to knowledge about flooding, increasing age was significantly associated with higher scores on fear, depression, and desperation measures.

Caucasian and African American older adults and younger survivors of a 1982 tornado in Texas were compared on differential vulnerability (Bolin & Klenow, 1988). A random sample was drawn from an American Red Cross survey of damaged residences, and participants from 431 families were interviewed. The findings presented only focused on the older adult survivors. A significantly higher proportion of Caucasian older adults considered themselves fully recovered at 8 months as compared with older African-Americans. This was measured using a single-item that asked survivors to assess their emotional well-being and recovery from the effects of the disaster. For older African-Americans, psychosocial recovery was predicted by eight variables: higher socioeconomic status, larger family size, marital status (i.e., having a spouse), availability of primary group members, number of aid sources received, social support, federal aid adequacy, and number of moves in temporary housing. For older Caucasians, all of those variables predicted psychosocial recovery except for family size and the number of aid sources received. Unlike Caucasians, many older African Americans were residing with extended family and had likely come to rely on extra familial networks for support.

Krause (1987) employed a synthetic cohort design with a random community survey of older adults to examine the length of time needed for physical and mental health symptoms to abate following the 1983 Hurricane Alicia in Southern Texas. As time since the natural disaster increased, older adults were less likely to describe their physical health in negative terms. The major effects of the storm diminished after 16 months; there were significant gender differences in the adjustment process. Women reported higher somatic symptoms than men at 9 months, but these differences seemed to disappear at 16 months. The authors surmised that although older women were more vulnerable to the effects initially, they had the social support resources to eventually adjust to this event.

Two related but separate studies that yielded numerous important findings on older adults and the effects of natural disasters were: (1) a large prospective panel investigation of more than 200 predominately Caucasian older adults (55 and older) interviewed before and after a severe flood in Kentucky in 1981 and 1984, and (2) a smaller follow-up study of a subset who had lived in one of the two counties flooded in 1981 or one of five adjacent counties. Participants were interviewed at approximate 6-month intervals over a period of 2 years, yielding five interview waves. The follow-up study yielded a sixth wave of interviews approximately 2 years later.

Findings from this dataset include that men, those with lower occupational status, and people aged 55 to 64 were at significantly greater risk for increases in psychological symptoms (Phifer, 1990). Among all three age groups (55–64, 65–74, and 75 and older), prior symptom level was the strongest predictor of current psychological symptoms. Anxiety, depression, and physical symptoms were still evident 16 to 18 months postflood. However, most symptoms were mild to moderate and did not meet criteria for clinical disorders. This study found a relative resilience of the older-old (75 and older), which was tentatively attributed to higher incidence of past resolved stressful experiences and low incidence of current unresolved stressful experiences.

Also utilizing data from this same sample, Phifer and Norris (1989) found that for each of the psychological measures (i.e., anxiety, depression, and general well-being) preflood symptom levels were the strongest predictor of postflood symptom levels. Personal loss was associated with short-term (up to 1 year) increases in negative affect and decreases in positive affect. When older adults experienced both personal loss and high levels of community destruction, their increased levels of psychological distress persisted for a minimum of 2 years postflood. Thus, personal loss was required for psychological distress, but concurrent level of community destruction established the durability of the symptoms. Controlling for preflood symptoms, there were modest flood effects on trait anxiety and weather-specific distress in those with no prior flood experience (Norris & Murrell, 1988). In those with previous flood experience, there were no effects of the flood. These findings support the inoculation hypothesis in that experience with a natural disaster earlier in life reduced the impact of a natural disaster experienced in later life, often referred to as direct tolerance.

Norris, Phifer, and Kaniasty (1994) reported that exposure to the Kentucky floods was related to a decline in physical health and social relations for these older adults as well. Namely, older adults reported increased difficulties in performing daily activities, greater fatigue, and more medical conditions. Except for fatigue, these physical effects appeared to be less strong and lasting than the effects on mental health. For each of the five measures of physical health, preflood health was found to be the strongest predictor, accounting for between 50% and 70% of the variance in physical health (Phifer et al., 1988). However, albeit weakly, these floods did impact physical health the first year following the flood, accounting for between 1% and 4%. The impact of physical health appears to be strongest for those who had experienced both high personal losses and high community destruction in the floods.

With regard to social support, older adults' expectations of how much help they would receive after a disaster was approximately three times higher than the actual amount of help received (Norris et al., 1994). The authors hypothesized that this may be because the need for support essentially surpassed its availability. This sample was obtained from a fairly impoverished area, with a disproportionate number of people living below the poverty line, high unemployment, and low educational attainment. It may be that older adults with higher resources might experience different nature, timing, duration, and course of symptoms after disasters than those sampled here.

The frequency and severity of PTSD was examined among younger and older adults selected from the general population one and a half years after the 1988 earthquake in Armenia (Goenjian et al., 1994). Although there was no difference in total mean symptoms, there was a significant difference in symptom profiles between younger and older adults, with older adults scoring higher on arousal symptoms and lower on intrusive symptoms.

Eight hundred and thirty-one adults from southeastern United States were interviewed 12, 18, and 24 months after the 1989 Hurricane Hugo regarding their related stressors and psychological functioning (Thompson et al., 1993). This large and heterogeneous sample was fairly evenly divided into young (19–39), middle-aged (40–59), and older (over 60) adults, with half of the sample African American, half female. Regarding the high impact group, there was a curvilinear interaction between postdisaster distress and age, with middle-aged adults having the highest level of symptoms. This was explained by the burden perspective, meaning that a disproportionate share of familial and social responsibilities already lies with this age group, and in the face of disasters they have the most stress with which to contend. Although the older adults in this sample were the least educated of the age groups, they were psychologically affected (except for somatic complaints) only if life threat or personal loss had occurred. In addition, this sample of older adults was particularly sheltered from financial loss, being the least likely to have these losses and the least affected by them when they did occur.

One year after the 1989 Hurricane Hugo struck Puerto Rico, St. Croix, South Carolina, and North Carolina, 1,000 disaster and nondisaster impacted community-dwelling residents were asked about social support they exchanged following the aftermath (Kaniasty & Norris, 1995). Although very high amounts of tangible, informational, and emotional support were received and provided by disaster survivors, help was not dispersed evenly across groups. Indeed, several factors (i.e., race, education, and age) moderated the impact of disaster exposure on receipt of postdisaster help. When older adults were faced with threats to their life and health, they were given high levels of tangible and informational assistance by their social networks. This was deemed a "pattern of concern." This same pattern did not emerge, however, in response to more material losses like property damage. In this case, older adults may experience a "pattern of neglect" (Kilijanek & Drabek, 1979).

A four-phase 2-year longitudinal investigation of community and patient/specialty populations (i.e., injured, displaced, owners of damaged businesses, and relief workers) was conducted in the aftermath of the 1989 Newcastle earthquake in Australia (Carr, Lewin, Webster, & Kenardy, 1997). Several specific community groups (e.g., older adults and non-English-speaking immigrants) were at risk for psychiatric morbidity. Namely, adults less than 65 years ($N = 2{,}371$) were compared with those aged 65 years and older ($N = 636$) (Ticehurst, Webster, Carr, & Lewin, 1996). Although older adults reported fewer disaster threat and disruption experiences and used fewer, general, and disaster-related support services, they endorsed higher PTSD and general distress than younger adults. Within the older group, those who had greater PTSD symptoms were more likely to be female and to use behavioral and avoidance coping styles. Those with high exposure levels of threat or disruption who completed at least three phases of the study were included in a follow-up investigation (Lewin, Carr, & Webster, 1998). Of the 515 who met inclusion criteria, psychological difficulties persisted longer in those who were older, female, and more introverted; had lower levels of education and a history of emotional problems; used more neurotic defenses; and reported higher levels of postdisaster life events.

An investigation of 248 evacuees of a volcanic eruption from Mt. Unzen in Japan that began in 1991 but continued to cause damage beyond 1992 was conducted longitudinally (Ohta et al., 2003). In contrast to younger evacuees whose reductions in psychological distress continued over time, middle-aged and older adults' distress decreased only after 44 months or remained high throughout the investigation. More specifically, high distress levels in the 50 to 59 and 60 to 69 age ranges persisted through the third wave of the survey at 24 months, with significant decreases occurring by the fourth wave at 44 months, while those 70 years and older had high distress levels throughout.

In needs assessment interviews with 58 older African American public housing residents in Miami, Florida, who were displaced from their homes after the 1992 Hurricane Andrew, Sanders, Bowie, and Bowie (2003) found that less than 30% had their physical health care needs met following relocation. Over 70% reported that they did not want to remain in their current housing arrangement, citing three main reasons: missed formal or informal support systems, substandard living conditions, and limited ability to perform independent activities of daily living in new surroundings (e.g., shopping, using public transportation). The authors noted that several respondents exhibited PTSD, but there was no mention of how this information was collected or the exact numbers of individuals experiencing these symptoms.

Pre- and post-1993 flood data was collected from 651 older persons in Iowa (Tyler & Hoyt, 2000). The overall level of depression did not increase significantly over time for the young-old (55–69 years) but was significantly higher for the old-old (70 and older). Depressive levels before the flood were predictive of depressive levels after the flood for both groups. Social support buffered the effects of disaster exposure on depression only in the young-old. The authors hypothesized that relative to other age-related stressors, the flooding may not have been severe enough to qualify as a stressor to the older adults.

Prepostdata on depression were examined for 166 adults aged 30 to 102 who experienced the 1994 Northridge earthquake in Los Angeles (Knight, Gatz, Heller, & Bengston, 2000). Postdata was collected 9 to 14 months following the earthquake. There was no significant elevation in depression over time, and neither neighborhood damage nor personal damage exposure affected depression. Controlling for preearthquake depression, greater prior earthquake exposure was associated with lower postearthquake depression scores, which is consistent with the inoculation hypothesis (i.e., prior exposure with disaster is protective in the event of future disasters). The old-old reported more earthquake-specific rumination than the two younger groups.

Posttraumatic symptoms were measured over a 5-week time period after the 1995 Hanshin-Awaji earthquake in Western Japan among younger (less than 60 years) and older (60 and older) shelter-residing evacuees (Kato & Kato, 1998). Three weeks after the earthquake, both age groups experienced significant sleep disturbances, depression, hypersensitivity, and irritability (Kato, Asukai, Miyake, Minakawa, & Nishiyama, 1996). At the second assessment 5 weeks later, the percentage of younger adults with PTSD symptoms did not decrease, while older adults showed a significant decrease in 8 of 10 PTSD symptoms. The investigators hypothesized that there were various reasons for this pattern, including that younger adults may have had the added psychological stress of rebuilding their lives (e.g., finding new jobs), while older adults were more likely to be retired and receiving a fixed pension. Additionally, older adults in Japan often have extensive social networks and previous disaster experiences, which might buffer the effects of natural disasters. A limitation of this study was that the sample was not random, and the interviews were conducted during the day while a large number of the shelter-residing evacuees were working or attempting to salvage their belongings.

More than half of the fatalities of the Hanshin-Awaji earthquake were among those over 60 years old; of these, female fatalities were almost double those of men (Tanida, 1996). While many younger survivors rebuilt and returned to their homes, many of the older adults remained in temporary accommodations. Approximately 40% of older families who were in provisional housing reported that reconstructing new relationships was difficult (Tanida, 1996).

As part of an ongoing longitudinal investigation, prepost data were collected from 68 Caucasian older adults who were exposed to the 1997 Red River flood in North Dakota (Ferraro, Morton, Knuston, Zink, & Jacobson, 1999). Reaction time and physical health symptoms increased for both women and men. Women used more medications following the flood and also spent more days away from home. There were no significant differences between flood-damaged groups (none, minimal, slight, moderate, or severe) on depression, vocabulary ability, and state or trait anxiety. There were significant differences between the groups on the number of physical symptoms, with increased self-reported problems as the flood damage magnitude increased. Follow-up data on self-rated health, depression, and vocabulary ability from

37 of these older adults were examined (Ferraro, 2003). There were no main or interaction effects regarding these variables by gender or by time. The author interpreted these findings to mean that many older adults appear to be resilient to some of the negative effects of natural disasters.

In a small qualitative investigation with six residents of Grand Forks, North Dakota, aged 26 to 77, 6 months after a flood in 1997, older adults were deemed especially vulnerable to emotional exhaustion (Keene, 1998).

Posttraumatic stress disorder symptoms in adults were examined 6 to 12 months after the 1992 Hurricane Andrew in the United States ($n = 270$), the 1997 Hurricane Paulina in Mexico ($n = 200$), and the 1997 flood in Poland ($n = 285$) (Norris, Kaniasty, Conrad, Inman, & Murphy, 2002). There was no one consistent effect of age. Among Americans, age had a curvilinear relation with PTSD (i.e., middle-aged adults were most distressed); among Mexicans, age had a linear and negative relation with PTSD (i.e., young adults were most distressed); and among Poles, age had a linear and positive relation with PTSD (i.e., older people were most distressed). The authors surmised that the greater distress levels in older Poles may be explained, in part, by the contribution of several societal factors (e.g., war, oppression, poor economic and social conditions). Clearly, Norris, Kaniasty, and colleagues' findings (2002) are seminal in highlighting the importance of context, including social, economic, cultural, and historical factors, in predicting mental health outcomes among disaster-stricken individuals.

Eight hundred residents of Tegucigalpa, Honduras, aged 15 years and over, who had high and low exposure to Hurricane Mitch in 1998 were assessed for their psychological functioning (Kohn, Levav, Garcia, Machuca, & Tamashiro, 2005). Older adults had prevalence rates of 14% for PTSD, 19% for depression, 4% for alcohol misuse, and 21% for "emotional distress." There were no significant differences in disaster exposure or psychological reactions between older, middle-aged, and younger adults. Among older individuals, prehurricane psychological difficulties and exposure intensity were associated with increased risk for PTSD, depression, and emotional distress.

More than a year and a half after the 1999 earthquake in Marmara Turkey, PTSD and depression were examined in 586 nontreatment seeking survivors living in temporary housing sites (Şalcıoğlu, Başoğlu, & Livavanou, 2003). More severe PTSD symptoms were related to greater fear during the earthquake, being female, older age, participation in rescue work, having been trapped under rubble, and past psychiatric illness. More severe depressive symptomatology was related to older age, loss of close ones, being single and female, having previous traumatic experience, and personal and family history of psychiatric illness.

Three months after the 1999 Chi-Chi earthquake in Taiwan, 663 victims were screened for psychiatric morbidity at a local general hospital (Yang et al., 2003). The most frequently reported symptoms of emotional distress were excessive worrying, nervousness, and insomnia, while the most frequently reported PTSD symptoms were intrusive recollections, flashbacks, difficulties sleeping, and impaired memory. Variables associated with the presence of psychiatric morbidity and posttraumatic symptoms included female gender, old age, financial loss, as well as obsessive and nervous traits.

In a longitudinal investigation of changes in depressive symptoms among older Taiwanese adults who were displaced in the Chi-Chi earthquake, depression was relatively high and did not change between 6 and 12 months (Watanabe, Okumura, Chiu, & Wakai, 2004). The effects of social support varied across time and source. Lower depressive symptoms at 6 months were related to higher child and extended family support levels, whereas lower depressive symptoms at 12 months were related to greater extended family and neighbor support as well as social participation.

Three months after a supercyclone hit Orissa, India, in 1999, data was collected from 130 individuals regarding anxiety, depression, and PTSD (Suar, Mishra, & Khuntia, 2007). Controlling for exposure, caste, and gender, there were linear effects of age on psychological distress.

Specifically, with increasing age, adults experienced more distress. There were no quadratic effects of age. The authors surmised that in India where older adults are culturally the custodian of family and community, they likely had a greater sense of resource loss after the cyclone, with little hope for regain.

Following the 2004 Florida hurricanes, older adults not only reported fewer symptoms of PTSD, depression, and generalized anxiety than younger adults, but also their psychological reactions were more closely connected to the economic consequences of disasters (Acierno, Ruggerio, Kilpatrick, Resnick, & Galea, 2006). Distinctively, postinsurance dollar losses and number of days displaced from one's home predicted distress in older adults but were unrelated to distress in younger individuals. The authors concluded that many older adults have fixed incomes and may not have the ability to increase their earnings to address unexpected postdisaster expenses.

A multistage, cluster, population-based mental health survey was conducted in random samples of displaced and nondisplaced survivors of the 2004 tsunami in southern Thailand (Van Griensven et al., 2006). Although old age was not a factor associated with higher prevalence of anxiety, it was significantly associated with increased symptoms of depression. In addition to old age, being female, hearing voices, having a family member who died or was missing, losing employment, and being injured as a result of the tsunami were also significant associates with depression.

Cherry, Galea, and Silva (2008) utilized data from 66 participants in the ongoing Louisiana Healthy Aging Study, a multidisciplinary study of the determinants of healthy aging, to examine the impact of the 2005 Hurricanes Katrina and Rita in middle-aged (45–64), young-old (65–84), and older-old (90 and older) samples across several domains of cognitive and psychosocial functioning. Almost 90% of the research participants lived outside the severely affected hurricane area (i.e., within a 40 mile radius of the devastated region), did not have to evacuate their place of residence, and had minimal direct trauma exposure. As they had relatives and friends who lived in the affected areas and some of their hometowns were shelters for the evacuees, they likely heard about property damage and community destruction; however, this exposure at most was indirect. It is also questionable whether these participants would even be considered "secondary victims" (Bolin, 1985) when they did not live in the affected area, likely did not witness the destruction, and were likely not "inconvenienced" by washed-out roads or bridges. Though hearing about the disaster experiences of family members and friends was likely upsetting, the majority of these study participants did not appear to meet diagnostic criteria for a traumatic event for PTSD, and it is questioned why PTSD was even assessed. It is certainly not surprising that utilizing this sample, the authors found that there were no negative significant changes in medications, life circumstances, depression, or generalized anxiety and that no one met criteria for PTSD. It may be misleading to categorize these individuals as "resilient" to the effects of the hurricanes when they were not primary or likely even secondary survivors of Hurricane Katrina and Rita.

Overall, the empirical literature on the effects of natural disasters such as floods, hurricanes, and earthquakes on the mental health of older adults is equivocal and varies according to a variety of factors.

14.2.2. Human-Made Disasters

Human-made disasters have an element of human intent, negligence, and error or involve failure of a system (e.g., terrorism, structural collapse, transportation accidents). Compared to natural disasters, much less is known about the effects of human-made catastrophes in the lives of older adults.

One year after the 1988 bombing explosion of Pan Am Flight 103 in midair over Lockerbie, Scotland, the mental health of 31 older adult survivors was compared with 24 younger adults (Livingston, Livingston, Brooks, & McKinlay, 1992). Although PTSD symptoms between the two groups were similar, older individuals had a high incidence of coexisting depression. Loss or injury to friends and the witnessing of human remains was associated with a diagnosis of PTSD in older but not younger adults. Neither material nor personal loss nor the witnessing of human remains was associated with a diagnosis of depression in older individuals, whereas material loss was associated with depression in the younger group. The findings from this sample may be limited by the fact that the individuals in this sample were seeking legal compensation and were the most severely distressed from the first wave of referrals from the solicitors.

Of the 33 older adults, 19 were reevaluated 1 year later (Livingston, Livingston, & Fell, 1994). Although there was a significant reduction in PTSD, 16% continued to meet full diagnostic criteria. PTSD was no longer associated with witnessing gruesome sights, loss of a partner, or destruction of personal property. Additionally, these older individuals had other persistent mental health problems, particularly other anxiety-related symptoms and major depression.

As part of a federally funded disaster mental health outreach program entitled Project Heartland, 45 Asian and Middle Eastern immigrants living in Oklahoma City at the time of the 1995 terrorist bombing were surveyed up to 2 years after the event (Trautman et al., 2002). Ninety-one percent reported some degree of PTSD associated with a prior trauma. These symptoms were the most robust predictor of current disaster-related PTSD symptoms. Additionally, disaster-related symptoms increased with current age, being highest in those over 50, and were inversely related to age at the time of prior trauma. There were several limitations of this study, including the small sample size; a mixed sample of immigrants differing in terms of history, religion, political beliefs, and acculturation; and the relatively low rates of physical and interpersonal exposure to the bombings in Oklahoma City. Nonetheless, these findings provide some indication about the vulnerabilities of previously traumatized older immigrants.

After 19 months of intense recurrent terrorist attacks in Israel beginning in September 2000, Bleich, Gelkopf, Melamed, and Solomon (2005) examined the psychological sequelae and coping methods in a national Jewish sample of young (18–64 years old), young-old (65–74 years old), and old-old (more than 74 years old) adults. Overall, there were no significant differences between the groups on traumatic exposure and stress symptoms, including probable PTSD. Both groups of older adults used cigarettes/alcohol and tranquilizers to cope with stress more often than young adults.

Over 2,000 New York City residents were interviewed shortly after the terror attacks of September 11, 2001, and then in subsequent follow-ups (Tracy & Galea, 2006). Of the three age groupings (18–34, 35–54, and 55 and over), the youngest age group experienced the highest cumulative prevalence of probable PTSD, while older adults had the lowest. In addition, older adults also had the lowest prevalence of probable depression, while the 35 to 54 age range had the highest depression level. In a multivariate model, lifetime stressors, ongoing stressors, education, and prior history of PTSD were significant predictors of probable PTSD among the older age group. For this same age group, ongoing traumatic events, poor physical health, and prior history of depression were significant predictors of depression.

Capitalizing on a 5-year longitudinal investigation of older adult vision rehabilitation applicants in New York City, Brennan, Horowitz, and Reinhardt (2003) examined the effects of the September 11th terror attacks on depression and life satisfaction. Data from 2 months before September 11th were compared to data from 2 months post–September 11th. Although there was a spike in depression in the 4 days immediately following September 11th, there were no other noticeable effects on depression or life satisfaction. Many of the participants apparently lived in close proximity to the former World Trade Center, but more specific details, such as whether these were residents of Manhattan who lived south of Canal Street, a line of geographical demarcation that has been related to increased psychopathology, were not provided. Additionally, the majority of the sample was Caucasian, and PTSD or other trauma-related symptoms were not assessed. Despite these limitations, this study provides some evidence of the resiliency of many older American citizens in the face of terrorist attacks.

Several focus groups were conducted to understand the economic, social, and psychological impact of the September 11th attacks on 51 older Chinese immigrants in Chinatown, an area in close proximity to the former World Trade Center (Chung, 2003). The age range of participants was from early sixties to mid-seventies and over two-thirds were female. Most reported that they remained by themselves in their apartments during the first week after the attacks due to closings of many business and stores and tight police surveillance. Their living conditions were severely affected, and their phone lines remained out of service for several weeks. Ten months after the attacks, nearly half reported that they still experienced frequent nervousness, including rapid heartbeat, shortness of breath, and dizziness. For many, this event triggered struggles and other losses associated with aging as well as their immigrant background and led to depressive symptoms of crying, sad affect, helplessness, and hopelessness. Many reported that they coped by utilizing senior center services and receiving emotional support from peers. In general, these older immigrants explained that they did not feel comfortable seeking traditional mental health counseling as their general way of coping was to adhere to Asian cultural norms, which include an emphasis on forgetting or pushing away painful feelings. The author also commented that the Chinese elders' language and socioeconomic barriers undermined their contact with accessing and receiving mental health services.

Lewis (2003) discussed the numerous post–September 11th difficulties for the large number of older adults with health problems or disabilities living within the frozen or red zone, an area surrounding the World Trade Center that was blocked off by police barricades for weeks. With communication breakdowns precipitated by the destruction of telephone and television cables and discontinuation of mail and newspaper delivery, these individuals were at an enormous risk for isolation as they could not find out what was happening and were unable to reach out to family, friends, and health care providers. Lewis explained that although several local and federal agencies were eventually able to provide emergency prescriptions, health care, and meal services to these elders, it took numerous days for this to occur. It was further noted that other issues, such as poor air and water quality, structural damage to apartments or homes, and electricity and hot water breakdowns, may have compromised the physical, mental, and social functioning of these older adults as well. Although PTSD and other trauma-related mental health symptoms were not measured in these individuals, it is highly likely that they experienced significant emotional distress, at least on a temporary or short-term basis.

The empirical literature regarding the mental health effects of human-made disasters on older adults is much like that related to natural disasters, as it does not reveal a consistent differential vulnerability associated with age.

14.2.3. Technological Disasters

Technological disasters can be caused by human error or major industrial accidents. They typically involve failure of a system (e.g., structural collapse) or unplanned release of nuclear energy, fires, or explosions from hazardous substances (e.g., chemical spill).

Six months after the Teton Dam in Idaho collapsed in 1976, 387 adult survivors who had contacted various aid agencies were interviewed over the telephone (Huerta & Horton, 1978). Over two-thirds of the sample were female, and most were married and living with their spouses. Compared with younger adults, older individuals coped well and reported few adverse psychological effects and feelings of deprivation. However, the authors noted that the adults in this sample over the age of 65 were physically, socially, and economically more advantaged than most of the older adults in the state or nation.

Green and colleagues (1997) provided a synthesis to a series of studies conducted over nearly two decades with survivors of the 1972 Buffalo Creek dam collapse and flood in West Virginia. The original study sample consisted of 381 adults and 207 children who were plaintiffs suing the mining company that built the dam for wrongful death, property damage, and psychic impairment. At the time of initial data collection, PTSD was not yet in the official psychiatric nomenclature, and thus survivors were interviewed regarding their depression, anxiety, belligerence, and alcohol abuse. Individuals between the ages of 25 and 54 evidenced the most severe pathology, particularly the middle-aged (40 to 54), with younger and older adults being less affected (Gleser, Green, & Winget, 1981). Over 120 adults were followed 14 years later. Clear-cut improvements over time were found but were unrelated to age. At the second follow-up, the two oldest groups demonstrated the fewest mental health symptoms (Green, Gleser, Lindy, Grace, & Leonard, 1996). These older groups reported that they turned to religion to cope with their disaster-related distress and that they spent more of their leisure time in church than younger adults. The findings regarding age were not entirely clear due to complicating factors. Namely, some of the older adults in the original group had died, and a number of the adults in the middle-aged group were now old. The authors suggested that current age rather than the age at which the traumatic event occurred may be a better indicator for identification of those at high risk for disaster-related mental health problems.

There were no significant differences in posttrauma stress symptoms, general health problems or coping between young, middle-aged, and older adults who had been exposed to two technological disasters (an aircraft crash in 1994 and a train collision in 1996) in the United Kingdom (Chung, Dennis, Easthope, Farmer, & Werrett, 2005; Chung, Werrett, Easthope, & Farmer, 2004). Across all three age groups, those exposed to the aircraft crash experienced significantly more intrusion and avoidance symptoms and general health problems and engaged in more confrontative coping than those exposed to the train collision.

14.2.4. Summary

There is inconsistent evidence of mental health vulnerability in older adults following disasters due to varying research methods; studies are characterized by differing definitions and inclusions of age groupings, with few including those over a certain age or those who do not live independently; insufficient sample sizes; various assessment measures; inconsistent time points at data collection; and cross-sectional design and lack of predisaster data, which complicate differentiation of cohort and age effects. Despite these limitations and taken together, there appears to be no differential vulnerability on the part of the general older adult population as compared with younger adults. The studies that show that older adults are more vulnerable are predominately either international studies or adults from industrialized countries with different ethnicities.

As evidenced by the research on older adults and disasters beginning in the late 1950s through the present, there has been a long history of interest in older adults as a potentially vulnerable population. Although some of the earlier, more sociological studies did not always measure mental health thoroughly or well, much progress has been made in the quality of research methodology. Like disaster mental health research on other populations, however, the research done in this area has typically been cross-sectional and after-only designs, used convenience sampling, and had relatively small samples (Norris, 2006).

In general, most studies examining the effects of disasters have not recruited sufficient numbers of older adults to examine age effects or have not included older adults at all. A further major limitation of many of the existing studies is that when they have included older adults, there are varying definitions of "older," and the number of participants who are in those "older" age categories is not always clear. Typically, those over 60 or 65 have often been relegated to a single older age category; potentially obfuscating age-related differences. Older adulthood encompasses at least a 25 to 30 year range in age, and the life experiences, health status, and functioning of these individuals may differ markedly. Thus, rather than simply combining together as "elderly" all those 60 or 65 and older, disaster mental health researchers and health care providers may benefit from categorizing older adults as young-old (65–74), middle-old (75–84), old-old (85 and older) (Neugarten, 1974), and centenarians (100 years of age and over) (He et al., 2005). As people progress through these chronological ages, they are more likely to experience physical and mental health compromises that may place them in a more vulnerable position for disaster mental health problems.

Almost all of the epidemiologic disaster studies that have focused on or included older adults have exclusively sampled community-dwelling, noninstitutionalized individuals. Thus, those older adults who are among the least healthy have been systematically excluded. This is noteworthy because not accounted for are those older adults who are likely the most vulnerable (e.g., physically or emotionally impaired, homebound, or long-term care residents). Therefore, any overarching statements that older individuals are the least likely to be effected by disaster are inaccurate and potentially misleading. A belief such as this could keep scarce clinical resources from older adults most in need.

These limitations have implications for future research. Unless the sample size is very large, researchers would need to oversample older adults to truly examine age differences. Future research should attempt to capture more representative samples and not those who are self-selected or chosen because of ease of access. Potentially vulnerable populations should be specifically targeted for inclusion (e.g., homebound or long-term care residents). In addition, longitudinal research is needed to elucidate the postdisaster vulnerability and resilience trajectories more clearly. Further, mental health is just one broad area of examination. Older adults' physical health, mobility, functioning, as well as greater risk of death are also important areas for future investigation and disaster planning.

Norris, Kaniasty, and colleagues (2002) advice against overgeneralizations regarding older adults as either the least or most vulnerable to mental health difficulties following disasters. Within the general adult population, age may not automatically and exclusively be a risk factor for vulnerability; rather, a host of individual (e.g., predisaster mental health, gender), social (e.g., psychosocial resources and social support), economic, and disaster-related variables may interact with age or age-related variables like physical health, functional status, and caregiving status to predict vulnerability (Elmore & Brown, 2007; Fernandez, Byard, Lin, Benson, & Barbera, 2002; Norris, Kaniasty, et al., 2002). Additionally, disaster impact may be greatest when two of the following are present: (1) widespread damage, (2) serious and ongoing community financial difficulties, (3) high prevalence of trauma from injuries, threat to life, and loss of life, and (4) disaster caused by human intent (Norris et al., 2002).

In regards to the differential age vulnerabilities for individuals from industrialized countries in the face of disasters, this may also be dependent, in part, on the type and severity of stressors/trauma to which an individual was exposed at an earlier time (Cook, 2001). Older adult survivors of less severe trauma, such as natural disasters, have displayed both direct and cross-tolerance (Knight et al., 2000; Norris & Murrell, 1988), suggesting that disasters may reduce the impact of same and different stressors. However, there is some evidence from both Holocaust survivors and combat veterans to support the vulnerability perspective (Danieli, 1997). Older adult survivors of severe trauma appear to have a heightened vulnerability to subsequent stressors (Yehuda et al., 1995).

Regarding the four existing explanations of potential differential effects of age (i.e., the resource, exposure, inoculation, and burden perspectives), these may also be contingent on other factors. For example, the burden hypothesis, which explains that middle-aged individuals are the most effected by disaster, and the inoculation perspective, which suggests that older adults are least effected, may be true for primarily Caucasian, middle income individuals from industrialized countries or those who experienced non-interpersonal trauma in earlier life. The resource and exposure perspectives may hold true for those who experienced severe and prolonged trauma earlier in life, and those who are psychologically compromised or those from various disadvantaged minority groups who have few social and financial resources in late life. Clearly constructing an assessment battery to include such models into future research investigations would help to build a stronger and more theoretical foundation for work in this area.

14.3. ADDRESSING DISASTER MENTAL HEALTH PREPAREDNESS AND RESPONSE CHALLENGES FOR OLDER ADULTS

The disaster mental health literature provides some important insights regarding ongoing preparedness and response challenges. Unique experiences and lessons learned from several large-scale disasters may highlight ways to prepare for and respond to the needs of the growing aging population in future disasters.

14.3.1. Preparedness and Planning

Perhaps the most significant lesson from past disasters is the importance of preparedness and planning. Rather than waiting for large-scale disasters to occur before beginning the response planning process, efforts must be made to develop preventive measures, public education and preparation, and psychological support services for older adults well before disasters occur. To ensure that the unique needs of older adults are addressed, a variety of aging and mental health stakeholders should be active partners throughout the preparedness and response processes at the local, state, and federal level (Elmore & Brown, 2007).

14.3.2. Identifying, Locating, and Accessing Older Adults in Disasters

An important part of prevention and emergency preparedness involves the identification of potentially vulnerable individuals who may require assistance in safely sheltering in place or evacuating. Vulnerable individuals may include those with physical, functional, emotional, or socioeconomic challenges. Identification of those particularly at risk among the older adult population is imperative to prioritize public health resources that are often limited during times of disaster (Johnson & Langlieb, 2005).

Some studies suggest that older adults may be less likely to evacuate, to heed warnings, and to acknowledge danger before a disaster (Myers, 1990). These behaviors and choices may be guided by a variety of circumstances and beliefs. Ostroff (2002) articulated a number of suggestions that are particularly relevant to the unique emergency preparedness needs of older adults and individuals with disabilities, including that older adults might need more time to make necessary preparation; disaster warnings need to include a variety of formats to reach those with impairments, including closed captioning, audio alerts, and additional visual cues; people with impaired mobility are often concerned about being dropped, and thus appropriate transfer techniques should be utilized by emergency workers; because of various impairments, some older individuals may not be able to remember and/or communicate their individualized medication or treatment regimes.

Timely access for older adults in need of assistance has proven to be a significant challenge in past disasters. O'Brien (2003) identified the need for a rapid system to identify and locate elders among the four most significant shortcomings of the current emergency preparedness system for older adults. In particular, older adults living semiindependently but with chronic health conditions and functional disabilities may have greater needs during a disaster. Both Lewis (2003) and O'Brien (2003) elaborated on the difficulties encountered in accessing many older adults who lived in the frozen zone around the former World Trade Center immediately and shortly after the terror attacks of September 11th. Health care workers other than emergency personnel could not gain access to the area near the disaster, and thus many older people waited for up to 7 days for ad hoc medical teams to rescue them. Meal service, dressing changes, and needed supplies, such as oxygen, were unable to be delivered/provided.

During disasters, federal agencies (e.g., Federal Emergency Management Agency) and national organizations (e.g., American Red Cross) should partner with state and local health, aging, and social service organizations to develop specific coordinated plans to locate and assist older adults who may be in need (Lewis, 2003). In addition, the use of census reports or hazard mapping to identify at-risk geographic and social areas with a high concentration of older adults and using neighborhood organizations to locate buildings where large numbers of elders live may also be helpful (O'Brien, 2003; Somasundaram & Van de Put, 2006). It is critical to enlist the assistance of the local professional aging services network that provides regular support to older adults in the community (e.g., senior centers, adult day care centers, home and community-based nutrition and health agencies). Further outreach efforts will likely also be necessary to reach those older adults who are not currently known by the aging services network (Brown, Norris, Bryant, & Schinka, 2007). In addition, a system must be developed to identify health professionals and permit their entry into a disaster area in times of need (O'Brien, 2003).

Older adults must also be encouraged to self-identify and assist in their own disaster preparedness efforts. An official emergency telephone hotline should be established for older adults to access information and assistance. Elders living with chronic health conditions and functional disabilities and their caregivers should be provided with a list of emergency items that should be kept in the home, including battery radios, 3-day supplies of water, flashlights, and a list of prescriptions, health care providers and family members (Lewis, 2003).

14.3.3. Maintaining Physical and Mental Health and Well-Being

Among the most significant challenges for many older adults during disasters is maintaining their health and well-being. Vulnerable older adults were substantially overrepresented among the dead in Hurricane Katrina (Bourque, Siegel, Kano, & Wood, 2006). In fact, it is estimated that those 60 years and older constituted 74% of hurricane-related deaths (Simerman, Ott, & Mellnik, 2005).

Those who survived Hurricane Katrina often faced significant barriers to meeting their basic physical and mental health needs. Rudowitz, Rowland, and Shartzer (2006) discussed the availability of health and support services in New Orleans after the hurricane and challenges for reconstruction. In general, there was overcrowding and long waits at hospitals. Even though health services were made available via mobile clinics, there was limited staff, supplies, and hours of operation. Further, there were difficulties finding pharmacies, reconnecting with previous health care providers or findings new ones, and paying for care. For those who were physically capable and without major functional limitations, there was little available transportation or finances to facilitate evacuation. In addition, many residents either did not have bank accounts or available credit cards or lacked access to these resources.

Studies of the evacuees that took shelter at the Reliant Astrodome Complex in Houston, Texas, following Hurricane Katrina suggest that individuals aged 65 years and older accounted for 56% of those seen in the medical unit (Baylor College of Medicine and the American Medical Association, 2006). Further evidence suggests that many of these older adults had significant physical, mental, and functional impairments (Baylor College of Medicine and the American Medical Association, 2006). The loss of connections with family and loved ones was particularly traumatizing for many older adult survivors of Hurricane Katrina (Perry, Dulio, Artiga, Shartzer, & Rousseau, 2006).

Similar challenges were faced by many with chronic health problems in the aftermath of Hurricane Charley, which struck Florida in 2004. A rapid needs assessment of older adults conducted by the Centers for Disease Control and Prevention in 2004 following this disaster found that many experienced reduction in quality of life, exacerbation of medical conditions due to inability to receive medical care for preexisting conditions, and disruption in social support networks.

Efforts must be made to prepare for and address the mental health needs of older adult disaster survivors. While psychological first aid and crisis counseling may be all that many individuals will require following a disaster, those with more severe mental health needs should be referred to more appropriate and comprehensive mental health services (Somasundaram & van de Put, 2006). Those requiring ongoing mental health care may seek assistance in a variety of sectors and settings, including state offices of mental health, Department of Veterans Affairs, hospital emergency rooms, schools, social service agencies, private practices, primary care settings, churches or other religious institutions, and self-help groups (Siegel, Laska, & Meisner, 2004). It is extremely important that those involved in early disaster intervention help to facilitate the transition of those in need to the appropriate level of mental health care (Everly & Parker, 2005).

A variety of clinical interventions are thought to be effective in the aftermath of disasters, including cognitive-behavioral treatments, anxiety management, supportive therapy, or pharmacological interventions (Norris et al., 2002). Like younger populations, there needs to be a restoration of livelihood and social support networks and a return to routine for older adults to prevent and diminish mental health problems.

14.3.4. Exploitation and Abuse

Older adults are among the subgroups of the population that may be vulnerable to exploitation and abuse in the wake of disasters (Ehrenreich & McQuaide, 2001; Oriol, 1999). Following the September 11th terror attacks, there were warnings from numerous private and government agencies urging older adults to be wary of criminals who were masquerading as representatives of charitable organizations to convince elders to donate money (Salerno & Nagy, 2002). Emergency shelter settings may also pose a danger to older adults, particularly those with physical, mental, and cognitive impairments (Baylor College of Medicine and the American Medical Association, 2006). Efforts must be made to educate older adults, their caregivers, and their health care providers regarding the dangers of exploitation and abuse (Elmore & Brown, 2007 and policies must be put in place to deter those who may exploit older adults during disaster emergencies.

14.3.5. Access to and Utilization of Resources

Studies indicate that once a disaster occurs, older adults often underutilize disaster support services as compared with other age groups (Ticehurst et al., 1996). There are many factors that can influence an individual's ability to respond to and seek assistance during a disaster, including current physical health and functional limitations, current and past mental health, lack of economic and social resources, and available social support systems. Massey (1997) articulated the unique difficulties that may influence the response of older adults with sensory impairments and functional limitations during disasters. For example, eye glasses and hearing aids may not be on, and canes or other assistive devices may not be easily within reach. She pointed out that if these corrective devices are not found immediately postdisaster, an older individual may have trouble adapting and may experience difficulties in reading and filling out forms for needed services or referrals. It is crucial for caregivers, disaster health care providers, and relief workers to be sensitive to these types of age-related challenges.

Additional impediments to seeking or engaging fully in services might include struggling with thoughts of starting over again. Relocating or rebuilding a home may seem insurmountable; precious heirlooms or keepsakes may be destroyed, and thus critical connections to the past may no longer be available. In addition, older adults who fear losing their independence or being placed in a nursing home may be more hesitant to reach out for assistance and resources.

Emergency response resources are not just relevant for older adults with significant physical, mental, and cognitive impairments. Depending on level of functioning, older adults may need assistance with activities of daily living (e.g., feeding, dressing, toileting) or instrumental activities of daily living (e.g., shopping, using public transportation, paying bills). Grocery stores, pharmacies, or other important places of business might be closed in the aftermath of a disaster, and thus older adults may not be able to easily obtain essential items. Transportation access to these types of services is imperative for many.

Experts suggest that in circumstances where older adults find themselves competing with others for resources, they may require support or protection to access the services they need (HelpAge International, 2000). In addition, older adults may more positively receive outreach efforts if those who are familiar with the community make them and if they maintain a focus on the practical needs of the older adults whom they are trying to assist (Chung, 2003; Phifer, 1990).

14.3.6. Nursing Facilities and Institutional Care

Evidence from past disasters suggests that older adults residing in institutional settings, such as nursing homes or assisted living facilities, may be particularly vulnerable during disasters. According to the Center on Aging of Florida International University (2005), 1 week after Hurricane Katrina, 34 older adults were found dead at St. Rita's Nursing Home in Chalmette, Louisiana, after reportedly being abandoned by staff and administrators. Another account suggests that a group of older adults had been evacuated from a nursing home only later to be found abandoned at a school that suffered damage from flooding (Blytheway, 2007). Those living in nursing homes, assisted living facilities, or senior housing depend on the staff to provide safety, protection and care, and yet the evacuation and relocation process for older adults with chronic health conditions and functional limitations does not often occur in an orderly and timely manner.

In many ways, the problems and lack of solutions for the nursing facilities during Hurricane Katrina was a larger scale repeat of history. Saliba, Buchanan, and Kington (2004) surveyed Los Angeles County nursing facility administrators after the 1994 Northridge earthquake. Seventy-eight percent of the facilities sustained severe damage, 5 closed and 72 lost vital services. Numerous additional problems were noted, including staff absences, phone equipment not working; difficulty in immediate movement and evacuation of residents; and insufficient water, emergency fuel, and other supplies (e.g., flashlights, blankets, food, linens). Surprisingly, increased admissions to the facility among those who were previously community-dwelling were also noted. These individuals apparently were displaced from affordable housing, became frightened of living alone, or found themselves unable to function when their physical support systems (e.g., respirators, oxygen, and electric wheelchair) were disrupted. Unfortunately, there was no central clearinghouse that organized the information regarding facility needs, bed availability, and community resources.

Following the differential loss of life due to Hurricane Katrina, representatives from long-term care facilities in Alabama, Florida, Louisiana, Mississippi, Georgia, and Texas evaluated disaster preparedness, response, and recovery in their provider networks (Hyer, Brown, Berman, & Polivka-West, 2006). Before Katrina, and unlike hospitals, long-term care facilities often were not incorporated into the emergency response systems. This meant that restoration of public utility services such as electricity, telephones, elevators, water, and other basic services was not given priority.

A number of recommendations to address these problems were made: a more efficient and effective tracking system to identify residents, monitor their evacuation and streamline the transfer (i.e., universal patient-identification systems with a centralized tracking system); data management systems that track the transport of needed products (e.g., medical equipment, medical records, disposables, food and water); more sophisticated ways to monitor electrical, structural, and water problems; development of effective communication systems (e.g., telephone and computers are typically unavailable during disasters and ham radios or satellite phones are often needed); and coordinated systems to provide updates on bed availability (Hyer et al., 2006).

14.3.7. Growing Diversity in the Aging Population

There is increasing heterogeneity in racial, ethnic, cultural and linguistic diversity in the growing aging population. This diversity is accompanied by an increasing need to be aware of culture-specific belief systems and coping mechanisms for dealing with disaster, loss, and death (e.g., seeing ghosts or hearing voices of deceased in people from Southeast Asia) and to deliver culturally and linguistically competent mental health interventions (Van Griensven et al., 2006).

Regarding her work with older adults in New York City's Chinatown after September 11th, Chung (2003) advised that cultural organizations, such as churches, temples, or senior centers, could be used as hosts or providers for therapeutic discourse. In addition, she suggested that bilingual mental health providers should visit these organizations and try to engage those who might benefit from individual or group services. She further commented that due to the increasing number of those from ethnic minority populations losing close ties to families and community due to acculturation, recreation of a kinship network might prove beneficial in the healing process.

14.3.8. Older Adults as a Disaster Response Resource

Clearly not all members of the older adult population are vulnerable and in need of assistance during disasters. In fact, many older adults are physically and mentally healthy and thus could serve as untapped resources in helping to provide a variety of disaster-related services (e.g., community canvassing, house sitting, child care, and meal preparation) (Thompson et al., 1993; Zeiss, Cook, & Cantor, 2003). Indeed, Lopes estimated (as cited in Oriol, 1999) that 65% of disaster volunteers for the American Red Cross are 55 years of age and older.

14.3.9. Federal Policy Initiatives

A variety of federal emergency and disaster preparedness efforts in aging have recently taken place or are currently underway. In fact, disaster preparedness for older adults was among the top 50 recommendations of the 2005 White House Conference on Aging. This conference, which included a group of 1,200 appointed delegates from around the country, cited the following recommendation among its priorities, "encourage the development of a coordinated federal, state, and local emergency response plan for seniors in the event of public health emergencies or disasters" (White House Conference on Aging, 2006, p. 26). As part of the 2006 reauthorization of the Older Americans Act, Congress added new provisions to federal law to improve disaster preparedness and response. These new Older Americans Act provisions require the preparedness plans of state and area agencies to include information on how they intend to coordinate activities and develop long-term emergency preparedness plans (O'Shaughnessy & Napili, 2006). Another federal policy initiative worthy of special mention is the Geriatric Education Centers (GEC) initiative related to bioterrorism and emergency preparedness in aging. Funded through Title VII of the Public Health Service Act, the GECs are collaborating on a multicenter initiative to develop, evaluate, and disseminate curricula to assist health care providers in responding to the needs of older adults during disasters (Johnson et al., 2006).

14.3.10. Resources to Assist Older Adults during Disasters

Similar to randomized controlled trials examining efficacy of psychotherapy for PTSD from a broad range of traumas, there are no treatment studies that primarily focus on older adults, and rarely are there ones that include them (for reviews of trauma/PTSD treatments in older adults, see Cook & Niederehe, 2007; Cook & O'Donnell, 2005). This makes it difficult to understand what interventions might be most efficacious for psychiatrically distressed older individuals following a disaster. It may be that psychological first-aid and case management may be helpful and effective for those who are mildly to moderately symptomatic and have compromised resources (e.g., financial, social). For those who are the most psychologically impaired, it is likely they could benefit from cognitive-behavioral, problem-solving type interventions. Definitive conclusions cannot be drawn until more systematic investigations and randomized clinical trials have been conducted.

There are numerous suggestions for fostering resilience in older adults in response to terrorism/disasters (Zeiss et al., 2003). These include the importance of maintaining a routine, taking good care of oneself, engagement in pleasurable activities, and finding supportive people. In addition, those older individuals who are able may benefit themselves and their communities by engaging in disaster relief efforts.

REFERENCES

Acierno, R., Ruggiero, K. J., Kilpatrick, D. G., Resnick, H. S., & Galea, S. (2006). Risk and protective factors for psychopathology among older versus younger adults following the 2004 Florida hurricanes. *American Journal of GeriatricPsychiatry, 14*, 1051–1059.

Baylor College of Medicine, & The American Medical Association. (2006). *Recommendation for best practices in the management of elderly disaster victims*. (July 3, 2007); http://www.ama-assn.org/ama1/pub/upload/mm/415/best_prac_elderly.pdf

Bell, B. D. (1978). Disaster impact and response: Overcoming the thousand natural shocks. *The Gerontologist, 18*, 531–540.

Bell, B., Kara, G., & Batterson, C. (1978). Service utilization and adjustment patterns of elderly tornado victims in an American disaster. *Mass Emergencies, 3*, 71–81.

Bleich, A., Gelkopf, M., Melamed, Y., & Solomon, Z. (2005). Emotional impact of exposure to terrorism among young-old and old-old Israeli citizens. *American Journal of Geriatric Psychiatry, 13*, 705–712.

Blytheway, B. (2007). *The evacuation of older people: The case of hurricane Katrina*. Retrieved (July 3, 2007); http://understandingkatrina.ssrc.org/Bytheway/

Bolin, R., & Klenow, D. J. (1982–1983). Response of the elderly to disaster: An age-stratified analysis. *International Journal of Aging and Human Development, 16*, 283–296.

Bolin, R. C. (1985). Disaster characteristics and psychosocial impacts. In B. J. Sowder (Ed.), *Disasters and mental health: Selected contemporary perspectives*. Rockville, MD: National Institute of Mental Health.

Bolin, R. C., & Klenow, D. J. (1988). Older people in disaster: A comparison of black and white victims. *International Journal of Aging and Human Development, 26*, 29–43.

Bourque, L. B., Siegel, J. M., Kano, M., & Wood, M. M. (2006). Weathering the storm: The impact of hurricanes on physical and mental health. *Annals of the American Academy of Political and Social Science, 604*, 129–151.

Brennan, M., Horowitz, A., & Reinhardt, J. P. (2003). The September 11th attacks and depressive symptomatology among older adults with vision loss in New York City. *Journal of Geronotological Social Work, 40*, 55–71.

Brown, L. M., Norris, F., Bryant, C., & Schinka, J. A. (2007, July). Pilot study of disaster mental health service use by older adults. Presented at the meeting of the 19th NIMH Conference on Mental Health Services Research, Washington, DC.

Carr, V. J., Lewin, T. J., Webster, R. A., & Kenardy, J. A. (1997). A synthesis of the findings from the Quake Impact Study: A two-year investigation of the psychosocial sequelae of the 1989 Newcastle earthquake. *Social Psychiatry and Psychiatric Epidemiology, 32*, 123–136.

Center on Aging of Florida International University. (2005). *Disaster planning for older adults in Palm Beach County*. (July 3, 2007) http://www.fiu.edu/~coa/downloads/long%20term%20care/PBC.pdf

Centers for Disease Control and Prevention. (2004). *Rapid assessment of the needs and health status of older adults after Hurricane Charley - Charlotte, DeSoto and Hardee Counties, Florida, August 27–3, 2004*. www.cdc.gov/mmwr/preview/mmwrhmtl/mm5336a.htm

Cherry, K. E., Galea, S., & Silva, J. L. (2008). Successful aging and natural disasters: Role of adaptation and resiliency in late life. In M. Hersen & A. M. Gross (Eds.), *Handbook of clinical psychology* (pp. 810–833). Hoboken, NJ: John Wiley & Sons.

Chung, I. (2003). The impact of the 9/11 attacks on the elderly in NYC Chinatown: Implications for culturally relevant services. *Journal of Gerontological Social Work, 40*, 37–53.

Chung, M. C., Dennis, I., Easthope, Y., Farmer, S., & Werrett, J. (2005). Differentiating posttraumatic stress between elderly and younger residents. *Psychiatry, 68*, 164–173.

Chung, M. C., Werrett, J., Easthope, Y., & Farmer, S. (2004). Coping with post-traumatic stress: Young, middle-aged and elderly comparisons. *International Journal of Geriatric Psychiatry, 19*, 333–343.

Cohen, E. S., & Poulshock, S. W. (1979). Societal response to mass dislocation of the elderly. *The Gerontologist, 17*, 262–268.

Cook, J. M. (2001). Post-traumatic stress disorder in older adults. *National Center for PTSD Research Quarterly, 12*, 1–7.

Cook, J. M., & Niederehe, G. (2007). Trauma in older adults. In M. J. Friedman, T. M. Keane, & P. A. Resick (Eds.), *PTSD science & practice: A comprehensive handbook*. New York: Guilford Press.

Cook, J. M., & O'Donnell, C. (2005). Assessment and psychological treatment of Posttraumatic Stress Disorder in older adults. *Journal of Geriatric Psychiatry and Neurology, 18*, 61–71.

Danieli, Y. (1997). As survivors age: An overview. *Journal of Geriatric Psychiatry, 30*, 9–26.

Ehrenreich, J. H., & McQuaide, S. (2001). Coping in disasters: A guidebook to psychosocial intervention. (July 3, 2007); http://www.mhwwb.org/CopingWithDisaster.pdf

Elmore, D. L., & Brown, L. M. (2007). Emergency preparedness and response: Health and social policy implications for older adults. *Generations. 31*(4), 66–74.

Everly, G. S., & Parker, C. L. (Eds.). (2005). *Mental health aspects of disaster: Public health preparedness and response*. Baltimore, MD: Johns Hopkins Center for Public Health Preparedness.

Fernandez, L. S., Byard, D., Lin, C. C., Benson, S., & Barbera, J. A. (2002). Frail elderly as disaster victims: Emergency management strategies. *Prehospital and Disaster Medicine, 17*, 67–74.

Ferraro, F. R. (2003). Psychological resilience in older adults following the 1997 flood. *Clinical Gerontologist, 26*, 139–143.

Ferraro, F. R., Morton, M., Knuston, S., Zink, J., & Jacobson, B. (1999). Impact of the 1997 flood on cognitive performance in the elderly. *Clinical Gerontologist, 20*, 79–82.

Friedsam, H. (1961). Reactions of older persons to disaster-caused losses. *The Gerontologist, 1*, 34–37.

Gleser, G., Green, B., & Winget, C. (1981). *Prolonged psychological effects of disaster: A study of Buffalo Creek*. New York: Academic Press.

Goenjian, A. K., Najarian, L. M., Pynoos, R. S., Steinberg, A. M., Manoukian, G., Tavosian, A., et al. (1994). Posttraumatic stress disorder in elderly and younger adults after the 1988 earthquake in Armenia. *American Journal of Psychiatry, 151*, 895–901.

Green, B. L., Gleser, G. C., Lindy, J. D., Grace, M. C., & Leonard, A. (1996). Age-related reactions to the Buffalo Creek dam collapse: Effects in the second decade. In P. Ruskin & J. Talbott (Eds.), *Aging and posttraumatic stress disorder*. Washington, DC: American Psychiatric Press.

Green, B. L., Kramer, T. L., Grace, M. C., Gleser, G. C., Leonard, A. C., Vary, M. G., et al. (1997). Traumatic events over the life span: Survivors of the Buffalo Creek disaster. In T. W. Miller (Ed.), *Clinical disorders and stressful life events*. Madison, CT: International Universities Press.

Hansson, R. O., Noulles, D., & Bellovich, S. J. (1982). Knowledge, warning and stress: A study of comparative roles in an urban floodplain. *Environment and Behavior, 14*, 171–185.

He, W., Sengupta, M., Velkoff, V. A., & DeBarros, K. A. (2005). *65+ in the United States: 2005* (Current Population Reports P23–209). Washington, DC: U.S. Government Printing Office

HelpAge International. (2000). *Older people in disasters and humanitarian crises: Guidelines for best practice*. (March 3, 2007); http://www.reliefweb.int/library/documents/HelpAge_olderpeople.pdf

Huerta, F., & Horton, R. (1978). Coping behavior of elderly flood victims. *The Gerontologist, 18*, 541–546.

Hyer, K., Brown, L. M., Berman, A., & Polivka-West, L. (2006). Establishing and refining hurricane response systems for long-term care facilities. *Health Affairs*, 25, 407–411.

Johnson, A., Howe, J. L., McBride M. R., Palmisano, B., Perweiler, E. A., Roush, R. E., et al. (2006). Bioterrorism and emergency preparedness in aging (BTEPA): HRSA-funded GEC collaboration for curricula and training. *Gerontology & Geriatrics Education, 26*, 63–86.

Johnson, S., & Langlieb, A. (2005). Mental health needs of special and vulnerable populations in a disaster. In G. S. Everly & C. L. Parker (Eds.), *Mental health aspects of disaster: Public health preparedness and response*. Baltimore, MD: Johns Hopkins Center for Public Health Preparedness.

Kaniasty, K. Z., & Norris, F. H. (1995). In search of altruistic community: Patterns of social support mobilization following Hurricane Hugo.

American Journal ofCommunity Psychology, 23, 447–477.

Kato, H., Asukai, N., Miyake, Y., Minakawa, K., & Nishiyama, A. (1996). Post-traumatic symptoms among younger and elderly evacuees in the early stages following the 1995 Hanshin-Awaji earthquake in Japan. *Acta Psychiatrica Scandinavica, 93,* 477–481.

Kato, H. & Kato, H. (1998). Posttraumatic symptoms among victims of the great Hanshin-Awaji earthquake in Japan. *Psychiatry and Clinical Neurosciences, 52,* S59-S65.

Keene, E.P. (1998). Phenomenological study of the North Dakota flood experience and its impact on survivors' health. *International Journal of Trauma Nursing, 4,* 79–84.

Kilijanek, T.S., & Drabek, T.E. (1979). Assessing long-term impacts of a natural disaster: A focus on the elderly. *The Gerontologist, 19,* 555–566.

Knight, B.G., Gatz, M., Heller, K., & Bengston, V.L. (2000). Age and emotional response to the Northridge earthquake: A longitudinal analysis. *Psychology and Aging, 15,* 627–634.

Kohn, R., Levav, I., Donaire Garcia, I., Machuca, M.E., & Tamashiro, R. (2005). Prevalence, risk factors and aging vulnerability for psychopathology following a natural disaster in a developing country. *International Journal of Geriatric Psychiatry, 20,* 835–841.

Krause, N. (1987). Exploring the impact of a natural disaster on the health and psychological well-being of older adults. *Journal of Human Stress, 13,* 61–69.

Lewin, T.J., Carr, V.J., & Webster, R.A. (1998). Recovery from post-earthquake psychological morbidity: Who suffers and who recovers? *Australian and New Zealand Journal of Psychiatry, 32,* 15–20.

Lewis, M. (2003). *The frail and hardy seniors of 9/11: The needs and contributions of Older Americans.* www.upmc-biosecurity.org/pages/events/peoplesrole/lewis/lewis.html

Lister, S. A. (2005, September 21). Hurricane Katrina: The public health and medical response (Congressional Research Service Report No. RL33096). Retrieved March 3, 2007, from http://fpc.state.gov/documents/organization/54255.pdf

Livingston, H.M., Livingston, M.G., Brooks, D.N., & McKinlay, W.W. (1992). Elderly survivors of the Lockerbie air disaster. *International Journal of Geriatric Psychiatry, 7,* 725–729.

Livingston, H.M., Livingston, M.G., & Fell, S. (1994). The Lockerbie disaster: A 3-year follow-up of elderly victims. *International Journal of Geriatric Psychiatry, 9,* 989–994.

Logue, J.N., Hansen, H., & Struening, E. (1981). Some indications of the long-term health effects of a natural disaster. *Public Health Reports, 96,* 67–79.

Massey, B.A. (1997). Victims or survivors?: A three-part approach to working with older adults in disaster. *Journal of Geriatric Psychiatry, 30,* 193–202.

Melick, M.E., & Logue, J.N. (1985–1986). The effect of disaster on the health and well-being of older women. *International Journal of Aging and Human Development, 21,* 27–38.

Mokdad, A.H., Mensah, G.A., Posner, S.F., Reed, E., Simoes, E.J., Engelgau, M.M., et al. (2005). When chronic conditions become acute: Prevention and control of chronic diseases and adverse health outcomes during natural disasters. *Preventing Chronic Disease: Public Health Research, Practice, and Policy, 2,* 2–4.

Myers, D. (1990). *Older adults reactions to disaster.* Sacramento: California Department of Mental Health.

Neugarten, B.L. (1974). Age groups in American society and the rise of the young-old. *Annals of the American Academy of Political and Social Science, 415* (Political Consequences of Aging), 187–198.

Norris, F., & Murrell, S. (1988). Prior experience as a moderator of disaster impact on anxiety symptoms in older adults. *American Journal of Community Psychology, 16,* 665–683.

Norris, F.H. (2006). Disaster research methods: Past progress and future directions. *Journal of Traumatic Stress, 19,* 173–184.

Norris, F.H., Friedman, M.J., & Watson, P.J. (2002). 60,000 disaster victims speak: Part II. Summary and implications of the disaster mental health research. *Psychiatry, 65,* 240–260.

Norris, F.H., Friedman, M.J., Watson, P.J., Byne, C.M., Diaz, E., & Kaniasty, K. (2002). 60,000 disaster victims speak: Part I. An empirical review of the empirical literature, 1981–2001. *Psychiatry, 65,* 207–239.

Norris, F.H., Kaniasty, K.Z., Conrad, M.L., Inman, G.L., & Murphy, A.D. (2002). Placing age differences in cultural context: A comparison of the effects of age on PTSD after disasters in the United States, Mexico, and Poland. *Journal of Clinical Geropsychology, 8,* 153–173.

Norris, F.H., Phifer, J.F., & Kaniasty, K.Z. (1994). Individual and community reactions to the Kentucky floods: Findings from a longitudinal study of older adults. In R. J. Ursano, B. G. McCaughey, & C. S. Fullerton (Eds.), *Individual and community responses to trauma and disaster: The structure of human chaos.* Cambridge: Cambridge University Press.

O'Brien, N. (2003). *Emergency preparedness for oder people*. International Longevity Center-USA, 1–6.

Ohta, Y., Araki, K., Kawasaki, N., Nakane, Y., Honda, S., & Mine, M. (2003). Psychological distress among evacuees of a volcanic eruption in Japan: A follow-up study. *Psychiatric and Clinical Neurosciences, 57*, 105–111.

Oriol, W. (1999). *Psychosocial issues for oder adults in disasters* (DHHS Publication No. ESDRB SMA 99-3323). Washington, DC: U.S. Government Printing Office.

O'Shaughnessy, C., & Napili, A. (2006, December 11). The older Americans act: Programs, funding, and 2006 Reauthorization (P.L. 109-365) (Congressional Research Service Report No. RL31336). (July 3, 2007);http://www.ncoa.org/attachments/CRSOAAReport.pdf

Ostroff, S. (February, 2002). *The CDC and emergency preparedness for the elderly and disabled*. Testimony before the Senate Special Committee on Aging – NY Field Hearing. February 11, 2002.

Perry, M., Dulio, A., Artiga, S., Shartzer, A., & Rousseau, D. (2006). *Voices of the storm: Health experiences of low-income Katrina survivors*. (August 3, 2007) http://www.kff.org/uninsured/upload/7538.pdf

Phifer, J. (1990). Psychological distress and somatic symptoms after natural disaster: Differential vulnerability among older adults. *Psychology and Aging, 5*, 412–420.

Phifer, J. F., & Norris, F. H. (1989). Psychological symptoms in older adults following natural disaster: Nature, timing, duration, and course. *Journals of Gerontology: Social Sciences, 44*, S207–217.

Phifer, J. F., Kaniasty, K. Z., & Norris, F. H. (1988). The impact of natural disaster on the health of older adults: A multiwave prospective study. *Journal of Health and Social Behavior, 29*, 65–78.

Poulshock, S. W., & Cohen, E. S. (1975). The elderly in the aftermath of a disaster. *The Gerontologist, 15*, 357–361.

Rudowitz, R., Rowland, D., & Shartzer, A. (2006). Health care in New Orleans before and after Hurricane Katrina. *Health Affairs, 25*, 393–406.

Salcioglu, E., Basoglu, M., & Livavanou, M. (2003). Long-term psychological outcome for non-treatment-seeking earthquake survivors in Turkey. *Journal of Nervous and Mental Disease, 191*, 154–160.

Salerno, J. A., & Nagy, C. (2002). Terrorism and aging. *Journal of Gerontology: Medical Sciences, 57A*, M552–M554.

Saliba, D., Buchanan, J., & Kington, R. S. (2004). Function and response of nursing facilities during community disaster. *American Journal of Public Health, 94*, 1436–1441.

Sanders, S., Bowie, S. L., & Bowie, Y. D. (2003). Lessons learned on forced relocation of older adults: The impact of hurricane Andrew on health, mental health, and social support of public housing residents. *Journal of Gerontological Social Work, 40*, 23–35.

Siegel, C. E., Laska, E., & Meisner, M. (2004). Estimating capacity requirements for mental health services after a disaster has occurred: A call for new data. *American Journal of Public Health, 94*, 582–585.

Simerman, J., Ott, D., & Mellnik, T. (2005, December 30). Katrina affected elderly the most: Analysis: Assumptions on victims were incorrect. *The Charlotte observer*. (February 14, 2006); http://www.charlotte.com/mld/charlotte/news/13513079.htm

Somasundaram, D. J., & Van de Put, W. A. C. M. (2006). Management of trauma in special populations after a disaster. *Journal of Clinical Psychiatry, 67*(Suppl. 2), 64–73.

Suar, D., Mishra, S., & Khuntia, R. (2007). Placing age differences in the context of the Orissa supercyclone: Who experiences psychological distress? *Asian Journal of Social Psychology, 10*, 117–122.

Tanida, N. (1996). What happened to elderly people in the great Hanshin earthquake? *British Medical Journal, 313*, 1133–1135.

Thompson, M. P., Norris, F. H., & Hanacek, B. (1993). Age differences in the psychological consequences of hurricane Hugo. *Psychology and Aging, 8*, 606–616.

Ticehurst, S., Webster, R. A., Carr, V. J., & Lewin, T. J. (1996). The psychosocial impact of an earthquake on the elderly. *International Journal of Geriatric Psychiatry, 11*, 943–951.

Tracy, M. & Galea, S. (2006). Post-traumatic stress disorder and depression among older adults after a disaster: The role of ongoing trauma and stressors. *Public Policy & Aging Report, 16*, 16–19.

Trautman, R., Tucker, P., Pfefferbaum, B., Lensgraf, S. J., Doughty, D. E., Buksh, A., et al. (2002). Effects of prior trauma and age on posttraumatic stress symptoms in Asian ad Middle Eastern immigrants after terrorism in the community. *Community Mental Health Journal, 38*, 459–474.

Tyler, K., & Hoyt, D. R. (2000). The effects of an acute stressor on depressive symptoms among older adults: The moderating effects of social support and age. *Research on Aging, 22*, 143–164.

Van Griensven, F., Somchai Chakkraband, M. L., Thienkrua, W., Pengjuntr, W., Lopes Cardozo, B., Tantipiwatanaskul, P., et al. (2006). Mental health problems among adults in tsunami-affected areas in Southern Thailand. *Journal of the American Medical Association*, *296*, 537–548.

Watanabe, C., Okumura, J., Chiu, T., & Wakai, S. (2004). Social support and depressive symptoms among displaced older adults following the 1999 Taiwan earthquake. *Journal of Traumatic Stress*, *17*, 63–67.

White House Conference on Aging. (2006). *The booming dynamics of aging: From awareness to action.* (July 3, 2007); http://www.whcoa.gov/press/05_Report_1.pdf

Yang, Y. K., Yeh, T. L., Chen, C. C., Lee, C. K., Lee, I. H., Lee, L. C., et al. (2003). Psychiatric morbidity and posttraumatic symptoms among earthquake victims in primary care clinics. *General Hospital Psychiatry*, *25*, 253–261.

Yehuda, R., Kahana, B., Schmeidler, J., Southwick, S., Wilson, S., & Giller, E. (1995). Impact of cumulative lifetime trauma and recent stress on current posttraumatic stress disorders symptoms in Holocaust survivors. *American Journal of Psychiatry*, *152*, 1815–1818.

Zeiss, A. M., Cook, J. M., & Cantor, D. W. (2003). Fact sheet: Fostering resilience in response to terrorism: For psychologists working with older adults. *Report to American Psychological Association Task Force on Resilience in Response to Terrorism.*

15 The Effects of Disaster on the Mental Health of Individuals with Disabilities

LAURA M. STOUGH

15.1. INTRODUCTION

Hemingway and Priestley (2006) report that "specific vulnerabilities arise at the intersections of disability, class, gender, and ethnicity" and conclude that people with disabilities "are disproportionately vulnerable to natural hazards primarily as a consequence of social disadvantage, poverty, and structural exclusion" (p. 54). However, while a limited number of studies have examined the physical and social impacts of disaster on individuals with disabilities, the extent to which disasters affect the mental health of individuals with disabilities is rarely addressed. In this chapter, I review results from studies that have systematically studied the effects of disaster on individuals with disabilities and whose results contribute to our understanding of the psychological impact of disaster on this population.

15.1.1. Defining Disability

Individuals with disabilities represent a significant portion of the population, accounting for 19.3% of the total U.S. population (Bault, 2008). The percent of population considered to have a disability varies geographically; in general, poorer communities and most of the U.S. southern states report higher disability rates. The National Organization on Disability estimated that over 23% of the population in New Orleans affected by Hurricane Katrina were individuals with a disability (National Organization on Disability, 2005a) and reported that it was "clear that a disproportionate number of [hurricane-related] fatalities were people with disabilities" (National Organization on Disability, 2005b). Statistics released support these observations and suggest that of those deaths directly attributable to Katrina, a disproportionate number were elderly or individuals with preexisting disabilities (Aldrich & Benson, 2008; Bourque, Siegel, Kano, & Wood, 2006). Disability is present in significant numbers in both developed and developing countries but is strongly correlated with poverty: Up to 80% of the world population of individuals with disabilities lives in low-income countries, often in disaster-prone areas of the world (World Health Organization, 2005).

"Disability" is not a consistently defined term; Mashaw and Reno (1996) document over 20 definitions of disability used either for purposes of entitlement to governmental services, income support programs, or statistical analysis. "Disability" is most commonly used to refer to individual functioning that is impaired relative to a normative standard of physical, sensory, or cognitive intellectual functioning. Certain chronic diseases, such as multiple sclerosis, are also considered to be disabling conditions, as are some forms of mental illness, particularly when the individual's ability to perform everyday tasks or to live independently is compromised, as may be the case with schizophrenia or major depression. The International Classification of Functioning, Disability and Health (ICF), created by the World Health Organization (2008) provides perhaps the most ecumenical definition of disability and uses a "biopsychosocial" approach to disability. The ICF classification defines disability "as a dynamic interaction between health conditions (diseases, disorders, injuries, traumas, etc.) and contextual factors" (p. 8). Activity limitations and participation restrictions to individual functioning according to the ICF classification can include learning and applying knowledge; general tasks and demands; communication, mobility, self-care, domestic life, interpersonal interactions, and relationships; major life areas; and community, social, and civic life. These domains cut across traditionally held categories of disability.

15.2. DISASTERS AND VULNERABLE POPULATIONS

Demographic differences shape the risks that people encounter, how they prepare for disasters, and how people are affected when disasters occur (Mileti, 1999). Most fatalities and physical injuries are among those who have lower incomes, have chronic diseases, are elderly or very young, are ethnic minorities, or who are not a member of the language majority (Jonkman & Kelman, 2005). Much of the difference in how natural disasters affect these demographic groups is due to the contributing variable of poverty. Individuals living in poverty tend to live in substandard housing and lack transportation that would allow them to evacuate in a timely manner, which places them at risk in most disaster situations. Resources such as health and education can decrease vulnerability, and people with disabilities typically have less access to these types of resources. Other situational variables, such as living uninsured in flood plains or being a renter, also contribute to vulnerability (Morrow, 1999; Phillips & Morrow, 2007), and individuals with disabilities, given their disparate economic status in most areas of the United States, are more likely to live in housing that is at risk in disaster situations.

In an examination of people at risk for earthquake hazards, Tierney, Petak, and Hahn (1988) pointed out that people with disabilities have situational characteristics that may place them at risk for the effects of earthquake. Several factors that they noted were that individuals with disabilities tended to have lower incomes than their nondisabled peers, to be more likely to live in older buildings and near urban centers, and to experience social distancing associated with their label of "disabled." In their sample, 14% of people with disabilities lived alone and outside of any type of caregiver institution, suggesting that many would not only need assistance following disaster but would need assistance during an evacuation preceding disaster.

Phillips and Morrow (2007) suggest that each additional disabling condition, whether situational, demographic, or material, that affects an individual increases their level of vulnerability to a disaster. Individuals with disabilities are at risk for many of these factors, potentially making them one of the groups most vulnerable to the economic and psychological effects of a disaster. Individuals with disabilities and their families are disproportionately poor and thus more likely to live in areas where housing and rental properties are less expensive, such as flood-prone areas. In addition, disasters can cause disabilities through injury, conflict, or the disruption of health-care services following a disaster (International Federation of Red Cross and Red Crescent Societies, 2007).

Most of the reports on the vulnerability of individuals with disabilities have come from anecdotal, media, and policy reports and most of these same reports have been published in the last three years. Interest within the disability community on the affects of disaster on individuals with disabilities was intensified when the Special Needs Assessment for Katrina Evacuees (SNAKE), commissioned and designed by the National Organization on Disability (2005a), investigated shelters along the Gulf Coast following Katrina and found numerous inequities and barriers that affected a wide range of people with disabilities. Policy makers' attention also was drawn to the particular vulnerabilities of individuals with disabilities following Hurricane Katrina. One of the most horrifying incidences occurred at the Santa Rita nursing facility, where 35 elderly individuals with mobility and health impairments died from drowning as a direct result of the flooding following the hurricane. Hurricane Rita, which followed 3 weeks later, resulted in the death of 23 elderly people being evacuated from a nursing home when their improperly maintained bus caught fire. The SNAKE report findings, supplemented by anecdotal reports circulated throughout the disability community, generated interest from researchers in effects of disaster on disability, and the majority of currently published research is a direct by-product of this interest following the storm.

Most reports and articles, however, have focused on the support services needs of individuals with disabilities during and following disaster, rather than upon their psychological needs. Psychologically, nonminorities and households with higher socioeconomic status tend to cope better with the effects of disaster, while female heads-of-households, people of low socioeconomic status, and members of minority groups are at risk for a number of negative psychological and economic outcomes (Gladwin & Peacock, 2002; Norris et al., 2002; Norris, Kaniasty, Conrad, Inman, & Murphy, 2002; Tobin & Whiteford, 2002). It is thus important to distinguish between those demographic variables that place individuals at risk for physical harm and those that place people at risk for psychiatric illness. As an example, a number of studies have documented higher adverse physical risk for those who are elderly (e.g., Bourque et al., 2006; Perry & Lindell, 1997) while studies on psychological outcomes have found the elderly to be psychologically resilient postdisaster (Norris & Murrell, 1988; Norris, Kaniasty, et al., 2002).

In the following sections, research that has focused primarily on the effects of disaster on individuals with disabilities will be summarized and findings that have implications for the mental health of individuals with disabilities will be highlighted. For the purposes of summarization, this discussion is organized around the types of disabling conditions identified by the researchers as the target population in their studies.

15.3. PEOPLE WITH MOBILITY IMPAIRMENTS

The Centers for Disease Control and Prevention (2006) estimates that 21.2 million people in the United States have a condition that limits basic physical activities such as walking, climbing stairs, reaching, lifting, or carrying objects. Those with mobility impairments are particularly at risk during disaster as they may be physically unable to escape disasters (National Council on Disability [NCD], 2005). Most evacuation plans presuppose the ability of individuals to run, walk, climb, and use alternate forms of egress to escape from the built environment (Christensen, Blair, & Holt, 2007; National Council on Disability, 2005). For individuals who have mobility impairments, these plans are often inadequate.

The Nobody Left Behind project at the University of Kansas, led by Glen White, has focused a series of studies on the effects of disaster on individuals with physical disabilities. In the first of their published studies (Fox, White, Rooney, & Rowland, 2007) 30 emergency managers were surveyed to determine the extent to which their county emergency management plan contained procedures to assist people with mobility impairments during disaster. Also assessed was the level of knowledge of these emergency managers on the needs of individuals with disabilities during disaster response. Only 27% of the participating county emergency managers reported that they had completed training through the FEMA Emergency Planning and Special Populations course, and only 20% had specific guidelines in place in their counties on how to assist people with disabilities. Perhaps more shocking, 67% had no intention of modifying their emergency management guidelines to accommodate the needs of people with mobility impairments. The study did not, however, address psychological factors associated with mobility impairments.

In a second study, Rowland and colleagues (Rowland, White, Fox, & Rooney, 2007) interviewed a group of 12 emergency services managers and firefighters in Kansas. They found that none of the agencies represented by the participants had policies, guidelines, or practices that were specifically designed to assist people with mobility impairments. All of the participating emergency administrators expressed uncertainty about how to address the needs of people with mobility impairments in the future population of their studies. Again, none mentioned psychological supports that these individuals with disabilities might need.

Rooney and White's (2007) study of consumers with mobility impairments is one of the few that have obtained data directly from individuals with disabilities. A total of 56 people with mobility impairments completed an eight-question, online survey on their experiences following disaster. Survey participants resided in 20 different states and in 47 cities. The largest percentage of disasters experienced by the group were, in order of reported frequency, hurricane, earthquake, flooding, severe storms, fire, bomb threat, blackouts, tornadoes, and power outages. Analysis of the results found three common themes regarding what respondents believed was helpful for survival, including preplanning and preparedness measures, personal networks, and help from first responders during and after the disaster. Six problem areas identified by these respondents included (1) lack of worksite or community evacuation plans, (2) being left behind when people without disabilities were evacuated, (3) inaccessible shelters and options for accessible temporary housing, (4) disaster relief personnel who were unaware of disaster relief options for people with disabilities, (5) inadequate infrastructures, such as power, public transportation systems, and access to potable water, elevators, and air conditions, and (6) difficulties returning to daily routines. Eight key informants (13%) reported some type of postdisaster emotional trauma including fear, grief, nightmares, and generalized stress. It should be noted, however, that these were self-reports of emotions experienced after these events and not the results of a clinical assessment of the mental health of these participants.

Extending the previously summarized studies, White, Fox, Rooney, and Cahill (2007) conducted a fourth study on gaps in services and barriers for people with disabilities following Hurricane Katrina. The researchers surveyed directors of Centers for Independent Living (CILs), which create programs and supports for individuals with disabilities that live in the community, and again surveyed emergency managers. Findings supported those found previously in that emergency managers were inadequately trained on the needs of people with disabilities during and following disaster. The study also included focus groups with 18 people with uncategorized disabilities, along with nine in-depth interviews. In their analysis of this data, the researchers reported that emotional stress and depression were experienced by all of the participants. In some cases, the participants stated that this stress had an impact on their physical health as well. Diagnosis of psychological status pre- and postdisaster was not performed, nor was mental health one of the primary categories identified in the results. The researchers did report on the concern these individuals had about their social relationships, as well as upon their appreciation for and reliance on family members as supports during evacuation.

Brodie, Weltzien, Altman, Blendon, and Benson (2006) conducted a survey of 680 people staying in one of two large shelters after Hurricane Katrina. Sixteen percent of the sample responded positively when asked, "Has your doctor ever told you that you have a physical disability?" Although this survey did not focus specifically on the needs of individuals with disabilities, responses pertaining to the reasons why these individuals did not evacuate are of interest. A full 22% responded that they were "physically unable to leave," while 23% responded, "I had to care for someone who was physically unable to leave." In all, 12% of those surveyed named one of these two reasons as their primary reason for not evacuating in advance of the hurricane.

In a similar survey conducted by the Harvard School of Public Health (2007) on over 5,000 adults living in counties along the Gulf coastline, 15% of respondents reported that either they themselves or a member of their household had a chronic illness or disability that would require assistance in the case of a disaster, yet only 58% had planned for assistance in the case that they did have to evacuate. Of those individuals who had lived in a community that was damaged by a major hurricane in the last 3 years, 6% responded that they had experienced problems during and immediately following the disaster because they were disabled or chronically ill. An additional

8% responded that they had problems caring for a disabled, chronically ill, or elderly member of their household. The survey did not ask about the mental health of the respondents.

Research on the elderly is addressed in another chapter of this volume; however, the needs of people who are elderly often appear to intersect with those of individuals with disabilities. McGuire and colleagues (2007) surveyed 529 adults over age 65 in southern Louisiana and asked, "Are you limited in any way in any activities because of physical, mental, or emotional problems?" They found that nearly one-third (31.6%) met the criteria for having some type of disability and that 16.6% of the total sample reported using an assistance device such as a cane, wheelchair, special bed, or telephone. The authors emphasized that in disaster situations, individuals with disabilities need additional assistance preparing for an evacuation and during an evacuation but did not detail particular psychological or cognitive supports needed by this population.

None of these studies was designed to examine the mental health aspects of disaster; their reports of psychological factors were coincidental, rather than central, in their results. When individuals experience additional barriers following disaster it seems logical to assume that these hardships would negatively affect their mental health; however, none of these studies presented evidence that details the extent or type of psychological consequences experienced by the participants in these studies.

15.4. PEOPLE WITH SENSORY DISABILITIES

Individuals with sensory disabilities include those who are visually impaired or blind, representing approximately 3% of the U.S. population (American Foundation for the Blind, 2008), and those who are auditorally impaired or deaf, represent approximately 2.4% of the U.S. population (Galludet Research Institute, 2004). Few published articles exist on the experience of individuals with sensory impairments during and following disaster; however, Barbara White (2006) provides an autobiographical narrative of her experiences as both a member of the Deaf community and as a researcher. She details her experiences in a shelter in Houston, where she was assisting individuals with hearing impairments, then as an evacuee from a shelter, in anticipation of Hurricane Rita. White emphasizes the inequitable access to communication experienced by the deaf community – announcements about the coming hurricanes were only available on selected television stations, translators were not available in shelters, information from FEMA or Red Cross was not communicated in sign language or in another accessible manner. However, while White related the emotional stress and confusion of members of the deaf community in shelters in Houston, she did not focus on the mental health needs of this population following disaster.

The SNAKE Report from the National Organization on Disability (NOD) (2005a) identified the Deaf or hard of hearing population as being the most underserved group in shelters following Hurricane Katrina. The report noted that

> Less than 30% of the shelters had access to American Sign Language interpreters, 80% did not have TTYs, and 60% did not have TVs with caption capability. Only 56% of shelters had areas where oral announcement were posted so people who are deaf, hard of hearing or out of hearing range could go to a specified area to get or read the content of announcements. This meant that the deaf or hard of hearing had no access to the vital flow of information. (pp. 8–9)

The SNAKE report also stated that some individuals with visual disabilities were separated from their assistance dogs or durable medical equipment (e.g., canes) during evacuation but did not provide a count of these cases. The SNAKE Report noted that mental health services were not consistently available across shelters but did not report systematically on the psychological needs of individuals with disabilities in these shelters.

Barile, Fichten, Ferraro, and Judd (2006) compared the experiences of individuals with disabilities to those of their nondisabled peers during and following the 1998 ice storm in Canada. In their study, two individuals reported a hearing impairment, and six reported having a visual impairment. The researchers asked participants, "Compared to most others, how do you feel you coped psychologically during the ice storm period?" and "Compared to most others, how do you feel you coped physically during the ice storm period?" Participants with and without disabilities had similar ratings on their experiences during the ice storm; in fact, while participants with disabilities had physically fared somewhat worse than their counterparts without disabilities they reported coping slightly better psychologically. The researchers also asked participants to report on symptoms of anxiety or depression experienced during the ice storm but found no difference between participants with and without disabilities. They also found no differences in self-reported feelings of anxiety and depression before the storm as when compared to feelings after the storm. The authors suggested that individuals with disabilities are accustomed to encountering barriers in their lives and that these experiences may provide them with psychological resilience to the impacts of disaster.

15.5. PEOPLE WITH COGNITIVE DISABILITIES

Individuals with cognitive disabilities include those individuals who are labeled as having autism, developmental disabilities, traumatic brain injury, learning disabilities, or intellectual disabilities (formally referred to as mental retardation). Depending on the definition, 15% to 20% of the population can be said to have some type of cognitive disability, with the largest category being a specific learning disability.

Christ and Christ (2006) reported on the academic and behavior reactions of four children with learning disabilities whose firefighter fathers had died in the September 11, 2001, World Trade Center attack in New York City. They compared the reactions of these children to their same aged peers and found that the two groups exhibited somewhat different reactions. Following an initial grief reaction, most of the children with disabilities seemed to "tune out the painful reminders and focus on less painful topics more rapidly than their siblings or other children whose father was killed" (p. 71). The researchers concluded that a strong protective factor was support from their special education teachers and related school supports. In addition, the children in the study experienced a change in status at their school as a child who had lost a father who was a hero, rather than their previous primary status as a child with a disability.

In addition to this published work, several conference papers have reported on the experiences of individuals with intellectual disabilities. Joseph Scotti, Stevens, Cavender, Morford and his colleagues at Western Virginia University (2007) have studied the responses to emergency events by 405 individuals with intellectual disabilities and related developmental disabilities. Over 30% of the caretakers of these individuals reported that they became distressed during emergency situations and had stressed responses to emergency related stimuli, including sirens/bells (37%), fire drills (22%), flashing lights (22%), strangers (18%), and emergency personnel (10%). These findings suggested that cues used to signal looming disasters may actually trigger stress reactions in individuals with cognitive disabilities, rather than assist them in appropriately preparing for evacuation or sheltering. Most family members similarly reported that these individuals displayed notable emotional reactions to these events, including fear, helplessness, and horror. Interestingly, the number of traumatic events reported was positively correlated with the number of medical and behavioral problems as well as the severity of the medical problems that had been reported by the family member. Distress ratings were negatively correlated with the age of the individual, their level of independence, the extent to which they responded positively to strangers, and their level of independence following instructions from strangers.

A second study by Scotti, Stevens, Cavender, Jacoby and colleagues (2007) analyzing the same database examined the prevalence and impact of traumatic events, including disasters. Primary caretakers of individuals with intellectual disabilities reported that their wards had experienced an average of two to three types of potentially traumatic events over their lifetime. Reactions to traumatic events included reexperiencing, hyperarousal, avoidance, and changes in sleep patterns. The researchers concluded that persons with mental retardation and developmental disabilities appear to exhibit symptoms and distress that resemble posttraumatic stress disorder (PTSD) when exposed to traumatic events, but they noted that the clinical differentiation of PTSD from behavioral problems in this population would be challenging.

Stough and Sharp (2007) conducted a study of the long-term recovery of 31 individuals with disabilities who had been directly affected by Hurricane Katrina. Individuals with disabilities or their family members participated in one of five focus groups that were conducted in the Gulf States. Seven of the participants or their family members had a cognitive disability, while over half (a total of 16) reported having more than one disability. Participants overwhelmingly identified family members and friends as their primary sources of support following the disaster. In response to the question "What has prevented your recovery from Hurricane Katrina?" not one of the participants believed that they and their family had "recovered," although these focus groups took place nearly two years following the disaster. In addition, almost all of the participants made a negative statement about their current level of depression or stress, even though the prompt was not designed to elicit this information. Over half of the participants believed that these self-identified feelings of depression or despair had negatively affected their ability to search for services, obtain employment, and to recover from the disaster.

15.6. PSYCHIATRIC DISABILITIES

Mental illness is not considered disabling in most instances, and while adverse situational variables certainly may contribute to psychological distress following disaster, they do not necessarily lead to psychiatric illness. In keeping with the World Health Organization's definition, the Americans with Disabilities Act considers a mental illness disabling only if it "substantially limits one or more of the major life activities" (U.S. Equal Employment Opportunity Commission, 1990). According to American Psychiatric Association (APA) (2000), a disorder must interfere markedly with social, occupational, or school functioning to be considered a severe mental illness. Diagnoses included under the category of severe mental illness generally include schizophrenia or its related psychotic disorders, bipolar affective disorder, autism, major depression, obsessive-compulsive disorder (OCD), and panic disorder (Reggeri, Leese, Thornicroft, Bisoffi, & Tansella, 2000). It is estimated that 2.8% of the population has a severe mental illness (Narrow et al., 2000). PTSD is the most frequent diagnosis assessed by researchers following disaster exposure but is not, when presented on its own, usually considered a severe mental illness.

Bromet, Schulber, and Dunn (1982), in an early study on disaster and individuals with severe mental illness, assessed a group of 151 outpatients with psychiatric illnesses living near the Three Mile Island nuclear facility during the 1979 disaster. The group's postdisaster mental health status was compared with a group of similarly diagnosed individuals living near a nonaffected nuclear plant. The researchers assessed the two groups for stress, depression, and anxiety at three different time points following the Three Mile Island disaster. While they found increased levels of anxiety or depressive episodes in both groups following the disaster, they found no difference between the two groups on these measures.

Three studies have examined institutionalized populations with severe mental illness exposed to disasters, which allowed for verification of clinical diagnosis both pre and postdisaster. In the first study, Godleski, Luke, DiPreta, Kline, and Carlton (1994) reported on a group of 22 patients at a chronic rehabilitation unit that experienced a direct impact from Hurricane Iniki. The clinical status of the patients was assessed at three time periods during the storm, beginning

1 week after the storm and up to 12 months afterward. The researchers reported that following the disaster none of the patients met the criteria for PTSD, none required an increase in medications, and there was no additional decompensation of the mental health status of the patients. The second study, by Stout and Knight (1990), was conducted on 15 adolescents receiving inpatient treatment in a facility that was flooded. In contrast to results the adolescents were found to use positive coping mechanisms following the disaster, and the researchers noted no increase in psychopathology and PTSD. A third study by Bystritsky, Vapnik, Maidment, Pynoos, and Steinberg (2000) examined the reaction of two groups of patients with anxiety disorders, one with OCD and the other with panic disorders, who were directly impacted by the Northridge earthquakes of 1994. Neither groups displayed an increase in their primary symptomatology following the disaster. Interestingly, measures of anxiety and depression significantly increased in the group with panic disorders but not in the group with OCD. It should be noted that the group with OCD was participating in a partial hospitalization program while the patients with panic disorder were participating in studies on panic disorder. Together, these three studies suggest that individuals with severe mental illness may be buffered from additional psychological impacts of disasters when they receive ongoing psychiatric care in a therapeutic environment.

Results from two other studies similarly suggest (although they did not statistically analyze the level of psychiatric functioning pre- and postdisaster) that intensive community treatment programs may prevent additional pathology in individuals with severe mental illness (Lachance, Santos, & Burns, 1994; McMurray & Steiner, 2000). The constant across these studies was continuity of mental health supports following disaster. Again, it may be that when ongoing psychological supports are available to individuals with severe mental illness, psychological deterioration is mitigated.

In contrast to these findings, Chubb and Bisson (1996) found that the majority (50%) of institutionalized victims, who were involved in a deadly vehicle collision, met criteria for PTSD following the accident. A higher level of morbidity was found in those with depression and anxiety postdisaster, but following the disaster victims with schizophrenia actually had lower scores on measures of depression, anxiety, and PTSD. In contrast results reported in the Bromet et al. (1982), and Bystritsky et al. (2000), and Godleski et al. (1994) studies, the victims in this study directly witnessed the deaths of family members and caretakers during the event, which may have affected the level of PTSD experienced by these participants.

Several other studies have examined populations with severe mental illness receiving institutionalized or outpatient psychiatric care following the attacks of September 11th (see DeLisi, Cohen, & Maurizio, 2004; Franklin, Young, & Zimmerman, 2002; Riemann, Braun, Greer, & Ullman, 2004; Taylor & Jenkins, 2004). However, the patients in these studies were not at physical risk during these disasters, were not directly impacted by the event, and were at substantial distance from any of the sites where the attacks occurred. In the study by DeLisi and colleagues, patients were institutionalized at Bellevue Hospital and had the opportunity to view the event distantly from windows at the hospital, which was three miles away from the Towers, but were not questioned if they actually had seen the event occur. However, no significant difference in increase in morbidity or occurrence of new symptoms was found between those patients who did and who did not have the opportunity to view the destruction. Person and Fuller (2007) give a more extensive review of this set of studies, as well as a detailed discussion of the psychological measures used in these and in several other studies.

Another group of studies have analyzed the results of disaster on large populations that included participants both with and without diagnosed mental health disorders. Robins (1986) interviewed 252 individuals affected by the multiple Times Beach disasters of flooding, radiation, tornados, and dioxin and matched them to a sample that had not been exposed. They found little evidence that these disasters had significant effects on mental health other than an increase in PTSD associated with the event. In addition, they found little evidence that these disasters caused the recurrence of mental illness or caused new mental illnesses. They concluded that most individuals, regardless of preexisting mental health status, are psychological resilient in the face of disaster.

Several studies have examined the association between severe mental illnesses and PTSD that has been diagnosed in relationship to disasters. Breslau, Davis, Andreski, and Peterson (1991) hypothesized that PTSD may lead to other psychiatric disorders, rather than the converse argument that prior disorders lead to PTSD vulnerability. McMillen, North, Mosley, and Smith (2002) empirically examined explanations for the high rates of psychiatric comorbidity that are typically associated with PTSD. They examined a sample of 162 survivors of the Great Midwest Floods using the Diagnostic Interview Schedule (DIS) and its Disaster Supplement. Thirty-five of their subjects met criteria for PTSD related to the flood, and the diagnosis of PTSD was frequently comorbid with other disorders. Although 10% of the sample developed a new, non-PTSD psychiatric disorder after the flood, these disorders were rare in the absence of PTSD symptoms. The results supported a model in which PTSD contributed to the development of other disorders following trauma but found no support for the hypothesis that other psychological disorders develop independently of PTSD following disaster.

In another study on the effects of the Midwest floods, North, Kawaskai, Spitznagel, and Hong (2004) examined a sample of 162 individuals, 44% of who had a predisaster psychiatric illness at sometime in their life. Only 25% of the sample reported any new somatoform symptom after the flood event, and for two-thirds of these individuals, the new illness was flood-related PTSD; flood-related PTSD developed three times as often in people with a preexisting psychiatric disorder. New somatization disorders and new alcohol or substance abuse were not observed results of the floods. Some participants did develop new somatoform symptoms (though not pathology), but these symptoms were associated with the presence of preflood psychiatric disorders. These large-scale studies suggest that the presence of postdisaster psychiatric illness is highly dependent on predisaster levels of illness and support other studies that have found that the majority of victims do not develop PTSD following disaster.

Individuals with preexisting psychiatric disorders may be at additional risk due to events that occur postdisaster. The National Council on Disability (2005) released a report following hurricanes Katrina and Rita that identifies a number of mental health concerns for people with psychiatric disabilities following disaster. One of these most basic identified needs was access to psychotropic medicines following the disaster as most individuals who evacuated did so without their medications or with only a limited supply. Shelters used in these two disasters were reported to lack psychiatric support, and hurricane victims therefore experienced disruption in their therapeutic treatment. NCD also reported inappropriate institutionalization of people with psychiatric disabilities postdisaster, and noted that institutionalization could have been avoided simply by refilling needed psychiatric medications.

In summary, studies on individuals with preexisting psychiatric illness suggest that continuity of psychological and other supports may mitigate the effects of disaster, that higher rates of PTSD occur in these individuals than in those without preexisting disorders following disaster, but that the development of new psychiatric disorders unrelated to PTDS symptomology is rare in most instances.

15.7. SUMMARY OF RESEARCH ON INDIVIDUALS WITH PREEXISTING DISABILITIES

The limited empirical research on the effects of disaster on individuals with disabilities, with the exception of the literature on preexisting mental health issues, focuses on physical or service barriers experienced during and following disaster rather than on the psychological impacts experienced by these individuals. The literature suggests that people with disabilities, including those with severe mental illness, have unequal access to information about impending disaster, are treated differently during the relief stage of disaster, and encounter additional barriers in recovering from disaster. Much less clear are the psychological effects of disaster on individuals with disabilities. Excluding the small collection of empirical studies on individuals with preexisting psychiatric illnesses, researchers have virtually ignored the psychological effects of disaster on individuals with intellectual disabilities, physical disabilities, or sensory impairments. In part, the lack of attention given to the mental health needs of individuals with nonpsychiatric disabilities can be attributed to the theoretical orientation of the researchers who have conducted this research: Most are researchers from the disability field rather than psychologists or psychiatrists. Thus, studies that do focus on the effects of disaster on people with disabilities tend to have a policy or social support focus rather than upon the mental health of this population. In addition, researchers have generally given limited attention to the mental health of individuals with disabilities, with the exception of a collection of studies on depression in individuals with mental retardation (e.g., Esbensen & Benson, 2006; Lunsky, 2004), and this same lack of attention can be noted in the disaster-related literature.

15.8. FUTURE RESEARCH

Two lines of research seem to be the most promising in examining the effects of disaster on people with disabilities. First is the question of whether the mental health of people with disabilities is *disproportionately* affected by disaster. Reliable measures of individual psychological functioning both before and after a disaster event will be needed to measure impact, as well as a comparison with individuals without disabilities. As it can be difficult to obtain reliable and valid measures of psychological functioning on many individuals with disabilities, researchers will be challenged to assess if disasters differentially affect the mental health status of people with disability or if psychological consequences are manifested differently than those in the nondisabled population.

The second line of research is on the psychosocial consequences of disaster for people with disabilities. The social and personal supports that surround individuals with disabilities are fragile and appear to be particularly susceptible to the type of disruption that disasters incur. Several studies have suggested that victims of disaster choose family and friends as their most frequent method for coping with disaster (Haines, Hurlbert, & Beggs, 1999). However, the extent to which these support systems are disrupted following disaster and whether these systems are more difficult for people with disabilities to reassemble has not been systematically examined.

We know that individuals with disabilities tend to have lower income, fewer people in their social networks, and lower rates of education – all of which are factors that place other vulnerable groups at physical risk following disaster (Bourque et al., 2006). The question for researchers, then, is if the loss of these supports places people at additional risk for psychological disorders following disasters. Theories that suggest that the loss of resources and psychosocial supports following disaster affect psychological hardiness, for example, Hobfall's (1989) theory of conservation of resources or Kaniasty and Norris' (1993) social support deterioration model, would be of most use in framing this line of research. However, the loss of supports available to individuals with disabilities may tell us more about how disaster exacerbates existing social inequalities than it does about the mental health effects of disaster on this population.

Acknowledgments

This work was supported by the National Institute of Mental Health Research Education in Disaster Mental Health (REDMH) mentoring program, Grant #5R25MH068298-04. The author would like to additionally thank Carol North for her guidance.

REFERENCES

Aldrich, N., & Benson, W. F. (2008). Disaster preparedness and the chronic disease needs of vulnerable older adults. *Preventing Chronic Disease, 5*(1), A27.

American Foundation for the Blind (2008). *Facts and figures on Americans with vision loss.* (September, 2008); http://www.afb.org/Section.asp?SectionID=15&DocumentID=4398

American Psychiatric Association. (2000). *Diagnostical and statistical manual of mental disorders 4th ed., Text Revision.* Washington, DC: American Psychiatric Association.

Barile, M., Fitchten, C., Ferraro, V., & Judd, D. (2006). Ice storm experiences of persons with disabilities: Knowledge is safety. *The Review of Disability Studies I, 2*(3), 35–48.

Bault, M. (2008). *Disability status and the characteristics of people in group quarters: a brief analysis of disability prevalence among the civilian noninstitutionalized and total populations in the American Community Survey. United States Census Bureau Report.* (February 2008); http://www.census.gov/hhes/www/disability/GQdisability.pdf

Bourque, L. B., Siegel, J. M., Kano, M., & Wood, M. M. (2006). Weathering the storm: The impact of hurricanes on physical and mental health. *The Annals of the American Academy, 604,* 129–151

Breslau, N., Davis, C. G., Andreski, P., & Peterson, E. L. (1991). Traumatic events and posttraumatic stress disorder in an urban population of young adults. *Archives of General Psychiatry, 48,* 216–222.

Brodie, M., Weltzien, E, Altman, D., Blendon, R. J., & Benson, J. M. (2006). Experiences of Hurricane Katrina evacuees in Houston shelters: Implications for future planning. *American Journal of Public Health, 96*(8), 1402–1408.

Bromet, E., Schulberg, H. C., & Dunn, I. (1982). Reactions of psychiatric patients to the Three Mile Island nuclear accident. *Archives of General Psychiatry, 39*(6), 725–730.

Bystritsky, M. D., Vapnik, R., Maidment, K., Pynoos, R. S., & Steinberg, A. M. (2000). Acute responses of anxiety disorder patients after a natural disaster. *Depression and Anxiety, 11,* 43–44.

Centers for Disease Control. (2006). *Disability.* (February 2008); http://www.cdc.gov/omhd/Populations/Disability/Disability.htm.

Christ G. H., & Christ, T. W. (2006). Academic and behavioral reactions of children with disabilities to the loss of a firefighter father: The New York World Trade Center attack 9/11/01. *The Review of Disability Studies, 2*(3), 68–77.

Christensen, K. M., Blair, M. E., & Holt, J. M. (2007). The built environment, evacuations, and individuals with disabilities: A guiding framework for disaster policy and preparation. *Journal of Disability Policy Studies, 17*(4), 249–253.

Chubb, H. L., & Bisson, J. I. (1996). Early psychological reactions in a group of individuals with pre-existing and enduring mental health difficulties following a major coach accident. *The British Journal of Psychiatry, 169*(4), 430–433.

DeLisi, L. E., Cohen, T. H., & Maurizio, A. M. (2004). Hospitalized psychiatric patients view the World Trade Center disaster. *Psychiatry Research, 129*(2), 201–207.

Esbensen, A. J., & Benson, B. A. (2006). Diathesis-stress and depressed mood. *American Journal on Mental Retardation, 111*(2), 100–112.

Fox, M. H., White, G. W., Rooney, C., & Rowland, R. L. (2007). Disaster preparedness and response for persons with mobility impairments: Results from the University of Kansas Nobody Left Behind Study. *Journal of Disability Policy Studies, 17*(4), 196–205.

Franklin, C. L., Young, D., & Zimmerman, M. (2002). Psychiatric patients' vulnerability in the wake of the September 11th terrorist attacks. *The Journal of Nervous and Mental Disease, 190*(12), 833–838.

Galludet Research Institute. (2004). *A brief summary of estimates for the size of the deaf population in the USA based on available federal data and published research.* (February 2008); http://gri.gallaudet.edu/Demographics/deaf-US.php

Gladwin, H., & Peacock, W. G. (2000). Warning and evacuation: A night for hard houses. In W. Peacock, B. Morrow, & H. Gladwin (Eds.), *Hurricane Andrew: Ethnicity, gender and the sociology of disasters.* Miami: International Hurricane Center.

Godleski, L. S., Luke, K. N., DiPreta, J. E., Kline, A. E., & Carlton, B. S. (1994). Responses of state hospital patients of Hurricane Iniki. *Hospital and Community Psychiatry, 45*(9), 931–933.

Haines, B. A., Hurlbert, J. S., & Beggs, J. J. (1999). The disaster framing of the stress process: A test of an expanded model. *International Journal of Mass Emergencies and Disasters, 17*(3), 367–397.

Harvard School of Public Health. (2007). *Hurricane readiness in high-risk areas.* (January 2008); http://www.hsph.harvard.edu/news/pressreleases/files/Hurricane_2007_Survey_state_results.doc

Hemingway, L., & Priestley, M. (2006). Natural hazards, human vulnerability and disabling societies: A disaster for disabled people? *The Review of Disability Studies: An International Journal, 2*(3), 57–67.

Hobfall, S. E. (1989). Conservation of resources: A new attempt at conceptualizing stress. *American Psychologist, 44,* 513–524.

International Federation of Red Cross and Red Crescent Societies. (2007). *World disasters report: Focus on discrimination*. Satigny/Verner, Switzerland: ATAR Roto Presse.

Jonkman S.N., & Kelman, I. (2005). An analysis of the causes and circumstances of disaster deaths. *Disasters, 29*(1), 75–97.

Kaniasty, K., & Norris, F.H. (1993). A test of the social support deterioration model in the context of natural disaster. *Journal of Personality and Social Psychology, 64*, 395–408.

Lachance, K.R., Santos, A.B., & Burns, B.J. (1994) The response of an assertive community treatment program following a natural disaster. *Community Mental Health Journal, 30*(5), 505–515.

Lunsky, Y. (2004). Suicidality in a clinical and community sample of adults with mental retardation. *Research In Developmental Disabilities, 25*(3), 231–243.

Martz, E., & Cook, D.W. (2001). Physical impairments as risk factors for the development of posttraumatic stress disorder. *Rehabilitation Counseling Bulletin, 44*(4), 217–221.

Mashaw, J., & Reno, V. (1996). *Balancing security and opportunity: The challenge of disability income policy. Report of the Disability Policy Panel*. Washington, DC: National Academy of Social Insurance.

McGuire, L.C., Ford E.S., & Okoro, C.A. (2007). Natural disaster and older U.S. adults with disabilities: Implication for evacuation. *Disasters, 31*(1), 49–56.

McMillen, C., North, C., Mosley, M., & Smith, E. (2002). Untangling the psychiatric comorbidity of postraumatic stress disorder in a sample of flood survivors. *Comprehensive Psychiatry, 43*(6), 478–485

McMurray, L., & Steiner, W. (2000). Natural disaster and service delivery to individuals with severe mental illness- Ice storm 1998. *Canadian Journal of Psychiatry, 45*(4), 383–385.

Mileti, D.S. (1999). *Disasters by design: A reassessment of natural hazards in the United States*. Washington, DC: John Henry Press.

Morrow, B.H. (1999). Identifying and mapping community vulnerability. *Disasters, 23*(1), 1–18.

Narrow, W.E., Regier, D.A., Norquist, G., Rae, D.S., Kennedy, C., & Arons, B. (2000). Mental health service use by Americans with severe mental illnesses. *Social Psychiatry and Psychiatric Epidemiology, 35*(4), 147–155.

National Council on Disability. (2005). *Saving lives: Including people with disabilities in emergency planning*. (February 2008); http://www.ncd.gov/newsroom/publications/2005/saving_lives.htm.

National Organization on Disability. (2005a). *Report on special needs assessment for Karina evacuees (SNAKE) Project*. Washington, DC (October 2005); http://www.nod.org/Resources/PDF/katrina_snake_report.pdf.

(2005b). *The Impact of Hurricanes Katrina and Rita on people with disabilities: A look back and remaining challenges*. (September 2007); http://www.ncd.gov/newsroom/publications/2006/hurricanes_impact.htm

Norris, F.H., Friedman, M.J., Watson, P.J., Byrne, C.M., Diaz, E., & Kaniasty, K. (2002). 60,000 Disaster Victims Speak: Part I. An empirical review of the empirical literature, 1981–2001. *Psychiatry, 65*(3), 207–239.

Norris, F. H., Kaniasty K., Conrad, M., Inman G., & Murphy, A. (2002). Placing age differences in cultural context: A comparison of the effects of age on PTSD after disasters in the U.S., Mexico, and Poland. *Journal of Clinical Geropsychiatry, 8*, 153–173.

Norris, F., & Murrell, S. (1988). Prior experience as a moderator of disaster impact on anxiety symptoms in older adults. *American Journal of Community Psychology, 16*, 665–683.

North, C.S., Kawaskai, A., Spitznagel, E.L., & Hong, B.A. (2004). The course of PTSD, major depression, substance abuse, and somatization after a natural disaster. *The Journal of Nervous and Mental Disease, 192*(12), 823–829.

Perry, R.W., & Lindell, M.K. (1997). Aged citizens in the warning phase of disasters. *International Journal of Aging and Human Development, 44*, 257–267.

Person, C., & Fuller, E.J. (2007). Disaster care for persons with psychiatric disabilities: Recommendations for policy change. *Journal of Disability Policy Studies, 17*(4), 238–248.

Phillips, B.D., & Morrow, B.H. (2007). Social science research needs: Focus on vulnerable populations, forecasting, and warnings. *Natural Hazards Review, 8*(3), 61–68.

Riemann, B.C., Braun, M.M., Greer, A., & Ullman, J.M. (2004). Effects of September 11 on patients with obsessive compulsive disorder. *Cognitive Behavior Therapy, 33*(2), 60–67.

Reggeri, M., Leese, M., Thornicroft, G., Bisoffi, G., & Tansella, M. (2000). Definition and prevalence of severe and persistent mental illness. *The British Journal of Psychiatry, 177*, 149–155.

Robins, L.N., Fischback, R.L., Smith, E.M., Cottler, L.B., Solomon, S.D., & Goldring, E. (1986). Impact of disaster on previously assessed mental health. In J.H. Shore (Ed.), *Disaster stress studies: New methods and findings*. Washington, DC: American Psychiatric Press, Inc.

Rooney, C., & White, G.W. (2007). Narrative analysis of a disaster preparedness and emergency response survey from persons with mobility impairments. *Journal of Disability Policy Studies, 17*(4), 206–215.

Rowland, J.L., White, G.W., Fox, M.H., & Rooney, C. (2007). Emergency response training practices for people with disabilities. *Journal of Disability Policy Studies*, *17*(4), 216–222.

Scotti, J.R., Stevens S., Cavender, A, Morford, M., Jacoby V., Freed, R., et al. (2007). Response of persons with mental retardation/developmental disabilities to emergency situation: Implications for disaster preparedness. Presented at the annual meeting of the International Society for Traumatic Stress Studies, Baltimore, MD.

Scotti, J.R., Stevens S., Cavender, A., Jacoby, V., Kalvitis, J., Morford, A., et al. (2007). Trauma in persons with mental retardation/developmental disabilities: Relation between trauma history, behavior problems, and functional level. Presented at the annual meeting of the International Society for Traumatic Stress Studies, Baltimore, MD.

Stout, C.E., & Knight, T. (1990). Impact of a natural disaster on a psychiatric inpatient population: Clinical observations. *The Psychiatric Hospital*, *21*(3), 129–135.

Stough, L.M., & Sharp, A.N. (2007). The recovery of individuals with disabilities following Hurricane Katrina. Presented at the annual meeting of the International Society for Traumatic Stress Studies, Baltimore, MD.

Taylor, M., & Jenkins, K. (2004). The psychological impact of September 11 terrorism on Australian inpatients. *Australiasian Psychiatry Bulletin of the Royal Australian and New Zealand College of Psychiatrists*, *12*(3), 253–255.

Tierney, K.J., Petak, W.J., & Hahn, H. (1988). *Disabled persons & earthquake hazards*. Boulder, CO: Institute for Social and Behavioral Science, Natural Hazards Research and Applications Information Center.

Tobin, G.A., & Whiteford, L.M. (2002). Community resilience and volcano hazard: The eruption of Tungurahua and evacuation of the faldas in Ecuador. *Disasters*, *26*(1), 28–48.

United States Equal Opportunities Commission. *The Americans with Disability Act*. (February 2008); http://www.eeoc.gov/types/ada.html

White, B. (2006). Disaster relief for deaf persons: Lessons from Hurricanes Katrina and Rita. *The Review of Disability Studies*, *2*(3), 49–56.

White, G.W., Fox, M.H., Rooney, C., & Cahill, A. (2007). *Assessing the impact of Hurricane Katrina on persons with disabilities*. Lawrence, KS: The University of Kansas, The Research and Training Center on Independent Living.

World Health Organization. (2005). *Disability, including prevention, management and rehabilitation*. (February 2008); http://www.who.int/gb/ebwha/pdf_files/WHA58/A58_17-en.pdf

(2008). *International classification of functioning, disability and health. Introduction*. (March 2008); http://www.who.int/classifications/icf/site/icftemplate.cfm?myurl=homepage.html&mytitle=Home%20Page.

16 Factors Associated with Exposure and Response to Disasters among Marginalized Populations

ALESIA O. HAWKINS, HEIDI M. ZINZOW, ANANDA B. AMSTADTER, CARLA KMETT DANIELSON, AND KENNETH J. RUGGIERO

16.1. INTRODUCTION

One of the greatest challenges in disaster-response efforts is to rapidly identify and assist individuals who have limited resources. Marginalized populations, most notably racial/ethnic minorities and individuals with low socioeconomic status (SES), are at heightened risk for disaster exposure and vulnerability to disaster-related mental health outcomes. The degree to which these marginalized populations are disproportionately affected by disasters has long been recognized as a topic of great importance by researchers, policy makers, public health officials, disaster-response personnel, and the media. While a significant number of studies have assisted in addressing this question, most have focused on a narrow range of variables and have isolated a specific phase of the disaster (i.e., pre-, peri-, or postdisaster). Additionally, much of the disaster literature has focused solely on risk factors associated with marginalized populations and has not adequately examined resilient and protective factors among marginalized populations.

This chapter attempts to summarize the current state of the literature relating to each of the disaster phases across a wide range of variables, including sociocultural factors and environment and community resources. Following an introductory section on definitions, the chapter is organized as follows: First, we briefly summarize disaster studies examining race/ethnicity, SES, and mental health outcomes. Second, major sections summarize the current state of the literature on sociocultural factors and environment and community resources. Within each of these sections, we discuss marginalized populations within the context of phases of disaster. Notably, some factors were identified in both the pre- and peridisaster phase in our review; therefore, these two phases were combined. Table 16.1 provides an overview of this structure and is a useful reference to help guide the reader through the major sections. Finally, we discuss implications for research, disaster-response efforts, and practice.

16.1.1. Definitions

Marginalized populations are most often defined by race/ethnicity, SES, geography, gender, age, and disability status. In disaster research, marginalized populations refer to individuals within these categories who are disproportionately affected by disaster and are most vulnerable to negative consequences of disaster. In this review, we focus primarily on race/ethnicity and SES because these factors have been found in clinical and epidemiologic research to account for a significant amount of variance in health outcomes. Heterogeneity exists across studies in how race and ethnicity are defined. Neither term has a clear agreed-upon scientific definition. Generally, *ethnicity* refers to the characterization of a group of people who see themselves and are seen by others as having a common ancestry, shared history, shared traditions, and shared cultural traits, such as language, beliefs, and values; whereas, *race* more often refers to a characterization of a group of people believed to share physical characteristics such as skin color, facial features, and other hereditary traits or biological origin (Cokley, 2007). Consistent with many disaster studies, we

Table 16.1. Factors associated with pre-, peri-, and postdisaster exposure and response among marginalized populations

	Predisaster [a] and Peridisaster [b]	Postdisaster
Sociocultural factors	Decision to evacuate[a]	Help-seeking behavior
	Risk perception[a]	Discrimination/racism
	Cultural attitudes and beliefs and acculturative stress[a,b]	Social support
	Prior trauma	Religious/spiritual support
Environment and community resources	Financial resources and Infrastructure[a]	Access to evidence-based treatment
	Crisis preparation[a]	Economic hardship
	Decision to evacuate[a,b]	Job loss
	Emergency response[a,b]	Family displacement
		Crime

Notes:
[a] Variables associated with predisaster.
[b] Variables associated with peridisaster.

will combine the two terms and refer to "race/ethnicity."

16.2. MENTAL HEALTH OUTCOMES

Reviews of disaster studies have concluded that large-scale traumatic events significantly increase psychological problems in the short term and can have long-lasting negative mental health consequences such as anxiety, depression, and, most notably, posttraumatic stress disorder (PTSD) (e.g., Brewin, Andrew, & Valentine, 2000; McMillen, North, & Smith, 2000). A variety of factors have been identified as increasing individuals' vulnerability to negative postdisaster mental health consequences: race/ethnicity, SES, severity of exposure, prior trauma experiences, and a variety of psychosocial resources all appear to play a role, including interactions among these factors (Norris, Friedman, & Watson, 2002). Some researchers suggest that racial/ethnic minorities and individuals with lower SES tend to endure greater trauma exposure during disasters than mainstream populations, including life threat, damage to property, injury, and death of friends and family members (Fothergill, Maestas, & Darlington, 1999; Perilla, Norris, & Lavizzo, 2002).

Findings from a limited number of disaster studies reporting on race/ethnicity suggest that racial/ethnic minorities are at a heightened risk for experiencing more distress postdisaster (e.g., Jones, Frary, Cunningham, Weddle, & Kaiser, 2001; Perilla et al., 2002), while other disaster studies do not find racial/ethnic group differences (e.g., Adams & Boscarino, 2005; Garrison et al., 1995; Shannon, Lonigan, Finch, & Taylor, 1994). Norris and colleagues' (2002) review found that 8 out of 11 studies reporting on race/ethnicity and disaster outcomes showed racial/ethnic minorities fared worse after disaster. Similarly, Perilla, Norris, and LaVizzo (2002) found that Hispanics and African Americans were more adversely affected by Hurricane Andrew than Caucasians. However, these racial/ethnic groups also reported more exposure to other traumas than Caucasians in that study. Perilla and colleagues argued that the severity of exposure to stressful or traumatic events may have accounted for racial/ethnic differences. These findings suggest identification as a racial/ethnic minority, in and of itself, does not place an individual at risk for adverse psychological sequelae; instead, an interaction among various factors contributes to this group's vulnerability in the face of disaster.

Very few studies have examined SES and disaster effects. When SES was examined, poverty or lower SES (e.g., Dew & Bromet, 1993; Ginexi, Weihs, Simmens, & Hoyt, 2000; Phifer, 1990) was associated with a higher risk for experiencing more distress postdisaster. In fact,

Norris and colleagues' (2002) review of disaster studies found that in 13 of the 14 disaster studies reporting SES status, lower SES was consistently associated with greater postdisaster distress. In addition to limited studies examining SES, methodological constraints have been identified as a challenge to better understanding the effects of SES on postdisaster mental health (Norris et al., 2002). For instance, Norris and colleagues noted that for most studies examining income and other SES indicators, SES was tested as a main effect rather than as a variable that may potentially modify the impact of disaster exposure. Additionally, due to the nature of disaster, participants in many of the disaster studies were of the same or similar occupation (e.g., Holen, 1991; McFarlan, 1989) or income level (e.g., McMillen et al., 2000) limiting statistical comparisons of postdisaster effects across a range of SES levels.

16.3. SOCIOCULTURAL FACTORS

16.3.1. Predisaster and Peridisaster

16.3.1.1. Decision to Evacuate

Both differential exposure and differential vulnerability to disasters appear to play a role in the heightened impact of disaster among marginalized populations. One significant factor accounting for these populations' greater disaster exposure is that racial/ethnic minority and low-income groups are the least likely and able to evacuate during disasters (Curtis, Mills, & Leitner, 2007; Elliott & Pais, 2006; Gladwin & Peacock, 1997; Peacock, 2003; Riad, Norris, & Ruback, 1999; Sattler et al., 1995). Spence and colleagues (2007) found that 64.5% of African American and 82.9% of other non-White respondents reported evacuating before Hurricane Katrina, as compared with 85.5% of the Caucasian respondents. Racial/ethnic differences in evacuation decisions before Hurricane Andrew were also reported, revealing that evacuation was lowest among African Americans and Hispanics (Gladwin & Peacock, 1997; Peacock, 2003; Sattler et al., 1995).

Multiple reasons have been offered as to why marginalized populations are less likely or unable to evacuate in response to disasters. Some studies have indicated that they are less likely than majority populations to be prepared for evacuation or to be educated about what is required to prepare or evacuate (Faupel, Kelley, & Petee, 1992; Fothergill et al., 1999; Gladwin & Peacock, 1997; Turner, Nigg, Paz, & Young, 1980). Marginalized populations may be mistrustful of the government and authorities due to prior negative experiences and therefore less likely to consider evacuation warnings from these sources as credible (Eisenman, Cordasco, Asch, Golden, & Glik, 2007; Fothergill et al., 1999; Henkel, Dovidio, & Gaertner, 2006; Morrow, 1997; Phillips & Ephraim, 1992).

Social networks among racial/ethnic minority cultures can be a significant protective factor against adverse mental health consequences, and the emphasis on social networks among many racial/ethnic minority cultures appears to also influence evacuation efforts. One qualitative study of a sample of primarily African American Hurricane Katrina survivors indicated that evacuation decisions were influenced by extended family and other members of participants' social networks either facilitating or, in some cases, inhibiting evacuation. Their findings suggest responsibilities for family may have weighed heavily on their decision whether to evacuate or not (Eisenman et al., 2007). Research has shown that racial/ethnic minorities tend to consider interpersonal channels as more important sources of information (Morrow, 1997; Peacock & Mushkatel, 1986; Perry & Greene, 1982; Perry & Lindell, 1991; Perry & Nelson, 1991; Peguero, 2006). However, networks of intense ties may communicate less new information (Eisenman et al., 2007). Large social networks have also been associated with perceiving the impending disaster as less threatening, which may hinder evacuation (Aguirre, 1988; Riad et al., 1999). Further, because families tend to evacuate as a unit, people with extended family units may exhibit delayed responses to evacuation warnings. For example, Hispanic survivors of disaster have reported that accounting for extended family members delayed responses to disaster warnings (Perry & Mushkatel, 1986). Moreover, obligations to relatives who are less likely to evacuate, such as the elderly, may cause individuals to remain behind (Eisenman et al., 2007). Large family units may also stretch limited resources, further affecting their ability to evacuate (Blaikie, Cannon, Davis, & Wisner, 1994; Morrow, 1999). However, other researchers have found that those with larger social support networks were less likely to cite low resources as affecting their evacuation decision and were more likely to evacuate (Riad et al., 1999). These findings underscore the necessity of including immediate and extended family and close social networks in crisis preparation.

16.3.1.2. Risk Perception

Differences in risk perception between minority and majority populations also may contribute to differences in disaster exposure. For example, a large, comprehensive survey of Hurricane Katrina survivors found that African Americans were less likely to evacuate than Caucasians before the storm primarily because they were less likely to believe that the storm would be as devastating as it was (Elliott & Pais, 2006). Similarly, Mexican American flood victims were found to identify risks as high less frequently than Anglo-Americans, despite living in equally hazardous areas (Lindell et al., 1980). In contrast, other studies have reported conflicting findings. For example, one study found that Mexican immigrants had heightened risk perception in comparison to other earthquake victims; however, this appeared to be due their prior experience with earthquakes in Mexico (Aptekar, 1990). A study of flood victims found no differences among racial/ethnic groups in terms of risk perception (Ives & Furseth, 1983).

Research also has mixed insights in regards to the relationship of income to risk perception. Flynn, Slovic, and Mertz (1994) found individuals with lower SES experienced heightened levels of risk perception. Flynn and colleagues argued that this finding may be due to lower SES individuals' lacking financial resources to recover (e.g., damaged property) from a disaster, thus, having more to lose in the face of disaster than individuals with higher income. In contrast, Vaughan (1995) suggested that individuals with lower SES experienced lower levels of risk perception, finding that lower SES status was associated with denial or minimization of risk. These findings may be due to lower SES individuals' previous involvement in high-risk or hazardous occupations, and thus, they are more likely to employ coping mechanisms to deal with daily risks they face (Fothergill & Peek, 2004). Further research is necessary using standardized assessments of risk perception, controlling for factors such as prior disaster experience and determining the impact of risk perception on evacuation and subsequent mental health outcomes.

16.3.1.3. Cultural Attitudes and Beliefs and Acculturative Stress

A variety of cultural beliefs appear to affect individuals in pre- and peridisaster phases. Emphasis on collectivism, or group identity, is a particular strength among African American, Hispanic, and Asian American cultures. Collectivist beliefs particularly associated with Hispanic culture include familism, or an emphasis on familial interconnectedness, and simpatia, which emphasizes respect and subordinating individual needs to the group (Sabogal, Marin, Otero-Sabogal, Marin, & Perez-Stable, 1987; Triandis, Marin, Lisansky, & Betancourt, 1984). There is a tendency for members of certain racial/ethnic groups to rely on family to prepare for disaster; for instance, African Americans and Hispanics are more likely to have been helped by relatives in preparing for disaster (Morrow, 1997). Family assistance during disaster has also been found among Hispanics (Kaniasty & Norris, 2000). Overall, collectivist values maintained in marginalized communities have a positive effect on their psychological well-being. However, at times these values may engender some reluctance among minority disaster survivors to burden family members by seeking support from them (de Bocanegra & Brickman, 2004; Kaniasty & Norris, 2000). For example, one study of World Trade Center survivors after the September

11th terrorist attacks described how the value that Asian Americans placed on forbearance, or sacrificing one's own needs so as not to burden others, caused them to refrain from discussing the event with other members of the family (Constantine, Alleyne, Caldwell, McRae, & Suzuki, 2005). Emphasis on family obligations also could lead to increased stress among disaster survivors (Norris et al., 2002).

Another set of beliefs associated with Hispanic and African American cultures involves fatalism, or the tendency to view events as controlled by external factors versus being controlled by the individual (Perilla et al., 2002; Turner et al., 1980). A few studies have found a strong sense of fatalism associated with failure to evacuate, increased disaster-related distress, and greater risk for PTSD among minority populations (Elliott & Pais, 2006; Perilla et al., 2002; Pole, Best, Metzler, & Marmar, 2005). Self-blame coping has been associated with Hispanic survivors' possible increased risk for PTSD, perhaps in part because of religious beliefs where negative events could be interpreted as punishment for one's sins (Pole et al., 2005).

Individuals of Hispanic descent generally report higher levels of peritraumatic dissociation and panic attacks in comparison to other racial/ethnic groups, which has been found to relate to their heightened risk for PTSD (Galea et al., 2004; Pole et al., 2005). In general, the fear and distress experienced during a disaster has been found to be highest among Hispanic women, particularly those of lower income and educational levels (Goltz, Russell, & Bourque, 1992). Emphasis on masculinity found in some cultures may affect disaster-related coping. For example, Mexicans who placed emphasis on masculinity exhibited the greatest gender differences in PTSD (with women reporting more symptoms than men) in comparison to Caucasian and African American participants in a sample of Hurricane Andrew and Hurricane Paulina survivors (Norris, Perilla, & Murphy, 2001).

Among Native Americans, traditions and cultural practices often demand a positive interaction and harmony with the forces of nature. These value systems, as well as subsistence activities and traditional practices tied to the land, can be disrupted in the context of disasters. Some researchers hypothesize disruption can lead to exacerbated distress among Native American populations (Markstrom & Charley, 2003; Palinkas, Downs, Petterson, & Russell, 1993). Furthermore, Native American culture tends to stress communicating in a contained, respectful, and careful manner, which may inhibit expressions of distress and help-seeking in the context of disasters (Markstrom & Charley, 2003). Researchers speculate that cultural norms for emotional expression and beliefs about mental health symptoms among various cultural groups may mediate their responses.

Conflicts in values between dominant and marginalized cultures can occur, resulting in acculturative stress among racial and ethnic minority populations (see Rudmin, 2003). At least one study has demonstrated a significant relationship between acculturative stress and increased PTSD symptoms among hurricane survivors (Perilla et al., 2002). Additionally, immigrants may experience the added stress of resettling and being removed from a familiar culture that provided a meaning system for understanding exposure to traumatic events (De Vries, 1996); such stressors can be significant factors in exacerbating PTSD in minority populations exposed to disaster (Markstrom & Charley, 2003; Trautman et al., 2002).

16.3.1.4. Prior Trauma

Individuals from marginalized populations are likely to have had other prior trauma experiences that increase their vulnerability to disaster-related psychological problems. For example, women are more likely to have experienced prior interpersonal violence in comparison to men, and immigrants have often been exposed to stressors such as war, violence, and malnutrition before relocation (Trautman et al., 2002; Wolfe & Kimerling, 1997). Prior PTSD symptoms and violent life events have been associated with increased symptomatology and negative self-health assessments among minority and immigrant disaster survivors (Cheever & Hardin, 1999; Galea et al., 2004;

Trautman et al., 2002). Thus, prior trauma exposure among marginalized populations, combined with underutilization of mental health services to address these experiences, may increase vulnerability to adverse psychological functioning in the face of disaster.

16.3.2. Postdisaster

16.3.2.1. Help-Seeking Behavior

Several factors have an impact on marginalized populations' postdisaster mental health outcomes. While some factors (e.g., perceived discrimination, negative stigma about mental health services, unfamiliarity with available services) negatively affect marginalized communities, others (e.g., reliance on informal social support and on religious or spiritual activities) may have a beneficial effect on individuals' mental health postdisaster (Bauer, Rodriguez, Quiroga, & Flores-Ortiz, 2000; Constantine, Myers, Kindaichi, & Moore, 2004; Solberg, Ritsma, Davis, Tata, & Jolly, 1994). These factors may influence marginalized populations seeking formal mental health services.

Discrimination/Racism. Postdisaster researchers suggest that, because of their experiences with prejudice and discrimination, racial and ethnic minority disaster survivors may perceive that they were "left behind," that more could have been done to protect their neighborhood from the effects of the disaster, or that emergency response and community rebuilding was delayed because of their minority status (Bourque, Siegel, Kano, & Wood, 2006; Eisenman et al., 2007; Phillips, 1993; Weems et al., 2007). Negative media images that associate racial and ethnic minorities with disvalued groups, such as looters, may contribute to these negative perceptions (Fothergill et al., 1999; Weems et al., 2007). Furthermore, racial tension can escalate during a disaster, leading to conflict between victims and disaster-response personnel (Weems et al., 2007). Such experiences can have significant mental health implications, since adverse race-related events and perceived discrimination among racial and ethnic minority group members have been associated with increased risk for negative mental health outcomes such as PTSD (Loo, Fairbank, & Chemtob, 2005; Pole et al., 2005; Ruef, Litz, & Schlenger, 2000). Moreover, prior discriminatory experiences and discrimination from disaster responders may hinder accessing formal mental healthcare.

Social Support. Social support among racial and ethnic groups can be a significant protective factor against adverse mental health consequences. Kaniasty and Norris (2000) found many similarities among racial and ethnic groups when comparing comfort with emergency help-seeking among a sample of Hispanics, African Americans, and Caucasians. All three groups felt most comfortable seeking help from family than friends or outside support. In addition, all three racial/ethnic groups felt more comfortable seeking emotional and informational help as opposed to seeking tangible (material) help.

Researchers also suggest that there may be racial/ethnic differences in receiving social support (Kaniasty & Norris, 2000). Although some research suggest that racial and ethnic minorities have been found to seek similar levels of social support, they appear less likely than White Americans to receive social support after disasters (Galea et al., 2004; Kaniasty & Norris, 1995, 2000). This lack of support may have a particularly negative impact on collectivist cultures, which is underscored by findings that low social support among Hispanic participants partially accounts for their heightened risk of PTSD (Pole et al., 2005). One explanation that may account for this finding may be displacement after a disaster. In disaster-stricken settings, social ties are often disrupted and victims are unable to reach their social networks (Perilla et al., 2002; Weems et al., 2007). As social support can buffer traumatic stress reactions, disruption of social support can place victims at higher risk for adverse mental health outcomes.

Religious and Spiritual Support. The use of religious and spiritual support has been studied among racial and ethnic minority groups

(Bjorck, Cuthbertson, Thurman, & Lee, 2001; Culver, Arena, Wimberly, Antoni, & Carver, 2004). For example, prayer is one of the most important religious behaviors identified among African Americans and serves as a mechanism for coping with personal tragedy or adverse personal circumstances for many in this group (Taylor, Chatters, & Levin, 2004). Some studies examining social support indicated that African Americans were more likely to report relying on their religious or spiritual faith after disaster, while Caucasians were more likely to rely on family and friends (e.g., Elliot & Pais, 2006). In a study of African American, Hispanic, and Asian American respondents surveyed after September 11th, African American and Hispanic respondents used more religious coping strategies, such as prayer and attending church services, in comparison to other racial/ethnic groups (Constantine et al., 2005). The findings from social support literature regarding postdisaster outcomes indicate that mental health professionals should be aware of the nature and function of social and faith-based support networks (Constantine et al., 2005) in facilitating mental health treatment. In addition, mental health professionals should be aware of the beneficial role religiosity and spirituality has for certain racial and ethnic groups.

16.4. ENVIRONMENT AND COMMUNITY RESOURCES

16.4.1. Pre- and Peridisaster

16.4.1.1. Financial Resources and Infrastructure

One of the reasons that minority and low-income populations experience heightened exposure to disaster and its effects is a lack of financial and physical resources. Marginalized populations have a greater likelihood of living in poorly constructed, at-risk homes in communities with inadequate infrastructure (Bolin & Stanford, 1991; Quarantelli, 1994). Many racial and ethnic minorities live in older apartment buildings with unreinforced masonry, which is more susceptible to damage during disaster (Fothergill et al., 1999). In addition, marginalized populations are often more likely to live in hazardous areas (Bolin & Stanford, 1991; Curtis et al., 2007; Cutter, Boruff, & Shirley, 2003); for example, the site of many indigent neighborhoods during Hurricane Katrina made them more vulnerable to flooding (Curtis et al., 2007). Furthermore, poor infrastructure in these communities can result in lack of access to proximal medical and emergency services.

16.4.1.2. Crisis Preparation

Studies regarding crisis preparation for disasters suggest racial and ethnic minority and lower income groups are less likely to receive disaster instruction, such as making structural home improvements to mitigate damage, stockpiling emergency supplies, or developing an emergency plan to prepare for a disaster-related crisis (Fothergill et al., 1999). Language and communication problems also have been identified as barriers to receiving crisis preparation education from local governments (Gladwin & Peacock, 1997; Lindell & Perry, 2004; Peguero, 2006). Historically, many disaster and hazard warnings have been broadcast only in English, leaving many non-English speaking persons more susceptible to danger (Perry & Lindell, 1991; Perry & Mushkatel, 1986). Glik and colleagues (2004) investigated the accessibility of preparation education for primarily Spanish-speaking Hispanics in a national bioterrorism preparedness study. Hispanic participants in the study reported that there were no locally available crisis preparedness resources printed in Spanish, that they did not know where to receive Spanish language materials, and that they were concerned their needs would not get met in case of a bioterrorist attack. Owing to such barriers in communication, some racial and ethnic minority groups may rely on friends and family for disaster information rather than on the local government (Perry & Greene, 1982; Perry & Lindell, 1991).

Although they may be less likely to receive disaster education, some studies have found that racial and ethnic minorities tend to be more prepared for disasters. For example, Eisenman and colleagues (2006) analyzed data from the Los Angeles County Health Survey to examine crisis preparedness among racial and ethnic groups. African Americans and Latinos were significantly more likely to adopt preparedness actions after the September 11th attacks. This is consistent with Torabi and Seo's (2004) study showing that after the September 11th attack, African Americans were more likely than Caucasians to report gathering emergency supplies as part of a crisis preparation plan.

16.4.1.3. Emergency Response and Decision to Evacuate

Disparities in emergency response during a disaster can impact marginalized populations. For instance, there is a paucity of bilingual personnel among emergency response workers (Phillips & Ephraim, 1992), and forms and information are often distributed solely in the English language, contributing to disparity in access to relief. Furthermore, emergency personnel may be culturally insensitive, and the interactions between relief workers and victims can come to replicate larger social problems (Beady & Bolin, 1986; Katayama, 1992). For example, one hurricane study found that response workers restored power in African American communities only after restoring power in Caucasian communities and that African American communities received less shelter, food, and assistance (Beady & Bolin, 1986). Racial tension can also escalate during a disaster, leading to conflict between victims and disaster-response personnel (Weems et al., 2007). Another factor that contributes to disparities in emergency response involves the tendency of media to focus on wealthier areas, which leads to fewer volunteers and less assistance being directed toward disadvantaged neighborhoods (Rodrigue & Rovai, 1994).

With regard to decision to evacuate, in addition to factors such as disaster preparation, social support, and risk perception that were discussed earlier, lack of resources can also shape evacuation practices. Limited economic resources, in addition to lack of transportation and shelter options, hinder marginalized populations' ability to evacuate before and during a disaster. For example, Elliot and Pais (2006) found that New Orleans residents with household income in the $40,000 to $50,000 range were nearly twice as likely as those in the $10,000 to $20,000 range to evacuate before the storm as opposed to after the storm. The residents with the lowest income were most likely not to evacuate the city at all. After Hurricane Katrina, one of the most frequent reasons cited for not evacuating among shelter residents was a lack of resources or resource means (Curtis et al., 2007). In another study of hurricane survivors, almost one in ten nonevacuees cited low resources as a contributing factor, with Latinos being the most likely group to report this barrier (Riad et al., 1999).

16.4.2. Postdisaster

16.4.2.1. Availability and Accessibility of Services

Psychosocial resources play a central role in protecting disaster victims' mental health (Norris et al., 2002), and there are striking discrepancies in the use of mental health care among marginalized populations. Racial and ethnic minority groups, in particular, have been found to delay seeking mental health services until symptoms are more severe and turn to informal sources of support (e.g., family, religious support) instead of mental health care providers. Research examining health disparities among racial and ethnic minority groups has offered explanations for these discrepancies in utilizing mental health services. Pre- and postdisaster strain because of unemployment or job loss, loss of primary financial contributor in the family, and lack of health insurance has contributed to difficulties accessing mental health care (Hargraves & Hadley, 2003). Sue and colleagues (2006) add that the limited availability of culturally competent psychotherapists and culturally responsive services has significantly contributed to marginalized populations' underutilization of mental health care.

16.4.2.2. Crime

Although disaster studies have not examined the relation between race and ethnicity and postdisaster violence, it is clear that criminal violence increases after disaster. Looting behavior in the disaster aftermath is a common concern, and family violence and sexual assault incidents can increase after some disasters. For example, following Hurricane Andrew in Miami, domestic violence calls to the local community helpline increased by 50% (Laudisio, 1993), and over one-third of 1,400 surveyed residents reported that someone in their home had lost verbal or physical control in the 2 months since the hurricane (CDC, 1992). Researchers suggest that displacement of women and children from other family members, significant strain due to disaster effects on family, and women left alone without support are among the contributing factors.

16.5. IMPLICATIONS FOR RESEARCH, RESPONSE EFFORTS, AND PRACTICE

16.5.1. Gaps in Disaster Research

Our review highlights critical gaps in disaster research examining marginalized populations, specifically racial and ethnic minorities and individuals from lower income populations. Examination of the literature on sociocultural factors suggests differential use of social support among racial and ethnic groups. Assessments of how coping mechanisms such as religiosity are differentially utilized and perhaps have a different impact for various populations are warranted. Future research studies should examine how specific culture-bound beliefs affect disaster preparedness and response to disaster. Additional studies are needed to examine unique culture-specific variables that may be a protective factor pre-, peri-, and postdisaster. For example, several of the sociocultural factors noted in the chapter, such as social support (e.g., emphasis on extended family), are strengths among racial/ethnic minority communities and can serve as a protective factor in the face of disasters. Perceived discrimination and racism also may impact marginalized populations' preparedness and response, as well as help-seeking behavior. In addition, our review of environmental and community resources suggests that limited or lack of resources appears to significantly impact disaster-response in marginalized populations. Future studies should investigate how resource – or lack thereof – contributes to increased risk for exposure and delayed recovery.

Another area of disaster research where additional attention is warranted is the examination of biological factors associated with mental health sequelae. From a biologic perspective, important differences in DNA sequences (the basic unit of heredity) are found in the population in the United States, and elsewhere. These differences may have important implications for understanding psychiatric risk and resilience in response to disaster, as many prevalent postdisaster mental health problems have high heritability (Koenen, Nugent, & Amstadter, 2008). The literature is inconclusive with regards to the role of genetic risk or resilience factors and the extent to which these factors may be distributed across racial and ethnic groups. However, one consistent finding from genetics research in the field of traumatic stress is the striking inequality in racial representation among the existing genetic studies' samples. For example, six of the ten published PTSD candidate gene studies involve exclusively male samples, specifically non-Hispanic veterans. Our review suggests that studies of disasters need to include women, other racial and ethnic groups, and age groups in adequate number (e.g., by oversampling) to have adequate power to detect any potential meaningful findings or differences and to improve the generalizability of such studies. Overall, this review underscores the need for future studies to utilize a multifactor approach to disaster research examining marginalized populations to understand the complex interplay between variables and inform disaster efforts and treatment.

16.5.2. Disaster-Response Efforts

Development of a special needs assessment may significantly contribute to disaster response, especially for marginalized populations. The purpose of such an assessment is to help communities understand which citizens in their community have special needs, the risks they face from natural disasters, and strategies to help citizens with special needs prepare for, respond to, and recover from disasters (Bollig & Lynn, 2006). To use a special needs assessment as a tool for communities to prepare at-risk populations for natural disasters, Bollig and Lynn (2006) recommend identifying vulnerable populations and understanding the risks faced by special needs populations and what their needs are in relation to disaster management, design and direct emergency management, communication strategies, education and outreach processes, and risk reduction efforts.

16.5.3. Treatment Efforts

The disparities in access to and quality of care for marginalized populations are well documented, with marginalized communities throughout the United States tending to underutilize formal mental health services in comparison to majority populations. Mental health care practices should be informed by empirical knowledge and should include formal evaluation (Rosen, Young, & Norris, 2006), and treatment efforts should address the psychological, environmental, and social needs of marginalized populations (Norris et al., 2002). The lack of evidence-based interventions for disaster-affected communities and delivery to those most vulnerable to significant mental health outcomes has hampered treatment efforts.

Our review highlights the need for developing evidence-based and culturally informed interventions and educational resources that incorporate culturally specific issues salient to marginalized populations (e.g., emphasis on family vs. individually based techniques) and improve accessibility of care to these communities. This may require new, innovative methods of service delivery by mental health personnel. For example, the development of self-help resources and telehealth-based interventions may reduce financial and accessibility barriers identified in marginalized communities. Recent findings have demonstrated the feasibility of delivering empirically supported Web-based interventions to disaster survivors (Ruggiero et al., 2006).

16.6. CONCLUSIONS

In general, findings from studies examining disaster effects suggest that marginalized populations are at higher risk for problematic mental health outcomes than the mainstream. While it appears that race/ethnicity and SES may play an important role in the experience and consequences of disaster (Stamm & Friedman, 2000; Stamm, Stamm, Hudnall, & Higson-Smith, 2004), our review instead suggests that adverse mental health outcomes of disaster-exposed marginalized communities may be accounted for by the interaction of various risk factors before, during, and after disaster and have little to do with racial/ethnic status and SES independently. More research is necessary to shed light into how vulnerable populations are when affected by disasters and what can be done to prevent or alleviate any resulting adverse mental health outcomes.

REFERENCES

Adams, R. A., & Boscarino, J. A. (2005). Differences in mental health outcomes among Whites, African Americans, and Hispanics following a community disaster. *Psychiatry*, *68*, 250–265.

Aguirre, B. E. (1988). Evacuation in Cancun during Hurricane Gilbert. *International Journal of Mass Disasters*, *9*, 31–45.

Aptekar, L. (1990). A comparison of the bicoastal disasters of 1989. *Behavioral Science Research*, *24*, 73–104.

Bauer, H., Rodriguez, M., Quiroga, S., & Flores-Ortiz, Y. (2000). Barriers to health care for abused Latina and Asian immigrant women. *Journal of Health Care for the Poor and Underserved*, *11*, 33–44.

Beady, C. H., & Bolin, R. C. (1986). *The role of the black media in disaster reporting to the black community. working paper no. 56.* Institute for Behavioral Science, Boulder: University of Colorado.

Blaikie, P., Cannon, T., Davis, I., & Wisner, B. (1994). *At risk: Natural hazards, people's vulnerability, and disasters.* New York: Routledge.

de Bocanegra, H., & Brickman, E. (2004). Mental health impact of the World Trade Center attacks on displaced Chinese workers. *Journal of Traumatic Stress, 17,* 55–62.

Bolin, R., & Stanford, L. (1991). Shelter, housing, and recovery: A comparison of US disasters. *Disasters, 15,* 24–34.

Bollig, S., & Lynn, K. (2006). *Guidelines for conducting a special needs emergency management assessment.* Resources Innovations, University of Oregon Institute for a Sustainable Environment.

Bourque, L., Siegel, J., Kano, M., & Wood, M. (2006). Weathering the storm: The impact of hurricanes on physical and mental health. *The Annals of the American Academy of Political and Social Science, 604,* 129–151.

Bjorck, J. P., Cuthbertson, W., Thurman, J. W., & Lee, Y. S. (2001). Ethnicity, coping, and distress among Korean Americans, Filipino Americans, and Caucasian Americans. *Journal of Social Psychology, 141,* 421–442.

Brewin, C. R., Andrews, B., & Valentine, J. D. (2000). Meta-analysis of risk factors for posttraumatic stress disorder in trauma-exposed adults. *Journal of Consulting and Clinical Psychology, 68,* 748–766.

Center for Disease Control. (1992). *Post-Hurricane Andrew assessment of health care needs and access to health care in Dade County, Forida.* EPI-AID 93–09. Miami: Department of Health and Rehabilitative Services.

Cheever, K., & Hardin, S. (1999). Effects of traumatic events, social support, and self-efficacy on adolescents' self-health assessments. *Western Journal of Nursing Research, 21,* 673–684.

Cokley, K. (2007). Critical issues in the measurement of ethnic and racial identity: A referendum on the state of the field. *Journal of Counseling Psychology, 54,* 224–234.

Constantine, M., Alleyne, V., Caldwell, L., McRae, M., & Suzuki, L. (2005). Coping responses of Asian, Black, and Latino/Latina New York City residents following the September 11, 2001 terrorist attacks against the United States. *Cultural Diversity and Ethnic Minority Psychology, 4,* 293–308.

Constantine, M., Myers, L., Kindaichi, M., & Moore, J. (2004). Exploring indigenous mental health practices: The roles of healers and helpers in promoting well-being in people of color. *Counseling and Values, 48,* 110–126.

Culver, J. L., Arena, P. L., Wimberly, S. R., Antoni, M. H., & Carver, C. S. (2004). Coping among African-Americans, Hispanic, and non-Hispanic White women recently treated for early stage breast cancer. *Psychology & Health, 19,* 157–166.

Curtis, A., Mills, J., & Leitner, M. (2007). Katrina and vulnerability: The geography of stress. *Journal of Health Care for the Poor and Underserved, 18,* 315–330.

Cutter, S., Boruff, B. J., & Shirley, W. L. (2003). Social vulnerability to environmental hazards. *Social Science Quarterly. 84,* 243–261.

Dew, M., & Bromet, E. (1993). Predictors of temporal patterns of psychiatric distress during 10 years following the nuclear accident at Three Mile Island. *Social Psychiatry and Psychiatric Epidemiology, 28,* 49–55.

De Vries, M. (1996). Trauma in cultural perspective. In van der Kolk, B., McFarlane, A., & Weisath, L. (Eds.), *Traumatic stress.* New York: Guilford Press.

Eisenman, D., Cordasco, K., Asch, S., Golden, J., & Glik, D. (2007). Disaster planning and risk communication with vulnerable communities: Lessons learned from Hurricane Katrina. *American Journal of Public Health, 97,* S109–S115.

Eisenman, D., Wold, C., Fielding, J., Long, A., Setodji, C., Hickey, S., et al. (2006). Differences in individual-level terrorism preparedness in Los Angeles county. *American Journal of Preventive Medicine, 30,* 1–6.

Elliott, J., & Pais, J. (2006). Race, class, and Hurricane Katrina: Social differences in human responses to disaster. *Social Science Research, 35,* 295–321.

Faupel, C., Kelley, S., & Petee, T. (1992). The impact of disaster education on household preparedness for Hurricane Hugo. *International Journal of Mass Emergencies and Disasters, 14,* 33–56.

Flynn, J., Slovic, P., & Mertz, C. K. (1994). Gender, race, and perception of environmental health risk. *Risk Analysis, 14,* 1101–1108.

Fothergill, A., Maestas, E., & Darlington, J. (1999). Race, ethnicity and disasters in the United States: A review of the literature. *Disasters, 23,* 156–173.

Fothergill, A., & Peek, L. A. (2004). Poverty and disaster in the United States: A review of recent sociological findings. *Natural Hazards, 32,* 89–110.

Galea, S., Vlahov, D., Tracy, M., Hoover, D., Resnick, H., & Kilpatrick, D. (2004). Hispanic ethnicity and post-traumatic stress disorder after a disaster: Evidence from a general population survey after September 11, 2001. *Annals of Epidemiology, 14,* 520–531.

Garrison, C., Bryant, E., Addy, C., Spurrier, P., Freedy, J., & Kilpatrick, D. (1995). Posttraumatic stress disorder in adolescents after Hurricane Andrew.

Journal of the American Academy of Child and Adolescent Psychiatry, 34, 1193–1201.

Ginexi, E., Weihs, K., Simmens, S., & Hoyt, D. (2000). Natural disaster and depression: A prospective investigation of the reactions to the 1993 Midwest floods. *American Journal of Community Psychology, 28,* 495–518.

Gladwin, H., & Peacock, W. (1997). Warning and evacuation: A night for hard houses. In W. Peacock, B. Morrow, & H. Gladwin (Eds.), *Hurricane Andrew: Ethnicity, gender, and the sociology of disasters.* New York: Routledge.

Glik, D., Harrison, K., Davoudi, M., & Riopelle, D. (2004). Public perceptions and risk communications for botulism. *Biosecurity and Bioterrorism: Biodefense Strategy, Practice, and Science, 2,* 216–223.

Goltz, J., Russell, L., & Bourque, L. (1992). Initial behavioral response to a rapid onset disaster: A case study. *International Journal of Mass Emergencies and Disasters, 10,* 43–69.

Hargraves, J., & Hadley, J. (2003). The contribution of insurance coverage and community resources to reducing racial/ethnic disparities in access to care. *Health Services Research, 38,* 809–829.

Henkel, K., Dovidio, J., & Gaertner, S. (2006). Institutional discrimination, individual racism, and Hurricane Katrina. *Analyses of Social Issues and Public Policy, 6,* 99–124.

Holen, A. (1991). A longitudinal study of the occurrence and persistence of post-traumatic health problems in disaster survivors. *Stress Medicine, 7,* 11–17.

Ives, S. M., & Furseth, O. J. (1983). Immediate response to headwater flooding in Charlotte, North Carolina. *Environment and Behavior, 15,* 512–525.

Jones, R., Frary, R., Cunningham, P., Weddle, J., & Kaiser, L. (2001). The psychological effects of Hurricane Andrew on ethnic minority and Caucasian children and adolescents: A case study. *Cultural Diversity and Ethnic Minority Psychology, 7,* 103–108.

Kaniasty, K., & Norris, F. (1995). In search of altruistic community: Patterns of social support mobilization following Hurricane Hugo. *American Journal of Community Psychology, 23,* 447–477.

(2000). Help-seeking comfort and receiving social support: The role of ethnicity and context of need. *American Journal of Community Psychology, 28,* 545–581.

Katayama, T. (1992). *Aftermath of the Loma Prieta earthquake: How radio responded to the disaster.* INCEDE Report No. 2.

Koenen, K.C., Nugent, N.R., & Amstadter, A.B. (2008). Posttraumatic stress disorder: A review and agenda for gene-environment interaction research in trauma. *European Archives of Psychiatry and Clinical Neuroscience, 258,* 82–96.

Laudisio, G. (1993). Disaster aftermath: Redefining response-Hurricane Andrew's impact on I & R. *Alliance of Information and Referral Systems, 15,* 13–32.

Lindell, M., & Perry, R. (2004). *Communicating environmental risk in multiethnic communities.* Thousand Oaks, CA: Sage.

Loo, C. M., Fairbank, J. A., & Chemtob, C. M. (2005). Adverse race-related events as a risk factor for posttraumatic stress disorder in Asian-American Vietnam veterans. *The Journal of Nervous and Mental Disease, 193,* 455–463.

Markstrom, C., & Charley, P. (2003). Psychological effects of technological/human-caused environmental disasters: Examination of the Navajo and uranium. *American Indian & Alaska Native Mental Health Research, 11,* 19–45.

McFarlane, A. (1989). The aetiology of posttraumatic morbidity: Predisposing, precipitating and perpetuating factors. *British Journal of Psychiatry, 154,* 221–228.

McMillen, J. C., North, C. S., & Smith, E. S. (2000). What parts of PTSD are normal: Intrusion, avoidance or arousal? Data from the Northridge, California Earthquake. *Journal of Traumatic Stress, 13,* 57–75.

Morrow, B. (1997). Stretching the bonds: The families of Andrew. In W. Peacock, B. Morrow, & H. Gladwin (Eds.), *Hurricane Andrew: Ethnicity, gender, and the sociology of disasters.* New York: Routledge.

Morrow, B. (1999). Identifying and mapping community vulnerability. *Disasters, 23,* 11–18.

Norris, F., Friedman, M., & Watson, P. (2002). 60,000 disaster victims speak: Part II. Summary and implications of the disaster mental health research. *Psychiatry, 65,* 240–260.

Norris, F., Perilla, J., & Murphy, A. (2001). Postdisaster stress in the United States and Mexico: A cross-cultural test of the multicriterion conceptual model of posttraumatic stress disorder. *Journal of Abnormal Psychology, 110,* 553–563.

Palinkas, L., Downs, M., Petterson, J., & Russell, J. (1993). Social, cultural, and psychological impacts of the Exxon Valdez oil spill. *Human Organization, 52,* 1–13.

Peacock, W. (2003). Hurricane mitigation status and factors influencing mitigation status among Florida's single-family homeowners. *Natural Hazards Review, 4,* 149–158.

Peacock, W., & Mushkatel, A. (1986). *Minority citizens in disasters.* Athens: University of Georgia Press.

Peguero, A. (2006). Latino disaster vulnerability: The dissemination of hurricane mitigation information among Florida's homeowners. *Hispanic Journal of Behavioral Sciences, 28,* 5–22.

Perilla, J., Norris, F., & Lavizzo, E. (2002). Ethnicity, culture, and disaster response: Identifying and explaining ethnic differences in PTSD six months after Hurricane Andrew. *Journal of Social and Clinical Psychology, 21*, 20–45.

Perry, R., & Greene, M. (1982). The role of ethnicity in the emergency decision-making process. *Sociological Inquiry, 52*, 306–334.

Perry, R., & Lindell, M. (1991). The effects of ethnicity on decision-making. *International Journal of Mass Emergencies and Disasters, 9*, 47–68.

Perry, R., & Mushkatel, A. H. (1986). *Minority citizens in disaster*. Athens: University of Georgia.

Perry, R., & Nelson, L. (1991). Ethnicity and hazard information dissemination. *Environment Management, 15*, 581–587.

Phifer, J. (1990).Psychological distress and somatic symptoms after natural disaster: Differential vulnerability among older adults. *Psychology and Aging, 5*, 412–420.

Phillips, B. (1993). Cultural diversity in disasters: Sheltering, housing, and long-term recovery. *International Journal of Mass Emergencies and Disasters, 11*, 99–110.

Phillips, B., & Ephraim, M. (1992). *Living in the aftermath: Blaming processes in the Loma Prieta earthquake*. Working Paper No. 80. IBS, Natural Hazards Research and Applications Information Center, University of Colorado, Boulder.

Pole, N., Best, S., Metzler, T., & Marmar, C. (2005). Why are Hispanics at greater risk for PTSD? *Cultural Diversity and Ethnic Minority Psychology, 11*, 144–161.

Quarantelli, E. (1994). *Future disaster trends and policy implications for developing countries*. Newark, DE: Disaster Research Center.

Riad, J., Norris, F., & Ruback, R. (1999). Predicting evacuation in two major disasters: Risk perception, social influence, and access to resources. *Journal of Applied Social Psychology, 29*, 918–934.

Rodrigue, C. M., & Rovai, E. (1994). *Social construction of vulnerability: The "Northridge" earthquake*. Natural Hazards Workshop, Boulder, CO.

Rosen, C., Young, H., & Norris, F. (2006). On a road paved with good intentions, you still need a compass: Monitoring and evaluating disaster mental health services. In C. Ritchie, P. Watson, & M. Friedman (Eds.), *Mental health intervention following disasters or mass violence*. New York: Guilford Press.

Rudmin, F. (2003). Critical history of the acculturative psychology of assimilation, separation, integration, and marginalization. *Review of General Psychology, 7*, 3–37.

Ruef, A., Litz, B., & Schlenger, W. (2000). Hispanic ethnicity and risk for combat-related posttraumatic stress disorder. *Cultural Diversity and Ethnic Minority Psychology, 6*, 235–251.

Ruggiero, K. J., Resnick, H. S., Acierno, R., Coffey, S. F., Carpenter, M. J., Ruscio, A. M., et al. (2006). Internet-based intervention for mental health and substance use problems in disaster-affected populations: A pilot feasibility study. *Behavior Therapy, 37*, 190–205.

Sabogal, F., Marín, G., Otero-Sabogal, R., Marín, B., & Perez-Stable, E. (1987). Hispanic familism and acculturation. *Hispanic Journal of Behavioral Sciences, 9*, 397–412.

Sattler, D., Sattler, J., Kaiser, C., Hamby, B., Adams, M., Love, L., et al. (1995). Hurricane Andrew: Psychological distress among shelter victims. *International Journal of Stress Management, 2*, 133–143.

Shannon, M., Lonigan, C., Finch, A., & Taylor, C. (1994). Children exposed to disaster: I. Epidemiology of post-traumatic symptoms and symptom profile. *Journal of the American Academy of Child and Adolescent Psychiatry, 33*, 80–93.

Solberg, J., Ritsma, S., Davis, B., Tata, S., & Jolly, A. (1994). Asian-American students' severity of problems and willingness to seek help from university counseling centers: Role of previous counseling experience, gender, and ethnicity. *Journal of Counseling Psychology, 41*, 275–279.

Spence, P. R., Lachlan, K. A., & Griffin, D. R. (2007). Crisis communication, race, and natural disasters. *Journal of Black Studies, 37*, 539–554.

Stamm, B., & Friedman, M. (2000). Cultural diversity in the appraisal and expression of trauma exposure. In A. Halev, R. Yehuda, & A. McFarlane (Eds.), *International handbook of human response to trauma*. NY: Plenum Press.

Stamm, B., Stamm, H., Hudnall, A., & Higson-Smith, C. (2004). Considering a theory of cultural trauma and loss. *Journal of Loss and Trauma, 9*, 89–111.

Sue, S., Zane, N., Levant, R. F., Silverstein, L. B., Brown, L. S., Olkin, R., et al. (2006). How well do both evidence-based practices and treatment as usual satisfactorily address the various dimensions of diversity? In J. C. Norcross, L. E. Beutler, R. F. Levant, (Eds.), *Evidence-based practices in mental health: Debate and dialogue on the fundamental questions*. Washington DC: American Psychological Association.

Taylor, R. J., Chatters, L. M., & Levin, J. (2004). *Religion in the lives of African Americans: Social, psychological, and health perspectives*. Thousand Oaks, CA: Sage Publications.

Torabi, M. R., & Seo, D. (2004) National study of behavioral and life changes since September 11. *Health Education & Behavior, 31*, 179–192.

Trautman, R., Tucker, P., Pfefferbaum, B., Lensgraf, S., Doughty, D., Buksh, A., et al. (2002). Effects of prior trauma and age on posttraumatic stress symptoms in Asian and Middle Easter immigrants after terrorism in the community. *Community Mental Health Journal, 38*, 459–474.

Triandis, H., Marin, G., Lisansky, J., & Betancourt, H. (1984). Simpatia as a cultural script of Hispanics. *Journal of Personality and Social Psychology, 54*, 323–338.

Turner, R., Nigg, J., Paz, D., & Young, B. (1980). *Community response to earthquake threat in southern California*. Institute for Social Science Research, University of California, Los Angeles.

Vaughan, E. (1995). The significance of socioeconomic and ethnic diversity for the risk communication process. *Risk Analysis, 15*, 169–180.

Weems, C., Watts, S., Marsee, M., Taylor, L., Costa, N., Cannon, M. F., et al. (2007). The psychosocial impact of Hurricane Katrina: Contextual differences in psychological symptoms, social support, and discrimination. *Behaviour Research and Therapy, 45*, 2295–2306.

Wolfe, J., & Kimerling, R. (1997). Gender issues in the assessment of posttraumatic stress disorder. In J. Wilson & T. Keane (Eds.), *Assessing psychological trauma and PTSD*. New York: Guilford Press.

17 Journalism and Media during Disasters

ELANA NEWMAN, BRUCE SHAPIRO, AND SUMMER NELSON

17.1. INTRODUCTION

On Boxing Day 2004, Kimina Lyall, a newspaper reporter for *The Australian*, was on the Golden Buddha Beach, off Thailand's west coast, with her partner, when the water changed. "It hit our ears first. A roar, louder than an ascending jet, broke the blue and froze us all into stunned silence ... Way out to sea, impossibly far, a cloud of white water forming" (Lyall, 2007). Lyall was separated from her partner and witnessed friends and neighbors carried out to sea. She was one of the hundreds of thousands caught up in one of the great disasters of the contemporary era. But she was also by profession a journalist. "The fact that I was part of the tsunami story did not alter my responsibility as the Southeast Asia correspondent for *The Australian*. Within hours of the wave hitting, the acting editor was on the phone, checking to see if I was OK to get on the reporting task" (Lyall, 2005). She answered yes. Over the next week Lyall filed numerous stories recounting her community's wait for rescue and the wider impact in neighboring provinces. She visited dozens of morgues and 10 hospitals, writing longhand and dictating by often-interrupted telephone connections.

In a disaster, no sector of civil society bears more responsibility than the news media. Before, during, and after a disaster, news media are the essential vehicle for public perception of risk, preparedness, scope of disaster, the impact on victims and survivors, and lines of accountability. During a disaster, news media are the essential channel for information from government and rescue agencies, and these sources communicate potent images that stir the emotions of news consumers far from the disaster zone. Journalists themselves are often-overlooked first responders, rushing toward danger and immersing themselves in the lives of survivors along with rescue workers, humanitarian aid agencies, and military units.

This chapter reviews the role of journalists and news media during disasters, the challenges they face as professional witnesses, and reporters' risk and resiliency with respect to trauma-related psychopathology. After focusing on journalists themselves, the evidence regarding the impact of journalists' work upon the public is presented. This chapter concludes with recommendations for future scholarship, research, and practice.

17.2. JOURNALISTS AND MEDIA'S ROLE IN DISASTERS

At the time of a disaster, news reports serve as the public's eyes and ears, providing immediate information about the unfolding events. For example, a national phone survey less than a week after the September 11th attacks in New York City and Washington, D.C., indicated that American adults reported watching an average of 8.1 hours of television coverage of the events on that day, with 18% of respondents watching 13 hours or more (Schuster et al., 2001). In the 3 weeks after a tsunami affected Thailand, Indonesia, Sri Lanka, India, and the Maldives, over a third (34%) of a representative sample of Hong Kong residents reported watching more than 10 media reports of the event, with the entire sample reporting an average of 9.48 exposures, consisting of mostly televised or radio reports (Lau, Lau, Kim, & Tsui, 2006). Given technological advances such as satellite news gathering and Internet capacities to transmit information and images (Friend, 2006, p. xviii), journalists provide information about disasters in real time, often as information is being gathered about the cause, extent of damage and loss, and its implications.

The role of the media in disasters is complex. For purposes of discussing recent research it is helpful to separate that role into two overlapping components: (1) journalists in their professional role, as fact-finders, image-collectors, and narrators of first resort and (2) media in its institutional or corporate role, as a powerful and trusted medium for communication in civil society. With respect to journalists as those individuals who produce and transmit information, the term "journalist" not only refers to the reporters or photographers or videographers assigned to the disaster scene (or who, like Kimina Lyall, find themselves there by happenstance) but also describes managers and support staff generally invisible to news consumers: editors, producers, technicians, and other behind-the-scenes newsroom gatekeepers and personnel, who shape raw reports and choose how stories and images are presented. What is commonly known as "the first draft of history" is a team effort. This team of journalists has a narrative responsibility in democratic society – independently assessing significant events in the life of a community and ensuring accountability for the causes of and responses to disaster. Sometimes the search for narrative (if not always legal) accountability for disaster begins well after the fact, but it nonetheless shapes the perceptions of victims, surviving family members, and the broader public.

In their institutional capacity during disasters, print and online media often serve as direct, barely mediated channels for official government information (how to evacuate, where to find refuge or get help, what services are available, etc.) and for nongovernmental organizations such as the Red Cross or Red Crescent. In this institutional role, media can serve as a powerful "bulletin board," directly connecting individuals and families. In this sense, the media are the essential vehicle for crisis communication. For example, broadcast media conveyed information about safety, transportation routes, and volunteer needs in the immediate aftermath of the September 11th attacks. Such information about the crisis site and emergency response may prevent nonessential personnel from congregating around the disaster scene and interfering with the work of acute emergency responders. News media can also provide improvised mechanisms of communication that can help officials and survivors in the immediate aftermath of disaster. For instance, after the Oklahoma City bombing in 1995, the *Daily Oklahoman* created a column, "Searching for Survivors," which helped the State Health Department ascertain and contact survivors of the bombing in the days following the event (Simpson & Cote, 2006, p. 225). In 1992, the *Miami Herald* created a bulletin board for the community to communicate with each other during and after Hurricane Andrew, which affected much of South Florida (Clark, Sept. 11, 2001). Similarly, E-mails sent to the Web site of the *Times-Picayune* for the first 2 weeks after Hurricane Katrina provided rescue teams with the locations of stranded people around the city and facilitated communication among survivors. This public dialog also served to promote community engagement about disaster-related experiences.

17.3. JOURNALISM AS NARRATIVE

One of the consequences of technological change, a 24-hour news cycle, and immediate communication about disaster is that journalists can create the initial memories and images of these events for bystanders and, in some cases, even family members. Friend (2006) emphasizes that the public used to ask, "where were you when you heard about Kennedy's assassination?" rather than now, "where were you when you saw the World Trade Towers collapse?" While he focuses on the movement from sound to images, he is also describing a change in how events are communicated and apprehended. One may have "heard about" Kennedy's assassination from a neighbor, a school teacher, a coworker, and a newscast. By contrast, one could only "see" the World Trade Center collapse in two ways: as an eyewitness, or, far more commonly, through broadcast news images. The implication is that changes in technology have made such news images a nearly universal mediator of catastrophic events.

Once the basic information is relayed, such new stories and images provide vehicles for the community to create a collective narrative that delineates community strengths and vulnerabilities, and sets volunteer and civic action in motion. During Hurricane Katrina, staff at the New Orleans *Times-Picayune* achieved this as they remained in the shattered city, continuing to cover the news exclusively online until they could resume print format 4 days later. The public viewed this news outlet as a lifeline for reliable information on food, water, clothing, and information on missing relatives. Further, it helped people scattered across the country feel connected and begin to consider issues of reentry (Folkenflik, 2007). Researchers have found that social embeddedness is one of the strongest protective factors from psychological and physical distress postdisaster (Norris & Elrod, 2006, p. 34). The *Times-Picayune*'s efforts may have fostered such resiliency. Future studies need to examine what groups find what types of narratives about the event helpful and/or beneficial to public health and which are resented and/or harmful.

17.4. CHALLENGES OF REPORTING

Reporting on breaking news about disaster and catastrophe is no easy task, and journalists are faced with multiple challenges in obtaining and communicating verified information, especially as the event is unfolding. Often journalists and photojournalists arrive on the scene before rescue personnel, which not only may place them in physical danger but also can provoke ethical dilemmas about whether to intervene or document the situation (Simpson & Cote, 2006, p. 143). Key people with the most information are typically immersed in directly responding to the situation at hand, leaving little time to talk to reporters in the midst of a crisis response. Often disasters compromise communication systems (e.g., cellular phones, telephone, Internet, facsimiles) upon which journalists rely to exchange information.

While journalists' accounts of disaster may incorporate official information, health and science advice, or recommendations from officials, their main function is to provide an accurate picture of what is happening. This narrative function depends heavily on reporters' sources and location. It is not scientific. It requires rapidly assimilating journalists' own eyewitness accounts, interviews with witnesses or survivors, official and unofficial conjecture, images collected both professionally and by amateurs, and rumors. Lyall (2005) says of the Boxing Day tsunami: "on this assignment, everything was difficult. In the week I covered the tsunami story from the affected Thai provinces, I did not read a single newspaper, listen to a radio report in English, connect to the internet, or see international television coverage. I knew nothing about the story beyond what was written in my own notebook." In addition, in the context of a disaster, sources often cannot be phoned for verification and fact-checking as the story unfolds; hence, the quality of information may be problematic. For example, reports of extensive looting, assaults, and atrocities in New Orleans after Hurricane Katrina were simply inaccurate, although a few cases have been verified (Thevenot & Russel, 2005). Responsible journalists and news organizations publicly reexamine their own reporting in an effort to correct misinformation.

Disaster reporting itself challenges reporters' craft. Media professionals, at all levels, make difficult decisions about the content and format of news they impart. Picture editors must review multiple gory images, making decisions about what pictures to show the public, size and placement of images, whether and how to warn consumers about those images, and how to solicit and respond to public responses to those images. Nowhere is this balancing act more evident than in terrorism-related disaster, when timely and accurate information must be conveyed in a manner that does not further the terrorists' goal of producing widespread panic (Bull & Newman, 2002). Decision making may be very different for local journalists whose audience and needs differ from nonlocal journalists who need to communicate to people outside the community.

Compounding such difficulties, the newsroom itself may be compromised. For example, during Hurricane Katrina flood waters blocked the *Times-Picayune* building, including its newsroom and presses. The staff fled at the height of the storm, eventually relocating to Baton Rouge, some 80 miles away, working at first from a state university and then an improvised newsroom in a shopping mall. While a small team of reporters returned to the city across flooded roads, the news was provided exclusively online until paper editions began to be printed at another newspaper 40 miles from New Orleans (Romenesko, 2005). Similarly during September 11th, the *Wall Street Journal* had to relocate offices to an emergency back-up location to produce the newspaper, and radio and television broadcasters were forced to find alternative transmitters to the World Trade Center's aerial.

Reporting can also become personal as news staff cope with their own responses to calamity. Perspectives and professional boundaries get blurred when the tragedies covered directly affect journalists' workplace, home, community, and loved ones (e.g., Gilbert, Hirschkorn, Murphy, Walensky, & Stephens, 2002). New Orleans *Times-Picayune* reporters covering Hurricane Katrina lost housing, and many were separated from their families while doing their job. Kimina Lyall has written powerfully of the conflict between professional responsibility and commitment to her partner in the aftermath of the Boxing Day tsunami (Lyall, 2006).

In addition, most journalists receive no preparatory training in covering violence, interviewing victims, or experiencing the potential impact of traumatic stress on their own lives. Until recently, no newsroom managers were trained to support journalists on these difficult assignments. This situation is gradually changing. The first systematic approach to newsroom trauma support was developed in 2002 by the British Broadcasting Corporation, in conjunction with the Dart Center for Journalism and Trauma, as part of the news department's preparation for the Iraq war (Rees, 2007). Recent events in the United States, among them the Columbine school shootings, the Oklahoma City bombing, September 11th, and Hurricane Katrina, have persuaded news organizations to provide briefings for their staff. Two leading journalism training centers – the Poynter Institute and the American Press Institute – have sponsored well-attended seminars, and the Dart Center for Journalism and Trauma attracts prominent journalists from the United States and abroad to its annual Dart Center Ochberg Fellows Program. In Australia, the Australian Broadcasting Corporation is training all of its regional news bureaus in trauma awareness. Journalism educators now are showing growing interest in trauma-related curricula (e.g., Cane, n.d; Dworznik & Grubb, 2007). A pilot study suggests journalism students increased their short-term knowledge about traumatic stress and trauma-related reporting from such specialized curriculum, but it is unknown how long this information was retained (Mills et al., 1999). Existing methods to prepare journalists to be safe and resilient in the face of dangerous or traumatic work assignments need to be evaluated systematically. Similarly, more comprehensive industry-wide standards must be developed and evaluated.

17.5. REPORTERS AS WITNESSES

As professional witnesses of trauma, reporters and staff are directly and indirectly exposed to events that qualify as traumatic stressors. For example, journalists are often first on the scene of mass disasters, where they are exposed to direct danger and bear witness to death, injury, and destruction. In fact, like other first responders, 86% to 100% of journalists report high rates of exposure to potentially traumatic events (e.g., Newman, Simpson, & Handschuh, 2003; Pyevich, Newman, & Daleiden, 2003; Simpson & Boggs, 1999). A few general conclusions can be drawn from this emerging area of study despite the many methodological limitations of the current database. Rates of probable posttraumatic stress disorder (PTSD) among specialized war correspondents are high (i.e., more than one in four, or as many as 28%), whereas rates of probable PTSD among other groups of journalists range from average to low (between 4% and 13%; Newman et al., 2003; Pyevich et al., 2003; Teegen & Grotwinkel, 2001). Research on the impact of bearing witness on office-based presenters, researchers, production, and technical staff who select and process words and/or images; newsroom managers; and editors is sorely lacking. Future studies require studying groups that are representative of all journalists (or carefully defined subgroups of journalists) rather than self-selected or convenience samples. Future studies should transcend simply studying journalists' psychopathology; instead, a focus upon problems and concerns that are not in the clinical range, but that may affect journalists' quality of life, relationships, and their views about the world, would be far more instructive.

17.5.1. Risks

A subgroup of journalists, particularly war correspondents, appear to be at risk for PTSD, depression, and substance abuse problems (Feinstein, Owen, & Blair, 2002; Newman et al., 2003; Pyevich et al., 2003; Simpson & Boggs, 1999). Clearly, PTSD and related disorders are occupational hazards for journalists who cover stories that involve the pain and suffering of others. Potential risk factors that have been identified for increased risk and level of PTSD symptomatology among journalists include repeated exposure to both personal and professional traumatic events; low perceived social support/organizational support; and personality traits of neuroticism, anger, and hostility (e.g., Marais & Stuart, 2005; McMahon, 2001; Newman et al., 2003; Pyevich et al., 2003; Teegen & Grotwinkel, 2001). With respect to years in the field, there are inconsistent results. In studies that simultaneously analyze trauma exposure and years in the field (e.g., Newman et al., 2003; Pyevich et al., 2003) experience drops out as a meaningful risk factor, but in studies where experience is analyzed separately, years in the field remains as a risk factor for PTSD symptoms (McMahon, 2001; Simpson & Boggs, 1999).

Furthermore, good coverage of trauma requires empathetic engagement with the pain of others (Simpson & Cote, 2006), a task that has been shown in other responder groups to contribute to posttraumatic risk (Regher, Goldberg, & Hughes, 2002) but has never been examined among journalists. Given that journalists are seldom taught how to empathetically engage with others and simultaneously protect themselves psychologically, it is likely that this is a potential risk factor.

To understand the role of traumatic stressors, the overall role of occupational stressors in journalism needs examination. A qualitative study of 54 British reporters covering the Iraq war suggested that inadequate organizational support from management and inability to control aspects of the work were associated with stress and poor job satisfaction (Greenberg, Thomas, Murphy, & Dandeker, 2007). Since it is likely that the same is true for disaster reporting, future studies of journalists' occupational risk need to include both traumatic and daily stressors and outcomes such as absenteeism, turnover, and economic instability in the news industry. The impact of technology also deserves investigation, since technological changes enhancing remote reporting (e.g., personal computers, digital cameras, and cell phones) have also created a 24-hour work cycle, which may reduce collegial interactions.

17.5.2. Resiliency

Given the high level of traumatic events and pain they witness, journalists appear extremely resilient (Newman et al., 2003; Pyevich et al., 2003). Commitment to the mission of telling stories of the exploited and the opportunity to put their experiences into narrative may aid in resiliency. Furthermore, training and support from management and colleagues may assist journalists in resiliency (e.g., Greenberg et al., 2007). Several pilot studies suggest positive outcomes that lead to personal growth (McMahon, 2004, 2005). Therefore, future research should investigate potential signs of resiliency in the face of stress by journalists, measuring such factors as job performance indices (e.g., dependability, productivity of reporting, independent recognition such as awards for quality of reporting), job commitment, and the longitudinal trajectory of journalists' careers.

Understanding journalists' symptomatic and attitudinal responses to covering traumatic stories, including risk and protective factors, is a vital area of continued study. Beyond simple indicators of psychiatric morbidity and/or occupational problems and success, research focusing on the role that journalists' personal responses may have on the quality of disaster coverage is a necessary area of future scholarly attention (Newman, Davis, & Kennedy, 2006).

17.6. MEDIA'S EFFECT ON NEWS CONSUMERS AND THE PUBLIC

The often graphic nature of news reports and images following incidents of terrorism and disaster is undeniable, raising questions about the effect that news coverage of terrorism and disasters has on the public. What is the actual effect that these news stories – especially powerful broadcast images – have on the public? While a handful of studies, nearly all connected to television viewing, have been done to answer this question, the relationship is not yet fully understood.

17.6.1. Adults

In laboratory experiments, immediate increases in distress or anxiety have been correlated with viewing terrorism-related news, although none of these reactions were in the clinical range (Slone, 2000). Similarly, of 1,200 American adults surveyed from September 13th to the 17th of 2001, 92% of the sample reported experiencing feelings of sadness, 77% reported feelings of fright, and 45% reported feeling "tired out" while watching broadcast news about the attacks of September 11th (Pew Research Center, 2001). Such responses to television news coverage of disasters and terrorism are not necessarily pathological or even abnormal – these responses may be empathetic and appropriate reactions to upsetting events (Newman et al., 2006), unrelated to the way such news is presented. Moreover, the public often perceives disasters, especially those created or intensified by human design, as personal attacks or reminders of personal vulnerability rather than distant events affecting only those who were injured or killed (e.g., Dixon, Rehling, & Shiwach, 1993; Schuster et al., 2001).

Clearly learning about mass casualties is upsetting, but does it cause problems beyond these normal levels of distress? Among adults, there is a correlation between viewing news coverage and exhibiting symptoms of posttraumatic stress or complicated grief, especially those with direct disaster exposure. Three to five days after the September 11th attacks, a trend between number of broadcast images viewed and prevalence of trauma-related and depressive symptoms was noted among a sample of 1,008 adults in Manhattan (Ahern et al., 2002). This association was strongest for those experiencing direct losses or witnesses of the image of people plummeting from the towers. However, 5 to 8 weeks after the September 11th attacks, the association between number of viewed images of people jumping or falling from the World Trade Center towers and symptoms of PTSD and depression existed only among those who were directly exposed to the tragedy (Ahern et al., 2002). Among those who experienced a September 11th loss, adults who retrospectively (2–3 years later) reported watching the September 11th attacks live on television were those more likely to endorse symptoms consistent with complicated grief (Neria et al., 2007). In contrast, in a sample of New York City residents both directly and indirectly involved in the attacks, amount of broadcast news watched was correlated with the number of posttraumatic stress symptoms endorsed 2 months after the event, but specific imagery was not found to distinguish the symptomatic from the nonsymptomatic (Schlenger et al., 2002). Further examination of amount, type, and content of news, as well as survivor status and symptomatic distress, needs clarification; to date, it does appear that symptomatic survivors of disaster report more consumption of disaster-related news than nonsymptomatic survivors.

Nonetheless, studies have not conclusively demonstrated the presence of this same relationship in adults who are not directly affected by the disaster. A national phone survey conducted less than a week after the September 11th attacks noted a connection between heavy news exposure and symptoms of distress 3 to 5 days after the event (Schuster et al., 2001), as did a representative sample of Hong Kong households (who were not directly exposed) 2 to 4 weeks after the tsunami (Lau et al., 2006). However, a study 6 months after the 1995 bombing of the Alfred P. Murrah Federal Building in Oklahoma City did not identify a significant relationship between media exposure and distress about the event (Tucker, Pfefferbaum, Nixon, & Dickson, 2000).

Multiple explanations have been proposed to explain why this relationship may be more common in survivors. Continued exposure to reminders of the traumatic event by television news may prevent individuals from recovery by sustaining the initial high levels of psychological and physiological arousal (McFarlane, 1986; Newman et al., 2006). Televised news may serve to further consolidate conditioning between the events and emotional distress and/or trigger distressing memories or thoughts (Bernstein et al., 2007). The International Society for Traumatic Stress Studies (ISTSS) suggests that "media reminders that occur without warning are particularly troublesome for survivors because they contribute to a sense of helplessness, emotional imbalance, and lack of control" (ISTSS, 2002). Perhaps individuals affected by the event seek out media reports for information, solace, understanding, or other reasons. Alternatively, symptomatic survivors may selectively recall watching more terrorism-related news.

To further complicate the matter, the effects of anniversary coverage are not well understood, and thus far only one research team has examined its impact. With respect to the 1 year anniversary coverage of the September 11th attacks, people who reported watching more than 12 hours of televised anniversary coverage were three times more likely to develop probable PTSD; this relationship was especially strong among those who previously endorsed at least one PTSD symptom within the first week of the event (Bernstein et al., 2007).

17.6.2. Children

Although the research on children has many methodological flaws, it does appear that in comparison to adults, children report more symptomatic reactivity in response to disaster-related news (Nader, Pynoos, Fairbanks, Al-Ajeel, & Al-Asfour, 1993; Otto et al., 2007; Pfefferbaum et al., 1999, 2001; Saylor, Cowart, Lipovsky, Jackson, & Finch, 2003; Schuster et al., 2001). In contrast to their adult counterparts, both child survivors and nonsurvivors appear to report a relationship between terrorism-related news consumption and distress (Otto et al., 2007; Pfefferbaum et al., 1999, 2001; Schuster et al., 2001).

Less than a week after the attacks of September 11th, parents reported in telephone interviews that on September 11th their children had watched, on average, 3 hours of news coverage of the attacks, with older children tending to watch more (Schuster et al., 2001). While this amount of television exposure was less than the average amount of time adults had spent viewing news of the attacks, there was a relationship between the amount of reported television exposure and the number of symptoms parents reportedly observed in their children (Schuster et al., 2001). Another study also found a strong relationship between parents' reports regarding amount of their child's news consumption and PTSD symptoms for children under the age of 10 (Otto et al., 2007). Parental report, however, may be unreliable, representing parental distress and recall rather than the child's experience.

Other studies have discovered similar connections, determining that viewing disaster-related news is connected to symptoms of posttraumatic stress 4 to 8 weeks after the actual event (Nader et al., 1993; Pfefferbaum et al., 1999, 2001; Saylor et al., 2003; Terr et al., 1999). For example, two studies following the Oklahoma City bombing determined that there was a relationship between children's reported exposure to bomb-related television coverage and reported symptoms of posttraumatic stress 7 weeks after the bombing (Pfefferbaum et al., 1999, 2001). This held true for children who were not physically or emotionally connected to the events (Pfefferbaum et al., 2001). Similarly, children who watched the Space Shuttle Challenger disaster on television reported symptoms of posttraumatic stress, even without seeing the events first hand (Terr et al., 1999).

While studies demonstrate a relationship between children's reported exposure to news coverage and their symptoms of posttraumatic stress, explanations are sorely lacking. First, no evidence proves that viewing television coverage actually causes the posttraumatic stress symptoms in children. While it might be tempting to suggest that these stress responses are because of the news coverage itself, it is likewise possible that viewing news coverage of terrorism and disasters is a symptom of a distress and not the cause. In other words, children who exhibit these negative reactions could be more likely to seek out and view more coverage of disasters, perhaps to gather information and/or decrease their fears (Pfefferbaum et al., 1999, 2001). Owing to developmental differences between adults and children, children's emotional transient reactions may also be expressed more behaviorally than verbally as seen in adults.

Finally, research has yet to identify what types of news coverage are most associated with negative reactions in children. Most of the current research has focused on exposure to television news, ignoring, for the most part, news found in newspapers, on the radio, and on the Internet. One study did find that children who were exposed to Internet news exhibited more symptoms of posttraumatic stress than those who had been exposed to television and print news (Saylor et al., 2003). A possible explanation for this finding is that children could have had access through the Internet to forums where discussions of the events were more unfiltered than what one would find on television (Saylor et al., 2003). In examining children's reactions to war-related coverage, graphic images were more likely to be upsetting to younger children (aged 5–8), while older children (aged 13–17) were more likely to be frightened by the more abstract concepts in the news stories themselves (Smith & Moyer-Gusé, 2006). Determining whether this same relationship exists with coverage of disaster and terrorism would be useful.

17.6.3. Gaps in Knowledge

Overall it appears that news consumption is related to temporary increases in anxiety in the general public, both for adults and for children. For adults, only direct victims evidence an association between amount of accessed televised news coverage and PTSD symptoms. For children and adolescents, amount of broadcast news of the disaster appears related to distress regardless of their involvement in the disaster. Nevertheless, despite the correlation between news and distress, lasting symptoms for the majority of news consumers have not been documented (Michels, 2002).

More sophisticated research is needed. Rather than solely focusing on the relationship between televised news and distress, other forms of news media require attention. Furthermore, future research might directly measure actual news consumption rather than rely solely on self-report. Finally, few studies have examined the extent and duration of distress directly emanating from news coverage of disasters, an area that deserves greater attention.

Further clarity is needed to determine whether news reports of tragedy are a part of the stressor itself or part of the response to the stressor. Specifically, are media portrayals an actual part of the disaster, an additive malevolent stressor, a buffer to the event, a response indicator of distress, and/or an indicator of preexisting tendencies (e.g., seeking out news, avoidance)? Conceptual precision in research and analysis can help us understand more about the role and effects of media portrayal of tragedy on the public.

17.7. CONCLUSION

Knowledge about the impact of disaster reporting and images on the public needs to be addressed through more systematic and long-term research that can then inform the choices of news organizations, disaster planners, and individual news professionals. In addition, the impact of disaster reporting on individual journalists and the efficacy of training and support methods need careful evaluation. Such research needs to employ better sampling strategies, clearer definitions of phenomenon, and varied methodology. Such research can improve the journalists' own quality of life and ensure that these skilled and courageous professionals can maintain their resilience, judgment, and narrative capacity in the face of catastrophic events.

Journalists and the news media are an essential thread in the fabric of disaster response. While relief agencies and clinicians sometimes hold an understandable skepticism or even hostility toward the media, the powerful and complex role of journalists and news media before, during, and after catastrophic events needs to be understood as central to the mobilization of civil society, to the social ratification of the experiences of witnesses and survivors, and to the apprehension of traumatic events by survivors, witnesses, and the broader public. Maintaining an appreciation and understanding for the role of journalists, including their need for information to make autonomous decisions about the disaster and disaster response, will help all stakeholders in these events. As demonstrated throughout this book, disaster response requires a multidisciplinary response; journalists are indeed important responders.

REFERENCES

Ahern, J., Galea, S., Resnick, H., Kilpatrick, D., Bucuvalas, M., Gold, J., et al. (2002). Television images and psychological symptoms after the September 11 terrorist attacks. *Psychiatry, 65*(4), 289–300.

Bernstein, K. T., Ahern, J., Tracy, M., Boscarino, J. A., Vlahov, D., & Alea, S. (2007). Television watching and the risk of incident probable posttraumatic stress disorder: A prospective evaluation. *Journal of Nervous and Mental Disease, 195*, 41–47.

Bull, C., & Newman, E. (2002). *Covering terrorism*. Retrieved on September 30, 2007, from http://www.dartcenter.org/training/selfstudy/2_terrorism/text_00.html.

Cane, M. (n.d). *Covering trauma: UW curriculum offers important training for students*. Retrieved September 30, 2007, from http://www.dartcenter.org/training/teachers/covering_trauma.html.

Clark, R. (2001, September 11). *Advice from a veteran of disaster coverage*. Retrieved September 27, 2007, from http://www.poynter.org/content/content_view.asp?id=6296.

Dixon, P., Rehling, G., & Shiwach, R. (1993). Peripheral victims of the Herald of Free Enterprise disaster. *British Journal of Medical Psychology, 66*, 193–202.

Dworznik, G., & Grubb, M. (2007). Preparing for the worst: Making a case for trauma training in the journalism classroom. *Journalism and Mass Communication Educator, 62*(2), 190–210.

Feinstein, A., Owen, J., & Blair, N. (2002). A hazardous profession: War, journalists, and psychopathology. *American Journal of Psychiatry, 159*(9), 1570–1575.

Folkenflik, D. (2007, September 1). Katrina marked a turning point for 'Times Picayune'. *National Public Radio*. Retrieved September 27, 2007, from http://www.npr.org/templates/story/story.php?storyId=13984564&ft=1&f=1093.

Friend, D. (2006). *Watching the world change: The stories behind the images of 9/11*. New York: Picador.

Gilbert, A., Hirschkorn, P., Murphy, M., Walensky, R., & Stephens, M. (2002). *Covering catastrophe: Broadcast journalists report September 11th*. Chicago, IL: Bonus Books.

Greenberg, N., Thomas, S., Murphy, D., & Dandeker, C. (2007). Occupational stress and job satisfaction in media personnel assigned to the Iraq war (2003): A qualitative study. *Journalism Practice, 1*(3), 356–371.

International Society for Traumatic Stress Studies. (2002). *What does the news industry need to know about the science related to survivors, the public and news consumption?* Retrieved September 30, 2007, from http://www.istss.org/resources/news_consumption.cfm.

Lau, J. T. F., Lau, M., Kim, J. H., & Tsui, H. Y. (2006). Impacts of media coverage on the community stress level in Hong Kong after the tsunami on 26 December 2004. *Journal of Epidemiology and Community Health, 60*, 675–682.

Lyall, K. (2005, March). *The emotional toll of disaster reporting*. Retrieved September 30, 2007, from http://www.dartcenter.org/articles/personal_stories/lyall_kimina.html.

(2007). *Out of the blue: Facing the Tsunami*. Sydney, Australia: ABC Books.

Marais, A., & Stuart, A.D. (2005). The role of temperament in the development of post-traumatic stress disorder amongst journalists. *Psychological Society of South Africa*, *35*(1), 89–105.

McFarlane, A.C. (1986). Victims of trauma and the news media. *Medical Journal of Australia*, *145*, 664.

McMahon, C. (2001). Covering disaster: A pilot study into secondary trauma for print media journalists reporting on disaster. *Australian Journal of Emergency Management*, *16*(2), 52–56.

(2004, November). Journalists and trauma: The parallel world of growth and pathology through the 'salutogenic lens'. Presentation given at the International Society of Traumatic Stress Studies, New Orleans.

(2005). Journalists and Trauma: The parallel worlds of posttraumatic growth and posttraumatic stress – preliminary findings. *Proceedings of the 40th. APS Annual Conference, Melbourne, 188–192.*

Michels, R. (2002). Exposure to traumatic images: Symptoms or cause? *Psychiatry*, *64*, 304–305.

Mills, L.J., Simpson, R., Newman, E., Reynolds-Ablacas, P., Scherer, M., Maxson, J., et al. (1999). Examining the effectiveness of a trauma training program for journalists, presentation in F. Ochberg's Journalism and Trauma Symposium, 15th Annual Convention of the International Society for Traumatic Stress Studies, Miami.

Nader, K., Pynoos, R., Fairbanks, L., Al-Ajeel, M., & Al-Asfour, A. (1993). A preliminary study of PTSD and grief among the children of Kuwait following the Gulf crisis. *British Journal of Clinical Psychology*, *32*, 407–416.

Neria, Y., Gross, R., Maguen, S., Insel, B., Seirmarco, G., Rosenfeld, H., et al. (2007). Prevalence and psychological correlates of complicated grief among bereaved adults 2.5–3.5 years after September 11th attacks. *Journal of Traumatic Stress*, *20*, 251–262.

Newman, E., Davis, J., & Kennedy, S. (2006). Journalism and the public during catastrophes. In Y. Neria, R. Marshall, & E. Susser (Eds.), *9/11: Mental health in the wake of terrorist attacks*. Cambridge: Cambridge University Press.

Newman, E., Simpson, R., & Handschuh, D. (2003). Trauma exposure and post-traumatic stress disorder among photojournalists. *News Photographer*, *58*(1), 4–13.

Norris, F., & Elrod, C. (2006). Psychosocial consequences of disaster: A review of past research. In F. Norris, S. Galea, M. Friedman, & P. Watson (Eds.), *Research methods for studying mental health after disasters and terrorism: Community and public health approaches*. New York: Guilford Press.

Otto, M.W., Henin, A., Hirshfeld-Becker, D.R., Pollack, M.H., Biederman, J., & Rosenbaum, J.F. (2007). Posttraumatic stress disorder symptoms following media exposure to tragic events: Impact of 9/11 on children at risk for anxiety disorders. *Journal of Anxiety Disorders*, *21*, 888–902.

Pew Research Center. (2001, September 19). *American psyche reeling from terrorist attacks*. Retrieved September 30, 2007, from http://people-press.org/reports/display.php3?ReportID=3.

Pfefferbaum, B., Nixon, S.J., Tivis, R.D., Doughty, D.E., Pynoos, R.S., Gurwitch, R.H., et al. (2001). Television exposure in children after a terrorist incident. *Psychiatry*, *64*(3), 202–211.

Pfefferbaum, B., Nixon, S.J., Tucker, P.M., Tivis, R.D., Moore, V.L., Gurwitch, R.H., et al. (1999). Posttraumatic stress responses in bereaved children after the Oklahoma City bombing. *Journal of the American Academy of Child and Adolescent Psychiatry*, *38*(11), 1372–1379.

Pyevich, C., Newman, E., & Daleidan, R. (2003). The relationship among cognitive schemas, job-related traumatic exposure, and PTSD symptoms in journalists. *Journal of Traumatic Stress*, *16*, 325–328.

Rees, G. (2007, January 4). *From stigma to support: Fighting stress the royal marines' way*. Retrieved September 30, 2007, from http://www.dartcenter.org/articles/special_features/rees_trim.html.

Regher, C., Goldberg, G., & Hughes, J. (2002). Exposure to human tragedy, empathy, and trauma in ambulance paramedics. *American Journal of Orthopsychiatry*, *72*(4), 505–513.

Romenesko, J. (2005, September 1). *Times-Picayune* to resume printing. Message posted to http://poynter.org/forum/view_post.asp?id=10210

Saylor, C.F., Cowart, B.L., Lipovsky, J.A., Jackson, C., & Finch, A.J. (2003). Media exposure to September 11: Elementary school students' experiences and posttraumatic symptoms. *American Behavioral Scientist*, *46*(12), 1622–1642.

Schlenger, W.E., Caddell, J.M., Ebert, L., Jordan, B.K., Rourke, K.M., Wilson, D., et al. (2002). Psychological reactions to terrorist attacks: Findings from the national study of Americans' reactions to September 11. *Journal of the American Medical Association*, *288(5)*, 581–588.

Schuster, M.A., Stein, B.D., Jaycox, L.H., Collins, R.L., Marshall, G.N., Elliott, M.N., et al. (2001). A national survey of stress reactions after the September 11, 2001, terrorist attacks. *New England Journal of Medicine*, *345*(20), 1507–1512.

Simpson, R.A., & Boggs, J.G. (1999). An exploratory study of traumatic stress among newspaper journalists. *Journalism and Communication Monographs*, *1*(1), 1–26.

Simpson, R., & Cote, W. (2006). *Covering violence: A guide to ethical reporting about victims and trauma*. New York: Columbia University Press.

Slone, M. (2000). Responses to media coverage of terrorism. *Journal of Conflict Resolution*, *44*(4), 508–522.

Smith, S., & Moyer-Gusé, E. (2006). Children and the war on Iraq: Developmental differences in fear responses to television news coverage. *Media Psychology*, *8*(3), 213–237.

Teegen, F., & Grotwinkel, M. (2001). Traumatische erfahrungen und posttraumatische belastrungsstorung bei jounalisten: eine internet basierte studie. *Psychotherapeutic*, *46*(3), 169–175.

Terr, L. C., Block, D. A., Beat, M. A., Shi, H., Reinhardt, J. A., & Metayer, S. (1999). Children's symptoms in the wake of Challenger: A field study of distant-traumatic effects and an outline of related conditions. *American Journal of Psychiatry*, *156*, 1536–1544.

Thevenot, B., & Russel, G. (2005, September 26). Rumors of deaths greatly exaggerated. *The Times-Picayune*. Retrieved September 30, 2007, from http://www.nola.com/newslogs/tporleans/index.ssf?/mtlogs/nola_tporleans/archives/2005_09_26.html#082732.

Tucker, P., & Pfefferbaum, B., Nixon, S. J., & Dickson, W. (2000). Predictors of post-traumatic stress symptoms in Oklahoma City: wExposure, social support, peri-traumatic responses. *Journal of Behavioral Health Services and Research*, *27*(4), 406–416.

18 Uniformed Rescue Workers Responding to Disaster

SHANNON E. MCCASLIN, SABRA S. INSLICHT, CLARE HENN-HAASE, CLAUDE CHEMTOB, THOMAS J. METZLER, THOMAS C. NEYLAN, AND CHARLES R. MARMAR

18.1. INTRODUCTION

This chapter aims to impart an understanding of the potential impact of disaster response on uniformed first responders, including police officers and firefighters. This population deserves unique consideration as they are often asked to respond to disaster against the backdrop of an occupation that inherently places them at greater risk of trauma exposure. In the following pages we will review and discuss the prevalence of posttraumatic stress disorder (PTSD) and other psychiatric disorders and reactions, individual differences in risk and vulnerability for posttraumatic distress, and the prevention and treatment of posttraumatic distress in uniformed first responders.

Both human-made and natural disasters, such as the terrorist attacks of September 11, 2001, and Hurricane Katrina in 2005, can cause overwhelming destruction and tax the coping resources of survivors and disaster responders. In these situations we depend on first responders (e.g., police officers and firefighters) to take action and to aid those in need. At times these services are taken for granted without a great deal of consideration for the toll that such sacrifice can take on an individual responder or the overall agency. Although certain characteristics may cause first responders to be uniquely resilient (e.g., selection and training), long hours and repeated exposure to potentially traumatic stressors in the context of disaster place first responders at heightened risk for psychological distress (McCaslin et al., 2006; Weiss et al., 1999).

It has been recognized for decades that disaster workers may experience negative psychological effects following disaster response. In 1977, Heffron observed stress reactions in helpers responding to a massive flood and attributed these reactions to the helpers being "continually faced with the tragic reality of the disaster, encountering deteriorating situations where they felt frustrated and unable to help and the feelings of being continually emotionally drained" (Heffron, 1977, pp. 103–111). Raphael and colleagues (1983) observed and attempted to quantify stress reactions in relief workers responding to the Granville rail disaster in 1977, when a commuter train in a Sydney suburb derailed and crashed into the stanchions of a concrete bridge, which then collapsed on the train. Seventy percent of the relief workers responding to this disaster reported psychological distress related to the magnitude of the disaster, mutilation of the bodies, anguish of the victims' relatives, the pressure of working under emergency conditions, and uncertainty about how active a role they should take in the disaster response. In particular, many disaster workers expressed that they experienced feelings of helplessness. Another study in 1983 reported that rescue workers experienced symptoms such as repeated intrusive memories, sadness, anxiety, and startle reactions following response to the sudden collapse of two skywalks in a hotel lobby in 1981, in which 114 people were killed and 200 were injured (Wilkinson, 1983).

Following these initial studies, Raphael and Middleton (1987, p. 1336) concluded that, "there is a need to look at the 'hidden' victims of disaster, the relief workers themselves." Other investigators were also calling for increased attention to this area (Bartone, Ursano, Wright, & Ingraham, 1989; Durham, McCammon, & Allison, 1985; Jacobs, 1995; Wright, Ursano, Bartone, & Ingraham, 1990). Since that time, the field of trauma research has experienced a rapid growth in investigations and awareness concerning the increased risk for acute and chronic stress reactions among first responders and disaster workers following disaster-related experiences.

18.2. PREVALENCE OF POSTTRAUMATIC DISTRESS IN UNIFORMED FIRST RESPONDERS

As is true in the general population, the majority of uniformed first responders will experience little or no lasting impairment following exposure to a potentially traumatizing experience. However, a minority of responders may continue to experience psychological distress following disaster response, including symptoms of PTSD, depression, alcohol use, and other anxiety disorders. The majority of research in this area, though, has focused on rates of PTSD and associated problems. The general prevalence of PTSD has been estimated to be 7% to 18.2% among emergency services personnel (Marmar, Weiss, Metzler, Ronfeldt, & Foreman, 1996; McFarlane, 1988c; Robinson, Sigman, & Wilson, 1997; Stein, Walker, Hazen, & Forde, 1997; Ursano, Fullerton, Kao, & Bhartiya, 1995; Wagner, Heinrichs, & Ehlert, 1998, Weiss, Marmar, Metzler, & Ronfeldt, 1995) and has been reported to be as high as 26% among police officers who witnessed traumatic victimization of others (Martin, McKean, & Veltkamp, 1986). Many estimates for first responders are relatively higher than the 3.5% one-year prevalence (Kessler, Chiu, Demler, Merikangas, & Walters, 2005) and the 6.8% lifetime prevalence (Kessler et al., 2005) estimates of PTSD among adults (aged 18 to over 60 years) in the general population, 9.2% among adults belonging to an urban health maintenance organization (Breslau, Davis, Andreski, & Peterson, 1991), and 12.3% among a nationally representative sample of women (Resnick, Kilpatrick, Dansky, Saunders, & Best, 1993).

Rates of PTSD among first responders exposed to disaster, whether human-made or natural, vary considerably. Most of the studies in this area have been cross-sectional studies surveying first responders following disaster response, an understandable methodology given the ethical issues surrounding the study of disaster survivors and responders. However, in one of the few studies to have collected pre- and post-disaster data, Marmar and colleagues (2003) surveyed 553 New York City and 194 Bay Area police officers approximately 1.5 years before the September 11th World Trade Center attacks and conducted a follow-up survey approximately 18 months after the attacks with the New York City Police Department (NYPD) officers, asking specifically about how disaster response had impacted their mental health. Sudden and by human design, the terrorist attacks of September 11th were overwhelming in scale, causing horror and sadness throughout the United States. The fear and chaos in New York City, a primary target of this disaster, was particularly palpable. Police and firefighters responding to the disaster that day were hailed as heroes, facing intense needs from survivors and victims and losing colleagues who rushed to provide aid. Before the attacks, 3.5% of the officers met criteria for current PTSD and 3.5% for partial PTSD. Following the attacks, 8.8% of the NYPD officers met criteria for current PTSD and 15.0% for subsyndromal PTSD. A rate of 6.2% of police officers with PTSD was reported by Perrin and colleagues (2007) in their study of first responders who provided aid following the September 11th attacks. Both estimates compare strikingly with a rate of 0.6% for current PTSD and 4.7% for subsyndromal PTSD in a demographically representative sample of adult residents of Manhattan living south of 110th Street surveyed 6 months after the attacks (Galea et al., 2003).

Several other researchers have also reported relatively high rates of PTSD and associated symptoms among first responders following disaster response. North, Tivis, McMillen, Pfefferbaum, Spitznagel and colleagues (2002) reported on a sample of 181 firefighters responding to the Oklahoma city bombing; 13% were diagnosed with PTSD, a high rate but lower than that for the primary survivors (23%). In the firefighter group, 38% met criteria for at least one postdisaster psychiatric disorder. Higher rates of alcohol disorders (24% postdisaster) were seen among the disaster workers than among the primary survivors; however, the onset of the alcohol disorders in the workers occurred predominately before the disaster and was more common in those who also had predisaster psychopathology.

Hurricane Katrina, that hit the Gulf Coast, including New Orleans, in 2005 was devastating in scope, with even higher rates of PTSD and other mental health symptoms reported 7 to 13 weeks afterward (Centers for Disease Control and Prevention [CDC], 2006). This natural disaster required police and firefighters to respond amid concerns for their own families and homes as well as hostility and aggression directed at police and other responders in some communities; in addition, the responders worked long hours and experienced sleep deprivation. In a sample of 525 firefighters, 114 (22%) reported symptoms consistent with PTSD, and 133 of 494 (27%) reported major depressive symptoms. Among 912 police officers, 19% (170) reported PTSD symptoms, and 26% (227 of 888) reported symptoms of major depression. In another study conducted after a natural disaster, 21% of 84 firefighters responding to an earthquake in Taiwan had posttraumatic distress 5 months subsequent to the disaster (Chang et al., 2003).

Thompson (1993) reported on a survey of 28 police officers and 40 ambulance workers involved in body recovery duties during several different disasters. The police officers were found to score lower on measures of PTSD and general health symptoms than ambulance workers, with PTSD scores being only slightly higher than normal comparison. However, 16% of police officers did endorse posttraumatic distress, with 3% in the moderate to severe category.

Other studies have found relatively lower rates of PTSD and other distress in this population. Three percent of firefighters (N = 1,996) responding to an air disaster in Amsterdam reported a moderate to severe traumatic reaction (Witteveen et al., 2007). Although a smaller proportion endorsed symptoms in the moderate to severe range, many experienced associated disturbances and symptoms such as anxiety symptoms (12%), somatic complaints (17%), sleep disturbances (23%), and fatigue (17%). They reported significantly higher levels of PTSD, anxiety, depression, somatic complaints, sleep disturbances, and PTSD symptoms than non–disaster exposed police officers also assessed.

Gabriel and colleagues (2007) interviewed three different samples, survivors (N=127), general population (N=485), and police officers involved in rescue efforts (N=153), who had been exposed to the March 11, 2004, terrorist bomb attacks on commuter trains in Madrid on average 2 months following the event. In this study, it was striking that only 1.3% of police officers met criteria for PTSD, whereas rates were 44.1% among those injured and 12.3% among the residents of the city. Similarly, the prevalence of major depression was 31.5% among the injured, 8.5% among the general population, and 1.3% among police officers. The low reported rates in the police officers may represent resilience or reluctance to disclose emotional distress because of stigma and concerns about career impact.

18.2.1. Additional Psychiatric Reactions to Disaster Response

Trauma-exposed first responders are also at risk of developing other psychiatric symptoms and conditions such as depression, substance abuse, and other anxiety disorders (Duckworth, 1986; Ersland, Weisaeth, & Sund, 1989; Fullerton, Ursano, & Wang, 2004; Jones, 1985; Marmar et al., 1996; Weiss et al., 1995). Generally, other mental health problems such as dysphoria, peritraumatic dissociation, and subjective poor mental health have been estimated to occur at a rate of 9% to 32% among emergency responders (Duckworth, 1986; Ersland et al., 1989; Jones, 1985; Marmar et al., 1996; Weiss et al., 1995). Liao and colleagues (2002) measured psychological distress in 1,104 rescue workers who provided aid after a major earthquake in 1999. Severe psychological distress was reported by

137 (16.4%) subjects. Of those reporting severe psychological distress, the types of symptoms most commonly reported were phobic-anxiety (18.7%), hostility (17.6%), obsessive-compulsive symptoms (16.2%), depression (14.9%), paranoid ideation (14.2%), interpersonal sensitivity (13.3%), psychoticism (11.9%), anxiety (10.8%), and somatization (6.2%).

Conditions such as depression and substance use are highly comorbid with PTSD. Wagner and colleagues (1998) investigated the presence of other disorders among firefighters (both those with and those without PTSD) and reported that 39.7% suffered from depressive mood, 60.3% displayed social dysfunction, and 19.0% were substance abusers. In a subsequent study of firefighters who had responded to an Australian bushfire, McFarlane and Papay (1992) reported that only 16 out of a total of 147 participants diagnosed with PTSD did not meet criteria for an additional disorder. Among those with PTSD, 51% were also diagnosed with major depressive disorder (MDD), 39% with generalized anxiety disorder, 37% with panic disorder, 33% with a phobic disorder, 13% with obsessive-compulsive disorder, and 8% with a manic episode. In the study of NYPD police officers following September 11th exposure, in addition to increased PTSD symptoms, the officers showed a significant increase in general psychiatric symptoms, anxiety, and depression, and significantly decreased quality of life, social adjustment and support, and quality of sleep from before September 11th (Marmar et al., 2003).

In addition to mental health symptoms, disaster-related experiences can impact responders' health, quality of life, and functioning. Slottje and colleagues (2008) examined the use of health care by 1,468 police officers after an air disaster in Amsterdam that took place in 1992. The questionnaire assessment took place on average 8.5 years postdisaster. Eight hundred and thirty-four of the officers reported engagement in disaster-related tasks and 634 were not exposed. Involved police officers were found to use health care (e.g., a general practitioner, medical specialist, paramedical specialist, privately practicing psychologist, or psychiatrist) more often and also reported more frequent self-initiated use of drugs (as opposed to prescribed use) and of sleeping pills or tranquillizers. Prescribed use of drugs and hospitalization was not increased for the involved officers. Increased self-initiated rather than prescribed medication use may reflect the understandable reluctance of police officers to ask for assistance from medical professionals. Forty-one percent of the involved police officers with physical or psychological health complaints attributed these to the air disaster in Amsterdam, including its aftermath. Firefighters who had responded to the disaster also reported a significantly lower health-related quality of life (e.g., physical functioning, bodily pain) than those who did not respond. Police officers exposed to the disaster work also reported significantly poorer physical health and mental health-related quality of life than nonexposed police officers.

Gross and colleagues (2006) examined the relationship between mental health and physical health symptoms in 1,131 workers who participated in the clean-up effort following the September 11th World Trade Center attacks. In addition to reporting significant psychological symptoms (13.5% probable PTSD, 16.1% major depression, 7.2% panic disorder, 6.8% alcohol use), these workers also reported significant physical health concerns (73% current cough, 84% current wheezing, and 19.8% past or present asthma). All estimates of mental and physical health problems were significantly greater than for those in a group of unexposed workers. Interestingly, probable PTSD was associated with respiratory problems, highlighting the impact that each problem may have on the other.

A greater increase in the number of sick days during the first year after disaster response has been shown among responders with psychological problems, such as PTSD and burnout (Morren, Dirkzwager, Kessels, & Yzermans, 2007). PTSD has also been shown to be associated with reduced job satisfaction and functional impairment (North et al., 2002).

There are many reasons why rates of PTSD and other psychological disorders may vary across studies. Factors contributing to lower reports of mental health symptoms or resilience among first responders include (1) strictness of screening procedures, (2) underreporting of symptoms because of stigma and fear of how one may be judged as able to do his/her job (Perrin et al., 2007), (3) uniqueness of the study sample (e.g., Gabriel and colleagues [2007] had studied an elite corps of police officers with extensive training in the handling of terrorist attacks), (4) career selection, (5) preparedness and training, (6) fewer injuries incurred during the work (North, Tivas, McMillen, Pfefferbaum, Spitznagel et al., 2002), (7) good management and organization (e.g., encouraged to take a break if needed) (Thompson, 1993), and (8) postdisaster mental health interventions (education and debriefings) (North, Tivas, McMillen, Pfefferbaum, Spitznagel, et al., 2002). Factors contributing to reports of greater levels of symptoms may include environmental factors such as civil disobedience, hostility, and aggression toward law enforcement, as in the case of Hurricane Katrina (CDC, 2006), and participation in response activities for which the responder was not trained (CDC, 2006; Marmar et al., 1996).

18.2.2. Symptom Course

The traumatic stress symptoms experienced by rescue workers can be quite chronic in nature. One of the worst disasters to hit the San Francisco Bay Area in decades was the 1989 Loma Prieta earthquake. This magnitude 7.1 earthquake wreaked havoc on buildings and roads and caused a major freeway collapse. Emergency service workers deployed to the disaster faced personal threat as aftershocks rolled through the Bay Area, and many were not even sure if their own loved ones were safe or their homes were intact. Approximately 1 year following this tragedy, Marmar and colleagues (1996) surveyed responders to the I-880 freeway collapse (i.e., police, firefighters, emergency medical technician [EMT]/paramedics, and California Department of Transportation [Caltrans] road workers), and two other groups of first responders: (1) emergency services personnel residing in the Bay Area but not deployed to the freeway collapse and (2) responders residing in San Diego at the time of the earthquake. The groups were very similar with regards to demographics, experience, and level of current posttraumatic stress symptoms (9%). However, the responders to the I-880 freeway collapse reported greater stress exposure, greater immediate threat appraisal at the time of the incident, and more sick days.

Over 3 years later, follow-up assessment of 322 of the rescue workers who responded to the Loma Prieta earthquake freeway collapse revealed that those who had moderate to high levels of trauma-related distress at the initial assessment continued to report chronic symptomatic distress (Marmar et al., 1996, 1999). The sample as a whole reported modest improvements in intrusive and avoidant symptoms of PTSD and improved work and interpersonal functioning. There were marginally greater levels of general psychiatric symptoms and no change in hyperarousal symptoms.

McFarlane and colleagues (McFarlane, 1986, 1988c; McFarlane & Papay, 1992) conducted several studies on the impact of responding to the Ash Wednesday bushfire on over 400 volunteer firefighters. The bushfire occurred in South Australia in 1983 and caused destruction to 2,804 square kilometers that included national park land and orchards. Several thousand trained volunteer firefighters were exposed to extreme and unrelenting danger for many hours. Three were killed and many injured, and some sustained losses of their homes, stock, and farms. The researchers found that 31% of firefighters qualified for a diagnosis of PTSD at 4 months, 27% at 11 months, and 30% at 29 months, with the majority of those highest in distress at 4 months remaining highly symptomatic at 29 months. Fifty-six percent of those who had been diagnosed with PTSD immediately after the bushfire remained symptomatic 42 months later (McFarlane & Papay, 1992). When reassessed 8 years after the disaster, only 4% met full criteria for a diagnosis of PTSD (McFarlane, 2000); however, 60% continued to report significant intrusive and hyperarousal symptoms as reported earlier at 42 months. It was suggested that the relatively smaller proportion of firefighters meeting diagnostic criteria for PTSD at 8 years was accounted for by subthreshold avoidant symptoms. Symptoms were found to fluctuate significantly over time in approximately half of the firefighters with chronic PTSD.

Additional studies have provided further evidence for the long-lasting nature of such symptoms. In a 4-year longitudinal study of disaster workers responding to the explosion of a fireworks depot in the Netherlands in May 2000, Morren and colleagues (2007) found that the negative effects of disaster may last for years and that some effects may have delayed onset of a year or more after the event. Approximately one-third of police officers who had responded to an aviation disaster at a California shopping mall reported moderate to high distress 6 months following the disaster (Foreman & Eranen, 1999). At 12- and 18-month follow-up, the authors found little change in levels of symptomatology. Forty-one police officers were surveyed 18 months after providing aid during a discotheque fire in 1998 with the intention to determine the occurrence of PTSD (Renck, Weisaeth, & Skarbo, 2002). The researchers found that after 18 months several of the 41 officers continued to experience posttraumatic stress symptoms and general distress symptoms. Only one officer had an IES-R intrusion score that suggested a stress reaction of clinical significance. However, 19 were still at a medium level on the intrusion subscale. Seven percent had a high level of psychological distress, and most of the officers showed various degrees of reduced social functioning.

At least first responders study has not provided support for the chronic nature of symptoms. Alexander (1993) surveyed body handlers responding to an oil platform disaster, where the police officers duties included retrieval and identification of human remains. The officers were surveyed initially several months following the disaster and again at a 3-year follow-up. At neither point of time did results suggest that officers experienced an adverse reaction, and most did not develop long-term psychiatric morbidity. Indeed, symptoms of anxiety significantly *declined* at each point of time. The authors emphasized the role of good organizational preparation and "sensitive staff management" in the mental health of the responders. Optimizing the work environment may mitigate the psychological risks to disaster-exposed responders (Liberman et al., 2002; Maguen et al., 2007).

18.3. INDIVIDUAL DIFFERENCES IN RISK AND VULNERABILITY FOR POSTTRAUMATIC DISTRESS

Given the complex nature of stressor exposure in rescue workers, the potentially chronic course of symptoms, and the degree to which symptoms may contribute to adjustment problems in social, family, and work settings (Stein et al., 1997; Zatzick et al., 1997), screening and early intervention are vital. To develop targeted interventions, it is necessary to understand the variables that predispose a rescue worker to be more vulnerable to developing mental health symptoms following critical incident exposure. Although the risk of stress reactions is higher among emergency responders than in the general population, as we can see from the earlier studies cited, there remains considerable variability in who will develop such reactions following exposure to a highly stressful event. A number of pretraumatic, peritraumatic, and posttraumatic individual differences likely act together to impact one's vulnerability or resilience to developing distress following traumatic exposure.

Factors that predict posttraumatic distress in the general population are also important in predicting which responders will go on to develop significant mental health symptoms following disaster work. These variables include female gender (Renck et al., 2002); preexisting psychopathology (North, Tivas, McMillen, Pfefferbaum, Spitznagel, et al., 2002); minority status (Pole et al., 2001); prior negative life events (McFarlane, 1988a, 1989); psychological traits, such as adjustment, locus of control, and general dissociative tendencies (Marmar et al., 1996); personality traits, including greater neuroticism (Hodgins, Creamer, & Bell, 2001); greater peritraumatic dissociation and peritraumatic emotional distress (Marmar et al.,

1994, 1996); degree of exposure to the trauma (Marmar et al., 1996); lower social support (Fullerton, McCarroll, Ursano, & Wright, 1992; Lazarus & Folkman, 1984; Marmar et al., 1999; Solomon, Mikulincer, & Avitzur, 1988; Terry, 1994); and coping style (e.g., escape-avoidance coping, distancing) (Chang et al., 2003).

Preexisting negative beliefs about oneself, the world, and others may also predispose both civilian and first responders to distress following trauma exposure. Bryant and Guthrie (2007) reported that pretrauma negative self-appraisals were a risk factor for PTSD in firefighters assessed during training and reassessed 4 years later. In addition to the factors listed earlier, there are a number of variables unique to the work of emergency responders that influence the risk of experiencing distress related to disaster response. These include the type of exposure, with perceived threat to the life of responders increasing risk (McCaslin et al., 2006); degree of identification with the injured or deceased; other compounding life events; training and experience; and organizational factors.

18.3.1. Trauma Exposure

Perhaps the most important risk factor is simply that responders are likely to experience higher exposure to traumatic and stressful events than individuals in the general population. Within police work, for example, Beaton and colleagues (1998) sampled 173 firefighters/EMTs who ranked the stressfulness of 33 actual and/or potential duty-related incident stressors and reported how often they had experienced these stressors within the past 6 months. Results suggested that these workers encounter the following categories of stressors quite often: catastrophic injury to self or coworker (40%), gruesome victim incidents (10%), rendering aid to seriously injured and vulnerable victims (5%), minor injury to self (4%), and exposure to the dead and dying (4%).

The risk of exposure to trauma and stressors among first responders increases during disaster response. Uniformed emergency service personnel are frequently among the first to arrive at the scene of an event and not only are often responsible for caring for the victims, but also are subject to the circumstances surrounding the scene of the event. For example, a police officer may not only need to aid a victim of a violent crime, but he or she may also confront a scene that may be directly traumatizing. Experiences such as witnessing dead bodies and destroyed buildings, and enduring a sense of possible future danger for themselves, their families, or community, can cause a scene to be particularly stressful. In addition to frequently placing themselves in dangerous situations and being confronted with and providing aid to those who are suffering or are traumatized, responders also have to contend with the added challenge of high levels of routine work and organizational stressors.

Specific disaster-related experiences have been linked to mental health symptoms in much previous research. In a study of volunteer firefighters responding to a firework depot explosion in the Netherlands, disaster-related experiences such as fire extinguishing and rescuing victims or recovering bodies were related to PTSD subscale and total scores (Morren, Yzermans, van Nispen, & Wevers, 2005). Chang and colleagues (2003) reported that contact with dead bodies, not overall trauma exposure, was related to psychiatric symptoms. Following the September 11th terrorist attacks, Perrin and colleagues (2007) found that risk of PTSD among responders, with the exception of firefighters, was increased if the responder had been involved in evacuating individuals from one of the World Trade Center towers. Lower health-related quality of life among firefighters responding to an air disaster was reported to be related to exposure to rescuing people and clean-up of the disaster area (Slottje et al., 2007). Exposure variables related to psychological symptoms among police officers responding to this disaster included supporting injured victims and workers or having close ones affected by the disaster.

Events that are characterized by a high level of personally relevant threat, including threat of serious injury or death to oneself or a close associate (e.g., fellow officer, have been shown to place emergency services personnel at greater risk for PTSD symptoms (McCaslin et al., 2006). Indeed, Perrin and colleagues (2007) reported that sustaining an injury while responding to the September 11th terrorist attacks was the only within-disaster experience that increased risk among all occupations studied and was the strongest risk factor for all occupations except police and construction/engineering workers.

18.3.2. Identification with the Deceased or Survivors

Another important factor that appears to place emergency responders and disaster workers at higher risk of traumatic stress is the extent to which they begin to identify with the deceased or with those they are helping. Ursano and colleagues (1999) examined the role of identification with the deceased as one of the mechanisms of PTSD occurrence in a group of 54 disaster workers who participated in the body recovery and identification of sailors left dead after a gun turret explosion on the USS Iowa (Ursano, Fullerton, Vance, & Kao, 1999). Three types of identification with the dead were delineated: (1) identification with the deceased as oneself, (2) identification with the deceased as a friend, and (3) identification with the deceased as a family member. PTSD symptoms were assessed 1, 4, and 13 months after the disaster. Results indicated that identification occurs in nearly 75% of disaster workers exposed to deceased victims. Disaster workers who reported identification with the deceased as a friend were more likely to have PTSD than those who did not. Disaster workers who reported identification with the deceased as a family member had greater intrusive symptoms 1 month after the disaster than those who did not. Overall, identification with the dead as a friend or family member was associated with increased rates of PTSD, greater disaster-related intrusive and avoidant symptoms, and general symptoms (including depression, anxiety, hostility, and somatization). Losing comrades in the disaster or during the disaster work, such as during the World Trade Center attacks, may also impact later distress (Perrin et al., 2007).

Degree and type of interaction with survivors and bereaved family members has also been linked to the level of distress among rescue workers. Bartone and colleagues (1989) found degree of exposure to bereaved people among health workers providing assistance to family members of deceased soldiers was related to mental and physical stress symptoms such as headaches, tenseness, difficulty in sleeping, and depressed mood. A relationship between worker distress and degree of involvement with survivors was also found following the Ash Wednesday bushfire (Berah, Jones, & Valent, 1984). Intense and intimate involvements between helpers and survivors led to increased muscle tension, fatigue, and sleep disturbances.

18.3.3. Peritraumatic Reactions

While the characteristics of the incident, such as degree of life threat or identification with the deceased, influence trauma responses, perhaps even more important are the psychological and biological responses experienced during and immediately following exposure. Peritraumatic reactions have been shown to be strongly associated with PTSD symptoms (Brunet et al., 2001; Marmar et al., 1996; Marmar, Metzler, & Otte, 2004). Indeed, peritraumatic dissociation was found to be the strongest predictor of PTSD symptoms in a meta-analysis of risk factors for PTSD (Ozer, Best, Lipsey, & Weiss, 2003). Differences in reactions at the time of trauma exposure may help to explain why much research fails to find a simple dose-response relationship between frequency and severity of stressor exposure and the risk for psychopathology (Pitman, Shalev, & Orr, 2000). Peritraumatic emotional distress and dissociation may be a mediator of this relationship.

Greater paniclike reactions during exposure (e.g., sweating, shaking, heart racing, fear of dying, and fear of losing emotional control) are associated with greater adrenergic activation, a biomarker of peritraumatic panic and dissociation. Sustained fear-related adrenergic activation may lead to PTSD by triggering greater fear conditioning and overconsolidation of traumatic memories, resulting in the persistence of hyperarousal symptoms (Ozer et al., 2003). In turn, the persistence of hyperarousal symptoms has been found to be predictive of chronic PTSD symptoms (Carlier, Lamberts, & Gersons, 1997; Schell, Marshall, & Jaycox, 2004). However, as mentioned previously, reactions at the time of the experience will interact with personal and environmental resources in the recovery environment, including new stressful life events in the year after exposure and more negative work environments, in determining posttraumatic adjustment.

18.3.4. Personal Life Events

Negative personal life change following on the heels of critical incident exposure can result in compounded levels of distress – possibly interfering with the recovery process for rescue workers (e.g., Marmar et al., 2006; McCaslin et al., 2005; Morren et al., 2005; Renck et al., 2002) – and in a more chronic form of distress (e.g., Dougall, Herberman, Delahanty, Inslicht, & Baum, 2000; Epstein, Fullerton, Ursano, 1998; Maes, Mylle, Delmeire, & Janca, 2001). This is particularly germane during large-scale disasters when rescue workers are often required to cope with both the disaster response and the impact of the disaster on their personal life. For example, during the September 11th terrorist attacks, rescuers not only were managing the usual demands of response but were also encountering daily threats to their safety (e.g., the anthrax attacks that took place shortly after September 11th) and an uncertainty of what might happen next (e.g., that there may be more terrorist attacks).

18.3.5. Training and Experience

The value of preparation for responding to disaster should not be underestimated. Adequate preparation for a stressful event can minimize the impact of the event and may even protect affected individuals from the development of traumatic stress symptoms (Bartone et al., 1989; Chemtob, Bauer, Neller, & Hamada, 1990; Deahl & Bisson, 1995). Preparation for an event, through reduction in uncertainty can increase a sense of control and may strengthen coping skills, making them more likely to be effective during a stressful event (Shalev, 1996).

Indeed, the process of preparing for an event may be even more valuable than the actual content of a training program (Shalev, 1996). For example, Hytten (1989) surveyed military personnel who had been trained in airplane rescue maneuvers and had later responded to an airplane crash. The author reported that the personnel had perceived the training exercises as helpful even though the rescue maneuvers actually executed during the event differed significantly from those learned and rehearsed during training. It was suggested by the author that these results indicated that preparatory training may be more effective in preventing negative mental health consequences than relying only on a specific protocol to follow during the event. It was further suggested that any relevant preparatory training protocol may be useful because it would provide a schema or background for the response. In another investigation, Lundin and Bodegard (1993) examined the psychological impact of responding to an earthquake on 50 Swedish rescue workers. The rescue workers with more prior experience endorsed significantly greater feelings of having managed well than those who were less experienced, even though none had prior experience specific to working with earthquake victims.

Additional studies conducted with emergency responders provide further evidence that level of experience is an important factor in adjustment. Robinson and colleagues (1997) examined the effects of duty-related stress on 100 police officers. Officers with 11 or fewer years of experience reported more PTSD and somatic complaint symptoms. In another sample of emergency service workers who responded to damage caused by a large-scale earthquake, less preparation for the tasks that they confronted was predictive of greater distress approximately 1 to 4 years after their response (Marmar et al., 1996). In this study, Caltrans workers responding to a freeway collapse with multiple casualties reported greater distress than professionally trained emergency services personnel. While prior training seems to be helpful even if training exercises are not identical to what is experienced on the job, there is some evidence that the further removed the task is from one's training background, the higher the risk of later distress. Perrin and colleagues (2007) reported strong associations between level of PTSD and duty assignment, noting that these associations were the strongest for those who had performed tasks that were uncharacteristic of their job. For example, PTSD risk among police and emergency medical services/medical/disaster personnel increased twofold when they had engaged in firefighting, and for firefighters, engaging in light construction was the only task associated with PTSD symptoms.

While prior experience and training may be helpful when confronting a new disaster situation, there is also evidence to suggest that longer duration of work provides more opportunity for trauma exposure and, in this way, may contribute to greater psychological distress. Longer time on the job and higher number of distressing assignments have been shown to be predictive of higher reports of PTSD symptoms (Alexander & Klein, 2001; Wagner et al., 1998). Chang and colleagues (2003) found longer job experience to be a significant predictor of posttraumatic symptoms among 84 firefighters who had responded to an earthquake in Taiwan. The authors proposed that cumulative exposure over more years of service may have resulted in residual symptoms from previous events that then predisposed them to greater psychiatric distress following later disaster response. Finally, Corneil and colleagues (1999) reported that having more than 15 years of service contributed significantly to the development of PTSD in a sample of 625 Canadian firefighters. However, it was noted that this relationship was not present in a comparable sample of 203 U.S. firefighters. It is possible that, depending upon the circumstances and mediating factors, level of experience may serve as either a protective or a vulnerability factor.

Further, accumulation of negative personal life events before response to a critical incident puts some workers at risk. McFarlane's study (McFarlane, 1988b, 1989) of the impact of response to a large-scale bush fire on volunteer firefighters found that at 29 months after the disaster, negative life events that occurred before the critical incident exposure were a significant contributor to persistent and chronic stress.

18.3.6. Organizational Stress

Additional stressors unique to the role of emergency service workers responding to disaster include organizational stressors such as long work hours (Maguen et al., 2007; Perrin et al., 2007; Williams, Solomon, & Bartone, 1988) and coordination of a multiple-agency response that can increase confusion and cause stress in workers at the disaster site (Williams et al., 1988). Long work hours under extreme conditions can lead to severe fatigue and physical exhaustion (Fullerton et al., 1992). In their study of Red Cross volunteers who had responded to the 1989 Loma Prieta earthquake in the San Francisco Bay Area, Armstrong and colleagues (1998) found that workers commonly complained of stressors including long work shifts, sickness, fatigue, guilt for not doing more for the victims, conflicts among staff, and concern about personal safety (Armstrong et al., 1998). These complaints about coordination and organizational issues were echoed by Red Cross workers who had responded to a fire in the Oakland-Berkeley California Hills in 1991 (Armstrong, Lund, McWright, & Tichenor, 1995). Violanti and Aron (1993) found that among a sample of 103 police officers, police organizational stressors increased psychological distress 6.3 times more than stressors unique to police work when mediated by job satisfaction and goal orientation.

Liberman and colleagues (2002) found that among 733 police officers, exposure to routine work stressors (e.g., management and administration, supervisors, shift work, boredom, role conflict) significantly predicted general psychological distress and posttraumatic stress symptoms following the officer's most traumatic incident during his/her career (Liberman et al.,

2002). The effects for routine work stressors were independent of, and greater than, the effects of cumulative critical incident exposure. It was proposed that routine occupational stress exposure was a significant risk factor for both psychological distress and posttraumatic stress symptoms. Furthermore, as noted previously, if the critical incident or disaster hits close to home, occupational stressors may be further compounded by the workers' concerns for their own families and friends as a result of the disaster; separation from family and friends; and concern about damage to personal residences (Marmar et al., 1996). In summary, the organizational and other such work-related stressors of disaster response should not be underestimated.

18.4. PREVENTION AND TREATMENT OF POSTTRAUMATIC DISTRESS IN UNIFORMED FIRST RESPONDERS

There are a number of avenues through which posttraumatic distress reactions following disaster response may be minimized or prevented. Research strongly emphasizes the role of the workplace in providing support and anticipating the needs of the responders (Maguen et al., 2007). For example, ensuring that police officers and firefighters are supported by their organization (e.g., encouraged to take breaks when needed, provided with support resources such as someone with whom to discuss the stressful experiences they are encountering if necessary) is very important in buffering the impact of disaster work. Those in leadership positions must ensure that the organizational aspects of the response are helpful rather than harmful to the individual responders (e.g., avoid applying an autocratic leadership style in a situation that requires more flexibility [Paton, 1994]). To this end, it may be helpful to provide additional training and education regarding leadership needs in various situations. At the individual level, first responders may benefit from psychoeducation regarding signs of stress and healthy coping and from learning basic anxiety management skills that can be easily employed in the field. Furthermore, because disaster scenarios can vary so widely, preparation for disaster work should include training and practice in handling a diverse range of situations. While it is impossible to prepare for every possible scenario, preparation in handling a range of different disaster scenarios and problems may help the responder to feel more prepared and confident and may lessen the negative effects of disaster response (Paton, 1994).

Until fairly recently, critical incident stress debriefing (CISD) was the treatment of choice for first responders who had been exposed to a critical incident or traumatic stressor. CISD is a single session, individual or group intervention that provides education about common trauma reactions and encourages the expression of thoughts and feelings about the traumatic experience. CISD is usually conducted in a group setting and involves having the participants discuss the event and their feelings about it. Although anecdotal evidence supported the use of such debriefings when researchers began to collect data on their effectiveness, it became apparent that oftentimes the debriefings were not helpful (Conlon, Fahy, & Conroy, 1999; Hobbs, Mayou, Harrison, & Worlock, 1996), and some studies suggested that they could even result in more symptomatology (Mayou, Ehlers, & Hobbs, 2000). It may be that requesting an individual to discuss the trauma in detail immediately following the event, when a sense of threat may still be present and the memory has not been completely consolidated, may actually reinforce a sense of threat and danger, resulting in increased fear conditioning and overconsolidation of the traumatic memory. Thus, new models have been proposed for immediate intervention that does not require that the individual processes the experience in detail during or immediately following it.

Recent studies suggest that the administration of propranolol, a centrally acting adrenaline-blocking medication that reduces anxiety arousal, immediately following traumatic exposure and for the subsequent 1 to 2 weeks may reduce the likelihood of developing PTSD symptoms (Pitman et al., 2002; Vaiva et al., 2003). However, there are many individuals who may refuse medication, and pharmacologic interventions may be stigmatizing or may compromise cognitive and physical performance in the midst of a disaster response. Promising early behavioral interventions are aimed at controlling arousal in the immediate aftermath of traumatic exposure through providing anxiety management and calming techniques without the requirement of discussing the event.

There have been few randomized trials of treatment for PTSD and associated symptoms in first responders for symptoms occurring in the months and years following disaster response. In one of the first studies, Difede and colleagues (2007) reported findings from a controlled clinical trial of cognitive-behavioral therapy (CBT) for utility disaster workers and clean-up operations responding to the World Trade Center attacks. In this study, participants were randomly assigned to a 12-week cognitive-behavioral exposure treatment ($N = 15$) or a treatment-as-usual (TAU) ($N = 16$) condition. The CBT condition included psychoeducation, breathing exercises, imaginal and graduated in vivo exposure, and cognitive reprocessing. The participants receiving the CBT treatment showed a significantly greater decline in PTSD symptoms, with large effect sizes. These findings are important in demonstrating that provision of such an intervention in the aftermath of disaster is indeed feasible and can be helpful.

Although a significant number of first responders may experience mental health symptomatology following disaster response and might benefit from receiving psychiatric services, there unfortunately are substantial barriers to receiving care. In a study related to that cited previously (Difede et al, 2007), Jayasinghe et al. (2006) examined 328 male utility disaster workers' responses to referral for psychotherapy to address symptoms related to their work following the World Trade Center attacks. Among those offered such referrals during psychological screening, approximately 48% chose to accept, 28% chose to only consider, and 24% chose to decline referral. These findings emphasize the importance of addressing stigma of mental illness among first responders.

18.5. SUMMARY

Uniformed first responders are both uniquely resilient, by virtue of selection and training, and particularly vulnerable because of repeated exposure to critical incident stressors in the context of a highly stressful work environment. Episodically, they face the additional risks of extreme events including large-scale natural and human-made disasters. Factors associated with greater vulnerability include lack of preparation for the specific roles needed to respond to an incident, personal histories of childhood and lifetime traumatic stress exposure outside of work responsibilities, personal and family history of psychiatric disorders, higher ongoing levels of stress in their personal lives, less cohesive and supportive work environments, and isolation from important social supports in their personal life. Despite the challenges, only a minority of first responders develop PTSD and related emotional disorders, with overall rates of PTSD variable but higher in the weeks and months following major traumatic events. Promising strategies for immediate management of acute stress disorders include the use of adrenaline-blocking medications and cognitive behaviorally informed antipanic interventions for peritraumatic distress. Prevention strategies should aim to build long-term career resilience and include improved training procedures, inoculation to ecologically valid stressors, flexible training exercises that will result in skills that generalize across disaster response scenarios, team building for greater cohesion and support, leadership training emphasizing communication and collaboration, and institutional support for recognition and management of emotional problems.

REFERENCES

Alexander, D. A. (1993). Stress among police body handlers: A long-term follow-up. *British Journal of Psychiatry, 163*, 806–808.

Alexander, D. A., & Klein, S. (2001). Ambulance personnel and critical incidents: Impact of accident and emergency work on mental health and emotional well-being. *British Journal of Psychiatry, 178*, 76–81.

Armstrong, K., Lund, P., McWright, L., & Tichenor, V. (1995). Multi-stressor exit debriefing and the American Red Cross: The East Bay Hills fire experience. *Social Work Journal, 40*, 83–90.

Armstrong, K., Zatzick, D., Metzler, T., Weiss, D.S., Marmar, C.R., Garma, S., et al. (1998). Debriefing of American Red Cross personnel: Pilot study on participants' evaluations and case examples from the 1994 Los Angeles earthquake relief operation. *Social Work in Health Care, 27*(1), 33–50.

Bartone, P.T., Ursano, R.J., Wright, K.M., & Ingraham, L.H. (1989). The impact of a military air disaster on the health of assistance workers: A prospective study. *Journal of Nervous and Mental Disease, 177*(6), 317–328.

Beaton, R., Murphy, S., Johnson, C., Pike, K., & Corneil, W. (1998). Exposure to duty-related incident stressors in urban firefighters and paramedics. *Journal of Traumatic Stress, 11*(4), 821–828.

Berah, E.F., Jones, H.J., & Valent, P. (1984). The experience of a mental health team involved in the early phase of a disaster. *Australian and New Zealand Journal of Psychiatry, 18*(4), 354–358.

Breslau, N., Davis, G.C., Andreski, P., & Peterson, E. (1991). Traumatic events and Posttraumatic Stress Disorder in an urban population of young adults. *Archives of General Psychiatry, 48*(3), 216–222.

Brunet, A., Weiss, D.S., Metzler, T.J., Best, S.R., Neylan, T.C., Rogers, C., et al. (2001). The Peritraumatic Distress Inventory: A proposed measure of PTSD criterion A2. *American Journal of Psychiatry, 158*(9), 1480–1485.

Bryant, R.A., & Guthrie, R.M. (2007). Maladaptive self-appraisals before trauma exposure predict posttraumatic stress disorder. *Journal of Consulting and Clinical Psychology, 75*(5), 812–815.

Carlier, I.V.E., Lamberts, R.D., & Gersons, B.P.R. (1997). Risk factors for posttraumatic stress symptomatology in police officers: A prospective analysis. *Journal of Nervous and Mental Disease, 185*(8), 498–506.

CDC. (2006). Health hazard evaluation of police officers and firefighters after Hurricane Katrina – New Orleans, Louisiana, October 17–28 and November 30-December 5, 2005. *MMWR Morb Mortal Wkly Rep, 55*(16), 456–458.

Chang, C.M., Lee, L.C., Connor, K.M., Davidson, J.R., Jeffries, K., & Lai, T.J. (2003). Posttraumatic distress and coping strategies among rescue workers after an earthquake. *Journal of Nervous and Mental Disease, 191*(6), 391–398.

Chemtob, C.M., Bauer, G.B., Neller, G., & Hamada, R. (1990). Post-traumatic stress disorder among Special Forces Vietnam Veterans. *Military Medicine, 155*(1), 16–20.

Conlon, L., Fahy, T.J., & Conroy, R. (1999). PTSD in ambulant RTA victims: A randomized controlled trial of debriefing. *Journal of Psychosomatic Research, 46*(1), 37–44.

Corneil, W., Beaton, R., Murphy, S., Johnson, C., & Pike, K. (1999). Exposure to traumatic incidents and prevalence of posttraumatic stress symptomatology in urban firefighters in two countries. *Journal of Occupational Health Psychology, 4*(2), 131–141.

Deahl, M., & Bisson, J.I. (1995). Dealing with disasters: Does psychological debriefing work? *Journal of Accident and Emergency Medicine, 12*(4), 255–258.

Difede, J., Malta, L.S., Best, S., Henn-Haase, C., Metzler, T., Bryant, R., et al. (2007). A randomized controlled clinical treatment trial for World Trade Center attack-related PTSD in disaster workers. *Journal of Nervous and Mental Disease, 195*(10), 861–865.

Dougall, A.L., Herberman, H.B., Delahanty, D.L., Inslicht, S.S., & Baum, A. (2000). Similarity of prior trauma exposure as a determinant of chronic stress responding to an airline disaster. *Journal of Consulting and Clinical Psychology, 68*(2), 290–295.

Duckworth, D.H. (1986). Psychological problems arising from disaster work. *Stress Medicine, 2*, 315–323.

Durham, T.W., McCammon, S.L., & Allison, E.J. (1985). The psychological impact of disaster on rescue personnel. *Annals of Emergency Medicine, 14*, 664–668.

Epstein, R.S., Fullerton, C.S., & Ursano, R.J. (1998). Posttraumatic stress disorder following an air disaster: A prospective study. *American Journal of Psychiatry, 155*(7), 934–938.

Ersland, S., Weisaeth, L., & Sund, A. (1989). The stress upon rescuers involved in an oil rig disaster: "Alexander L. Kielland": 1980. *Acta Psychiatrica Scandinavica, 80* (Suppl. 355), 38–49.

Foreman, C., & Eranen, L. (1999). Trauma of world policing: Peacekeeping duties. In J. M. Violanti & D. Paton (Eds.), *Police trauma: Psychological aftermath of civilian combat* (pp. 189–200). Springfield, IL: Charles C. Thomas.

Fullerton, C.S., McCarroll, J.E., Ursano, R.J., & Wright, K.M. (1992). Psychological responses of rescue workers: Fire fighters and trauma. *American Journal of Orthopsychiatry, 62*(3), 371–378.

Fullerton, C.S., Ursano, R.J., & Wang, L. (2004). Acute stress disorder, posttraumatic stress disorder, and depression in disaster or rescue workers. *American Journal of Psychiatry, 161*(8), 1370–1376.

Gabriel, R., Ferrando, L., Corton, E.S., Mingote, C., Garcia-Camba, E., Liria, A.F., et al. (2007).

Psychopathological consequences after a terrorist attack: An epidemiological study among victims, the general population, and police officers. *European Psychiatry*, *22*(6), 339–346.

Galea, S., Vlahov, D., Resnick, H., Ahern, J., Susser, E., Gold, J., et al. (2003). Trends of probable post-traumatic stress disorder in New York City after the September 11 terrorist attacks. *American Journal of Epidemiology*, *158*(6), 514–524.

Gross, R., Neria, Y., Tao, X., Massa, J., Ashwell, L., Davis, K., et al. (2006). Posttraumatic Stress Disorder and other psychological sequelae among World Trade Center clean up and recovery workers. *Annals of the New York Academy of Sciences*, *1071*, 495–499.

Heffron, E. F. (1977). Project Outreach: Crisis intervention following natural disaster. *Journal of Community Psychology*, *5*(2), 103–111.

Hobbs, M., Mayou, R., Harrison, B., & Worlock, P. (1996). A randomised controlled trial of psychological debriefing for victims of road traffic accidents. *British Medical Journal*, *313*(7070), 1438–1439.

Hodgins, G. A., Creamer, M., & Bell, R. (2001). Risk factors for posttrauma reactions in police officers: A longitudinal study. *The Journal of Nervous and Mental Disease*, *189*(8), 541–547.

Hytten, K. (1989). Helicopter crash in water: Effects of simulator escape training. *Acta Psychiatrica Scandinavia Supplement*, *355*, 73–78.

Jacobs, G. A. (1995). The Development of a National Plan for Disaster Mental Health. *Professional Psychology: Research and Practice*, *26*(6), 543–549.

Jayasinghe, N., Giosan, C., Difede, J., Spielman, L., & Robin, L. (2006). Predictors of responses to psychotherapy referral of WTC utility disaster workers. *Journal of Traumatic Stress. Special issue: Innovations in trauma research methods*, *19*(2), 307–312.

Jones, D. R. (1985). Secondary disaster victims: The emotional effects of recovering and identifying human remains. *American Journal of Psychiatry*, *142*(3), 303–307.

Kessler, R. C., Berglund, P., Demler, O., Jin, R., Merikangas, K. R., & Walters, E. E. (2005). Lifetime prevalence and age-of-onset distributions of DSM-IV disorders in the National Comorbidity Survey Replication. *Archives of General Psychiatry*, *62*(6), 593–602.

Kessler, R. C., Chiu, W. T., Demler, O., Merikangas, K. R., & Walters, E. E. (2005). Prevalence, severity, and comorbidity of 12-month DSM-IV disorders in the National Comorbidity Survey Replication. *Archives of General Psychiatry*, *62*(6), 617–627.

Lazarus, R., & Folkman, S. (1984). *Stress, appraisal, and coping*. New York: Springer.

Liao, S. C., Lee, M. B., Lee, Y. J., Weng, T., Shih, F. Y., & Ma, M. H. (2002). Association of psychological distress with psychological factors in rescue workers within two months after a major earthquake. *Journal of the Formosan Medical Association*, *101*(3), 169–176.

Liberman, A., Best, S., Metzler, T., Fagan, J., Weiss, D., & Marmar, C. (2002). Routine occupational stress and psychological distress in police. *Policing: An International Journal of Police Strategies and Management*, *25*(2), 421–439.

Lundin, T., & Bodegard, M. (1993). The psychological impact of an earthquake on rescue workers: A follow-up study of the Swedish group of rescue workers in Armenia, 1988. *Journal of Traumatic Stress*, *6*(1), 129–139.

Maes, M., Mylle, J., Delmeire, L., & Janca, A. (2001). Pre- and post-disaster negative life events in relation to the incidence and severity of post-traumatic stress disorder. *Psychiatry Research*, *105*(1), 1–12.

Maguen, S., Metzler, T. J., McCaslin, S. E., Inslicht, S., Henn-Haase, C., Neylan, T. C., et al. (2007). Routine work environment stress and PTSD symptoms in police officers. *The International Society for Traumatic Stress 23rd Annual Meeting*. Baltimore, MD.

Marmar, C., Best, S., Metzler, T., Chemtob, C. M., Gloria, R., Killeen, A., et al. (2003). *Impact of the World Trade Center attacks on New York City police officers; A prospective study, invited address*. Paper presented at the 34th Annual Meeting of the International Society of Psychoneuroendocrinology, New York.

Marmar, C., Weiss, D., Metzler, T. J., & Delucchi, K. L. (1996). Characteristics of emergency services personnel related to peritraumatic dissociation during critical incident exposure. *American Journal of Psychiatry*, *153*(7), 94–102.

Marmar, C. R., McCaslin, S. E., Metzler, T. J., Best, S., Weiss, D. S., Fagan, J., et al. (2006). Predictors of posttraumatic stress in police and other first responders. *Annals of the New York Academy of Sciences*, *1071*, 1–18.

Marmar, C. R., Metzler, T. J., & Otte, C. (2004). The peritraumatic distress inventory: A proposed measure of PTSD criterion A2. In J. Wilson & T. Keane (Eds.), *Assessing psychological trauma and PTSD* (pp. 144–167). New York: Guilford Press.

Marmar, C. R., Weiss, D. S., Metzler, T. J., Delucchi, K. L., Best, S. R., & Wentworth, K. A. (1999). Longitudinal course and predictors of continuing distress following critical incident exposure in emergency services personnel. *Journal of Nervous and Mental Disease*, *187*(1), 15–22.

Marmar, C. R., Weiss, D. S., Metzler, T. J., Ronfeldt, H. M., & Foreman, C. (1996). Stress responses of emergency services personnel to the Loma Prieta earthquake interstate 880 freeway collapse and control traumatic incidents. *Journal of Traumatic Stress*, *9*(1), 63–85.

Marmar, C. R., Weiss, D. S., Schlenger, W. E., Fairbank, J. A., Jordan, B. K., Kulka, R. A., et al. (1994). Peritraumatic dissociation and posttraumatic stress in male Vietnam theater veterans. *American Journal of Psychiatry*, *151*(6), 902–907.

Martin, C. A., McKean, H. E., & Veltkamp, L. J. (1986). Post-traumatic stress disorder in police and working with victims: A pilot study. *Journal of Police Science and Administration*, *14*, 98–101.

Mayou, R. A., Ehlers, A., & Hobbs, M. (2000). Psychological debriefing for road traffic accident victims. Three-year follow-up of a randomised controlled trial. *British Journal of Psychiatry*, *176*, 589–593.

McCaslin, S. E., Rogers, C. E., Metzler, T. J., Best, S. R., Weiss, D. S., Fagan, J. A., et al. (2006). The impact of personal threat on police officers' responses to critical incident stressors. *Journal of Nervous and Mental Disease*, *194*(8), 591–597.

McCaslin, S., Jacobs, G., Johnson-Jimenez, E., Metzler, T., & Marmar, C. (2005). How does negative life change following disaster response impact distress among Red Cross responders? *Professional Psychology: Research and Practice*, *36*(3), 246–253.

McFarlane, A. C. (1986). Long-term psychiatric morbidity after a natural disaster. Implications for disaster planners and emergency services. *Medical Journal of Australia*, *145*(11–12), 561–563.

(1988a). The longitudinal course of posttraumatic morbidity. The range of outcomes and their predictors. *Journal of Nervous and Mental Disease*, *176*(1), 30–39.

(1988b). The phenomenology of posttraumatic stress disorders following a natural disaster. *Journal of Nervous and Mental Disease*, *176*(1), 22–29.

(1988c). Relationship between psychiatric impairment and a natural disaster: The role of distress. *Psychological Medicine*, *18*(1), 129–139.

(1989). The aetiology of post-traumatic morbidity: Predisposing, precipitating, and perpetuating factors. *British Journal of Psychiatry*, *154*, 221–228.

(2000). Posttraumatic stress disorder: A model of the longitudinal course and the role of risk factors. *Journal of Clinical Psychiatry*, *61* (Suppl. 5), (15–20), 21–13.

McFarlane, A. C., & Papay, P. (1992). Multiple diagnoses in posttraumatic stress disorder in the victims of a natural disaster. *Journal of Nervous and Mental Disease*, *180*(8), 498–504.

Morren, M., Dirkzwager, A. J., Kessels, F. J., & Yzermans, C. J. (2007). The influence of a disaster on the health of rescue workers: A longitudinal study. *CMAJ*, *176*(9), 1279–1283.

Morren, M., Yzermans, C. J., van Nispen, R. M., & Wevers, S. J. (2005). The health of volunteer firefighters three years after a technological disaster. *Journal of Occupational Health*, *47*(6), 523–532.

North, C. S., Tivis, L., McMillen, J. C., Pfefferbaum, B., Cox, J., Spitznagel, E. L., et al. (2002). Coping, functioning, and adjustment of rescue workers after the Oklahoma City bombing. *Journal of Traumatic Stress*, *15*(3), 171–175.

North, C. S., Tivis, L., McMillen, J. C., Pfefferbaum, B., Spitznagel, E. L., Cox, J., et al. (2002). Psychiatric disorders in rescue workers after the Oklahoma City bombing. *American Journal of Psychiatry*, *159*(5), 857–859.

Ozer, E., Best, S. R., Lipsey, T. L., & Weiss, D. S. (2003). Predictors of posttraumatic stress disorder and symptoms in adults: A meta-analysis. *Psychological Bulletin*, *129*(1), 52–73.

Paton, D. (1994). Disaster relief work: An assessment of training effectiveness. *Journal of Traumatic Stress*, *7*(2), 275–288.

Perrin, M. A., DiGrande, L., Wheeler, K., Thorpe, L., Farfel, M., & Brackbill, R. (2007). Differences in PTSD prevalence and associated risk factors among World Trade Center disaster rescue and recovery workers. *American Journal of Psychiatry*, *164*(9), 1385–1394.

Pitman, R. K., Sanders, K. M., Zusman, R. M., Healy, A. R., Cheema, F., Lasko, N. B., et al. (2002). Pilot study of secondary prevention of Posttraumatic Stress Disorder with propranolol. *Biological Psychiatry*, *51*(2), 189–192.

Pitman, R. K., Shalev, A. Y., & Orr, S. P. (2000). Posttraumatic Stress Disorder: Emotion, conditioning, and memory. In M. D. Corbetta & M. S. Gazzaniga (Eds.), *The new cognitive neurosciences* (pp. 687–700). New York: Plenum Press.

Pole, N., Best, S., Weiss, D., Metzler, T., Liberman, A., Fagan, J., et al. (2001). Effects of gender and ethnicity on duty-related Posttraumatic Stress symptoms among rrban police officers. *Journal of Nervous and Mental Disease*, *189*(7), 442–448.

Raphael, B., & Middleton, W. (1987). Mental health responses in a decade of disasters: Australia, 1974–1983. *Hospital and Community Psychiatry*, *38*(12), 1331–1337.

Raphael, B., Singh, B., Bradbury, L., & Lambert, F. (1983). Who helps the helpers? The effects of a disaster on the rescue workers. *Omega: Journal of Death and Dying*, *14*(1), 9–20.

Renck, B., Weisaeth, L., & Skarbo, S. (2002). Stress reactions in police officers after a disaster rescue operation. *Nordic Journal of Psychiatry*, *56*(1), 7–14.

Resnick, H. S., Kilpatrick, D. G., Dansky, B. S., Saunders, B. E., & Best, C. J. (1993). Prevalence of civilian trauma and Posttraumatic Stress Disorder in a representative national sample of women. *Journal of Consulting and Clinical Psychology, 61*(6), 984–991.

Robinson, H. M., Sigman, M. R., & Wilson, J. P. (1997). Duty-related stressors and PTSD symptoms in suburban police officers. *Psychological Reports, 81*(3, Pt. 1), 835–845.

Schell, T., Marshall, G., & Jaycox, L. (2004). All symptoms are not created equal: The prominent role of hyperarousal in the natural course of posttraumatic psychological distress. *Journal of Abnormal Psychology, 113*, 1115–1119.

Shalev, AY (1996). Stress versus traumatic stress: From acute homeostatic reactions to chronic psychopathology. In B. A. van der Kolk, A. C. McFarlane, & L. Weisaeth (Eds.), *Traumatic stress: The effects of overwhelming experience on mind, body, & society* (pp. 77–101). New York, NY: The Guilford Press.

Slottje, P., Twisk, J. W., Smidt, N., Huizink, A. C., Witteveen, A. B., van Mechelen, W., et al. (2007). Health-related quality of life of firefighters and police officers 8.5 years after the air disaster in Amsterdam. *Quality of Life Research, 16*(2), 239–252.

Slottje, P., Witteveen, A. B., Twisk, J. W., Smidt, N., Huizink, A. C., Mechelen, W. V., & Smid, T. (2008). Post-disaster physical symptoms of firefighters and police officers: Role of types of exposure and post-traumatic stress symptoms. *British Journal of Health Psychology, 13*(2), 327–342.

Solomon, Z., Mikulincer, M., & Avitzur, E. (1988). Coping, locus of control, social support, and combat-related posttraumatic stress disorder: A prospective study. *Journal of Personality and Social Psychology, 55*(2), 279–285.

Stein, M., Walker, J., Hazen, A., & Forde, D. (1997). Full and partial Posttraumatic Stress Disorder: Findings from a community survey. *American Journal of Psychiatry, 154*, 1114–1119.

Terry, D. J. (1994). Determinants of coping: The role of stable and situational factors. *Journal of Personality and Social psychology, 66*(5), 895–910.

Thompson, J. (1993). Psychological impact of body recovery duties. *Journal of the Royal Society of Medicine, 86*(11), 628–629.

Ursano, R. J., Fullerton, C. S., Kao, T. C., & Bhartiya, V. R. (1995). Longitudinal assessment of Posttraumatic Stress Disorder and depression after exposure to traumatic death. *Journal of Nervous & Mental Disease, 183*(1), 36–42.

Ursano, R. J., Fullerton, C. S., Vance, K., & Kao, T. (1999). Posttraumatic Stress Disorder and identification in disaster workers. *American Journal of Psychiatry, 156*(3), 353–359.

Vaiva, G., Ducrocq, F., Jezequel, K., Averland, B., Lestavel, P., Brunet, A., et al. (2003). Immediate treatment with propranolol decreases Posttraumatic Stress Disorder two months after trauma. *Biological Psychiatry, 54*(9), 947–949.

Violanti, J. M., & Aron, F. (1993). Sources of police stressors, job attitudes, and psychological distress. *Psychol Rep, 72*(3, Pt. 1), 899–904.

Wagner, D., Heinrichs, M., & Ehlert, U. (1998). Prevalence of symptoms of Posttraumatic Stress Disorder in German professional firefighters. *American Journal of Psychiatry, 155*(12), 1727–1732.

Weiss, D. S., Brunet, A., Metzler, T. J., Best, S., Fagan, J., Liberman, A., et al. R. (1999). *Critical incident exposure in police officers: Frequency, impact and correlates.* Paper presented at the Paper presented at the International Society for Traumatic Stress Studies, 15th Annual Meeting., Miami, FL.

Weiss, D. S., Marmar, C. R., Metzler, T. J., & Ronfeldt, H. M. (1995). Predicting symptomatic distress in emergency services personnel. *Journal of Consulting and Clinical Psychology, 63*(3), 361–368.

Wilkinson, C. (1983). Aftermath of a disaster: The collapse of the Hyatt Regency Hotel skywalks. *American Journal of Psychiatry, 140*(9), 1134–1139.

Williams, C. L., Solomon, S. D., & Bartone, P. (1988). Primary prevention in aircraft disasters. Integrating research and practice. *American Psychologist, 43*(9), 730–739.

Witteveen, A. B., Bramsen, I., Twisk, J. W., Huizink, A. C., Slottje, P., Smid, T., et al. (2007). Psychological distress of rescue workers eight and one-half years after professional involvement in the Amsterdam air disaster. *Journal of Nervous and Mental Disease, 195*(1), 31–40.

Wright, K. M., Ursano, R. J., Bartone, P. T., & Ingraham, L. H. (1990). The shared experience of catastrophe: An expanded classification of the disaster community. *American Journal of Orthopsychiatry, 60*(1), 35–42.

Zatzick, D. F., Marmar, C. R., Weiss, D. S., Browner, W., Metzler, T., Golding, J. M., et al. (1997). Posttraumatic Stress Disorder and functioning and quality of life outcomes in a nationally representative sample of male Vietnam veterans. *American Journal of Psychiatry, 154*(12), 1690–1695.

PART FIVE

Interventions and Health Services

19 Mental Health Treatments in the Wake of Disaster

RICHARD A. BRYANT AND BRETT LITZ

19.1. INTRODUCTION

There is overwhelming evidence that disasters can lead to a range of posttraumatic mental health problems. The aim of this chapter is to review the evidence for psychological and pharmacological approaches to treating people with adverse psychological reactions after disaster; specifically, we focus on interventions that can be provided in the short and intermediate phases after disaster. First we review common postdisaster psychiatric disorders. We then turn to describing and outlining the evidence for psychological approaches to treatment. Next we review pharmacological treatments for posttraumatic conditions. Finally, we comment on factors that influence the management of psychological approaches in the acute postdisaster environment.

19.2. PSYCHOLOGICAL EFFECTS OF DISASTERS

There is convergent evidence that an array of psychiatric disorders arise after disasters. Posttraumatic stress disorder (PTSD) is the most commonly identified, and the disorder is characterized by three clusters of symptoms, including reexperiencing of the traumatic event, avoidance and numbing, and hyperarousal. Symptoms need to be present for at least 1 month and cause clinically significant distress or impairment in functioning to fulfill criteria for PTSD. Rates of PTSD were reported in 34% of survivors of the Oklahoma City bombing (North et al., 1999) and 53% after Australian bushfires (McFarlane, 1986). Across studies, the prevalence of PTSD is higher among direct victims (30%–40%) than rescue personnel (10%–20%; Neria, Nandi, & Galea, 2007). It is important to note, however, that other disorders also commonly occur both with PTSD and independently of PTSD. Depression is the second most commonly observed psychological disorder in survivors of disasters followed by various problems with anxiety (Norris et al., 2002). For example, after the Oklahoma City bombing, 22% of people suffered depression, 7% suffered panic disorder, 4% had generalized anxiety disorder, 9% had alcohol use disorder, and 2% had drug use disorder; overall, 30% of people had a psychiatric disorder other than PTSD (North et al., 1999).

19.3. TIMING OF INTERVENTIONS

Prevalence estimates of mental disorders, and especially PTSD, after disaster is heavily reliant on when the assessment is made. Generally, rates of PTSD are high in the initial months after a disaster, but most become noncases in the subsequent months. For example, Galea and colleagues (2002) surveyed residents of New York City to gauge their response to the September 11, 2001, terrorist attacks. Five to eight weeks after the attacks, 7.5% of a random sample of adults living south of 110th Street in Manhattan had developed PTSD, and of those living south of Canal Street, 20% had PTSD. In February 2002, Galea's group did a follow-up study on another group of adults living south of 110th Street and found that only 1.7% of the sample had PTSD related to the attacks (Galea et al., 2003). A similar pattern was found in Thailand after the 2004 tsunami, where 12% of displaced people had PTSD 2 months after the tsunami, but this rate dropped to 7% at 9 months (van Griensven et al., 2006). This study also reported that depression decreased from 30% to 25%, and anxiety decreased from 37% to 17%. These patterns indicate that most disaster survivors eventually regain functioning on their own without formal mental health intervention, which has implications for when treatments are offered after disasters.

Short-term and intermediate-term interventions can be distinguished by their intention. Short-term interventions are primarily designed to promote safety, assist coping, and stabilize the individual and their environment. In contrast, intermediate interventions are designed to prevent or treat psychopathological responses that have begun to emerge after the disaster. However, it is important to note that the decision to introduce a short- or intermediate-term intervention is not based simply on a formula of days or weeks after the disaster. The decision to implement an intervention will depend largely on the extent that immediate threat has subsided and a degree of stability has returned to the survivor's environment. If a disaster is discrete and the effects are short lived, then a short-term intervention may occur within days and an intermediate intervention within a month. In the aftermath of a more extreme disaster that has long-lasting effects, it may not be appropriate to consider an intermediate intervention until several months have passed. Following Hurricane Katrina, for example, many people's lives were massively disrupted for lengthy periods because of relocation, lack of housing, and loss of basic infrastructures that would allow normal living routines.

Two critical issues that are important for deciding the appropriateness of an intervention are (1) the extent to which threat still exists for the survivor and (2) the extent to which the survivor has sufficient resources to manage the intervention. A disaster survivor who is homeless, unemployed, and unaware of the well-being of a family member several months after a massive disaster may still not be an appropriate candidate for intermediate-phased intervention because he is still underresourced to manage daily stressors. It is only when an individual has secured safety and an adequate sense of security and resources that one should consider intermediate-phased interventions.

19.4. SHORT-TERM INTERVENTIONS FOR ALL DISASTER SURVIVORS

19.4.1. Psychological Debriefing

Over the past two decades, psychological debriefing has been the model approach to reducing the risk for chronic PTSD after disasters. The modern form of debriefing has been popularized by Mitchell (1983), who termed the intervention critical incident stress debriefing (CISD). Although CISD is not the only form of debriefing, it is the most commonly used and is conceptually very similar to other debriefing practices that are currently available (Raphael & Wilson, 2000). According to Mitchell, a single debriefing session "will generally alleviate the acute stress responses which appear at the scene and immediately afterward and will eliminate, or at least inhibit, delayed stress reactions" (Mitchell, 1983, p. 36). Although this approach was initially developed for emergency service personnel, it has been proposed to be effective for a wide variety of victims of trauma (Everly & Mitchell, 1999). A CISD session typically occurs within 48 hours of the event and involves education about trauma reactions, requires participants to describe what occurred and their cognitive and emotional responses to the event, enquires about psychological or physical symptoms, and provides suggestions for stress reduction.

Proponents of CISD claim that it is an effective means of reducing stress reactions (Mitchell & Bray, 1990). Across many studies, there are reports that people typically enjoy receiving CISD and endorse it in post-CISD surveys. It is important to distinguish between strategies after a disaster that are perceived favorably and those that actually assist longer-term adaptation. Over the past decade, a series of studies have compared trauma survivors who received CISD with those who did not receive the intervention (Bisson, Jenkins, Alexander, & Bannister, 1997; Conlon, Fahy, & Conroy, 1999; Hobbs, Mayou, Harrison, & Worlock, 1996; Rose, Brewin, Andrews, &

Kirk, 1999). Systematic reviews of these studies indicate that people who receive CISD do not enjoy better outcomes than those who do not receive CISD (Rose, Bisson, & Wessely, 2001; van Emmerik, Kamphuis, Hulsbosch, & Emmelkamp, 2002). Specifically, CISD does not prevent PTSD.

Some have argued that debriefing may have a toxic effect by impairing the natural recovery that typically occurs following trauma exposure. This concern has arisen because of findings from several studies that indicated that people who receive CISD, especially those who are highly distressed, have slightly higher PTSD levels at follow-up than those who do not receive CISD (e.g., Hobbs et al., 1996). It is possible that requiring people to ventilate their emotions within days of trauma exposure may hasten arousal and strengthen their trauma memories, which may impede natural recovery (McNally, Bryant, & Ehlers, 2003). It should be noted that the evidence that initial debriefing may be harmful for some people is not strong, and it requires replication of properly randomized studies to validate this concern. Nonetheless, the adage that providers' first goal is to "do no harm" has raised serious concerns about early debriefing and has led the field to consider other interventions that may be viable alternatives to debriefing.

19.4.2. Alternatives to Psychological Debriefing

In the wake of increasing evidence that CISD does not prevent PTSD, there has been a shift in thinking about what to offer disaster survivors in the immediate aftermath of their trauma. A recent commentary has summarized current conceptualizations about immediate disaster response by noting five key principles that are important in facilitating adaptation after disaster (Hobfoll et al., 2007). The first principle is promoting a sense of safety for survivors. This step is imperative because of the overwhelming evidence that one of the strongest predictors of subsequent problems is the sense that one is under persistent threat (Mikulincer & Solomon, 1988) and that enhancing safety is associated with reductions in adverse mental health outcomes (Ozer, Best, Lipsey, & Weiss, 2003). Safety can be promoted at individual, group, organizational, and community levels; the common messages across these contexts are that practical steps to increase actual safety are useful, enhancing the perception that immediate threat has subsided and teaching that trauma reminders are not actually harmful. The second goal is promoting calming, which aims to reduce the hyperarousal that is frequent after disaster. This principle emerges from evidence that hyperarousal in the acute aftermath of trauma is strongly predictive of subsequent PTSD (Bryant, 2006; Shalev & Freedman, 2005). As noted earlier, one argument against the utility of CISD has been that it potentially increases arousal immediately after trauma exposure, and this may impair adaptation (Hobfoll et al., 2007). The range of strategies that can be issued to calm an individual includes relaxation training, breathing control, problem solving, and adaptive self-talk. The third principle involves promoting a sense of self-efficacy, which refers to the belief that one's actions will lead to a positive outcome. This perception is often lost in the aftermath of disasters, so it is important to encourage individuals and communities to regain a sense of control over their environment. Problem solving is a core strategy in this goal because it allows individuals to develop the skills to successfully overcome their immediate problems. The fourth goal is promoting connectedness because of the very strong evidence that social support is one of the strongest buffers against problems after trauma exposure (Norris et al., 2002). The fifth goal is instilling hope because optimism can be an important predictor of successful outcomes after trauma (Antonovsky, 1979). Optimism can be achieved at an individual level by cognitive reframing of one's expectations so they are not overly negative and at a community level by public activities that focus on adaptation, recovery, and problem solving.

19.4.3. Psychological First Aid

Building on many of the principles highlighted by Hobfoll and colleagues (2007), the most common alternative to CISD is psychological first aid (PFA; Young, 2006). PFA has three major goals. The first goal is to facilitate adaptive coping and problem solving for disaster survivors, which is met by establishing the survivor's safety through ensuring that the survivor has shelter, food, water, medical supplies, and other essential resources. The second goal of PFA is to reduce acute stress reactions. This goal is met by reducing the postdisaster stressors that the survivor may be exposed to (e.g., limiting exposure to grotesque sights, restricting exposure to trauma reminders) and by providing a tool-kit of potential strategies that may limit stress reactions. The latter includes techniques to reduce physiological arousal and encourage adaptive appraisals about the postdisaster environment, including muscle relaxation procedures, education to normalize reactions, and cognitive reframing techniques to reduce overly negative judgments about one's response to the disaster. The third major goal of PFA is to guide the survivor to additional resources that may enhance their coping. This strategy is based on the notion that an important ingredient in the adaptation process is to regain control over one's environment. Simply encouraging a survivor to access agencies that assist in rebuilding one's house may decrease one's sense of helplessness and loss of control because it places the survivor in a position of successful problem solving. Importantly, PFA does not encourage ventilation of the trauma experience (which is prescribed in CISD), although it permits discussion of the event if the individual wishes to talk about the experience. In this way, PFA attempts to enhance coping skills in the immediate aftermath of a disaster without causing undue distress by directing the survivor to revisit the traumatic experience.

It should be noted that PFA has not yet been subjected to empirical scrutiny, so it is premature to conclude that it is the appropriate response. In the absence of studies, expert consensus meetings have endorsed PFA (National Institute of Mental Health, 2002). One of the interesting challenges for studies of PFA is to define the target measures that attempt to measure the success of PFA because it does not explicitly prevent PTSD or other mental health disorders. Accordingly, there is a need to determine the appropriate outcomes of PFA, which at this point in time are adaptive coping skills in the postdisaster environment. In the meantime, PFA appears to be a promising approach to managing immediate reactions to disasters, and it has been adopted by numerous government agencies (for full details of PFA, see National Child Traumatic Stress Network and National Center for PTSD, 2006).

19.5. INTERMEDIATE INTERVENTIONS AFTER DISASTER

This section reviews the available evidence on treating posttraumatic disorders that can arise in the intermediate phase after a disaster. Intermediate interventions refer to treatments that occur after the initial phase has finished, the survivor is safe and has sufficient resources to allocate to a formal intervention, and there is a determined problem that the intervention will address. Unfortunately, there is very little empirical evidence pertaining to the treatment of disaster-affected people. Although there is a substantial literature on efficacious treatments of PTSD and comorbid conditions, this literature is nearly exclusively focused on survivors of discrete civilian trauma or military trauma. It seems reasonable to extrapolate from these studies to posttraumatic disorders after disasters, although as we discuss in the subsequent text, there may be reasons to consider that disaster-affected people may respond differently to established treatments.

19.5.1. Cognitive-Behavior Therapy

There is little doubt that the treatment of choice for all posttraumatic disorders is cognitive-behavior therapy (CBT). The treatment components that typically constitute CBT depend on the nature of the psychological disorder experienced by the disaster survivor, but here we describe the more common strategies used in CBT programs. Virtually all CBT programs commence with psychoeducation about common reactions following a disaster. This component aims to legitimize the individual's reactions, help the individual to develop a formulation of his/her problems, and to establish a rationale for the treatment. Anxiety management strategies are often employed to provide individuals with coping skills to assist them in gaining a sense of mastery over their fear, to reduce arousal levels, and to assist them when engaging in exposure to traumatic memories. Anxiety management approaches often include stress inoculation training that follows Meichenbaum's (1975) program of psychoeducation, relaxation skills, thought stopping, and self-talk. Cognitive therapy strategies are also employed to counteract maladaptive appraisals pivotal in the development and maintenance of a range of posttraumatic adjustment problems (Ehlers & Clark, 2000). Cognitive therapy involves teaching individuals to identify and evaluate the evidence for negative automatic thoughts, as well as helping patients to evaluate their beliefs about the trauma, the self, the world, and the future (Beck, Rush, Shaw, & Emery, 1979).

Exposure is a CBT procedure that targets avoidance of feared memories and reminders of traumatic events. Prolonged imaginal exposure requires the individual to vividly imagine the trauma for prolonged periods. The therapist assists the patient to provide a narrative of their traumatic experience in a way that emphasizes all relevant details, including sensory cues and affective responses. In an attempt to maximize the sense of reliving the experience, the individual may be asked to provide the narrative in the present tense, speak in the first person, and ensure that there is focus on the most distressing aspects. Prolonged exposure typically occurs for at least 50 minutes and is usually supplemented by daily homework exercises. Variants of imaginal exposure involve requiring clients to repeatedly write down detailed descriptions of the experience (Resick & Schnicke, 1993) and implementing exposure with the assistance of virtual reality paradigms via computer-generated imagery (Rothbaum, Hodges, Ready, Graap, & Alarcon, 2001). Most exposure treatments supplement imaginal exposure with in vivo exposure that involves live graded exposure to the feared trauma-related stimuli.

19.5.2. CBT for Disaster-Related PTSD

There is now consistent evidence that CBT is an efficacious intervention for PTSD (see Foa, 2000; Harvey, Bryant, & Tarrier, 2003). There is also limited evidence that the same techniques are useful for survivors of disasters who develop PTSD. In a series of studies, Başoğlu and colleagues (Başoğlu, Livanou, Şalcioğlu, & Kalender, 2003; Başoğlu, Şalcioğlu, & Livanou, 2007) demonstrated that a single session of CBT with earthquake survivors was effective in decreasing PTSD, and survivors who received repeated assessments had decreased fear of subsequent earthquakes. This intervention did not involve cognitive restructuring but focused on teaching participants to engage in self-exposure to fear-evoking situations with an emphasis on self-control during these reexposures. Despite the apparent utility of this approach, these studies treated survivors of earthquakes years after they were exposed to the major quake. Accordingly, this evidence does not relate directly to intermediate interventions. Currently, our best indirect evidence comes from intermediate interventions after nondisaster traumatic events.

19.6. EARLY INTERVENTION FOR PTSD

19.6.1. Identification of People Who Are at High Risk for PTSD

The evidence that most people will adapt in the months after a disaster poses a difficult challenge for possible early intervention strategies. In the early aftermath of disasters, it is often imprudent and logistically infeasible to provide expert care. In addition, as clinician resources are limited, it is inappropriate to case a wide net because most people do not require intervention; they either have little impairments, or they will soon adapt on the basis of their own resourcefulness. Apart from possibly wasting limited health resources, we also need to be concerned about respecting and not interfering with natural recovery processes. The fact remains, however, that a significant minority of people will have persistent psychological problems after disaster, and a major challenge shortly after a traumatic event is how to accurately discriminate between these people and the majority of people who are displaying a transient stress reaction.

The fourth edition of the *Diagnostic and statistical manual of mental disorders* (DSM-IV; American Psychiatric Association, 1994) introduced the acute stress disorder (ASD) diagnosis to describe stress reactions in the initial month after a trauma. One goal of the diagnosis was to identify people shortly after trauma exposure who would subsequently develop PTSD (Koopman, Classen, Cardeña, & Spiegel, 1995). The DSM-IV stipulates that ASD can occur after a fearful response to experiencing or witnessing a threatening event. The requisite symptoms to meet criteria for ASD include three dissociative symptoms, one reexperiencing symptom, marked avoidance, marked anxiety or increased arousal, and evidence of significant distress or impairment. The disturbance must last for a minimum of 2 days and a maximum of 4 weeks, after which time a diagnosis of PTSD should be considered. The primary difference between the criteria for ASD and PTSD is the timeframe and the former's emphasis on dissociative reactions to the trauma. The diagnosis of ASD requires that the individual has at least three of the following: (1) a subjective sense of numbing or detachment, (2) reduced awareness of one's surroundings, (3) derealization, (4) depersonalization, or (5) dissociative amnesia.

There are now many prospective studies that have prospectively assessed in adults the relationship between ASD in the initial month after trauma and development of subsequent PTSD (Brewin, Andrews, Rose, & Kirk, 1999; Bryant & Harvey, 1998; Creamer, O'Donnell, & Pattison, 2004; Difede et al., 2002; Harvey & Bryant, 1998, 1999, 2000; Holeva, Tarrier, & Wells, 2001; Kangas, Henry, & Bryant, 2005; Murray, Ehlers, & Mayou, 2002; Schnyder, Moergeli, Klaghofer, & Buddeberg, 2001; Staab, Grieger, Fullerton, & Ursano, 1996). In terms of people who meet criteria for ASD, a number of studies have found that approximately three-quarters of trauma survivors who display ASD subsequently develop PTSD (Brewin et al., 1999; Bryant & Harvey, 1998; Difede et al., 2002; Harvey & Bryant, 1998, 1999, 2000; Holeva et al., 2001; Kangas et al., 2005; Murray et al., 2002). Compared to the expected remission of most people who display initial posttraumatic stress reactions, these studies indicate that the ASD diagnosis is performing reasonably well in predicting people who will develop PTSD. It should be noted that many people develop PTSD without initially displaying ASD, apparently because many people develop PTSD without initial dissociative symptoms (Bryant, 2003). Similar patterns have been found across several studies of children after traumatic events (Bryant, Salmon, Sinclair, & Davidson, 2007; Kassam-Adams & Winston, 2004; Meiser-Stedman, Yule, Smith, Glucksman, & Dalgleish, 2005). The limited capacity for ASD to optimally identify most people who are at high risk of developing PTSD has led others to look for alternate means to identify people who are at high risk (see Bryant, 2003). Consequently, some commentators have suggested that assessing severity of PTSD symptoms in the period after trauma exposure may be the best way to identify people who will develop chronic PTSD (Brewin, 2005).

19.6.2. Early Intervention for PTSD

There have been attempts to prevent PTSD by administering CBT several weeks after trauma exposure. Foa and colleagues (1995) provided an abridged version of CBT several weeks after trauma. Each participant received four sessions and was then assessed by blind providers at 2 months posttreatment and 5 months follow-up. Whereas 10% of the CBT group met criteria for PTSD at 2 months, 70% of the control group met the criteria; there were no differences between the groups at 5 months, although the CBT group was less depressed. In a subsequent study, Foa, Zoellner, and Feeny (2002) randomly allocated survivors of assault who met criteria for PTSD in the initial weeks after the assault to 4 weekly sessions of CBT, repeated assessment, or supportive counselling. At posttreatment, patients in the CBT and repeated-assessment conditions showed comparable improvements. Supportive counseling was associated with greater PTSD severity and greater general anxiety than the CBT group. At 9-month follow-up, approximately 30% of participants in each group met criteria for PTSD.

Despite the limitations of the ASD diagnosis, there is good evidence that people with ASD are more likely to develop chronic PTSD, and therefore these people provide a more stringent test of early intervention strategies (Bryant, 2003). In an initial study of ASD participants, Bryant and colleagues (1998) randomly allocated motor vehicle accident or nonsexual assault survivors with ASD to either CBT or supportive counseling. Both interventions consisted of five 1.5-hour weekly individual therapy sessions. CBT included education about posttraumatic reactions, relaxation training, cognitive restructuring, and imaginal and in vivo exposure to the traumatic event. The supportive counseling condition included trauma education and more general problem-solving skills training in the context of an unconditionally supportive relationship. At the 6-month follow-up, there were fewer participants in the CBT group (20%) who met diagnostic criteria for PTSD compared with supportive counseling control participants (67%). In a subsequent study that dismantled the components of CBT, 45 civilian trauma survivors with ASD were randomly allocated to five sessions of (1) CBT (prolonged exposure, cognitive therapy, anxiety management), (2) prolonged exposure combined with cognitive therapy, or (3) supportive counseling (Bryant, Sackville, Dang, Moulds, & Guthrie, 1999). This study found that at the 6-month follow-up, PTSD was observed in approximately 20% of both active treatment groups compared with 67% of those receiving supportive counseling. The utility of this intervention has been replicated in two subsequent studies by the same team (Bryant, Moulds, Guthrie, & Nixon, 2003, 2005; Bryant, Moulds, Guthrie, Dang, & Nixon, 2003). It should be noted that follow-up of participants who completed these treatment studies indicated that the treatment gains of those who received CBT were maintained up to 4 years after treatment (Bryant, Moulds, & Nixon, 2003; Bryant et al., 2006).

19.7. A STRUCTURE FOR PROVIDING MENTAL HEALTH INTERVENTIONS

Any intervention after a disaster needs to consider the timing of the intervention and the context in which the intervention may occur. It is often misleading to formalize timelines for interventions because the contextual circumstances are variable across disasters. Instead, interventions should be planned in response to the needs and resources of the individual affected by the disaster, taking into account the nature of the postdisaster context. For example, it would be inappropriate to implement exposure therapy 2 months after a hurricane for a woman who has lost her husband, is living in a temporary shelter, and is highly concerned about where she will live with her young children. Despite suffering PTSD and complicated grief, it is likely that the demands being placed on this woman result in her being unable to adequately utilize exposure therapy, and it could place excessive burdens on her and exacerbate her condition. Alternatively, a clinician may decide that it is more useful to focus on problem-solving approaches that address her immediate needs for making decisions about housing and her children and possibly employ non–exposure-based CBT approaches to assist her to come to terms with her husband's death. This woman would benefit from an active CBT program for her PTSD and complicated grief months later when her social situation has settled and she has the resources to allocate to therapy. In another case, however, it may be appropriate to offer CBT a month after the disaster because the individual has the resources to manage the demands of therapy and the therapist feels that the individual would benefit.

Figure 19.1 provides a general schema for planning interventions after a disaster. We suggest that the first step should involve psychological first aid. Although this strategy is not a formal mental health intervention, it allows people in the disaster area to provide the support and assistance that can facilitate coping in the immediate phase after the event. In this context, it is possible to assess immediate psychiatric and physical needs. At this stage, people requiring

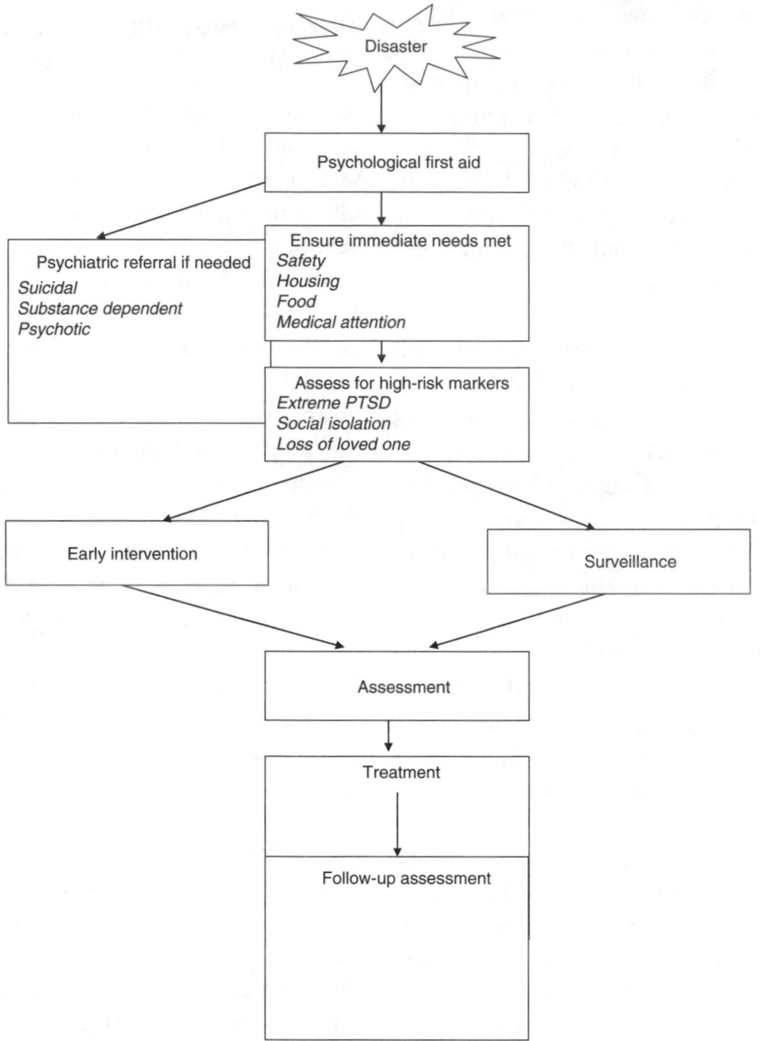

Figure 19.1. Diagram for managing postdisaster mental health needs.
Note: PTSD, posttraumatic stress disorder.

urgent psychiatric assistance, such as addressing suicidal intent, substance dependence, psychosis, or other urgent psychological need, should be referred to available mental health services. Any physical need can be addressed at the same time. The individual may urgently need medical attention, short-term housing, and assistance in connecting with family and friends or other practical issues that could compound the individual's psychological reaction if they are not addressed.

The next stage can involve assessment of people who are at high risk for developing subsequent psychiatric disorder. At this stage, the only body of research that exists pertains to identifying people who may develop PTSD or depression. If the individual is safe and has adequate resources, it is appropriate to provide early intervention (CBT) if that person is displaying initial signs of chronic PTSD or depression. Typically in a disaster context, methods of identifying people who are at high risk for subsequent disorder are error prone, and accordingly, it is useful to implement surveillance methods to identify people months after the disaster to determine if they require mental health interventions. At that point, clinical assessment should be conducted and appropriate evidence-based treatments provided. It is important to follow up disaster survivors over time because many problems may not resolve after treatment, relapse can occur, and ongoing stressors can contribute to new problems that were not initially apparent.

19.8. ADDITIONAL ISSUES FOR PROVIDING MENTAL HEALTH INTERVENTIONS AFTER DISASTERS

19.8.1. Grief

It is not uncommon for survivors of disasters to lose loved ones in the course of the disaster. Whereas grief is the normal response to the loss of a loved one, complicated grief refers to those reactions that persist over time. Complicated grief involves yearning for the deceased, bitterness about the loss, inability to proceed with life, preoccupation with the loss, hopelessness about the future, and preoccupation with sorrow (Lichtenthal, Cruess, & Prigerson, 2004). The available research suggests that complicated grief persists in approximately 10% of bereaved people (Bonanno & Field, 2001). Although previous reviews of grief counseling approaches have shown them to be largely ineffective (Kato & Mann, 1999), recent treatments that have incorporated CBT strategies, including exposure and cognitive therapy, have been shown to be effective. Shear and colleagues (2005) compared a form of CBT with interpersonal psychotherapy to treat complicated grief. The CBT comprised (1) grief reduction by imaginal and in vivo exposure, (2) communicating unresolved issues with the deceased, (3) increasing activity schedules, and (4) distress tolerance. Imaginal exposure focused on the death scene, and in vivo exposure focused on avoided situations. This study found that CBT performed more effectively than interpersonal psychotherapy, with more patients recovering after receiving CBT (51%) than interpersonal psychotherapy (28%). This approach has been replicated in independent trials of CBT for people suffering complicated grief (Boelen, Keijser, van den Hout, & van den Bout, 2007).

19.8.2. Ongoing Stressors

It is very common in the aftermath of a disaster that survivors will experience a range of ongoing stressors that can compound their reaction. Relocation, loss of employment, pain, physical injury, legal procedures, and financial loss are some of the common burdens that disaster survivors endure. There is considerable evidence that posttraumatic stress is compounded by the presence of stressors occurring in the posttraumatic phase (Bryant & Harvey, 1995; King, King, Fairbank, & Keane, 1996); therefore, it is important to consider the current demands on disaster survivors when planning any intervention. Many therapies are very taxing on the individual, especially those using exposure-based strategies, and it is often premature to offer more effortful therapy programs to survivors if they are currently dealing with marked stressors in the wake of the disaster. For example, a person in New Orleans who lost his/her house in Hurricane Katrina and still is struggling to find housing and employment may not be able to focus on trauma-focused therapy because there are other more pressing concerns that need to be addressed. In such cases, it may be more appropriate to offer problem-solving strategies that assist the person in managing immediate needs before commencing with other therapy modalities that address PTSD or related conditions.

In this sense, very often the best "mental health" interventions may be practical strategies that alleviate current stress and facilitate return to prior routines and functioning. The importance of practical assistance as the most important form of mental health intervention has been noted for many years, and there are many instances of how practical assistance has assisted disaster survivors' mental health (Gist & Lubin, 1989). Typifying the role of practical input, anecdotal reports after the Asian tsunami indicated that one of the most beneficial steps taken to alleviate depression in southern Thailand was the rebuilding of fishing, which allowed men to resume fishing and ensure that the economies of fishing villages were sustained (Bryant & Njenga, 2006). Practical input that meets survivors' daily needs is a cornerstone of PFA and has also been noted as one of the key principles of managing postdisaster mental health (Hobfoll et al., 2007).

19.8.3. Ongoing Threat

Many treatment programs for PTSD presume that the threat has passed and that treatment is occurring in a context of relative safety. In the wake of many disasters, however, it is possible that realistic threats persist when therapy is commencing. Aftershocks may occur after an earthquake, housing may collapse after a hurricane, or subsequent attacks may occur in the context of terrorist attacks. For example, after the September 11th terrorist attacks in New York City, there was a concern about anthrax circulating in a number of cities. Although concern about realistic threat can be adaptive, many studies have shown that people with anxiety disorders exaggerate the likelihood of harmful events happening to them, and this pattern clearly impedes adequate functioning (Dunmore, Clark, & Ehlers, 2001; Ehlers, Mayou, & Bryant, 1998; Warda & Bryant, 1998). Thus, there is a need to encourage adaptive appraisals about safety while not encouraging dysfunctional behaviors.

Recent commentaries have noted that cognitive therapy approaches need to be modified to accommodate the particular needs of people living under conditions of potential threat. Marshall and colleagues (2007) proposed a series of steps in teaching appropriate risk appraisals with survivors of terrorist-related disasters. The first step is to clarify the person's belief; it is essential to determine whether the belief is rational or is excessive in the light of available evidence. Second, one should empathically challenge the validity of the belief by discerning between what is "likely risk" and "acceptable risk." Most people accept certain levels of risk on a daily basis, such as driving a car in traffic, because it reaps certain rewards. This is an important step to avoid the common problem of seeking zero levels of risk, which can never be attained, and objectively determining that the likelihood of threat is a useful exercise. For example, Marshall and colleagues (2007) cite the example of helping a person understand the risk of traveling on a subway. They calculated that an attack similar to the London subway bombings would kill 40 persons/4,500,000 daily riders, which resulted in the likelihood of 1 death in 100,000 on that day. On the basis that one attack occurs per year, the risk was estimated at 1 in 30 million, or essentially zero. The third step involves highlighting the benefits and losses associated with a belief that threat is imminent. Take, for example, a New Yorker who decided to avoid Manhattan and any high-rise buildings after September 11th; although this strategy may have provided short-term relief of anxiety, it could also have led to loss of job, career advancement, and social interaction, and financial losses. Engaging in motivational interviewing about the benefits and losses of ascribing to a particular belief can assist a disaster survivor in deciding that accepting a reasonable level of risk is in their best interest (Walitzer, Dermen, & Conners, 1999). Finally, the fourth step is to test these beliefs by engaging in experiments that allow the person to learn that their fear is not justified. These steps can be useful in helping people to learn that despite some level of potential threat, they can still function in a way that is reasonably safe.

19.8.4. Mass Violence

One of the major issues after a large-scale disaster is the limited resources for mental health services available to those who are affected by the event. The sudden increase in need for mental health services typically overwhelms most mental health agencies. The numbers of people affected by recent events such as the September 11th terrorist attacks, Hurricane Katrina, and the Asian tsunami highlight that governments do not have the resources to provide mental health services to those who seek them, and there are limited numbers of personnel who are trained in treating posttraumatic disorders. There is also abundant evidence that most people with PTSD do not seek treatment (Boscarino, Galea, Ahern, Resnick, & Vlahov, 2002; Hoge, Auchterlonie, & Milliken, 2006; Kulka & Schlenger, 1990; Smith,

Christiansen, & Hann, 1999). Taken together, these factors point to the need for novel means to disseminate effective treatment programs to the thousands of people who require mental health assistance but do not receive this help from traditional services.

The World Wide Web is providing some promising avenues to provide CBT to people who cannot access formal mental health services. The Web is useful because many CBT strategies can be taught without the direct input from a therapist, it disseminates treatment to people in remote regions, it can provide therapy to people who avoid formal treatment services, and it provides anonymity to people who are reluctant to disclose their need for treatment (Litz, Williams, Wang, Bryant, & Engel, 2004). Several recent studies demonstrated the potential for the Web to assist people after disaster. A feasibility study was conducted in New York City after the September 11th terrorist attacks, in which 285 out of 1,035 participants accepted an invitation to participate in the program. This program contained modules that were based on CBT principles and addressed PTSD/panic, depression, worry, alcohol use, marijuana use, drug use, and cigarette use. The acceptance rate was encouraging, and many participants reported greater knowledge of these areas after completing the modules. More recently, a randomized controlled trial was conducted with military personnel who were in the Pentagon when it was attacked and provided them with an initial single therapy session followed by either a Web-based CBT program or a Web-based program in which they wrote about their daily concerns (Litz, Engels, Bryant, & Papa, 2007). The CBT consisted of self-monitoring of situations that triggered trauma-related distress, stress management strategies, self-guided in vivo exposure, and writing about the trauma. The program led to one-third of participants achieving high-end state functioning compared with none of the participants in the control condition.

These finding needs to be considered in the context of other Web-based programs that have successfully reduced symptoms of grief (Wagner, Knaevelsrud, & Maercker, 2006) and depression (Christensen, Leach, Barney, Mackinnon, & Griffiths, 2006). Together, there is initial evidence to suggest that Web-based programs have a role to play in reducing disaster-related psychological problems. Although it is probable that Web-based programs will not be as effective as personal therapy programs, the Web can ensure that therapy can be provided to disaster survivors who would otherwise not receive any therapeutic intervention.

19.9. CONCLUDING COMMENT

Disasters can be profoundly disruptive. A person, a family, a community, or an entire culture can lose the things that otherwise contribute to well-being and quality of life. Substantial physical resources and livelihoods can be lost, and the emotional residue can linger for months and years. PFA is recommended for mental health professionals wanting to help survivors in the immediate aftermath of disasters. It is an informal conversational approach to care that is sensitive to timing and context, respects individuals' ability to recover, and is based on their culture and their resources. It is also a useful prelude to formal secondary prevention interventions, of which CBT is the prescriptive form of care.

REFERENCES

American Psychiatric Association. (1994). *Diagnostic and statistical manual of mental disorders, 4th ed.* Washington, DC: American Psychiatric Association.

Antonovsky, A. (1979). *Health, stress, and coping.* San Francisco, CA: Jossey-Bass.

Başoğlu, M., Livanou, E., Şalcioğlu, E., & Kalender, D. (2003). A brief behavioural treatment of chronic post-traumatic stress disorder in earthquake survivors: Results from an open trial. *Psychological Medicine, 33*, 647–654.

Başoğlu, M., Şalcioğlu, E., & Livanou, E. (2007). A randomized controlled study of single-session behavioural treatment of earthquake-related post-traumatic stress disorder using an earthquake simulator. *Psychological Medicine, 37*, 203–213.

Beck, A. T., Rush, A. J., Shaw, B. F., & Emery, G. (1979). *Cognitive therapy of depression.* New York: Guilford Press.

Bisson, J. I., Jenkins, P. L., Alexander, J., & Bannister, C. (1997). Randomised controlled trial of psychological debriefing for victims of acute burn trauma. *British Journal of Psychiatry*, *171*, 78–81.

Boelen, P. A., de Keijser, J., van den Hout, M. A., & van den Bout, J. (2007). Treatment of complicated grief: A comparison between cognitive-behavioral therapy and supportive counseling. *Journal of Consulting and Clinical Psychology*, *75*, 277–284

Bonanno, G. A., & Field, N. P. (2001). The varieties of grief experience. *Clinical Psychological Review*, *21*, 705–734.

Boscarino, J. A., Galea, S., Ahern, J., Resnick, H., & Vlahov, D. (2002). Utilization of mental health services following the September 11th terrorist attacks in Manhattan, New York City. *International Journal of Emergency Mental Health*, *4*, 143–155.

Brewin, C. R. (2005). Systematic review of screening instruments for adults at risk of PTSD. *Journal of Traumatic Stress*, *18*, 53–62

Brewin, C. R., Andrews, B., Rose, S., & Kirk, M. (1999). Acute stress disorder and posttraumatic stress disorder in victims of violent crime. *American Journal of Psychiatry*, *156*, 360–366.

Bryant, R. A. (2003). Early predictors of posttraumatic stress disorder. *Biological Psychiatry*, *53*, 789–795.

(2006). Longitudinal psychophysiological studies of heart rate: Mediating effects and implications for treatment. In R Yehuda. (Ed.), *Psychobiology of PTSD: A decade of progress. Annals of the New York Academy of Sciences*. Wiley-Backwell.

Bryant, R. A., & Harvey, A. G. (1995). Psychological impairment following motor vehicle accidents. *Australian Journal of Public Health*, *19*, 185–188.

(1998). Relationship of acute stress disorder and posttraumatic stress disorder following mild traumatic brain injury. *American Journal of Psychiatry*, *155*, 625–629.

Bryant, R. A., Harvey, A. G., Dang, S. T., Sackville, T., & Basten, C. (1998). Treatment of acute stress disorder: A comparison of cognitive behavior therapy and supportive counseling. *Journal of Consulting and Clinical Psychology*, *66*, 862–866.

Bryant, R. A., Moulds, M. L., Guthrie, R. M., Dang, S. T., & Nixon, R. D. V. (2003). Imaginal exposure alone and imaginal exposure with cognitive restructuring in treatment of posttraumatic stress disorder. *Journal of Consulting and Clinical Psychology*, *71*, 706–712.

Bryant, R. A., Moulds, M. L., Guthrie, R., & Nixon, R. D. V. (2003). Treating acute stress disorder after mild brain injury. *American Journal of Psychiatry*, *160*, 585–587.

Bryant, R. A., Moulds, M. L., Guthrie, R. M., & Nixon, R. V. (2005). The additive benefit of hypnosis and cognitive behavior therapy in treating acute stress disorder. *Journal of Consulting and Clinical Psychology*, *73*, 334–340.

Bryant, R. A., Moulds, M. A., & Nixon, R. (2003). Cognitive behaviour therapy of acute stress disorder: A four-year follow-up. *Behaviour Research and Therapy*, *41*, 489–494.

Bryant, R. A., Moulds, M. L., Nixon, R. V., Mastrodomenico, J., Felmingham, K., & Hopwood, S. (2006). Hypnotherapy and cognitive behaviour therapy of acute stress disorder: A three year follow-up. *Behaviour Research and Therapy*, *44*, 1331–1335.

Bryant, R. A., & Njenga, F. (2006). Cultural sensitivity: making assessment and treatment plans culturally relevant. *Journal of Clinical Psychiatry*, *67*(Supp. 2), 74–79.

Bryant, R. A., Sackville, T., Dang, S. T., Moulds, M., & Guthrie, R. (1999). Treating acute stress disorder: An evaluation of cognitive behavior therapy and counselling techniques. *American Journal of Psychiatry*, *156*, 1780–1786.

Bryant, R. A, Salmon, K., Sinclair, E., & Davidson, P. (2007). The relationship between acute stress disorder and posttraumatic stress disorder in injured children. *Journal of Traumatic Stress*, *20*, 1075–1079.

Christensen, H., Leach, L. S., Barney, L., Mackinnon, A. J., & Griffiths, K. M. (2006). The effect of web based depression interventions on self reported help seeking: Randomised controlled trial. *BMC Psychiatry*, *6*(1), 13.

Conlon, L., Fahy, T. J., & Conroy, R. (1999). PTSD in ambulant RTA victims: A randomized controlled trial of debriefing. *Journal of Psychosomatic Research*, *46*, 37–44.

Creamer, M. C., O'Donnell, M. L., & Pattison, P. (2004). The relationship between acute stress disorder and posttraumatic stress disorder in severely injured trauma survivors. *Behaviour Research and Therapy*, *42*, 315–328.

Difede, J., Ptacek, J. T., Roberts, J. G., Barocas, D., Rives, W., Apfeldorf, W. J., et al. (2002). Acute stress disorder after burn injury: A predictor of posttraumatic stress disorder. *Psychosomatic Medicine*, *64*, 826–834.

Dunmore, E., Clark, D. M., & Ehlers, A. (2001). A prospective investigation of the role of cognitive factors in persistent Posttraumatic Stress Disorder (PTSD) after physical and sexual assault. *Behaviour Research and Therapy*, *39*, 1063–1084.

Ehlers, A., & Clark, D. (2000). A cognitive model of posttraumatic stress disorder. *Behaviour Research and Therapy*, *38*, 319–345.

Ehlers, A., Mayou, R.A., & Bryant, B. (1998). Psychological predictors of chronic PTSD after motor vehicle accidents. *Journal of Abnormal Psychology, 107*, 508–519.

Everly, G.S., Jr., & Mitchell, J.T. (1999). *Critical incident stress management (CISM): A new era and standard of care in crisis intervention, 2nd ed.* Ellicott City, MD: Chevron.

Foa, E.B. (2000). Psychosocial treatment of posttraumatic stress disorder. *Journal of Clinical Psychiatry, 61* (Suppl. 5), 43–48.

Foa, E.B., Hearst-Ikeda, D., & Perry, K.J. (1995). Evaluation of a brief cognitive behavioral program for the prevention of chronic PTSD in recent assault victims. *Journal of Consulting and Clinical Psychology, 63*, 948–955.

Foa, E.B., Zoellner, L.A., & Feeny, N.C. (2002). An evaluation of three brief programs for facilitating recovery after assault. *Journal of Traumatic Stress, 19*, 29–43.

Galea, S., Ahern, J., Resnick, H., Kilpatrick, D., Bucuvalas, M., Gold, J., et al. (2002). Psychological sequelae of the September 11 terrorist attacks. *New England Journal of Medicine, 346*, 982–987.

Galea, S., Vlahov, D., Resnick, H., Ahern, J., Susser, E., Gold, J., et al. (2003). Trends of probable posttraumatic stress disorder in New York City after the September 11 terrorist attacks. *American Journal of Epidemiology, 158*, 514–524.

Gist, R., & Lubin, B. (1989). *Psychosocial aspects of disaster.* Oxford: John Wiley & Sons.

Harvey, A.G., & Bryant, R.A. (1998). Relationship of acute stress disorder and posttraumatic stress disorder following motor vehicle accidents. *Journal of Consulting and Clinical Psychology, 66*, 507–512.

(1999). A two-year prospective evaluation of the relationship between acute stress disorder and posttraumatic stress disorder. *Journal of Consulting and Clinical Psychology, 67*, 985–988.

(2000). A two-year prospective evaluation of the relationship between acute stress disorder and posttraumatic stress disorder following mild traumatic brain injury. *American Journal of Psychiatry, 157*, 626–628.

Harvey, A.G., Bryant, R.A., & Tarrier, N. (2003). Cognitive behaviour therapy of posttraumatic stress disorder. *Clinical Psychology Review, 23*, 501–522.

Hobbs, M., Mayou, R., Harrison, B., & Worlock, P. (1996). A randomised controlled trial of psychological debriefing for victims of road traffic accidents. *British Medical Journal, 313*, 1438–1439.

Hobfoll, S.E., Watson, P., Bell, C.C., Bryant, R.A., Brymer, M.J., Friedman, M.J., et al. (2007). Five essential elements of immediate and mid-term mass trauma intervention: Empirical evidence. *Psychiatry, 70*, 283–315.

Hoge, C.W., Auchterlonie, J.L., & Milliken, C.S. (2006). Mental health problems, use of mental health services, and attrition from military service after returning from deployment to Iraq or Afghanistan. *JAMA, 295*, 1023–1032.

Holeva, V., Tarrier, N., & Wells, A. (2001). Prevalence and predictors of acute stress disorder and PTSD following road traffic accidents: Thought control strategies and social support. *Behavior Therapy, 32*, 65–83.

Kangas, M., Henry, J.L., & Bryant, R.A. (2005). The relationship between acute stress disorder and posttraumatic stress disorder following cancer. *Journal of Consulting and Clinical Psychology, 73*, 360–364.

Kassam-Adams, N., & Winston, F.K. (2004). Predicting child PTSD: The relationship between acute stress disorder and PTSD in injured children. *Journal of the American Academy of Child & Adolescent Psychiatry, 43*, 403–411.

Kato, P.M., & Mann, T. (1999). A synthesis of psychological interventions for the bereaved. *Clinical Psychology Review, 19*, 275–296.

King, L.A., King, D.W., Fairbank, J.A., & Keane, T.M. (1996). Resilience-recovery factors in posttraumatic stress disorder among female and male Vietnam veterans: Hardiness, postwar social support, and additional stressful life events. *Journal of Personality and Social Psychology, 74*, 420–434.

Koopman, C., Classen, C., Cardeña, E., & Spiegel, D. (1995). When disaster strikes, acute stress disorder may follow. *Journal of Traumatic Stress, 8*, 29–46.

Kulka, R.A., & Schlenger, W.E. (1990). *The national Vietnam veterans readjustment study.* New York: Brunner/Mazel.

Lichtenthal, W.G., Cruess, D.G., Prigerson, H.G. (2004). A case for establishing complicated grief as a distinct mental disorder in DSM-V. *Clinical Psychology Review, 24*, 637–662.

Litz, B., Engels, C., Bryant, R.A., & Papa, A. (2007). A randomized controlled proof of concept trial of an internet-based therapist-assisted self-management treatment for posttraumatic stress disorder. *American Journal of Psychiatry, 164*, 1676–1684.

Litz, B.T., Williams, L., Wang, J., Bryant, R.A., & Engel, C.C. (2004). The development of an Internet-based program to deliver therapist-assisted self-help behavioral treatment for traumatic stress. *Professional Psychology: Science and Practice, 35*, 628–634.

Marshall, R.D., Bryant, R.A., Amsel, L., Cook, F., Suh, E.J., & Neria, Y. (2007). Relative risk perception and 9/11-related PTSD in the context of ongoing threat. *American Psychologist*, *62*, 304–316.

McFarlane, A. C. (1986). Posttraumatic morbidity of a disaster. *Journal of Nervous and Mental Disease*, *174*, 4–14.

McNally, R. J., Bryant, R. A., & Ehlers, A. (2003). Psychological debriefing and its alternatives: A critique of early intervention for trauma survivors. *Psychological Science in the Public Interest*, *4*, 45–79.

Meichenbaum, D. (1975). Self-instructional methods. In F. H. Kanfer & A. P. Goldstein (Eds.), *Helping people change*. New York: Pergamon.

Meiser-Stedman, R., Yule, W., Smith, P., Glucksman, E., & Dalgleish, T. (2005). Acute stress disorder and posttraumatic stress disorder in children and adolescents involved in assaults or motor vehicle accidents. *American Journal of Psychiatry*, *162*, 1381–1383.

Mikulincer, M., & Solomon, Z. (1988). Attributional style and combat-related posttraumatic stress disorder. *Journal of Abnormal Psychology*, *97*, 308–313.

Mitchell, J. T. (1983). When disaster strikes…The Critical Incident Stress Debriefing process. *Journal of Emergency Medical Services*, *8*, 36–39.

Mitchell, J., & Bray, G. (1990). *Emergency services stress*. Englewood Cliffs, NJ: Prentice-Hall.

Murray, J., Ehlers, A., & Mayou, R. A. (2002). Dissociation and post-traumatic stress disorder: Two prospective studies of road traffic accident survivors. *British Journal of Psychiatry*, *180*, 363–368.

National Child Traumatic Stress Network, and National Center for PTSD. (2006). *Psychological first aid: Field operations guide, 2nd ed.*; http://www.nctsn.org.

National Institute of Mental Health. (2002). *Mental health and mass violence – Evidence based early psychological intervention for victims/survivors of mass violence: a workshop to reach consensus on best practices* (NIH Publication No. 02–5138). Washington, DC: U.S. Government Publishing Office.

Neria, Y., Nandi, A., & Galea, S. (2007). Post-traumatic stress disorder following disasters: A systematic review. *Psychological Medicine*, *38*, 467–480.

Norris, F. H., Friedman, M. J., Watson, P. J., Byrne, C. R., Diaz, E., & Kaniasty, K. (2002). 60,000 disaster victims speak: Part I. An empirical review of the empirical literature, 1981–2001. *Psychiatry*, *65*, 207–239

North, C. S., Nixon, S. J., Shariat, S., Mallonee, S., McMillen, J. C., Spitznagel, E. L., et al. (1999). Psychiatric disorders among survivors of the Oklahoma City bombing. *JAMA*, *282*, 755–762.

Ozer, E. J., Best, S. R., Lipsey, T. L., & Weiss, D. S. (2003). Predictors of posttraumatic stress disorder and symptoms in adults: A meta-analysis. *Psychological Bulletin*, *129*, 52–73.

Raphael, B., & Wilson, J. P. (Eds.). (2000). *Psychological debriefing: Theory, practice and evidence*. Cambridge, England: Cambridge University Press.

Resick, P.A., & Schnicke, M. K. (1993). *Cognitive processing therapy for rape victims: a treatment manual*. London: Sage.

Rose, S., Bisson, J., & Wessely, S. (2001). *Psychological debriefing for preventing posttraumatic stress disorder (PTSD)* (Cochrane Library, Issue 3). Oxford, England: Update Software.

Rose, S., Brewin, C. R., Andrews, B., & Kirk, M. (1999). A randomized controlled trial of individual psychological debriefing for victims of violent crime. *Psychological Medicine*, *29*, 793–799.

Rothbaum, B. O., Hodges, L. F., Ready, D., Graap, K., & Alarcon, R.D. (2001). Virtual reality exposure therapy for Vietnam veterans with posttraumatic stress disorder. *Journal of Clinical Psychiatry*, *62*, 617–22.

Schnyder, U., Moergeli, H., Klaghofer, R., & Buddeberg, C. (2001). Incidence and prediction of posttraumatic stress disorder symptoms in severely injured accident victims. *American Journal of Psychiatry*, *158*, 594–599.

Shalev, A. Y., & Freedman, S. (2005). PTSD following terrorist attacks: A prospective evaluation. *American Journal of Psychiatry*, *162*(6), 1188–1191.

Shear K. M., Frank, E., Houck, P. R., Reynolds, C. F. 3rd. (2005). Treatment of complicated grief: A randomized controlled trial. *JAMA*, *293*, 2601–2608.

Smith, D. W., Christiansen, E. H., & Hann, N. E. (1999). Population effects of the bombing of Oklahoma City. *Journal of the Oklahoma State Medical Association*, *92*, 193–198.

Staab, J. P., Grieger, T. A., Fullerton, C. S., & Ursano, R. J. (1996). Acute stress disorder, subsequent posttraumatic stress disorder and depression after a series of typhoons. *Anxiety*, *2*, 219–225.

van Emmerik, A. A. P., Kamphuis, J. H., Hulsbosch, A. M., & Emmelkamp, P. M. G. (2002). Single session debriefing after psychological trauma: A meta-analysis. *Lancet*, *360*, 766–771.

van Griensven, F., Chakkraband, M. L., Thienkrua, W., Pengjuntr, W., Lopes Cardoza, B., Tantipiwatanaskul, P., et al. (2006). Mental health problems among adults in tsunami-affected areas in Southern Thailand. *JAMA*, *296*, 537–548.

Wagner, B., Knaevelsrud, C., & Maercker, A. (2006). Internet-based cognitive behavioral therapy for complicated grief: A randomized controlled trial. *Death Studies*, *30*, 429–453

Walitzer, K. S, Dermen, K. H., & Conners, G. J. (1999). Strategies for preparing clients for treatment: A review. *Behavior Modification, 23*, 129–151.

Warda, G., & Bryant, R. A. (1998). Cognitive bias in acute stress disorder. *Behaviour Research and Therapy, 36*, 1177–1183.

Young, B. H. (2006). The immediate response to disaster: Guidelines for adult psychological first aid. In E. C. Ritchie, P. J., Watson, & M. J. Friedman (Eds.), *Interventions following mass violence and disasters: Strategies for mental health practice*. New York: Guilford.

20 Evidence-Based Long-Term Treatment of Mental Health Consequences of Disasters among Adults

JoAnn Difede and Judith Cukor

20.1. INTRODUCTION

Disasters come in the form of natural events such as earthquakes, accidents or technological failures such as airplane crashes, and human-generated incidents such as terror attacks (Norris et al., 2002). Such disparate events share a common feature – the swift, most often unanticipated, infliction of harm and damage (Neufeldt & Guralnik, 1989). Statistics on the scope of disasters underscore the challenge of developing and delivering effective mental health care worldwide. For natural disasters alone, between 1991 and 2005, approximately 3,470,162,961 people were affected worldwide while another 960,502 individuals were killed. In 2005, the most recent year for which statistics were available, there were 360 natural disasters worldwide, killing almost 100,000 people and affecting more than 150 million others (United Nations, 2005).

Communities recovering from the aftermath of disasters may have to come to terms with members threatened or actual injury and loss of life, disruption of social relations and networks, loss of property and resources, and increased uncertainty about the future (Norris et al., 2002). Though the impact of disaster usually reverberates throughout a social group (e.g., a family, a community), the focus of empirical study and the locus of intervention is typically the individual. Psychiatric nosology refers to disorder in the individual, and most of what is categorized and quantified concerns the individual, whether the individual is the index trauma patient or a family member.

A review of articles based on studies of 80 disasters worldwide point to five key outcomes of disaster on individuals and communities: (1) "psychological problems," such as posttraumatic stress disorder (PTSD) and major depressive disorder (MDD); (2) "nonspecific distress"; (3) "health problems," such as somatic complaints, increased substance use, and sleep disruption; (4) "chronic problems in living," such as increased interpersonal, occupational, and financial stressors; and (5) "psychosocial resource losses," including reductions in perceived social support and social embeddedness (Norris et al., 2002). The bulk of empirical support for these outcomes is drawn from research on direct victims.

In its consideration of evidence-based treatments, this chapter focuses primarily on the first outcome, "psychological problems." Multiple studies of myriad disasters have documented high rates of PTSD, MDD, and substance abuse or dependence (Norris et al., 2002). Though rates vary by the type of disaster and the methodology employed in each study, it is given that a substantial minority of people who experience a disaster firsthand will develop PTSD, which is the most common disorder following any type of trauma. In an extensive review of the literature, Norris and colleagues (2002) found that PTSD was the most common outcome following disaster, reported in 109 of the 160 studies (68%) published between 1981 and 2001.

In the remainder of this chapter we discuss the evidence base for long-term treatment of the most common outcomes following disaster and the gaps in that knowledge base. The discussion of treatment focuses primarily on psychological interventions and closes with two case studies presented to illustrate symptom presentation, implementation of empirically validated treatments as the standard of care, and barriers to treatment.

20.2. THE LONG-TERM TREATMENT OF PTSD FOLLOWING A DISASTER AMONG ADULTS: THE EVIDENCE BASE

In the past decade or two there has been a growing body of research on psychological interventions for the treatment of PTSD following disaster. Randomized clinical trials have established the efficacy of cognitive-behavioral therapy (CBT) for the treatment of PTSD following many types of trauma (Harvey, Bryant, & Tarrier, 2003).

20.2.1. What Is the Long Term?

For a multitude of reasons, empirical studies of the effects of disaster tend to be restricted to the first year posttrauma. In a review of 160 empirical studies of disaster survivors across the globe, published between 1981 and 2002, Norris and colleagues (2002) concluded that half of the samples in the longitudinal studies were only reassessed within the first year of the disaster. It is remarkable that despite the large numbers of people affected by trauma worldwide every year, few studies have examined its effects beyond the first 2 or 3 years. These limitations appear to be epistemiological, fiscal, and logistical. One problem concerns what the scientific and clinical community is willing to accept as knowledge. With the zeitgeist in psychiatry turning from the presentation of clinical or phenomenological data toward the empirical, there is little interest in the long-term effects (i.e., beyond the first few years) of disasters. Funding for the study of the very long term using empirical methods is also seriously limited, and logistical issues inherent in organizing after a disaster serve as further obstacles.

It is not surprising, then, that as the time frame for the study of the effects of disaster is so short, the time frame for the assessment of treatment outcome studies is even shorter. The prototypical treatment outcome study offers weekly treatment sessions for approximately 12 weeks and then follows participants for 6 months posttreatment (Bisson et al., 2007; Bradley, Greene, Russ, Dutra, & Westen, 2005). Thus, our knowledge regarding long-term efficacy of treatment interventions is limited.

20.2.2. The Evidence for the Treatment of PTSD

In general, there is a substantial evidence base for the psychological treatment of PTSD. A recent report issued by the Institute of Medicine found that exposure therapy was the only treatment for PTSD with substantial empirical support (Institute of Medicine, 2006). A meta-analysis by Bradley and colleagues (2005) reviewed 26 treatment outcome studies following diverse trauma. They concluded that the preponderance of evidence supports CBTs, but more studies are required as the relatively small number of studies prohibited the comparison of specific modes of treatment. Another meta-analysis by Bisson and colleagues (2007) reviewed 38 studies, concluding that individual CBT that focused on the memory of the traumatic event and its meaning was significantly more effective than waitlist or usual care groups in improving symptoms of PTSD, and there was limited evidence that it was even effective in improving symptoms of depression and other anxiety. Eye movement desensitization and reprocessing (EMDR) also showed clinical effectiveness, but the evidence base for EMDR was not as strong as that for CBT with a focus on the traumatic memory. Stress management/relaxation and group CBTs showed success on some measures. Other therapies, including supportive therapy/nondirective counseling, psychodynamic therapies, and hypnotherapy, did not show clinically significant effects on PTSD symptoms.

Within CBTs for PTSD, an impressive evidence base supports the use of prolonged imaginal exposure as a specific therapeutic technique. Over the past decade a multitude of controlled studies (Bryant, Moulds, Guthrie, Dang, & Nixon, 2003; Davis, 2002; Foa et al., 1999; Fecteau & Nicki, 1999; Resick, Nishith, Weaver, Astin, & Feuer, 2002; Rothbaum et al., 1995; Rothbaum,

Hodges, Watson, Kessler, & Opdyke, 1996) have demonstrated positive outcomes for exposure-based treatment in which patients are gradually and systematically exposed to cues likely to elicit memories of the traumatic event (Rothbaum, Meadows, Resick, & Foy, 2000). Consequently, expert treatment guidelines for PTSD were published for the first time in 1999, recommending that CBT with exposure therapy should be the first-line treatment (Foa, Davidson, & Frances, 1999). The current PTSD treatment literature demonstrates the efficacy of CBT, including stress inoculation training, cognitive processing therapy, and exposure therapy, in alleviating symptoms (Rothbaum et al., 2000).

The efficacy of prolonged exposure with disaster victims has been demonstrated in the treatment of 91 individuals who experienced a car bombing in Ireland (Gillespie, Duffy, Hackmann, & Clark, 2002). An average number of eight sessions in this community sample resulted in significant improvement in PTSD symptoms. However, studies specifically for postdisaster are sparse. In our own study of survivors of the World Trade Center (WTC) attacks (Difede, Cukor et al., 2007), we evaluated a CBT protocol using exposure enhanced by a virtual environment. A comparison of the treatment and a waitlist control group showed significant improvement of PTSD symptoms for those treated with the CBT protocol with a large between-group posttreatment effect size. Another study by our group assessing a 12-week CBT protocol for disaster workers following the WTC attacks (Difede, Malta, et al., 2007) found that CBT treatment was effective in reducing PTSD symptoms in this specialized sample following a disaster as well.

Cognitive therapy has also been demonstrated to be an effective treatment technique for PTSD (Resick et al., 2002) and has been used specifically for disaster victims (Difede & Eskra, 2002). Studies comparing the relative gains of imaginal exposure and cognitive restructuring have found comparable rates of improvement on symptoms of PTSD (Marks, Lovell, Noshirvani, Livanou, & Thrasher, 1998; Tarrier, Pilgrim, & Sommerfield, 1999), though Tarrier and Sommerfield (2004) found more significant gains in the cognitive restructuring group on symptoms of PTSD at a 5-year follow-up. Bryant and colleagues (2003) reported that a combined imaginal exposure and cognitive processing treatment was more effective than imaginal exposure alone in improvement of symptoms of PTSD and maladaptive cognitive styles at 6-month follow-up.

20.2.3. Limitations of the PTSD Treatment Outcome Literature

There are several limitations of the PTSD treatment literature. Germane to our topic, very few of the randomized controlled trials (RCTs) have enrolled disaster survivors. Perhaps this is not surprising given the logistical difficulties of organizing a treatment outcome study in the aftermath of disaster (Difede, Cukor, Jayasinghe, & Hoffman, 2006), particularly those disasters that encompass an entire community or geographic region (e.g., the 2006 Hurricane Katrina in the United States). Thus, it is unclear how well the results of RCTs, which carefully define the inclusion criteria of study participants, will translate into the community. In general, there is a paucity of PTSD treatment dissemination studies, and barriers to effective dissemination remain to be addressed (Bradley et al., 2005; Cahill, Foa, Hembree, Marshall, & Nacash, 2006).

Although exposure therapy alone and in combination with cognitive techniques has an unparalleled success rate in treating PTSD, as is the case with most treatments for psychiatric conditions, a substantial minority of patients show only limited benefit. A recent meta-analysis reviewed studies (Bradley et al., 2005) where patients were treated by well-trained clinicians within RCTs with strict inclusion criteria. By the end of the treatment, PTSD did not remit in 17% to 42% of subjects who completed prolonged exposure conditions; the disorder persisted in 25% to 41% of subjects who completed imaginal and/or in vivo exposure conditions; and PTSD persisted in 13% to 50% of those who completed CBT conditions that included some form of exposure therapy. In addition, convergent evidence from multiple studies suggests that less than 50% of PTSD patients improve on serotonin reuptake inhibitors (Foa, Franklin, & Moser, 2002), the only class of medication that has FDA approval for the treatment of PTSD, suggesting that alternative approaches to pharmacotherapy for PTSD should be pursued as well.

Therefore, the collected research suggests that clinical scientists should continue to investigate ways to improve upon current treatments for the consequences of disaster.

20.3. THE TREATMENT OF DISORDERS COMORBID WITH PTSD: MAJOR DEPRESSIVE DISORDER AND SUBSTANCE ABUSE

Comorbidity of major depression and substance abuse with PTSD has been well documented (Jacobsen, Southwick, & Kosten, 2001; Kessler, Sonnega, Bromet, Hughes, & Nelson, 1995).

20.3.1. Major Depressive Disorder

The National Comorbidity Survey (Kessler et al., 1995) reports that 48% of men and 49% of women with PTSD have lifetime major depression, making it the most common comorbidity with PTSD. The relationship between the disorders is unclear. Brady, Killeen, Brewerton, and Lucerini (2000) point out that there are many overlapping symptoms between the two disorders, complicating the issue of differential diagnosis, yet there is also evidence that PTSD and MDD may be independent and common sequelae of exposure to a trauma. Others maintain that depression and PTSD develop as interwoven disorders (Deering, Glover, Ready, Eddleman, & Alarcon, 1996). Prospective studies tracking the onset of the symptoms would help clarify the nature of comorbidity (Deering et al., 1996). Of most relevance to our topic, despite the high rates of comorbid PTSD and depression, the use of therapies in populations with comorbidity has not been explored (Brady et al., 2000). Although a recent meta-analysis of PTSD outcome studies suggests that these treatments may also improve symptoms of depression (Bisson et al., 2007), this is far from a certainty. Given the incidence of MDD following disasters, the paucity of treatment outcome studies focusing on MDD postdisaster is a glaring omission in the disaster studies literature and one that it is imperative to redress in the very near term.

20.3.2. Substance Abuse and Dependence

Multiple studies have found increased use of alcohol as well as prescription and street drugs following disasters (Adams, Boscarino, & Galea, 2006; Joseph, Yule, Williams, & Hodgkinson, 1993; Pfefferbaum & Doughty, 2001; Stewart, Mitchell, Wright, & Loba, 2004; Vlahov et al., 2006). Comorbidity of PTSD and substance abuse ranges from 22% to 43% among civilians (Jacobsen et al., 2001), and rates of comorbidity of alcohol or substance abuse in veteran samples have been cited as high as 75% (Jacobsen et al., 2001). The National Comorbidity Survey reported that among participating men with PTSD, over 51% met criteria for alcohol abuse/dependence, and over 34% met criteria for drug abuse/dependence, while rates among women were 27% for alcohol abuse/dependence and over 26% for drug abuse/dependence (Kessler et al., 1995).

There is controversy in the clinical literature as to how to approach the dual problem of PTSD and substance use. Recent evidence suggests that PTSD and substance use disorder should be treated concurrently. If the substance problem is ignored, any gains made in the PTSD treatment hour might be mitigated by substance abuse. If the substance abuse is treated first, the patient is likely to relapse because the PTSD symptoms, such as intrusive imagery, are cues for drinking (Najavits, 2002). Though the prevailing clinical wisdom is to engage patients in a plan to quit their substance use, premature adoption of this strategy may lead to treatment failures (Ouimette, Brown, & Najavits, 1998) as patients are not offered an adequate substitute to ease their suffering.

It appears as if the controversy as to whether comorbid treatment is ethically and scientifically justifiable has impeded the progress of clinical science in this area. The vast majority of PTSD treatment outcome studies have excluded substance abuse or dependence (Bradley et al., 2005), and few studies have been funded to examine comorbid treatment of PTSD and substance use. Fortunately, those that exist do show promising results. Najavits (2002) has developed a treatment for PTSD and comorbid substance abuse in those with a childhood history of sexual abuse that has documented efficacy; however, there are no published studies of PTSD and comorbid substance use or dependence following disaster. Again, given the psychological, social, and economic costs of excessive drug and alcohol use, this shortcoming in the clinical literature is troubling. Advocacy for funding for treatment outcome studies addressing these comorbidities should be a priority in the disaster studies community.

20.4. DISSEMINATION OF EVIDENCE-BASED TREATMENTS AND THE TRAINING AND CREDENTIALING OF MENTAL HEALTH PROVIDERS

Gaps in the treatment outcome literature are compounded by problems with the dissemination and acceptance of the clinical science literature by both patients and mental health practitioners in the community.

20.4.1. Dissemination of Knowledge: Implementing Empirically Validated Treatments in the Community

The field has to date been focused on empirical trials, but the next phase in communicating the knowledge base for disaster trials is dissemination to the community at large. The dissemination of exposure therapy in the community is dependent partly on the tolerability of the treatment for the broad population. Exposure therapy itself has not been associated with a greater percentage of treatment dropouts in RCTs; however, there is some evidence that RCTs underestimate the dropout rates in "real world" clinical settings (Leon, Demirtas, & Hedeker, 2007). A study of PTSD outpatients at a clinic that specialized in exposure therapy found a treatment completion rate of only 28%, far below that of RCTs (Leon et al., 2007). However, in this study patients who initiated exposure therapy were actually more likely to complete treatment than those who did not, and the authors suggested that expectations about exposure therapy may have affected treatment completion more than the actual experience of exposure therapy. Zayfert and colleagues (2005) suggested that researchers should continue to explore ways to increase the appeal of exposure therapy to clients. The results of a study on factors that influence PTSD treatment choice suggest that further enhancing treatment efficacy while reducing any perceived negative side effects could be one way to do this (Zoellner, Feeny, Cochran, & Pruitt, 2003).

20.4.2. Use of Treatments by Practitioners

Beyond the appeal of exposure therapy for clients, there is reluctance on the part of clinicians to use the treatment. Becker, Zayfert, and Anderson (2004) found that only 17% of 217 licensed psychologists surveyed reported using exposure therapy to treat PTSD. Inadequate training was the most common reason for not utilizing the therapy. However, even among those with training, over one-third (38%–46%) did not utilize exposure therapy. In addition to disinclination to use manualized treatments, clinicians expressed the concern that patients would decompensate, despite there being equivocal evidence for any lasting symptom exacerbation from exposure therapy (Feeny, Hembree, & Zoellner, 2003; Foa, Zoellner, Feeny, Hembree, & Alvarez-Conrad, 2002). These results were confirmed by Cahill and colleagues (2006) who trained a large cohort of psychologists to use prolonged exposure therapy for PTSD related to the WTC attacks of September 11th. They found implementation of treatment was hindered by discomfort in using exposure and cognitive restructuring techniques, concerns about decompensation, and a disinclination to use manualized treatments. On the basis of their findings, the researchers proposed that experts in PTSD treatment outcomes train people who will supervise the implementation of exposure treatments in their community clinics. We successfully implemented a similar model in our own WTC screening and treatment program, in which clinical faculty using exposure therapy to treat PTSD had weekly supervision with the program director, an experienced clinical research psychologist, as well as a weekly peer case conference (Difede et al., 2006).

20.4.3. Other Barriers to Treatment: Cultural Factors

Another barrier to treatment utilization remains the challenge of the initial engagement of clients into therapy. Jayasinghe and colleagues (2005) found that ethnicity predicted engagement in treatment, as Caucasian WTC disaster workers were more likely than minorities to enroll and attend at least one treatment session. Consistent with this finding, Difede and colleagues (Difede, Malta, et al., 2007) found in a RCT of CBT for disaster workers with WTC-related PTSD that minority disaster workers and those with fewer years of formal education were more likely to drop out of therapy. These findings suggest a need for psychoeducation regarding the course of PTSD with and without treatment and the need to address the stigma of treatment among certain ethnic groups.

20.4.4. Training and Credentialing

Finally, a standardization of training for specialists in trauma treatment with possible credentialing should be considered. Effective treatment of PTSD must occur in a therapeutic manner and environment clearly differentiated from the patient's own ruminations about the trauma. Principles of trauma treatment are unique, and without proper training, therapists may cause more harm than good. Harm may be visible through an exacerbation of symptoms or may manifest more subtly – a patient who is not improving because of the therapist's lack of training may perceive an implicit message that treatment will not help, causing the patient not to pursue specialized treatment and sustaining the PTSD symptoms indefinitely.

20.5. THE INTERPERSONAL EFFECTS OF DISASTER

While psychiatric nosology has an extensive system of classification and categorization for disorders of the individual, the system fails to capture the experience or "dis-orders" of the family system or couple that are often consequences of trauma. This is a serious gap, since the power of disaster strikes with such force that the reverberations, like the aftershock in an earthquake, are often felt throughout the family system for years afterward. As a general rule, the longer the time from the trauma to initiation of treatment for the survivor, the more likely that individual members of the family will have been adversely affected by the survivor's trauma, psychiatric symptoms, and consequent behaviors, and will be in need of treatment as well.

The symptoms of PTSD are known to be associated with interpersonal conflict. Studies suggest rates of marital conflict leading to divorce at approximately 9% and impairment of close relationships as high as 40% (North et al., 1999); domestic violence is not uncommon (Mechanic et al., 2000). Indeed, in the WTC screening program, participants frequently reported that the interpersonal problems were more troubling than the PTSD symptoms (Difede et al., 2006). These problems are further compounded in the presence of a comorbid major depression or substance abuse disorder, as both of these diagnoses have been shown independently to affect interpersonal functioning (Herr, Hammen, & Brennan, 2007; Lipsey, Wilson, Cohen, & Derzon, 1997).

In an article describing the effects of PTSD on interpersonal relationships, McFarlane, Bookless, and Air (2001) identify a number of pathways through which PTSD contributes to dysfunctional family interactions. First, they state there is an intensification of attachments to others who have shared the trauma with the individual. This can significantly affect closeness with a spouse if the disaster was not a shared experience. Furthermore, the specific symptoms of PTSD contribute to dysfunctional interactions; normal conflict in a relationship can spark the irritability common in PTSD. At the same time, the numbing typical of PTSD can create detachment and lack of affect and contribute to a decrease in wider social interactions, which can compound the disruption of homeostasis in the family. PTSD also affects intimacy and sexuality. One study found that 8 months after the 1983 Ash Wednesday bushfires in Australia, 80% of the firefighters still reported being more irritable with their families, 50% reported spending less time with their families, and 65% reported avoiding discussing their problems (McFarlane & Bookless, 2001). Two and a half years later problems with intimacy were still reported by 31% of married firefighters. It is notable that change in sexual functioning is not assessed formally in research studies, though it is commonly reported by PTSD patients as a problem (independent of psychotropic medication usage) (Difede et al., 2006).

Studies of combat veterans with PTSD have identified negative effects of the disorder on spousal and family interactions that result in high conflict levels in families (Solomon, Mikulincer, Fried, & Wosner, 1987), psychological distress in wives (Solomon et al., 1992), impaired marital and family interactions (Solomon et al., 1992), impaired marital and family adjustment (Jordan et al., 1992), caregiver psychological distress (Calhoun, Beckham, & Bosworth, 2002), and caregiver dysphoria and anxiety (Beckham, Lytle, & Feldman, 1996). Similar problems in family interactions have been cited in individuals with PTSD resulting from a motor vehicle accident (Blanchard et al., 1995). Another study showed that almost 20% of children of emergency medical technicians displayed symptoms of probable PTSD 6 months after the WTC attacks of 2001 (Duarte, Hoven, & Wu, 2006). However, with the exception of the final two studies just described, descriptive studies of the long-term effects of PTSD on family members outside of military populations are severely lacking.

There is an acknowledgment of the importance of including family members and their interactions in the PTSD treatment process (Catherall, 1999; Harkness & Zador, 2001). One pilot study (Monson, Schnurr, Stevens, & Guthrie, 2004) described the results of a sample of Vietnam veterans with PTSD treated in a couple's modality with cognitive-behavioral couple's treatment (CBCT) for PTSD. However, we found limited other work devoted to examining the efficacy of treatment involving family members. In light of the established effects of PTSD on interpersonal functioning, this represents a true deficiency in the field that must be addressed in future research.

20.6. IMPLEMENTATION OF EMPIRICALLY VALIDATED TREATMENT FOLLOWING DISASTERS: TWO CASE STUDIES

To illustrate the clinical presentation of symptoms and the development of treatment plans several years after a trauma, the following narratives of two families are presented. To protect the identities of the individuals, a composite of several families and their disaster experiences has been created to illustrate the substantive clinical and scientific issues.

20.6.1. Case 1: The Jones Family

Mr. Jones had been an officer in the New York Fire Department for 20 years at the time of the WTC attacks. On the morning of September 11, 2001, he was in the lobby of the South tower when it collapsed. Mr. Jones was buried in rubble, sustaining multiple injuries, until he was freed by fellow firefighters. Over the course of the next days and weeks, Mr. Jones learned of dozens of colleagues and friends who were killed in the attacks. While the attacks were occurring, Mrs. Jones sat watching the news and waiting for any word of her husband, anticipating he may likely have been killed. She finally received a telephone call that her husband had been hospitalized with multiple fractures and was in critical condition. Mrs. Jones then took a shower and fixed her hair before driving to the hospital. The Jones's had three children impacted by this event and its effects on their parents.

Mr. Jones initially presented for treatment 2 years following the event. He reported symptoms consistent with a diagnosis of PTSD and comorbid major depression. He was experiencing intrusive thoughts of the attacks and frequent nightmares, and he avoided situations in which he felt his movements could be constrained and public places that he felt were in danger of attack. Mr. Jones reported symptoms of emotional numbing and estrangement from his family and friends. He was experiencing severe sleep difficulty, anger outbursts, and trouble with irritability and concentration. Mr. Jones also described feelings of depression accompanied by anhedonia. At the time of his initial interview he acknowledged that his marriage was failing. His wife had recently threatened to leave him, citing a long list of troubling behaviors, including his irritability and possessiveness, yet apparent indifference to her and their children.

As the discussion of his marital problems progressed, evidence emerged suggesting that his wife was also suffering from symptoms of anxiety and depression as a consequence of the effects the WTC attacks had had on her husband, their marriage, and their children. Mrs. Jones experienced frequent ruminations about September 11th and the events that led to the significant change in her husband's physical and mental health. She too began to avoid friends and social situations and decreased her involvement in pleasurable activities. She experienced significant anxiety, irritability, and chronic feelings of depression.

Two of the children also appeared to be having problems. Abe was a 12-year-old boy who had been a straight-A student until the WTC attacks. In the year following the attacks his grades began to slip and he began to fight with his parents. Bill was a 19-year-old young man who was living at home at the time of the attacks, working, and trying to "get his life together." His parents described him as "very angry," getting into fist fights at a local bar and on one occasion with his father, who then asked him to leave the house. Their daughter, Cindy, was a 15-year-old sophomore in high school at the time of the attacks. She was also a straight-A student engaged in many extracurricular activities, including the high school orchestra and soccer team, and was exhibiting no outward signs of adjustment difficulties.

Despite the symptoms exhibited by Mrs. Jones and two of her children, she was resistant to treatment for herself or her family. Mrs. Jones firmly believed that their difficulties stemmed from her husband's behaviors and their effects on the family, and that the family problems would resolve if her husband could control his symptoms.

20.6.1.1. The Family Treatment Plan

When Mr. Jones was in treatment for several weeks, ample evidence accrued to confirm the initial impression that each member of the family needed treatment for the effects of the trauma. Referrals were provided for individual and couple's therapy; however, only Mr. Jones entered treatment. The patient attributed this in part to logistical issues and in part to his wife's perception that the family problems would resolve with her husband's symptom improvement. Our program then received funding to treat couples and family members of trauma patients, and the spouse, two of the children, and the couple all gradually accepted treatment.

The treatment for Mr. Jones consisted of cognitive behavioral techniques, including relaxation techniques to target irritability and hyperarousal symptoms, in vivo exposure targeting avoided situations, and imaginal exposure therapy addressing his trauma memories. Cognitive restructuring focused on feelings of guilt and traumatic grief related to the death of close friends and colleagues. Cognitive techniques were also used to address his increased sense of vulnerability and perceived danger. Treatment also focused on improving interactions and communication with his wife and family and coping with current responsibilities.

The treatment for Mrs. Jones was geared toward coping with her own reactions to the trauma as well as adjusting to the changes in her husband. Prolonged exposure targeted Mrs. Jones's memories of September 11th and her perceived loss of her husband on September 11th in the moments she thought he was dead and learned he was in critical condition. Further treatment focused on coping with the life changes and the "loss" of her husband "as she knew him" brought on by her husband's medical condition, subsequent retirement, and the changes in role and relationship she perceived were caused by his symptoms. Behavioral activation focused on increasing her social and enjoyable activities and garnering resources to cope with her strained relationship. Finally, cognitive restructuring targeted her maladaptive thoughts about her husband's symptoms, their stressful relationship, and her statements of attribution regarding the changes that had occurred in the family.

Couple's counseling began later in the course of treatment and greatly enhanced the work done in individual treatment. The couple's sessions allowed Mr. and Mrs. Jones to address their marital problems as a team with the guidance of a therapist who was allied with them as a couple. Themes of couple's therapy included understanding each others' experiences and symptoms, increasing expressions of affection, improving effective communication, discussing perceived imbalances in responsibility and parenting, and improving the sexual relationship.

Finally, family therapy allowed the children and parents to interact in a neutral environment where they could process their experiences and address ongoing problems. The children were able to speak with their father about their fears on September 11th – a topic he had avoided for the past 2 years. They were able to express their own needs while learning to appreciate those of their parents. Perceived vulnerability and fears for each other's safety, as well as feelings of anger and resentment, were finally brought to light and could be addressed in a constructive manner instead of festering beneath the surface.

Though treatment began 2 years following the trauma, this specialized treatment plan was effective in improving symptoms for all the individuals and relationships for the entire family. Most notably, marital satisfaction improved, and the couple no longer talked of separating. Indeed, with time they seemed to forge a stronger bond and present a united front against future adversities.

20.6.2. Case 2: The Brown family

The Browns were a family with two teenage boys and one girl who presented to our clinic 6 years after their trauma for evaluation services. Owing to an earthquake that reverberated throughout their neighborhood, a fire had broken out in their home. When Mrs. Brown heard the smoke detectors and smelled the fire, she immediately roused Mr. Brown, and he went to investigate, while she called 911. Their son, Eddie, was already up and following the family's fire plan, but the location of the fire prevented Mr. Brown from reaching the rooms of his 12-year-old daughter, Dana, and his 15-year-old son, Frank. Firefighters arrived within minutes, but Dana's room was already engulfed in flames. Frank escaped by climbing out the window of his second floor bedroom, sustaining multiple fractures.

Mr. Brown presented with PTSD and major depression and continued to suffer from traumatic bereavement as a direct consequence of his daughter's death. Mr. Brown reported intrusive images of the fire and the lifeless body of his daughter and frequent emotional upset. Mr. Brown avoided thinking and talking about the fire, news programming, and places that reminded him of the fire. He described feeling distant, cut off, and sometimes numb, which contributed to his interpersonal difficulties. Mr. Brown reported hyperarousal symptoms, including frequent feelings of anger and irritability, as well as difficulty concentrating. Preexisting sleep problems had worsened since the fire. Mr. Brown also suffered from recurrent major depression of moderate severity, reporting depressed mood, anhedonia, and feelings of helplessness and hopelessness. In addition, Mr. Brown's grief over the death of his daughter was all-consuming; his symptoms hindered his ability to function effectively as a parent to his two sons or as a marital partner to his wife. Mr. Brown believed his symptoms would improve on their own and agreed to the evaluation only because his wife had recently threatened to leave him.

Mrs. Brown was diagnosed with moderate PTSD and a comorbid major depression, which was in partial remission at the time of her evaluation. Mrs. Brown complained of psychological distress when reminded of the fire and stated that she had become emotionally volatile since the fire, which had interfered with her ability to make and maintain friendships. She reported avoiding thoughts, feelings, activities, places, and people that reminded her of the fire and said that she had grown distant from her husband. She reported very few symptoms of autonomic arousal, likely because these symptoms were palliated by psychotropic medication, which she had been taking since the fire. Mrs. Brown also suffered from recurrent major depression; she indicated that during the past month she felt good but noted that "when I feel happy, I feel like I am dishonoring Dana," suggestive of survivor's guilt. Though she was functioning well at work, Mrs. Brown no longer tended to chores at home and did not engage emotionally with her husband or her sons. Indeed, she preferred to avoid coming home, stating that her home felt like a cold and empty place. The presence of these symptoms despite her psychotropic medication regimen suggested that Mrs. Brown needed more intensive treatment than she was currently receiving.

Frank presented with mild PTSD, which represented a significant improvement in his PTSD symptoms. Shortly after the fire, Frank was hospitalized for angry outbursts at home. He had received intensive psychotherapy and medication in a psychiatric treatment facility for 3 months, followed by supportive therapy from a clinician who did not specialize in trauma treatment, but he was no longer seeing her on a regular basis. At the time of the interview, Frank continued to report residual symptoms. He worried that "bad things" might happen to him and felt generally apathetic. Frank also had substantial survivor's guilt, saying that he would trade places with Dana if he could and that Dana "had more to offer the world" than himself.

20.6.2.1. The Family Treatment Plan

The Browns presented to our clinic 6 years after their trauma after being referred by Mrs. Brown's new employee assistance program psychiatrist. Before this time, each member of the family had been in individual counseling with a clinician known to the family but who did not have specialized training in trauma and bereavement, and their symptoms had persisted years after the trauma. This experience reflects many of the problems that beset anyone attempting to access optimal mental health care in the United States today. At best, the Browns received mediocre care, prior to presenting at our specialized clinic, for a multitude of reasons: (1) inadequate medical insurance, (2) lack of knowledge that their problems could have been addressed with specialized psychiatric services, (3) "normalization" of symptoms by both the family members and their medical (i.e., nonpsychiatric) providers, caused by the failure of both survivors and medical professionals to distinguish between "normal distress" (i.e., symptoms of grief, trauma, and shock) and the pernicious symptoms of chronic PTSD and major depression, (4) failure of the treating clinicians to recognize that each family member would benefit from treatment with a specialist, and (5) lack of acceptance and use of empirically validated treatments for PTSD among mental health providers.

The ideal treatment plan would incorporate comprehensive psychiatric treatment for each member of the family on an individual basis, supplemented by couple's counseling and family therapy, from a team of trauma specialists. Consistent with the Expert Consensus Guidelines (Foa, Davidson, et al., 1999), Mr. and Mrs. Brown's individual treatment should include prolonged exposure therapy for PTSD and pharmacotherapy for major depression.

Mr. Brown's prognosis is fair, given that 6 years after the fire there has been little improvement; a major challenge is to engage Mr. Brown in treatment. During his assessment, he rightly noted that no mental health intervention could resolve the existential pain and suffering consequent to the loss of his daughter. The challenge of working with someone like Mr. Brown is to convey to him that psychiatric treatment could improve his symptoms of PTSD and depression, the quality of his life, and his relationship with his wife and sons, making it worth the effort required to engage in treatment. This reflects the importance of being able to instill hope within an individual whose hopelessness is endemic to his symptomatology and the lack of success of previous treatment.

With optimal therapy over the course of 2 to 3 years, Mrs. Brown is likely to see her PTSD and major depression remit and learn to cope more effectively with her grief and guilt over the death of her daughter and the destruction of her family. However, due to the severity of this trauma, Mrs. Brown will remain vulnerable to relapses for the duration of her life whenever she is under stress or if she experiences further trauma.

Frank would benefit from individual therapy with a trauma specialist focused on his traumatic bereavement. Frank was a troubled teenager at the time of the fire and was very much in need of the continued guidance of his parents and community; the fire destroyed this foundation at a critical juncture in his development. His grief and survivor's guilt, which are part of a traumatic bereavement syndrome, could likely adversely impact his future development (e.g., as a potential spouse or parent and as a wage-earner) and need to be addressed in treatment.

Mr. and Mrs. Brown would also benefit from couple's therapy, which may help repair their marriage. Trauma survivors often misinterpret their own changes in feelings and behaviors, misattributing problems that are most likely consequent to their trauma to more obvious and common causes. For example, a spouse may conclude that she is no longer in love with her mate rather than acknowledge that being close to a partner is too emotionally painful and reminiscent of their pretrauma life together. It is not uncommon for parents to separate after the death of a child because by staying together each partner is reminded of the deceased child; thus, separation can be an avoidant strategy and part of the trauma syndrome. In addition, the entire family would benefit from family therapy with a therapist experienced in working with severe trauma survivors. Family therapy would allow each member of the family to address the death of Dana, their own physical impairments, and the changes in the family in a more constructive manner that could allow for improved communication, role functioning, and resolution of the chronic complicated bereavement patterns embedded in the family system.

20.7. FUTURE DIRECTIONS

There are numerous challenges confronting the disaster research community concerning treatment, training, and dissemination of scientific findings to the larger clinical and political community concerned with disasters. The empirical literature underscores the paucity of research on the treatment of all comorbid outcomes following disaster, except PTSD. The dearth of treatment studies in these other areas is compelling given the number of disasters that occur worldwide each year.

Additional challenges to researchers in this area are (1) to develop studies that are designed to follow participants prospectively for the long term (e.g. 5–10 years) to evaluate relapse rates and the course of symptomatology posttreatment and (2) to develop and employ measurement strategies that capture the psychiatric problems of the individual, whether the index patient, another member of the immediate family, or a significant other, as well as the family, couple, or other immediate social group as a unit.

In sum, significant strides have been made in postdisaster research. However, in light of the rates of disaster and the horrific nature of its consequences, strong efforts are warranted to fill in the sizeable gaps in our current knowledge base.

REFERENCES

Adams, R.E., Boscarino, J.A., & Galea, S. (2006). Alcohol use, mental health status and psychological well-being 2 years after the World Trade Center attacks in New York City. *American Journal of Drug and Alcohol Abuse, 32*(2), 203–224.

Beckham, J.C., Lytle, B.L., & Feldman, M.E. (1996). Caregiver burden in partners of Vietnam War veterans with posttraumatic stress disorder. *Journal of Consulting and Clinical Psychology, 64*(5), 1068–1072.

Becker, C.B., Zayfert, C., & Anderson, E. (2004). A survey of psychologists' attitudes towards and utilization of exposure therapy for PTSD. *Behavioral Research and Therapy, 42*(3), 277–292.

Bisson, J.I., Ehlers, A., Matthews, R., Pilling, S., Richards, D., & Turner, S. (2007). Psychological treatments for chronic post-traumatic stress disorder. Systematic review and meta-analysis. *British Journal of Psychiatry, 190*, 97–104.

Blanchard, E.B., Hickling, E.J., Vollmer, A.J., Loos, W.R., Buckley, T.C., & Jaccard, J. (1995). Short-term follow-up of post-traumatic stress symptoms in motor vehicle accident victims. *Behavioral Research and Therapy, 33*(4), 369–377.

Bradley, R., Greene, J., Russ, E., Dutra, L., & Westen, D. (2005). A multidimensional meta-analysis of psychotherapy for PTSD. *American Journal of Psychiatry, 162*(2), 214–227.

Brady, K.T., Killeen, T.K., Brewerton, T., & Lucerini, S. (2000). Comorbidity of psychiatric disorders and posttraumatic stress disorder. *Journal of Clinical Psychiatry, 61*(Suppl. 7), 22–32.

Bryant, R.A., Moulds, M.L., Guthrie, R.M., Dang, S.T., & Nixon, R.D. (2003). Imaginal exposure alone and imaginal exposure with cognitive restructuring in treatment of posttraumatic stress disorder. *Journal of Consulting and Clinical Psychol, 71*(4), 706–712.

Cahill, S.P., Foa, E.B., Hembree, E.A., Marshall, R.D., & Nacash, N. (2006). Dissemination of exposure therapy in the treatment of posttraumatic stress disorder. *Journal of Traumatic Stress, 19*(5), 597–610.

Calhoun, P.S., Beckham, J.C., & Bosworth, H.B. (2002). Caregiver burden and psychological distress in partners of veterans with chronic posttraumatic stress disorder. *Journal of Traumatic Stress, 15*(3), 205–212.

Catherall, D.R. (1999). Family as a group treatment for PTSD. In B. H. Young & D. D. Blake (Eds.), *Group treatments for post-traumatic stress disorder*. Philadelphia: Brunner/Mazel.

Davis, M. (2002). Role of NMDA receptors and MAP kinase in the amygdala in extinction of fear: Clinical implications for exposure therapy. *European Journal of Neuroscience, 16*(3), 395–398.

Deering, C.G., Glover, S.G., Ready, D., Eddleman, H.C., & Alarcon, R.D. (1996). Unique patterns of comorbidity in posttraumatic stress disorder from different sources of trauma. *Comprehensive Psychiatry, 37*(5), 336–346.

Difede, J., Cukor, J., Jayasinghe, N., & Hoffman, H. (2006). Developing a virtual reality treatment protocol for posttraumatic stress disorder following the World Trade Center attack. In M. J. Ray (Ed.), *Novel approaches to the diagnosis and treatment of PTSD*. IDS Press.

Difede, J., Cukor, J., Jayasinghe, N., Patt, I., Jedel, S., Spielman, L., et al. (2007). Virtual reality exposure therapy for the treatment of posttraumatic stress disorder following September 11, 2001. *Journal of Clinical Psychiatry, 68*(11), 1639–1647.

Difede, J., & Eskra, D. (2002). Adaptation of Cognitive Processing Therapy for the treatment of PTSD following terrorism: A case study of a World Trade Center (1993) survivor. *Journal of Trauma Practice, 1*(3/4), 155–165.

Difede, J., Malta, L.S., Best, S., Henn-Haase, C., Metzler, T., Bryant, R., et al. (2007). A randomized controlled clinical treatment trial for World Trade Center attack-related PTSD in disaster workers. *Journal of Nervous and Mental Diseases, 195*(10), 861–865.

Duarte, C.S., Hoven, C.W., Wu, P., Bin, F., Cotel, S., Mandell, D.J., et al. (2006). Posttraumatic stress in children with first responders in their families. *Journal of Traumatic Stress, 19*(2), 301–306.

Fecteau, G., & Nicki, R. (1999). Cognitive behavioural treatment of post traumatic stress disorder after motor vehicle accident. *Behavioural and Cognitive Psychotherapy, 27*, 201–214.

Feeny, N.C., Hembree, E. A., & Zoellner, L. (2003). Myths regarding exposure therapy for PTSD. *Cognitive and Behavioral Practice, 10*, 85–90.

Foa, E.B., Dancu, C.V., Hembree, E.A., Jaycox, L.H., Meadows, E.A., & Street, G.P. (1999). A comparison of exposure therapy, stress inoculation training and their combination for reducing posttraumatic stress disorder in female assault victims. *Journal of Consulting and Clinical Psychology, 67*(2), 194–200.

Foa, E.B., Davidson, R.T., & Frances, A. (1999). Expert Consensus Guideline Series: Treatment of posttraumatic stress disorder. *Journal of Clinical Psychiatry, 60*, 5–76.

Foa, E.B., Franklin, M.E., & Moser, J. (2002). Context in the clinic: How well do cognitive-behavioral therapies and medications work in combination? *Biological Psychiatry, 52*(10), 987–997.

Foa, E.B., Zoellner, L.A., Feeny, N.C., Hembree, E.A., & Alvarez-Conrad, J. (2002). Does imaginal exposure exacerbate PTSD symptoms? *Journal of Consulting and Clinical Psychology, 70*(4), 1022–1028.

Gillespie, K., Duffy, M., Hackmann, A., & Clark, D.M. (2002). Community based cognitive therapy in the treatment of posttraumatic stress disorder following the Omagh bomb. *Behavioral Research and Therapy, 40*(4), 345–357.

Harkness, L., & Zador, N. (2001). Treatment of PTSD in families and couples. In J.P. Wilson M.J. Friedman, & J.D. Lindy (Eds.), *Treating psychological trauma and PTSD*. New York: Guilford Press.

Harvey, A.G., Bryant, R.A., & Tarrier, N. (2003). Cognitive behaviour therapy for posttraumatic stress disorder. *Clinical Psychology Review, 23*(3), 501–522.

Herr, N.R., Hammen, C., & Brennan, P.A. (2007). Current and past depression as predictors of family functioning: A comparison of men and women in a community sample. *Journal of Family Psychology, 21*(4), 694–702.

Institute of Medicine. (2006). *Posttraumatic stress disorder: Diagnosis and assessment*. Washington, DC; http://www.nap.edu/catalog/11674.html

Jacobsen, L., Southwick, S., & Kosten, T. (2001). Substance use disorder in patients with posttraumatic stress disorder: A review of the literature. *American Journal of Psychaitry, 158*, 1184–1190.

Jayasinghe, N., Spielman, L., Cancellare, D., Difede, J., Klausner E.J., & Giosan, C. (2005). Predictors of treatment utilization in World Trade Center attack disaster workers: Role of race/ethnicity and symptom severity. *International Journal of Emergency Mental Health, 7*(2), 91–99.

Jordan, B.K., Marmar, C.R., Fairbank, J.A., Schlenger, W.E., Kulka, R.A., Hough, R.L., et al. (1992). Problems in families of male Vietnam veterans with posttraumatic stress disorder. *Journal of Consulting and Clinical Psychology, 60*(6), 916–926.

Joseph, S., Yule, W., Williams, R., & Hodgkinson, P. (1993). Increased substance use in survivors of the Herald of Free Enterprise disaster. *British Journal of Medical Psychology, 66*(Pt. 2), 185–191.

Kessler, R.C., Sonnega, A., Bromet, E., Hughes, M., & Nelson, C.B. (1995). Posttraumatic stress disorder in the National Comorbidity Survey. *Archives of General Psychiatry, 52*(12), 1048–1060.

Leon, A.C., Demirtas, H., & Hedeker, D. (2007). Bias reduction with an adjustment for participants' intent to dropout of a randomized controlled clinical trial. *Clinical Trials, 4*(5), 540–547.

Lipsey, M.W., Wilson, D.B., Cohen, M.A., & Derzon, J.H. (1997). Is there a causal relationship between alcohol use and violence? A synthesis of evidence. In M. Galanter (Ed.), *Recent developments in alcoholism, Vol. 13: Alcohol and violence: Epidemiology, neurobiology, psychology, family issues*. New York: Plenum Press.

Marks, I., Lovell, K., Noshirvani, H., Livanou, M., & Thrasher, S. (1998). Treatment of posttraumatic stress disorder by exposure and/or cognitive restructuring: A controlled study. *Archives of General Psychiatry, 55*(4), 317–325.

McFarlane, A.C., & Bookless C. (2001). The effect of PTSD on interpersonal relationships: Issues for emergency service workers. *Sexual and Relationship Therapy, 16*(3), 261–267.

McFarlane, A.C., Bookless, C., & Air, T. (2001). Posttraumatic stress disorder in a general psychiatric inpatient population. *Journal of Traumatic Stress, 14*(4), 633–645.

Mechanic, M. B., Uhlmansiek, M. H., Weaver, T. L., & Resick, P. A. (2000). The impact of severe stalking experienced by acutely battered women: an examination of violence, psychological symptoms, and strategic responding. *Violence and Victims, 15*(4), 443–458.

Monson, C.M., Schnurr, P.P., Stevens, S.P., & Guthrie, K. (2004). Cognitive-behavioral couple's treatment for posttraumatic stress disorder: Initial findings. *Journal of Traumatic Stress, 17*(4), 341–344.

Najavits, L. M. (2002). *Seeking Safety: a Treatment Manual for PTSD and Substance Abuse*. New York, NY: The Guilford Press.

Neufeldt, V., & Guralnik, D.B. (1989). *Webster's new world dictionary*, 3rd ed. New York: Prentice Hall.

Norris, F.H., Friedman, M.J., Watson, P.J., Byrne, C.M., Diaz, E., & Kaniasty, K. (2002). 60,000 disaster victims speak: Part I. An empirical review of the empirical literature, 1981–2001. *Psychiatry, 65*(3), 207–239.

North, C. S., Nixon, S. J., Shariat, S., Mallonee, S., McMillen, J. C., Spiznagel, E. L., et al., (1999). Psychiatric disorders among survivors of the Oklahoma City bombing. *Journal of the American Medical Association, 282*(8), 755–762.

Ouimette, P.C., Brown, P.J., & Najavits, L.M. (1998). Course and treatment of patients with both substance use and posttraumatic stress disorders. *Addictive Behavior, 23*(6), 785–795.

Pfefferbaum, B., & Doughty, D. E. (2001). Increased alcohol use in a treatment sample of Oklahoma City bombing victims. *Psychiatry, 64*(4), 296–303.

Resick, P.A., Nishith, P., Weaver, T.L., Astin, M.C., & Feuer, C.A. (2002). A comparison of cognitive-processing therapy with prolonged exposure and a waiting condition for the treatment of chronic posttraumatic stress disorder in female rape victims. *Journal of Consulting and Clinical Psychology, 70*(4), 867–879.

Rothbaum, B.O., Hodges, L.F., Kooper, R., Opdyke, D., Williford, J.S., & North, M. (1995). Virtual reality graded exposure in the treatment of acrophobia: A case report. *Behavioral Therapy, 26*, 547–554.

Rothbaum, B., Hodges, L, Watson, B.A., Kessler, G.D., Opdyke, D. (1996). Virtual reality exposure therapy in the treatment of fear of flying: A case report. *Behavioral Research and Therapy, 34*(5–6), 477–481.

Rothbaum, B. O., Meadows, E. A., Resick, P. A., & Foy, D. W. (2000). Cognitive-Behavioral Therapy. In E. B. Foa T. M. Keane, & M. J. Friedman (Eds.), *Effective treatments for PTSD*. New York: The Guilford Press.

Solomon, Z., Mikulincer, M., Fried, B., & Wosner, Y. (1987). Family characteristics and posttraumatic stress disorder: A follow-up of Israeli combat stress reaction casualties. *Family Process, 26*(3), 383–394.

Solomon, Z., Waysman, M., Levy, G., Fried, B., Mikulincer, M., Benbenishty, R., et al. (1992). From front line to home front: A study of secondary traumatization. *Family Process, 31*(3), 289–302.

Stewart, S., Mitchell, T. L., Wright, K. D., & Loba, P. (2004). The relations of PTSD symptoms to alcohol use and coping drinking in volunteers who responded to the Swissair Flight 1111 airline disaster. *Anxiety Disorders, 18*(1), 51–68.

Tarrier, N., Pilgrim, H., Sommerfield, C., Faragher, B., Reynolds, M., Graham, E., et al. (1999). A randomized trial of cognitive therapy and imaginal exposure in the treatment of chronic posttraumatic stress disorder. *Journal of Consulting and Clinical Psychology, 67*(1), 13–18.

Tarrier, N., & Sommerfield, C. (2004). Treatment of chronic PTSD by cognitive therapy and exposure: 5-year follow-up. *Behavior Therapy, 35*(2), 231–246.

United Nations. (2005). 2005 Disaster in Numbers. (2008); http://www.unisdr.org/disaster-statistics/pdf/2005-disaster-in-numbers.pdf

Vlahov, D., Galea, S., Ahern, J., Rudenstine, S., Resnick, H., Kilpatrick, D., et al. (2006). Alcohol drinking problems among New York City residents after the September 11 terrorist attacks. *Substance Use and Misuse, 41*(9), 1295–1311.

Zayfert, C., Deviva, J. C., Becker, C. B., Pike, J. L., Gillock, K. L., & Hayes, S. A. (2005). Exposure utilization and completion of cognitive behavioral therapy for PTSD in a "real world" clinical practice. *Journal of Traumatic Stress, 18*(6), 637–645.

Zoellner, L. A., Feeny, N. C., Cochran, B., & Pruitt, L. (2003). Treatment choice for PTSD. *Behavioral Research and Therapy, 41*(8), 879–886.

21 Mental Health Care for Children in the Wake of Disasters

JESSICA MASS LEVITT, KIMBERLY EATON HOAGWOOD, LINDSAY GREENE, JAMES RODRIGUEZ, AND MARLEEN RADIGAN

21.1. INTRODUCTION

When disaster strikes, whether it is terrorism, war, a natural event, or a human-made or technological accident, children and adolescents are especially vulnerable. Abundant evidence exists to document the adverse mental health consequences that trauma exposure can have on youth (Silva, 2004; Silverman & LaGreca, 2002); yet, the research literature on psychosocial treatments for traumatized children and adolescents is very limited. Even less is known about disaster-traumatized youth; indeed, research on postdisaster trauma treatment for children and adolescents is still in its infancy (Cohen, Berliner, & Mannarino, 2000; Taylor & Chemtob, 2004). This is especially noteworthy when compared to the size of the research literature on treatments for other types of child mental health issues. Further, the few research studies that have been conducted to develop and evaluate postdisaster trauma treatments for children and adolescents are quite limited in terms of scientific rigor, making it difficult to identify optimal treatments for youth who have experienced a disaster. Efficacy research is needed to identify specific treatment approaches that improve outcomes for disaster-traumatized youth, and effectiveness studies that address issues of transportability, implementation, and dissemination are also needed to examine how these treatments work when used in the community.

The goal of this chapter is to consider how existing knowledge about postdisaster trauma treatments for children and adolescents can be best used to inform clinical practice and ensure that the highest quality services are available in the community. The chapter will first review the research literature on postdisaster trauma treatments for children and adolescents and describe the progress made in identifying efficacious treatments for sexually abused youth. Next, the chapter will examine issues of effectiveness when moving efficacious treatments to the community for use in the wake of disasters. Finally, the chapter will discuss challenges in conducting postdisaster treatment research and conclude with suggestions for future research that will move the field forward.

21.2. POSTDISASTER TRAUMA TREATMENTS FOR CHILDREN AND ADOLESCENTS

Both efficacy and effectiveness research are needed to identify treatment approaches that will be useful in community practice (Chorpita, 2003; Schoenwald & Hoagwood, 2001). Efficacy research is generally defined to include studies that are conducted under highly controlled conditions, including careful selection of patients, use of highly trained therapists, and intensive supervision of therapists by experts. Designs often include random assignment of patients to either a treatment or control condition (Hoagwood, Burns, Kiser, Ringeisen, & Schoenwald, 2001). Current standards for a treatment to be considered efficacious require one or two independent randomized controlled treatment studies (RCTs) with specific types of comparison conditions and other characteristics (Chambless & Hollon, 1998; Task Force on Promotion and Dissemination of Psychological Procedures, 1995).

Efficacy research, however, is not enough to justify using a treatment in community practice. It is well known that treatments that work in highly controlled research settings may not generalize to community practice. This is because it is extremely difficult to deliver clinical care in the same way in community practice as is done in efficacy research trials (Schoenwald & Hoagwood, 2001; Weisz, 2000; Weisz, Donenberg, Han, & Kauneckis, 1995; Weisz, Donenberg, Han, & Weiss, 1995). Consequently, there has been increasing interest among funding agencies to promote and support effectiveness research. Effectiveness research includes studies that use practicing clinicians, routine service settings for delivery, and a range of design options including RCTs, preference-based designs, and mixed methods (Hoagwood et al., 2001). While efficacy research trials are on the one hand equipped to provide the highest quality services to every patient participating in the study and to exclude patients who do not meet research criteria, community practice, on the other hand, rarely has these advantages. Instead, the quality of services provided in community practice is often influenced by patient volume, staff availability, referral sources, financial arrangements, and availability of other resources. Thus, it is important to determine whether efficacious treatments can be made to work in the real world of practice. To address this issue, effectiveness research examines issues of transportability, implementation, and dissemination of the treatment to community practice.

Research on postdisaster trauma treatments for children and adolescents have not yet been subjected to this careful progression of research studies. The majority of existing research studies can be considered to be preliminary work that, at best, indicates promising treatment approaches in need of efficacy and effectiveness studies. A small number of RCTs have been conducted, which might be considered a first step in establishing efficacy of certain treatment approaches, yet clearly more research is needed to accomplish this goal.

21.2.1. Randomized Controlled Trials of Postdisaster Trauma Treatments

According to an extensive literature search of the Medline (1950 to January 2008) and PsychInfo (1806 to January 2008) databases, and recent review articles (Cohen et al., 2000; Taylor & Chemtob, 2004), only three randomized controlled studies and one quasirandomized controlled study have been published that specifically investigate treatments for children or adolescents exposed to disaster (Berger, Pat-Horencyk, & Gelkopf, 2007; Chemtob, Nakashima, & Carlson, 2002; Chemtob, Nakashima, & Hamada, 2002; Field, Seligman, Scafedi, & Schanberg, 1996). These four studies describe four different psychosocial treatments, each with positive outcomes in some important areas. For example, treatments were shown to reduce trauma-related symptoms, anxiety symptoms, or depressive symptoms. Three of the studies include youth exposed to devastating hurricanes, and one study involved children exposed to a series of terrorist attacks.

The literature search indicates that Field, Seligman, Scafidi, and Schanberg (1996) conducted the earliest randomized controlled study of treatments for children or adolescents exposed to disaster. This study compared massage therapy, conceptualized as a stress reduction treatment, to a video attention control group among 60 grade-school children (grades one to five) who showed increased physical contact and excessive clinging behavior as well as severe posttraumatic stress symptoms 4 weeks following Hurricane Andrew. Notably, Hurricane Andrew was the second most destructive hurricane in history, devastating areas in Florida and Louisiana in 1992 and causing approximately $26.5 billion in damage and 65 deaths. Four weeks after exposure to this hurricane, child participants were randomly assigned to receive massage therapy twice a week over a 1 month period ($N = 30$) or to the video attention control group ($N = 30$) in which children watched an animated film for the same period of time as the massage group. As compared with the video control group, children who received massage therapy reported being happier and less anxious and had lower salivary cortisol levels after therapy. In addition, the massage group showed decreased anxiety and depressive symptoms and was observed to be more relaxed.

Chemtob and colleagues (2002) have conducted two randomized controlled studies of treatments for youth who were exposed to Hurricane Iniki, the most powerful hurricane to strike the Hawaiian Islands in recorded history. Hurricane Iniki caused approximately $1.8 billion in damage and six deaths. In their first study, Chemtob, Nakashima, and Carlson (2002) evaluated the effectiveness of Eye Movement Desensitization and Reprocessing (EMDR) Therapy (Shapiro, 1995) for 32 treatment-resistant children, ages 6 to 12, who continued to meet PTSD criteria 1 year following the hurricane and initial interventions. Children were randomly assigned to a wait-list control condition or to three sessions of EMDR provided by trained doctoral level therapists. The treatment condition included two groups, with 1-month delayed treatment for the second group. EMDR incorporates elements of psychodynamic and cognitive-behavioral treatments while using specific eye movements to reprocess traumatic events. Children who received EMDR reported significant reductions in trauma symptoms as well as a decrease in anxiety and depressive symptoms compared to the wait-list control group.

In a second RCT, Chemtob, Nakashima, and Hamada (2002) evaluated the efficacy of a cognitive-behavioral intervention for children who reported high levels of trauma-related symptoms ($N = 248$) 2 years after Hurricane Iniki. Children were selected from 10 public elementary schools on Kauai attending second through sixth grade. On the basis of the screening, 88% of children entering the study met DSM criteria for self-reported posttraumatic stress disorder (PTSD). Children were then randomly assigned to one of three consecutively treated cohorts. Those children awaiting treatment served as the control group. Within each cohort, children were randomly assigned to individual ($N = 73$) or group treatment (four to eight children per group; $N = 176$), both lasting four sessions. Intervention was provided by specially trained, school-based counselors and included restoring a sense of safety, grieving losses and renewing attachments, adaptively expressing anger, and achieving closure about the disaster to move forward. Though there was no difference in efficacy between the group and individual cohorts, treated children reported significant reductions in trauma-related symptoms compared with children waiting to be treated.

Most recently, a quasi-RCT investigating a universal, school-based intervention for children or adolescents exposed to terrorism was conducted by Berger, Pat-Horencyk, and Gelkopf (2007). This study took place in 2003 within a public elementary school in Hadera, Israel, a city that suffered five terror attacks in the 30 months preceding the study. Ten classrooms were randomly assigned to either the universal school-based intervention, or a wait-list control group. Although all children in each classroom participated in the intervention or control condition, parental consent for assessment could only be obtained for 43% of students. This low rate of parental consent limits the effects of classroom randomization and raises concerns that the sample may be biased. Despite this limitation, the study included a rather large sample: 142 second to sixth graders from the randomly assigned classrooms. Half of this sample had been exposed to a terrorist incident by being either present or knowing someone else who was injured or killed. Although only 11 children (7.8%) met DSM symptom criteria for PTSD, the authors report that the overall majority of children reported at least one PTSD symptom. Approximately one quarter described at least mild functional impairment. The intervention, developed by the Israel Trauma Center, included psychoeducational material and skills training with meditative practices, bioenergy exercises, art therapy, and narrative techniques for reprocessing traumatic experiences. Eight 90-minute sessions included homework review, experiential group activity, psychoeducational presentation, practical coping skills training, and a closure exercise. Two months after the study, the intervention group reported significant improvement in PTSD symptoms.

The three RCTs utilize the most scientifically rigorous research design available by randomly assigning children to either a treatment or no treatment comparison group. This design provides confidence that any outcomes obtained are a result of the treatments and not any alternative factors. In particular, the three aforementioned RCTs describe some important positive outcomes for children exposed to disasters as a result of the investigated treatments, and they demonstrate that these treatment approaches are better than no treatment at all. The quasi-experimental study also showed positive outcomes for children in the treatment group. Although potential sample bias cannot be ruled out as an explanation for observed differences between groups posttreatment, it is encouraging that the universal intervention was successful for such a large number of children whose parents provided consent. Finally, it is important to note that all four studies compared an active treatment to a wait-list or placebo condition rather than to an active treatment condition. Limitations to these kinds of studies have been described by Jensen and colleagues (2005) who point out that these studies cannot provide any evidence about whether the tested treatments are better than other active treatments. Further research is needed to examine this question.

There appears to be some similarities in the treatments tested in the randomized and quasi-randomized trials, although they are all different treatment approaches. For instance, all of the treatments evaluated include some aspects of cognitive-behavioral therapy (CBT), such as relaxation training, the development of coping skills, or exposure to and reprocessing of memories of the traumatic experience. Yet, only one treatment is identified explicitly as a cognitive-behavioral treatment (Chemtob et al., 2002; Taylor & Chemtob, 2004). Although the studies are not designed to test the effectiveness of cognitive-behavioral treatment components, the fact that these elements are common across successful treatments suggests that these components may be an important aspect of treatment for youth exposed to disasters. In addition, the age range of the children across the studies was narrow: 6 to 12 years old. None of the randomized or quasi-randomized studies was conducted with teenagers, suggesting another area in need of further study. It is also important to note that the majority of treatments were conducted with children exposed to hurricanes, and one study included children exposed to terrorism. Further research is needed to examine the efficacy of treatments for youth exposed to other types of disasters.

Despite some similarities, these studies did vary in terms of the number of children included in the research, the amount of treatment provided (e.g., duration and intensity), the severity of children's posttraumatic stress, the structure of the treatment itself (e.g., individual vs. group treatments), focus (e.g. universal vs. targeted), timing, and role of the implementer (e.g., teacher, counselor, therapist). These variations across studies make it impossible to generalize findings from one study to the next and emphasize the need for more rigorous studies to provide information about treatment efficacy and to answer specific questions, such as who is appropriate for specific treatments, when should specific treatments be provided, who should provide specific treatments, and so on.

21.2.2. Nonrandomized Studies of Postdisaster Trauma Treatments

With so few RCTs focusing on treatments for child and adolescent victims of disaster, the majority of our current knowledge about postdisaster treatments comes from nonrandomized studies. Importantly, the literature contains many more nonrandomized studies investigating postdisaster trauma treatments for youth. Results from nonrandomized studies must be interpreted with caution because they are unable to determine whether observed differences between groups can be attributed solely to the effects of treatment or if some other factor(s) may be responsible. However, nonrandomized studies are valuable in suggesting the potential benefits of treatment approaches.

For example, Wolmer and colleagues (2003; 2005) conducted a series of nonrandomized studies that support use of a treatment including cognitive-behavioral strategies with child and adolescent victims of disaster. The authors investigated the effectiveness of a classroom-based intervention combining psychoeducational modules and cognitive-behavioral techniques following a catastrophic 1999 earthquake in Turkey, which killed approximately 15,000 people, injured approximately 23,000, and left 800,000 living on the streets. Four to five months after the earthquake, 215 students from a school near the damaged city received treatment from teachers who were trained, supervised, and supported by the study authors. The intervention consisted of eight 2-hour meetings over the course of 4 weeks. Assessments of the children were collected before intervention and again 6 weeks after (Wolmer, Laor, & Yazgan, 2003); the assessments gathered information regarding exposure and risk, symptoms of trauma, grief, and dissociation. Results showed that the severity of posttraumatic and dissociative symptoms following treatment decreased significantly. Importantly, the percentage of children with a PTSD diagnosis dropped from 32% to 17% after treatment.

Three years later, Wolmer and colleages (Wolmer, Laor, Dedeoglu, Siev, & Yazgan, 2005) followed up with a subset of the original treatment group (*N* = 67). The authors also evaluated an additional 220 earthquake-exposed children, aged 9 to 17, who had not received the prior intervention. All children were evaluated in terms of traumatic grief and dissociative symptoms, as well as adaptive functioning. Results show that, approximately 4 years after the earthquake (and 3 years after the initial intervention), the severity of traumatic symptoms between the two groups was comparable, but children who had participated in the teacher-mediated treatment were rated significantly higher than the untreated group in terms of adaptive functioning. These findings suggest that although the intervention did not impact long-term trauma symptoms, it was successful for promoting adaptive functioning 4 years after the earthquake.

A trauma/grief-focused, group CBT (Layne, Saltzman, Savjak, & Pynoos, 1999) has been developed and examined in a series of studies. The group protocol consists of 20 semistructured sessions, divided into four modules. The modules aim to build group cohesion and coping skills, process traumatic events, promote adaptive grieving, and promote normal developmental progression. Groups meet once a week for approximately 20 weeks and generally last 50 minutes. The treatment has been investigated in three studies with different populations of trauma-exposed adolescents (earthquake, war, community violence).

Goenjian and colleagues (1997; 2005) investigated the effectiveness of this treatment among adolescents exposed to the 1988 Spitak earthquake in Armenia, which caused the destruction of four cities and 350 villages, killing at least 25,000 people. One and half years after the earthquake, 64 early adolescent students from four schools were evaluated for PTSD symptoms and then assigned to treatment (*N* = 35) or no treatment (*N* = 29) groups on the basis of the location of their school. Approximately 52% to 60% of early adolescents enrolled in the study met DSM criteria for PTSD. Trained therapists provided the trauma/grief-focused treatment, which included four classroom group sessions and two individual sessions of psychotherapy over a 3-week period. The most symptomatic subjects received up to four individual sessions.

Outcomes were assessed at 18 months (Goenjian et al., 1997) and 42 months (Goenjian et al., 2005) after study entry (3 years and 5 years after the earthquake, respectively). At the 18-month assessment (Goenjian et al., 1997), treated children reported a significant decrease in the severity of their posttraumatic stress symptoms, while untreated children reported significant increases. Despite the significant reduction in treated children's posttraumatic stress symptom severity, treated children remained somewhat symptomatic, suggesting that additional intervention was needed. At the 42-month assessment (Goenjian et al., 2005), the treated group continued to show improvement; decreases in posttraumatic stress symptom scores was three times that of the untreated comparison group, despite the fact that posttraumatic stress symptoms among untreated children also decreased significantly. Importantly, the untreated group reported significant increases in depressive symptoms at 42 months while the treated group did not have any change in depressive symptoms.

Layne and colleagues (2001) further studied the effectiveness of trauma/grief focused group psychotherapy (Layne et al., 1999) with war-traumatized adolescents in Bosnia and Hercegovina. The 4-year war in Bosnia and Hercegovina (1992–1995) caused a massive amount of loss of human life (approximately 200,000 dead, including 16,000 children) and disrupted much of the country's basic services, especially those supporting women and children. Participants included 55 students, aged 15 to 19, from ten Bosnian secondary schools, who reported clinical levels of trauma, depression, and grief symptoms after significant war exposure. School counselors provided treatment. Adolescents completed pretreatment and posttreatment self-report measures of posttraumatic stress, depression, and grief symptoms and posttreatment measures of psychosocial adaptation and group satisfaction. Participation in the treatment was associated with significant reductions in posttraumatic stress, depression, and grief symptoms. In addition, reductions in distress symptoms were associated with higher levels of psychosocial adaptation, such as classroom rule compliance, school interest, and peer relationships. Finally, focus group data showed that both student and leader evaluations of the groups were positive (Cox et al., 2007).

Saltzman and colleagues (2001) further examined this treatment in southern California with adolescents exposed to community violence. Participants consisted of 26 students, aged 11 to 14, who reported high levels of traumatic symptoms and significant functional impairment following their trauma exposure. Of the 26 youth, 14 had initial levels of PTSD in the severe to very severe range. Five groups were formed according to the primary treatment issue (trauma vs. traumatic death, the severity of trauma, and general developmental level); each group included five to seven students and two trained clinician group leaders. Consistent with previous research conducted with youth exposed to disaster, the results showed that participation in the group treatment was associated with improvements in posttraumatic stress, grief symptoms, and academic performance.

These are examples of published studies using nonexperimental designs that suggest that treatments including cognitive-behavioral strategies may be beneficial for child and adolescent victims of disaster. While it is not possible to make any firm conclusions about the differential effectiveness of these treatment approaches, it is clear that postdisaster treatments, including cognitive-behavioral strategies, have shown promising results and consequently deserve further development and more sustained and rigorous testing.

21.2.3. Randomized Controlled Studies of Nondisaster Trauma Treatments

Randomized controlled studies of treatments for children who have experienced nondisaster related traumas provide evidence that cognitive-behavioral treatment can be efficacious. Treatments for children who have been sexually abused have received the most research attention (see Finkelhor & Berliner, 1995; Saywitz, Mannarino, Berliner, & Cohen, 2000). In particular, the results of several pre-post investigations (Deblinger, McLeer, & Henry, 1990; Stauffer & Deblinger, 1996) and at least five RCTs (Cohen, Deblinger, Mannarino, & Steer, 2004; Cohen & Mannarino, 1996, 1998; Deblinger, Lippmann, & Steer, 1996; Deblinger, Mannarino, Cohen, & Steer, 2006; Deblinger, Stauffer, & Steer, 2001) demonstrate the efficacy of trauma-focused CBT (TF-CBT) (Cohen, Mannarino, & Deblinger, 2006) for treating sexually abused children. Specifically, studies have shown TF-CBT to be more effective in improving PTSD symptoms, depression, anxiety, shame, and behavior problems than other supportive treatments and no treatment. TF-CBT has also been shown to be effective in improving parental distress, parental support, and parental depression. There is also evidence that TF-CBT is effective in treating childhood traumatic grief (Cohen, Mannarino, & Staron, 2006). Independent research teams have replicated the efficacy of TF-CBT and other similar cognitive-behavioral treatment approaches with children who have experienced sexual abuse (King et al., 2000) as well as children who experienced single-incident traumas (Amaya-Jackson et al., 2003; March, Amaya-Jackson, Murray, & Schulte, 1998).

The TF-CBT treatment model is based on effective interventions for adult PTSD and non-PTSD child anxiety disorders as well as on cognitive and learning theories about the development of PTSD in children. The model is meant to address symptoms and features of PTSD, depression, and anxiety, as well as to address secondary behavioral issues. The treatment is designed to be provided flexibly and sequentially with each session building on skills and progress from previous sessions. The first half of TF-CBT focuses on psychoeducation and skill building, including the development of stress management, emotional regulation, problem solving, and cognitive restructuring skills. The second half concentrates on creating a trauma narrative, which is an exercise designed to promote gradual exposure and cognitive processing of the traumatic experience(s). Parental involvement is an important aspect of the treatment and is used to promote improved communication with children, to provide education about personal safety and healthy sexuality, to address parenting skills, and to allow the parent and child to discuss the trauma narrative together in a healthy manner.

Recent reviews of the child sexual abuse literature have found that TF-CBT has the most rigorous empirical support for its effectiveness in treating sexually abused children who have PTSD and related problems (American Academy of Child and Adolescent Psychiatry, 1998; Putnam, 2003; Saunders, Berliner, & Hanson, 2004; SAMHSA Model programs, 2008). Owing to the support for using TF-CBT with sexually abused youth, the model has been applied to children who have suffered a variety of other types of traumatic experiences, including exposure to physical abuse, terrorism, or community or domestic violence (Cohen et al., 2006). Results of much of the research using TF-CBT in these populations have not yet been reported. In addition, TF-CBT has also been implemented in community service settings, and early data suggest that the model is feasible for use in the community to treat children and adolescents who have been exposed to disaster (CATS Consortium, 2007; Hoagwood et al., 2006; Hoagwood, Vogel, Levitt, D'Amico, & Paisner, 2007) and other types of trauma (North et al., 2008).

21.3. EFFECTIVENESS OF POSTDISASTER TRAUMA TREATMENTS IN COMMUNITY PRACTICE

Despite the fact that efficacious treatments for children and adolescents exposed to disaster have not yet been clearly identified, there is still a great need for providing services to youth who have been affected by disasters. Importantly, there is some indication that TF-CBT or other treatments including cognitive-behavioral strategies may be helpful for youth exposed to disaster. However, little is known about the effectiveness of these approaches when deployed into real-world service settings (Schoenwald & Hoagwood, 2001). This problem is not unique to the trauma field. In fact, there is very little treatment research, in general, examining the kinds of adaptations necessary to feasibly transport treatments into community settings. Nor is there much research investigating strategies for implementing treatments in such contexts or guidance about methods that are best able to evaluate the performance of the intervention under naturalistic conditions (for exceptions see Storch &

Crisp, 2004). Studies examining these issues are extremely valuable; one such project has been conducted with youth exposed to terrorism and offers some important insights.

21.3.1. The Child and Adolescent Trauma Treatments and Services Consortium

The Child and Adolescent Trauma Treatments and Services (CATS) is a project that provided two trauma-specific cognitive-behavioral treatments to children and adolescents affected by the terrorist attacks on the World Trade Center in New York City on September 11, 2001. Although the two treatments had not previously been studied among youth exposed to terrorism, the project examined issues of transportability, implementation, and dissemination of these treatment approaches when deployed in community practice settings. Through a competitive grant process, nine provider organizations spanning 45 clinical and school sites were selected to adopt a common cross-site assessment and treatment protocol. Given the strength of the research evidence supporting the efficacy of TF-CBT with sexually abused children and adolescents, the CATS project selected this treatment for use with children who were affected by the disaster. For adolescents the Trauma/Grief-focused Group Psychotherapy Program (Layne, Saltzman, & Pynoos, 2002) was selected. The treatment developers adapted this treatment to be delivered in an individual format for this particular program. By the end of the project, a total of 173 clinical staff had been trained on both interventions.

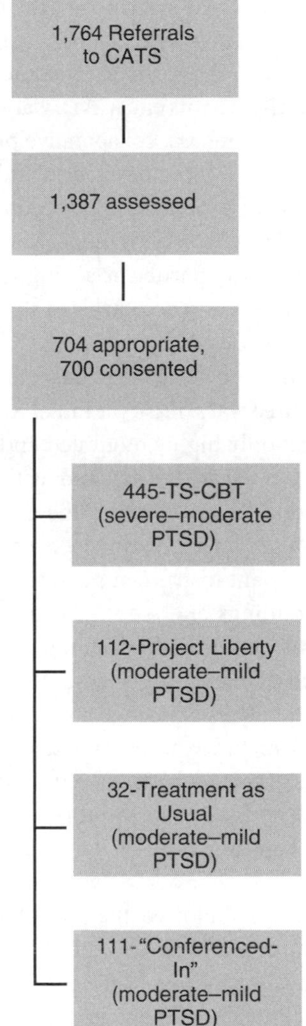

Figure 21.1. Flow of participants into the CATS project.

As depicted in Figure 21.1, a total of 1,764 children and youth were referred for clinical services. Of these, 1,387 were assessed and 700 consented to participate in the evaluation arm of the project. Two thirds of the children and families in the project were of Latino/Hispanic descent, and almost half of the youth were from very low-income families (e.g., below $15,000 per year). Baseline data indicated that the children in this project had very high levels of posttraumatic symptoms, anxiety, and depression. (For a more thorough history of the project see, CATS Consortium, 2007; Hoagwood et al., 2007.) The recruitment, outreach, and engagement methods for sample selection have been described previously (CATS Consortium, 2007), and results of the evaluation itself are available (Hoagwood et al., 2006).

21.3.1.1. Transportation of Trauma Treatments into Community Settings

When transporting research-based treatments into community settings, it is necessary to figure out how to fit the treatment into the existing system and how to adjust the system to fit the treatment. Therefore, engaging organizations, clinical staff, and families with the particular treatment models is a first priority. To this end, CATS was structured from the beginning as a collaborative project that engaged both treatment developers and community health care provider organizations to work together to design a service model that would be feasible within the particular settings participating in the project and acceptable to the clinicians and families involved in treatment.

Engagement of organizations was accomplished in three ways. First, the initial RFP process ensured that only highly motivated and prepared organizations would be involved with the program. Second, once selected, the participating organizations formed committees to select appropriate assessment instruments and treatments, to schedule trainings and work with the treatment developers to coordinate planning, and to provide consultation and guidance on the evaluation of the project. Third, once the project was underway, CATS included a structured communication process (via weekly conference calls, group E-mail lists, and site visits by project staff), which enabled a constant flow of information among treatment developers, CATS staff, and the Steering Committee. This allowed the project to remain flexible and responsive to site-specific needs while simultaneously adhering to the core components of the two clinical treatment models.

To address the need for high-quality training, clinicians were trained directly by the manual developers themselves. The manual developers each provided 2 full days of training on their respective trauma treatment manuals. As the project progressed, the manual developers returned to provide "booster training" sessions for the sites. This direct booster session training consisted of 1 full day, wherein each site had 2 hours to discuss the challenges specific to their setting and patient population.

In addition to the in-person trainings, clinicians and their supervisors attended monthly clinical consultation phone calls performed by the manual developers and the Ph.D.-level CATS clinical training director over an 18-month period. The calls consisted of case presentations with feedback on issues ranging from how to specifically apply the interventions specified in the manuals to how to modify the interventions for specific cases, problems, or populations to broader issues concerning how to adapt the manuals for specific settings (e.g., conducting trauma- or grief-focused interventions in school settings). "Specialty" consultation calls included additional didactic training on topics such as bereavement, sexual abuse, and supervision of clinicians. The consultation calls were also tailored to respond to clinicians' initial attitudes toward manualized treatments as having value only insofar as they could be used as practical tools in their clinical practice (Murray et al., in press). Thus, a major focus of the consultation calls became emphasizing the value of the skills and techniques as clinical tools. To provide additional supports for clinician- and organization-specific issues, the clinical training director visited with site clinicians and supervisors regularly to provide local site-specific consultation. Much of this consultation focused on fidelity to the treatment models and problem solving around implementation challenges.

Qualitative data gathered during the study indicated that this training and consultation model successfully engaged clinicians in overcoming some of the obstacles noted at the beginning of the project (Murray et al., in press). In particular, clinicians' reports of their success in working with traumatized children became more positive toward the end of the project, indicating their perception that use of the trauma-specific treatments was helping children to get better. In addition, clinicians' initial skepticism around use of the trauma treatments lessened over time, suggesting that the actual use of the trauma treatments with specific cases may have led clinicians to change their attitudes about the treatments. Finally, during the in-person trainings, some clinicians expressed some resistance to the use of the trauma narrative technique itself, yet during the consultation calls, it was observed that as clinicians used the gradual exposure with success, they showed a significant increase in confidence and buy-in. It is plausible that clinicians may alter their opinions about research-based treatments within the process of implementing them (Murray et al., in press).

Finally, engaging families in treatment is a critical component of transporting research-based treatments into community settings. The CATS project undertook an extensive outreach program to increase the visibility of the treatments that were offered (see CATS Consortium, 2007). In addition, to improve outreach, initial contact, and retention of families and youth in clinical services, an empirically validated and manualized engagement protocol (McKay, Pennington, Lynn, & McCadam, 2001) was incorporated into the project. All key intake staff (e.g., receptionists, aides, intake workers, clinical staff) at each of the nine provider sites were trained on this protocol by McKay and the CATS staff over a period of 6 months. Each site had "booster sessions" with McKay and CATS staff during which site-specific difficulties with engagement were discussed and solutions developed. The engagement protocol focused on clarifying the roles of key staff and of intake and on creating a foundation for collaborative working relationships.

Incorporation of this strategy was successful. Of the 445 youth eligible for either the TF-CBT or the trauma/grief group treatment, 385 (86%) received some treatment with a range from 1 to 36 sessions. Across the nine CATS provider organizations, rates of engagement ranged from 67% to 95% (Rodriguez et al., 2009). These engagement rates are considerably higher than what is found in community-based services where no-show rates over 50% are common (McKay, McCadam, & Gonzales, 1996; McKay, Stoewe, McCadam, & Gonzales, 1998). Among the treatment engagers, 65% of youth attended at least eight sessions or more (Rodriguez et al., 2009).

21.3.1.2. Flexible Implementation of Trauma Treatments in the Community

A major aim of CATS was to study the process involved with implementing research-based treatments in community settings. As previously mentioned, monthly consultation calls were held with the treatment developers to assist clinicians in applying the interventions with specific cases under specific circumstances. Two broad issues emerged during these consultations that ultimately can be considered adaptations of the trauma treatments.

The first issue was that the treatments specifically targeted children who had been exposed to single-incident traumas (such as the September 11th terrorist attack) rather than children who had experienced multiple traumas, which are common in New York City. This topic consequently became a focus of many of the consultation calls and booster sessions. Many participating clinicians observed substantial therapeutic improvements in their child and adolescent cases even when the youth had experienced multiple traumatic events. These direct "first hand" observations appeared to dissipate many of their initial concerns.

A second issue involved cultural adaptations to the treatments. The majority of clients included in the CATS project were low income, urban, Latino youth and families. This necessitated adaptation and flexibility in the treatment model, and the treatment developers responded in several ways. First, the training and consultations were amended to include more examples that reflected the cultural diversity of the population. Second, the developers emphasized how the CBT model was a Components Based Therapy to emphasize the need to fit the model to the family and not the family to the clinical model. They also encouraged flexibility in introducing different components, ordering of components, reviewing previously mastered components, and the possible lack of synchrony between child and parent components at different points in therapy. Third, the developers highlighted commonalities and overlaps between the trauma-specific CBT models and the models to which many therapists had prior allegiances and experiences in tailoring to the population being treated.

21.3.1.3. Evaluation of the Trauma Treatments under Naturalistic Conditions

Another major objective of CATS was to study outcomes associated with delivery of the trauma-specific CBT treatments in community practice settings. However, ethical concerns precluded use of random assignment. The magnitude of the terrorist attack necessitated a quick response and delivery of some treatment to all children in need. Therefore a quasi-experimental design, called a regression discontinuity (RD) design, was used (Cappelleri & Trochim, 1995). (For more details, see Hoagwood et al., 2006.)

The RD analyses were augmented with a mixed effects regression model, which enabled a more fine-grained analysis of differences between groups, inclusion of data collected at multiple time points, and methods for accommodating missing values (see CATS Consortium, 2007). Changes in child and adolescent scores on the PTSD Reaction Index (Steinberg, Brymer, Decker, & Pynoos, 2004) during the CATS project are displayed in Figure 21.2. The findings from the RD analyses showed that the majority of youth across both the experimental and comparison groups experienced a decrease in trauma symptoms over time, yet the mixed effects model indicated that the rate of improvement over time was greater for the trauma-specific CBT group than the comparison group. Specifically, the estimated improvement over time for children in the trauma-specific CBT group was 9.7 points per 6-months versus 3.8 points per 6 months for the comparison group (p <0.001). Thus, the study suggests that while children in both groups improved, the slope of improvement was greater for the trauma-specific CBT group, despite the fact that they began with a considerable disadvantage. Importantly, this group had significantly higher baseline levels of severe trauma, multiple traumas, and numerous family stressors. Despite these disadvantages, the children receiving the CBT treatments experienced significant improvements.

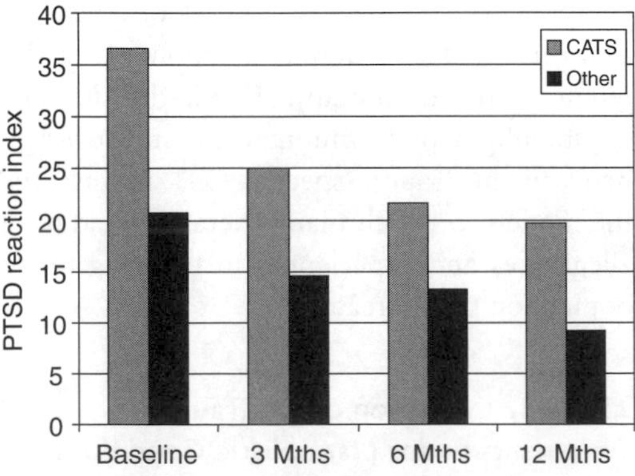

Figure 21.2. Changes in child and adolescent scores on the PTSD Reaction Index during the CATS project.

21.3.2. Summary

Studies examining the transportability of efficacious treatments into community settings point to the vast differences between research and practice conditions (CATS Consortium, 2007; Mufson, Dorta, Olfson, Weissman, & Hoagwood, 2004; Schoenwald, Halliday-Boykins, & Henggeler, 2003). Despite the variability in conditions and the challenges of transportation, it is possible for research-based treatments to work in community practice so that children benefit. These studies provide the beginning of a knowledge base that can be used to inform and motivate future study. The next generation of studies, however, needs to find ways to employ a range of alternative and rigorous research designs to provide more definitive answers about optimal treatments for children and adolescents exposed to disasters. Further research should systematically compare different strategies for implementing psychotherapy treatments in community practices to ensure that treatments retain their effectiveness when provided in the community.

21.4. LIMITATIONS OF POSTDISASTER TREATMENT RESEARCH

Given the logistical issues involved in mounting research studies in the wake of unforeseen disaster situations, it is commendable that any research studies have been conducted at all. Postdisaster research is challenging because of the time needed to develop an adequate research infrastructure, including securing funding, obtaining relevant approvals for research with human subjects and other approvals, developing a recruitment network, and assembling a cadre of adequately trained mental health treatment providers. In some cases, the damage done by the disaster may make transportation difficult and restrict access to resources. Ethical concerns about assigning participants to no treatment or wait-list controls and a general skepticism by the public toward conducting research after a mass disaster event can also constrain options (CATS Consortium, 2007). The small amount of research that has been conducted despite these obstacles provides a valuable foundation for our knowledge about the consequences of trauma for children and provides useful information for the development of effective treatments. However, the challenge of conducting research in a postdisaster environment has led to a variety of methodological sacrifices in most of the reported studies.

21.5. CONCLUSION

Research on treatments for children and adolescents who have been traumatized by disasters is still in its infancy. Studies are needed to identify efficacious treatments specifically for youth exposed to disasters and to determine how best to implement these treatments in community settings after a disaster has occurred. A major obstacle to the growth of this field is the numerous challenges in providing services and conducting research in the wake of unforeseen disaster events. No one knows when a disaster will strike, and once it does, each disaster involves unique circumstances and consequences. It is difficult to plan research in advance that can contend with all of the possible scenarios.

However, the field is moving forward. Organizational structures and collaborative networks, such as the National Child Traumatic Stress Network (R. Pynoos, Director), are established and can be accessed in the wake of a disaster to facilitate the start-up of disaster research projects. At the onset, disaster research projects will need to create their own infrastructure to support information sharing and ongoing communication (via E-mail, conference calls, site visits) for efficient management of the project. Further work is needed to help researchers obtain quick funding for research when disasters occur and to help obtain human subjects and other approvals in an expeditious manner.

There is also progress in the identification of treatments that are likely to be effective for children and adolescents exposed to disasters. The randomized controlled studies of TF-CBT with sexually abused children and the nonrandomized studies supporting cognitive-behavioral treatments suggest promising approaches for children affected by other types of trauma. The CATS project extended these findings by demonstrating that these trauma-specific cognitive-behavioral approaches can be successful with youth exposed to a mass disaster. In addition, the study suggests that community clinicians can be trained effectively on CBT approaches even in postdisaster situations. When conducting research-based treatments in community settings, it is important to expect that the treatments will need some degree of adaptation to the specific conditions of the disaster and the community. In addition, strategic attention to engaging families and youth in services is likely to be needed. Even if treatments are offered free of charge, help-seeking will need to be actively facilitated. Despite the progress that has been made using trauma-specific cognitive-behavioral treatments, further research is still needed to replicate and extend studies of the efficacy and effectiveness of these approaches with children and adolescents exposed to disasters.

To more fully advance the field of study, future investigations must find ways to employ a range of rigorous research designs that can provide some flexibility for examining delivery of targeted mental health interventions in postdisaster environments. Studies contrasting different active treatments within community settings are especially needed. In addition, there is a great need for studies that examine barriers to and strategies for deploying evidence-based clinical services into routine practice. Studies such as CATS provide valuable descriptive information about obstacles to implementing a research-based treatment in community settings and the methods used to overcome them. Additional work is needed to develop and elaborate on possible strategies for managing implementation difficulties and to then systematically test different strategies in community settings.

ACKNOWLEDGMENTS

The CATS Consortium is a cooperative multisite treatment study performed by nine independent teams in collaboration with the New York State Office of Mental Health. The New York State collaborators are Kimberly Eaton Hoagwood, Ph.D., Chip Felton, M.S.W., Sheila Donahue, M.A., Anita Appel, M.S.W., James Rodriguez, Ph.D., Laura Murray, Ph.D., David Fernandez, M.A., Jessica Mass Levitt, Ph.D., Joanna Legerski, B.S., Michelle Chung, B.A., Jacob Gisis, B.S., Jennifer Sawaya, B.A., Marleen Radigan, Dr. P.H., Sudha Mehta, M.P.H. Jameson Foster, M.S. The Principal investigators and co investigators from the nine sites are Robert Abramowitz, M.D., (JIFFS), Reese Albright, M.D., (St. Vincent's Hospital), Peter D'Amico, (North Shore/ Long Island Jewish), Giuseppe Constantine, Ph.D., (Lutheran Hospital), Carrie Epstein, I.E.-R., (Safe Horizon), Jennifer Havens, M.D., (Columbia University), Sandra Kaplan, M.D., (North Shore/LIZ), Jeffrey Newcorn, M.D., (Mount Sinai School of Medicine), Moises Perez, Ph.D., (Alianza Dominicana), Raul Silva, M.D., (NYU/Bellevue), Heike Thiel de Bocanegra, Ph.D., (Safe Horizon), Juliet Vogel, Ph.D., (North Shore/LIZ). The Scientific Advisors to the project are Leonard Bickman, Ph.D., (Vanderbilt University), Peter S. Jensen, M.D., (Reach Institute), Mary McKay, Ph.D., (Mount Sinai School of Medicine), Susan Essock, Ph.D., (Columbia University), Sue M. Marcus, Ph.D., (Mount Sinai School of Medicine), Wendy Silverman, Ph.D. (Florida International University), Robert Pynoos, M.D. (University of California, Los Angeles); Allan Steinberg, Ph.D. (University of California, Los Angeles); Lawrence Palinkas, Ph.D., (University of California at San Diego); and Joseph Cappelleri, Ph.D., (Pfizer Corporation). The Treatment Developers and Scientific Consultants to the project are: Judy Cohen, M.D., (Allegheny General Hospital), Anthony Mannarino, Ph.D., (Allegheny General Hospital), Christopher Layne, Ph.D., (Brigham Young University), William Saltzman, Ph.D., (UCLA).

REFERENCES

Amaya-Jackson, L., Reynolds, V., Murray, M.C., McCarthy, G., Nelson, A., Cherney, M.S., et al. (2003) Cognitive-behavioral treatment for pediatric posttraumatic stress disorder: Protocol and application in school and community settings. *Cognitive and Behavioral Practice, 10*(3), 204–213.

American Academy of Child and Adolescent Psychiatry. (1998). Practice parameters for the diagnosis and treatment of posttraumatic stress disorder in children and adolescents. *Journal of the American Academy of Child and Adolescent Psychiatry, 37*(Suppl. 10), 4S–26S.

Berger, R., Pat-Horencyk, R., & Gelkopf, M. (2007). School-Based intervention for prevention and treatment of elementary-students' terror-related distress in Israel: A quasi-randomized controlled trial. *Journal of Traumatic Stress, 20*(4), 541–551.

Cappelleri, J.C., & Trochim, W.M. (1995). Ethical and scientific features of cutoff-based designs of clinical trials: A simulation study. *Medical Decision Making, 15*(4), 387–394.

CATS Consortium. (2007). Implementing CBT for traumatized children and adolescents after September 11th: Lessons learned from the child and adolescent trauma treatments and services (CATS) project. *Journal of the American Academy of Child and Adolescent Psychiatry, 36*(4), 581–592.

Chambless, D.L., & Hollon, S.D. (1998) Defining empirically supported theories. *Journal of Consulting and Clinical Psychology, 66*, 7–18.

Chemtob, C.M., Nakashima, J., & Carlson, J.G. (2002). Brief treatment for elementary school children with disaster-related posttraumatic stress disorder: A field study. *Journal of Clinical Psychology, 58*, 99–112.

Chemtob, C.M., Nakashima, J.P., & Hamada, R.S. (2002). Psychosocial intervention for postdisaster trauma symptoms in elementary school children: A controlled community field study. *Archives of Pediatrics & Adolescent Medicine, 156*, 211–216.

Chorpita, B. (2003). The frontier of evidence-based practice. In A. E. Kazdin & J. R. Weisz (Eds.), *Evidence-based psychotherapies for children and adolescents*. New York, NY: The Guilford Press.

Cohen, J.A., Berliner, L., & Mannarino, A.P. (2000). Treating traumatized children: A research review and synthesis. *Trauma, Violence, & Abuse, 1*(1), 29–46.

Cohen, J.A., Deblinger, E., Mannarino, A.P., & Steer, R.A. (2004). A multisite, randomized controlled trial for children with sexual abuse-related PTSD symptoms. *Journal for the American Academy of Child & Adolescent Psychiatry, 43*(4), 393–402.

Cohen, J. A., & Mannarino, A. P. (1996). A treatment outcome study for sexually abused preschool children: Initial findings. *Journal of the American Academy of Child & Adolescent Psychiatry, 35*, 42–50.

(1998). Interventions for sexually abused preschool children: Initial treatment findings. *Journal of the Academy of Child and Adolescent Psychiatry, 35*, 42–50.

Cohen, J. A., Mannarino, A. P., & Deblinger, E. (2006). *Treating trauma and traumatic grief in children and adolescents*. New York: The Guilford Press.

Cohen, J. A., Mannarino, A. P., & Staron, V. R. (2006) A pilot study of modified cognitive-behavioral therapy for childhood traumatic grief (CBT-CTG). *Journal of the American Academy of Child & Adolescent Psychiatry, 45*(12), 1465–1473.

Cox, J., Davies, D. R., Burlingame, G. M., Campbell, J. E., Layne, C. M., & Katzenbach, R. J. (2007). Effectiveness of a trauma/grief focused group intervention: A qualitative study with war-exposed Bosnian adolescents. *International Journal of Group Psychotherapy, 57*(3), 319–345.

Deblinger, E., Lippman, J., & Steer, R. (1996). Sexually abused children suffering posttraumatic stress symptoms: Initial treatment outcome findings. *Child Maltreatment, 1*, 310–321.

Deblinger E., Mannarino, A. P., Cohen, J. A., & Steer, R. A. (2006). A follow-up study of a multisite, randomized, controlled trial for children with sexual abuse-related PTSD symptoms. *Journal of the American Academy of Child & Adolescent Psychiatry, 45*(12), 1474–1484.

Deblinger, E., McLeer, S. V., & Henry, D. (1990). Cognitive behavioral treatment for sexually abused children suffering posttraumatic stress: Preliminary findings. *Journal of the American Academy of Child and Adolescent Psychiatry, 29*, 747–752.

Deblinger, E., Stauffer, L. B., & Steer, R. A. (2001). Comparative efficacies of supportive and cognitive behavioral group therapies for young children who have been sexually abused and their nonoffending mothers. *Child Maltreatment, 6*(4), 332–343.

Field, T., Seligman, S., Scafedi, F., & Schanberg, S. (1996). Alleviating posttraumatic stress in children following Hurricane Andrew. *Journal of Applied Developmental Psychology, 17*, 35–50.

Finkelhor, D., & Berliner, L. (1995). Research on the treatment of sexually abused children: A review and recommendations. *Journal of the American Academy of Child & Adolescent Psychiatry, 34*(11), 1408–1423.

Goenjian, A. K., Karayan, I., Pynoos, R. S., Minassian, D., Najarian, L. M., Steinberg, A., et al. (1997). Outcome of psychotherapy among early adolescents after trauma. *American Journal of Psychiatry, 154*(4), 536–542.

Goenjian, A., Walling, D., Steinberg, A. M., Karayan, I., Najarian, L. M., & Pynoos, R. (2005) A prospective study of posttraumatic stress and depressive reactions among treated and untreated adolescents 5 years after a catastrophic disaster. *American Journal of Psychiatry, 162*(12), 2302–2308.

Hoagwood, K., Burns, B. J., Kiser, L., Ringeisen, H., & Schoenwald, S. K. (2001) Evidence-based practice in child and adolescent mental health services. *Psychiatric Services. 52*(9), 1179–1189.

Hoagwood, K., Radigan, M., Rodriguez, J., Levitt, J. M., Fernandez, D., Foster, J., et al. (2006). *Final report on the Child and Adolescent Trauma Treatment Consortium (CATS) Project*. Rockville, MD: Substance Abuse and Mental Health Services Administration, U.S. Department of Health and Human Services Administration.

Hoagwood, K. E., Vogel, J. M., Levitt, J. M., D'Amico, P. J., & Paisner, W. I. (2007). Implementing an evidence-based trauma treatment in a state system after September 11: The CATS Project. *American Academy of Child and Adolescent Psychiatry, 46*(6), 773–779.

Jensen, P. S., Weersing, R., Hoagwood, K. E., Goldman, E. (2005) What is the evidence for evidence-based treatments? A hard look at our soft underbelly. *Mental Health Services Research, 7*(1), 53–74.

King, N., Tonge, B., Mullen, M., Myerson, N., Heyne, D., Rollings, S., et al. (2000). Treating sexually abused children with posttraumatic stress symptoms: A randomized clinical trial. *American Academy of Child and Adolescent Psychiatry, 39*, 1347–1155.

Layne, C. M., Pynoos, R. S., Saltzman, W. R., Arslanagic, B., Black, M., Savjak, N., et al. (2001). Trauma/grief focused group psychotherapy school-based postwar intervention with traumatized Bosnian adolescents. *Group Dynamics: Theory, Research and Practice, 5*(4), 227–290.

Layne, C. M., Saltzman, W. R., & Pynoos, R. S. (2002). Trauma/grief focused group psychotherapy program. Manuscript submitted for publication.

Layne, C. M., Saltzman, W. R., Savjak, N., & Pynoos, R. S. (1999). *Trauma/grief-focused group psychotherapy manual*. Sarajevo, Bosnia: UNICEF Bosnia & Hercegovina.

March, J. S., Amaya-Jackson, L., Murray, M. C. & Schulte A. (1998). Cognitive-behavioral psychotherapy for children and adolescents with posttraumatic stress disorder after a single-incident stressor. *Journal of the American Academy of Child & Adolescent Psychiatry, 37*(6), 585–593.

McKay, M. M., McCadam, K., & Gonzales, J. J. (1996). Addressing the barriers to mental health services for inner city children and their caretakers. *Community Mental Health Journal, 32*, 353–361.

McKay, M. M., Pennington, J., Lynn, C. J., & McCadam, K. (2001). Understanding urban child mental health service use: Two studies of child, family, and environmental correlates. *Journal of Behavioral Health Services and Research, 28*, 475–483.

McKay, M. M., Stoewe, J., McCadam, K., & Gonzales, J. (1998). Increasing access to child mental health services for urban children and their care givers. *Health and Social Work, 23*, 9–15.

Mufson, L. H., Dorta, K. P., Olfson, M., Weissman, M. M., & Hoagwood, K. (2004). Effectiveness research: Transporting interpersonal psychotherapy for depressed adolescents (IPT-A) from the lab to school-based health clinics. *Clinical Child Family Psychology Review, 7*(4), 251–261.

Murray, L. K, Radigan, M., Rodriguez, J., Frimpong, E., Legerski, J., Mass-Levitt, J., et al. (under review). Clinician attitudes on the implementation of trauma-focused evidence-based treatments within the CATS Project. *Journal of Traumatic Stress*.

North, M. S., Gleacher, A. A., Radigan, M., Greene, L., Levitt, J. M., Chassman, J., et al. (2008). Evidence-based Treatment and Dissemination Center (EBTDC): Bridging the research-practice gap in New York State. *Report on Emotional & Behavioral Disorders in Youth, 8*(1), 9–16.

Putnam, F. W. (2003). Ten year research update review: Child sexual abuse. *Journal of the American Academy of Child and Adolescent Psychiatry, 42*, 269–278.

Rodriguez, J. A., Gopalan, G., Radigan, M., Foster, J., McKay, M., Chung, M., et al. (2009). The impact of evidence-based engagement strategies on the participation of youth in trauma treatments post-9/11. Manuscript submitted for publication.

Saltzman, W. R., Pynoos, R. S., Layne, C. M., Steinberg, A. M., & Aisenberg, E. (2001). Trauma- and grief-focused intervention for adolescents exposed to community violence results of a school based screening and group treatment protocol. *Group Dynamics: Theory, Research and Practice, 5*(4), 291–303.

SAMHSA Model Programs: Effective substance abuse and mental health programs for every community. (February, 2008). modelprograms.samhsa.gov.

Saunders, B. E., Berliner, L., & Hanson, R. F. (Eds.). (2004). *Child physical and sexual abuse: Guidelines for treatment (Revised Report: April 26, 2004)*. Charleston, SC: National Crime Victims Research and Treatment Center.

Saywitz, K. J., Mannarino, A. P., Berliner, L., & Cohen, J. A. (2000). Treatment for sexually abused children and adolescents. *American Psychologist, 55*, 1040–1049.

Schoenwald, S. K., Halliday-Boykins, C. A., & Henggeler, S. W. (2003). Client-level predictors of adherence to MST in community service settings. *Family Process, 42*(3), 345–359.

Schoenwald, S. K., & Hoagwood, K. E. (2001). Effectiveness, transportability, and dissemination of interventions: What matters when? *Psychiatric Services, 52*, 1190–1197.

Shapiro, F. (1995). *Eye movement desensitization and reprocessing: Basic principles, protocols and procedures* (1st ed.). New York: Guilford Press.

Silva, R. (2004). *Posttraumatic stress disorders in children and adolescents: Handbook*. New, York: W W Norton & Co.

Silverman, W. K., & La Greca, A. M. (2002). Children experiencing disasters: Definitions, reactions, and predictor of outcomes. In A. La Greca, W. Silverman, E. Silverman, & M. Roberts (Eds.), *Helping children cope with disasters and terrorism*. Washington, DC: American Psychological Association.

Stauffer, L. B., & Deblinger, E. (1996). Cognitive behavioral groups for nonoffending mothers and their young sexually abused children: A preliminary treatment outcome study. *Child Maltreatment, 1*, 65–76.

Steinberg, A. M., Brymer, M. J., Decker, K. B., & Pynoos, R. S. (2004). The University of California at Los Angeles Post-traumatic Stress Disorder Reaction Index. *Current Psychiatry Reports, 6*, 96–100.

Storch, E. A., & Crisp, H. L. (2004). Taking it to the schools: Transporting empirically supported treatments for childhood psychopathology to the school setting. *Clinical Child and Family Psychology Review, 7*(4), 191–267

Task Force on Promotion and Dissemination of Psychological Procedures, Division of Clinical Psychology, American Psychological Association. (1995). Training in and dissemination of empirically-validated psychological treatments: report and recommendations. *The Clinical Psychologist, 48*, 3–23.

Taylor, T. L., & Chemtob, C. M. (2004). Efficacy of treatment for child adolescent traumatic stress. *Archives of Pediatrics & Adolescent Medicine, 158*, 786–791.

Weisz, J. R. (2000) President's message: Lab-clinic differences and what we can do about them: I. The clinic-based treatment development model. *Clinical Child Psychology Newsletter, 15*(1), 1–3,10.

Weisz, J. R., Donenberg, G. R., Han, S. S., & Kauneckis, D. (1995). Child and adolescent psychotherapy outcomes in experiments versus clinics: Why the disparity? *Journal of Abnormal Child Psychology, 63*, 688–701.

Weisz, J. R., Donenberg, G. R., Han, S. S., & Weiss, B. (1995). Bridging the gap between laboratory and clinic in child and adolescent psychotherapy. *Journal of Counseling and Clinical Psychology, 63*, 688–701.

Wolmer, L., Laor, N., Dedeoglu, C., Siev, J., & Yazgan, Y. (2005). Teacher-mediated intervention after disaster: A controlled three-year follow-up of children's functioning. *Journal of Child Psychology and Psychiatry, 46*(11), 1161–1168.

Wolmer, L., Laor N., & Yazgan Y. (2003). School reactivation programs after disaster: Could teachers serve as clinical mediators? *Child & Adolescent Psychiatric Clinics of North America, 12*(2), 363–381.

22 Utilization of Mental Health Services after Disasters

JON D. ELHAI AND JULIAN D. FORD

22.1. INTRODUCTION

This chapter deals with the use of mental health care among individuals affected by disasters. First, we present background literature on correlates of mental health care use among victims of traumatic events and theoretical models used to explain treatment utilization. Second, we review the literature on correlates of mental health care use among disaster-affected persons in particular. Finally, we discuss methodological and statistical issues and advances in examining mental health treatment use in the disaster-affected population.

22.2. BACKGROUND ON TRAUMA-RELATED MENTAL HEALTH CARE UTILIZATION

Traumatic event exposure, especially when resulting in posttraumatic stress disorder (PTSD), is associated with a serious mental health toll, including substantial emotional impairment, risk of suicide, and enormous societal costs (Kessler, 2000). Thus, trauma victims and PTSD-diagnosed persons should be more likely than both nonvictims and non–PTSD-diagnosed persons to need and utilize mental health treatment (including a greater frequency of visits). Consistent with this view, studies demonstrate greater mental health care seeking for trauma victims (compared with nonvictims) among large-scale community samples (Lewis et al., 2005; Sorenson & Siegel, 1992). Evidence from national community samples of civilians (Greenberg et al., 1999; Lewis et al., 2005) and military personnel (Elhai, Richardson, & Pedlar, 2007) also supports a relationship between both PTSD diagnosis and severity with mental health care utilization.

Additionally, among trauma-exposed samples, a large body of research demonstrates significant correlates of mental health care use including the female gender, the extent of previous trauma, and PTSD (reviewed in Elhai, North, & Frueh, 2005; Gavrilovic, Schutzwohl, Fazel, & Priebe, 2005; Walker, Newman, & Koss, 2004). Furthermore, these correlates were revealed in studies including diverse types of traumatized samples, such as war veterans and survivors of assault or disaster. Finally, PTSD's robust association with treatment use does not seem to be accounted for by the disorder's substantial psychiatric comorbidity (i.e., having more than one mental disorder) that could potentially also affect the use of treatment (Brown, Stout, & Mueller, 1999; Schnurr, Friedman, Sengupta, Jankowski, & Holmes, 2000).

It should be noted that in an early relevant investigation, Schwarz and Kowalski (1992) found that PTSD symptom severity was associated with a *decreased* likelihood of mental health treatment seeking. These authors suggested that the effortful avoidance of trauma-related reminders in PTSD (e.g., preferring not to discuss the trauma, becoming distressed when reminded of the trauma) may interfere with treatment seeking. However, subsequent research has not corroborated a relationship between PTSD's avoidance symptoms and treatment use (Elhai, Jacobs, et al., 2006; Goto, Wilson, Kahana, & Slane, 2002; Marshall, Jorm, Grayson, Dobson, & O'Toole, 1997).

22.3. MODELS EXPLAINING MENTAL HEALTH TREATMENT UTILIZATION

Several models explaining *health care* utilization have been proposed, including the Illness

Behavior Model, Health Belief Model, and others, all of which are relevant to *mental health care* utilization (reviewed in Bruce, Wells, Miranda, Lewis, & Gonzalez, 2002). Perhaps the most accepted and validated model of health care use is Andersen's Behavioral Model (Andersen & Newman, 1973), which has garnered decades of empirical support (Andersen, 1995) and has been validated in studies of trauma victims (e.g., Koenen, Goodwin, Struening, Hellman, & Guardino, 2003).

The Behavioral Model theorizes that three personal factors can account for an individual's use of health care. First, *predisposing* variables are historical or sociodemographic characteristics dating before one's current health condition. Predisposing variables can include demographic features, such as gender and racial background; personality or attitudinal characteristics, such as attitudes toward treatment; historical stressors, such as trauma exposure history; and social network variables, such as social support or family structure. Second, *enabling* variables are characteristics involving access to and availability of treatment resources. Enabling variables can include availability factors, such as whether one lives in a geographical area void of mental health care (e.g., a remote rural setting), and treatment access variables, such as employment and health insurance. Third and most important for determining mental health care use (Bland, Newman, & Orn, 1997; Elhai & Ford, 2007), are *need* or illness variables related to one's health condition. Need can include subjective perceptions of illness, such as self-perceived need for treatment, and objective indices, such as a clinician-assigned PTSD diagnosis or psychiatric disability (Andersen, 1995). On the basis of these three factors, the Behavioral Model can be useful in defining equitable access to treatment (i.e., when need is more important than predisposing or enabling variables). It can also elucidate potential inequitable treatment access disparities (i.e., when predisposing or enabling variables overshadow need) (Andersen, 1995).

Given the acceptance of and empirical support for the Behavioral Model of health-care use, we will now review the literature detailing correlates of disaster-affected individuals' mental health care use, organized around this model.

22.4. REVIEW OF POSTDISASTER MENTAL HEALTH CARE UTILIZATION

22.4.1. Disaster-Related Study Types

Despite the extensive research literature on mental health care use correlates among trauma victims, relatively fewer studies have examined this issue specifically in disaster-affected individuals. We now discuss three types of these studies, defined on the basis of the characteristics of their samples. These investigations studied (1) individuals directly exposed and/or in close proximity to a disaster (e.g., Manhattan residents surveyed after the New York City September 11, 2001, terrorist attacks), (2) disaster relief workers (e.g., Red Cross personnel providing services to disaster victims), and (3) individuals not directly exposed to disaster, but living within a driving distance and queried about their disaster-related experiences (e.g., Connecticut residents after the September 11th New York City attacks).

22.4.2. Studies Included in This Review

Through searching bibliographic databases (i.e., Medline, PsycINFO), we located 25 studies of disaster-affected individuals that investigated formal mental health care use. Of these investigations, we included in our review subsequently only those that sampled at least one of the types of disaster-affected groups mentioned earlier and that statistically explored correlates of some form of professional/formal mental health care use. Thus, we excluded one study (Fishbain, Aldrich, Goldberg, & Duncan, 1991) that purported to examine disaster victims (witnesses to a riot) where the "disaster" is not traditionally defined as such in the traumatic stress literature. We excluded two papers that did not present data analysis test statistics (Covell et al., 2006; Stuber, Galea, Boscarino, & Schlesinger, 2006), thus limiting our ability to draw conclusions from their findings while quantifying a reasonable margin of error. An additional two studies were eliminated because utilization of mental health-related and other medical treatment was not distinguished (de Bocanegra & Brickman, 2004; Franklin, Young, & Zimmerman, 2002). We excluded one study that examined the prediction of follow-up crisis counseling sessions and thus did not fit well with this intended review's focus on predicting overall receipt of treatment (Donahue, Covell, Foster, Felton, & Essock, 2006). Two additional studies were sorted out because their mental health care use outcome variable involved the offer and acceptance of a referral to additional, enhanced mental health services among crisis counseling participants (Covell, Essock, Felton, & Donahue, 2006; Norris et al., 2006); we cannot infer from those data whether the additional services were actually used.

The remaining 17 reports explored the relationship of a wide variety of variables with mental health care use among disaster-affected persons. The vast majority of these studies examined whether participants used mental health treatment (a dichotomous "use"/"nonuse" variable) as the outcome. The definition of "mental health treatment" varied across investigations, where some only included mental health specialists (e.g., mental health counseling), and others included mental health care delivered in any service sector (e.g., clergy, primary care physician). Nearly all of these studies assessed mental health care use by participant self-report rather than on the basis of medical records. Participants were initially assessed in these investigations as early as 2 weeks after the disaster, with some following them longitudinally for up to 4 years later. Studies varied in how mental health problems were assessed; most of the New York-conducted September 11th studies used structured diagnostic interviews, while the remaining studies used self-report measures, and one used only records-based diagnoses (Dorn, Yzermans, Kerssens, Spreeuwenberg, & van der Zee, 2006).

With two exceptions (Adams, Ford, & Dailey, 2004; Ford, Adams, & Dailey, 2006), these studies did not use a conceptual framework to guide service use analyses. However, many of the variables studied fit well within the Behavioral Model's framework. Some investigations used an error rate (p value) >0.05 to judge significant associations, but only p values ≤ 0.05 will be interpreted as significant in this review to minimize conclusions on the basis of potentially spurious findings. Samples ranged in size from over 1,000 participants in epidemiological studies to mostly in the 200 to 600 range for remaining nonepidemiological examinations; only one study had less than 100 subjects (thus compromising statistical power to detect true associations).

When a particular study included predictor models of several different types of services used (e.g., mental health specialists, overall mental health care), we report here on analyses detailing overall mental health care received. Additionally, two papers presented analyses predicting both general mental health care utilization, and utilization specifically related to the disaster (Boscarino, Adams, & Figley, 2004; Boscarino, Adams, Stuber, & Galea, 2005); we report only the latter analyses, which should be more sensitive in explaining service use patterns. Finally, some studies reported correlates of informal, in addition to formal, mental health care use (Adams et al., 2004; Ford et al., 2006), but we only discuss analyses of formal care in this paper. These methodological issues are specified in Tables 22.1 through 22.3 and will be discussed later in this chapter.

22.4.3. Correlates of Mental Health-Care Use among Directly Exposed Disaster Victims

Eleven studies examined mental health care use correlates among victims directly exposed to disaster. Most of these investigations sampled New York City residents after the September 11th attacks (ranging from 5 to 8 weeks to 18 months after the attacks) (Boscarino, Adams, et al., 2004; Boscarino et al., 2005; Boscarino, Galea, et al., 2004; Boscarino, Galea, Ahern, Resnick, & Vlahov, 2002, 2003; DeVoe, Bannon, & Klein, 2006; Stuber et al., 2002). The remaining studies sampled Gulf Coast residents living in counties affected by Hurricane Katrina several months after the disaster (Wang et al., 2007), evacuees 1 year after a volcano eruption

Table 22.1. Determinants of mental health service use in directly exposed disaster victims

Sample (Citation)	Service Use Criterion	Criterion Type	Time Frame Assessed	Service Data Type	Predictors
1,008 randomly sampled community subjects living near World Trade Center during 9/11 attacks (sampled within 2 months. post -9/11) (Boscarino et al., 2002)	Increase in MH	D	1 month post versus 1 month before 9/11	SR	*Bivariate results*: (+) younger age, female gender, unmarried couple, previous trauma, close associate killed, recent stressful events, rescue operation involvement, peridisaster panic attack, current depression, current PTSD; (0) race, education, residence's proximity to WTC, displaced, believed could be killed, social support, witnessed attacks, post media exposure, income, health insurance, lost work, alcohol consumption postdisaster *Significant multivariate results*: (+) younger age, female gender, previous trauma, recent stressful events, some rescue operation involvement, highest income, peridisaster panic attack
1,008 randomly sampled community subjects living near World Trade Center during 9/11 attacks (sampled within 2 months post -9/11) (Boscarino, et al., 2003)	New Psych Med	D	1 month post versus 1 month before 9/11	SR	*Significant multivariate results*: female gender, two or more past traumas, health insurance, peridisaster panic attack, PTSD
122 parents of child in home, among 1,008 randomly sampled community subjects living near World Trade Center during 9/11 attacks (sampled within 2 months post-9/11) (Stuber, et al., 2002)	Disaster-Related Child MH	D	Since 9/11 (past 1–2 months)	SR	*Bivariate results (child characteristics unless otherwise noted)*: (+) unmarried parents, residence's proximity to WTC, saw parents cry about disaster, current parent disaster-related PTSD; (0) age, gender, race, siblings in home, away from home during disaster, location of school/daycare, parent witnessed disaster, parent lost close associate, knew someone lost in disaster, time until reunited with parents, parental concern about child's safety during disaster, displaced, parent lost possessions, parent lost job, TV exposure, parent income, difficulties with other children, concentration problems, depression, recent parent depression, parent peridisaster panic attack, parent MH visit since disaster *Significant multivariate results (child characteristics)*: male gender, sibling in home, current PTSD

(*continued*)

Table 22.1 *(continued)*

Sample (Citation)	Service Use Criterion	Criterion Type	Time Frame Assessed	Service Data Type	Predictors
2,011 randomly sampled community subjects living in New York City (sampled 4–5 months post -9/11) (Boscarino, Galea, et al., 2004)	MH Psych Med	D	Past month	SR	*MH Bivariate results*: (+) middle-aged, graduate school versus < high school education, closer distance to WTC, two or more previous traumas, one or more recent stressors, had primary care provider, increased alcohol use, peridisaster panic attack, current PTSD, depression; (–) African American race, Hispanic ethnicity *MH significant multivariate results*: non-African American, non-Hispanic, 4 or more past traumas, two or more recent stressors, current PTSD, depression Psych Med bivariate results: (+) age 25+, previously married, two or more past traumas, one or more recent stressors, had primary care provider, health insurance, peridisaster panic attack, increased alcohol use, current PTSD, depression; (0) social support, one past trauma; (–) African American race, Hispanic ethnicity *Psych Med significant multivariate results*: Caucasian, Asian, age 25–64, one or more recent stressors, had primary care provider, current depression
180 parents of children (less than age 5 on 9/11), recruited in childhood centers in New York City in summer 2002 (DeVoe, et al., 2006)	Child MH	D	Since 9/11 attacks	SR	*Bivariate results (child characteristics unless otherwise noted)*: (+) saw WTC attack in person, less 9/11 media exposure, PTSD, afraid of new things, parent anxiety, parent depression, parent sought MH treatment for self; (0) more aggressive since disaster, clingy/dependent, upset when separated, parent PTSD, sleep difficulty *Significant multivariate final model results (child characteristics unless otherwise noted)*: afraid of new things, witnessed attack in person, less 9/11 media exposure, parent depression, parent MH treatment for self
2,368 randomly sampled community subjects living in New York City near World Trade Center during 9/11 attacks (sampled 1 year post-9/11) (Boscarino, Adams, et al., 2004)	Disaster-Related MH Disaster-Related Psych Med	D	Past year	SR	*Disaster-related MH multivariate results*: (+) younger age, college education, at least moderate disaster exposure, two or more negative life events, peridisaster panic attack, higher anxiety, low to moderate self-esteem, past-year PTSD, past-year depression; (0) gender, marital status, previous trauma, income, health insurance, had primary care doctor; (–) African American race, low social support

					Disaster-related Psych Med multivariate results: (+) middle-aged, female gender, high disaster exposure, two or more negative life events, higher anxiety, low self-esteem, past-year PTSD, past-year depression; (0) education, marital status, social support, previous trauma, income, health insurance, had primary care doctor, peridisaster panic attack; (–) African American race
473 participants diagnosed with PTSD or major depression, among 2,368 randomly sampled community subjects living in New York City near World Trade Center during 9/11 attacks (sampled 1 year post-9/11) (Boscarino, et al., 2005)	Disaster-Related MH Disaster-Related Psych Med	D	Past year	SR	*Disaster-related MH bivariate results*: (+) at least moderate disaster exposure, had regular primary care doctor, peridisaster panic attack; (0) gender, age, health insurance, borough of residence; (–) African American race *Significant disaster-related MH multivariate results*: non-African American race, at least moderate disaster exposure, had regular primary care doctor, peridisaster panic attack *Disaster-related Psych Med bivariate results*: (+) middle-aged, at least high disaster-related exposure, had regular primary care doctor, peridisaster panic attack; (0) borough of residence, gender, health insurance; (–) African American race Significant disaster-related Psych Med multivariate results: non–African American race, middle-aged, peridisaster panic attack
1,034 adult residents of counties affected by Hurricane Katrina, randomly sampled on the basis of random digit dialing and from those individuals seeking disaster relief assistance (evaluated 4–6 months posthurricane) (Wang, et al., 2007)	MH	D	Since Hurricane Katrina	SR	*Multivariate results for postdisaster treatment use, controlling for clinical variables*: (+) middle-aged, married at some point in life *Multivariate results for current treatment use, controlling for clinical variables*: (+) Caucasian race, low or high education level, married at some point in life, own home without a mortgage remaining, current health insurance *Multivariate results for dropping out of treatment (among those reporting some treatment use postdisaster), controlling for clinical variables*: (+) Hispanic race, other race/ethnicity (aside from Caucasian, African American, Hispanic), not previously married, own home with a current mortgage

(*continued*)

Table 22.1 *(continued)*

Sample (Citation)	Service Use Criterion	Criterion Type	Time Frame Assessed	Service Data Type	Predictors
231 adults evacuated from homes after volcano eruption (evaluated 1 year post) (Goto, et al., 2002)	MH	C	Past year	SR	(+) Older age, PTSD's intrusion and hyperarousal symptoms, depression severity, help sought from physician predisaster; (0) educational level, years resided at home, help sought by MH professional predisaster, PTSD's avoidance symptoms
286 fire victims, 802 victims' family members, 3,722 community control subjects from family medical practices, 10,230 patients from a national reference population (Dorn, et al., 2006)	MH to family practitioner	C	1 year prefire, and 3 years postfire	REC	(+) victim group, time period postfire, uninjured victims, loss of a child
662 affected residents of fireworks explosion, assessed 2–3 weeks after, at 18 months, and at 4 years. Comparison group was included starting at 18 months (Van der Velden, et al., 2006)	MH	D	Past year	SR	(+) affected group across time points, affected group with severe depression across time points (compared with comparison group with severe depression), affected group with severe anxiety in first 12 months only (compared with comparison group with severe anxiety)

Notes: For *criterion type*, C, continuous (intensity of services used); D, dichotomous (presence or absence of services used). For *service data type*, REC, records-based; SR, self-report. For *predictors*, statistically significant (at least as stringent as $p < 0.05$) relationships (where criterion variable reference category is presence of or increased service use) are noted as significant positive association (+), significant negative association (−), and no significant relationship (0). When *time frame assessed* was not specified in article, this information was obtained by contacting the author. Psych Med, psychiatric medication use; MH, mental health treatment use; PTSD, posttraumatic stress disorder; WTC, World Trade Center.

Table 22.2. Determinants of mental health service use in disaster relief Workers

Sample (Citation)	Service Use Criterion	Criterion Type	Time Frame Assessed	Service Data Type	Predictors
3,015 Red Cross disaster workers 1 year after 9/11 attacks (Elhai, Jacobs, et al., 2006)	MH	D	Past year	SR	*Multivariate final results controlling for MH use before 9/11*: (+) younger age, previously married, posttraumatic intrusion and hyperarousal symptoms; (0) gender, race, education, number of previous disaster responses, visited disaster site, contact with families of victims, posttraumatic avoidance; (−) previous MH use
174 disaster utility workers from 9/11 attacks accepting psychotherapy referral (Jayasinghe, et al., 2005)	MH	D	Past year since 9/11	REC	*Bivariate results*: (+) non-Hispanic Caucasians, PTSD severity; (0) age, education, marital status, previous trauma, prior MH treatment, past mental disorder (depression, panic or generalized anxiety disorder), witnessed disaster, knew someone in WTC, knew someone killed in WTC, attended funeral/memorial, worked at WTC, number of days worked at WTC, experienced danger at WTC, saw dead bodies, current PTSD diagnosis, current other diagnosis (depression, panic or generalized anxiety disorder), depression severity, distress severity *Significant multivariate results*: race/ethnicity, PTSD severity, race × PTSD severity interaction
207 disaster/rescue workers exposed to an airplane crash, and 421 nonexposed control disaster/rescue workers, assessed 2, 7, and 13 months after (Fullerton, et al., 2004)	MH	D	Past 2 months, past 7 months, past 13 months	SR	(+) exposed group (at each time point)
54 disaster workers working in a mortuary after an explosion on a U.S. naval ship, assessed 1, 1–4, and 4–13 months after (Ursano, et al., 1999)	MH	D	Past month, past 1–4 months, past 4–13 months	SR	(0) identification with the victim as oneself, friend or family member

Notes: For *criterion type*, C, continuous (intensity of services used); D, dichotomous (presence or absence of services used). For *service data type*, REC, records-based; SR, self-report. For *predictors*, statistically significant (at least as stringent as $p < 0.05$) relationships are noted as significant positive association (+), significant negative association (−), and no significant relationship (0). When *time frame assessed* was not specified in article, this information was obtained by contacting the author. MH, mental health treatment use; PTSD, posttraumatic stress disorder; WTC, World Trade Center.

Table 22.3. Determinants of mental health service use in other affected individuals of a disaster

Sample (Citation)	Service Use Criterion	Criterion Type	Time Frame Assessed	Service Data Type	Predictors
Random phone survey of 1,762 Connecticut residents, within first 3 mos of 9/11 attacks (Adams, et al., 2004)	MH	D	Since 9/11 attacks	SR	*Bivariate results*: (+) victim status, smoker, at least one poor physical health day in past month, at least one poor mental health day in past month, at least one mental health problem, sleep problems, increased substance use; (0) gender, age, race, 9/11 location, alcohol use, health insurance, attended 9/11 funeral *Significant multivariate results*: relationship to victim, sleep problems, increased substance use, informal help used
Random phone survey of 4,640 Connecticut residents, 5–15 mos after 9/11 attacks (Ford, et al., 2006)	MH	D	Since 9/11 attacks	SR	*Bivariate results for formal help received:* (+) unmarried, unemployed, disabled, smokes, nondrinker, 1 or more poor physical health days in past month, 1 or more poor mental health days in past month, depression, one or more days of worry in past month, increased smoking; (0) date assessed, gender, age, race, ethnicity, health insurance, sleep problems, increased alcohol use *Significant multivariate results for formal help received*: number of poor mental health days

Notes: For *criterion type*, C, continuous (intensity of services used); D, dichotomous (presence or absence of services used). For *service data type*, REC, records-based; SR, self-report. For *predictors*, statistically significant (at least as stringent as $p < 0.05$) relationships are noted as significant positive association (+), Significant Negative Association (–), and no significant relationship (0). When *time frame assessed* was not specified in article, this information was obtained by contacting the author. MH, Mental health treatment use; Mos, months.

(Goto et al., 2002), fire victims 3 years later (Dorn et al., 2006), and fireworks explosion victims 2 to 3 weeks later and at intervals up to 4 years afterward (Van der Velden et al., 2006).

Mental health treatment use prevalence was reported in the September 11th studies, ranging from 19% for services and 12% for medication specifically in the weeks after the September 11th attacks (Boscarino et al., 2002), falling to roughly 8% for medication and services use after 4 to 5 months (Boscarino, Galea, et al., 2004), with services climbing back up to 20% and medication use stabilizing at 8% after 1 year (Boscarino, Adams, et al., 2004). Mental health care use prevalence within 4 to 6 months after Hurricane Katrina among those affected was 16%, mostly involving the general medical service sector (11% of the entire sample) and pharmacotherapy exclusively without combined psychotherapy (9% of the entire sample). It is important to note, however, that these rates of treatment use are not higher than recent estimates from the general population (20%, Wang et al., 2007).

For each of these studies, Table 22.1 describes the samples, methods, and associations with mental health care use. Several correlates of mental health care utilization are apparent across these studies, in terms of both mental health care use and psychiatric medication use. Three predisposing variables were consistently related to treatment use. First, younger age was consistently associated with a greater likelihood of mental health care use in studies of adults that examined age as a potential correlate. Younger age is in fact a consistently demonstrated predictor of mental health care use in general adult community samples (e.g., Kessler, Olfson, & Berglund, 1998), and in fact recent work demonstrates progressively more positive attitudes toward such treatment in both more recent decades and generational cohorts (Mojtabai, 2007). However, age has been found to be variably related to postdisaster distress across nationalities and cultures (Norris, Kaniasty, Conrad, Inman, & Murphy, 2002), so it may be that older adults are more willing than young or midlife adults to seek mental health care in some populations (e.g., Goto et al., 2002). Four of the studies of postdisaster mental health care found that midlife adults were most likely to report utilization (Boscarino et al., 2005; Boscarino, Adams, et al., 2004; Boscarino, Galea, et al., 2004; Wang et al., 2007), consistent with prior findings that postdisaster distress has been associated with midadulthood rather than younger or older adulthood (Norris, Friedman, et al., 2002). Thus, midlife adults appear to both experience and acknowledge the most severe distress following disaster, and some evidence suggests that this age group is more willing than others to seek treatment for distress or mental health concerns in the wake of disaster.

Second, African-Americans were less likely than Caucasians to report mental health care use, with Hispanic ethnicity also associated with a lower likelihood of utilization in one study (Boscarino, Galea, et al., 2004) and increased likelihood of treatment drop-out in another (Wang et al., 2007) as well as possibly in a third study that grouped all "non-Caucasian" respondents (Boscarino et al., 2005). A greater likelihood and intensity of mental health care use by Caucasians, with comparably less use by racial minorities, has been consistently demonstrated in community samples of adults as well (e.g., Kessler, Chiu, Demler, & Walters, 2005). Third, the extent of exposure to the disaster was consistently associated with the likelihood of mental health care utilization. The postdisaster exposure-treatment use relationship is consistent with the results of previous reports for other types of trauma exposure (Sorenson & Siegel, 1992; Walker et al., 1999) and thus extends findings on this relationship to now include disaster exposure as well. Little evidence was found for enabling variables as correlates of mental health care use. This lack of a potent relationship for enabling characteristics supports recent work demonstrating that need overshadows such enabling variables (Elhai & Ford, 2007).

Consistently demonstrated need-related correlates of treatment use included panic attacks during the disaster, and diagnoses of major depressive disorder and PTSD, supporting previous findings of a robust association between mental health care use and the presence of anxiety and mood disorders (Elhai & Ford, 2007; Parslow & Jorm, 2000). PTSD was particularly associated (across studies) with mental health treatment use in our review. PTSD is not as often studied as other disorders or symptoms of psychological distress in general epidemiological studies for correlates of mental health care utilization. The results of the postdisaster studies that we reviewed suggest that PTSD should be considered a robust need factor in directly exposed populations with regard to mental health care utilization. Given recent evidence for PTSD's role in mediating the relationship between disaster exposure and physical health problems (Norris, Slone, Baker, & Murphy, 2006), PTSD also may warrant further investigation in postdisaster studies as a potential mediator of the relationship between disaster exposure and mental health care utilization.

Two studies investigated mental health care use by children (as reported by their parents) following the New York City September 11th terrorist attacks. In the first 2 months after the disaster, correlates of mental health care utilization by children included exposure (i.e., proximity of residence to the World Trade Center) but also largely related to their parents' relational stability (i.e., unmarried parents were more likely to seek help for their child) and posttraumatic stress or grief reactions (Stuber et al., 2002). Several months later (9–11 months postdisaster) these two factors again were associated with mental health care use by children but with different specific indicators: exposure to the disaster involved directly witnessing the events; parental difficulties included depression and seeking mental health treatment for oneself (DeVoe et al., 2006). Factors associated with parents' seeking of mental health care for their child in the wake of disaster warrants further study in relation to other types of disaster, but in the wake of the September 11th terrorist attacks, exposure and parental acute distress or persistent depression appeared to be key correlates of child mental health care use. This pattern of findings is consistent with a robust empirical literature demonstrating that parental reactions and coping in the aftermath of children's exposure to psychological trauma is a key influence on their child's risk for posttraumatic problems (Aisenberg & Ell, 2005).

Interestingly, associations for the need-based predictor variables (e.g., PTSD, depression, panic attacks) remained stable across the longitudinal time points examined across investigations. However, ethnoracial minority background began appearing as a significant treatment use correlate only at the 1-year time point (with one exception finding minority status as a significant correlate of medication use at 4 to 5 months after September 11th [Boscarino, Galea, et al., 2004]). Other predisposing (e.g., gender, unmarried status) and need (e.g., increased alcohol use) factors were associated with mental health care utilization in the first months after disaster but not at later time points. Systematic research is needed to identify factors associated with mental health care use that are stable over time and those that are associated with specific phases in the wake of disaster.

22.4.4. Correlates of Mental Health Care Use among Disaster Relief Workers

Four studies examined mental health treatment correlates among disaster relief workers. Two of these papers sampled disaster workers 1 year after responding to the September 11th attacks (Elhai, Jacobs, et al., 2006; Jayasinghe et al., 2005). Other studies sampled disaster workers longitudinally for up to 13 months postdisaster in response to an airplane crash (Fullerton, Ursano, & Wang, 2004) and a naval ship explosion (Ursano, Fullerton, Vance, & Kao, 1999). Mental health care use prevalence 1 year postdisaster ranged from 11% among Red Cross workers responding to the September 11th attacks (Elhai, Jacobs, et al., 2006) to 15% among exposed relief workers responding to an airplane crash (Fullerton et al., 2004). Across these investigations, PTSD severity was the strongest and most consistent correlate of mental health care use. As discussed previously, younger age and Caucasian race were also associated with mental health care utilization, but the pattern of findings was not as consistent as that for PTSD. Little support was found for any other predisposing or enabling variables as correlates of mental health care use (see Table 22.2).

Relief workers vary greatly in not only their personal characteristics but also their extent of preparation (i.e., ranging from no training for utility workers, to brief training for some Red Cross workers, to extensive technical training for professional rescue teams and experienced Red Cross responders) and exposure to psychological trauma. However, of the four studies with disaster relief workers, only two systematically assessed such a range of potential correlates. Thus, much more research is needed to empirically examine and establish the factors associated with mental health care use following disasters by relief workers.

22.4.5. Correlates of Mental Health-Care Use among Other Affected Individuals of a Disaster

Two studies examined mental health care use correlates among affected individuals residing outside of New York City but within driving distance of the World Trade Center during the September 11th attacks. These papers sampled Connecticut residents within the first 3 months of the attacks (Adams et al., 2004) and subsequently at 5 to 15 months after the attacks (Ford et al., 2006). A small proportion of respondents (<5%) either were directly exposed (i.e., in New York City at the time of the attacks) or were family members of, or personally knew, a deceased victim. Mental health care use prevalence ranged from 6% (3% for formal treatment) in the first 3 months to 9% after 5 to 15 months.

In these studies, sleep difficulty – which can be a symptom of PTSD – was consistently related to mental health care utilization. Consistent support was also found for an increased likelihood of mental health care utilization as the number of days of self-reported poor health or mental health in the past month increased (see Table 22.3). In the first 3 months following the terrorist attack, direct exposure to the attack or having a personal relationship with a deceased victim and increased alcohol use were associated with an increased likelihood of mental health care use. During the following year, poor overall mental health was the only unique correlate of mental health care use. Thus, acute postdisaster mental health care utilization appeared to be associated primarily with immediate need due to exposure or sleep or alcohol use problems, while mental health-care use over the longer term appeared to be primarily related to general mental health problems.

To the extent that the brief subjectively reported mental health variables assessed in these studies are related to more objective mental health indices (e.g., clinician-assigned diagnoses based on structured diagnostic interviews), these results suggest that acute posttraumatic distress related to disaster exposure is critical to mental health care utilization even in a population in which most persons were not directly affected. Furthermore, general mental health problems (which are more accurately assessed by objective diagnostic indices) may become the primary correlate of mental health care utilization a year or more after the disaster. As with disaster relief workers, more research is needed to replicate findings of the few studies that have been conducted with the at-risk but less intensely disaster-affected populations.

22.4.6. Result Trends across Studies of Disaster-Affected Individuals' Mental Health-Care Use

Across the three study types of disaster-affected individuals, we find that need (especially PTSD) variables were consistently related to mental health treatment use. Enabling variables were infrequently associated with mental health care utilization. Additionally, although some predisposing variables were consistently related to mental health care use among adults (e.g., age, race), other variables expected to be related on the basis of general community study findings (e.g., female gender and nonmarried status [Bland et al., 1997; Kessler et al., 2005]) in fact were inconsistently (and generally only in the acute postdisaster period) related to mental health care utilization among disaster-affected individuals.

Odds ratios reported in these studies can inform the reader about the magnitude of associations with mental health care use, with an odds ratio of 2.5 indicating that the positive presence of the characteristic of interest (e.g., presence of PTSD) is associated with a 150% increased likelihood of treatment use (approximating a medium effect size). Across investigations, need variables, especially depression, anxiety, and PTSD (and increased alcohol use in the acute postdisaster period) tended to be associated with the largest odds ratios, typically exceeding 3.0. Aside from age, stressful life events, trauma and disaster exposure, which also tended to possess respectable odds ratios, other predisposing and enabling variables did not appear to be strongly related to mental health care use.

22.5. METHODOLOGICAL AND STATISTICAL ISSUES IN EXAMINING DISASTER-AFFECTED INDIVIDUALS' MENTAL HEALTH CARE UTILIZATION

Several methodological issues are important in exploring mental health care use, specifically in trauma victims, as detailed elsewhere (Elhai et al., 2005). Furthermore, the statistical analysis of mental health care utilization data is associated with several sensitive issues that are often difficult to overcome, limiting previous investigations' findings (Elhai, Calhoun, & Ford, 2008). These methodological and statistical issues are discussed next.

22.5.1. Methodological Issues in Examining Disaster-Affected Individuals' Mental Health-Care Use

Inquiring about mental health treatment utilization first requires that the investigator and respondent are in agreement about what is meant by both mental health "*problems*" and "*treatment*." Thus, the investigator should ideally use questions that are as behaviorally specific as possible, without leaving ambiguity about what these terms mean. Fortunately, many of the studies included in the earlier review defined mental health problems using several possible terms ("emotional problems," "family problems," "mental health problems"), orienting the respondent to answer about treatment received for such specific problems.

We have recommended specifying to respondents examples of the types of providers visited to ensure that respondents accurately recall and report their previous visits to providers of interest to the investigators (Elhai et al., 2005). For example, an investigator may ask about mental health care from a "psychiatrist, other physician, psychologist, counselor, social worker, clergy, or other health professional." An even more sophisticated approach would involve providing a list of such providers so that respondents can indicate previous service use (and recent visit frequency) for each individual type of provider. This issue is important, since people have various preferences about the types of health care sectors in which they prefer to obtain mental health care (e.g., primary care, mental health specialty sector, clergy), with different sets of correlates found for various sectors (Elhai & Ford, 2007; Wang et al., 2006). Thus, asking more globally about mental health treatment, without respect to specific providers, can potentially lose important information when examining service utilization predictor models. Many of the studies reviewed here provided examples of the types of providers inquired about, and some inquired about visits to several specific types of providers using questions adapted from the National Comorbidity Survey's service use items (Kessler et al., 1999).

Providing a time frame for self-reported previous service use is crucial as well. Prior research has discovered that inquiring about shorter time frames (e.g., past month) is associated with substantially more accurate recall than longer time frames (e.g., past year) when validating self-reported use and frequency of use against medical records as many respondents underestimate their actual previous services used (Roberts, Bergstralh, Schmidt, & Jacobsen, 1996; Wallihan, Stump, & Callahan, 1999). Several of the studies reviewed in this chapter inquired about service use using short time frames (e.g., 1 month); however, a minority implemented time frames of longer than 1 year. Even more sophisticated, but rarely found within our review, is the use of records to define services used; however, such records-based data are time-consuming to extract and are generalizable only to the clinic or provider network to which the individual presented. The use of continuous time sampling designs (Adams et al., 2004; Ford et al., 2006) provides a more complete description of trends and factors in mental health care use over time following disaster, but the most informative design, a fully prospective study with repeated pre- and postdisaster assessments, has not as yet been reported in this research area.

Most of the investigations reviewed here inquired about mental health services used in general. However, some studies inquired about such services specifically related to one's disaster experience (Boscarino, Adams, et al., 2004; Boscarino et al., 2005). Services may be sought at any time because of a variety of precipitating factors; thus, disaster research should attempt to link one's mental health care use specifically to the disaster being studied for more precise and sensitive (and less error-prone) modeling of service utilization.

Two studies inquired about informal sources of help as well as formal mental health care services, revealing different patterns of correlates for these types of services (Adams et al., 2004; Ford et al., 2006). Further study of the full range of supports and services from which people receive help for mental health problems will provide a fuller understanding of where, when, and how people seek help for the emotional impact of disaster as well as for preexisting mental health needs.

Only two studies reviewed here inquired about barriers to seeking or continuing mental health treatment among disaster victims (Boscarino et al., 2005; Wang et al., 2007). Wang et al. (2007) found that among participants who dropped out of treatment postdisaster, the most common reasons cited included factors related to decreased need for treatment (52%) and factors related to inadequate resources to continue treatment, such as lack of adequate finances or transportation (42%). Additionally, Boscarino et al. (2005) found that the most frequently reported treatment barrier in their study was the belief that one did not have a problem needing treatment, endorsed by nearly three-quarters of those victims diagnosed with PTSD or major depressive disorder. Thus, aside from those papers' findings, little is known about disaster-affected individuals' barriers to either initiating treatment or continuing treatment once started. One advantage of Boscarino and colleagues' (2005) study is that they used open-ended questions to inquire about potential barriers to treatment, and thus their results may have less bias than previous studies on treatment barriers among the general population (e.g., Wells, Robins, Bushnell, Jarosz, & Oakley-Browne, 1994). In both quantitative and qualitative studies, it will be important in the future to distinguish between people who intended to but did not or could not access mental health care from people who neither intended to nor actually utilized mental health care. These are very different subgroups of nonutilizers who may have distinguishing predisposing, access, or need characteristics that can facilitate the development of approaches to enhancing access by overcoming barriers to the access of services.

One limitation of the disaster studies reviewed is the way in which PTSD was analyzed as a correlate variable of service use. First, many of these studies examined PTSD as a dichotomous diagnostic variable (diagnostic "presence" or "absence") and thus neglected to capture the dimensionality (i.e., severity) of the disorder's symptoms. Furthermore, even those studies measuring PTSD dimensionally tended to examine the disorder as a global PTSD construct, without further analyzing specific PTSD symptom clusters that may be more or less associated with treatment use. Finally, two studies separately analyzed PTSD's intrusion, avoidance, and hyperarousal symptom clusters (Elhai, Jacobs, et al., 2006; Goto et al., 2002), but recent research suggests that the avoidance cluster is best conceptualized by splitting its symptoms into effortful avoidance and emotional numbing (passive avoidance) symptoms (Asmundson, Stapleton, & Taylor, 2004).

22.5.2. Statistical Issues in Examining Disaster-Affected Individuals' Mental Health-Care Use

Nearly all studies reviewed in this chapter examined disaster-affected persons' use versus nonuse of treatment. However, classifying individuals into crude "use"/"nonuse" categories neglects to capture the dimensionality that can be associated with mental health care utilization. Importantly, it classifies an individual with only one recent treatment visit into the same category as someone with weekly or daily visits. Thus, while this review derived conclusions on the correlates of use versus nonuse of treatment among disaster-affected persons, little is known about correlates of the intensity of disaster-related treatment use.

In fact, until recently it was highly problematic to model the frequency of mental health care visits. Mental health visit count variables quite often possess substantial heteroscedasticity (i.e., error variance is unequally distributed across participants), a positive skew with most participants falling on the low end of the frequency distribution and many zero values (since many subjects have not sought any mental health care in a recent time-frame) (Elhai et al., 2008). Thus, using traditional general linear model analyses (e.g., linear regression) is contraindicated for modeling such an outcome variable because results would produce biases in regression coefficient standard errors, test statistic values, and effect size estimates (Gardner, Mulvey, & Shaw, 1995). Even conducting a two-step approach, first modeling use from nonuse (e.g., using logistic regression) and then modeling the continuum of service use among only those with at least one visit (e.g., with linear regression), is problematic because of the resulting substantially skewed distribution of those participants with at least one visit.

Other solutions to such complexly distributed visit count data can be just as problematic. Arbitrarily assigning visit counts to categories (e.g., "no visits," "one to nine visits," "ten or more visits"), while providing richer information than a simpler dichotomous "use"/"nonuse" variable, still loses important information, as such continuous variable dichotomization has undesirable effects, such as loss of power and biased significance levels and effect size estimates (MacCallum, Zhang, Preacher, & Rucker, 2002). Previously, the best possible solution was to conduct data transformations on the outcome variable (e.g., square root, logarithmic, or inverse transformation), but transformations can lead to uninterpretable regression coefficients, and more importantly, mental health visit counts are often too skewed for any transformation to result in a successfully normalized distribution (Elhai et al., 2008).

More recently, however, statistical methods specifically designed for count data (e.g., visit counts) have been developed. Poisson and negative binomial regression are basic count regression analyses, using the *generalized* rather than *general* linear model, and assume data distributions that more closely resemble visit count data, including Poisson and gamma distributions, respectively. These methods function by linearizing the nonlinear visit count outcome variable and using maximum likelihood estimation to model the outcome. More applicable to mental health visit counts are zero-inflated versions of Poisson and negative binomial regression, which account for the substantial proportion of zero values in visit counts by modeling use versus nonuse and weighing cases accordingly in Poisson/negative binomial analyses. (Perhaps less relevant, but worth mentioning, are the zero-truncated versions of Poisson/negative binomial regression, designed for instances where no zero values are present, such as when modeling the continuum of visit counts among individuals who already visited a clinic at least once.) For a review of such statistical analyses, see Elhai and colleagues (2008).

In fact, such contemporary analytic methods are effective in modeling zero-laden data (Hall & Zhengang, 2004; Long, 1997) and have outperformed other statistical analyses in modeling mental health visit counts in particular (Bao, 2002; Elhai et al., 2008). Finally, recent evidence indicates that modeling mental health care use *intensity* with such analyses results in different findings than when modeling "use"/"nonuse" of treatment (Elhai & Ford, 2007), suggesting that additional information can be gained by adding the exploration of service use intensity to service use investigations.

Thus, such contemporary analyses represent a promising method of more comprehensively examining models of treatment use intensity among disaster victims. Furthermore, recent studies have implemented these methods in modeling the relation of mental health care use with both trauma victimization and PTSD (Elhai, Patrick, Anderson, Simons, & Frueh, 2006; Elhai et al., 2007; Elhai & Simons, 2007). Elhai and colleagues (2008) offer additional descriptions of these analyses and current software packages that implement them.

22.6. CONCLUSION

This chapter reviewed empirical findings on the correlates of mental health care use among disaster victims, organized within the Behavioral Model of health care use. Among samples of individuals directly affected by disaster, disaster relief personnel, and other individuals living near disasters, need variables (especially PTSD) appear most consistently related to the use of mental health care, with some predisposing variables such as age and racial background also demonstrating some consistent relationships.

Methodological issues that should be considered when reviewing this literature or conducting future relevant studies include the use of behaviorally specific definitions of mental health problems and services (including distinguishing specific types of mental health treatment providers), distinction between use in the acute and subsequent postdisaster periods, and the inclusion of longer time frames and prospective research designs when surveying mental health care use, querying service use specifically related to the disaster in question, and assessing PTSD dimensionally and its symptom clusters and comorbid problems and disorders (e.g., depression, substance abuse). Statistical issues that should be considered in future research include analyzing the continuum of visit counts and using contemporary analytic methods designed for such complexly distributed data. Extant research on the correlates of mental health care utilization in the wake of disaster provides a small but solid foundation for more methodologically sophisticated studies that can identify the prospective predictors of mental health care utilization in the wake of a range of types of disaster.

ACKNOWLEDGMENTS

We thank Gerard A. Jacobs, Ph.D., for his valuable comments on an earlier draft of this chapter.

REFERENCES

Adams, M.L., Ford, J.D., & Dailey, W.F. (2004). Predictors of help seeking among Connecticut adults after September 11, 2001. *American Journal of Public Health, 94*, 1596–1602.

Aisenberg, E.F., & Ell, K. (2005). Contextualizing community violence and its effects: An ecological model of parent-child interdependent coping *Journal of Interpersonal Violence, 20*, 855–871.

Andersen, R.M. (1995). Revisiting the behavioral model and access to medical care: Does it matter? *Journal of Health and Social Behavior, 36*, 1–10.

Andersen, R.M., & Newman, J.F. (1973). Societal and individual determinants of medical care utilization in the United States. *Milbank Quarterly, 51*, 95–124.

Asmundson, G.J.G., Stapleton, J.A., & Taylor, S. (2004). Are avoidance and numbing distinct PTSD symptom clusters? *Journal of Traumatic Stress, 17*, 467–475.

Bao, Y. (2002). Predicting the use of outpatient mental health services: Do modeling approaches make a difference. *Inquiry, 39*, 168–183.

Bland, R.C., Newman, S.C., & Orn, H. (1997). Help-seeking for psychiatric disorders. *Canadian Journal of Psychiatry, 42*, 935–942.

Boscarino, J.A., Adams, R.E., & Figley, C.R. (2004). Mental health service use 1-year after the World Trade Center disaster: Implications for mental health care. *General Hospital Psychiatry, 26*, 346–358.

Boscarino, J.A., Adams, R.E., Stuber, J., & Galea, S. (2005). Disparities in mental health treatment following the World Trade Center disaster: Implications for mental health care and health services research. *Journal of Traumatic Stress, 18*, 287–297.

Boscarino, J.A., Galea, S., Adams, R.E., Ahern, J., Resnick, H., & Vlahov, D. (2004). Mental health service and medication use in New York City after the September 11, 2001, terrorist attack. *Psychiatric Services, 55*, 274–283.

Boscarino, J.A., Galea, S., Ahern, J., Resnick, H., & Vlahov, D. (2002). Utilization of mental health services following the September 11th terrorist attacks in Manhattan, New York City. *International Journal of Emergency Mental Health, 4*, 143–156.

Boscarino, J.A., Galea, S., Ahern, J., Resnick, H., & Vlahov, D. (2003). Psychiatric medication use among Manhattan residents following the World Trade Center disaster. *Journal of Traumatic Stress, 16*, 301–306.

Brown, P.J., Stout, R.L., & Mueller, T. (1999). Substance use disorder and posttraumatic stress disorder comorbidity: Addiction and psychiatric treatment rates. *Psychology of Addictive Behaviors, 13*, 115–122.

Bruce, M.L., Wells, K.B., Miranda, J., Lewis, L., & Gonzalez, J.J. (2002). Barriers to reducing burden of affective disorders. *Mental Health Services Research, 4*, 187–197.

Covell, N.H., Donahue, S.A., Allen, G., Foster, M.J., Felton, C.J., & Essock, S.M. (2006). Use of Project Liberty counseling services over time by individuals in various risk categories. *Psychiatric Services, 57*, 1268–1270.

Covell, N.H., Essock, S.M., Felton, C.J., & Donahue, S.A. (2006). Characteristics of Project Liberty clients that predicted referrals to intensive mental health services. *Psychiatric Services, 57*, 1313–1315.

de Bocanegra, H.T., & Brickman, E. (2004). Mental health impact of the World Trade Center attacks on displaced Chinese workers. *Journal of Traumatic Stress, 17*, 55–62.

DeVoe, E.R., Bannon, W.M., & Klein, T.P. (2006). Post-9/11 helpseeking by New York City parents on behalf of highly exposed young children. *American Journal of Orthopsychiatry, 76*, 167–175.

Donahue, S.A., Covell, N.H., Foster, M.J., Felton, C.J., & Essock, S.M. (2006). Demographic characteristics of individuals who received Project Liberty crisis counseling services. *Psychiatric Services, 57*, 1261–1267.

Dorn, T., Yzermans, C.J., Kerssens, J.J., Spreeuwenberg, P.M.M., & van der Zee, J. (2006). Disaster and subsequent healthcare utilization: A longitudinal study among victims, their family members, and control subjects. *Medical Care, 44*, 581–589.

Elhai, J.D., & Ford, J.D. (2007). Correlates of mental health service use intensity in the National Comorbidity Survey and National Comorbidity Survey Replication. *Psychiatric Services, 58*, 1108–1115.

Elhai, J.D., & Simons, J.S. (2007). Trauma exposure and posttraumatic stress disorder predictors of mental health treatment use in college students. *Psychological Services, 4*, 38–45.

Elhai, J.D., Calhoun, P.S., & Ford, J.D. (2008). Statistical procedures for analyzing mental health services and costs data. *Psychiatry Research, 160*, 129–136.

Elhai, J.D., Jacobs, G.A., Kashdan, T.B., DeJong, G.L., Meyer, D.L., & Frueh, B.C. (2006). Mental health service use among American Red Cross disaster workers responding to the September 11, 2001 U.S. terrorist attacks. *Psychiatry Research, 143*, 29–34.

Elhai, J.D., North, T.C., & Frueh, B.C. (2005). Health service use predictors among trauma survivors: A critical review. *Psychological Services, 2*, 3–19.

Elhai, J.D., Patrick, S.L., Anderson, S., Simons, J.S., & Frueh, B.C. (2006). Gender- and trauma-related predictors of use of mental health treatment services among primary care patients. *Psychiatric Services, 57*, 1505–1509.

Elhai, J.D., Richardson, D., & Pedlar, D. (2007). Predictors of general medical and psychological treatment use among a national sample of peacekeeping veterans with health problems. *Journal of Anxiety Disorders, 21*, 580–589.

Fishbain, D.A., Aldrich, T.E., Goldberg, M., & Duncan, R.C. (1991). Impact of a human made disaster on the utilization pattern of a psychiatric emergency service. *Journal of Nervous and Mental Disease, 179*, 162–166.

Ford, J.D., Adams, M.L., & Dailey, W.F. (2006). Factors associated with receiving help and risk factors for disaster-related distress among Connecticut adults 5–15 months after the September 11th terrorist incidents. *Social Psychiatry & Psychiatric Epidemiology, 41*, 261–270.

Franklin, C.L., Young, D., & Zimmerman, M. (2002). Psychiatric patients' vulnerability in the wake of the September 11th terrorist attacks. *Journal of Nervous and Mental Disease, 190*, 833–838.

Fullerton, C.S., Ursano, R.J., & Wang, L. (2004). Acute stress disorder, posttraumatic stress disorder, and depression in disaster or rescue workers. *American Journal of Psychiatry, 161*, 1370–1376.

Gardner, W., Mulvey, E.P., & Shaw, E.C. (1995). Regression analyses of counts and rates: Poisson, overdispersed Poisson, and negative binomial models. *Psychological Bulletin, 118*, 392–404.

Gavrilovic, J.J., Schutzwohl, M., Fazel, M., & Priebe, S. (2005). Who seeks treatment after a traumatic event and who does not? A review of findings on mental health service utilization. *Journal of Traumatic Stress, 18*, 595–605.

Goto, T., Wilson, J.P., Kahana, B., & Slane, S. (2002). PTSD, depression and help-seeking patterns following the Miyake Island volcanic eruption. *International Journal of Emergency Mental Health, 4*, 157–172.

Greenberg, P.E., Sisitsky, T., Kessler, R.C., Finkelstein, S.N., Berndt, E.R., Davidson, J.R.T., et al. (1999). The economic burden of anxiety disorders in the 1990s. *Journal of Clinical Psychiatry, 60*, 427–435.

Hall, D.B., & Zhengang, Z. (2004). Marginal models for zero inflated clustered data. *Statistical Modelling, 4*, 161–180.

Jayasinghe, N., Spielman, L., Cancellare, D., Difede, J., Klausner, E.J., & Giosan, C. (2005). Predictors of treatment utilization in World Trade Center attack disaster workers: Role of race/ethnicity and symptom severity. *International Journal of Emergency Mental Health, 7*, 91–100.

Kessler, R.C. (2000). Posttraumatic stress disorder: The burden to the individual and to society. *Journal of Clinical Psychiatry, 61*(Suppl. 5), 4–12.

Kessler, R.C., Chiu, W.T., Demler, O., & Walters, E.E. (2005). Prevalence, severity, and comorbidity of 12-month DSM-IV disorders in the National Comorbidity Survey Replication. *Archives of General Psychiatry, 62*, 617–627.

Kessler, R.C., Olfson, M., & Berglund, P.A. (1998). Patterns and predictors of treatment contact after first onset of psychiatric disorders. *American Journal of Psychiatry, 155*, 62–69.

Kessler, R.C., Zhao, S., Katz, S.J., Kouzis, A.C., Frank, R.G., et al. (1999). Past-year use of outpatient services for psychiatric problems in the National Comorbidity Survey. *American Journal of Psychiatry, 156*, 115–123.

Koenen, K.C., Goodwin, R., Struening, E., Hellman, F., & Guardino, M. (2003). Posttraumatic stress disorder and treatment seeking in a national screening sample. *Journal of Traumatic Stress, 16*, 5–16.

Lewis, S.F., Resnick, H.S., Ruggiero, K.J., Smith, D.W., Kilpatrick, D.G., Best, C.L., et al. (2005). Assault, psychiatric diagnoses, and sociodemographic variables in relation to help-seeking behavior in a national sample of women. *Journal of Traumatic Stress, 18*, 97–105.

Long, J.S. (1997). *Regression models for categorical and limited dependent variables*. Thousand Oaks, CA: Sage Publications.

MacCallum, R.C., Zhang, S., Preacher, K.J., & Rucker, D.D. (2002). On the practice of dichotomization of quantitative variables. *Psychological Methods, 7*, 19–40.

Marshall, R.P., Jorm, A.F., Grayson, D.A., Dobson, M., & O'Toole, B.I. (1997). Help-seeking in Vietnam veterans: Post-traumatic stress disorder and other predictors. *Australian and New Zealand Journal of Public Health, 21*, 211–213.

Mojtabai, R. (2007). Americans' attitudes toward mental health treatment seeking: 1990–2003. *Psychiatric Services, 58*, 642–651.

Norris, F.H., Donahue, S.A., Felton, C.J., Watson, P.J., Hamblen, J.L., & Marshall, R.D. (2006). A psychometric analysis of Project Liberty's adult enhanced services referral tool. *Psychiatric Services, 57*, 1328–1334.

Norris, F.H., Friedman, M.J., Watson, P.J., Byrne, C.M., Diaz, E., & Kaniasty. (2002). 60,000 disaster victims speak: Part I. An empirical review of the empirical literature, 1981–2001. *Psychiatry, 65*, 207–239.

Norris, F.H., Kaniasty, K.Z., Conrad, M.L., Inman, G.L., & Murphy, A.D. (2002). Placing age differences in cultural context: A comparison of the effects of age on PTSD after disasters in the United States, Mexico, and Poland. *Journal of Clinical Geropsychology, 8*, 153–173.

Norris, F.H., Slone, L.B., Baker, C.K., & Murphy, A.D. (2006). Early physical health consequences of disaster exposure and acute disaster-related PTSD *Anxiety, Stress and Coping, 19*, 95–110.

Parslow, R.A., & Jorm, A.F. (2000). Who uses mental health services in Australia?: An analysis of data from the National Survey of Mental Health and Wellbeing. *Australian and New Zealand Journal of Psychiatry, 34*, 997–1008.

Roberts, R.O., Bergstralh, E.J., Schmidt, L., & Jacobsen, S.J. (1996). Comparison of self-reported and medical record health care utilization measures. *Journal of Clinical Epidemiology, 49*, 989–995.

Schnurr, P.P., Friedman, M.J., Sengupta, A., Jankowski, M.K., & Holmes, T. (2000). PTSD and utilization of medical treatment services among male Vietnam veterans. *Journal of Nervous and Mental Disease, 188*, 496–504.

Schwarz, E.D., & Kowalski, J.M. (1992). Malignant memories: Reluctance to utilize mental health services after a disaster. *Journal of Nervous and Mental Disease, 180*, 767–772.

Sorenson, S.B., & Siegel, J.M. (1992). Gender, ethnicity, and sexual assault: Findings from a Los Angeles study. *Journal of Social Issues, 48*, 93–104.

Stuber, J., Fairbrother, G., Galea, S., Pfefferbaum, B., Wilson-Genderson, M., & Vlahov, D. (2002). Determinants of counseling for children in Manhattan after the September 11 attacks. *Psychiatric Services, 53*, 815–822.

Stuber, J., Galea, S., Boscarino, J.A., & Schlesinger, M. (2006). Was there unmet mental health need after the September 11, 2001 terrorist attacks? *Social Psychiatry & Psychiatric Epidemiology, 41*, 230–240.

Ursano, R. J., Fullerton, C. S., Vance, K., & Kao, T. (1999). Posttraumatic stress disorder and identification in disaster workers. *American Journal of Psychiatry, 156*, 353–359.

Van der Velden, P. G., Grievink, L., Kleber, R. J., Drogendijk, A. N., Roskam, A.-J. R., Marcelissen, F. G. H., et al. (2006). Post-disaster mental health problems and the utilization of mental health services: A four-year longitudinal comparative study. *Administration and Policy in Mental Health and Mental Health Services Research, 33*, 279–288.

Walker, E. A., Newman, E., & Koss, M. P. (2004). Costs and health care utilization associated with traumatic experiences. In P.P. Schnurr & B.L. Green (Eds.), *Trauma and health: Physical health consequences of exposure to extreme stress* (pp. 43–69). Washington, DC: American Psychological Association.

Walker, E. A., Unützer, J., Rutter, C., Gelfand, A., Saunders, K., VonKorff, M., et al. (1999). Costs of health care use by women HMO members with a history of childhood abuse and neglect. *Archives of General Psychiatry, 56*, 609–613.

Wallihan, D. B., Stump, T. E., & Callahan, C. M. (1999). Accuracy of self-reported health services use and patterns of care among urban older adults. *Medical Care, 37*, 662–670.

Wang, P. S., Demler, O., Olfson, M., Pincus, H. A., Wells, K. B., & Kessler, R. C. (2006). Changing profiles of service sectors used for mental health care in the United States. *American Journal of Psychiatry, 163*, 1187–1198.

Wang, P. S., Gruber, M. J., Powers, R. E., Schoenbaum, M., Speier, A. H., Wells, K. B., et al. (2007). Mental health service use among Hurricane Katrina survivors in the eight months after the disaster. *Psychiatric Services, 58*, 1403–1411.

Wells, J. E., Robins, L. N., Bushnell, J. A., Jarosz, D., & Oakley-Browne, M. A. (1994). Perceived barriers to care in St. Louis (USA) and Christchurch (NZ): Reasons for not seeking professional help for psychological distress. *Social Psychiatry and Psychiatric Epidemiology, 29*, 155–164.

PART SIX

Case Studies

23 The Mental Health Impact of the Southeast Asia Tsunami

BARBARA LOPES CARDOZO, FRITS VAN GRIENSVEN, WARUNEE THIENKRUA, BENJAPORN PANYAYONG, M.L. SOMCHAI CHAKKRABAND, AND PRAWATE TANTIPIWATANASKUL

23.1. INTRODUCTION

In this chapter we describe the mental health impact of the 2004 tsunami in Southeast Asia. The tsunami had a profound impact on the livelihood of the affected populations, which in itself had an effect on the mental health of the people. Differences between people and cultures from the affected countries may have influenced how tsunami survivors coped with its consequences. Certain segments of the affected populations were more vulnerable during the tsunami, particularly women and children. The mental health consequences, interventions, and programs are described, and we offer some lessons learned from the tragic experience.

23.2. BACKGROUND

On December 26, 2004, a massive undersea earthquake in the waters northwest of Sumatra, Indonesia, with a magnitude of 9.3 on the Richter scale, triggered a giant ocean shockwave, or tsunami, that devastated the shorelines of Indonesia, Sri Lanka, India, Thailand, the Maldives, and several other countries. At least five million people were directly affected by the tsunami, and the death toll exceeded 280,000 people, making it one of the deadliest natural disasters in history. Over one million people were displaced as a result of the destruction (Ghodse & Galea, 2006). The psychological and social consequences of the tsunami are substantial and are likely to be felt for years to come. In addition to the countries directly affected by the tsunami, there were tens of thousands of citizens from other countries traveling in the region and on holiday. Sweden, for instance, lost more than 500 citizens to the tsunami (Lamberg, 2005).

The impact of the tsunami was compounded in some of the affected areas by political strife. Two areas in particular – the province of Aceh (in Indonesia) and Sri Lanka – had been sites of turmoil and armed conflict. In these settings, the psychological impact of the tsunami may have been aggravated by the ongoing political violence (Silove, 2004). Existing studies indicate that war-affected populations are at higher risk for trauma-related mental illness (Lopes Cardozo et al., 2005; Lopes Cardozo, Vergara, Agani, & Gotway, 2000). In addition, conflict areas often suffer from a diminished or overburdened public health infrastructure, which can make mental health resources scarce. Further, the political situation presented potential security and logistical problems for rescue operations and post-tsunami assistance.

23.3. IMPACT OF THE TSUNAMI

The impact of the tsunami on the environment and economic systems was profound and widespread. The loss of livelihoods, homes, and the devastation of entire community networks, which normally would help one recover from loss, all aggravated the psychological impact of the tsunami.

Evidence from Thailand indicates that economic losses – particularly the loss of livelihood – had a significant impact on mental health (van Griensven et al., 2006). That may well be the case for the entire tsunami-affected area. It is also possible that psychological distress among large parts of the population made economic recovery more difficult. As a result, the mental health consequences of the disaster contributed to the tsunami's impact on the economies of the affected areas.

The loss of livelihood in southern Thailand was extensive. The affected coastal areas were heavily dependent on the fishing and tourism industries, which came to an almost complete standstill after the disaster. In a survey conducted by the Centers for Disease Control and Prevention (CDC) and the Department of Mental Health of the Royal Thai Government in the tsunami-affected regions in Thailand, almost half of the people in the most affected area, Phang Nga province, had lost their livelihood; among people surveyed in less affected areas, the estimate was almost 20%. An important finding from this survey was that loss of livelihood was significantly associated with symptoms of posttraumatic stress disorder (PTSD), anxiety, and depression in the adult population (van Griensven, et. al., 2006).

Similarly, in a study in Tamil Nadu, India, researchers found that the odds of PTSD were higher among individuals who had no household incomes (Kumar et al., 2007). Extensive damage occurred in India due to the giant waves from the tsunami, affecting the coastal districts of Tamil Nadu, Kerala, and Andhra Pradesh, as well as the Union Territories of Pondicherry and Andaman and Nicobar Islands. Seawater that washed up to 3 km inland affected approximately 2,260 km of the coastline and all of the islands in the Nicobar district of Andaman and Nicobar Islands. Fishermen (and women) working and living within the first few hundred meters of the sea were the main victims. The industry of catering to tourists and pilgrims – another key source of income for the area – was also seriously hampered by the tsunami (Krishnamoorthy, Harichandrakumar, Krishna Kumar, & Das, 2005).

In Indonesia's Aceh province, the hardest hit economic sectors were agriculture and fishing. These losses were not confined only to the areas immediately adjacent to the sea. In some places, the tsunami wave reached farther than 5 km inland, destroying crops and killing livestock as well as sweeping through houses (Bappenas, 2005). Throughout the affected region, economic losses were far reaching. According to one report, 83% of affected families in Indonesia, 59% in Sri Lanka, and 47% in India had experienced a decrease in their income of more than 50% (Fritz Institute, 2005).

23.4. MENTAL HEALTH CONSEQUENCES

The magnitude of the tsunami's impact on mental health has been documented in a number of studies and surveys in different parts of the affected region. These studies have consistently shown widespread psychological trauma associated with the disaster, generally consistent with what had been found in the wake of other major natural disasters (Basoglu, Kilic, Salcioglu, & Livanou, 2004; Chang, Connor, Lai, Lee, & Davidson, 2005; Wang et al., 2000).

Following a natural disaster, psychological problems can include acute stress reactions among a subset of the exposed population within the first month after the event. PTSD can occur after 1 month, depression, anxiety, and grief reactions may also be present (Carballo, Heal, & Hernandez, 2005).

Studies in the tsunami-affected areas showed increases in the prevalence of PTSD, anxiety, and depression. Many people died during this disaster, and in some cases, whole villages or communities were destroyed and lost much of their population. Surviving family members lost many persons in one family, including children or parents, and close friends. Grief reactions might have been expected in this situation, but these are less well documented than PTSD and depression. Acute stress reaction was also not measured because surveys and studies to capture these reactions are not usually conducted within 1 month of the occurrence of the disaster.

In the tsunami-affected areas in Thailand, a multistage cluster, population-based mental health survey was conducted by the CDC-Thai Collaboration. The time frame for determining symptoms of PTSD, depression, and anxiety was 4 weeks. The survey found PTSD in 12% (*N* = 371) of displaced and 7% (*N* = 322) of nondisplaced persons in Phang Nga (the most affected province) and in 3% (*N* = 368) of nondisplaced persons in Krabi and Phuket (less affected provinces). The Harvard Trauma Questionnaire was used to assess PTSD (Mollica, Caspi-Yavin, Bollini, Truong, Tor, & Lavelle, 1992). PTSD was defined as a score of three or four on at least one of the four reoccurring symptoms, at least three of the seven avoidance and numbing symptoms, and at least two of five arousal symptoms. We used the Hopkins symptom Checklist-25 to detect symptoms of anxiety and depression. Mean cumulative symptom scores higher than 1.75 indicated the presence of anxiety and depression and have been found to be valid in predicting clinical diagnoses of these disorders (Derogatis et al., 1974). Anxiety was reported by 37% (*N* = 371) of displaced and 30% (*N* = 322) of nondisplaced persons in Phang Nga and 22% (*N* = 368) of nondisplaced persons in Krabi and Phuket. Depression was reported by 30% (*N* = 371) of displaced and 21% (*N* = 322) of nondisplaced persons in Phang Nga and 10% (*N* = 368) of nondisplaced persons in Krabi and Phuket. In the 9-month follow-up survey of 270 (73%) displaced and 250 (80%) nondisplaced participants in Phang Nga, prevalences of PTSD, anxiety, and depression among displaced persons decreased to 7%, 24.8%, and 16.7%, respectively, and among nondisplaced persons, decreased to 2.3%, 25.9%, and 14.3%, respectively (van Griensven et al., 2006). The prevalence for post-tsunami PTSD in Thailand was relatively low compared to other populations in countries that have been affected by natural disasters. This may be due to certain cultural differences and other protective factors such as the Buddhist religion in Thailand (van Griensven et al., 2006).

In Sri Lanka, a separate study also found a measurable psychological impact from the tsunami. Using the less rigorous method of convenience sampling, investigators found a 56% prevalence of PTSD among people displaced by the tsunami (Ranasinghe & Levy, 2004). A study conducted in Tamil Nadu, India, 2 months after the disaster by the National Institute of Epidemiology, Indian Council of Medical Research, Chennai, surveyed adults aged 18 years or older in an affected coastal village using structured interviews and the Harvard Trauma Questionnaire. The study found that the prevalence of PTSD was 12.7% (95% CI = 9.4%–17.1%), and it observed that the risk for PTSD was higher among individuals with no household income, females, and those injured during the tsunami (Kumar et al., 2007).

23.5. CULTURAL FACTORS

Cultural differences may influence how survivors of the tsunami interpreted the event and how they coped with its consequences. For example, in Thailand and Sri Lanka, where a large portion of the population is Buddhist, elements of that belief system came into play (de Silva, 2006). A central tenet of Buddhism is the concept of *Karma*, a belief that events in this life are to some degree predetermined by individual actions in a previous life (Mulder, 2000; U.S. Library of Congress, LePoer, 1987). This belief helped provide something of an explanation for the event and a protective effect against anxiety and depression. This is consistent with previous studies (Holtz, 1998; Shrestha, Sharma, & van Ommeren, 1998). The Thai belief system also holds that a supernatural power rules over every space, including air or water (Mulder, 2000; U.S. Library of Congress, LePoer, 1987). The territory of those supernatural powers must be respected, and they must be informed and pleased before they will share the space. Anecdotal evidence indicates that some of those affected by the tsunami believed that the spirits sought revenge for human exploitation of the sea. It is possible that by providing an understandable explanation to an otherwise incomprehensible natural disaster, the belief system makes the events less of a random occurrence and even gives the individual and the community a sense that they have a certain level of control, however, limited.

Cultural differences help to explain certain phenomena that by Western standards might be construed as pathology. For example, tsunami survivors in Thailand reported seeing ghosts or hearing voices. Before categorizing this as a mental disorder, it is important to note that within Thai culture it is imperative to conduct appropriate rituals for the dead in order for the ghosts of the deceased to come to rest. After the tsunami, however, many of the victims' bodies, necessary for conducting the rituals, were never found or could not be identified. Thai tradition dictates that improperly performed rituals can result in the dead reincarnating as malevolent ghosts *(phii)*. Hence, in most cases this phenomenon should be interpreted in the context of the local belief system and as a culturally specific way of coping with death and reincarnation rather than a symptom of mental illness.

All these examples show that cultural understanding and sensitivity are important for the assessment of mental illness, the interpretation of psychological problems, and the implementation of mental health programs (Bryant, 2006).

23.6. VULNERABLE POPULATIONS

As in other disasters and complex emergencies, certain sectors of the population experienced a greater psychological impact from the disaster (Lopes Cardozo et al., 2005). That was particularly true for women and children affected by the Southeast Asia tsunami. For women, the increased impact of the tsunami was due to a variety of reasons and was not restricted to mental health: Women were four times more likely to be killed than men (MacDonald, 2005; Oxfam, 2005). Women were more likely to have been in the villages running household errands and taking care of the children, whereas, most of the men in the affected area are employed as subsistence fishermen who go out daily or work on ships located on fishing grounds for extended periods of time. There is also anecdotal evidence that women perished in the waves while trying to save their children. Other reasons for the higher mortality rates among women varied from country to country. According to Oxfam, the tsunami hit during a time of the week when men tend to be away from home, while women remained in their houses, closer to the sea. In India, according to the same report, women were waiting on the shore for the fishermen to return when the wave pushed ashore (Oxfam, 2005). In Sri Lanka, the tsunami struck during the time when women were bathing in the sea (MacDonald, 2005).

After the event, women encountered new sources of trauma. In camps for displaced persons, women were victims of sexual violence and physical harassment by men (Rees, Pittaway, & Bartolomei, 2005; U.S. Department of State, 2005). Obtaining relief supplies was more difficult for women than for men because of cultural issues and relative physical strength. Problems were compounded for pregnant women due in part to the absence of reproductive health services and the general shortcomings of the available facilities (MacDonald, 2005).

In a survey conducted in Sri Lanka, 147 (56%) individuals of a convenience sample, showed symptom profiles consistent with PTSD. Women showed a higher prevalence (63.7%) than men (41.7%), and they had at least twice the risk for experiencing PTSD (Ranasinghe & Levy, 2004). Several other studies have shown that women are more likely to experience PTSD and depression than men after disasters or complex emergencies (van Griensven et al., 2006).

Children also experienced mental health consequences from the tsunami (Thienkrua et al., 2006). In Thailand, our study showed prevalence of PTSD symptoms of 13% among children living in camps, 11% among children from affected villages, and 6% among children from unaffected villages (camps vs. unaffected villages, $p = 0.25$); for depression symptoms, the prevalence was 11%, 5%, and 8%, respectively ($p = 0.39$). In multivariate analyses of the first assessment, having had a delayed evacuation, having felt one's own or a family member's life was in danger, and having felt extreme panic or fear were significantly associated with PTSD symptoms. Older age and having felt that one's own or a family member's life was in danger were significantly associated with depression symptoms. About 72% (151/210) of children from Phang Nga participated in a follow-up survey. Prevalence of symptoms of PTSD and depression among these children did not decrease significantly over time (Thienkrua et al., 2006).

In Sri Lanka, a study conducted 3 to 4 weeks after the tsunami disaster examined PTSD prevalence among children living in three severely affected communities. Across all communities, 87% of the children reported one or more traumatic events before the tsunami. Previous traumatic exposure was high in the civil war affected Tamil region and in the Sinhalese region. Depending on location, between 4.6% and 8.5% of children had PTSD unrelated to the tsunami. Another 13.9% to 38.8% of children fulfilled the preliminary diagnosis of tsunami-related PTSD (Neuner, Schauer, Catani, Ruf, & Elbert, 2006).

An assessment conducted among 87 elderly people in Ban Nam Khem Community, Thailand, showed that 6 months after the disaster, this population still had increased psychological, physical, and socioeconomic problems (Prueksaritanond & Kongsakol, 2007). Most of participants lived alone because of missing family members; some had to raise the surviving children and had no identification cards to qualify for official support, such as the government elderly scheme. The prevalence of depression in this group was 24.1%. Risk factors associated with depression were female gender, being 65 years and over, living alone, loss of income, loss of family members, and having hypertension.

23.7. INTERVENTIONS AND PROGRAMS

A number of programs have been implemented to address the psychological and social needs of tsunami victims (Chandra, Pandav, & Bhugra, 2006). In India, the state government of Tamil Nadu organized a support program for victims that included provision of psychological first aid and identification of people in need of referrals for additional psychological or psychiatric assistance. In Indonesia, the Ministry of Health organized a mental health task force. In addition, a large number of nongovernmental organizations on the scene offered counseling services. The government of the Maldives quickly organized community-based mental health programs, using individuals already trained in counseling. The Psychological Unit at the National Disaster Management Center launched a program of media outreach, psychological first aid, and a helpline for public information. The effort was strengthened by the fact that the volunteers were locals, with good knowledge of language and cultural issues. A 2-day training program bolstered the pool of volunteers for "Emotional Support Brigades" to fan out across all the affected islands. Another program designated one teacher from each island for training as a point person for psychological support at the school level (Chandra et al., 2006). In Sri Lanka, members of the College of Psychiatrists, along with other mental health professionals, organized training for health workers. International organizations also provided trainings focusing on psychosocial support. Another program, organized by a religious nongovernmental organization (NGO), provided psychosocial support training to approximately 100 Buddhist monks in four different regions, guiding them in ways to provide support to the traumatized community (Chandra et al., 2006).

The response in Thailand was perhaps the most elaborate in the affected region. The country already had a strong health care infrastructure, and authorities quickly mobilized to provide a response. Within days of the event, mobile mental health teams were already visiting affected communities. As people gathered in the areas designated for identifying the remains of victims, psychological support tents were set up to help the survivors. Beyond those centralized locations, an extensive network of village volunteers was at work. Each volunteer – trained by the Department of Mental Health – was responsible for a number of families in his or her village. The work of the trained mental health volunteers was supported by regular visits by mobile mental health units, which included a psychiatrist, counselor, psychiatric nurse, pharmacists, and a psychiatric social worker. Mobile units arrived on a predetermined and regular schedule, providing the needed health care, including medication, to those in need. This combination of a large system of trained volunteers residing in the affected locations along with regular visits from more highly trained professionals provided a strong network of support for populations affected by the tsunami.

For the longer term, the government established a Mental Health Recovery Center in Phang Nga, the most severely affected area. The Center's purpose is to coordinate the work of public health organizations; to continue providing training to health workers, teachers and NGO workers; to establish mental health surveillance systems; and to support the work of community mental health workers and volunteers.

To date, the effectiveness of all these interventions has not been studied, and evaluations are urgently needed.

23.8. LESSONS LEARNED

The tragic experience from the Southeast Asia tsunami in 2004 provided a number of important lessons that should be considered in advance of future natural disasters.

23.8.1. Preparedness

Disaster preparedness is imperative. Planning for disaster after the event takes place is too late. The countries and regions that were able to respond quickly were the ones that had planned ahead (Yule, 2006). Other places scrambled to put together a plan even as the victims stood waiting for help. Mental health and psychosocial support programs should be integrated in all disaster preparedness plans (WHO SEARO, 2007). Identification of resources, personnel, training, and ongoing support/supervision are part of comprehensive a disaster preparedness plan (Mollica et al., 2004).

23.8.2. Coordination

A good disaster preparedness plan also includes an established coordination mechanism (Ganesen, 2006). Coordination of mental health and psychosocial support programs during the emergency phase and postemergency phase of a disaster is imperative to ensure effective, efficient, and appropriate planning and implementation of interventions. Following a major natural disaster, the establishment of a mental health coordination group with all key representatives from key government ministries, United Nations agencies, and NGOs can be helpful and is recommended (Inter-Agency Standing Committee (IASC), 2007). An established system also allows outside help to work more effectively. When international NGOs arrive at a scene where there is no preparedness plan in place, their efforts are haphazard, often duplicative, and even counterproductive (Silove, 2005). Further, outside assistance, while well-intentioned, often suffers from a lack of cultural sensitivity and knowledge (Bryant & Njenga, 2006; Weiss, van Ommeren, Saxena, & Saraceno, 2005). When outsiders can rely on the guidance of local personnel, their help can be more effectively integrated into a larger plan of action.

23.8.3. Interventions

Psychological support is an essential part of disaster response (Chakrabhand, Panyayong, & Sirivech, 2006). Mental health is part of public health; thus, public health structures must recognize that mental health is an integral component of health services (Davidson, 2006). Mental health services are best provided in these settings through a community mental health system (WHO SEARO, 2007). In many places, mental health resources are extremely limited during normal times (Lamberg, 2005); when the need increases due to a natural disaster, the system simply cannot cope. As a key component to increasing the availability of specialized mental health services, primary health care providers must have training to recognize mental illness and be able to provide basic mental health services. Similarly, all first aid programs should include psychological first aid as a component (Weine, Danieli, Silove, van Ommeren, Fairbank, Saul, 2002), and all training for emergency services must include mental health considerations. A culturally sensitive, collaborative, and participatory approach with local people and established systems for coordinating how people from outside the culture provide assistance after disasters is recommended (Carballo et al., 2005).

The focus of mental health interventions after disasters should be on the most vulnerable people (Ghodse & Galea, 2006). In the early phases of a disaster, it is crucial to identify the vulnerable populations and target them for specifically needed services. Previous disasters have demonstrated that women, children, the elderly (Prueksaritanond & Kongsakol, 2007), the disabled, and the mentally ill (Silove, Ekblad, & Mollica, 2000)) are at greater risk, and may also find it more difficult to obtain the services available to other victims. Outreach services may be required to contact and help vulnerable populations.

Ensuring continued livelihood is key. The evidence from several studies conducted after the tsunami clearly indicated that being able to make a living is key to regaining mental health. In many cases, it may be more cost-effective to provide the tools to reestablish a livelihood than to develop complicated mental health structures: Distributing fishing nets may do more for mental health than building a new mental health clinic.

Providing support for those caring for survivors of disasters is also a key consideration in interventions. Many of the primary health care personnel who assisted after the tsunami had little training in mental health issues and were themselves victims of the tsunami. Support strategies for aid workers and health staff may include preventive measures of self-care and organizational support systems to prevent burnout (Inter-Agency Standing Committee, 2007; Lopes Cardozo, 2004).

23.8.4. Research

Little research has been done to investigate which psychological support framework or services are the most effective in preventing adverse mental health outcomes among populations affected by natural disasters or staff providing assistance. Outcome evaluations of programs and interventions are urgently needed (Lopes Cardozo, 2008). Some interventions may be ineffective, take up much needed resources, or may even be harmful. One example is the use of single-session debriefings, which were initially utilized in Nagapattinam district in India. After the teams learned that, at best, there was no evidence that these types of psychological interventions were effective, these efforts were discontinued (Tharyan, Clarke, & Green, 2005).

More longitudinal studies and surveys are necessary to provide information on addressing mental health consequences of disasters in both survivors and those providing aid.

REFERENCES

Bappenas. (2005). Indonesia, preliminary damage and loss assessment, the December 26, 2004 Disaster. (2008). http://www.adb.org/media/Articles/2005/6618_tsunami_impact_Indonesia/Aceh_Joint_Government_Donor_Damage_Assessment.pdf.

Basoglu, M., Kilic, C., Salcioglu, E., & Livanou, M. (2004). Prevalence of posttraumatic stress disorder and comorbid depression in earthquake survivors in Turkey: An epidemiological study. *Journal of Trauma Stress, 17*, 133–141.

Bryant, R. (2006). Recovery after the tsunami: Timeline for rehabilitation. *Journal of Clinical Psychiatry, 67*(Suppl. 2), 50–55.

Bryant, R., & Njenga, F. (2006). Cultural sensitivity: Making trauma assessment and treatment plans culturally relevant. *Journal of Clinical Psychiatry, 67*(Suppl. 2), 74–79.

Carballo, M., Heal, B., & Hernandez, M. (2005). Psychosocial aspects of the Tsunami. *Journal of the Royal Society of Medicine, 98*(9), 396–399.

Chakrabhand, S., Panyayong, B., & Sirivech, P. (2006). Mental health and psychosocial support after the tsunami in Thailand. *International Review of Psychiatry, 18*(6), 599–605.

Chandra, V., Pandav, R., & Bhugra, D. (2006). Mental health and psychosocial support after the tsunami: Observations across affected nations. *International Review of Psychiatry, 18*(3), 205–211.

Chang, C.M., Connor, K.M., Lai, T.J., Lee, L.C., & Davidson, J.R. (2005). Predictors of posttraumatic outcomes following the 1999 Taiwan earthquake. *Journal of Nervous and Mental Disease, 193*, 40–46.

Davidson, J.R.T. (2006). After the tsunami: Mental health challenges to the community for today and tomorrow. *Journal of Clinical Psychiatry, 67*(Suppl. 2), 3–79.

Derogatis L. R., Lipman R. S., Rickels K., Uhlenhuth E. H., & Covi L. (1974). The Hopkins Symptom Checklist (HSCL): A self-report symptom inventory. *Behavioral Science, 19*, 1–15.

Fritz Institute. (2005). *Recipient Perceptions of Aid Effectiveness: Rescue, Relief and Rehabilitation in Tsunami Affected Indonesia, India and Sri Lanka.* (2008); http://www.fritzinstitute.org/PDFs/findings/NineMonthReport.pdf.

Ganesen, M. (2006). Psychosocial response to disasters-some concerns. *International Review of Psychiatry, 18*(3), 241–247.

Ghodse, H., & Galea, S. (2006). Tsunami: Understanding mental health consequences and the unprecedented response. *International Review of Psychiatry, 18*(3), 289–297.

Holtz, T.H. (1998). Refugee trauma versus torture trauma: A retrospective controlled cohort study of Tibetan refugees. *Journal of Nervous and Mental Disease, 186*, 24–34.

Inter-Agency Standing Committee (IASC) (2007). *IASC Guidelines on Mental Health and Psychosocial Support in Emergency Settings. Geneva: IASC.* (2008); http://www.who.int/hac/network/interagency/news/iasc_guidelines_mental_health_psychososial_text.pdf.

Krishnamoorthy, K., Harichandrakumar, K.T., Krishna Kumar, A., & Das, P.K. (2005). Years of life lost and productivity loss due to tsunami in India. *Current Science, 89*(5), 735.

Kumar, M., Murhekar, M., Hutin, Y., Subramanian, T., Ramachandran, V., & Gupte, M. (2007). Prevalence of posttraumatic stress disorder in a coastal fishing village in Tamil Nadu, India, after the December 2004 tsunami. (2007). *American Journal of Public Health, 97*(1), 99–101.

Lamberg, L. (2005). As tsunami recovery proceeds, experts ponder lessons for future disasters. *JAMA, 294*(8), 889–890.

Lopes Cardozo, B. (2004). Burnout among humanitarian aid workers and human service providers in post-conflict societies. In R. F. Mollica (Ed.), *Project 1 billion – book of best practices: trauma and the role of mental health in post-conflict recovery.* Cambridge, Rome; Tipolitografia Rocografica, Roma.

Lopes Cardozo, B., Bilukha, O., Gotway, C., Shaikh, I., Wolfe, M., Gerber, M., et al. (2005). Mental Health of women in postwar Afghanistan. *Journal of Women's Health, 14*(4), 285–293.

Lopes Cardozo, B., Vergara, A., Agani, F., Gotway, C. (2000). Mental health, social functioning and attitudes of Kosovar Albanians following the war in Kosovo. *JAMA, 284*(5), 569–577.

Lopes Cardozo, B. (2008). IASC guidelines need a more evidence-based approach: a commentary on the guidelines on mental health and psychosocial support in emergency settings. *Intervention: The International Journal of Mental Health, Psychosocial Work and Counselling in Areas of Armed Conflict, 6*, 252–254.

MacDonald, R. (2005). How women were affected by the Tsunami: A perspective from Oxfam. *PLoS Medicine, 2*(6), e178.

Mollica, R.F., Caspi-Yavin, Y., Bollini, P., Truong, T., Tor, S., & Lavelle, J. (1992). The Harvard Trauma Questionnaire: Validating a crosscultural instrument for measuring torture, trauma, and posttraumatic stress disorder in Indochinese refugees. *Journal of Nervous and Mental Disease, 180*, 111–116.

Mollica, R. F., Lopes Cardozo, B., Osofsky, H. J., Raphael, B., Ager, A., & Salama, P. (2004). Mental health in complex emergencies. *Lancet, 364*, 2058–2067.

Mulder, N. (2000). *Inside Thai society: Religion, everyday life, change.* Chiang Mai, Thailand: Silkworm Books.

Neuner, F., Schauer, E., Catani, C., Ruf, M., & Elbert, T. (2006). Post-tsunami stress: A study of posttraumatic stress disorder in children living in three severely affected regions in Sri Lanka. *Journal of Traumatic Stress, 19*(3), 339–347.

Oxfam (2005). The tsunami's impact on women, Oxfam Briefing Note. (March 2005); http://www.oxfam.org.uk/what_we_do/issues/conflict_disasters/downloads/bn_tsunamI_women.pdf. Last accessed Jan 17, 2008.

Prueksaritanond, S., & Kongsakol, R. (2007). Biopsychosocial impacts on the elderly from a Tsunami-affected community in southern Thailand. *Journal of the Medical Association of Thailand, 90*(8), 1501–1505.

Ranasinghe, P., & Levy, B. (2004). Prevalence of and sex disparities in posttraumatic stress disorder in an internally displaced Sri Lankan population 6 months after the 2004 tsunami. *Disaster Medicine and Public Health Preparedness, 1*, 34–43.

Rees, S., Pittaway, E., & Bartolomei, E. (2005). Waves of violence – women in post-tsunami Sri Lanka. *The Australasian Journal of Disaster and Trauma Studies, 2.* Retrieved January 17, 2008, from, http://www.massey.ac.nz/~trauma/issues/2005-2/rees.htm.

Silove, D. (2004). The challenges facing mental health programs for post conflict and refugee communities. *Prehospital Disaster Medicine, 19*, 90–96.

Silove, D. (2005). Translating compassion into psychosocial aid after the tsunami. *The Lancet, 365*, 269–271.

Silove, D., Ekblad, S., & Mollica, R. (2000). The rights of the severely mentally ill in postconflict societies. *Lancet, 355*, 1548–1549.

Shrestha, N. M., Sharma, B., van Ommeren, M., Regmi, S., Makaju, R., Komproe, I., et al. (1998). Impact of torture on refugees displaced within the developing world: Symptomatology among Bhutanese refugees in Nepal. *JAMA, 280*, 443–448.

Tharyan, P., Clarke, M., & Green, S. (2005). How the Cochrane Collaboration is responding to the Asian Tsunami. *PLoS Medicine, 2*(6), e169.

Thienkrua, W., Lopes Cardozo, B., Chakkraband, M., Guadamuz, T., Pengjuntr, W., Tantipiwatanaskul, P., et al. (2006). Tsunami-related post-traumatic stress disorder and depression among children in southern Thailand. *JAMA*, *296*, 549–559.

U.S. Department of State. (2006). Sri Lanka, Country Reports on Human Rights Practices, 2005. Bureau of Democracy, Human Rights, and Labor. (2008). Retrieved January 17, 2008, from, http://www.state.gov/g/drl/rls/hrrpt/2005/61711.htm.

U.S. Library of Congress. Buddhist doctrine and popular religion. (1987). In B. L. LePoer (Ed.), *Thailand: A country study*. Washington: GPO for the Library of Congress; http://countrystudies.us/thailand/55.htm.

van Griensven, F., Chakkraband, M., Thienkrua, W., Pengjuntr, W., Lopes Cardozo, B., Tantipiwatanaskul, P., et al. (2006). Rapid assessment of post-tsunami mental health problems among adults in southern Thailand. *JAMA*, *296*, 537–548.

Wang, X, Gao, L., Shinfuku, N., Zhang, H., Zhao, C., & Shen, Y. (2000). Longitudinal study of earthquake related PTSD in a random selected community sample in North China. *American Journal of Psychiatry*, *157*, 1260–1266.

Weiss, M, van Ommeren, M, Saxna, S., & Saraceno, B. (2003). Mental health in the aftermath of disasters: Consensus and controversy. *Journal of Nervous and Mental Disease*, *191*, 611–615.

Weine, S., Danieli, Y., Silove, D., van Ommeren, M., Fairbank, J. A., & Saul, J. (2002). Guidelines for international training in mental health and psychosocial interventions for trauma exposed populations in clinical and community settings. *Psychiatry*, *65*, 156–164.

WHO SEARO. (2007) The Mental health and psychosocial aspects of disaster preparedness. Report of an intercountry meeting Khao Lak, Thailand, June 20–23, 2006.

Yule, W. (2006). Theory, training and timing: Psychosocial interventions in complex emergencies. *International Review of Psychiatry*, *18*(3), 259–264.

24 Advances in Our Understanding of Earthquake Trauma and Its Treatment: a Self-Help Model of Mental Health Care for Survivors

METIN BAŞOĞLU, EBRU ŞALCIOĞLU, AND MARIA LIVANOU

24.1. INTRODUCTION

Earthquakes are among the most common natural disasters, causing widespread destruction and casualties and exposing millions of people to a wide range of severe traumatic events. Indeed, earthquakes are almost unique in their ability to cause large-scale human suffering and property loss (U.S. Geological Survey, 1999). On the basis of figures provided by the National Earthquake Information Center (2006) and considering only earthquakes that killed over a thousand people, approximately 2.4 million people have died in 117 earthquakes since the beginning of the twentieth century. Of these earthquakes, 91 occurred in developing countries, accounting for 81% of total number of deaths worldwide. Earthquakes often cause greater devastation and casualties in developing countries because of the generally low quality of buildings, lack of disaster preparedness, and inadequate rescue and relief efforts.

The August 1999 Marmara earthquake in Turkey illustrated the extent of devastation and casualties caused by major earthquakes in developing countries. This earthquake, measuring 7.4 on the Richter scale, occurred in Marmara, the most densely populated region of Turkey, with its epicenter near the town of Gölcük. According to official estimates (U.S. Geological Survey, 1999), 17,123 people died and 43,953 were injured; an estimated 214,000 residential units were reduced to rubble or suffered structural damage, leaving more than 250,000 people homeless. On the 12th of November that same year a second earthquake (7.2 on the Richter scale) took place in Düzce (a town approximately 100 km southeast of Gölcük), causing an additional death toll of 832, injuring approximately 4,950 people, and destroying 13,000 buildings (Government Crisis Center, 1999). The traumatic impact of these earthquakes was aggravated by hundreds of aftershocks that lasted for more than a year afterwards, and expectations of yet another major earthquake predicted to occur near Istanbul in the next 25 years.

Following the August 1999 earthquake we launched a 6-year project to provide specialized psychological care for survivors, serving a catchment area of 60,000 in the disaster region. Inundated by demands for help from thousands of survivors, we quickly realized the need for brief interventions that could be delivered on a self-help basis with as little therapist contact as possible. Accordingly, we set out to develop a new mental health care model based on brief assessment and largely self-help treatments. We developed this model through extensive research into the psychological effects of the disaster, mechanisms of traumatic stress, and effective treatment methods for survivors. This work included four field surveys and three epidemiological studies (altogether involving over 6,200 survivors), a phenomenological study of earthquake trauma, two uncontrolled and two randomized controlled treatment studies (altogether involving 331 survivors), nine questionnaire development studies, and eight single-case experimental treatment studies. We also tested this model extensively during routine outreach work with more than 12,000 survivors.

This chapter presents an overview of our work. A detailed review of the literature on earthquake survivors is beyond the scope of this chapter, but we draw on relevant literature evidence in discussing our model. It is worth noting that our efforts represent a rather unique attempt to develop a new intervention model based on experimental models of traumatic stress. As such, it circumvents the most serious methodological shortcoming that characterizes much of the work with disaster survivors, that is, lack of a sound theoretical basis. Among the theories used in explaining the mechanisms of traumatic stress, the learning model of anxiety and fear is probably the most extensively investigated, particularly in animals (see review by Mineka & Zinbarg, 2006; see also Başoğlu & Mineka, 1992, for a detailed review of experimental models of traumatic stress and their relevance to human behavior under duress). Because this theoretical model explores the "universal" mechanisms of traumatic stress that cut across not only human cultures but also species, it is probably the most useful in understanding how humans develop and recover from traumatic stress in their natural environment and what this implies for effective interventions.

In this chapter we first briefly review the evidence on the prevalence of traumatic stress problems after major earthquakes and examine whether the current status of knowledge in trauma treatment sufficiently informs us in effectively dealing with the mental health consequences of major earthquakes. We then examine earthquake trauma from a learning theory perspective, the role of unpredictable and uncontrollable stressors in earthquake-induced traumatic stress, cognitive and behavioral strategies for coping with earthquake stressors, research findings pointing to possible evolutionary processes that facilitate natural recovery from trauma, and their implications for effective treatment of disaster survivors. We then present a self-help model of mental health care based on learning theory formulations of earthquake trauma, examine the evidence of its effectiveness, and briefly review possible modes of cost-effective treatment dissemination. Finally, we review the implications of our studies for developing and industrialized countries, prevention and treatment of PTSD secondary to other traumas, and clinical applications of cognitive-behavioral treatment of PTSD. A full review of our mental health care model, its evidence base, and guidelines in its implementation in mass trauma settings can be found in a forthcoming book (Başoğlu & Şalcıoğlu, in press).

24.2. MENTAL HEALTH EFFECTS OF EARTHQUAKES AND ASSOCIATED FACTORS

Studies using probability sampling show that exposure to devastating earthquakes in developing countries is associated with elevated prevalences of posttraumatic stress disorder (PTSD) and depression. The reported levels range from 12% to 50% for PTSD (Armenian et al., 2000; Başoğlu, Kılıç, Şalcıoğlu, & Livanou, 2004; Durkin, 1993; Kılıç & Ulusoy, 2003; Lai, Chang, Connor, Lee, & Davidson, 2004; Önder, Tural, Aker, Kılıç, & Erdoğan, 2006; Wang et al., 2000) and 8% to 52% for depression (Armenian et al., 2002; Başoğlu et al., 2004; Durkin, 1993; Kılıç & Ulusoy, 2003; Lai et al., 2004; Önder et al., 2006; Wang et al., 2000). Such variability reflects differences in sampling, assessment measures used, and time since the earthquake. These rates are generally higher than those reported from industrialized countries. Although longitudinal studies are scarce, available evidence suggests that earthquake-related PTSD runs a chronic course (Carr et al., 1997; Wang et al., 2000). This is also supported by our field surveys, which showed stable rates of PTSD over time (around 40% at 8, 20, and 40 months postdisaster) among relocated survivors in the epicenter region (Başoğlu, Şalcıoğlu, & Livanou, 2002; Şalcıoğlu, Başoğlu, & Livanou, 2003, 2007a).

As few studies have examined the entire range of psychiatric disorders after earthquakes, we know relatively less about the association between earthquake exposure and psychiatric conditions other than PTSD and depression. During our routine outreach program we examined this issue in a convenience sample of 387 survivors with high trauma exposure, involving both treatment-seeking (e.g., those referred to our community center) and nontreatment-seeking (e.g., those contacted through house visits) survivors (Şalcıoğlu, 2004). The most common psychiatric disorders in these groups were current PTSD (52% and 31%), at least one anxiety disorder other than PTSD (47% and 25%), and major depression (42% and 21%). All other psychiatric disorders were found in less than 11% of treatment-seekers and 7% of non-treatment-seekers. In the whole sample, 53% of the cases with PTSD also had major depression, and 49% had at least one anxiety disorder (most commonly panic disorder and agoraphobia). The select nature of this sample involving survivors with high trauma exposure (e.g., being trapped under rubble, loss of close ones, participation in rescue work, etc.) limits the generalizability of the findings. Nevertheless, this study gives some idea about the psychiatric conditions that need priority attention in any outreach treatment delivery program implemented in a disaster region. The association between high trauma exposure and high rates of anxiety/depression is also consistent with a learning theory formulation of earthquake trauma, as will be detailed later.

Although there are reports of a wide range of risk factors for traumatic stress in earthquake survivors, they will not be reviewed here, mainly because of the difficulty in assessing their generalizability. Most studies examined risk factors in a post hoc fashion, without prior theoretical formulation of earthquake-induced traumatic stress, making it difficult to interpret what the findings imply for effective intervention. Moreover, relatively little attention has been given to the problem of intercorrelated predictor variables. Traumatic stressors often occur concurrently in clusters, leading to correlated independent variables in research studies (Şalcıoğlu, Başoğlu, & Livanou, 2008). For example, collapse of one's house during an earthquake is not only a traumatic stressor in itself but also might mean loss of close ones and resources, as well as relocation. In our studies we attempted to circumvent such methodological problems by selectively focusing on risk factors that provide useful insights into the mechanisms of traumatic stress in earthquake survivors. Using detailed measures specifically designed to examine the traumatic processes both during the earthquake and in its aftermath, we obtained data on the subjective impact (e.g., perceived distress) of a wide range of earthquake stressors. In addition, we used multiple regression analyses to examine the unique effects of individual risk factors and cross-validated the results several times in different samples. We will review only the most important findings here.

Survivors often report that a major earthquake is an intensely frightening experience. Curiously, however, very few studies have examined fear as a risk factor for earthquake-related PTSD. In all of our field surveys the intensity of fear experienced during the earthquake consistently emerged as the most important predictor of PTSD (Başoğlu et al., 2002, 2004; Livanou, Başoğlu, Şalcıoğlu, & Kalender, 2002; Şalcıoğlu et al., 2003, 2007a). It explained far greater variance in PTSD (and comorbid depression) than any other risk factor, including demographic variables, personal and family psychiatric history, past history of trauma, proximity to the epicenter, and other earthquake stressors (e.g., collapse of a house, being trapped under rubble, witnessing grotesque scenes, loss of close ones and resources). A phenomenological study showed that loss of control over anticipatory fear of future earthquakes (e.g., aftershocks) was an even stronger predictor of PTSD than fear during the initial major shock (Şalcıoğlu, 2004). Similar findings were also reported by other studies (Bergiannaki, Psarros, Varsou, Paparrigopoulos, & Soldatos, 2003; Kılıç & Ulusoy; 2003; Livanou et al., 2005; Sümer, Karancı, Berument, & Güneş, 2005; Tural et al., 2004). These findings suggest that fear accounts for much of the traumatic stress responses in earthquake survivors and thus needs to be the focus of attention in any mental health care approach. Further evidence on the association between fear and traumatic stress reactions will be reviewed later.

24.3. CURRENT STATUS OF KNOWLEDGE IN TREATMENT OF DISASTER SURVIVORS

Our findings pointing to fear of earthquakes as a far more important risk factor than direct exposure to the devastating impact of an earthquake imply that when an earthquake occurs in a densely populated area, such as the Marmara region of Turkey (population 25 million), large numbers of people, perhaps millions, are likely to develop PTSD because of exposure to earthquake tremors alone. The enormity of such a problem clearly poses a major challenge for current knowledge in trauma treatment.

This challenge becomes more obvious when one considers the fact that effective handling of a problem of this magnitude requires interventions that are (1) based on sound theory, (2) proven to be effective, (3) brief, (4) easy to train therapists in their delivery, (5) practicable in different cultural settings, and (6) suitable for dissemination on a self-help basis through media other than a therapist (Başoğlu & Şalcıoğlu, in press). A theoretical framework is essential in understanding the mechanisms of disaster-induced traumatic stress and the interventions likely to reverse this process. The interventions need to be proven to be effective, given that ineffective treatments lead to waste of time and valuable resources. They need to be brief because cost-effectiveness of care is an important issue, particularly for low-income countries. They also need to be relatively easy to administer, without requiring lengthy and costly training. The sixth requirement is arguably the most important. Given the large numbers of people that need help after major disasters, even the most effective and briefest interventions are of limited value if they are not suitable for dissemination as self-help treatments.

Judged against these criteria, none of the currently available trauma treatments have the potential to meet the demands of postdisaster circumstances. Among these treatments, only exposure-based interventions (e.g., cognitive-behavioral treatment (CBT)) and Eye Movement Desensitization and Reprocessing (EMDR) have been reported to be effective in PTSD (Bradley, Greene, Russ, Dutra, & Westen, 2005; Van Etten & Taylor, 1998). The theoretical basis of EMDR is unclear, and its reported efficacy might well be explained by imaginal exposure to trauma memories, which is essentially a behavioral technique. Indeed, eye movements do not appear to be essential for improvement (Boudewyns & Hyer, 1996; Devilly, Spence, & Rapee, 1998; Pitman et al., 1996; Renfrey & Spates, 1994). Most importantly, EMDR is not suitable for dissemination as a self-help intervention. CBT, on the other hand, often involves a mixture of various interventions, including imaginal exposure, cognitive restructuring, and various anxiety management techniques, such as relaxation training, coping skills training, breathing training, thought stopping, and guided self-dialogue. Its delivery takes an average of 15 weekly sessions (Van Etten & Taylor, 1998), and treatment often involves monitoring, diary keeping, troubleshooting with regard to problems encountered, and encouragement and verbal praise for progress. It is difficult to ascertain which of these therapy ingredients are essential for improvement, how they effect change, and whether the therapist is essential for this process. Evidence showing that exposure alone is as effective as cognitive restructuring in reducing PTSD (Foa et al., 2005; Marks, Lovell, Noshirvani, Livanou, & Thrasher, 1998; Paunovic & Öst, 2001) and achieving cognitive change (Foa & Rauch, 2004; Paunovic & Öst, 2001) suggests that the latter therapy element is redundant. Furthermore, most therapy elements are elaborate procedures that rely heavily on therapist skills and are thus difficult to deliver on a self-help basis. The fact that there are so far two failed attempts (Ehlers et al., 2003; Scholes, Turpin, & Mason, 2007) to develop a CBT-based self-help tool for PTSD reflects the difficult nature of this task. Clearly, there is need for a much simpler intervention for self-management of PTSD.

Ideally, a mental health care model should involve interventions that can be used in both prevention and treatment of posttraumatic stress, as well as in increasing people's resilience against the traumatic effects of future disasters. Psychological debriefing, the only early intervention available, does not offer much prospect in prevention, given the recent evidence of its ineffectiveness (McNally, Bryant, & Ehlers, 2003). In view of the current status of our knowledge, is such a mental health care model conceivable? In our view, the answer to this question probably lies in our evolutionary heritage in coping with trauma. Trauma is as old as human history itself, and it is plausible to assume that the survival process has taught us effective ways of dealing with it. Indeed, this might well explain why many trauma survivors recover without any treatment. It should be possible, at least in theory, to identify the mechanisms of natural recovery processes and incorporate them in a mental health care model. In the following section we will examine the prospects of such a model, based on a learning theory formulation of earthquake trauma and natural recovery processes.

24.4. MECHANISMS OF TRAUMATIC STRESS AND NATURAL RECOVERY IN EARTHQUAKE SURVIVORS

Since the 1960s, substantial experimental work with animals suggests that unpredictable and uncontrollable stressors play an important role in the development of anxiety and fear responses. Exposure to unpredictable and uncontrollable stressors (e.g., inescapable shocks) is associated with certain associative, motivational, and emotional deficits in animals that closely resemble the effects of traumatic stress in humans (see reviews by Başoğlu & Mineka, 1992; Mineka & Zinbarg, 2006). While much of the evidence on the role of unpredictable and uncontrollable stressors in anxiety is based on animals, evidence that emerged in the last 15 years is suggestive of close parallels between animal and human response to such stressors. In a series of studies we demonstrated a strong association between perceived uncontrollability of traumatic stressors and PTSD and depression in survivors of war (Başoğlu et al., 2005), torture (Başoğlu, Livanou, & Crnobarić, 2007; Başoğlu, Mineka, Paker, Aker, Livanou, & Gök, 1997), and earthquakes (Şalcıoğlu, 2004). Another study showed that sense of control over torture events had a protective effect against PTSD in torture survivors (Başoğlu et al., 1997), consistent with animal experiments showing that prior exposure to controllable aversive events may immunize the animals against the deleterious effects of subsequent exposure to uncontrollable aversive events (e.g., Seligman & Maier, 1967; Williams & Maier, 1977). In these studies, impact of trauma on beliefs about self and others (e.g., loss of faith or trust in people, sense of injustice, etc.) was not associated with posttrauma outcome. These findings are also consistent with evidence from studies of other anxiety disorders pointing to an association between sense of control and anxiety (Başoğlu, Marks, Kılıç, Brewin, & Swinson, 1994; Livanou et al., 2002; Sanderson, Rapee, & Barlow, 1989).

Our work with Marmara earthquake survivors provided extensive evidence in support of a learning theory formulation of earthquake-related traumatic stress. A personal experience of the earthquake and its aftermath and naturalistic observations of individual and collective responses to the disaster provided valuable insights into how earthquakes traumatize people. Such observations generated hypotheses that we subsequently tested in a series of field surveys and phenomenological and treatment studies. Using an Exposure to Earthquake Stressors Scale (EESS), we obtained data on the relative stressfulness of more than 50 earthquake-related stressors during the acute trauma phase (Şalcıoğlu, 2004). The acute phase stressors included (1) stressors during the initial major shock; (2) stressors in the early postearthquake phase, such as being trapped under rubble, losing close ones, witnessing grotesque scenes, having survival problems, and experiencing loss of resources (e.g., loss of property or occupation, relocation to shelters); and (3) stressors from the ongoing aftershocks that lasted for more than a year. Thus, it is important to note that we regard the acute phase of earthquake trauma as involving not just the initial shock and its immediate aftermath but all the other traumatic events that follow, most importantly the numerous aftershocks that often follow the initial major earthquake. The period following the cessation of aftershocks constitutes the posttrauma or chronic phase. This definition is important to bear in mind in interpreting our research findings, particularly those from the treatment studies, some of which took place during the acute phase.

24.4.1. The Initial Major Shock

As noted earlier, exposure to earthquake tremors is an intensely frightening experience, which may indeed explain the increased rates of myocardial infarction, abortions, premature births, and normal deliveries after earthquakes (Noji, 1997). In our phenomenological study of 387 survivors, 76% described severe/very severe fear, and 40% marked total loss of control during the earthquake (on the basis of the global ratings of fear and loss of control during the earthquake) (Şalcıoğlu, 2004). A significant association between the latter ratings suggests that the intensity of fear during an earthquake was associated with perceived uncontrollability of the stressors.

What is it about earthquakes that make them so frightening? The EESS data show that three groups of stressors are most distressing: visual and auditory stimuli (sight of moving walls, sound of moving objects, the rumbling noise that come from under the ground, sound of buildings collapsing) and loss of postural control (e.g., being thrown about by the tremors). Perceptually, a moving physical environment is quite an extraordinary phenomenon, well outside the range of ordinary human experience. This is perhaps because spatial or proprioceptive orientation in humans (and possibly in other subhuman living organisms) is defined in reference to a stable physical environment (Başoğlu & Şalcıoğlu, in press). The extremely alien nature of this perceptual experience might indeed explain why earthquake survivors have a very high rate (74%) of reexperiencing symptoms (e.g., nightmares, flashbacks, intrusive thoughts) that involve such visual images in the early aftermath of the disaster (Başoğlu et al., 2001). The distressing nature of this experience might be further enhanced by equally alien auditory stimuli, such as the rumbling noise that comes from under the ground and the noise made by moving structures and objects in the environment. Loss of postural control is also a particularly distressing situation because it makes any self-protective action very difficult. Indeed, survivor accounts of an experience at the epicenter of a 7.4-magnitude earthquake indicate that it is quite difficult to stand up, walk, and engage in any meaningful self-protective action during the tremors. Our epidemiological study suggests that while earthquake tremors are most frightening in the epicenter region, they also evoke comparable levels of fear in people located at a distance of 100 kilometers from the epicenter (Başoğlu et al., 2004).

24.4.2. Stressors in the Early Postearthquake Phase

Postearthquake stressors broadly fall into two categories: those that involve exposure to grotesque scenes (e.g., sights of injured people, rescue work, dead bodies, people trapped under rubble, etc.) and those that involve events concerning close ones, such as witnessing them being trapped under rubble and dying, having to wait helplessly near rubble unable to save them, or seeing their bodies being recovered from rubble. The EESS data show that the latter events are among the most distressing. The fact that "having to wait helplessly near the rubble unable to save close ones" was rated as the most distressing stressor points to the role of helplessness in appraisal of this event as highly distressing. Other stressors, such as perceptions of delayed efforts in rescuing people, rescue teams not making sufficient efforts to save people, or people's indifference to close ones being trapped under rubble, were also highly distressing because such events are likely to aggravate feelings of helplessness. These findings provide further evidence that the intensity of distress during a traumatic event is closely associated with the uncontrollability of stressors.

24.4.3. Aftershocks

There are striking similarities between repeated exposures to earthquakes and inescapable shock experiments in animals; both situations involve repetitive stressors that are unpredictable and uncontrollable and lead to similar psychological responses, that is, anxiety, fear, and helplessness (Başoğlu & Şalcıoğlu, in press). Several factors contribute to appraisal of threat and consequent anticipatory fear in survivors. First, the initial shock demonstrates the nature and extent of devastation that can be caused by major earthquakes. People whose houses collapse during the earthquake are directly exposed to the devastating impact of the earthquake, while others are indirectly affected by witnessing its destructive effects on other people. Everyone knows the same events could happen again. Second, the aftershocks, although, usually much less strong than the initial shock, demonstrate that further devastation is possible, however limited it might be. Third, there is always a risk of further major earthquakes in a seismologically active region and not necessarily in the too distant future. Finally, aftershocks occur at variable intervals in an unpredictable fashion. They can catch people while they are asleep, in the bathroom, having sexual intercourse, or in an enclosed space from which escape is difficult during an earthquake. Thus, "protection" from a possible earthquake requires high levels of constant vigilance. Prolonged exposure to such unpredictable and uncontrollable aftershocks (and consequent helplessness/hopelessness responses) might indeed explain the increased suicide rates reported in some survivor populations (Chou et al., 2003; Yang, Xirasagar, Chung, Huang, & Lin, 2005).

24.4.4. Attempts to Gain Control over Earthquake Stressors

Earthquakes provide fascinating examples of various cognitive and behavioral strategies that people use in an attempt to gain control over their fear. These include (1) search for information about the safety of their house (e.g., its structural quality) and employment of various safety measures (e.g., strengthening the house, moving to relatively safer locations), (2) tendency to underestimate danger (e.g., "I am safe because my house sits on solid ground," or "I live in upper floors nearer the roof or lower floors from which escape is easy," or "The contractor who built the house told me it was safe," etc.), (3) reliance on "safety signals" (e.g., the absence of threat signals, such as birds making a noise or dogs barking, a particular color of the sea, clear visibility of the stars at night, or an unusually hot and windless day) to estimate the probability of an impending earthquake, (4) a tendency to believe in frequent rumors about an earthquake expected to occur on a particular date (possibly as an attempt to reduce anxiety by making an unpredictable stressor more predictable and, therefore, more controllable), (5) fatalistic thinking (e.g., "it will happen if it is God's will"), which possibly acts as an ultimate form of control over anxiety by attributing power of control to a higher being and relinquishing all attempts to maintain control over future threats, (6) avoidance of situations that signal threat, and (7) attempts to gain control over fear by not avoiding feared situations (e.g., self-exposure to fear cues) (Başoğlu & Şalcıoğlu, in press). These observations provide remarkable examples of human responses to unpredictable and uncontrollable stressors. For example, reliance on safety signals is consistent with findings from experimental work with animals. When given a choice, animals generally show a strong preference for predictable or signaled aversive events in comparison to unpredictable or unsignaled aversive events (Badia, Harsh, & Abbott, 1979). According to Seligman's safety signal theory (Seligman, 1968; Seligman & Binik, 1977; Weiss, 1977), preference for predictability derives from the fact that having a signal when the event is going to happen also means, functionally, that when the signal is not on, the organism can relax and feel safe. If the organism is in a context where aversive events are occurring unpredictably, this means that they may be in a state of chronic fear. Evidence in support of the safety signal theory has largely been drawn from clinical cases with anxiety disorders, such as agoraphobia (Rachman, 1984). What is interesting about our observations is that this theory appears to be able to account for a social phenomenon or the collective behavior of large masses of people.

Another common response to recurring earthquakes is avoidance of various earthquake-related situations. Avoidance relates to two types of situations: (1) those that signal danger in case of a future earthquake and (2) those that act as distressing reminders of the past earthquake. The most common example of the first type is avoidance of concrete buildings. Many survivors avoid entering buildings even when they know that a particular building is safe. It is worth noting that 58% of the 15,000 survivors in Turkey who were living in shelters 6 months after the earthquake had a safe and inhabitable house (Committee for Tent Cities in Kocaeli, 2000). Other evidence (Şalcıoğlu et al., 2008) showed that avoidance was the strongest predictor of relocation to shelters. Other commonly avoided situations include staying alone at home, staying in the dark, taking a shower, getting undressed before going to bed, sleeping with lights off, sleeping with the bedroom door closed, sleeping before 3:00 a.m. (the time of the night when the earthquake happened), having sexual intercourse, or being in places from which escape during an earthquake would be difficult. Some people could not go near the sea because parts of the land near the sea had sunk during the earthquake, causing many people to drown. Many people devised a rotation at home to have a family member stay awake and keep vigil during the night, while the others slept. This type of avoidance, often associated with significant social and occupational disability, clearly reflects a state of constant vigilance caused by the unpredictable nature of aftershocks.

The second type of avoidance behaviors reflects conditioned fears in relation to a wide range of trauma reminders. For example, some people avoided sleeping in the room where they had experienced the earthquake. Others avoided sights of rubble or destroyed buildings. Some stopped reading newspapers or watching TV news to avoid being reminded of the earthquake. Conditioned fears often generalized to a wide range of situations. For example, some people avoided the clothes they were wearing during the earthquake. A woman who was brushing her teeth during the earthquake had to change her toothbrush and the brand of her toothpaste because they evoked fear. Many people avoided places where they experienced shaking sensations, such as hung floors in shops that shake when people walk over them or other places where the vibrations created by passing trucks could be felt.

24.4.5. The Role of Fear, Avoidance, and Helplessness in PTSD

Several lines of evidence suggest that fear and avoidance play an important role in the development of PTSD in earthquake survivors. As noted earlier, our field surveys consistently revealed strong associations between fear and PTSD. In addition, the rates of behavioral avoidance and PTSD in the early months of the disaster (70% and 40%, respectively) (Başoğlu et al., 2001, 2004) remained fairly high at 40 months post-disaster (50% and 40%, respectively) (Şalcıoğlu et al., 2007a), pointing to an association between the two. This was also confirmed by another study showing strong correlations among measures of fear, avoidance, helplessness cognitions, PTSD, and depression (Şalcıoğlu, 2004).

Further evidence comes from factor analyses of PTSD symptoms, which consistently revealed a clustering of various hyperarousal and reexperiencing symptoms and behavioral and cognitive avoidance (with emotional numbing, detachment, sense of foreshortened future, amnesia loading on a depression factor) (Başoğlu et al., 2002; Livanou, Başoğlu, Şalcıoğlu, 2002; Şalcıoğlu et al., 2003, 2007a). Such a PTSD symptom profile was quite characteristic of earthquake trauma, as hypervigilance, startle, and avoidance reflected the effects of anticipatory fear of earthquakes, while the reexperiencing symptoms were often associated with the stressors experienced during and immediately after the earthquake. This symptom constellation is also consistent with the two types of most commonly avoided situations reviewed earlier (e.g., those that signal danger in case of an earthquake and those that act as distressing reminders of the past earthquake).

24.4.6. Fear of Earthquakes and Coping with Fear: an Evolutionary Perspective

The high rates of fear and avoidance might perhaps reflect an evolutionarily determined response geared toward self-preservation. It is long known that defensive responses, such as heightened vigilance, fight or flight, and avoidance of threat, have played a fundamental role in the survival of the species for millions of years (Marks, 1987). There are close parallels between human and animal responses to earthquakes. Snarr (2005) has noted that animal responses to earthquakes have been observed as far back as 3,000 years ago, including responses before, during, and after the earthquake. Among the documented responses of nonhuman primates to earthquakes are increased restlessness and changes in space utilization in chimpanzees (Shaw, 1977), "freezing" responses in langur monkeys (*Presbytis entellus*) (Krusko et al., 1986), and stress, nervousness, and fear in orangutans (Antilla, 2001).

Further evidence comes from experimental work with animals. It has been suggested that primates may have a preparedness to acquire fear of certain kinds of objects or situations that have evolutionary significance (Öhman, Dimberg, & Öst, 1985; Seligman, 1971). Mineka and Zinbarg (2006) noted that people are more likely to have phobias of snakes, water, heights, and enclosed spaces than of bicycles, guns, or cars, even though the latter objects may be as likely to be associated with trauma. This might be related to a selective advantage in the course of evolution for primates who rapidly acquired fear of certain objects or situations that posed threats to humans' early ancestors. The authors also noted that prepared fears are not inborn or innate but rather very easily acquired and especially resistant to extinction. Given that earthquakes go far back in human history, this theory might also explain why people respond to earthquakes with such intense fear, why they rapidly acquire conditioned fears and avoidance in relation to a wide range of situations or activities, and why such fear is resistant to extinction in the long term (Başoğlu & Şalcıoğlu, in press). Furthermore, certain observations concerning the irrational nature of fear of earthquakes are consistent with the evidence reviewed by Mineka and Öhman (2002) showing that fear learning with fear-relevant stimuli is more impenetrable to conscious cognitive control than is fear learning with fear-irrelevant stimuli. For example, many survivors in camps displayed intense fear during aftershocks, rushing out of their tents in panic or running around in the field aimlessly. When asked about why they were frightened later, they were often unable to state a plausible reason for their fear and acknowledged the irrational nature of their behavior. Another example is the fear that survivors experience in an earthquake simulator, even when they know that there is no real danger involved. Thus, while cognitive factors, such as perceived threat to safety, may play a role in fear during an earthquake, they do not explain fear in a relatively safe environment or conditioning of fear to various objects or situations that pose no real threat.

In a review of the evidence on the role of evolutionarily determined defensive responses in PTSD, Cantor (2005, p. 143) noted that vigilant avoidance was the most commonly used strategy early in our evolutionary history, because of reptilian energy limitations. The use of this strategy, however, is said to be dependent on an appraisal of the relative costs and benefits of avoidance behavior or the "cost-benefit ratio" (Kavaliers & Choleris, 2001). In other words, avoidance has a survival value in animals as long as it does not interfere with feeding and mating opportunities. There is indeed evidence (Lima, 1998) to suggest that animals are prepared to take greater risk of predators when they are hungry.

This theory would predict that avoidant survivors for whom the costs of avoidance outweigh its benefits would be more likely to engage in risk-taking behaviors and eventually stop avoiding situations that signal threat to safety (e.g., concrete buildings) (Başoğlu & Şalcıoğlu, in press). Evidence from a study (Şalcıoğlu, 2004) supports this prediction. In this study the mean time for resettlement at home after the August 17th earthquake was 126 days (SD = 162, range 1–905). Thus, resettlement in most cases coincided with the onset of the particularly harsh winter of 1999. The most commonly stated reason for resettlement (67%) was the hardships of living in shelters. We also observed that many survivors with inhabitable houses needed to enter their house at some stage to fetch various essential items (e.g., clothes, blankets, electric heaters, etc.) or to take a shower, even though that meant taking a risk. Eighty percent of the survivors entered their house for the first time within the first week and 95% within 1 to 4 weeks afterward, times when the aftershocks were most frequent.

Some survivors made systematic attempts to overcome their fear by entering their homes in a graduated fashion. Realizing that living under difficult conditions was too high a price to pay for the relative safety of shelters, these survivors eventually came to the conclusion that they needed to do something to overcome their fear. Such cognitive change, sometimes accompanied by a fatalistic acceptance of risks, did not necessarily reduce fear initially. Faced with intense fear at the first attempt, many successfully used a graduated approach in moving back to their house in much the same way that would be prescribed by a behavior therapist.

Some survivors discovered the beneficial effects of confronting fear after an unintended or inevitable exposure to a particular feared situation and then went on to use this strategy intentionally to overcome their fear of other situations. Indeed, total avoidance of all earthquake-related cues is practically impossible because of the pervasiveness of these cues, which affect almost every aspect of life. Avoidance of sexual intercourse for fear of being caught up naked in an earthquake, a common problem in earthquake survivors, is a case in point. Social and occupational obligations that necessitate certain activities (e.g., traveling, visiting friends or relatives in their homes, etc.) also render total avoidance difficult. Such activities provide opportunities for testing risk-taking behaviors, which may then lead to the discovery of exposure as an effective strategy for overcoming fear. In some cases, this strategy might even be used to overcome earthquake-unrelated fears. For example, a survivor, after overcoming her fear of earthquakes, successfully treated her snake phobia using the same strategy.

Another finding from the same study highlighted the role of sense of control in natural recovery from fear of earthquakes. Sixty percent of the survivors reported some decrease (slight to very much) in their fear since the initial major shock. Decrease in fear (and associated traumatic stress symptoms) was associated with learning to cope with aftershocks and gaining sense of control over fear during the tremors. In some cases, rapid reduction in fear was associated with previous experience of repeated exposures to shaking sensations in particular situations (e.g., frequent sea traveling, living near a highway used by heavy trucks). This is consistent with anecdotal reports by some survivors (e.g., sailors) suggesting that being used to shaking sensations reduces fear during an earthquake. The protective effect of prior exposure to shaking environments accords with findings from stress immunization experiments, which showed that animals (dogs or rats) that were first exposed to a short series of escapable (controllable) shocks before receiving a long series of inescapable shocks did not show the learned helplessness deficits (e.g., Seligman & Maier, 1967; Williams & Maier, 1977). Interestingly, in the Williams and Maier experiment, these immunization effects occurred even when different kinds of aversive stimuli were used in the immunization and helplessness induction phases (e.g., an experience of escaping from cold water immunized rats against the effects of exposure to uncontrollable foot shocks). This might indeed explain why repeated exposures to shaking, which bears only some resemblance to real earthquake tremors, was sufficient in producing a protective effect against fear of real earthquakes. This implied that exposure to simulated tremors (e.g., in an earthquake simulator) might increase resilience against the traumatic effects of earthquake tremors. Indeed, it was this consideration that led to the development of earthquake simulation treatment reviewed in the next section.

To summarize, mainly three factors were responsible for increased risk-taking behavior among avoidant survivors: (1) the need for items essential for survival, (2) inevitable exposure to fear cues, leading to the discovery of this exposure as an effective strategy in overcoming fear, and (3) intentional use of exposure in fighting back fear and taking control over life. These naturally occurring processes support the theory that total avoidance of real or perceived risks posed by earthquakes is neither possible nor compatible with survival. This implies that risk-taking behaviors play an important role in natural recovery processes and immunization against traumatic stress. Evidence showing that PTSD in survivors improves after they resettle in concrete houses indeed supports this point (Şalcıoğlu et al., 2007a).

24.5. DEVELOPMENT OF A CONTROL-FOCUSED BEHAVIORAL INTERVENTION FOR TRAUMATIC STRESS

The foregoing analysis inevitably raises the question of why some survivors can overcome their fear, while others cannot. This might be explained by helplessness and hopelessness cognitions associated with prolonged exposure to uncontrollable stressors. This is a testable hypothesis, which implies that interventions designed to enhance sense of control over fear would remove the "blockage" caused by helplessness cognitions, thereby facilitating the natural recovery process. We developed such an intervention (control-focused behavioral treatment – CFBT) to test this hypothesis. It involves three steps: (1) identifying avoidance behaviors most closely associated with helplessness responses; (2) helping the survivor understand how fear and avoidance contribute to traumatic stress, helplessness, depression, and impairment in social, work, and family functioning; and (3) encouraging self-exposure to fear cues. In presenting the treatment rationale, fear is personified by presenting it as an adversary that the individual needs to fight. Avoidance is presented as a form of "surrender," and the survivor is presented with a choice between fighting fear to take control over life or surrendering to a life in fear and helplessness.

CFBT is fundamentally different from traditional exposure treatment in its focus on sense of control over fear cues (e.g., "confront your fear until you feel in control") rather than on habituation (e.g., "stay in a feared situation until your anxiety subsides"). Thus, exposure does not have to result in reduction of fear; increased sense of control over fear suffices. This is particularly important in situations where the stressor involves a realistic threat to safety (e.g., being in a building during an earthquake). In such situations complete habituation to the stressor may neither be possible nor desirable. This characteristic of CFBT also distinguishes it from traditional cognitive therapy, which also aims at fear reduction. In addition, CFBT involves minimal cognitive interventions, primarily geared towards enhancing motivation for self-exposure.

24.5.1. Treatment Studies

CFBT was tested by a series of treatment studies, altogether involving 331 survivors with PTSD (and delivered to more than 5,000 survivors in our routine outreach program). In an open clinical trial, 76% of the survivors improved after one and 88% after two sessions (Başoğlu et al., 2003). Improvement was maintained in the long term, despite further exposure to numerous aftershocks during the acute trauma phase, suggesting increased resilience. These findings were confirmed by a randomized controlled clinical trial, which found an improvement rate of 83% at 1 to 2-year follow-up (Başoğlu, Şalcıoğlu, Livanou, Kalender, & Acar, 2005). This study showed that CFBT could be reduced to a single session without undermining its effectiveness.

In the second study, participants with more severe fear, PTSD, and depression improved less, mainly because of their difficulty in initiating self-exposure, providing indirect support for the hypothesis that helplessness cognitions block recovery process. We conducted another randomized controlled study to investigate whether sense of control over fear could be enhanced at the outset of therapy by a single session of exposure to simulated earthquake tremors in an earthquake simulator (Earthquake Simulation

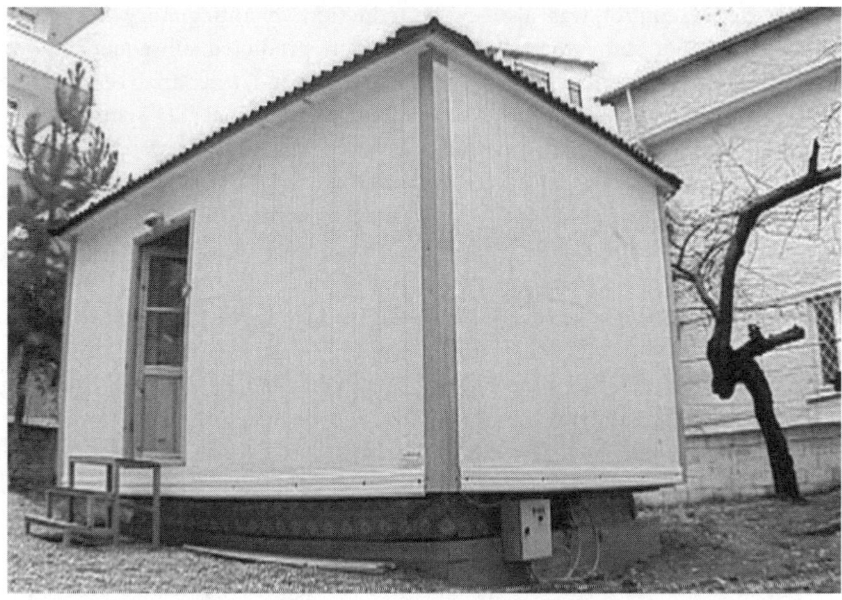

Figure 24.1. View of the earthquake simulator from the outside.

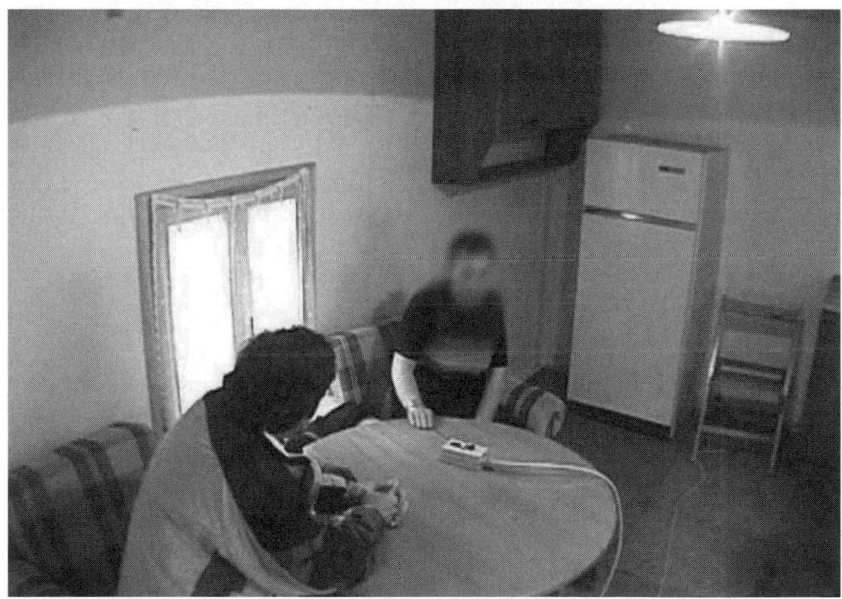

Figure 24.2. View of the earthquake simulator from the inside (photograph taken during a treatment session).

Treatment) specifically designed and constructed for this purpose (see Figure 24.1). A mobile control switch allowed the survivors to control the intensity and duration of the tremors from the inside (see Figure 24.2). Combining CFBT with Earthquake Simulation Treatment indeed achieved greater reduction in PTSD and better end-state functioning than CFBT alone (79% vs. 59%, respectively), thus providing further evidence of the role of increased sense of control in recovery (Başoğlu, Şalcıoğlu, & Livanou, 2007). The potent effect of Earthquake Simulation

Treatment on sense of control was also evidenced by an earlier pilot study that showed that the intervention leads to reduced behavioral avoidance and eventual improvement in PTSD, even when no explicit self-exposure instructions are given at postsession (Başoğlu, Livanou, & Şalcıoğlu, 2003).

These findings attest to the remarkable potency of CFBT in facilitating the recovery process, even when delivered in a single session. To facilitate a comparison of CFBT with other treatments in terms of effectiveness, the mean effect size obtained in our four studies and the mean effect sizes reported in a meta-analysis of treatment studies in PTSD (Bradley et al., 2005) are presented in Figure 24.3. The mean effect size on PTSD in our studies was substantially larger than the mean effect sizes reported in other studies. In all other studies the average length of treatment was 15.64 hours (SD = 10.52, range 3–52), compared with 60 minutes for CFBT.

Can the efficacy of a single session of CFBT be attributed to increased sense of control? First, in our study of Earthquake Simulation Treatment, improvement at follow-up was associated with increased sense of control (as measured by a Sense of Control Scale) (Başoğlu, Şalcıoğlu, et al., 2007). Furthermore, postsession reduction in anticipatory fear of earthquakes strongly predicted subsequent improvement in PTSD. Second, finer analyses of the sequence of improvement in PTSD symptoms showed that behavioral avoidance was the first symptom to improve early in treatment (reflecting increased sense of control), followed by improvement in other PTSD and depression symptoms (Şalcıoğlu, Başoğlu, & Livanou, 2007b). Reduction in avoidance thus appeared to be the critical factor in improvement. Third, Earthquake Simulation Treatment led to reduced behavioral avoidance, even when the survivors were not given explicit self-exposure instructions (Başoğlu et al., 2003), suggesting increased sense of control over fear. Fourth, in all our studies treatment improved not only PTSD but also depression, which reflected the helplessness effects of recurring earthquakes in most survivors. Earthquake Simulation Treatment was particularly effective in reducing the depressive symptoms of PTSD (Başoğlu, Şalcıoğlu, et al., 2007). Fifth, treatment appeared to enhance resilience against earthquake stressors, as suggested by remarkably low relapse rates in our studies (only three cases), despite further exposure to intermittent aftershocks in some cases. In the last study (Başoğlu, Şalcıoğlu, et al., 2007), 11 of the 13

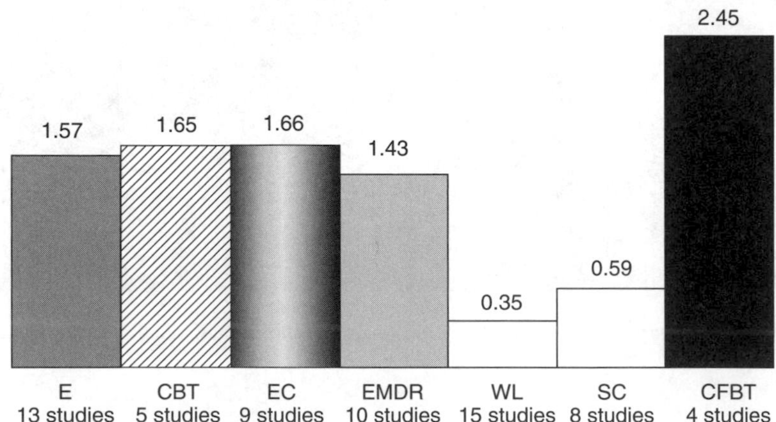

Figure 24.3. Comparison of mean treatment effect sizes on PTSD obtained by control-focused behavioral treatment and other psychological treatments.
Notes: CBT, cognitive behavioral therapy; CFBT, control-focused behavioral treatment; E, exposure; EC, exposure and cognitive restructuring; EMDR, eye movement desensitization reprocessing; SC, supportive control; WL, waiting list.

survivors who experienced an earthquake some time after the treatment reported much less fear and loss of control than usual during the tremors. This could reflect the immunizing effects of Earthquake Simulation Treatment, which may be explained by the fact that this intervention involves exposure not only to conditioned fear stimuli (e.g., earthquake reminders), but also to unconditioned stimuli (e.g., earthquake tremors), albeit in simulated form. In addition, an experience of a simulated version of the original trauma in a controllable environment where the stressors can be initiated or stopped at will might have reduced perceived uncontrollability of earthquake tremors, perhaps leading to an illusion of control over them. Sixth, a remarkably high rate of compliance (90%) with self-exposure instructions without subsequent therapist monitoring and reinforcement might well reflect the motivational impact of increased sense of control. Lack of compliance with exposure treatment in some patients is a problem well known to behavior therapists. Finally, minimal therapist contact may have enhanced sense of control by facilitating attributions of improvement to personal efforts, consistent with evidence that internal attributions of control consolidate treatment effects and reduce the risk of relapse in trauma survivors (Livanou, Başoğlu, Marks, et al., 2002), as well as in patients with panic disorder and agoraphobia (Başoğlu et al., 1994).

In summary, the evidence reviewed so far shows that learning theory of traumatic stress provides a very useful framework in understanding the mechanisms of traumatic stress in earthquake trauma, natural processes involved in natural recovery, and interventions that are likely to reduce traumatic stress. These findings have important implications for a wide range of issues, including but not limited to theory and treatment of trauma and care of disaster survivors. Such knowledge also enhances our understanding of anxiety disorders in general (Mineka, Watson, & Clark, 1998; Mineka & Zinbarg, 2006) and possibly some other psychiatric disorders, such as depression. In the following sections we will focus only on some of the most important implications of our findings.

24.6. IMPLICATIONS FOR A SELF-HELP MODEL OF MENTAL HEALTH CARE

Evidence from our studies implies that a self-help model of mental health care for earthquake survivors is conceivable. Considering that therapist involvement in treatment is limited to an initial assessment, explanation of treatment rationale, and self-exposure instructions, CFBT qualifies as a "predominantly self-help" treatment, as defined in the literature on self-help treatments (Newman, Erickson, Przeworski, & Dzus, 2003). The critical component of treatment is self-administered, except in a few cases where a single-session, therapist-assisted exposure might be needed to facilitate self-exposure. Less than 20% of the survivors require therapist contact and monitoring more than once.

The high rate of compliance with self-exposure instructions delivered in a single session without further therapist contact raises the prospect of treatment dissemination through other media. We have indeed explored this possibility by delivering treatment through a highly structured self-help manual. In a series of eight experimental (multiple baseline) single-case studies (Başoğlu, Şalcıoğlu, & Livanou, 2009), all survivors complied with self-exposure instructions and seven markedly improved at 3- and 6-month follow-up. Treatment effect sizes were comparable to those achieved by therapist-delivered treatment. This finding, though preliminary at this stage, suggests that CFBT can be administered on an entirely self-help basis.

Figure 24.4 illustrates a CFBT-based mental health care model (Başoğlu & Şalcıoğlu, in press) that can be used in postdisaster outreach programs targeting survivor shelters, schools, work places, or any other survivor group in the community. As can be noted from the representation of this model in Figure 24.4, the underlying idea is to deliver care with minimum therapist input to as many survivors as possible, while reserving relatively longer treatment programs for nonresponders to self-help. The model involves four stages: (1) assessment using a brief diagnostic screening instrument (Traumatic Stress Symptom Checklist[TSSC], Başoğlu et al., 2001)

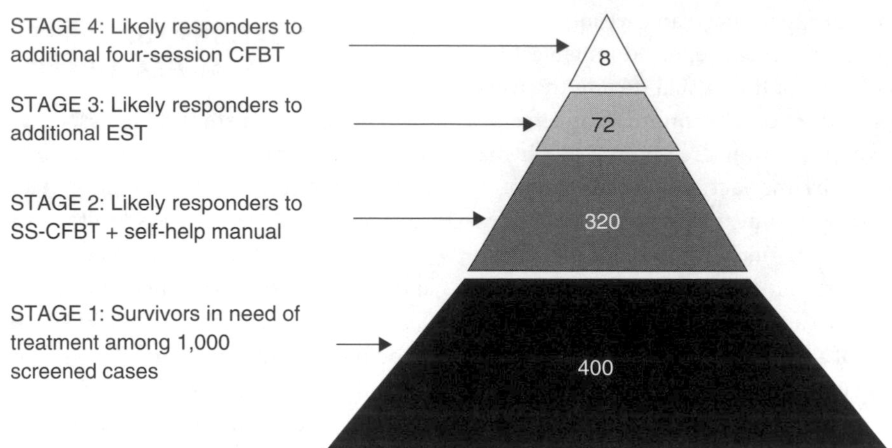

Figure 24.4. An outreach self-help model of mental health care: Probable numbers of survivors in need of treatment (per 1,000 screened cases) and recovered cases at each intervention stage.
Notes: CFBT, control-focused behavioral treatment; EST, earthquake simulation treatment; SS-CFBT, single-session control-focused behavioral treatment.

to identify cases in need of help, (2) single-session CFBT and self-help manual, (3) single-session Earthquake Simulation Treatment, and (4) four-session CFBT. Figure 24.4 also shows the likely response rates at each stage in a survivor population of 1,000, on the basis of our treatment studies. Our field surveys show that at least 400 out of 1,000 epicenter survivors are likely to need treatment. The likely response rate at stage two is 80%, thus leaving 80 nonresponders in need of stage three intervention. The expected improvement rate at stage three is 90% (Başoğlu, Şalcıoğlu, et al., 2007), which means only eight cases would need stage four treatment. Survival analyses show that the probability of improvement (defined as 60% reduction in PTSD) with full-course CFBT after four sessions is 100% (Başoğlu, Livanou, Şalcıoğlu, et al., 2003). Thus, using this model, only eight cases need full-course treatment, which corresponds to 0.8% of the targeted survivor population of 1,000 or 2% of those identified as in need of treatment after screening. In our experience, this small group is likely to include bereaved survivors with prolonged grief problems and other complicated cases. Treatment for prolonged grief involves a variant of CFBT, which will not be discussed here. It is also worth noting that this model substantially reduces the need for antidepressant treatment for cases with comorbid depression because treatment improves both PTSD and depression. Indeed, evidence shows that antidepressants confer no additional advantage when used with CFBT (Başoğlu, Livanou, Şalcıoğlu, et al., 2003).

The cost-effectiveness of this model could be further improved by developing dissemination methods that do not require professional therapists. If further research confirms the usefulness of the self-help manual when distributed to survivors as a stand-alone tool, therapist involvement at stage two could be further reduced. Such a finding would also raise the prospect of treatment dissemination to large survivor populations through mass media, such as television, radio, and the Internet – an issue well worth exploring in future research. Furthermore, our experience suggests that CFBT could also be disseminated through lay people, including the survivors themselves. Many survivors who recover with treatment tend to spread the word to friends and neighbors, encouraging them to conduct self-exposure. Some survivors who recovered using our self-help manual (distributed to more than 1,000 survivors in the disaster region) actually photocopied and distributed it to their relatives, friends, or neighbors. In another example, an 8-year-old girl who was living in a survivor camp with her family and who had recovered after a single treatment session later urged her traumatized father to overcome his fear of buildings so that the family could return home. She actually led him by hand several times to a building site where he practiced exposure and eventually recovered. These observations led us to recruit recovered survivors as "lay therapists" in survivor shelters. To utilize such potential in treatment dissemination, we developed a Treatment Delivery Manual for previously untrained health professionals (e.g., general practitioners, nurses, social workers, etc.) or lay people with an adequate educational background (e.g., schoolteachers, army personnel, religious leaders, etc.)(Başoğlu & Şalcıoğlu, in press).

Finally, prevention of chronic traumatic stress is an important issue that needs to be addressed by any mental health care model for disaster survivors. CFBT appears to reduce traumatic stress by increasing resilience against earthquake stressors. This implies that it has the potential to prevent chronic traumatic stress problems when used in the very early phases of a disaster. Furthermore, Earthquake Simulation Treatment appears to be a highly potent resilience-building intervention and could thus prove to be valuable in preparing people for future disasters in earthquake-prone countries. These issues deserve further research.

24.7. IMPLICATIONS FOR ASSESSMENT OF EARTHQUAKE SURVIVORS

A mental health care model for disaster survivors requires an assessment strategy consistent with the underlying theory. A learning theory model of earthquake trauma requires assessment of (1) the most important risk factors for traumatic stress, including the intensity of fear during the earthquake and common earthquake-related traumatic stressors (e.g., damage to house, being trapped under rubble, loss of close ones, material loss, participation in rescue work); (2) avoidance behaviors; (3) the most common mental health outcomes after earthquakes (e.g., PTSD, depression, and anxiety disorders); and (4) treatment outcome. We have developed two screening instruments for this purpose: the self-rated Screening Instrument for Traumatic Stress in Earthquake Survivors (SITSES) (Başoğlu et al., 2001) and Fear and Avoidance Questionnaire (FAQ).

The SITSES includes a Survivor Information Form (SIF), TSSC, and a Social Disability Scale (SDS) that assesses the extent of distress and social impairment caused by the traumatic stress problems. The SIF provides information that is useful in identifying cases at risk of PTSD and depression. The TSSC estimates the diagnoses of PTSD and comorbid depression with a certainty of 81% and 77%, respectively. The SDS also includes a question regarding whether the survivor feels the need for professional help, which is useful in identifying potential help-seekers in the community. Evidence from our treatment studies shows that both the TSSC and the FAQ are sensitive to clinical change and thus could be used as outcome measures in evaluation of treatment outcome. More detailed instruments for assessment of earthquake trauma (e.g., Semi-structured Interview for Survivors of Earthquakes) and prolonged grief have also been developed for research purposes but details will not be provided here.

24.8. IMPLICATIONS FOR DEVELOPING COUNTRIES

Our work is highly relevant to earthquake-prone developing countries. While it may be particularly suited to those who share similar sociocultural and postdisaster characteristics with Turkey, CFBT also is likely to have cross-cultural applicability, given that the underlying theoretical model focuses on the universals in human behavior. Fear in the face of life-threatening stressors is a universal human response, even though its manifestations might vary across cultures. Another strength of the model for postdisaster, resource-poor settings is that the relative simplicity of the intervention makes it fairly easy to deliver to survivors. Minimal reliance on cognitive interventions confers a distinct advantage in work with survivors of lower socioeducational status, as cognitive interventions require a reasonably well-differentiated cognitive structure and capacity for introspection on the part of the client. Therapist training could be completed within a few days with the help of a Treatment Delivery Manual.

Our experience demonstrates that it is possible to develop an effective mental health care approach for disaster survivors without depending on interventions "imported" from Western countries. Uncritical acceptance and use of treatments developed in Western countries is a common problem in developing countries (reflecting a cultural tendency to view everything coming from the West as "good") and thus deserve some attention here. In Turkey, for example, psychological debriefing and EMDR were among the commonly used interventions after the disaster, despite the considerable controversy surrounding the usefulness of debriefing (McNally et al., 2003) and the limited usefulness of EMDR in postdisaster work noted earlier. Such choice of treatment reflects not only a lack of understanding of the underlying mechanisms of stress in earthquake trauma but also the influence of foreign "trauma experts" who rush to the disaster scene to make their "expertise" available to the local professionals. Care providers in developing countries need to understand that experience in the Western world with the kind of large-scale disasters that occur in developing countries is rather limited and that their Western colleagues, however well intentioned they might be, might not always have the answers to their problems. Thus, local care providers need to rely on their own resources and develop their own assessment and treatment methods while also adapting the available knowledge to the cultural realities and the circumstances of the local setting.

Mental health professionals in developing countries also need to be aware of the fact that an evidence-based approach is not yet the norm in all areas of trauma work in Western countries. In Turkey we observed that most psychosocial aid projects executed, guided, or advised by Western groups (some funded by respectable international organizations) lacked a sound theoretical basis and did not involve outcome evaluation. Such projects are not only unlikely to yield useful outcomes, but also may have harmful effects for survivors. Similar concerns have also been voiced about the work of international psychosocial aid groups in developing countries after the tsunami disaster in Southeast Asia (Ganesan, 2006). This issue has important implications for governments in developing countries; the establishment of a national advisory body that reviews and vets all proposals for psychosocial aid projects and also coordinates and monitors them is worth serious consideration. Projects need to be assessed in terms of whether the proposed work has a basis in sound theory, demonstrated effectiveness, and a plan for outcome evaluation (Başoğlu, 2006). Funding organizations also need to adopt these criteria in their consideration of proposals to avoid wasting resources on potentially useless or even harmful projects. We have indeed observed significant amounts of financial resources wasted on such projects during our work in Turkey, and in former Yugoslavia countries.

24.9. IMPLICATIONS FOR INDUSTRIALIZED COUNTRIES

Earthquakes are generally not considered to be a priority problem among Western trauma researchers, mainly because earthquakes in industrialized countries, such as the United States or Japan, do not cause as extensive devastation and casualties as they do in developing countries. While this has been generally true so far, our findings show that earthquakes have the potential to lead to extensive conditioned fear responses and related traumatic stress problems in the community even in the absence of such devastation. Studies in industrialized countries support this point as well. For example, in a study (McMillen, North, & Smith, 2000) of 130 survivors of the 1994 Northridge California earthquake, while 13% met the criteria for PTSD, 48% had reexperiencing and arousal symptoms despite the fact that this earthquake caused relatively little devastation. In a study (Livanou et al., 2005) of 157 survivors of the 1999 Parnitha earthquake in Greece, which caused limited devastation and 143 deaths, 25% of survivors still had traumatic stress problems (most commonly hyperarousal and reexperiencing symptoms) 4 years after the disaster. Furthermore, a study (Carr, Lewin, et al., 1997) of the 1989 Newcastle earthquake in Australia (Richter scale magnitude 5.6), which caused 13 deaths, estimated that 18.3% of survivors exposed to high levels of threat were at risk of developing PTSD. Such findings largely reflect the traumatic effects of mere exposure to tremors.

Another important point is that studies focusing on PTSD diagnosis alone might not reflect the true extent of the mental health problems in the community. Our work suggests that studies also need to explore rates of depression and other anxiety disorders, most notably panic disorder with or without agoraphobia, specific phobias, and phobic fear of earthquakes. Furthermore, prevalence estimates of PTSD might create a seriously misleading impression of the actual proportion of the survivor population in need of care. In our fieldwork, of the 1,500 survivors who sought treatment from our community center in the epicenter region, 37% did not meet the criteria for PTSD, with mean TSSC scores (15.5, SD = 6.2) substantially lower than the cut off of 25 required for the diagnosis of probable PTSD. Most of these cases had subthreshold PTSD and other fear-related stress problems.

It is also worth questioning the general belief that earthquakes do not pose as serious a threat to life and property in industrialized countries as in developing countries. A report by the U.S. Geological Survey (2000) that reviewed the implications of the Marmara earthquake for the United States is quite sobering in this regard. According to this report, much of the building stock in the United States was constructed before the importance of ductility (the ability to deform without loss of strength) was fully understood. Consequently, large numbers of reinforced concrete structures in the eastern United States, including buildings and bridges, are vulnerable to catastrophic collapse during the oscillatory motions of large earthquakes because they have little or no ductility. The report also noted that a magnitude 7.2 earthquake on the San Francisco Peninsula would displace more than 100,000 people from their homes, while a magnitude 7.3 on the Hayward fault in California would displace 150,000 people. Recent forecasts indicate that the probability of a 6.7 magnitude earthquake in the San Francisco Bay region in the next 30 years is 70%, while the probability of an earthquake with a magnitude greater than or equal to that of the 7.4 Marmara earthquake is 13%. Pointing to the fact that the Marmara earthquake led to the collapse of more than 20,000 houses (and over 17,000 deaths) and displaced over 250,000 people, the report concluded that tragedies of comparable scale are possible in the United States.

24.10. IMPLICATIONS FOR PREVENTION AND TREATMENT OF PTSD

Our results suggest that CBFT is likely to be effective in cases of PTSD where fear is the prominent feature. Such cases are likely to constitute the majority of trauma survivors, considering that most traumatic events involve a threat to safety or life. In some cases fear might be related to a continuing realistic threat to safety (e.g., as in people exposed to war violence or torture survivors facing further risk of arrest and torture), while in others it might be maintained by reexperiencing symptoms and overestimated likelihood of reliving the same event (e.g., as in survivors of rape, road traffic accidents, etc.).

Several lines of evidence from our work with survivors of torture, war, and earthquake imply that traumatic events of human design are as likely to respond to CFBT as natural disaster trauma. First and most importantly, these trauma events seem to share the same mechanisms of traumatic stress. Second, cognitive responses to trauma (e.g., impact of trauma on beliefs about self and others, attributions of responsibility for trauma, appraisal of impunity for those held responsible for trauma, and associated emotional responses of anger, guilt, loss of faith in people, sense of injustice, etc.) (Şalcıoğlu, 2004) were remarkably similar across various survivor groups, suggesting that PTSD induced by traumas of human design is not by definition more severe and complicated than that caused by natural disasters. Third, cognitive effects of trauma were not associated with PTSD and depression in any of these studies, suggesting that such effects are merely epiphenomena of traumatic stress. Although we have not yet had an opportunity to test CFBT with war survivors, evidence from case studies with torture survivors suggests that it is no less effective in torture than in earthquake survivors (Başoğlu & Aker, 1996; Başoğlu, Ekblad, Baarnhielm, & Livanou, 2004).

The effects of CFBT appear to be mediated through exposure to trauma cues that evoke distress, anxiety, or fear. While such cues are often associated with behavioral avoidance, the latter may not be present in a small proportion of cases. In such cases exposure could involve distressing trauma reminders. In our phenomenological study, 91% of the survivors with PTSD had behavioral avoidance, 83% had cognitive avoidance, and 96% had distress when reminded of the trauma (Şalcıoğlu, 2004). Thus, distress- or fear-evoking trauma cues (with or without associated behavioral avoidance) could be identified in 99% of the cases. This does not appear to be unique to earthquake survivors, given the remarkably similar findings from our study of war trauma, which involved combat veterans, torture survivors, refugees, internally displaced people, and civilians exposed to aerial bombardment (Başoğlu, Livanou, et al., 2005). In that study, 73% of the cases with PTSD had behavioral avoidance, 87% had cognitive avoidance, and 93% had distress when reminded of the trauma; 97% had either behavioral avoidance or distress when reminded of the trauma. Thus, CFBT could be used in the large majority of cases with war-induced PTSD, though its relative efficacy in cases without overt behavioral avoidance remains to be explored further. In cases where emotions other than fear (e.g., guilt or anger) are the prominent features of PTSD, exposure to cues that trigger such emotions might be useful, but this also needs to be confirmed by future research.

The resilience-enhancing effects of CFBT suggest that the intervention could be used in the acute phase of traumatic stress to prevent the development of chronic problems in the long-term. This is also supported by other evidence showing the preventive effects of exposure-based interventions delivered in the early aftermath of traumatic events (e.g. Bryant, Sackville, Dang, Moulds, & Guthrie, 1999). Considering that currently there are no other brief interventions available to care providers, it is worth exploring the usefulness of CFBT as an early-phase intervention in future studies.

24.11. IMPLICATIONS FOR COGNITIVE-BEHAVIORAL TREATMENT OF PTSD

The effectiveness of live exposure alone inevitably raises questions about the need for certain commonly used interventions in CBT programs, such as imaginal exposure, cognitive restructuring, and various anxiety management techniques including relaxation training, coping skills training, breathing training, thought stopping, and guided self-dialogue. Our findings are consistent with evidence suggesting that cognitive interventions (Foa et al., 2005; Marks et al., 1998; Paunovic & Öst, 2001) or anxiety management techniques (Foa et al., 1999) do not confer additional benefits when used in combination with exposure. Imaginal exposure might not be as potent as live exposure (Devilly & Foa, 2001). Indeed, in examining the effect sizes achieved by exposure-based treatments in PTSD (reviewed by Bradley et al., 2005), we noted that the mean effect size for interventions involving imaginal exposure combined with live exposure was twice as large as that for imaginal exposure alone (1.78 vs. 0.91)(Şalcıoğlu et al, 2007b). Imaginal exposure might reduce the distress associated with trauma memories, but such improvement might not adequately generalize to behavioral avoidance without live exposure. Indeed, a study of this issue (Keane, Fairbank, Cadell, & Zimmering, 1989) found no effect of imaginal exposure on behavioral avoidance. Our results suggest that CBT could be refined into a more effective and cost-effective intervention by giving priority to live exposure and using the other techniques (and therapist-aided exposure) only when the patient is having difficulty in conducting exposure.

24.12. CONCLUSIONS

Perhaps the most important lesson we have learned from work with survivors of the Marmara earthquake is that nature has endowed humans with a remarkable potential to recover from traumatic stress by using cognitive and behavioral coping strategies. It follows naturally from this insight that interventions emulating natural recovery processes are likely to be most effective. The remarkable effectiveness of a relatively simple and largely self-help intervention is simply a validation of this logical conclusion. Our mental health care model obviously requires further work, as noted earlier. Nevertheless, set against the current state of knowledge in the field, it represents a significant advance in dealing with disaster trauma. Indeed, we are at a stage where we can begin to conceive of delivery of care through mass media channels in the future. While this might perhaps come across to some as an optimistic vision at this stage, it is nonetheless a distinct prospect within our sight.

In closing, our work suggests that a learning theory formulation of traumatic stress provides a very useful framework for understanding the mental health effects of disasters and effective ways of dealing with them. Also worth noting is that experimental models of traumatic stress have largely been derived from work with animals, and their relevance to humans has not been substantiated with extensive evidence. Although much has been said about the parallels between animal and human responses to unpredictable and uncontrollable stressors (reviewed by Mineka & Zinbarg, 2006; see also Başoğlu & Mineka, 1992), evidence of the kind reviewed here was largely lacking. Thus, the lessons learned from the Marmara earthquake, with their implications for our understanding of human response to stress in general, go far beyond a case study of a particular disaster.

ACKNOWLEDGMENTS

The work reviewed in this chapter was supported by Spunk Fund, Inc., CORDAID, and the Bromley Trust.

REFERENCES

Antilla, A. (2001). Orangutans react to earthquake in Seattle. *Long Call, 6*, 4.

Armenian, H. K., Morikawa, M., Melkonian, A. K., Hovanesian, A., Akiskal, K., & Akiskal, H. S. (2002). Risk factors for depression in the survivors of the 1988 earthquake in Armenia. *Journal of Urban Health: Bulletin of the New York Academy of Medicine, 79*, 373–382.

Armenian, H. K., Morikawa, M., Melkonian, A. K., Hovanesian, A. P., Haroutunian, N., Saigh, P. A., et al. (2000). Loss as a determinant of PTSD in a cohort of adult survivors of the 1988 earthquake in Armenia: Implications for policy. *Acta Psychiatrica Scandinavica, 192*, 58–64.

Badia, P., Harsh, J., & Abbott, B. (1979). Choosing between predictable and unpredictable shock conditions: Sata and theory. *Psychological Bulletin, 86*, 1107–1131.

Başoğlu, M. (2006). Rehabilitation of traumatised refugees and survivors of torture. *British Medical Journal, 333*, 1230–1231.

Başoğlu, M., & Aker, T. (1996). Cognitive-behavioural treatment of torture survivors: A case study. *Torture, 6*, 61–65.

Başoğlu, M., & Mineka, S. (1992). The role of uncontrollable and unpredictable stress in post-traumatic stress responses in torture survivors. In M. Başoğlu (Ed.), *Torture and its consequences: Current treatment approaches*. Cambridge: Cambridge University Press.

Başoğlu, M., & Şalcıoğlu, E. *A Mental Health Care Model for Earthquake and Other Mass Trauma Survivors*. Cambridge: Cambridge University Press. In press.

Başoğlu, M., Ekblad, S., Baarnhielm, S., & Livanou, M. (2004). Cognitive-behavioral treatment of tortured asylum seekers: A case study. *Journal of Anxiety Disorders, 18*, 357–369.

Başoğlu, M., Kılıç, C., Şalcıoğlu, E., & Livanou, M. (2004). Prevalence of posttraumatic stress disorder in earthquake survivors in Turkey: An epidemiological study. *Journal of Traumatic Stress, 17*, 133–141.

Başoğlu, M., Livanou, M., & Crnobarić, C. (2007). Torture versus other cruel, inhuman and degrading treatment: Is the distinction real or apparent? *Archives of General Psychiatry, 64*, 277–285.

Başoğlu, M., Livanou, M., & Şalcıoğlu, E. (2003). A single session with an earthquake simulator for traumatic stress in earthquake survivors. *American Journal of Psychiatry, 160*, 788–790.

Başoğlu, M., Livanou, M., Crnobarić, C., Frančišković, T., Suljić, E., Đurić, D., et al. (2005). Psychiatric and cognitive effects of war in former Yugoslavia – the relationship between lack of redress for trauma and posttraumatic stress reactions. *Journal of the American Medical Association, 294*, 580–590.

Başoğlu, M., Livanou, M., Şalcıoğlu, E., & Kalender, D. (2003). A brief behavioural treatment of chronic posttraumatic stress disorder in earthquake survivors: results from an open clinical trial. *Psychological Medicine, 33*, 647–654.

Başoğlu, M., Marks, I. M., Kılıç, C., Brewin, C. R., & Swinson, R. (1994). Alprazolam and exposure for panic disorder with agoraphobia: Attribution of improvement predicts subsequent relapse. *British Journal of Psychiatry, 164*, 652–659.

Başoğlu, M., Mineka, S., Paker, M., Aker, T., Livanou, M., & Gök, Ş. (1997). Psychological preparedness for trauma as a protective factor in survivors of torture. *Psychological Medicine, 27*, 1421–1433.

Başoğlu, M., Şalcıoğlu, E., & Livanou, M. (2002). Traumatic stress responses in earthquake survivors in Turkey. *Journal of Traumatic Stress, 15*, 269–276.

(2007). A randomized controlled study of single-session behavioural treatment of earthquake-related post-traumatic stress disorder using an earthquake simulator. *Psychological Medicine, 37*, 203–214.

(2009). Single-case experimental studies of a self-help manual for traumatic stress in earthquake survivors. *Journal of Behavior Therapy and Experimental Psychiatry, 40*, 50–58.

Başoğlu, M., Şalcıoğlu, E., Livanou, M., Kalender, D., & Acar G. (2005). Single-session behavioral treatment of earthquake-related posttraumatic stress disorder: A randomized waitlist controlled trial. *Journal of Traumatic Stress, 18*, 1–11.

Başoğlu, M., Şalcıoğlu, E., Livanou, M., Özeren, M., Aker, T., Kılıç, C., et al. (2001). A study of the validity of a screening instrument for traumatic stress in earthquake survivors in Turkey. *Journal of Traumatic Stress, 14*, 491–509.

Bergiannaki, J. D., Psarros, C., Varsou, E., Paparrigopoulos, T., & Soldatos, C. R. (2003). Protracted acute stress reaction following an earthquake. *Acta Psychiatrica Scandinavica, 107*, 18–24.

Boudewyns, P. A., & Hyer, L. A. (1996). Eye movement desensitization and reprocessing (EMDR) as treatment for posttraumatic stress disorder (PTSD). *Clinical Psychology and Psychotherapy, 3*, 185–195.

Bradley, R., Greene, J., Russ, E., Dutra, L., & Westen, D. (2005). A multidimensional meta-analysis of psychotherapy for PTSD. *American Journal of Psychiatry, 162*, 214–227.

Bryant, R. A., Sackville, T., Dang, S. T., Moulds, M., & Guthrie, R. (1999). Treating acute stress disorder: An evaluation of cognitive behavior therapy and counselling techniques. *American Journal of Psychiatry, 156*, 1780–1786.

Cantor, C. (2005). *Evolution and posttraumatic stress: Disorders of vigilance and defence*. New York: Routledge.

Carr, V. J., Lewin, T. J., Kenardy, J. A., Webster, R. A., Hazell, P. L., Carter, G. L., et al. (1997). Psychosocial sequelae of the 1989 Newcastle earthquake: III. Role of vulnerability factors in post-disaster morbidity. *Psychological Medicine, 27*, 179–190.

Carr, V. J., Lewin, T. J., Webster, R. A., Kenardy, J. A., Hazell, P. L., & Carter, G. L. (1997). Psychosocial sequelae of the 1989 Newcastle earthquake: II. Exposure and morbidity profiles during the first 2 years post-disaster. *Psychological Medicine, 27*, 167–178.

Chou, Y-J., Huang, N., Lee, C-H., Tsai, S-L., Tsay, J-H, Chen, L-S., et al. (2003). Suicides after the 1999 Taiwan earthquake. *International Journal of Epidemiology, 32*, 1007–1014.

Committee for Tent Cities in Kocaeli. (2000). *Report on the status of tent cities in Kocaeli*.

Devilly, G. J., & Foa, E. B. (2001). The investigation of exposure and cognitive therapy: Comment on Tarrier, et al. (1999). *Journal of Consulting and Clinical Psychology, 69*, 114–116.

Devilly, G. J., Spence, S. H., & Rapee, R. M. (1998). Statistical and reliable change with eye movement desensitization and reprocessing: Treating trauma within a veteran population. *Behavior Therapy, 29*, 435–455.

Durkin, M. E. (1993). Major depression and posttraumatic stress disorder following the Coalinga and Chile earthquakes: A cross-cultural comparison. *Journal of Social Behavior and Personality, 8*, 405–420.

Ehlers, A., Clark, D. M., Hackmann, A., McManus, F., Fennell, M., Herbert, C., et al. (2003). A randomized controlled trial of cognitive therapy, a self-help booklet, and repeated assessments as early interventions for posttraumatic stress disorder. *Archives of General Psychiatry, 60*, 1024–1032.

Foa, E. B., Dancu, C. V., Hembree, E. A., Jaycox, L. H., Meadows, E. A., & Street, G. P. (1999). A comparison of exposure therapy, stress inoculation training, and their combination for reducing posttraumatic stress disorder in female assault victims. *Journal of Consulting and Clinical Psychology, 67*, 194–200.

Foa, E. B., Hembree, E. A., Cahill, S. P., Rauch, S. A. M., Riggs, D. S., Feeny, N. C., et al. (2005).

Randomized trial of prolonged exposure for posttraumatic stress disorder with and without cognitive restructuring: Outcome at academic and community clinics. *Journal of Consulting and Clinical Psychology*, *73*, 953–964.

Foa, E. B., & Rauch, S. A. M. (2004). Cognitive changes during prolonged exposure versus prolonged exposure plus cognitive restructuring in female assault survivors with posttraumatic stress disorder. *Journal of Consulting and Clinical Psychology*, *72*, 879–884.

Ganesan, M. (2006). Psychosocial response to disasters-some concerns. *International Review of Psychiatry*, *18*, 241–247.

Government Crisis Center. (1999). *Press Release December 22, 1999*. (February, 2001); http://www.basbakanlik.gov.tr/krizyonetimmerkezi/22aralikbasinbildirisi.htm.

Kavaliers, M., & Choleris, E. (2001). Antipredator responses and defensive behaviour: Ecological and ethological approaches for the neurosciences. *Neuroscience and Biobehavioural Reviews*, *25*, 577–586.

Keane, T. M., Fairbank, J. A., Cadell, J. M., & Zimmering, R. T. (1989). Implosive (flooding) therapy reduces symptoms of PTSD in Vietnam combat veterans. *Behavior Therapy*, *20*, 245–260.

Kılıç, C., & Ulusoy, M. (2003). Psychological effects of the November 1999 earthquake in Turkey: An epidemiological study. *Acta Psychiatrica Scandinavica*, *108*, 232–238.

Krusko, N., Dolhinov, P., Anderson, C., Bortz, W., Kastlen, J., Flesher, K., et al. (1986). Earthquake: Langur monkey's response. *Laboratory Primate Newsletter*, *25*, 6–7.

Lai, T. J., Chang, C. M., Connor, K. M., Lee, L. C., & Davidson, J. R. T. (2004). Full and partial PTSD among earthquake survivors in rural Taiwan. *Journal of Psychiatric Research*, *38*, 313–322.

Lima, S. L. (1998). Stress and decision-making under the risk of predation: Recent developments from behavioral, reproductive and ecological perspectives. *Advances in the Study of Human Behavior*, *27*, 215–290.

Livanou, M., Başoğlu, M., Marks, I. M., de Silva, P., Noshirvani, H., Lovell, K., et al. (2002). Beliefs, sense of control and treatment outcome in posttraumatic stress disorder. *Psychological Medicine*, *32*, 157–165.

Livanou, M., Başoğlu, M., Şalcıoğlu, E., & Kalender, D. (2002). Traumatic stress responses in treatment-seeking earthquake survivors in Turkey. *Journal of Nervous and Mental Disease*, *190*, 816–823.

Livanou, M., Kasvikis, Y., Başoğlu, M., Mytskidou, P., Sotiropoulou, V., Spanea, E., et al. (2005). Earthquake-related psychological distress and associated factors 4 years after the Parnitha earthquake in Greece. *European Psychiatry*, *20*, 137–144.

Marks, I. M. (1987). *Fears, phobias, and rituals*. Oxford: Oxford University Press.

Marks, I. M., Lovell, K., Noshirvani, H., Livanou, M., & Thrasher, S. (1998). Treatment of posttraumatic stress disorder by exposure and/or cognitive restructuring: A controlled study. *Archives of General Psychiatry*, *55*, 317–325.

McMillen, J. C., North, C. S., & Smith E. M. (2000). What parts of PTSD are normal: Intrusion, Avoidance or Arousal? Data from the Northridge, California, Earthquake. *Journal of Traumatic Stress*, *13*, 57–75.

McNally, R. J., Bryant, R. A., & Ehlers, A. (2003). Does early psychological intervention promote recovery from posttraumatic stress? *Psychological Science in the Public Interest*, *4*, 45–79.

Mineka, S., & Öhman, A. (2002). Phobias and preparedness: The selective, automatic and encapsulated nature of fear. *Biological Psychiatry*, *52*, 927 937.

Mineka, S., & Zinbarg, R. (2006). A contemporary learning theory perspective on the etiology of anxiety disorders – it is not what you thought it was. *American Psychologist*, *61*, 10–26.

Mineka, S., Watson, D., & Clark, A. L. (1998). Comorbidity of anxiety and unipolar mood disorders. *Annual Review of Psychology*, *49*, 377–412.

National Earthquake Information Center. (2006). *Earthquakes with 1,000 or more deaths from 900*. (May, 2006); http://wwwneic.cr.usgs.gov/neis/eqlists/eqsmajr.html.

Newman, M. G., Erickson, T., Przeworski, A., & Dzus, E. (2003). Self-help and minimal contact therapies for anxiety disorders: Is human contact necessary for therapeutic efficacy? *Journal of Clinical Psychology*, *59*, 251–274.

Noji, E. K. (1997). Earthquakes. In E. K. Noji (Ed.), *The public health consequences of disasters*. New York: Oxford University Press.

Öhman, A., Dimberg, U., & Öst, L. G. (1985). Animal and social phobias: biological constraints on the learned fear response. In S. Reiss & R. Bootzin (Eds.), *Theoretical Issues in Behavior Therapy*. New York: Academic Press.

Önder, E., Tural, Ü., Aker, T., Kılıç, C., & Erdoğan, S. (2006). Prevalence of psychiatric disorders three years after the 1999 earthquake in Turkey: Marmara Earthquake Survey (MES). *Social Psychiatry and Psychiatric Epidemiology*, *41*, 868–874.

Paunovic, N., & Öst, L. G. (2001). Cognitive-behavior therapy vs exposure therapy in the treatment of PTSD in refugees. *Behaviour Research and Therapy*, *39*, 1183–1197.

Pitman, R. K., Orr, S. P., Altman, B., Longpre, R. E., Poire, R. E., & Macklin, M. L. (1996). Emotional processing during eye movement desensitization and reprocessing (EMDR) therapy of Vietnam veterans with posttraumatic stress disorder. *Comprehensive Psychiatry, 37*, 419–429.

Rachman, S. (1984). Agoraphobia: A safety-signal perspective. *Behaviour Research and Therapy, 22*, 59–70.

Renfrey, G., & Spates, C.R. (1994). Eye movement desensitization: A partial dismantling study. *Journal of Behavior Therapy and Experimental Psychiatry, 25*, 231–239.

Sanderson, W., Rapee, R., & Barlow, D.H. (1989). The influence of an illusion of control on panic attacks induced via inhalation of 5.5% carbon dioxide-enriched air. *Archives of General Psychiatry, 46*, 157–162.

Scholes, C., Turpin, G., & Mason, S.A. (2007) Randomised controlled trial to assess the effectiveness of providing self-help information to people with symptoms of acute stress disorder following a traumatic injury. *Behaviour Research and Therapy, 45*, 2527–2536.

Seligman, M. (1971). Phobias and preparedness. *Behavior Therapy, 2*, 307–320.

Seligman, M.E.P. (1968). Chronic fear produced by unpredictable shock. *Journal of Comparative and Physiological Psychology, 66*, 402–411.

Seligman, M.E.P., & Binik, Y. (1977). The safety-signal hypothesis. In H. Davis, & H. Hurwitz (Eds.), *Operant-Pavlovian interactions.* Hillsdale, N.J: Erlbaum.

Seligman, M.E.P., & Maier, S.F. (1967). Failure to escape traumatic shock. *Journal of Experimental Psychology, 74*, 1–9.

Shaw, E. (1977). Can animals anticipate earthquakes? *Natural History, 86*, 14–20.

Snarr, K.A. (2005). Seismic activity response as observed in mantled howlers (Alouatta palliate), Cuedo y Salado wildlife refuge, Honduras. *Primates, 46*, 281–285.

Sümer, N., Karancı, A.N., Berument, S.K., & Güneş, H. (2005). Personal resources, coping self-efficacy, and quake exposure as predictors of psychological distress following the 1999 earthquake in Turkey. *Journal of Traumatic Stress, 18*, 331–342.

Şalcıoğlu, E. (2004). *The effect of beliefs, attribution of responsibility, redress and compensation on posttraumatic stress disorder in earthquake survivors in Turkey*. PhD Dissertation. University of London.

Şalcıoğlu, E., Başoğlu, M., & Livanou, M. (2003). Long-term psychological outcome in non-treatment-seeking earthquake survivors in Turkey. *Journal of Nervous and Mental Disease, 191*, 154–160.

(2007a). Posttraumatic stress disorder and comorbid depression in survivors of the 1999 earthquake in Turkey. *Disasters, 31*, 115–129.

(2007b). Effects of live exposure on symptoms of posttraumatic stress disorder: The role of reduced behavioral avoidance in improvement. *Behaviour Research and Therapy, 45*, 2268–2279.

(2008). Psychosocial determinants of relocation in survivors of the 1999 earthquake in Turkey. *Journal of Nervous and Mental Disease, 196*, 55–61.

Tural, Ü., Coşkun, B., Önder, E., Çorapçıoğlu, A., Yıldız, M., Kesepara, C., et al. (2004). Psychological consequences of the 1999 earthquake in Turkey. *Journal of Traumatic Stress, 17*, 451–459.

U.S. Geological Survey Circular 1193. (November 22, 1999) *Implications for earthquake risk reduction in the United States from Kocaeli, Turkey earthquake of August 17*, 1999. U.S. Department of the Interior and U.S. Geological Survey.

Van Etten, M.L., & Taylor, S. (1998). Comparative efficacy of treatments for posttraumatic stress disorder: A meta-analysis. *Clinical Psychology and Psychotherapy, 5*, 126–144

Wang, X., Gao, L., Shinfuku, N., Zhang, H., Zhao, C., & Shen, Y. (2000). Longitudinal study of earthquake-related PTSD in a randomly selected community sample in North China. *American Journal of Psychiatry, 158*, 1260–1266.

Weiss, J. (1977). Psychological and behavioral influences on gastrointestinal lesions in animal models. In J. Maser & M.E.P. Seligman (Eds.), *Psychopathology: Experimental models.* San Francisco: Freeman

Williams, J., & Maier, S. (1977). Transsituational immunisation and therapy of learned helplessness in the rat. *Journal of Experimental Psychology: Animal Behaviour Processes, 3*, 240–252.

Yang, C-H., Xirasagar, S., Chung, H-C., Huang, Y-T, & Lin, H-C. (2005). Suicide trends following the Taiwan earthquake of 1999: Empirical evidence and policy implications. *Acta Psychiatrica Scandinavica, 112*, 442–448.

25 Hurricane Katrina

RONALD C. KESSLER, SANDRO GALEA, MICHAEL J. GRUBER, NANCY A. SAMPSON, MARIA PETUKHOVA, AND PHILIP S. WANG

25.1. INTRODUCTION

Hurricane Katrina was one of the strongest and deadliest hurricanes ever to make landfall in the United States and the costliest hurricane in U.S. recorded history. Katrina first made landfall on August 23, 2005, in southwestern Florida. It then gained force and crossed into the Gulf Coast region of Alabama, Louisiana, and Mississippi. A substantial part of the destruction caused by Katrina was associated with the fact that the hurricane's storm surge overwhelmed the levee system in New Orleans, resulting in a massive flood and evacuation of several parishes in the New Orleans Metropolitan Area. More than 500,000 people were evacuated, and nearly 90,000 square miles were declared a disaster area. More than 1,600 people died either as a direct result of the hurricane or the flood (Rosenbaum, 2006). The destruction caused by Hurricane Katrina persisted much longer than after previous U.S. natural disasters. At the time of writing this chapter, nearly 3 years after the hurricane, large infrastructure damage remains in much of the hurricane area and questions linger about the adequacy of the repaired levees in New Orleans to protect against future hurricanes.

On the basis of the severity of the event, we would expect Hurricane Katrina's effects on mental health to be at the upper end of the range of U.S. disasters and for the time course of recovery to be more protracted than after most other U.S. disasters. Owing to the wide geographical dispersion of the population displaced by Hurricane Katrina, it was challenging to carry out a comprehensive assessment of the mental health of survivors. As a result, the first mental health needs assessment surveys of the affected population focused on small, but well-characterized, high-risk population segments that were relatively easy to survey even though they were not representative of the entire affected population (Abramson & Garfield, 2006; Centers for Disease Control and Prevention, 2006a, 2006b). These included a survey carried out shortly after the hurricane among the minority of New Orleans residents who did not evacuate, a survey of people in evacuation centers during the first month after the hurricane, and a survey of families with children still residing in trailers supplied by the United States Federal Emergency Management Agency (FEMA) or hotel rooms sponsored by FEMA in Louisiana 6 months after the hurricane.

While these surveys documented high levels of trauma-related emotional problems in the high-risk samples that were studied, the population segments represented by each of these surveys included less than 1% of the affected population. Recognizing that public health decisions cannot be based on such a narrow empirical foundation and that ongoing monitoring was needed to track the time course of psychological recovery, the United States National Institute of Mental Health funded a panel survey designed to provide broader coverage of the population affected by Hurricane Katrina and to evaluate the need for mental health treatment in that population. A "panel" survey interviews the same people repeatedly over time, and the current chapter presents an overview of results from the first two waves of this panel. The first survey wave was administered 5 to 7 months after the storm, while the second survey wave was administered approximately 12 months after the first survey. Results of the second survey are currently in the initial phases of analysis, so the results reported here on trends are only preliminary. We focus on the prevalence and correlates of trauma-related mental disorders as well as on initial patterns of treatment of these disorders.[1]

25.2. SURVEY METHODS

25.2.1. The Sample

The target population for the surveys was English-speaking adults (aged 18 years or older) who before the hurricane lived in the areas subsequently defined by FEMA as affected by Hurricane Katrina. This population included approximately 4,137,000 adult residents of Alabama, Louisiana, and Mississippi in the 2000 Census. Census data show that only approximately 1% of this population was unable to speak English, suggesting that the restriction of the sample to English speakers did not introduce major bias into the sample.

As noted in the introduction, it was challenging to develop a sampling scheme for this population because of the wide geographic dispersion of survivors after the hurricane. Ideally, mass screening of households, shelters, and hospitals throughout the country could have been carried out; however, money was a serious constraint, making it necessary to develop a compromise study design. The design we used featured multiple sampling frames, each of which yielded a probability sample, with merging of these samples to create a representative sample of the whole population. Four sampling frames were used to select the sample for the surveys. The first frame consisted of the list of telephone numbers (landlines and cell phones) of the roughly 1.4 million families that applied to the American Red Cross (ARC) for assistance after the hurricane. The second frame was the list of telephone numbers of the roughly 2.3 million families that applied to FEMA for assistance after the hurricane. The third frame was the set of prehurricane telephone numbers of all households in the areas affected by the hurricane. The fourth frame was the set of hotels that housed FEMA-supported evacuees after the hurricane. Taken together, these four frames were estimated to cover well over 90% of the people affected by Hurricane Katrina.

It is important to note that the four frames had considerable overlap in membership. Many of the people who applied to the ARC for help, for example, also applied to FEMA and had landline phone numbers in the hurricane area. For the sample to be representative of the population, each person in the population should have the same probability of selection into the sample, so we had to take into consideration between-respondent variation in membership in multiple frames. We used a combination of two approaches to do this. The first approach was to remove most of the overlap between the random digit dialing (RDD) frame and the ARC/FEMA frames by exclusively selecting landline numbers in the latter two frames that were outside the hurricane area. However, this approach was incomplete because we had no way of knowing before carrying out the interviews the current residential locations of people who provided the ARC or FEMA with cell phone numbers rather than landline numbers. We were also uncertain before the interviews about the geographic location of people in the RDD sample even though the landlines in this sample were linked to specific addresses because of the fact that the landline phone company in the region set up a call-forwarding service shortly after the hurricane that forwarded calls made to the prehurricane landline number to the posthurricane residence of the owner of that phone number no matter where in the country.

As a result, our second approach to deal with the problem that some respondents had a higher probability than others of selection into the sample was to collect information from each respondent in all four subsamples about whether they were in each of the other four sample frames; we used this information to weight the final survey

[1] The results reported here summarize those reported in more detail in a series of journal articles (Kessler, Galea, Jones, & Parker 2006; Kessler et al., 2008; Wang et al., 2007, 2008; Galea et al., 2007). The reader is referred to these articles for more detailed presentations of results.

data. In addition, the number of respondents selected from each of the four sample frames was carefully selected to make sure we did not oversample any one population segment. As there was uncertainty about just how big each population segment was before carrying out the interviews, though, an additional weighting adjustment for differential probability of selection across the four frames was made at the very end of data collection. Finally, as we oversampled prehurricane residents of the New Orleans Metropolitan Area because of the much greater devastation that occurred due to flooding in that area than in other areas affected by Katrina, we used a weight to correct for that oversampling in analyses of the total sample.

Although the use of RDD might seem impractical in a population where many people evacuated, evacuation was much more common in the New Orleans Metropolitan Area than in the other hurricane-affected areas. Furthermore, many evacuees had returned as of the time of the survey, and as noted earlier, we were also able to contact some people who moved outside the area through RDD because of call forwarding. The vast majority of evacuees, in comparison, applied to either the ARC or FEMA (or both) for assistance and could be traced through contact information provided in the ARC or FEMA applications.

As noted previously, the first survey was carried out between January 19 and March 31, 2006, 5 to 7 months after the hurricane. A total of 1,043 respondents completed the interview, representing an estimated 41.9% of the eligible households we attempted to contact and interview. The FEMA sample frame was not yet available to us at the time of this first survey. As a result, the sample was supplemented with close to 2,000 additional respondents once the FEMA frame was made available. We had great difficulty contacting predesignated households, and once the households were contacted we achieved a low cooperation rate. The latter was due, at least in part, to the fact that we required a commitment from respondents for long-term involvement in the study to participate in the baseline survey, as the main goal of the study was to track the progress of recovery over time. Disillusionment, anger, exhaustion at dealing with the aftermath of the hurricane, and lack of time were doubtlessly involved in other refusals.

For purposes of making it clear that the sample was to be involved in tracking surveys we named the sample The Hurricane Katrina Community Advisory Group (CAG). This name emphasized the fact that CAG respondents were being given a unique opportunity to provide information to government policy makers about the needs of survivors of Hurricane Katrina. During initial efforts to recruit the sample, we asked a few questions about hurricane exposure, emotional response, and basic sociodemographic characteristics of all people who were contacted to participate in the CAG, even if these people subsequently decided not to participate. Analysis of these responses showed that the people who decided not to participate were similar to CAG participants on all sociodemographic variables but had a somewhat higher level of self-reported hurricane-related stress exposure. A weight was applied to the baseline CAG data to adjust for these response biases. A within-household probability of selection weight was also used along with a weight to adjust for residual discrepancies between the CAG and the 2000 Census population on a range of social, demographic, and prehurricane housing variables. More details about sampling and weighting of the final sample are described elsewhere (Kessler, et al., 2006).

Detailed personal contact information (current and permanent addresses, landline and cell phone numbers, email addresses) and tracing information (contact information for three people who would know how to find the respondent if he or she moved) were obtained for all baseline CAG members. This information was used to find respondents for the follow-up survey carried out 1 year after the initial interview. Some 815 of the 1,043 baseline respondents in the first wave of interviews were successfully traced and interviewed in this follow-up survey (78.1% of the baseline sample). Minor differences in the composition of the follow-up sample compared with the baseline sample in sociodemographic characteristics, traumatic stress exposure, and mental health were adjusted for by using an additional weight. Comparable proportions of subsequent baseline waves were also interviewed in a follow-up survey.

To obtain some information about pre–post change in mental health problems in the CAG, we made use of the fact that a large, nationally representative mental health survey, the National Comorbidity Survey-Replication (NCS-R) (Kessler & Merikangas, 2004), had interviewed 826 people between February 2001 and February 2003 in the two Census Divisions later affected by Hurricane Katrina. Although the NCS-R interviews were carried out face-to-face rather than over the telephone, we felt that some sort of pre-post comparison data would be useful. As a result, the same screening measure of anxiety-mood disorders used in the NCS-R was used in the CAG surveys. For purposes of comparison, we obtained the raw NCS-R data and extracted the subsample of 826 respondents who resided in the hurricane area for comparison with the baseline CAG sample. Results of this comparison are described later in this chapter.

25.2.2. Alternative Sampling Schemes

The low sample response rate reported earlier was due partly to our inability to trace the respondents initially selected from the ARC and FEMA lists. By the time we had negotiated access to the lists, many of the people we sampled could no longer be reached at the phone numbers provided on the lists, and we could not get adequate tracing information from the people at those numbers to contact our target respondents by phone. Predisaster establishment of collaborations with ARC and FEMA will be needed in the future to prevent this problem from recurring in new disaster situations.

Another problem with our sampling scheme was exclusive reliance on telephone contact. This was necessary for financial reasons. An efficient way to address this problem in the future would be to piggyback screening efforts onto one or more of the existing ongoing large-scale nationally representative government omnibus health surveys, such as the CDC Behavioral Risk Factor Surveillance Survey (BRFSS) or National Health Interview Survey (NHIS). These two surveys combined carry out interviews in approximately 400,000 U.S. households each year. In the case of the BRFSS, a new nationally representative telephone sample is interviewed every month. In the case of the NHS, a new nationally representative face-to-face sample is interviewed every week. It would not be either difficult or expensive to screen for evacuees in these ongoing surveys by adding a small number of additional questions to the end of each interview.

By cross-checking the identity of Katrina evacuees recruited from these screening samples with the ARC and FEMA master lists, it would have been possible to reconstruct samples of initial residents of the affected areas who never signed up for ARC or FEMA assistance and those who signed up but subsequently could not be traced. Both of these population segments could be recruited through BRFSS and NHIS screening, while people on the ARC or FEMA lists who could be traced could be sampled from these lists. To make this kind of multiple-frame sample design work, though, it is necessary to develop interagency collaborations that were beyond our ability when we launched the CAG study. It would be very valuable for an interagency task force to be established to develop plans for collaboration of this sort in advance of the next large-scale natural (or human-made) disaster that could profit from the use of intersecting screening efforts of this sort.

25.2.3. Measures

25.2.3.1. Mental Disorder

The K6 scale of anxiety–mood disorders (Kessler et al., 2002) was used both in the CAG and in the earlier NCS-R to screen for anxiety and mood disorders occurring within 30 days of the interview. The K6 is the most widely used mental health screening scale in the U.S. scores on the scale range from 0 to 24, and based on previous K6 validation (Kessler et al., 2003), scores in the range 13 to 24 were classified probable serious mental illness; those in the range 8 to 12 were classified probable mild–moderate mental illness (MMI);

and those in the range 0 to 7 were classified probable noncases. A small clinical reappraisal study was carried out with five respondents selected randomly from each of the three categories (serious mental illness, mild–moderate mental illness, noncase). A trained clinical interviewer administered the nonpatient version of the Structured Clinical Interview for DSM-IV (SCID) (First, Spitzer, Gibbon, & Williams, 2002), blinded to the category of each of the 15 respondents. The syndromes assessed were DSM-IV major depressive episode, panic disorder, generalized anxiety disorder, posttraumatic stress disorder (PTSD), agoraphobia, social phobia, and specific phobia. Serious mental illness was defined as a DSM-IV diagnosis with a global assessment of functioning (Endicott, Spitzer, Fleiss, & Cohen, 1976) score of 0 to 60 and MMI as a DSM-IV diagnosis with a global assessment of functioning score of 61 or more. K6 classifications were confirmed for 14 of 15 respondents, the exception being a respondent classified as having severe mental illness (SMI) by the K6 but MMI by the structured interview (on the basis of a global assessment of functioning score of 65).[2]

Given the special importance of PTSD in trauma situations, a separate PTSD screen was included on the basis of the 12-item Trauma Screening Questionnaire (TSQ) (Brewin et al., 2002), a validated screen for PTSD (Brewin, 2005). Our version differed from the original TSQ in using dimensional response options rather than a simple yes–no response format to assess 30-day symptom frequency (never, less than once a week, about once a week, 2 to 4 days a week, and most every day). A clinical reappraisal study was carried out to calibrate TSQ responses to DSM-IV PTSD with 30 respondents judged possible cases and ten randomly selected others. A cut-point on the factor-based zero to 42 scale of TSQ responses (12 items, each scored 0 to 4) of 20+ was selected to approximate the SCID PTSD prevalence in the weighted (to adjust for oversampling of screened positives) clinical reappraisal sample. Sensitivity (0.89), specificity (0.93), and area under the receiver operating characteristic curve (0.91) were all excellent for this dichotomous screen.

It is worth commenting here on the fact that comparison of results across postdisaster epidemiological surveys is hampered by the fact that no consensus exists about the best scales to use to assess PTSD and other mental disorders. Our hope in calibrating the K6 and TSQ scales to the SCID was to address this problem by calibrating our screening measures against a widely accepted clinical gold standard. Calibration of whatever screening scales are used should be built into any mental health needs assessment survey, even when the screening scales include a scale as widely used as the K6, as there is no guarantee that the screening scales will perform the same way in specific trauma samples as they do in the general population. It is much more plausible to think that semistructured clinician-administered interviews will be able to elicit comparable data on disorder prevalence that can legitimately be compared across surveys. By carrying out calibrations in this way and selecting cut-points on the screening scales that match clinical thresholds in the calibration interviews, legitimate comparisons can be made across surveys even when the screening scales used are different in the different surveys.

25.2.3.2. Suicidality

Suicidality was assessed in the CAG with questions about the lifetime occurrence of suicidal

[2] The K6 was designed to be a short screening scale used in general health tracking surveys to monitor broad trends in the prevalence of anxiety and mood disorders (Kessler et al., 2002). The K6 is used in a wide range of government health tracking surveys in the United States and elsewhere in the world (Centers for Disease Control and Prevention, 2004; Substance Abuse and Mental Health Services Administration, 2003). The definition of a serious mental illness (SMI) was mandated by Congress as part of the ADAMHA Reconstruction Act. A more detailed discussion of this Act and the definition of SMI is presented elsewhere (Kessler et al., 2003). Mild–moderate mental disorders are defined as all DSM-IV disorders that do not meet the criteria for SMI. The Global Assessment of Functioning Scale (Endicott et al., 1976), which was used to operationalize the severity criterion in the definition of SMI in the clinical reappraisal studies of the K6, is the standard measure of overall clinical severity used in research on mental disorders.

thoughts ("seriously thinking about killing yourself"), plans, and attempts, age of first occurrence of each of these outcomes, and recency of each outcome. Respondents were classified as first-onset cases with respect to each of these outcomes if they reported that the outcome occurred for the first time in their life within the past 12 months. This time frame was used because the suicidality questions were taken from the NCS-R, and the 12-month time frame was the most recent one assessed in the NCS-R. The use of identical questions and an identical time frame as in the NCS-R allowed us to make before–after comparisons of suicidality in the population affected by Katrina.

25.2.3.3. Posttraumatic Growth

We also included measures of several dimensions of personal growth occurring after the hurricane that previous research has found to occur after exposure to trauma and to facilitate psychological adjustment by making sense of the trauma or finding some positive aspect to the trauma (Davis, Nolen-Hoeksema, & Larson, 1998; Dougall, Hyman, Hayward, McFeeley, & Baum, 2001). We focused on five such dimensions based on their presence in the most commonly used inventories of posttraumatic personal growth (Park, Cohen, & Murch, 1996; Tedeschi & Calhoun, 1996): posttraumatic increases in emotional closeness to loved ones, faith in one's ability to rebuild one's life, spirituality or religiosity, meaning or purpose in life, and recognition of inner strength or competence.

25.2.3.4. Hurricane-Related Stressors

The baseline CAG survey included 29 structured questions developed on the basis of pilot interviews about hurricane-related stressors. Some of these stressors occurred at the time of the hurricane (e.g., death of loved one, a life-threatening experience that occurred to the respondent), and others occurred in the aftermath of the hurricane (e.g., homelessness, physical adversity). Still others were chronic stressful experiences that occurred in the first 5 to 7 months after the hurricane (e.g., geographic dislocation, financial adversity). The latter set of questions was repeated in the second wave of the CAG survey in an effort to learn how persistent the stressors had become. In addition, respondents were asked to provide a quantitative rating of the overall stressfulness of their situation in both CAG surveys by reporting "how stressful overall" they would say their experiences related to the hurricane and aftermath were on a 0 to 10 scale "where 0 means not at all stressful and 10 means the most stressful thing you can imagine." On the basis of the finding that responses to the structured questions about specific stressors were strongly related to responses to the global rating question, we focus on trends in responses to the latter question in our discussion of stress exposure, distinguishing respondents who reported severe (9–10), serious (7–8), moderate (5–6), or mild (3–4) stress from respondents who reported essentially no stress (0–2).

25.2.3.5. Treatment

All respondents who received professional counseling for emotional problems since the hurricane were asked about the number of sessions received, the duration of these sessions, and the types of professional they saw. Professionals were classified as psychiatrists, other mental health specialists (psychologist, psychotherapist, and any form of mental health counselor), general medical providers (primary care doctor, other general medical doctor, nurse, any other health professional not previously mentioned), human services professionals (religious or spiritual advisor, social worker), and complementary–alternative medicine professionals (any other type of healer such as chiropractors, herbalist, or spiritualist). Respondents who received fewer than eight counseling sessions or sessions lasting an average of less than 30 minutes were classified as receiving "counseling," while those who received eight or more sessions lasting an average of at least 30 minutes were classified as receiving "psychotherapy." All respondents who received medication for emotional problems since the hurricane were asked the name of the medication and the length of time they took the medication.

Respondents who did not receive any professional counseling or medication for emotional problems since the hurricane were asked a series of questions about their reasons for failing to obtain treatment, including lack of need (i.e., not having any psychological distress, or having distress but not feeling a need for treatment), enabling factors (e.g., not having health insurance or other determinants of access to care), and predisposing factors (e.g., feeling embarrassed to seek treatment or perceiving treatment to be ineffective). Respondents with a prehurricane mental illness who reduced or stopped treatment because of the disaster were asked a comparable series of questions about their reasons for reduction/termination.

25.2.3.6. Sociodemographics

We examined associations of the mental health and treatment outcomes with a number of sociodemographic variables, including respondent age, sex, race-ethnicity, family income in the year before the hurricane, education, current health insurance coverage, and current living situation. Age was coded 18 to 39, 40 to 59, and 60 and over. Race-ethnicity was coded non-Hispanic White, non-Hispanic Black, and other (largely Hispanics and Asians). Family income was coded in quartiles, where low was defined as less than or equal to 0.5 of the population median on the ratio of pretax income to number of family members, while low–average was defined 0.5+ through 1.0 on the same ratio, high–average 1.0 through 3.0, and high 3.0 or more on this ratio. Years of education were coded in four categories: none to 11, 12 (high school graduate), 13 to 15, and 16 or more (college graduate). Health insurance was coded yes–no. Current living situation, finally, was coded in four categories: living in the same house as before the hurricane, in the same county/parish but not the same house, in the same state but not the same county/parish, and in a different state.

25.2.4. Analysis

Prevalence of mental disorders and suicidality and basic patterns of treatment were estimated using simple cross-tabulations applied to the weighted data. Differences in the estimated prevalence of mental illness and suicidality were also compared between the NCS-R and the first CAG survey using cross-tabulations, as were differences in the prevalence of PTSD, more general anxiety–mood disorders, and suicidality between the first and second CAG surveys. Patterns of treatment and reasons for failing to seek treatment among people estimated to have a DSM-IV anxiety–mood disorder were examined using the same simple approach. Sociodemographic variation in all these outcomes was studied as well.

The statistical significance of between-survey comparisons involving the NCS-R and the first CAG survey was carried out using pooled regression equations in which the outcomes were coded as yes–no mental health outcomes (e.g., presence vs. absence of suicidal ideation), and the predictor of main interest was a dichotomous variable that distinguished between the two surveys being compared (e.g., a variable coded zero for respondents in the NCS-R and one for respondents in the first CAG survey). A logistic link function was used in the regression analysis (Hosmer & Lemeshow, 2001). A significant association between this predictor and the outcome meant that there was significant change between the two surveys. Sociodemographic variables were also included as predictors in these equations. Interactions between the main predictor variable that distinguished between surveys and the sociodemographic variables were examined. Statistically significant interactions of this sort meant that the change in outcomes between surveys was greater in one sociodemographic segment of the population than in another. The statistical significance of between-survey comparisons involving the first and second CAG surveys was carried out in a different way because of the fact that the same people were interviewed in both surveys. We computed measures of within-person change in the presence of mental disorders and suicidality and studied correlates of these changes. The role of posttraumatic growth was examined, finally, in a subgroup analysis.

Because the surveys featured weighting and geographical clustering, the statistical analyses used the Taylor series linearization method to estimate statistical significance (Wolter, 1985) implemented in the SUDAAN software system (Research Triangle Institute, 2002). This is a method that takes weighting and clustering into consideration in calculating statistical significance. Multivariate significance was calculated using Wald χ^2 tests based on design-corrected coefficient variance–covariance matrices. Statistical significance was evaluated using two-sided 0.05 level tests.

25.3. RESULTS

25.3.1. Baseline Prevalence of Mental Illness and Suicidality

The proportion of respondents estimated to have SMI was significantly higher in the baseline CAG survey (11.3%) than in the NCS-R (6.1%; $\chi^2_1 = 10.9$; $p < 0.001$). The same was true for the proportion estimated to have MMI (19.9 vs. 9.7%; $\chi^2_1 = 22.5$; $p < 0.001$) and those estimated to have any mental illness (31.2 vs. 15.7%; $\chi^2_1 = 35.9$; $p < 0.001$). Odds-ratios (ORs) were in the range 2.0 to 2.4 (Table 25.1). An OR is a measure of relative prevalence defined as $(p_1/q_1)/(p_2/q_2)$, where p_n is the prevalence of the dichotomous outcome in sample n and q_n is the additive inverse of p_n.

The difference between the surveys in suicidality, in comparison, was not significant either for ideation (2.9 vs. 2.8%; $\chi^2_1 = 0.0$; $p = 0.96$), plans (0.7 vs. 1.1%; $\chi^2_1 = 0.4$; $p = 0.54$), or attempts (0.7 vs. 0.6%; $\chi^2 = 0.0$; $p = 0.88$). This was surprising to us, as we had expected high suicidality to accompany the high rates of mental disorder found in the CAG. More detailed analysis showed, however, that the conditional prevalence of suicidality given probable mental illness was actually *lower* among those in the first CAG survey than among those surveyed several years before the hurricane in the NCS-R. More detailed analysis found that this was especially true for the first onset of suicidality during the past year among respondents with probable mental illness (Table 25.2). These differences were significant for ideation (0.7 vs. 8.4%; $\chi^2_1 = 13.1$; $p < 0.001$) and plans (0.4 vs. 3.6%; $\chi^2_1 = 6.0$; $p < 0.014$) but not for attempts (0.8 vs. 2.3%; $\chi^2_1 = 1.9$; $p = 0.17$).

25.3.2. Sociodemographic Correlates of Baseline Mental Illness and Suicidality

Significant sociodemographic correlates of SMI among those in the first CAG survey included being non-Hispanic White, not married before the hurricane, and classified as having an "other" employment status (mainly unemployed and disabled) before the hurricane. However, the only one of these associations that differed significantly in the CAG sample compared to the NCS-R was a higher prevalence of SMI among people who were not married after Katrina than before. The OR for this association was 7.4 for the previously married and 8.8 for the never married (compared with the married). The other significant associations, as they were in existence with comparable magnitude to the CAG sample before the hurricane, could be excluded as predictors of onset of new episodes of mental disorder after the hurricane.

Suicidal ideation was the focus of subsequent analysis of suicidality because suicide plans and attempts were too rare to be studied with adequate statistical power. The only statistically significant sociodemographic correlates of ideation were age (being 18–39 years of age) and race/ethnicity (minorities having much lower odds than non-Hispanic Whites), but only the second of these two associations was significantly higher in the CAG than in the NCS-R. The OR for this association was 0.2 for non-Hispanic Blacks and 0.0 for Hispanics (compared with non-Hispanic Whites). It is important to note that these significant associations with changes in SMI (marital status) and suicidal ideation (race/ethnicity)

Table 25.1. The estimated 30-day prevalence of DSM-IV anxiety–mood disorders and 12-month prevalence of suicidality in the National Comorbidity Survey-Replication (NCS-R; February 2001–February 2003) and the first CAG survey (January–March, 2006)[a]

	Survey					
	NCS-R		CAG		CAG: NCS-R	
	%	(se)	%	(se)	OR	(95% CI)
I. Anxiety–mood disorders						
SMI[b]	6.1	(0.7)	11.3	(1.7)	2.0*	(1.3–3.0)
MMI[b]	9.7	(1.0)	19.9	(2.1)	2.3*	(1.6–3.3)
Any (SMI or MMI)	15.7	(1.2)	31.2	(2.4)	2.4*	(1.8–3.2)
II. Suicidality						
Ideation	2.8	(0.4)	2.9	(0.9)	1.0	(0.5–2.1)
Plan	1.1	(0.3)	0.7	(0.5)	0.6	(0.1–2.9)
Attempt	0.6	(0.2)	0.7	(0.5)	1.1	(0.2–5.3)
(n)	(826)		(1,043)		(1,869)	

Notes:

* Significant difference between the two surveys at the 0.05 level, two sided test.

[a] Prevalence estimates were based on K6 screening scale. See the text for details.

[b] The abbreviation SMI refers to serious mental illness. The abbreviation MMI refers to mild–moderate mental illness. See the text for definitions.

Source: Originally appeared in Kessler, R. C., Galea, S., Jones, R. T., & Parker, H. A. (2006). Mental illness and suicidality after Hurricane Katrina. *Bulletin of the World Health Organization*, *84*(12), 930–939. Reprinted with permission from *Bulletin of the World Health Organization*. Available at: http://www.who.int/bulletin/volumes/84/12/06-033019.pdf. © 2006 World Health Organization. Used with permission.

Table 25.2. The estimated 12-month incidence of first lifetime onset of suicidality during the past 12 months among respondents estimated to have 30-day DSM-IV anxiety–mood disorder in the National Comorbidity Survey-Replication (NCS-R; February 2001–February 2003) and the first CAG survey (January–March, 2006)[a]

	Survey							
	NCS-R[b]			Post-Katrina[b]			CAG: NCS-R	
	%	(n_1/n_2)	(se)	%	(n_1/n_2)	(se)	OR	(95% CI)
Ideation	8.4	(15/147)	(2.3)	0.7*	(4/255)	(0.4)	0.1*	(0.0–0.3)
Plan	3.6	(9/191)	(1.3)	0.4*	(2/287)	(0.3)	0.1*	(0.0–0.6)
Attempt	2.3	(5/183)	(1.2)	0.8	(4/285)	(0.5)	0.3	(0.1–1.6)

Notes:

* Significant difference between the two surveys at the 0.05 level, two-sided test.

[a] Prevalence estimates were based on the K6 screening scale. See the text for details.

[b] Values are the percentage (numerator/denominator) (standard error) of respondents who met criteria for the outcome described in the row heading among those estimated to have a 30-day DSM-IV anxiety–mood disorder and no lifetime history of the outcome before the last 12 months.

Source: Originally appeared in Kessler, R. C., Galea, S., Jones, R. T., & Parker, H. A. (2006). Mental illness and suicidality after Hurricane Katrina. *Bulletin of the World Health Organization*, *84*(12), 930–939. Reprinted with permission from *Bulletin of the World Health Organization*. Available at: http://www.who.int/bulletin/volumes/84/12/06-033019.pdf. © 2006 World Health Organization. Used with permission.

explain only a small part of the observed variation in prevalence of these outcomes. By far the most striking result is that these outcomes do not differ markedly in their distributions across the population on a wide range of sociodemographic variables. This means that the adverse mental health effects of Hurricane Katrina were widespread in the population rather than concentrated in any one segment of the population.

The lower effects of the hurricane on suicidality among racial/ethnic minorities bear some comment. Previous research has shown that one of the ways in which traumas have adverse psychological effects is by shattering previously comforting assumptions about the world regarding safety, fairness, and predictability (Janoff-Bulman, 1989; Wortman, Silver, & Kessler, 1993). This adverse effect of traumas on mental health mediated by the shattering of comforting worldviews is sometimes found to be less powerful in socially disadvantaged segments of society because these comforting illusions were less common among the disadvantaged before the trauma occurred (Bonanno et al., 2002). It is conceivable that this type of process explains why the effects of the hurricane on suicidality were more benign among minorities than in others in our sample.

25.3.3. Posttraumatic Growth and Suicidal Ideation

The vast majority of respondents in the first CAG survey reported numerous types of posttraumatic growth, including becoming closer to their loved ones (81.6%), developing faith in their own abilities to rebuild their lives (95.6%), becoming more spiritual or religious (66.8%), finding deeper meaning and purpose in life (75.2%), and discovering inner strength (69.5%). The probabilities of two of these types of posttraumatic growth were found to vary significantly with mental illness: a comparatively low probability of finding deeper meaning and purpose in life and a comparatively high probability of discovering inner strength.

Two dimensions of posttraumatic growth were also significantly related to low prevalence of suicidal ideation among people thought to have mental illness: belief in their own abilities to recover and discovery of inner strength. The lower prevalence of suicidal ideation in the first CAG survey than in the NCS-R, in fact, was entirely limited to CAG members who reported these two aspects of posttraumatic growth, among whom the OR compared to the NCS-R was a statistically significant 0.2. The prevalence of suicidal ideation among mentally ill post-Katrina respondents with neither of these cognitions, in comparison, did not differ significantly from the prevalence among comparable respondents in the NCS-R, with a statistically insignificant OR of 1.1.

25.3.4. Differences in Prevalence between Respondents in New Orleans and Other Areas

The estimated prevalence of any 30-day DSM-IV anxiety–mood disorder in the first CAG survey was significantly higher among prehurricane residents of the New Orleans Metropolitan Area (49.1%) than in the remainder of the sample (26.4%; z= 5.0; $p < 0.001$) (Table 25.3). The ratio of SMI to other anxiety–mood disorders did not differ meaningfully, however, in the New Orleans Metro subsample (0.53) compared with the remainder of the sample (0.59).

All respondents classified by the TSQ as having PTSD were also classified by the K6 as having an anxiety–mood disorder. The estimated prevalence of PTSD in the first CAG survey was 16.3% in the total sample, with a significantly higher prevalence estimate in the New Orleans Metro subsample (30.3%) than in the remainder of the sample (12.5%; z = 4.1; $p < 0.001$). The conditional estimated prevalence of PTSD given probable SMI was extremely high in both subsamples (98.1% in New Orleans Metro and 85.8% in the remainder of the sample; z = 0.6; $p = 0.54$). The conditional estimated prevalence of PTSD given probable MMI, in comparison, was considerably higher in the New Orleans Metro subsample

Table 25.3. The estimated 30-day prevalence of DSM-IV anxiety–mood disorders in the first CAG survey separately among respondents who were prehurricane residents of the New Orleans Metropolitan Area and in the remainder of the sample

	New Orleans Metro		Remainder of sample	
	%	(se)	%	(se)
I. Anxiety–mood disorders				
SMI[a]	17.0*	(2.6)	9.8	(2.1)
MMI[a]	32.0*	(3.7)	16.6	(2.4)
Any (SMI or MMI)	49.1*	(3.3)	26.4	(3.1)
II. PTSD[b]				
PTSD given MMI	42.5	(8.9)	24.8	(7.0)
PTSD given SMI	98.1	(1.0)	85.8	(7.6)
PTSD total	30.3*	(3.7)	12.5	(2.2)
(n)	(594)		(449)	

Notes:

* Significant difference between the two subsamples at the 0.05 level, two-sided test.

[a] The abbreviation SMI refers to serious mental illness. The abbreviation MMI refers to mild–moderate mental illness. See the text for definitions. Prevalence estimates were based on the K6 screening scale. See the text for details.

[b] Prevalence estimates were on the basis of the TSQ screening scale. See the text for details.

Source: Originally appeared in Galea, S., Brewin, C. R., Gruber, M., Jones, R. T., King, D. W., King, L. A., et al. (2007). Exposure to hurricane-related stressors and mental illness after hurricane Katrina. *Archives of General Psychiatry*, *64*(12), 1427–1434.

(42.5%) than in the remainder of the sample (24.8%; z = 1.6; $p = 0.12$).

25.3.5. Prevalence of Hurricane-Related Stressors

The vast majority of respondents both in the New Orleans Metro subsample (91.9%) and in the remainder of the sample (81.7%) reported experiencing at least one of the ten categories of hurricane-related stressors assessed in the first CAG survey (Table 25.4). New Orleans Metro respondents reported a higher prevalence of each stressor than respondents in the remainder of the sample. The two most frequently reported stressors were housing adversity (71.7% in the New Orleans Metro subsample and 34.1% in the remainder of the sample; z = 8.6; $p < 0.001$) and property loss (70.2 vs. 47.8%; z = 4.9; $p < 0.001$). Other stressors occurred to between 33.6% to 46.3% (physical adversity) and 0.9% to 1.1% (life-threatening experience) of respondents.

25.3.6. Associations of Hurricane-Related Stressors with Anxiety–Mood Disorders

As high intercorrelations among stressors made it difficult to assess the separate effects of individual stressors in predicting anxiety–mood disorders, we developed a series of logistic regression models that included additive and interactive effects of exposure to multiple stressors. The best-fitting model in this set showed that physical illness/injury and physical adversity were associated with increased odds of adverse mental health outcomes in the New Orleans Metro subsample (2.8–7.9), while financial loss was associated with increased odds in the remainder of the areas affected by the hurricane (2.8–5.6) (Table 25.5). The ORs for other stressors were 3.6 to 6.3 in the New Orleans Metro subsample and 1.5 to 1.8 in the remainder of the sample. The ORs were consistently higher in the New Orleans Metro subsample than in the remainder of the sample with the exception of a higher OR associated

Table 25.4. The estimated prevalence of exposure to hurricane-related stressors in the first CAG survey separately among respondents who were prehurricane residents of the New Orleans Metropolitan Area and in the remainder of the sample

	New Orleans Metro		Remainder of Sample	
	%	(se)	%	(se)
I. Number of stressors				
One	12.8*	(1.8)	31.7	(3.2)
Two	19.5	(2.2)	22.5	(2.8)
Three	16.4	(2.8)	9.9	(2.0)
Four	15.4	(2.8)	7.6	(1.6)
Five or more	27.8*	(4.3)	10.1	(2.3)
Any	91.9*	(1.6)	81.7	(2.4)
II. Traumas				
Life-threatening experience	1.1	(0.4)	0.9	(0.6)
Victimized	11.8	(3.6)	5.4	(1.5)
Death of loved one	21.3*	(3.1)	7.4	(1.7)
Loved one victimized	19.3*	(3.7)	9.3	(1.9)
Any trauma	39.2*	(4.3)	17.0	(2.5)
III. Other stressors				
Property loss	70.2*	(3.1)	47.8	(3.4)
Income loss	28.3	(2.9)	20.0	(2.5)
Physical illness or injury	21.5	(3.2)	15.9	(2.4)
Housing adversity	71.7*	(3.2)	34.1	(3.0)
Physical adversity	46.3*	(3.6)	33.6	(3.3)
Psychological adversity	29.2	(3.8)	21.1	(2.9)
Any other stressor	90.0*	(1.8)	79.0	(2.6)
(n)	(594)		(449)	

Notes:

* Significant difference between the two subsamples at the 0.05 level, two-sided test.

Source: Originally appeared in Galea, S., Brewin, C. R., Gruber, M., Jones, R. T., King, D. W., King, L. A., et al. (2008). Exposure to hurricane-related stressors and mental illness after hurricane Katrina. *Archives of General Psychiatry*. Reprinted with permission from *Archives of General Psychiatry, 64* (12), 1427–1434.

with property loss in predicting PTSD in the remainder of the sample.

25.3.7. Trends in Anxiety–Mood Disorders and Suicidality between the Two CAG Surveys

The prevalence of anxiety–mood disorders did not change significantly between the first and second CAG surveys (Table 25.6). The estimated prevalence of SMI, in comparison, was significantly higher in the second survey than in the first in the total sample (14.0 vs. 10.9%; $t= 2.4$; $p = 0.018$) and in the subsample of respondents who were not from the New Orleans Metropolitan Area (13.2 vs. 9.4%; $t = 2.1$; $p = 0.038$). This trend was not significant, in comparison, in the New Orleans Metro subsample (16.9 vs. 16.5%; $t = 0.1$; $p = 0.91$). The estimated prevalence of PTSD was significantly higher in the second CAG survey than in the first in the subsample exclusive of the New Orleans Metropolitan Area (20.0 vs. 11.8%; $z = 4.0$; $p < 0.001$), but not in the New Orleans Metro subsample (24.1 vs. 25.9%; $t = 0.4$; $p = 0.68$). Finally, the prevalence of suicidality was significantly higher in the second than in the first CAG survey both with regard to suicidal ideation (6.4 vs. 2.8%; $t = 2.3$; $p = 0.020$)

Table 25.5. Multivariate associations of hurricane-related stressors with 30-day DSM-IV anxiety–mood disorders in the first CAG survey (N = 1,043)[a]

	PTSD[b]		Other SMI or MMI[c]		Any SMI or MMI	
	OR	(95% CI)	OR	(95% CI)	OR	(95% CI)
I. New Orleans Metro[d]						
Physical Injury/illness	2.8*	(1.2–6.6)	7.4*	(2.8–19.5)	6.5*	(2.9–14.6)
Physical adversity	7.9*	(3.2–19.7)	3.2*	(1.4–7.2)	6.0*	(2.9–12.3)
Any other stressor[e]	3.6	(0.7–20.2)	6.3	(1.8–21.4)	5.5*	(2.0–15.0)
II. Remainder of sample[d]						
Property loss	5.6*	(1.8–17.8)	2.8*	(1.3–6.3)	4.2*	(2.0–8.9)
Any other stressor[e]	1.8	(0.6–5.2)	1.5	(0.5–4.3)	1.7	(0.7–4.0)

Notes:

* Significant association between the stressor and the outcome at the 0.05 level, two-sided test.

[a] Coefficient estimates were based on multivariate regression equations using a logistic link function. See the text for details.

[b] Prevalence estimates were based on the TSQ screening scale. See the text for details.

[c] The abbreviation SMI refers to serious mental illness. The abbreviation MMI refers to mild–moderate mental illness. See the text for definitions. Prevalence estimates were based on the K6 screening scale. See the text for details.

[d] Each predictor was a dichotomy coded 1 for respondents who experienced the stressor and 0 for respondents who did not experience the stressor.

[e] The dichotomy defining any other stressor included all stressors other than physical illness/injury and physical adversity in the New Orleans Metro subsample and all stressors other than property loss in the remainder of the sample.

Source: Originally appeared in Galea, S., Brewin, C. R., Gruber, M., Jones, R. T., King, D. W., King, L. A., et al. (2008). Exposure to hurricane-related stressors and mental illness after hurricane Katrina. *Archives of General Psychiatry*. Reprinted with permission from *Archives of General Psychiatry*. *64* (12), 1427–1434.

and suicide plans (2.5 vs. 1.0 t = 3.1; p = 0.002). These trends, unlike those for SMI and PTSD, were significant and relatively comparable in magnitude in both the New Orleans Metro subsample and in the remainder of the sample.

We cross-classified baseline and follow-up diagnoses to study the composition of the diagnoses with significant trends. The majority of respondents classified as having SMI at follow-up either already had SMI at baseline (39.9%) or progressed from baseline MMI to SMI (31.6%), while the remaining 28.5% were delayed onsets (i.e., no disorder at baseline) (Table 25.7, Part I). A similar pattern was found for PTSD, where the majority of follow-up cases either already had PTSD at baseline (47.3%) or progressed from baseline MMI or SMI to PTSD (25.9%), while the remaining 26.8% were delayed onsets (i.e., no disorder at baseline). The proportions of delayed onsets were comparable for suicidal ideation (24.1%) and somewhat higher for suicide plans (46.6%), while the proportions with persistence (16.6% and 26.0% for ideation and plans, respectively) were lower than for SMI and PTSD. The proportions that represented progressions (i.e., from baseline cases with mental disorder but not suicidality) were higher for suicidal ideation (59.3%) than for SMI or PTSD and comparable for suicide plans, SMI, and PTSD.

It is noteworthy that the majority of respondents with baseline SMI (51.1%) continued to have SMI at follow-up (51.1%), while 30.8% of those with baseline SMI improved (i.e., were classified as having MMI at follow-up), and only a relatively small minority (18.1%) recovered (i.e., no longer met criteria either for SMI or MMI) (Table 25.7, Part II). In the case of PTSD, 66.4% of baseline cases continued to have PTSD at follow-up, while an additional 16.9% were classified as having MMI or SMI but not PTSD at follow-up, and only 16.7% recovered. Persistence was somewhat lower for suicidal ideation (37.9%) but much higher for plans (69.8%). Improvement, in comparison, was comparatively

Table 25.6. Trends in the estimated 30-day prevalence of DSM-IV anxiety–mood disorders and of 12-month suicidality among respondents who participated in both the first and second CAG surveys

	New Orleans Metro				Remainder of the Sample				Total Sample			
	Baseline		Follow-up		Baseline		Follow-up		Baseline		Follow-up	
	%	(se)	%	(se)	%	(se)	%	(se)	%	(se)	%	(se)
I. Any anxiety–mood disorder												
SMI[a]	16.5	(2.6)	16.9	(2.6)	9.4	(2.2)	13.2	(2.5)	10.9	(1.8)	14.0*	(2.0)
MMI[a]	27.8	(3.1)	24.9	(3.0)	17.5	(2.7)	18.6	(2.9)	19.8	(2.3)	19.9	(2.4)
PTSD	25.9	(3.1)	24.1	(3.0)	11.8	(2.4)	20.0*	(3.0)	14.9	(2.0)	20.9*	(2.5)
Any (SMI or MMI)	44.3	(3.3)	41.8	(3.3)	26.9	(3.3)	31.7	(3.4)	30.7	(2.7)	33.9	(2.8)
II. Suicidality (12-Month)												
Ideation	3.1	(1.2)	7.9*	(2.0)	2.8	(1.2)	6.0*	(2.0)	2.8	(1.0)	6.4*	(1.6)
Plan	0.8	(0.7)	3.0*	(1.4)	1.0	(0.9)	2.4*	(1.3)	1.0	(0.7)	2.5*	(1.0)
Attempt	0.7	(0.7)	0.9	(0.8)	0.8	(0.8)	0.0	(0.0)	0.8	(0.7)	0.2	(0.2)
(n)	(472)				(343)				(815)			

Notes:

* Significant difference between the two surveys at the 0.05 level, two-sided test.

[a] The abbreviation SMI refers to serious mental illness. The abbreviation MMI refers to mild–moderate mental Illness. See the text for definitions.

Source: Originally appeared in Kessler, R. C., Galea, S., Gruber, M. J., Sampson, N. A., Ursano, R. J., & Wessely, S. (2008). Trends in mental illness and suicidality after Hurricane Katrina. *Molecular Psychiatry, 13*(4), 374–384. Reprinted with permission.

Table 25.7. Decomposition of estimated 30-day prevalence of DSM-IV SMI[1] and PTSD and of 12-month suicidality among respondents who participated in both the first and second CAG surveys

	SMI[a]		PTSD		Ideation		Plans	
	%	(se)	%	(se)	%	(se)	%	(se)
I. Profiles of follow-up cases[b]								
Persistence	39.9	(7.7)	47.3	(6.7)	16.6	(10.0)	26.0	(22.1)
Progression	31.6	(7.4)	25.9	(6.0)	59.3	(12.9)	27.4	(14.5)
Delayed onset	28.5	(7.3)	26.8	(6.1)	24.1	(11.0)	46.6	(22.0)
(n)	(92)		(130)		(37)		(11)	
II. Transitions among baseline cases[b]								
Persistence	51.1	(9.1)	66.4	(6.5)	37.9	(18.7)	69.8	(29.3)
Improvement	30.8	(8.7)	16.9	(4.9)	49.9	(18.5)	12.2	(16.0)
Recovery	18.1	(6.9)	16.7	(5.0)	12.2	(7.4)	18.0	(21.2)
(n)	(74)		(107)		(23)		(4)	

Notes:

[a] The abbreviation SMI refers to serious mental illness. See the text for a definition.

[b] See the text for definitions of the categories.

Source: Originally appeared in Kessler, R. C., Galea, S., Gruber, M. J., Sampson, N. A., Ursano, R. J., & Wessely, S. (2008). Trends in mental illness and suicidality after Hurricane Katrina. *Molecular Psychiatry, 13*(4), 374–384. Reprinted with permission.

high for suicidal ideation (49.9%), but not for suicide plans (12.2%). Lastly, recovery (i.e., no MMI, SMI, or suicidality at follow-up) was relatively uncommon for either suicidal ideation (12.2%) or plans (18.0%).

25.3.8. Sociodemographic Predictors of the Trends

Only three sociodemographic variables were significant predictors of trends in SMI, PTSD, or suicidal ideation: respondent age, family income, and current living situation. (Suicide plans, which also increased significantly over time, were too rare to be included in the analysis of sociodemographic predictors.) Respondent age significantly predicted increased prevalence of PTSD (highest increases among respondents ages 40–59) and suicidal ideation (highest increases among respondents ages 18–39). Low family income predicted increased prevalence of all three outcomes. Family living situation predicted increased prevalence of SMI (higher increases among respondents not living in the same town as before the hurricane, whether or not they lived in the same county/parish or state, compared with those living in the same town). While significant in statistical terms, these associations were not strong in substantive terms, as the significant ORs (in the range 0.2–5.7) explained only between 2.1 (PTSD) and 2.7% (SMI) of the variance in the outcomes.

25.3.9. The Effects of Hurricane-Related Stress on the Trends

One possible explanation for the significant increases in the prevalence estimates of SMI, PTSD, and suicidal ideation is that hurricane-related stresses might have increased over time due to the slow pace of infrastructure recovery. As it turns out, however, this was not the case. A significantly *lower* proportion of respondents reported hurricane-related stress in the follow-up survey than in the baseline survey both in the New Orleans Metro subsample (97.9 vs.

78.3%; t = 8.0; $p < 0.001$) and in the remainder of the sample (90.0 vs. 51.7%; t = 8.2; $p < 0.001$). In light of the fact that the SMI–PTSD increases were found only in the subsample exclusive of the New Orleans Metro Area, it is noteworthy that the decrease in hurricane-related stress was less pronounced in the New Orleans Metro subsample than in the remainder of the sample. This means that higher levels of residual hurricane-related stress cannot explain the fact that SMI–PTSD prevalence increased over time only among respondents who were not from the New Orleans Metro Area.

Another possibility is that the psychological effects of hurricane-related stresses increased over time even though the magnitude of the stresses themselves decreased. A comparison of the cross-sectional associations between hurricane-related stresses and the outcomes found some superficial support for this possibility with regard to SMI, as the ORs linking stress with SMI in the follow-up survey were consistently larger than the parallel ORs in the baseline survey. However, these differences were not statistically significant (χ^2_4 = 8.1; $p = 0.09$). Furthermore, the pattern was not more pronounced in the subsample exclusive of the New Orleans Metro Area. This means that heightened reactivity to hurricane-related stress did not account for the fact that the significant increase in SMI was confined to respondents in the subsample exclusive of the New Orleans Metro Area. Furthermore, the pattern of higher ORs at follow-up than at baseline did not hold either for PTSD or for suicidal ideation.

This analysis was expanded to study the effects of hurricane-related stresses on trends in SMI, PTSD, and suicidal ideation by adding a control for the baseline value of the outcome to the prediction equation along with measures of stress assessed in both surveys. Baseline stress was not a significant predictor of trends in either SMI (χ^2_4 = 4.3; $p = 0.37$) or PTSD (χ^2_4 = 8.0; $p = 0.09$), while stress at follow-up was significant in both equations (χ^2_4 = 31.5; $p < 0.001$; χ^2_4 = 13.0; p = 0.011). No significant interactions were found between baseline stress and follow-up stress or between subsample (i.e., New Orleans Metro vs. the remainder of the sample) and either measure of stress. On the basis of these results, the final model for trends in SMI and PTSD included stress in the follow-up sample as the only key predictor. Stress exposure in this model was associated with substantial variation in both SMI and PTSD at follow-up, with ORs for serious–severe stress in the range 35.8 to 42.2 for SMI and 12.8 to 20.3 for PTSD, after controlling for baseline SMI and sociodemographics.

A good way to grasp the substantive significance of these results is to examine standardized prevalence estimates of the outcomes SMI and PTSD at follow-up. The latter are prevalence estimates in which adjustments have been made to correct for the associations of stress with baseline values of the outcomes, sociodemographics, and subsample, so the effects of stress can be seen as distinct from the effects of other variables. These standardized prevalence estimates were 0.3% (SMI) and 1.4% (PTSD) among respondents with no residual hurricane-related stress compared to 29.5% to 30.6% (SMI) and 38.8% to 46.1% (PTSD) among respondents with moderate-to-severe stress. If we think of these associations as causal, the population attributable risk proportions of SMI and PTSD because of hurricane-related stress (i.e., the proportions of currently existing SMI and PTSD that would be expected to remit if all hurricane-related stress was resolved) were 89.2% for SMI and 31.9% for PTSD.

The best-fitting model was different for suicidal ideation, as baseline stress and stress at follow-up interacted to predict trends in suicidal ideation (χ^2_1 = 7.2; $p = 0.007$). The best-fitting model distinguished respondents with severe–serious hurricane-related stress in one or both surveys versus all others. An additional complication was that the effect of stress in this model differed significantly between the New Orleans Metro subsample and the remainder of the sample, with the OR substantially higher among respondents not from the New Orleans Metro Area (104.1) than from New Orleans Metro (2.2). The prevalence estimates of suicidal ideation at follow-up among respondents with severe–serious hurricane-related stress were 3.1% in the New Orleans Metro subsample and

13.0% in the remainder of the sample compared with 0.3% and 0.0% among respondents without severe hurricane-related stress. If we think of these associations as causal, the population attributable risk proportion of suicidal ideation associated with severe–serious hurricane-related stress was 61.6% in the total sample.

25.3.10. Treatment

Nearly half of respondents with SMI (46.5%) and nearly one-fourth of those with MMI (23.0%) obtained some type of treatment for emotional problems in the first 5 to 7 months after the hurricane. The general medical sector was by far the most commonly used sector (by 11.0% of respondents), followed by the mental health speciality (MHS) (by 4.4%), human services (HS) (2.9%), and complementary-alternative medical (CAM) (0.0%). This pattern of differential use across sectors held in all disorder severity groups (i.e., SMI, MMI, and PTSD). Data on patterns of treatment in the second CAG survey were not yet analyzed at the time of preparing this chapter, so the focus here is on reports about treatment in the first CAG survey.

The most common treatment in the first CAG survey was pharmacotherapy alone (used by 8.8% of respondents), followed by psychotherapy alone (used by 3.7%), and pharmacotherapy plus psychotherapy (used by 3.4%). Among respondents treated since the hurricane, only a minority were still receiving psychotherapy at the time of the first CAG survey. The number of psychotherapy visits obtained since the disaster was low, with only 8.9% of those who received psychotherapy receiving eight or more visits, and 63.8% receiving only one to two visits. In addition, nearly one-third of the psychotherapy received lasted less than 30 minutes. Given the existing evidence from controlled treatment effectiveness studies, it is unlikely that so few psychotherapy visits of such brief duration were effective in resolving clinically significant hurricane-related anxiety–mood disorders.

In comparison, the vast majority of patients who received pharmacotherapy since the hurricane were still receiving pharmacotherapy at the time of the first CAG survey. The most frequently used classes of psychotropic medications were antidepressants (used by 60.2% of those who received pharmacotherapy), followed by benzodiazepines (30.1%), mood stabilizers (5.8%), nonbenzodiazepine hypnotics (5.0%), and antipsychotics (2.7%). Generally monotonic relationships between disorder severity and use of individual drug classes existed for antipsychotics, mood stabilizers, and nonbenzodiazepine hypnotics but not for antidepressants or benzodiazepines.

The proportion of untreated respondents in the first CAG survey that felt they needed mental health care was 13.7%. This perception ranged from a high of 47.9% among respondents with untreated SMI to 5.0% among untreated respondents with no evidence of any anxiety–mood disorder. Among those perceiving a need for treatment, nearly two-thirds (64.1%) reported lack of enabling factors (e.g., available services, financial means, transportation) as a reason for not seeking care. This proportion was highest among respondents with untreated SMI (86.4%) and lowest among those without any evidence of an anxiety–mood disorder (35.8%). Low perceived need (i.e., thinking the problem was not severe enough to warrant treatment or that the problem would get better on its own), in comparison, was reported as a reason most often by respondents without any evidence of an anxiety–mood disorder (37.3%) and least often by respondents with untreated SMI (10.0%). Attitudinal factors (e.g., stigma, perceived ineffectiveness of treatment, wanting to handle the problem on one's own) were also reported most often by respondents without any evidence of an anxiety–mood disorder (27.4%) and least often by respondents with untreated SMI (19.8%), although these proportions varied less than those associated with enabling and need factors across the disorder severity gradient.

25.4. DISCUSSION

A number of CAG survey measurement and design limitations need to be noted in interpreting the aforementioned results. First, mental disorders were estimated with screening scales rather than with clinical interviews, although calibration was used to select clinical cut-points on the screening scales. Despite this calibration, screening scales are inevitably less precise than clinical interviews, introducing imprecision into estimates of prevalence and correlates. Second, the survey response rate was low, and the sampling frame excluded people who were unreachable by telephone, almost certainly resulting in under-representation of the most marginalized and perhaps the most seriously ill people in the population. These sample limitations presumably made the estimates of disorder and stressor prevalence conservative. Third, the assessment of disaster-related stressors was necessarily retrospective, raising concerns about recall bias related to mental illness at the time of interview and the possibility that the associations between stressors and mental disorders were overestimated. Fourth, the comparison of results from the first wave of the CAG survey with results from the NCS-R was an inexact way to estimate the initial mental health effects of Hurricane Katrina due to the fact that the NCS-R and the CAG surveys differed in many ways.

Notwithstanding these limitations, the fact that the estimated prevalence of anxiety–mood disorders was twice as high in the first CAG survey as in the NCS-R was consistent with other evidence that major natural disasters have substantial adverse mental health effects (Norris et al., 2002; Galea, Nandi, & Vlahov, 2005). The higher prevalence estimates of anxiety–mood disorders in the first CAG survey in the New Orleans Metro subsample than in the remainder of the sample is consistent with the fact that the New Orleans population was more severely affected than the remainder of the Katrina population. The high initial prevalence estimates of anxiety–mood disorders in the New Orleans Metro subsample were consistent with those found in previous studies of people in highly disaster-affected areas (Canino, Bravo, Rubio-Stipec, & Woodbury, 1990; David et al., 1996), while the lower prevalence estimates in the remainder of the sample were consistent with the results of previous studies in areas with lower disaster impact (Caldera, Palma, Penayo, & Kullgren, 2001; Kohn, Levav, Donaire, Machuca, & Tamashiro, 2005). The finding that suicidality was lower in the first CAG survey than in the NCS-R is consistent with previous evidence of decreases in suicidal behavior during some times of crisis, such as during World War II. This presumably is due to people in some crisis situations developing a sense of meaning and purpose that protects them against the suicidal behavior that is often associated with extreme distress.

The significant increases in SMI, PTSD, and suicidal ideation and plans in the second CAG survey were different from the patterns found in other longitudinal surveys of mental illness after natural disasters, where prevalence typically decreases or, in extreme cases, remains the same over time (Carr et al., 1997; McFarlane, 1988; Norris, Perilla, Riad, Kaniasty, & Lavizzo, 1999). The fact that the increases in SMI and PTSD were confined to respondents not from the New Orleans Metro Area is difficult to interpret in light of the higher levels of hurricane-related stress both at baseline and at follow-up in the New Orleans Metro subsample. It is possible to speculate post hoc that the much greater media attention directed at New Orleans than the other areas affected by Hurricane Katrina might have led to a greater sense of abandonment among affected people in areas other than the New Orleans Metro Area, but we have no data to evaluate this interpretation. Another possibility is that the increases in SMI and PTSD outside the New Orleans Metro Area are partly due to increases in stressors that might only be indirectly linked to the hurricane. This possibility is consistent with evidence from several longitudinal studies that low-intensity ongoing stressors significantly predict long-term PTSD, presumably because these nagging stressors erode the resistance resources that would otherwise promote recovery (Adams & Boscarino, 2006; Galea et al., 2008). However, it is unclear why such stressors might be more prevalent among people not from the New Orleans Metro Area.

The results regarding disorder prevalence and correlates lead to four conclusions. First, hurricane-related stress clearly played a critical role in the high prevalence of hurricane-related anxiety–mood disorders in the population affected by Hurricane Katrina. Second, the fact that the associations between these stresses and the mental health outcomes considered here were stronger among affected people from areas other than the New Orleans Metro Area suggests that undetermined stress and/or vulnerability factors were present among people from other areas, which should lead policy makers to focus special attention on the needs of these people. Third, the observation that these adverse effects were only weakly related to sociodemographic variables means that the adverse effects of Katrina were distributed across the full range of the sociodemographic spectrum of the affected population. It is noteworthy in this regard that the significant upward trends in SMI, PTSD, and suicidality were found to be unrelated to sex, race/ethnicity, education, and health insurance status. Fourth, the fact that hurricane-related stressors were still quite common in the population at the time of our follow-up assessment, which occurred nearly 2 years after the hurricane, and that high proportions of the outcomes at follow-up were attributable to these continuing stressors suggests that efforts to address the problem of increased mental illness and suicidal ideation plans among people affected by Hurricane Katrina require efficient provision of practical and logistical assistance to deal with the high remaining levels of stress. This may be particularly challenging when it comes to helping prehurricane residents of the affected areas who are now living elsewhere in the country, but it is especially important to reach these geographically displaced people because of their comparatively high risk of SMI.

Our findings regarding treatment were striking in that showed that only a minority of the people with hurricane-related mental disorders received any form of treatment in the first 5 to 7 months after the hurricane. Although there was a gradient between severity of disorder and mental health service use, fully half of even the most serious cases received no mental health care. Furthermore, many of the people in treatment received low intensity or frequency of care. The vast majority of ongoing treatment consisted exclusively of pharmacotherapy provided by general medical doctors. These results may not be surprising given that Katrina led to widespread loss of mental health care facilities, treatments, and personnel, as well as to loss of the employment, financial resources, and insurance needed to pay for treatment. The negative consequences of this widespread unmet need are uncertain but presumably large, as dysfunction, morbidity, and mortality are associated with untreated mental disorders (Stein, Walker, Hazen, & Forde, 1997; Marshall et al., 2001).

The fact that most Katrina survivors relied on the general medical sector for mental health care after the hurricane emphasizes the importance of ensuring that primary care personnel can deliver quality mental health treatments in disaster settings. The specialty sector could have played a more prominent role in facilitating primary care competence by providing consultation, but no system was put into place to implement a collaborative model of care. Before calling the mental health treatment system to task for this omission, though, it is important to recognize that mental health specialists were also needed to care for the increasing needs of the most seriously mentally ill who could not realistically be cared for adequately in general medical settings. The fact that need for care of seriously mentally ill people increased dramatically at the same time as the number of mental health treatment providers dramatically dropped meant that the remaining mental health professionals were overwhelmed by this increased demand for their services.

It would be unrealistic to think that local mental health professionals could successfully meet the dramatically increased needs of the many people with mental disorders after a disaster as severe as Hurricane Katrina. Creative solutions continue to be essential to address this problem. In devastated areas, emergency mental health units were created to deal with the most severe unmet need for treatment (Operation Assist, 2006). One idea to expand capacity is that these units can be expanded and staffed, if necessary, by members of the uniformed services medical corps if other medical personnel are not available. It might also be possible to use part-time volunteer psychiatrists from throughout the country to provide telephonic consultation to primary care doctors in the affected area in an effort to increase the effectiveness of primary care pharmacological treatment of mental disorders. Another possibility is to draw on a wider range of part-time volunteer mental health professionals from throughout the country to directly deliver services like cognitive behavioral therapy over the telephone. Telephonic interventions of this sort have been shown to be effective (Simon, Ludman, Tutty, Operskalski, & Von Korff, 2004). Evaluations of the effectiveness of any such novel intervention programs, finally, are necessary to begin building a knowledge base that can be drawn on to help guide service implementation efforts in future major disaster situations.

ACKNOWLEDGMENTS

The research reported here was supported by the U.S. National Institute of Mental Health (R01 MH070884-01A2), with supplemental support from the US Federal Emergency Management Agency (FEMA) and the Assistant Secretary for Planning and Evaluation of the US Department of Health and Human Services. A public use version of the survey data reported here is available through the Interuniversity Consortium for Political and Social Research (ICPSR) at the University of Michigan. For details on data acquisition, go to www.HurricaneKatrina.med.harvard.edu. The views and opinions expressed in this report are those of the authors and should not be construed to represent the view of any of the sponsoring organizations, agencies, or U.S. government.

REFERENCES

Abramson, D., & Garfield, R. (2006). *On the edge: Children and families displaced by hurricanes Katrina and Rita face a looming medical and mental health crisis*. New York: Columbia University, Mailman School of Public Health.

Adams, R. E., & Boscarino, J. A. (2006). Predictors of PTSD and delayed PTSD after disaster: the impact of exposure and psychosocial resources. *Journal of Nervous and Mental Disease, 194*(7), 485–493.

Bonanno, G. A., Wortman, C. B., Lehman, D. R., Tweed, R. G., Haring, M., Sonnega, J., et al. (2002). Resilience to loss and chronic grief: A prospective study from preloss to 18 months postloss. *Journal of Personality and Social Psychology, 83*(5), 1150–1164.

Brewin, C. R. (2005). Systematic review of screening instruments for adults at risk of PTSD. *Journal of Traumatic Stress, 18*(1), 53–62.

Brewin, C. R., Rose, S., Andrews, B., Green, J., Tata, P., McEvedy, C., et al. (2002). Brief screening instrument for post-traumatic stress disorder. *British Journal of Psychiatry, 181*(2), 158–162.

Caldera, T., Palma, L., Penayo, U., & Kullgren, G. (2001). Psychological impact of the hurricane Mitch in Nicaragua in a one-year perspective. *Social Psychiatry and Psychiatric Epidemiology, 36*(3), 108–114.

Canino, G., Bravo, M., Rubio-Stipec, M., & Woodbury, M. (1990). The impact of disaster on mental health: Prospective and retrospective analyses. *International Journal of Mental Health, 19*(1), 51–69.

Carr, V. J., Lewin, T. J., Webster, R. A., Kenardy, J. A., Hazell, P. L., & Carter, G. L. (1997). Psychosocial sequelae of the 1989 Newcastle earthquake: II. Exposure and morbidity profiles during the first 2 years post-disaster. *Psychological Medicine, 27*(1), 167–178.

Centers for Disease Control and Prevention. (2004). Serious psychological distress. Early release of selected estimates based on data from the January–March 2004 National Health Interview Survey (September 2005); http://www.cdc.gov/nchs/data/nhis/earlyrelease/200409_13.pdf.

(2006a). Assessment of health-related needs after Hurricanes Katrina and Rita – Orleans and Jefferson Parishes, New Orleans area, Louisiana, October 17–22, 2005. *Morbidity and Mortality Weekly Report, 55*(2), 38–41.

(2006b). Surveillance in hurricane evacuation centers – Louisiana, September–October 2005. *Morbidity and Mortality Weekly Report, 55*(2), 32–35.

David, D., Mellman, T. A., Mendoza, L. M., Kulick-Bell, R., Ironson, G., & Schneiderman, N. (1996). Psychiatric morbidity following Hurricane Andrew. *Journal of Traumatic Stress, 9*(3), 607–612.

Davis, C. G., Nolen-Hoeksema, S., & Larson, J. (1998). Making sense of loss and benefiting from the experience: Two construals of meaning. *Journal of Personality and Social Psychology, 75*(2), 561–574.

Dougall, A., Hyman, K., Hayward, M., McFeeley, S., & Baum, A. (2001). Optimism and traumatic stress: The importance of social support and coping. *Journal of Applied Social Psychology, 31*(2), 223–245.

Endicott, J., Spitzer, R.L., Fleiss, J.L., & Cohen, J. (1976). The Global Assessment Scale: A procedure for measuring overall severity of psychiatric disturbance. *Archives of General Psychiatry, 33*(6), 766–771.

First, M.B., Spitzer, R.L., Gibbon, M., & Williams, J.B.W. (2002). *Structured clinical interview for DSM-IV axis I disorders, research version, non-patient edition (SCID-I/NP)*. New York, NY: Biometrics Research, New York State Psychiatric Institute.

Galea, S., Ahern, J., Tracy, M., Cerda, M., Goldmann, E., & Vlahov, D. (2008). The determinants of post-traumatic stress in a population-based cohort study. *Epidemiology, 19*(1), 47–54.

Galea, S., Brewin, C.R., Gruber, M., Jones, R.T., King, D.W., King, L.A., et al. (2007). Exposure to hurricane-related stressors and mental illness after hurricane Katrina. *Archives of General Psychiatry, 64*(12), 1427–1434.

Galea, S., Nandi, A., & Vlahov, D. (2005). The epidemiology of post-traumatic stress disorder after disasters. *Epidemiologic Reviews, 27*(1), 78–91.

Hosmer, D.W., & Lemeshow, S. (2001). *Applied logistic regression, 2nd edition*. New York, NY: Wiley & Son.

Janoff-Bulman, R. (1989). The benefits of illusions, the threat of disillusionment and the limits of inaccuracy. *Journal of Social and Clinical Psychology, 8*(2), 158–176.

Kessler, R.C., & Merikangas, K.R. (2004). The National Comorbidity Survey Replication (NCS-R): Background and aims. *International Journal of Methods in Psychiatric Research, 13*(2), 60–68.

Kessler, R.C., Andrews, G., Colpe, L.J., Hiripi, E., Mroczek, D.K., Normand, S.L., et al. (2002). Short screening scales to monitor population prevalences and trends in non-specific psychological distress. *Psychological Medicine, 32*(6), 959–976.

Kessler, R.C., Barker, P.R., Colpe, L.J., Epstein, J.F., Gfroerer, J.C., Hiripi, E., et al. (2003). Screening for serious mental illness in the general population. *Archives of General Psychiatry, 60*(2), 184–189.

Kessler, R.C., Galea, S., Gruber, M.J., Sampson, N.A., Ursano, R.J., & Wessely, S. (2008). Trends in mental illness and suicidality after Hurricane Katrina. *Molecular Psychiatry, 13*(4), 374–384.

Kessler, R.C., Galea, S., Jones, R.T., & Parker, H.A. (2006). Mental illness and suicidality after Hurricane Katrina. *Bulletin of the World Health Organization, 84*(12), 930–939.

Kohn, R., Levav, I., Donaire, I., Machuca, M., & Tamashiro, R. (2005). Psychological and psychopathological reactions in Honduras following Hurricane Mitch: Implications for service planning. *Revista Panamericana de Salud Publica, 18*(4–5), 287–295.

Marshall, R.D., Olfson, M., Hellman, F., Blanco, C., Guardino, M., & Struening, E.L. (2001). Comorbidity, impairment, and suicidality in subthreshold PTSD. *American Journal of Psychiatry, 158*(9), 1467–1473.

McFarlane, A.C. (1988). The longitudinal course of posttraumatic morbidity. The range of outcomes and their predictors. *Journal of Nervous and Mental Disease, 176*(1), 30–39.

Norris, F.H., Friedman, M.J., Watson, P.J., Byrne, C.M., Diaz, E., & Kaniasty, K. (2002). 60,000 disaster victims speak: Part I. An empirical review of the empirical literature, 1981–2001. *Psychiatry, 65*(3), 207–239.

Norris, F.H., Perilla, J.L., Riad, J.K., Kaniasty, K., & Lavizzo, E.A. (1999). Stability and change in stress, resources, and psychological distress following natural disaster: Findings from Hurricane Andrew. *Anxiety, Stress, and Coping, 12*(4), 363–396.

Operation Assist. (2006). Responding to an emerging humanitarian crisis in Louisiana and Mississippi: urgent need for a health care "Marshall Plan". (April 17, 2006); http://www.childrenshealthfund.org/whatwedo/operation-assist/pdfs/On%20the%20Edge_Final.pdf.

Park, C.L., Cohen, L.H., & Murch, R.L. (1996). Assessment and prediction of stress-related growth. *Journal of Personality, 64*(1), 71–105.

Research Triangle Institute. (2002). *SUDAAN: Professional Software for Survey Data Analysis*. Research Triangle Park, NC: Research Triangle Institute.

Rosenbaum, S. (2006). US health policy in the aftermath of Hurricane Katrina. *Journal of the American Medical Association, 295*(4), 437–440.

Simon, G.E., Ludman, E.J., Tutty, S., Operskalski, B., & Von Korff, M. (2004). Telephone psychotherapy and telephone care management for primary care patients starting antidepressant treatment: A randomized controlled trial. *Journal of the American Medical Association, 292*(8), 935–942.

Stein, M.B., Walker, J.R., Hazen, A.L., & Forde, D.R. (1997). Full and partial posttraumatic stress disorder: Findings from a community survey. *American Journal of Psychiatry, 154*(8), 1114–1119.

Substance Abuse and Mental Health Services Administration. (2003). *National survey on drug use and health: Results, 2004*. Washington,

DC: United States Department of Health and Human Services.

Tedeschi, R. G., & Calhoun, L. G. (1996). The Post-traumatic Growth Inventory: measuring the positive legacy of trauma. *Journal of Traumatic Stress, 9*(3), 455–471.

Wang, P. S., Gruber, M. J., Powers, R. E., Schoenbaum, M., Speier, A. H., Wells, K. B., et al. (2007). Mental health service use among Hurricane Katrina survivors in the eight months after the disaster. *Psychiatric Services, 58*(11), 1403–1411.

Wang, P. S., Gruber, M. J., Powers, R. E., Schoenbaum, M., Speier, A. H., Wells, K. B., et al. (2008). Disruption of existing mental health treatments and failure to initiate new treatments after Hurricane Katrina. *American Journal of Psychiatry, 165*(1), 34–41.

Wolter, K. (1985). *Introduction to variance estimation.* New York, NY: Springer-Verlag.

Wortman, C. B., Silver, R. C., & Kessler, R. C. (1993). The meaning of loss and adjustment to bereavement. In M. S. Stroebe, W. Stroebe, & R. O. Hansson (Eds.), *Handbook of bereavement*. Cambridge, U.K.: Cambridge University Press.

26 The Long-Term Mental Health Impacts of the Chernobyl Accident

EVELYN J. BROMET AND JOHAN M. HAVENAAR

26.1. INTRODUCTION

Over 20 years have passed since the explosion at the Chernobyl nuclear power plant on the night of April 26, 1986, thus beginning the largest peacetime nuclear disaster ever. More than six million people were subsequently exposed to radioactive fall-out. The population residing in the 30-km zone around the plant was permanently evacuated, and the health of the evacuees and the cleanup workers (locally called *liquidators*) has been monitored thereafter (Hatch, Ron, Bouville, Zablotska, & Howe, 2005). At the twentieth anniversary of the event, the United Nations created an interagency body, The Chernobyl Forum, to review the cumulative health, mental health, and socioeconomic impacts of the accident (The Chernobyl Forum, 2006). Although the Forum concluded that the only significant physical health effect during the first 20 years was thyroid cancer among exposed children, the Forum also identified the psychological aftermath as the largest public health problem unleashed by the accident to date.

This chapter reviews the empirical evidence on the mental health impact of Chernobyl. We begin with a synopsis of the events of 1986 and a brief discussion of the historical and research contexts in which the subsequent mental health studies took place. We then evaluate the evidence regarding the psychiatric and neuropsychological aftermath of the Chernobyl disaster. The vast majority of the mental health studies focused on three issues: stress-related psychopathology in the general population directly or indirectly affected by the accident; cognitive and developmental effects of exposure to radiation in highly exposed infants; and cognitive and emotional effects of exposure and disaster-related stress in the cleanup workers.

26.2. THE CHERNOBYL DISASTER

The Chernobyl nuclear power plant was constructed in the 1970s in north-central Ukraine along the Dnipro River. The plant housed four reactors, the last of which was completed in 1983. On the night of April 26, 1986, a breach of safety procedures during a routine shut-down operation resulted in an explosion in Unit 4. Burning debris and sparks shot into the air above the reactor, fell onto the roof of the machine room, and started a massive fire that led to a complete meltdown. Hundreds of tons of radioactive dust were dispersed all over Europe. Initially, the Soviet authorities tried to conceal the accident from the public while at the same time mounting an extensive operation to control the damage. A 30-km exclusion zone around the plant was established, and everyone living within it, including the entire population of Pripyat, a nearby town built to house the workers and their families (~50,000 people), was evacuated in a matter of days. During the evacuation, pregnant women were told to have abortions although they were not given an explanation. Reportedly, most complied.

Estimates vary, but over 600,000 men and women were sent in as emergency or cleanup personnel (The Chernobyl Forum, 2006). Many were in the military or other state services. Most were given inadequate or no protective clothing. In the immediate aftermath, 134 emergency workers were treated for radiation sickness

(Hatch et al., 2005), and 31 died. At the same time, in an effort to maintain an impression of normalcy, the Soviet government went forward with the First of May celebrations, including in Ukraine's capital city of Kiev, located to the south of Chernobyl. However, rumors about the accident soon began to spread, and by June, news reports described Kiev as a city without children as parents sent them to live with relatives and friends in contaminated by radiation.

Although precise figures are not available, in 1986 thousands of evacuee families were sent to Kiev where, on the heels of a series of frightening experiences during the evacuation, they then had difficulty obtaining the residency permit (propiska) required by law during Soviet times. Kiev had a housing shortage, and the evacuees were given new apartments that had been previously promised to local residents. For many evacuees, especially those from Pripyat, the new accommodations were smaller and less comfortable. Like the survivors of Hiroshima and Nagasaki, the evacuees and their children were stigmatized, feared, and at times treated with overt hostility by the local population. Legislation was passed granting the evacuees special medical benefits, but these benefits were initially meager and not forthcoming. Thus, the evacuees struggled for basic necessities and government benefits on top of living with their own fears about the radiation exposure they received when the plant exploded.

When the Soviet Union collapsed in 1991, responsibility for the medical care of the cleanup workers and evacuees was transferred to the newly independent countries, which were facing mounting poverty and scarce economic resources. Basic infrastructure (water, heating, electricity, roads, etc.) was inadequate to meet the rapid changes taking place, and corruption was rampant. The level of poverty was staggering (World Bank, 2003); according to a study by the International Monetary Fund (Braithwaite & Hoopengardner, 1997), the official poverty rate in Ukraine in June 1995, 9 years after the Chernobyl accident, was 29.5%, with urban areas particularly short of food and clothing. In terms of the health status of the population, the breakup of the Soviet Union led to declines in life expectancy and standard of living and an increase in mortality, especially from cardiovascular disease, accidents, and other causes related predominantly to alcohol and smoking. The incidence of sexually transmitted diseases in adolescents increased from 194 per 10,000 in 1991 to 447 per 10,000 in 1995. Ukraine also experienced a severe outbreak of cholera in 1994 and 1995. The health and economic needs of populations affected by Chernobyl, especially the evacuee families and cleanup workers, contributed to the overall economic strain, particularly in Ukraine and Belarus, the republics most directly affected by the accident.

26.3. HISTORICAL CONTEXT OF RESEARCH ON THE CHERNOBYL DISASTER

Studies of mental health consequences of disasters require epidemiologic designs and standardized, nonbiased methods of assessing mental health (Bromet & Havenaar, 2002, 2006). Before 1986, Western concepts of epidemiology were not widely utilized by investigators in Eastern European countries. There were no population-based statistics on health or mental health apart from government statistical reports based on infectious disease surveillance data. Hence, before 1986, no credible baseline data existed on population health or mental health, suicide, or rates of mental hospitalization. Moreover, the Soviet Union largely was closed to outside investigators. Thus, when the accident happened, local researchers did not have the tools to undertake the type of postdisaster epidemiologic research conducted in other parts of the world, and it was difficult for Western researchers to establish transparent collaborations with local physicians. The first reports from the Soviet Union that Chernobyl exposure had led to an increase in thyroid cancer were treated with skepticism by the Western scientific community; these findings were later confirmed in Western laboratories (Baverstock & Williams, 2006). Regarding mental health outcomes, no reliable data on the acute- and short-term impact of Chernobyl were available during the first 6 years after the accident.

One issue that remains controversial is the amount of radioactivity absorbed by the population living nearby. According to the Chernobyl Forum (2006), the average effective dose received by people who were evacuated from the 30-km zone in the spring and summer of 1986 was approximately 33 mSv although some evacuees received considerably higher exposure. It is important to note that these estimates are based on dose reconstructions performed years later because reliable information about exposure was unavailable at the time of the accident.

Starting in the mid-1990s after the collapse of the Soviet Union, open, collaborative, population-based research began in Ukraine, Belarus, Russia, and other Soviet countries. To a large extent, this transformation occurred because of the need to understand the physical and mental health consequences of the accident. Indeed, our own investigations of Chernobyl's mental health impact in Belarus (Havenaar, Rumyantzeva, van den Brink, et al., 1997; Havenaar, Rumyantzeva, Kasyanenko, et al., 1997) and Ukraine (Bromet et al., 2000) were the first psychiatric epidemiologic studies in these countries. More recently, the International Centre for Health and Society at University College London (e.g., Nicholson, Bobak, Murphy, Rose, & Marmot, 2005) has conducted a number of health and mental health surveys in former Soviet countries, and these too changed the nature of psychosocial research in that part of the world.

Like epidemiology, Western concepts of mental health and psychiatric treatment were not accepted before Chernobyl and the break-up of the Soviet Union. Moreover, the authorities used psychiatry as a means of maintaining social control over the population, punishing political dissidents by hospitalizing them in mental institutions (Gluzman, 1991). Thus, psychiatric disorders were (and still are) highly stigmatized (Shulman & Adams, 2002). Therefore, when the Chernobyl disaster occurred, there was no infrastructure or common language from which to launch clinically meaningful mental health research. In 1991, the Ukrainian Psychiatric Association (UPA) was founded by Dr. Semyon Gluzman with the mission of adopting and promulgating Western concepts of psychiatric diagnoses and treatments. The founding of UPA opened a dialogue between psychiatrists in Ukraine and psychiatrists in the West (Gluzman & Kostyuchenko, 2006); open and transparent clinical research collaborations were made possible by the translation and free dissemination of European and North American textbooks and psychiatric journals under the auspices of UPA. Our study of the mental health impact of Chernobyl in Kiev (2000), conducted jointly with UPA, ultimately paved the way for a national survey of mental health in Ukraine (Bromet et al., 2005) funded by the U.S. National Institute of Mental Health as a site for the World Mental Health (WMH) Survey Consortium (Kessler & Üstün, 2004).

26.4. MENTAL HEALTH EFFECTS

Three areas of research on the mental health consequences of Chernobyl are reviewed: (1) stress effects in the general population; (2) cognitive and emotional effects in highly exposed infants; and (3) the cognitive and emotional effects in cleanup workers.

26.4.1. Population-Based Morbidity Studies

A number of general population mental health surveys were conducted shortly after the accident and published in Russian-language journals or presented at international conferences. These reports all indicated that the psychological impact of Chernobyl was substantial. However, the methodologies were at best unclear and at worst unsystematic with respect to sampling, assessment, and analysis. A number of other studies of *émigré* populations who moved from the Soviet Union to the United States and Israel were also published. Because the underlying population bias in both the exposed and nonexposed comparison groups places an inherent constraint on the generalizability of these findings, these reports are not covered in this section. Rather we review here the findings from mental health studies of local affected populations published in English-language, peer-reviewed journals. Altogether, five large, population-based studies were undertaken in the affected republics.

The first two studies were independently conducted 7 years after the accident. One was a collaboration between Finnish and Russian scientists in which the mental health of 325 people ages 15 to 54 residing in a contaminated village in Bryansk (western edge of Russia on the border of Ukraine) was compared with that of 278 controls living in an uncontaminated village in the same region (Viinamäki et al., 1995). Mental health was measured with the 12-item version of the General Health Questionnaire (GHQ-12) (Goldberg, McDowell, & Newell, 1996), a broad screening instrument widely used in mental health research conducted in primary care and community populations to detect current mood and anxiety symptoms and to estimate the prevalence of "minor mental disorder" using an internationally accepted cutoff score. The findings from this study indicated that the rate of minor mental disorder was significantly higher among exposed women compared with controls (48% vs. 34%), but no difference was found among men. In addition to sex, the risk factors for psychological impairment were not having a partner, financial inadequacy, self-rated poor health, and uncertainty about the future because of the Chernobyl accident. The fact that the epidemiologic risk factors were consistent with findings from Western epidemiologic studies suggested that Western tools could provide meaningful data in former Soviet countries. Risk perceptions – in this case uncertainty about the future – proved to play a pivotal role in all subsequent Chernobyl research.

The other study conducted 6–7 years after the accident involved a collaboration of Dutch, Belarussian, and Russian physicians. This study assessed 1,617 adults in Gomel, an area of Belarus that was very badly contaminated by radiation, and 1,427 controls in Tver, Russia, a demographically similar region that was not exposed to radiation (Havenaar et al., 1996; Havenaar, Rumyantzeva, Kasnayenko, et al., 1997; Havenaar, Rumyantezeva, van den Brink, et al.,1997; Havenaar, de Wilde, van den Bout, Drottz-Sjöberg, & van de Brink, 2003). The study design had two phases. In phase 1, the entire sample was administered the GHQ-12 along with other self-report measures. In phase 2, subsamples with high and low GHQ scores were administered a standardized psychiatric examination by psychiatrists and physical examinations by specially trained physicians. The Gomel respondents were significantly more symptomatic on the GHQ and other subclinical self-report scales, rated their physical health more poorly, and were more likely to utilize medical services than their counterparts in Tver. The risk factors for these negative self-reports included being female, having young children, relocation because of Chernobyl, and more extreme risk perceptions about Chernobyl (Havenaar et al., 1996; Havenaar et al., 2003). However, the differences in diagnosable mood and anxiety disorders and in physical health status determined during phase 2 were small and nonsignificant except in the subgroup of Gomel mothers with children under age 18, who had elevated rates of anxiety and mood disorders (Havenaar, Rumyantezeva, van den Brink, et al., 1997).

In 1997, 11 years after the accident, we conducted a two-stage study of the psychological and medical aftermath of the Chernobyl accident with families evacuated to Kiev who had infants or were pregnant at the time of the accident. The study was funded by the National Institute of Mental Health. Most of the evacuee families (80.7%) came from Pripyat, the town located 1 mile from Chernobyl that was built to house the workers and their families; the rest were from small villages in the 30-km zone. Modeled on our prior research after the accident at the Three Mile Island nuclear power plant (Bromet, Parkinson, & Dunn, 1990), we assessed 300 evacuee mother–child dyads and 300 gender-matched classmate dyads with a comprehensive interview battery that focused on depression, anxiety, posttraumatic stress, and somatic symptoms and epidemiologic and Chernobyl-related risk factors (Adams et al., 2002; Bromet, et al., 2000; Bromet, Gluzman, Schwartz, & Goldgaber, 2002; Litcher et al., 2000). The study also obtained reports from teachers about the behavior of the children and information from the schools on grades and absenteeism. Importantly, all of the children received physical examinations and basic blood tests. Eight years later, in 2005 and 2006, we conducted a follow-up of the sample to determine the mental health outcomes of the children at age 19 and the changes in mental health among the mothers. In all, 265 evacuees (88% of the initial sample) and 261 classmates (87% of the initial sample) participated, along with a new, representative, population-based control group from Kiev (*N* – 296 mother–child dyads). In this section, we provide a synopsis of the findings on the mothers (median age in 1997 was 39). In Section 26.4.2, we describe the findings for the children.

At each interview wave, compared with controls, the evacuee mothers were more symptomatic on all of the mental health measures, especially with respect to posttraumatic stress symptoms measured with the Impact of Events Scale (22-item version) (Weiss & Marmar, 1997) and somatization measured with the 12-item subscale of the SCL-90 (Derogatis, 1983). The evacuee mothers also had higher rates of diagnosable major depressive disorder on the basis of a structured diagnostic interview for DSM-IV (2000). When asked to rate their health, 39% of evacuee mothers and 23% of controls rated their health as poor in 1997 (Bromet et al., 2002); 32% of evacuees and 23% of controls rated their health as poor 8 years later (Adams, Bromet, Panina, & Golovakha 2007). Risk perceptions substantially increased the likelihood that mothers perceived their health as poor at both times. In 1997, for example, evacuee mothers were seven times as likely to rate their health as poor if they believed that Chernobyl had adversely affected them (OR = 7.0; 95% CI = 4.1–11.7), while among controls, the effect was smaller but still sizeable (OR = 3.3; 95% CI = 1.8–6.2).

All three of these studies were consistent in showing that Chernobyl exposure elevated the rate of psychological impairment and that Chernobyl risk perceptions were potent risk factors, even after adjustment for epidemiologic risk factors. Moreover, they all pointed to mothers of young children as an especially high-risk group. This pattern of results is consistent with mental health findings after other toxic disasters (Havenaar, Cwikel, & Bromet, 2002), including the nuclear power plant accident at Three Mile Island that occurred 7 years before Chernobyl on another continent entirely (Bromet et al., 1990). However, in each of the three studies, the respondents knew that they were being interviewed in connection with the Chernobyl accident, and the interviewers were aware of who was exposed and who was not. Indeed, we cautioned the Kiev interviewers during the training not to inquire about Chernobyl until the end of the interview, but respondents often volunteered that they were evacuees when the interviewer walked in the door. This is a general problem in disaster research that leads to overestimations of the differences between exposed and nonexposed populations and of the effects of risk perceptions.

Fortunately, we had two opportunities to evaluate the mental health aftermath of Chernobyl using a study design that did not have this built-in bias. The first opportunity occurred in 1998, when we incorporated questions about Chernobyl and self-assessed health into a routine national probability sample survey conducted by the Kiev International Institute of Sociology (KIIS). KIIS was established in 1992 and modeled on the Institute for Social Research at the University of Michigan. KIIS conducts sociological, economic, and political surveys, as well as periodic omnibus surveys. KIIS also was responsible for conducting the fieldwork for the WMH survey in Ukraine described earlier (Bromet et al., 2005). The 1998 omnibus survey sampled 1,600 adults. We added four questions: How do you rate your physical health in general? (excellent, good, fair, poor, very poor); How do you rate your mental health? (same scale); Were you relocated after the accident? (yes/no); Do you think your health was affected by Chernobyl? (no, yes somewhat, yes very). Three percent of the survey sample was relocated after the accident. Not surprisingly, they were far more likely to believe that Chernobyl had a major adverse effect on their health (44.8% vs. 17.8% of nonrelocated; $p < 0.001$). Moreover, those who thought that their health was affected by Chernobyl reported worse physical and mental health than those who did not maintain this belief. Specifically, among men, 73.4% who believed that their health was affected by Chernobyl rated their mental health as fair/poor (vs. 52.2% of others; $p < 0.001$), and 77.9% rated their physical health as fair/poor (vs. 57.4% of others; $p < 0.001$). Among women, 79.9% of those who believed that their health was affected rated their mental health as fair/poor (vs. 70.7% of others; $p < 0.001$), and 92.0% (vs. 77.2%; $p < 0.001$) rated their physical health as fair/poor.

The second opportunity to consider the effects of Chernobyl under conditions with minimal bias occurred when we participated in the WMH Survey Consortium (Bromet et al., 2005). The consent form described the purpose of the study as being "to further our understanding of the well-being of adults in Ukraine and the effects of stress on health and quality of life." In fact, Chernobyl exposure was asked as part of the demographic module, which was positioned after the screening module, in which the self-rating of health appeared, and after the diagnostic modules for depression, anxiety, alcohol, and intermittent explosive disorders. The question we then posed was whether the respondent ever lived in an area contaminated by Chernobyl. Fewer than 10% answered affirmatively (weighted estimate = 8.2% of 4,725). Those exposed to Chernobyl (weighted $N = 388$) were more likely to rate their health as fair/poor (75.5% vs. 65.5%; $p < 0.001$). Like the Gomel findings, they were only slightly more likely to have experienced an episode of depression since the accident (18.0% vs. 14.4%; $p = 0.05$). Contrary to expectations, both sets of associations were more striking and more significant for the men than for the women.

To conclude, population morbidity surveys found that exposed populations were significantly more likely to report depression and anxiety symptoms and to assess their physical health as fair/poor health compared with controls, and risk perceptions about Chernobyl were significantly associated with these outcomes. Although the associations were stronger in magnitude in studies focused specifically on Chernobyl than in general population surveys in which Chernobyl was not the target of the research, they were still in the expected direction and, for the most part, statistically significant in general population surveys.

26.4.2. Cognitive, Developmental, and Emotional Impairment in Children

In the aftermath of Chernobyl, substantial concern arose about the developing brain of children who were in utero when the accident occurred. Rumors about brain damage and child psychopathology, especially dementia and schizophrenia, proliferated even though the highest level of exposure in the contaminated regions was lower than the level associated with brain damage in the offspring of survivors of Hiroshima and Nagasaki (Imamura, Nakane, Ohta, & Kondo., 1999; Otake & Schull, 1984; Schull & Otake, 1999). The World Health Organization (WHO) undertook an elegantly designed study, the International Pilot Study of Brain Damage In-Utero, when the exposed children were 7 years old and concluded that the rates of mental retardation and emotional problems were not higher in radiation-exposed children compared with controls (World Health Organization, 1995). However, the WHO results were not published in a peer-reviewed format because of serious flaws in the execution of the fieldwork. Nevertheless, two extension studies of this research were undertaken by local investigators in Belarus and Ukraine that came to different conclusions. The Belarus study expanded the sample and added assessments at age 12; only slight differences were found in intellectual functioning between exposed and unexposed children, but significant differences were found in ICD-10 developmental and childhood psychiatric disorders (Kolominsky, Igumnov, &

Drozdovitch, 1999; Igumnov & Drozdovitch, 2000). In the absence of a dose–response effect, however, the authors did not attribute the findings to radiation exposure per se. The second study, conducted in Kiev by the Research Center for Radiation Medicine (RCRM), reported significantly higher rates of borderline intelligence, mental retardation, and emotional problems in exposed children from contaminated villages compared with controls from Kharkiv as well as a dose–response relationship for radiation exposure in a subsample (Nyagu, Loganovsky, & Loganovskaja, 1998). They attributed their results directly to radiation exposure. However, the sampling, testing, and dose reconstruction methods were problematic, the selection factors for the subsample used in the dose–response analysis were unclear, the controls were from an urban area while the exposed were mostly from villages, and parental intelligence and education were not adjusted in the analysis. Nevertheless, this study was widely and repeatedly reported in the Ukrainian media and has had a huge impact locally.

The children in Kiev participating in our research were given a battery of neuropsychological tests to assess intelligence, learning, and memory in 1997 when they were 11 years old (Litcher et al., 2000) and again in 2005 and 2006 when they were 19 years old (Taormina et al., 2008). Our findings at both waves supported the conclusions of the WHO report. That is, at each point in time, we found no significant differences in neuropsychological performance between the evacuee children and classmate controls, including in separate analyses of the in utero subsample (Litcher et al., 2000; Taormina et al., 2008). At age 11 there were no differences in school grades, and at age 19 there were no significant differences in the proportions attending university. Another large study conducted in Israel also found no differences in performance on the Ravens Progressive Matrices among children and adolescents from high exposure (Gomel), mild exposure (Kiev or Mogilev), and unexposed regions who were under age 4 or in utero at the time of the accident (Bar Joseph, Reisfeld, Tirosh, Silman, & Rennert, 2004).

As noted previously, the WHO-extension studies in Belarus and Kiev found evidence that exposed children had higher rates of childhood emotional disorders. Our initial study, when the children were similar in age, failed to confirm these findings (Bromet et al., 2000; Drabick, Gadow, Carlson, & Bromet, 2004). Our study included subclinical and diagnosis-level measures of depression and anxiety. However, a recent study conducted in Finland (Huizink et al., 2007) found elevated rates of depression and ADHD in adolescents exposed during the second and third trimester compared with controls although the rates of both disorders were extremely low.

In summary, the hypothesis that the radiation exposure from Chernobyl adversely affected the cognitive, developmental, or emotional functioning of children exposed to radiation from Chernobyl at a young age or in utero remains unproven. It is possible that future evidence will resolve the current lack of consensus on this important issue.

26.4.3. Mental Health of Cleanup Workers

Research on the mental health of cleanup workers has focused on (1) the associations of high levels of radiation exposure with subsequent cognitive impairment, neuropsychological dysfunction, and psychosis and (2) rates of emotional problems, including suicide, in general samples of cleanup workers.

Three studies conducted in Kiev and reported in English-language peer-reviewed journals found that highly exposed cleanup workers had excess rates of different types of cognitive impairments or psychosis relative to controls. The first study, based at RCRM, reported an increased rate of schizophrenia spectrum disorders in highly exposed cleanup workers (~5/10,000) compared with the general population of Ukraine (~1.1/10,000) (Loganovsky & Loganovskaja, 2000). This finding awaits independent verification of the clinical assessments and diagnoses. Moreover, it is likely that the classification of schizophrenia at RCRM, which participated in several European and American funded studies, differed from that given in mental hospitals throughout Ukraine. The second study, conducted at the Institute of Gerontology in Kiev, found that 86% of highly exposed workers sent to Chernobyl before September 1986 suffered from accelerated aging, or "radiation progeroid syndrome," a classification based on a set of psychological and cardiovascular tests, compared with 59% of less exposed men sent to Chernobyl after September 1986 (Polyukhov, Kobsar, Grebelnik, & Voitenko, 2000). Unfortunately, the method for assembling the sample was not described, and the raters were not blind to exposure status. The third report was based on a collaborative study undertaken by American and Ukrainian researchers in which a 1-hour neuropsychological test battery was administered annually from 1995 to 1998 to 127 volunteers from throughout Ukraine (Gamache, Levinson, Reeves, Bidyuk, & Brantley, 2005). The sample included a subgroup of cleanup workers, all of whom were tested at the RCRM. The cleanup workers performed more poorly at each time point than the remainder of the sample. However, their test taking conditions differed, and the analysis failed to adjust for age, education, and drinking status. Moreover, the average performance levels for the entire sample declined significantly across time, suggesting that the internal reliability of the testing might have been compromised. Thus, the evidence supporting the hypothesis that radiation caused cognitive impairment in highly exposed workers is weak.

The emotional consequences of working as a liquidator, especially during the first few months, have also been studied. Two studies produced negative results. Specifically, 10% of the Havenaar, Rumyantzeva, van den Brink et al. (1997) Gomel sample were cleanup workers; no differences were found between their GHQ and subjective health scores and scores for the rest of the sample. However, the level of radiation exposure, if any, in this group of cleanup workers is unknown. The RCRM sample included both low (<0.3 Sv; N = 54) and highly (N = 146) exposed workers. They performed similarly on the GHQ-12 and the Minnesota Multiphasic Personality Inventory (MMPI) (Loganovsky & Loganovskaja, 2000).

However, evidence from two other studies suggests that the stress of working as a liquidator has taken a large toll. In a mortality study conducted in Estonia, a significant excess in deaths from suicide was found among cleanup workers (N = 5,000) for the period from 1986 to 1993 (SMR = 1.52; 95% CI = 1.01–2.19), while no significant excess of deaths from other causes was detected (Rahu et al., 1997). These findings were confirmed when the follow-up period was extended through 2002 (Rahu, Rahu, Tekkel, & Bromet, 2006). The authors attributed the excess suicide rate to the forced recruitment of these workers, uncertainty about the radiation dose received and its potential harm, and fear about future radiation-related diseases.

Together with KIIS and RCRM, we compared the mental health of 295 male cleanup workers sent to Chernobyl between 1986 and 1990 and interviewed 18 years after the accident with 397 geographic-matched controls interviewed as part of the Ukraine-WMH Survey 16 years after the accident (Loganovsky et al., 2008). The WHO Composite International Diagnostic Interview was administered, along with supplemental symptom scales for the cleanup worker sample. The analyses adjusted for age in 1986 and mental health before the accident. Consistent with Rahu et al. (1997, 2006), significantly more of the cleanup workers were diagnosed with DSM-IV depression (18.0% vs. 13.1%) and reported suicide ideation (9.2% vs. 4.1%) after the accident. Current (past year) prevalence rates of depression (14.9% vs. 7.1%), PTSD (4.1% vs. 1.0%), and headaches (69.2% vs. 12.4%) were also elevated, but no differences were found in rates of alcoholism. We further examined whether workers with depression and PTSD had greater occupational impairment than others in the study. Most strikingly, the affected workers reported more work-loss days than affected controls or unaffected workers or controls. When the cleanup workers were stratified into high, moderate, and low exposure groups based on when they worked at Chernobyl and whether they were on the roof or close to the structure, a clear dose–response relationship was found for current somatization and PTSD symptomatology. Thus, this study provided compelling evidence that the stresses experienced by liquidators, especially the highly exposed group, had significant psychological consequences.

To summarize, the mental health impact of Chernobyl on the cleanup workers needs greater study, but the findings to date indicate that highly exposed cleanup workers constitute a high-risk group for psychiatric disorders, especially depression. The findings are consistent with mental health research on workers at the Three Mile Island nuclear power plant (Parkinson & Bromet, 1983) and on first responders (Benedek, Fullerton, & Ursano, 2007), including findings from responders to the World Trade Center (Centers for Disease Control and Prevention, 2004). Further clinical research is needed to evaluate the mental health of this group, including investigating the potential synergistic effects of radiation exposure and occupational stress as well as objective assessments of cognitive functioning and history of psychiatric illness.

26.5. CONCLUSION

Chernobyl was a complex, high-impact disaster, and its emotional toll was substantial and protracted. This toll primarily took the form of depression, anxiety, and somatic symptoms and increased use of medical services among the exposed population. There is also suggestive evidence that exposure to the disaster led to increased rates of diagnosable psychiatric disorders in high-risk groups, such as cleanup workers and mothers of young children evacuated from the zone around the plant at the time of the accident. There is no compelling evidence of organic brain involvement in exposed children, but the issue has been inadequately tested. The population findings are consistent with results from studies of survivors of other toxic exposures, including the Three Mile Island accident, the Japanese atomic bombing, Bhopal, the Tokyo gas attack, and other toxic events (Havenaar et al., 2002).

General population studies and research on cleanup workers indicate that anxiety, depression, psychosomatic symptoms, and posttraumatic stress symptoms endured for years. The first systematic studies of this issue fromcommunities in Russia and Belarus found elevated rates 7 years later. Our Ukraine research found elevated rates in mothers of young children and cleanup workers almost 20 years later. Although the differences between exposed and nonexposed populations were not as dramatic in surveys that were not directly about Chernobyl compared to studies that focused specifically on Chernobyl (an issue that would have been obvious to the respondents during the consenting process), the rates were still in the expected direction. Moreover, those who came to believe that their health was adversely affected by the radiation exposure were the most vulnerable of all. It would appear, then, that like other toxic events, Chernobyl has had a protracted psychological toll and that the Chernobyl Forum (2006) was correct that this issue should be regarded as a major public health concern. Whether the psychological toll is the largest public health issue is debatable because other than a handful of outcomes – namely, cataracts, thyroid cancer, and leukemia – other health outcomes, including stress-related cardiovascular disease, have not been systematically investigated.

The studies of cognitive and emotional consequences in the population who were in utero or infants at the time of exposure have not produced consistent findings. The WHO study and two independent studies conducted by Western teams found no significant impact, but local investigations and a recent study in Finland suggest that Chernobyl negatively affected the cognitive and emotional development of this population. The latter findings are well known to the exposed population. In fact, although our research found no differences in objective neuropsychological test performance of evacuees relative to controls, the mothers of the evacuees were far more likely to believe that their children had problems with their memory. Indeed, the mothers reported memory problems irrespective of whether their children were attending university. In 1997, after completing the first wave of our study, we presented the findings at a town hall style meeting in Kiev that was attended by several hundred people. We explained all of our major findings, including the fact that the evacuee children had similar grades in school and performed like their classmates on the neuropsychological measures. At the time, the mothers seemed very relieved to hear that their children performed the same as the comparison group and that there was no evidence that any child had schizophrenia or dementia. Nevertheless, 8 years later, the evacuee mothers still voiced concerns that their children had memory problems. Thus, the objective and subjective realities are incongruent and probably unresolvable. In part this reflects the mothers' overall worry about Chernobyl's effects on their children's health. It is unfortunate that sensational documentaries and media reports continue to appear because these reports have great salience and perpetuate the myths – and hence the fears – associated with Chernobyl.

In contrast to the variety of well-described postdisaster interventions in Western settings (e.g., Ursano, Fullerton, & Norwood, 2003), hardly any systematic descriptions of interventions to confront the post-Chernobyl psychological problems have been published. This does not imply that no efforts have been undertaken to deal with these issues. The Soviet Union, and later the independent republics of Ukraine, Russia, and Belarus, made large investments in rehabilitation actions, such as rehousing projects, hospitals, and invalidity pensions to which increasing numbers of people turned for support over time. These interventions were targeted at the practical and physical consequences of the disaster rather than the psychological effects, but several projects specifically aimed at relieving public anxiety and reducing the mental health burden also have been undertaken. For the most part, these were initiated by international agencies or foreign governments. Unfortunately, the effectiveness of these projects was not systematically evaluated, and hence the extent to which they successfully reduced the levels of psychological morbidity stemming from Chernobyl is open to speculation. The groups that would be of particular importance for such interventions include (1) medical professionals, who have no training in psychosomatic medicine or in recognizing and managing psychological problems in medical populations, (2) local research communities, who need training in epidemiologic and social science research methods and in communicating findings to the media and to their research populations, and (3) community groups, including cohorts currently participating in epidemiologic studies funded by the United States and Europe, who could potentially benefit from information on recognition and self-help treatment for anxiety and depression. Unfortunately, in spite of the enormity of the Chernobyl catastrophe, few resources are likely to be allocated to population-based psychological intervention programs in the foreseeable future.

The accident at Chernobyl left its mark on a population previously exposed to horrific events, including the artificial famine and gulags of the Stalin era, the programmatic extermination of the Jewish population during World War II, and the suffocating political controls that existed until Peristroika. Although the mental health impact of the disaster is likely to be felt for years to come, the affected countries do not have the financial or medical resources to undertake continuing needs assessments or to undertake cohort studies to determine the long-term consequences of the accident. Moreover, in the 20 years since the accident, a number of other tragic events have occurred in the United States, Europe, and elsewhere in the world. The people affected by Chernobyl sense that their plight is no longer of concern to the outside world. We fully support the view of Baverstock and Williams (2006) that the world community must ensure continuing study of the consequences of the accident, and we hope that the mental health consequences among survivors and their offspring will continue to be monitored and managed. Future research on exposed populations must continue to incorporate basic epidemiologic principles of systematic sampling, appropriate control groups, and unbiased measurement, and must consider a comprehensive set of explanatory factors, including epidemiologic risk factors and risk perceptions arising in the wake of Chernobyl. Exposure severity estimates must also be considered, as imprecise as they are likely to be. Toxic disasters such as Chernobyl have persistent effects. Long-term follow-up studies are therefore needed to understand how long these mental health effects endure, what factors are associated with persistence and remission, and what psychological problems, if any, will be encountered by future generations.

ACKNOWLEDGMENTS

This chapter and our research in Kiev was funded by the National Institute of Mental Health (MH51947). The ideas expressed in this chapter were influenced by our collaborations with Semyon Gluzman, founder of the Ukrainian Psychiatric Association, Evgenii Golovakha and Natalia Panina (deceased) of the Ukrainian Academy of Science Institute of Sociology, and Vlodymir Paniotto, founder and director of the Kiev International Institute of Sociology.

REFERENCES

Adams, R. E., Bromet, E. J., Panina, N., & Golovakha, E. (2007). The Chernobyl nuclear power plant disaster and the well-being of mothers with children 20 years later. Presented at the Society for the Study of Social Problems, New York City.

Adams, R. E., Bromet, E. J., Panina, N., Golovakha, E., Goldgaber, D., & Gluzman, S. (2002). Stress and well-being in mothers of young children 11 years after the Chornobyl nuclear power plant accident. *Psychological Medicine*, *32*, 143–156.

Bar Joseph, N., Reisfeld, D., Tirosh, E., Silman, Z., & Rennert, G. (2004). Neurobehavioral and cognitive performances in children exposed to low-dose radiation in the Chernobyl accident: The Israeli Chernobyl Health Effects Study. *American Journal of Epidemiology*, *160*, 453–459.

Baverstock, K., & Williams, D. (2006). The Chernobyl accident 20 years on: An assessment of the health consequences and the international response. *Environmental Health Perspectives*, *114*, 1312–1317.

Benedek, D. M., Fullerton, C., & Ursano, R. J. (2007). .First responders: Mental health consequences of natural and human-made disasters for public health and public safety workers. *Annual Review of Public Health*, *28*, 55–68.

Braithwaite, J., & Hoopengardner, T. (1997). Who are Ukraine's poor? In P. K. Cornelius & P. Lenain (Eds.), *Ukraine: Accelerating the transition to market*. Washington, D.C.: International Monetary Fund.

Bromet, E. J., Gluzman, S. F., Paniotto, V. I., Webb, C. P., Tintle, N. L., Zakhozha, V., Havenaar, J. M., et al. (2005). Epidemiology of psychiatric and alcohol disorders in Ukraine: Findings from the Ukraine World Mental Health Survey. *Social Psychiatry and Psychiatric Epidemiology*, *40*, 481–690.

Bromet, E. J., Gluzman, S., Schwartz, J. E., & Goldgaber, D. (2002). Somatic symptoms in women 11 years after the Chornobyl accident: Prevalence and risk factors. *Environmental Health Perspectives*, *110*(Suppl. 4), 625–629.

Bromet, E. J., Goldgaber, D., Carlson, G., Panina, N., Golovakha, E., Gluzman, S. F., et al. (2000). Children's well-being 11 years after the Chornobyl catastrophe. *Archives of General Psychiatry*, *57*, 563–571.

Bromet, E. J., & Havenaar J. M. (2002). Mental health consequences of disasters. In N. Sartorius, W. Gaebel, J. J. Ibor-Lopez, & M. Maj (Eds.), *Psychiatry in society*. London: Wiley.

(2006). Basic epidemiologic approaches to disaster research: value of face-to-face procedures. In F. H. Norris, S. Galea, M. J. Friedman, & P. J. Watson (Eds.), *Methods for disaster mental health research*. New York: Guilford Press.

Bromet, E. J., Parkinson, D. K., & Dunn, L. O. (1990). Long-term mental health consequences of the accident at Three Mile Island. *International Journal of Mental Health*, *19*, 48–60.

Centers for Disease Control and Prevention (CDC). (2004). Mental health status of World Trade Center rescue and recovery workers and volunteers – New York City, July 2002–August 2004. *Morbidity and Mortality Weekly Report*, *53*, 812–815.

Derogatis, L. R. (1983). *Symptom Checklist-90-Revised: Administration, scoring, and procedures manual-II*. Towson, MD: Clinical Psychometric Research.

Drabick, D. A. G., Gadow, K. D., Carlson, G. A., & Bromet, E. J. (2004). ODD and ADHD symptoms in Ukrainian children: External validators and comorbidity. *Journal of the American Academy of Child and Adolescent Psychiatry*, *43*, 735–743.

Gamache, G. L., Levinson, D. M., Reeves, D. L., Bidyuk, P. I., & Brantley, K. K. (2005). Longitudinal neurocognitive assessments of Ukrainians exposed to ionizing radiation after the Chernobyl nuclear accident. *Archives of Clinical Neuropsychology, 20*, 81–93.

Gluzman, S. F. (1991). Abuse of psychiatry: Analysis of the guilt of medical personnel. *Journal of Medical Ethics, 17, 19*–20.

Gluzman, S., & Kostyuchenko, S. (2006). Psychiatry in Ukraine. *Bulletin of the Board of International Affairs of the Royal College of Psychiatrists, 3*, 12–14.

Goldberg, D., McDowell, I., & Newell, C. (1996). *Measuring health: A guide to rating scales and questionnaires. 2nd ed.* New York: Oxford University Press.

Hatch, M., Ron, E., Bouville, A., Zablotska, L., & Howe, G. (2005). The Chernobyl disaster: Cancer following the accident at the Chernobyl nuclear power plant. *Epidemiologic Reviews, 27*, 56–66.

Havenaar, J. M., Cwikel, J., & Bromet, E. (Eds.). (2002). *Toxic turmoil: Psychological and societal consequences of ecological disasters.* New York: Plenum.

Havenaar, J. M., van den Brink, W., Kasyanenko, A. P., van den Bout, J., Meijler-Iljina, L. I., Poelijoe, N. W., et al. (1996). Mental health problems in the Gomel Region (Belarus). An analysis of risk factors in an area affected by the Chernobyl disaster. *Psychological Medicine, 26*, 845–855.

Havenaar, J. M., Rumyantzeva, G. M., van den Brink, W., Poelijoe, N. W., van den Bout, J., van Engeland, H., & Koeter, M. W. J. (1997). Long-term mental health effects of the Chernobyl disaster: An epidemiological survey in two former Soviet Regions. *American Journal of Psychiatry, 154*, 1605–1607

Havenaar, J. M., Rumyantzeva, G. M., Kasyanenko, A. P., Kaasjager, K., Westermann, A. M., van den Brink, W., et al. (1997). Health effects of the Chernobyl disaster: illness or illness behaviour? A comparative general health survey in two former Soviet Regions. *Environmental Health Perspectives, 105*(Suppl. 6), 1533–1537.

Havenaar, J. M., de Wilde, E. J., van den Bout, J., Drottz-Sjöberg, B.-M., & van de Brink, W. (2003). Perception of risk and subjective health among victims of the Chernobyl disaster. *Social Science and Medicine, 56*, 569–572.

Huizink, A. C., Dick, D. M., Sihvola, E., Pulkkinen, L., Rose, R. J., & Kaprio, J. (2007). Chernobyl exposure as stressor during pregnancy and behaviour in adolescent offspring. *Acta Psychiatrica Scandinavica, 116*(6), 438–446.

Igumnov, S., & Drozdovitch V. (2000). The intellectual development, mental and behavioral disorders in children from Belarus exposed in utero following the Chernobyl accident. *European Psychiatry, 15*, 244–253.

Imamura, Y., Nakane, Y., Ohta, Y., & Kondo, H. (1999). Lifetime prevalence of schizophrenia among individuals prenatally exposed to atomic bomb radiation in Nagasaki City. *Acta Psychiatrica Scandinavica, 100*, 344–349.

Kessler, R. C., & Üstün, T. B. (2004). The World Mental Health (WMH) Survey Initiative Version of the World Health Organization (WHO) Composite International Diagnostic Interview (CIDI). *International Journal of Methods in Psychiatric Research, 13*, 93–121.

Kolominsky, Y., Igumnov, S., & Drozdovitch, V. (1999). The psychological development of children from Belarus exposed in the prenatal period to radiation from the Chernobyl atomic power plant. *Journal of Child Psychology & Psychiatry, 40*, 299–305.

Litcher, L., Bromet, E. J., Carlson, G., Squires, N., Goldgaber, D., Panina, N., et al. (2000). School and neuropsychological performance of evacuated children in Kiev 11 years after the Chornobyl disaster. *Journal of Child Psychology and Psychiatry, 41*, 291–299.

Loganovsky, K., Havenaar, J.M., Tintle, N., Tung, L., Kotov, R.I., & Bromet E.J. (2008). The mental health of clean-up workers 18 years after the Chornobyl accident. *Psychological Medicine, 38*, 481–488.

Loganovsky, K. N., & Loganovskaja, T. K. (2000). Schizophrenia spectrum disorders in persons exposed to ionizing radiation as a result of the Chernobyl accident. *Schizophrenia Bulletin, 26*, 751–773.

Nicholson, A., Bobak, M., Murphy, M., Rose, R., & Marmot, M. (2005). Alcohol consumption and increased mortality in Russian men and women: A cohort study based on the mortality of relatives. *Bulletin of the World Health Organization, 83*, 812–819.

Nyagu, A. I., Loganovsky, K. N., & Loganovskaja, T. K. (1998). Psychophysiologic aftereffects of prenatal irradiation. *International Journal of Psychophysiology, 30*, 303–311.

Otake, M., & Schull, W. J. (1984). In utero exposure to A-bomb radiation and mental retardation: A reassessment. *British Journal of Radiology, 57*, 409–414.

Parkinson, D. K., & Bromet, E. J. (1983). Correlates of mental health in nuclear and coal-fired power plant workers. *Scandinavian Journal of Work, Environment and Health, 9*, 341–345.

Polyukhov, A. M., Kobsar, I. V., Grebelnik, V. I., & Voitenko, V. P. (2000). The accelerated occurrence of age-related changes of organism in Chernobyl workers: A radiation-induced progeroidsyndrome? *Experimental Gerontology*, *35*, 105–115.

Rahu, K., Rahu, M., Tekkel, M., & Bromet, E. (2006). Suicide risk among Chernobyl cleanup workers in Estonia still increased: An updated cohort study. *Annals of Epidemiology*, *16*, 917–919.

Rahu, M., Tekkel, M., Veidebaum, T., Pukkala, T., Hakulinen, A., Auvinen, A., et al. (1997). The Estonian study of Chernobyl clean-up workers: II. Incidence of cancer and mortality. *Radiation Research*, *147*, 653–657.

Schull, W. J., & Otake, M. (1999). Cognitive function and prenatal exposure to ionizing radiation. *Teratology*, *59*, 222–226.

Shulman, N., & Adams, B. (2002). A comparison of Russian and British attitudes towards mental health problems in the community. *International Journal of Social Psychiatry*, *48*, 266–278.

Taormina, D. P., Rozenblatt, S., Guey, L. T., Gluzman, S. F., Carlson, G. A., Havenaar, J. M., et al. (2008). The Chornobyl accident and cognitive functioning: A follow-up study of infant evacuees at age 19 years. *Psychological Medicine*, *38*, 489–497.

The Chernobyl Forum 2003–2005. (2006). *Chernobyl's legacy: Health, environmental, and socio-economic impacts*. Austria: IAEA.

Ursano, R. J., Fullerton, S., & Norwood, A. E. (Eds.). (2003). *Terrorism and disaster. Individual and community mental health interventions.* Cambridge: Cambridge University Press.

Viinamäki, H., Kumpusalo, E., Myllykangas, M., Salomaa, S., Kumpusalo, L., Kolmakov, S., et al. (1995). The Chernobyl accident and mental well-being – a population study. *Acta Psychiatrica Scandinavica*, *91*, 396–401.

Weiss, D. S., & Marmar, C. R. (1997). The Impact of Event Scale-revised. In J. P. Wilson & T. M. Keane (Eds.), *Assessing psychological trauma and PTSD.* New York: Guilford Press.

World Bank. (2003) *Ukraine country brief*. http://lnweb18.worldbank.org/eca/eca.nsf

World Health Organization. (1995). *Health consequences of the Chernobyl accident. Results of the IPHECA plot projects and related national programmes*. Geneva: World Health Organization.

27 The *Exxon Valdez* Oil Spill

LAWRENCE A. PALINKAS

27.1. INTRODUCTION

On Friday, March 24, 1989, at approximately 12:30 a.m., the 987-foot supertanker *Exxon Valdez* ran aground on Bligh Reef (approximately 25 miles from the city of Valdez, Alaska), spilling over 11 million gallons (260,000 barrels) of crude oil into the once-pristine environment of Prince William Sound. The oil spread more than 750 km to the southwest along the Kenai Peninsula, Kodiak Archipelago, and the Alaska Peninsula (Figure 27.1). After considerable delay, Exxon officials arrived on the scene and initiated a sequence of actions designed to contain and clean up the spill. Fishing vessels were hired to help lay containment booms; fish tenders were hired to transport equipment and to ferry refuse to disposal or transhipment sites; and entire communities were hired to protect their own beaches. To protect vital resources, local governments were drawn into the response, committing the use of local community facilities (offices, meeting places, equipment, services, etc.) to organize, coordinate, and perform cleanup.

Under the direction of Exxon and its prime contractor, VECO, thousands of residents and nonresidents were hired to participate in the cleanup effort. Beaches were scoured with high-pressure water hoses and countless numbers of rocks were scrubbed to remove surface oil. Hundreds of fishing vessels boomed floating oil slicks while larger vessels ("skimmers") siphoned off collected oil. The highly advertised wages ($17.69 per hour) attracted both employed and unemployed individuals – initially from within Alaska, but later drawing workers from all over the United States. Such high wages for unskilled workers made it difficult for local enterprises such as hotels, shops, restaurants, grocery stores, and canneries to retain their employees. A chain reaction had begun that was to affect virtually every aspect of social and economic relations in the region.

In the wake of the spill, the public; subsequent mitigation efforts by Exxon and federal, state, and local agencies; and eventual litigation over damages all primarily focused on the direct environmental and economic impacts. An estimated 1,000 to 2,800 sea otters died as a result of contact with the oil, along with an estimated 250,000 to 500,000 seabirds and 302 harbor seals; oiling of fur and feathers caused loss of insulating capacity and led to death from hypothermia, smothering, drowning, and inhalation or ingestion of toxic hydrocarbons (Peterson et al., 2003). Mass mortality also occurred among macroalgae and benthic invertebrates on oiled shores through a combination of chemical toxicity, smothering, and physical displacement during cleanup (Peterson et al., 2003). The elevated mortality of incubating pink salmon eggs in oiled streams for at least 4 years after the spill was attributed to exposure to polycyclic aromatic hydrocarbons (PAHs) from partially weathered oil (Bui, Sharr, & Seeb, 1998). Loss in revenues for the commercial fishing industry totaled over $155 million in the 2 years immediately following the spill (Cohen, 1995), largely because of the total collapse of the herring fishery and a significant decline in the pink salmon fishery (Spies, Rice, Wolfe, & Wright, 1996). Fortunately, more recent studies on levels of toxins in fish have painted a

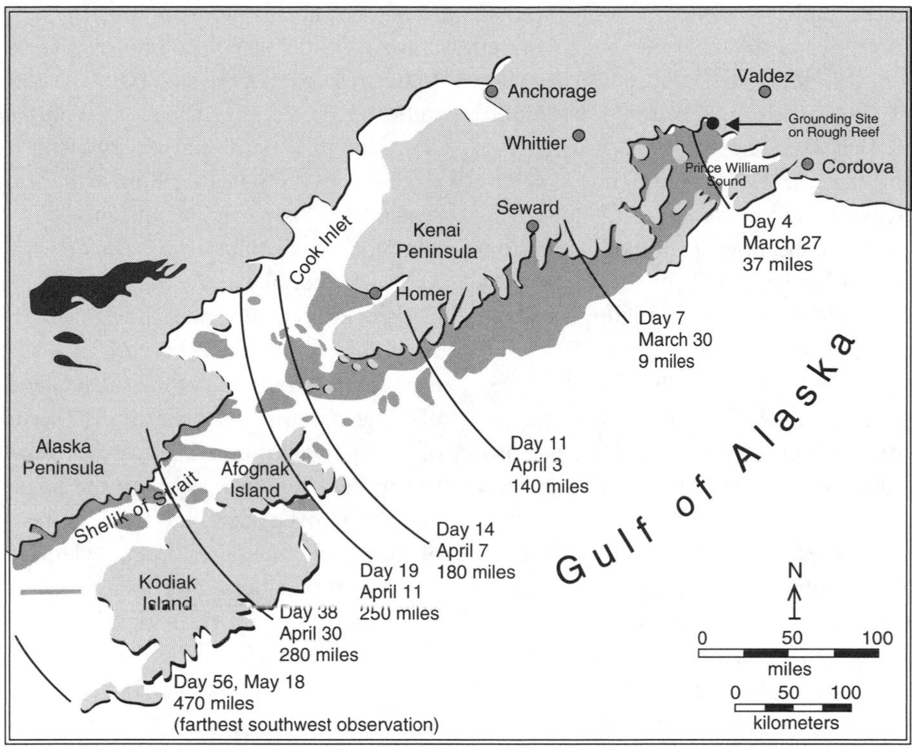

Figure 27.1. Map of the area affected by the *Exxon Valdez* oil spill, 1989.
Composite done by the *Exxon Valdez* Trustee Council from an original map by the Alaska Dept. of Environmental Conservation. It can be found on the site http://www.wholetruth.net/history.htm

somewhat hopeful picture of diminishing effects of the oil spill over time on the natural habitat of the region (Neff et al., 2006). Nevertheless, oil stranded by the spill has persisted in subsurface sediments of exposed shores for 16 years (Short et al., 2007). The remaining oil is in sufficient quantities and at toxic levels to induce chronic biological exposures with long-term impacts at the population level – especially among species associated with shallow sediments – and delayed population impacts from sublethal doses that compromise health, growth, and reproduction (Peterson et al., 2003).

Although the direct impacts of the oil spill on human health was believed to be minimal (Lord, 1997), there was also concern about the indirect social and psychological impacts. This concern stemmed from three distinct sources. The first was the largely anecdotal evidence of community conflict created by the unequal distribution of cleanup jobs and compensation for the use of boats and equipment owned by local residents and the influx of outsiders and resulting strain on community services (Dyer, Gill, & Picou, 1992; Impact Assessment, 1990; Minerals Management Service, 1993; Palinkas, Downs, Petterson, & Russell, 1993; Rodin, Downs, Petterson, & Russell, 1992). The second source of concern was the dramatic increase in visits to community clinics for primary care and mental health services reported throughout the affected region (Impact Assessment, 1990; Russell, Downs, Petterson, & Palinkas, 1996). The third was the evidence from earlier research that found significantly increased rates of physical health symptoms, psychiatric disorders, and disruption of social relations after other technological disasters, such as those that occurred at Three Mile Island, Bhopal, Chernobyl, and Love Canal (Baum & Fleming, 1993; Baum,

Gatchel, & Schaeffer, 1983; Bogard, 1989; Bromet, Gluzman, Schwartz, & Goldgaber, 2002; Bromet, Parkinson, Schulberg, & Dunn, 1980; Brown & Harris, 1979; Davidson & Baum, 1991; Houts, Cleary, & Hsu, 1988; Levine, 1982; Robins et al., 1986; Shrivastava, 1987). These impacts have been attributed to the uncertainty underlying the extent and consequences of biophysical contamination (Davidson & Baum, 1991; Erikson, 1991; Vyner, 1988), the protracted litigation over compensation for damages incurred (Brown & Mikkelsen, 1989; Picou & Rosebrook, 1993), and the emergence of a "corrosive" community context, which prolongs the recovery process (Freudenberg & Jones, 1991; Kroll-Smith & Couch, 1991, 1993).

The *Exxon Valdez* spill represents a specific type of technological disaster, one that impacted a population living in predominately natural or renewable resource communities, and one that did not result in a loss of human life but did result in a loss of social and material resources. A natural or renewable resource community is a population of individuals who live within a bounded area and whose primary cultural, social, and economic existences are based on the harvest and use of natural renewable resources (Dyer et al., 1992; Gill, 1994). Such a community is highly vulnerable to negative impacts from technological disasters because long-term environmental change may prevent the timely recovery of an established resource base, thus threatening core cultural traditions (Dyer et al., 1992). Disruption of these traditions can result in on-going social disruptions or secondary disasters (Erikson, 1976), leading to conflicts between friends and family, resentment toward neighbors who have been spared loss or perceived to have been overcompensated for loss, and anger and suspicion toward outsiders engaged in cleanup and recovery (Erikson, 1976). Such impacts represent a loss of social support, which can have significant consequences (Hobfoll, 1989).

However, the *Exxon Valdez* oil spill was more than an account of disaster-related psychosocial impacts. It was also an event of sociocultural change (Dyer, 1993; Gill & Picou, 1997; Minerals Management Service, 1993; Palinkas, Downs, et al., 1993). For both Native and non-Native residents of the small, rural communities in the affected region, the event represented the alteration of a traditional way of life in response to contact with the larger Euro-American social system. In this particular instance, this contact assumed two distinct forms. The first was the oil itself, whether physically during participation in cleanup efforts, culturally in terms of effects on traditional subsistence harvesting activities, or economically in terms of the subsequent closure of certain commercial fisheries. The second form of contact was the involvement of residents in the affected communities with the management and personnel of Exxon, VECO, representatives of numerous federal and state agencies, and a barrage of outsiders interested in participating in cleanup efforts for a variety of monetary or altruistic reasons.

27.2. PSYCHOSOCIAL IMPACTS

27.2.1. *Exxon Valdez* Oil Spill Studies

Although several studies of the psychosocial impacts of the oil spill were conducted (see Davis, 1996, for a review), only three studies provided any quantifiable estimates of the onset and persistence of psychiatric disorders. The first was the "Oiled Mayors" Study, conducted from 1989 to 1990 by Impact Assessment, Incorporated (Impact Assessment, 1990; McLees-Palinkas, 1994; Palinkas, Downs, et al., 1993; Palinkas, Petterson, Downs, & Russell, 2004; Palinkas, Petterson, Russell, & Downs, 1993; Palinkas, Russell, Downs, & Petterson, 1992; Rodin et al., 1992; Russell et al., 1996). In addition to methods for the assessment of fiscal and operations impacts on local governments and economic impacts on the private sector, the Oiled Mayors Study employed two different sets of methods in the assessment of social and psychological impacts of the oil spill. One was a qualitative analysis of data collected in 22 different communities by trained fieldworkers who conducted interviews with community leaders, health and social service workers, businessmen, and local residents.

The other set of methods used was a quantitative assessment of data collected from a survey of almost 600 randomly selected households located in 13 different communities between March 30 and May 15, 1990. Eleven of these communities ($N=437$ households) were in the region directly exposed to the oil spill itself. In addition, two communities in southeast Alaska far from the oil spill ($N=162$ households) served as a source of unexposed respondents. The impact of the oil spill on psychosocial outcomes was determined by classifying study participants by their exposure to the oil spill and subsequent events on the basis of responses to six different questions: (1) Did you or anyone in your household use, before the spill, areas along the coast that were affected by the spill? (2) Did you work on any of the shoreline or water cleanup activities of the oil spill? (3) Are there any other ways that you came into contact with the oil spill or cleanup activities, such as during recreation, hunting, fishing, or gathering activities? (4) Did you have any property that was lost or damaged because of the oil spill or cleanup? (5) Did the oil spill cause any damage to the areas you or other household members fish commercially? (6) Has the oil spill directly affected the hunting, fishing or gathering activities of any members of this household? Each response was coded 0 for a "no" response and 1 for a "yes"; the responses were then summed to provide a continuous measure of exposure with a range of 0 to 6 in an ordinal scale. The exposure index was found to have internal consistency reliability (Cronbach's alpha = 0.74) for this population. The mean exposure score for all study respondents was 1.97 (SD = 1.77).

Subjects were classified into three groups on the basis of maximum level of exposure. Residents in the study communities were classified as being either exposed or unexposed, depending on whether their exposure index score fell above or below the group median (2.00). Exposed residents were further dichotomized into low-exposed (exposure index scores = 2 or 3) and high-exposed (exposure index score = 4 and above) groups on the basis of a median split. Psychosocial outcomes assessed included depressive symptoms, using the Centers for Epidemiologic Studies-Depression (CES-D) Scale (Radloff, 1977), DSM-III diagnosis of Generalized Anxiety Disorder (GAD), and DSM-IIIR diagnosis of posttraumatic stress disorder (PTSD), using modules from the Diagnostic Interview Schedule (Robins, Helzer, Cottler, & Goldring, 1989; Robins, Helzer, Croughan, & Ratcliff, 1981) and questions relating to levels of and problems with drinking, drug abuse, and domestic violence since the spill and changes in social and family relations compared to the same period in the year before the spill (1988) (Impact Assessment, 1990). Both postspill (respondents' recollections of having experienced the symptoms within the past year – i.e., since the oil spill) and lifetime (recollections of ever having experienced these symptoms) prevalences of GAD and PTSD were calculated, and prevalence (symptoms experienced in the past week) of CES-D scores of 16 and above and 18 and above (the latter reflecting the need to increase the scale's specificity and reduce the positive misclassification rate in the face of observed ethnic differences in response patterns to the measure; see Palinkas et al., 1992) (Palinkas, Petterson, et al., 1993).

The second study was conducted by John Picou and colleagues from the University of South Alabama (Arata, Picou, Johnson, & McNally, 2000; Dyer, 1993; Dyer et al., 1992; Gill, 1994; Picou, Gill, & Cohen, 1997; Picou, Gill, Dyer, & Curry, 1992). Picou and associates collected data in Cordova, Valdez, and Petersburg, Alaska, in a series of studies beginning 4 and 1-half months after the oil spill and lasting until 1992. Study samples ranged from 125 (Arata et al., 2000) to 449 (Picou & Gill, 1996). Data were gathered through personal interviews with respondents, mail-out surveys, and telephone interviews. Petersburg was selected as a control community because of its similarity in demographic and economic characteristics to Cordova, while Valdez was selected because it represented a nonrenewable resource community also impacted by the oil spill. Alaskan Natives in Cordova were sampled using a network snowball sampling strategy, while non-Natives were sampled using a random household survey. Psychosocial impacts assessed included study participants' perceptions of changes in family, work, and community; measures of intrusive stress and avoidance behavior using the Impact of Events Scale (Horowitz, Milner, & Alvarez, 1979); and measures of anxiety, depression, and CR-PTSD using subscales from the SCL90-R (Arata, Saunders, & Kilpatrick, 1991).

Within a 12-month period after the oil spill itself, the Valdez Counseling Center conducted a survey of adult residents of the communities of Valdez ($N=64$) and Cordova ($N=53$) to determine the psychological impact of the *Exxon Valdez* oil spill for the purpose of mental health assessment and intervention planning (Donald, Cook, Bixby, Benda, & Wolf, 1990). Subjects were selected using a computer generated, simple random sample of registered voters. A second questionnaire was mailed to initial survey respondents approximately 8 months after the oil spill, and a third questionnaire was mailed approximately 12 months after the oil spill. Perceived social support was assessed using six items taken from the Interpersonal Support Evaluation List (ISEL) (Cohen & Hoberman, 1983). Depressive symptoms were measured using the CES-D scale described earlier. The 20-item Frederick Reaction Index (Frederick, 1987) was used to evaluate the level of stress response to the oil spill.

27.2.2. Psychiatric Disorders

The Oiled Mayors Study found that exposure to the oil spill and subsequent cleanup was significantly associated with the postspill prevalence of GAD, PTSD, and CES-D scores of 16 and above and 18 and above (Figure 27.2). When age, sex, and ethnicity were controlled, compared with the unexposed group, members of the high-exposed group were 3.7 times (95% CI = 2.0–7.0) as likely to have GAD, 2.6 times (95% CI = 1.2–5.7) as likely to have PTSD, 1.8 times (95% CI = 0.9–3.6) as likely to have a CES-D score of 16 and above, and 2.1 times (95% CI = 1.0–4.5) as likely to have a CES-D score of 18 and above. Members of the high-exposed group were also 2 times (95% CI = 1.0–3.6) as likely to have GAD as members

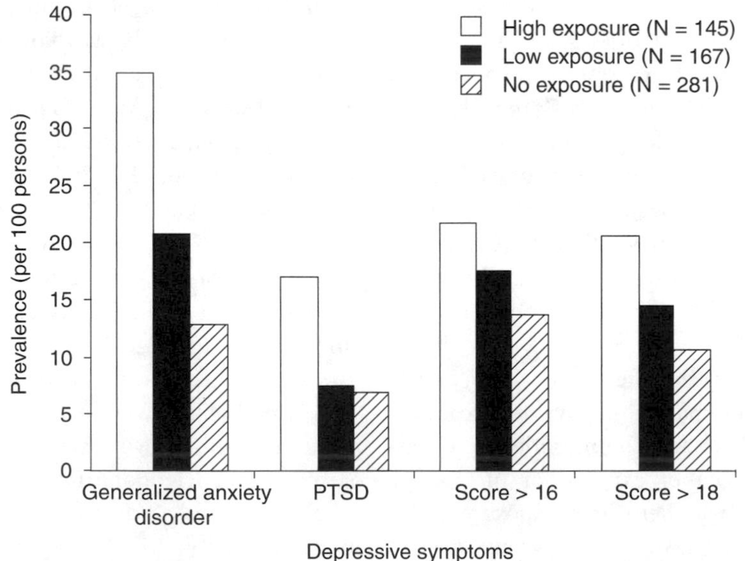

Figure 27.2. Prevalence of generalized anxiety disorder[a], PTSD[a], and depressive symptoms[b] in Oiled Mayors Study respondents ($N=593$) by exposure status, 1990.

Notes:

[a]One year after the spill.

[b]Centers for Epidemiologic Studies-Depression (CES-D) Scale scores within the past week.

of the low-exposed group who, in turn, were 1.9 times (95% CI = 1.0–3.6) as likely to have GAD as members of the unexposed group (Palinkas, Petterson, et al., 1993).

The high prevalence of psychiatric disorders revealed in the Oiled Mayors Study was confirmed by the results of the Picou et al. and the Valdez Counseling Center studies. Picou and colleagues (Picou et al., 1992; Dyer et al., 1992) identified significantly higher levels of intrusive stress and avoidance behavior in Cordova than in the control community of Petersburg 5 months after the spill and continuing over an 18-month period. Of the 43 Cordova respondents in the Valdez Counseling Center study, 36 (83%) reported symptoms consistent with the criteria for a diagnosis of PTSD. Of the Valdez sample, 65% reported symptoms consistent with PTSD at some point in the study (Donald et al., 1990).

Previous studies have found that comorbid conditions (the presence of more than one disorder in an individual) are more likely to occur after a disaster than single psychiatric disorders. For instance, Shore and his colleagues (Shore, Tatum, & Vollmer, 1986) found the presence of Mount St. Helen's Syndrome, which consisted of symptoms of depression, anxiety, and PTSD, in victims of the Mount St. Helen's disaster. A similar cluster of symptoms was reported by Smith and her colleagues (1990) among victims of a plane crash at a hotel. In the Oiled Mayors Study, household survey respondents in the high-exposed group were twice as likely to have at least one of the three psychiatric conditions ($\chi^2 = 21.7$, $p < 0.0001$), 2.4 times as likely to have more than one of the three psychiatric conditions ($\chi^2 = 12.0$, $p < 0.0001$), and 3.9 times as likely to have all three psychiatric conditions as individuals in the unexposed group ($\chi^2 = 8.6$, $p = 0.003$) (Figure 27.3).

Since the Oiled Mayors Study was cross-sectional, it was unable to determine the persistence of these symptoms over time. The Valdez Counseling Center, however, evaluated symptoms of PTSD and depression at three different points over a 1-year period following the oil spill itself (Donald et al., 1990). This study reported a decline in PTSD in Valdez from 50% 2 months after the spill, to 42% at 8 months after, to 30% at 12 months after. In Cordova, the prevalence of PTSD increased from 49% to 53.5% 8 months after the spill before declining to 44.2% at 12 months after the spill. In Valdez, the mean CES-D score increased from 6.5 two months after the spill to 10.2 at 8 months after, before declining slightly to 8.6 12 months after. In Cordova, mean CES-D scores remained relatively constant

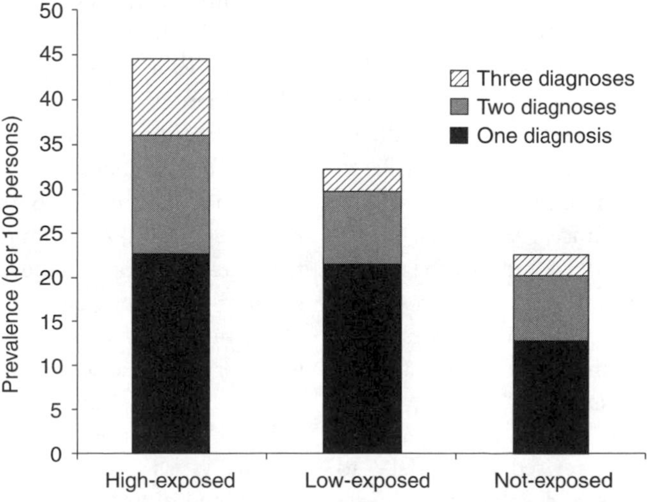

Figure 27.3. Prevalence of comorbid psychiatric disorders by exposure status, Oiled Mayors Study.

from 9.0 two months after the spill, to 8.9 at 8 months after, to 9.3 at 12 months after. In the Picou study, residents of Cordova did experience an overall reduction in the level of intrusive stress as measured by the IES but no change in the level of avoidance behavior 14 months later (Picou et al., 1992).

The findings of an association between exposure to the oil spill and increased prevalence of PTSD is noteworthy because it raises the issue of whether events that do not result in a loss of life are sufficiently traumatic to meet the Criterion A requirements for a diagnosis of PTSD. In DSM-IIIR, a traumatic event was defined as one that is

> outside the range of usual human experience and that would be markedly distressing to almost everyone, e.g., serious threat to one's life or physical integrity; serious threat or harm to one's children, spouse, or other close relatives and friends; sudden destruction of one's home or community; or seeing another person who has recently been, or is being, seriously injured or killed as the result of an accident or physical violence. (American Psychiatric Association, 1987, p. 250)

Many have argued that only the experience of death of others or the imminent threat of death to oneself is sufficient to warrant a diagnosis of PTSD. This argument was supported by research on combat veterans (Friedman, Schneiderman, & West, 1986) and victims of natural and man-made disasters (Shore, Vollmer, & Tatum, 1989; Green, Grace, & Gleser, 1985). Others have argued that the definition of an event as traumatic may vary from one culture to the next, from one individual to the next, and even from one experience to the next in the same individual (Davidson & Foa, 1993; Lindy, Green, & Grace, 1987; Neria, Nandi, & Galea, 2007; Norris, 1992) and that the definition of a traumatic event (Criterion A) should be broadened to allow for the empirical assessment of events that elicit symptoms of posttraumatic stress (Kilpatrick & Resnick, 1993).

In response to this debate, the criteria for a traumatic event was revised in DSM-IV to include both objective and subjective criteria and to eliminate the notion that the event must be "outside the range of normal human experience" (American Psychiatric Association, 1994, pp. 427–428). The revised criteria took into account the possibility that "different people can have profoundly different conceptions as to what constitutes a realistic 'threat'" (Young, 1995, p. 289). It also raised the possibility that an event or series of events may be sufficiently traumatic to warrant a diagnosis of PTSD – even in the absence of death or serious physical injury – if it threatens one's physical integrity or the physical integrity of others (Tomb, 1994).

It may also be argued that an event is sufficiently traumatic to warrant a diagnosis of PTSD if it threatens one's social integrity as well. Several studies have noted an association between PTSD and poor social support in military combat veterans (Fontana & Rosenheck, 1994; King, King, Foy, Keane, & Fairbank, 1999; Schnurr, Lunney, & Sengupta, 2004) and disaster victims (Acierno et al., 2007; Feng et al., 2007; Galea et al., 2002) and the loss of members of social networks in natural disasters and war (Kinzie et al., 1990; Norris, Baker, Murphy, & Kaniasty, 2005). A stressor is more likely to produce PTSD if, among other things, it is isolating or does damage to one's community or support systems (Tomb, 1994).

Finally, it may be argued that an event is sufficiently traumatic to warrant a diagnosis of PTSD if it threatens the integrity of the physical environment. In his Conservation of Resources Model, Hobfoll (1988) defines psychological stress as a reaction to the environment in which there is a net loss or threat of a net loss of resources – objects, personal characteristics, conditions, or energies that are valued by the individual. According to this conservation of resources model, environmental circumstances may threaten people's status, position, economic stability, loved ones, basic beliefs, or self-esteem. The actual or threatened loss of these resources is important because they have instrumental as well as symbolic value in that they help people define who they are.

Finally, as Neria and colleagues (2007) have noted, differences in the definition of the Criterion A between DSM-IV and DSM-IIIR, the latter being the basis for the assessment of PTSD in the Oiled Mayors Study, may influence rates, correlates, and course of PTSD, as documented across studies over time. Comparison of the results of this study with subsequent studies of other disasters would have to take these differences into account.

27.2.3. Substance Abuse

The oil spill resulted in a significant increase in alcohol and drug abuse as perceived by the respondents of the Oiled Mayors household survey. Individuals in the high-exposed group were significantly more likely to report an increase in drug and alcohol abuse in their community and among family and friends than individuals in the unexposed group (Palinkas, Downs, et al., 1993; Russell et al., 1996). In addition to a perceived increase in these activities, individuals in the high-exposed group were significantly more likely to report an increase in problems associated with drug and alcohol abuse in their community and among family and friends than individuals in the unexposed group (Palinkas, Downs, et al., 1992; Russell et al., 1996).

Self-reports of increases in alcohol and drug use were assessed in the Valdez Counseling Center study. However, only 3 of the 43 Cordova respondents and 1 of the 50 Valdez respondents indicated their alcohol consumption and/or illicit drug use had increased since the oil spill (Donald et al., 1990). In contrast to the Oiled Mayors Study, which asked respondents to describe patterns of substance use in others, this study asked respondents to describe their own patterns of use, which may account for the conflicting findings.

27.2.4. Disruption of Social Relations

Analyses of the data collected in the Oiled Mayors Study household survey found that exposure to the oil spill had a number of adverse effects on social relations both within and outside the household (Palinkas, Downs, et al., 1993; Russell et al., 1996). Compared with the unexposed group, individuals in the high-exposed group were significantly more likely to report an increase in fighting in their community and among family and friends, and an increase in problems associated with domestic violence in their community. A measure of social disruption (Palinkas et al., 2004) that included relations both within and outside the household was 4.6 times greater in high-exposed individuals than in unexposed individuals, and 2.8 times greater in low-exposed individuals than in unexposed individuals (Figure 27.4). Exposure to the oil spill and cleanup was significantly associated with reported declines in social relations with relatives not in the home, friends and neighbors, coworkers, and residents of other communities, compared to the same period in 1988 (Palinkas, Downs, et al., 1993; Russell et al., 1996). Individuals in the high-exposed group were also significantly more likely to report a conflict with outsiders and with friends since the spill than individuals in the unexposed group.

Picou and associates also found evidence of severe disruption in social relations within the family, the workplace, and the community in 1989 resulting from the oil spill (Dyer et al., 1992). In 1989, Cordova respondents were significantly more likely to report disruption in relations within the family, in the workplace, and within the community than their counterparts in Petersburg. Moreover, although the decline in the percentage reporting such disruption was greater in Cordova than Petersburg between 1989 and 1990, greater proportions of Cordova

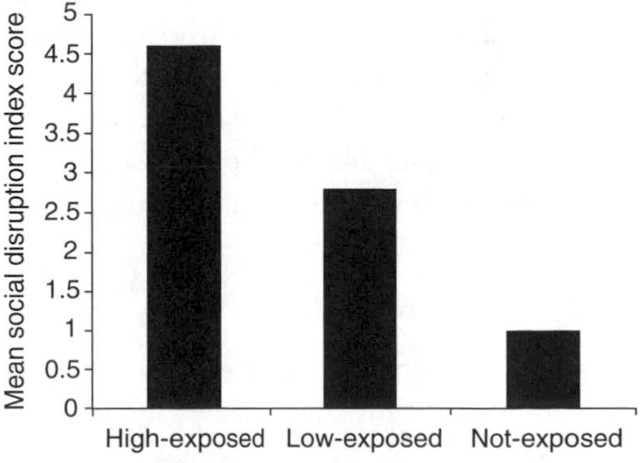

Figure 27.4. Mean social disruption index score by exposure status, Oiled Mayors Study, 1990.

respondents reported such declines in 1990 than their counterparts in Petersburg.

Although numerous studies have found social support to mediate the association between traumatic events and psychiatric disorders (Brewin, Andrews, & Valentine, 2000), it is also possible that the psychiatric disorders experienced by victims of the *Exxon Valdez* oil spill contributed to the disruption of social relations. Studies of PTSD and social support among a sample of Gulf War I veterans found that PTSD symptoms more strongly predicted subsequent social support than social support predicted subsequent PTSD (Keane, Marshall, & Taft, 2006). Kaniasty and Norris (2004) have observed a similar phenomenon among victims of disasters and acts of terrorism.

27.3. RISK AND PROTECTIVE FACTORS

Analyses of the psychosocial impacts of the oil spill described earlier revealed distinct subgroups or segments of the population that were especially vulnerable. For instance, women were particularly vulnerable to the effects of exposure to the oil spill and cleanup activities on the prevalence of GAD (OR = 1.4; 95% CI = 1.2–1.7), PTSD (OR = 1.4; 95% CI = 1.2–1.7), and CES-D scores of 18 and above (OR = 1.4; 95% CI = 1.1–1.6). Younger adults (18–44 years) were at increased risk of depressive symptoms (Palinkas, Petterson, et al., 1993). However, the increased risk of psychiatric disorders, substance abuse, domestic violence, and disruption of social relations was especially evident among five particular subgroups: local residents who participated in spill cleanup activities; residents who experienced loss of commercial, subsistence, and social resources; families and children; Alaska Natives; and participants in subsequent litigation.

27.3.1. Cleanup Participants

Studies of the *Exxon Valdez* oil spill suggested that individuals involved in cleanup activities were subjected to similar forms of stress for a number of reasons. These individuals were most exposed to the devastation resulting from the spill; they were able to observe firsthand the extent of the environmental damage resulting from the spread of oil and to grasp the significance of this damage in terms of its impact on their traditional way of life. They were also involved in the handling of remains of countless birds, otters, and other animals that were victims of the oil spill. They worked long hours attempting to halt the spread of oil and to remove it from affected shorelines and beaches. Despite the lucrative salaries offered by Exxon's contractor, VECO, the pace and intensity of work led to fatigue and increased stress in many of those involved in cleanup activities. For many of those living in areas directly exposed to the oil spill, participation in cleanup activities often required spending long periods away from the community and the family, the suspension of subsistence pursuits that otherwise form the basis for many important social ties and obligations, and separation of parents from their children.

Finally, the unequal distribution of cleanup jobs within and between communities led to feelings of bitterness and discontent such that cleanup workers were often subjected to criticism for having "sold out" to Exxon. In some instances, accepting these positions meant the risk of becoming social pariahs within the community and even within the family (Gill & Picou, 1997; Palinkas, Downs, et al., 1993). The Social Indicators Study also provided evidence that spill-related jobs were unequally distributed within the community, leading to tensions and hostility between those with jobs and those without. Survey respondents with relatively little work over the preceding year were less likely to have secured spill employment, and "moreover, tensions between those who accepted spill jobs and those who eschewed such jobs tended to disrupt customary social networks which are often key channels of mutual support and collaborative assistance, especially in small and predominately Native communities" (McNabb, 1991; p. 33).

Overall, a review of the available evidence on the effects of the *Exxon Valdez* oil spill suggests that participating in cleanup activities was associated with significantly increased rates of psychiatric disorder; a perceived decline in health status; increases in reported substance abuse and domestic violence within communities and among families and friends, and increased problems associated with these activities; and a decline in social relations and increase in levels of social conflict. Oil spill workers were 1.7 times more likely to report an increase in domestic violence in their community and 3.3 times more likely to report an increase in domestic violence among family and friends than individuals not employed as oil spill workers (Russell et al., 1996).

Community residents who worked on the oil spill cleanup experienced a decline in mental health. In the Oiled Mayors Study, when age, sex, and ethnicity were controlled, respondents who participated in cleanup activities ($N=148$) were 2.3 times (95% CI = 1.5–3.7) as likely to have GAD, 1.8 times (<1.0–3.4) as likely to have PTSD, 1.5 times (0.9–2.5) as likely to have a CES-D score of 16 and above, and 1.9 times (1.1–3.2) as likely to have a CES-D score of 18 and above as were members of the unexposed group ($N=445$). However, only the odds ratios for GAD and a CES-D score of 18 and above were statistically significant. This may be attributed to the fact that Native cleanup workers had higher rates of PTSD and a CES-D score of 16 and above than Natives not participating in cleanup; in contrast, non-Natives not participating in cleanup activities had higher rates of these disorders than non-Native cleanup workers. The Valdez Counseling Center study found that respondents who earned the most money from oil spill cleanup activities in Cordova also were most likely to experience symptoms of PTSD (Donald et al., 1990).

Reported declines in social relations with family members were also significantly associated with whether the parent participated in cleanup activities. Cleanup workers were 3.4 times more likely to report a decline in relations with spouse, 3.1 times more likely to report decline in relations with children, 5.6 times more likely to report a decline in relations with other relatives in the home, and 2.8 times more likely to report a decline in relations with relatives not in the home, as compared with individuals not involved in cleanup (McLees-Palinkas, 1994). Cleanup workers were also 2.4 times more likely to report arguments about the oil spill with family members and 1.6 times more likely to report arguments about the spill with others. The Social Indicators Study found that single parent households were especially affected by the decline in social relations because they were more likely to report being relocated for spill-related work (McNabb, 1991).

27.3.2. Resource Loss

Consistent with Hobfoll's (1989) Conservation of Resources Theory, individuals who reported loss of important economic, cultural, and social resources experienced significantly higher levels of psychological symptoms and prevalence of psychiatric disorders. In the Oiled Mayors Study, 47.9% of Alaska Natives and 35.3% of non-Natives participating in the Household Survey reported that the spill damaged commercial fishing areas they had used (Palinkas et al., 1992). Non-Native local residents who reported damage to commercial fishing areas reported significantly higher levels of depressive symptoms than non-Natives who did not report such damage (Palinkas et al., 1992). The prevalence of postspill PTSD was also significantly higher in Alaska Natives and non-Natives who reported damage to commercial fishing areas (19.8% and 14.3%, respectively) than their counterparts who reported no such damage (5.2% and 6.4%, respectively) (Palinkas et al., 2004). In the Picou study, individuals who experienced loss of income, despite taking on additional jobs to avoid loss, experienced significantly higher levels of depression, anxiety, and PTSD symptomatology (Arata et al., 2000). Another study by Picou and Gill (1996) found that IES measures of spill-related intrusive stress were significantly higher in the renewable resource community of Cordova than in the nonrenewable resource community of Valdez. Furthermore, this study found significantly higher levels of intrusive stress among commercial fishermen than in people who worked in other occupations in Cordova.

In the Oiled Mayors Study, exposure to the oil spill and participation in subsequent cleanup was significantly associated with reported declines in traditional subsistence activities. Compared to the same period in the year before the spill, between 60% and 90% of Alaska Natives and between 43% and 75% of non-Natives in the high-exposed group reported a decline in time spent hunting, fishing, and gathering, time normally spent with people from other households engaged in these activities, the amount of harvested resource foods shared with others and with elders, the amount of harvested resource foods received from others, number of household members engaged in these activities, and opportunities for children to learn hunting, fishing, and gathering (Palinkas, Downs, et al., 1993). Natives and non-Natives alike who reported that the spill and cleanup had affected their hunting, fishing, and gathering activities also reported significantly higher levels of depressive symptoms (Palinkas et al., 1992) and prevalence of PTSD (Palinkas et al., 2004) than those who reported no such effects.

As noted previously, the oil spill and subsequent cleanup also disrupted social relations both within the families and within and between affected communities. A decline in social relations was significantly associated with depressive symptoms and postspill prevalence of PTSD in both Alaska Natives and non-Natives in the Oiled Mayors Study (Palinkas et al., 1992, 2004). The postspill prevalence of PTSD was also associated with a decline in support from family members among Alaska Natives (Palinkas et al., 2004). Picou and colleagues (Dyer et al., 1992; Picou et al., 1992) found that 5 months after the spill, residents of Cordova experienced significant social disruption in personal, family, and work settings. Arata and colleagues (2000) found deterioration in relationships with others to be significantly associated with SCL90-R measures of depression, anxiety, and PTSD.

27.3.3. Families and Children

The Oiled Mayors Study also found a significant impact of the oil spill and subsequent cleanup on social relations within the family. Owing to spill-related disruptions, there was a reported decrease in time respondents spent visiting with other household members. According to the household survey data collected in the Oiled Mayors Study, in most communities 15% to 30% of the households reported decreases in time spent interacting with family members (Russell et al., 1996). In several native communities with high rates of cleanup involvement, 45% to 65% reported such decreases. Forty-five percent of those who worked on the cleanup reported less time spent with other household members, compared with 16% of those who did not work on the spill. Similarly, from 10% to 30% of the respondents in each of the affected communities indicated less time available for family vacations as a result of spill-related activities (Russell et al., 1996). As compared with individuals in the unexposed group, individuals in the high-exposed group were significantly more likely to report declines in socializing with other household members; sharing food, money, and other resources with family members; and overall household time together since the spill (McLees-Palinkas, 1994; Russell et al., 1996).

Some of the statements taken from Oiled Mayor Study participants (Impact Assessment, 1990, p. 45) are exemplary of the types of interpersonal disruptions the cleanup created in various communities:

> Yes, as a family we kind of lost it ... my husband ... we were so close. Then the oil spill came and he is drinking more and [we] separated.
>
> ... the loss of earnings of my husband [was bad] ... and the fact that he wasn't here this summer. It was a burden on our relationship.
>
> My husband's alcoholism got worse. He had quit before the spill. Now we're separated because of the spill.
>
> [The cleanup] contributed to my break-up with my fiancée. The spill caused lots of pressure for me to keep my business going – I was stressed and it affected my relationship.

In some instances, those who worked long hours on the spill simply had less time and energy to devote to their family relationships. In other instances, the cleanup created tensions related to family roles. For example, in Native communities where there was little child care available, the oldest child was often placed in charge of siblings as parents worked on the cleanup. When mothers and fathers returned home there were conflicts over the eldest child once again assuming a "child" rather than a caretaker role. These types of conflicts seemed small when viewed in isolation, but when viewed within the context of individual stress, coupled with community divisiveness and conflict and household disruptions, each additional stressor added to the overall disruption experienced by individuals, families, and communities (McLees-Palinkas, 1994). However, it is unclear whether these impacts were long term. Dyer and associates (1992) reported that 58% of Alaskan Natives noted disruptive changes in family relations in 1989, which declined to 25% in 1990. Nevertheless, the entire Cordova cohort was more likely to report disruptive changes in family relations in both 1989 and 1990 than their counterparts in Petersburg (Dyer et al., 1992).

The household survey data and ethnographic interviews obtained from the Oiled Mayors Study found that for children, increasing exposure to the oil spill event was significantly associated with a decline in school work and grades, greater fear of being left alone, fighting more with other children, and difficulty getting along with parents (McLees-Palinkas, 1994). Exposure to the oil spill was also significantly associated with the two global measures of children's behavioral dysfunction: parent's assessment that the oil spill had an effect on their children and scores on an index of children's behavioral disruption. These associations were independent of the gender, ethnicity, age of the parent, and the structure of the family. However, the association between exposure to the oil spill and reports of bedwetting being a new problem since the oil spill was greater in households with preschool children (infants to 5 years), reports of children's sleep problems was greater in households with school age children (6–12 years), reports of a decline in children's grades and school work was greater in households with adolescents. Although parental or adult reports of children's behavior referred to all children in the household, the results of this study indicated that parents or adults were more likely to report a certain dysfunctional behavior among children in the household if children of a particular age and, indirectly, level of emotional and cognitive development, were present in the household. These results thus confirmed the findings of other studies that indicate that level of cognitive and emotional development influences the types of symptom risk and symptom expression exhibited by children after a disaster.

In describing life for families during the cleanup, a resident of one of the affected communities commented:

> [the jobs] were not just 8 to 5 jobs. They were like to 7 or 12 [at night] and sometimes longer. They worked until midnight unloading boats, got home, slept three hours, and got up and went back to work. So that put a lot of stress on the families, because one person wasn't there … and the children were scared because they didn't realize what was happening, because the adults were all excited … so the children were real concerned about it, what was going on and not understanding why they weren't able to clean it up and be involved in some way. (Impact Assessment, 1990; p. 46)

The director of one of the day care facilities in Seward, who had extended periods of contact with children, described the behavioral changes she saw in children following the oil spill. Many were irritable and cried more frequently than usual, which the director attributed to feelings of anger and neglect because their parents were away from them for so many hours at a time. The director commented, "The kids had always used to color so nicely but since the oil spill they take a black crayon and cover everything black," which she believed was a manifestation of those feelings. In May 1989, 2 months after the spill, the kids were learning about and drawing pictures of sea life. All of the children reportedly drew the oil spill as part of their pictures even though the subject of the oil spill hadn't been raised at the day care (Impact Assessment, 1990).

In all but two communities, more than half of the parents indicated that their children exhibited separation anxiety. Summed for the entire sample of parents in the household survey ($N=326$), 73% indicated that their children did not like being left alone, a phenomenon they attributed to the effects of the spill and cleanup. The figures varied by site, with only 35% reporting separation anxiety at one Native village. In two other communities, Kodiak and Chignik, 85% of the parents reported such symptoms in their children. This is an important indicator of the disruptive effects of the spill and cleanup on children (Impact Assessment, 1990).

Another indicator of behavioral problems with children as a result of the spill was that 79% of all parents reported that they did not get along with their children as well as they did before the spill. There was some variation in responses between communities with a range of 47% to 95% reporting worsened child–parent relationships. The figures suggest that as a result of spill and cleanup-induced changes and disruptions, there was a general deterioration of child–parent relationships (Impact Assessment, 1990).

The lack of available day care, a typical problem in many communities, became exacerbated by the spill. Two-thirds of the parents in the household survey indicated they had problems with finding suitable child care services after the spill. However, there was significant variation between sites. In one Native village, only 11% indicated child care problems, while in another, 80% reported such problems. In non-Native communities, 40% to 70% of parents reported problems with day care availability (Impact Assessment, 1990). In part, these problems reflect the reduced day care services as a result of day care workers leaving their jobs to work at much higher wages on the spill cleanup. It also reflects the outside employment of family members who might otherwise stay at home and take care of children. As a consequence, children often were unsupervised for the periods of time that they were not in school. As one former day care worker from Cordova said, "[I] left my [day care] job because we couldn't keep enough people working there. Childcare is always a challenge but when $17 an hour is available rather than $6.00 an hour … The [day care] job is harder also because of stressed out kids, they are always away from [their] parents, the kids feel abandoned" (Impact Assessment, 1990; p. 48).

In the Oiled Mayors Study, the postspill prevalence of GAD, PTSD, and CES-D scores of 16 and above was significantly associated with exposure to the oil spill among parents but not among other adults (McLees-Palinkas, 1994). Household survey respondents reporting effects of the oil spill on the behavior of their children were more likely to have a psychiatric disorder than individuals not reporting effects of the spill on their children. The postspill prevalence of GAD, PTSD, and the prevalence of depressive symptoms were all significantly associated with reports of the following: children having problems sleeping, children getting upset when someone talks about the oil spill, bedwetting being a new problem for children in household, children's fear of being left alone, children in household fighting more with other children, and children in household fighting more with parents since the oil spill. Reports of problems finding child care for children since the oil spill were significantly associated with the postspill prevalence of GAD (OR = 3.5; 95% CI = 1.6–7.2), PTSD (OR = 3.7; 95% CI = 1.3–10.5), and CES-D scores of 16 and above (OR = 2.4; 95% CI = 1.1–5.5) among parents in the affected communities, independent of age, gender, ethnicity, exposure status, and level of family support (McLees-Palinkas, 1994).

27.3.4. Alaska Natives

While the oil spill affected Alaska Natives and non-Natives alike, the former were especially vulnerable to many of the psychosocial impacts described earlier. In the Oiled Mayors Study, 38.3% of the 189 Alaska Native participants reported participating in cleanup activities, compared with 19.1% of the 405 non-Native participants ($p < 0.001$) (Palinkas et al., 1992). Alaska Natives were also significantly more likely than non-Natives to report damage to commercial fishing areas (47.9% vs. 35.3%,

$p < 0.01$) and effects on hunting, fishing, and gathering (48.4% vs. 28.3%, $p < 0.001$). Natives were particularly vulnerable to the effects of exposure on the prevalence of CES-D scores of 16 and above (OR = 1.3; 95% CI = 1.1–1.5) (Palinkas, Petterson, et al., 1993) and the effects of participation in cleanup or other contact with oil and change in household income on mean CSD-D scores (Palinkas et al., 1992). Low family support, participation in spill cleanup activities, and a decline in subsistence activities were significantly associated with PTSD in Alaska Natives but not in Euro-Americans (Palinkas et al., 2004). Among Alaska Natives, PTSD was significantly associated with participation in cleanup activities, reports of property lost or damaged as a result of the spill, and effects on hunting, fishing, and gathering. Among Euro-Americans, PTSD was significantly associated only with effects on hunting, fishing, and gathering. Picou and colleagues reported that Alaska Natives living in Cordova reported higher levels of intrusive stress than non-Native commercial fishermen (Gill & Picou, 1997).

27.3.5. Litigation

As they are usually the result of human error, technological disasters are often followed by prolonged litigation that seeks to attribute blame to some person, persons, or institutions believed to be responsible for the disaster and to obtain compensation for the damages, both material and psychosocial, incurred as a result of the disaster (Picou, Marshall, & Gill, 2004). The *Exxon Valdez* oil spill was no exception to this pattern. As described by Hirsch (1996), within days if not hours of the spill, seemingly hundreds of lawyers descended on small towns and villages throughout Alaska. In 1994, an Anchorage jury awarded \$287 million for actual damages and \$5 billion for punitive damages to a group of plaintiffs that included 32,000 fishermen, Alaska Natives, landowners, and others whose livelihoods were gravely affected by the disaster. After several appeals by Exxon, the punitive damages award was eventually reduced to \$2.4 billion. To date, Exxon has yet to pay this amount to the plaintiffs (Lieff, Cabraser, Heimann, & Bernstein, 2008). Moreover, claims by Alaska Natives that the oil spill had irreparably damaged their traditional culture, largely through the destruction of local subsistence resources, were dismissed by the court on the grounds that such losses could not be quantified in monetary terms; this led to their further victimization by the oil spill (Gill & Picou, 1997). As a result, Picou and colleagues (2004) found that the status of litigant and the litigation stress were significant predictors of psychological stress 3 and 1½ years after the oil spill. They concluded that litigation is a critical characteristic of technological disasters that precludes timely community recovery and promotes chronic social and psychological impacts.

27.4. INTERVENTIONS AND MENTAL HEALTH SYSTEMS

The experience of the *Exxon Valdez* oil spill suggests that individuals living in communities impacted by technological disasters might benefit from interventions and programs in three specific areas: mental health services, postdisaster cleanup and recovery, and disaster-related litigation.

27.4.1. Mental Health Services

In the aftermath of the oil spill, locally available mental health services were scarce and overwhelmed by the number of local residents and transient workers seeking services (Donald et al., 1990; Impact Assessment, 1990). This was especially true in the smaller Alaska Native villages (Gill & Picou, 1997). What services were available either existed outside the region or were provided by outsiders with little knowledge of local culture and conditions. A quote from an Alaska Native in Cordova illustrates the difficulty of accessing services in remote communities in the aftermath of a disaster:

> The social service people are good at their jobs. [But] these people were damaged by the spill, just like everybody else. They tried to cope, their workload went up, but it was like the hurt helping the hurt. It was very difficult for them.

> And we would not accept at all a stranger coming in from Fairbanks or Juneau, or Nome, to be our social worker, and sit there and say: "Yes, I know how you feel." No, you don't know how I feel, because you were not there. You did not go through the scare, the trauma, the fright, the financial disaster. There was nothing that a social worker from anywhere else can say to help us. We have got to heal from within. (Dyer, 1993, pp. 82–83)

Services in the aftermath must be locally available and culturally competent. However, as the aforementioned quote illustrates, those services are themselves strained by the disaster as providers also experience traumatic symptoms. While there is no clear resolution to this dilemma, one solution would be the establishment of teams of mental health responders comprised of local service providers, peer counselors, and outside professionals who serve in an advisory capacity or whose main role is to provide treatment for local providers.

27.4.2. Cleanup and Recovery

In many respects, the *Exxon Valdez* oil spill provided a textbook case of what not to do in the aftermath to a technological disaster. As noted earlier, Exxon and its contractor VECO, were criticized for responding with "too little too late" and with developing hiring practices that contributed to an influx of outsiders that overwhelmed local services and facilities and resulted in an unequal distribution of income. One of the lessons learned from the cleanup experience is that companies and government agencies responsible for cleanup activities should pay greater attention to the health and well-being of those participating in such activity. This includes setting reasonable limits to the number of hours worked and making mental health services available to cleanup workers. The issue of an unequal distribution of resources is also important to prevent the formation of a corrosive community (Picou et al., 2004). Policies should be put into place that insure more equal distribution of employment and other economic opportunities to local residents affected by the disaster.

27.4.3. Litigation

When the process is relatively brief and the outcome relatively successful, litigation can provide numerous social and psychological benefits to those impacted by a technological disaster (Murphy & Keating, 1995). However, as illustrated by the *Exxon Valdez* oil spill, this is rarely the case. The stress associated by the uncertainty of ever achieving closure to the event may have been as profound as the initial shock of living in a world covered by oil. To address this stress and uncertainty, mental health providers should be working with representatives of the legal system to set realistic expectations for potential litigants by informing them of the process and likely outcomes of litigation, the role and value placed on negotiation in the litigation process, and the services available to litigants who are poorly equipped to deal with the intense demands placed on their time, privacy, and credibility.

27.4.4. Future Directions

Apart from the obvious need to conduct longitudinal research in the aftermath of technological disasters, the lessons of the *Exxon Valdez* oil spill suggest several avenues for research, policy, and planning to minimize the occurrence of adverse social and psychological outcomes in future oil spills. It is clear that natural renewable resource communities, such as those located in Prince William Sound, are especially vulnerable to mental health consequences of technological disasters that contaminate and destroy the natural environment. One reason is that for these communities, the natural environment plays a key role in the social environment and the personal and cultural identity of the community. Further, these communities typically lack the medical and mental health resources necessary to respond quickly in the aftermath of a large-scale disaster like the oil spill. Although timely efforts to provide counseling and referral are critical in such instances, it remains unclear as to whether specific programs and policies tailored to the needs of each community are necessary. For instance, empirically tested treatments for trauma, such as exposure therapy, cognitive therapy, and anxiety management techniques, may require modification to meet the needs of rural and predominately non-Euro-American communities. Similarly, community-based participatory research techniques might be applied in developing and evaluating interventions designed to prevent the deterioration of social support networks in the aftermath of an event like the oil spill. Such interventions might target families as well as individuals. Policies may be required to minimize the influx of outsiders involved in subsequent cleanup efforts to prevent local resources and infrastructure from being overwhelmed by their presence.

27.5. CONCLUSION

Although the oil spill did not place individuals in the affected communities in any immediate physical danger (i.e., apart from the potential long-term effects of prolonged exposure to aromatic hydrocarbons), as is the case in a natural disaster, it did threaten to destroy an entire way of life. For Alaskan Natives, that way of life revolved around the production and distribution of subsistence items harvested from the sea. The short-term and possibility of long-term destruction of the environment threatened the basis for individual identity, self-esteem, and social relations among Alaskan Natives throughout the affected community. For non-Natives living in the region, the possible destruction of the commercial fisheries that supported their economic livelihood proved to be equally devastating. Although the cleanup employment provided short-term relief, it did little to resolve long-term uncertainty and a sense of vulnerability to future oil spills. While this sense of the death of a way of life may have diminished over time, it produced social and psychological trauma that would not have been present had it not been for the spill of oil into Prince William Sound.

Efforts to clean up the damage caused by the oil spill proved to be as devastating, if not more so, to the mental health and well-being of the affected communities as the damage itself. Although Exxon may have acted with good intentions in offering substantial wages for cleanup jobs, the unequal distribution of these employment opportunities created or exacerbated preexisting conflicts within households, families, and communities. The availability of spill-related employment also disrupted services and threatened resources in communities faced with an influx of outsiders looking for work and the disappearance of key social service personnel (e.g., child care workers) as they left for higher paying spill-related cleanup jobs away from the community. The long hours devoted to cleanup work for the sake of short-term economic gain to balance the potential long-term economic losses also led to a decline in physical and mental health, a disruption of social activities and relationships, and a concern for the lack of adequate child care for children.

When the *Exxon Valdez* ran aground in Prince William Sound, it spilled oil into a social and a natural environment. That spill resulted in increased rates of depressive symptoms, anxiety, and PTSD, especially in women and Alaskan Natives. The spill also resulted in increased levels of alcohol and drug abuse, social conflict, disturbances in behavior of children, and a decline in perceived quality of life. Only further research will determine whether these impacts are transient or whether they are lasting consequences of permanent changes in the social, cultural, and economic fabric of these communities.

REFERENCES

Acierno, R., Ruggiero, K. J., Galea, S., Resnick, H. S., Koenen, K., Roitzsch, J., et al. (2007). Psychological sequelae resulting from the 2004 Florida hurricanes: Implications for postdisaster intervention. *American Journal of Public Health, 97*(Suppl. 1), S103–S108.

American Psychiatric Association. (1987). *Diagnostic and statistical manual of mental disorders* (3rd ed. rev.). Washingon, DC: American Psychiatric Association.

(1994). *Diagnostic and statistical manual of mental disorders* (4th ed.). Washington, DC: American Psychiatric Association.

Arata, C. M., Picou, J. S., Johnson, G. D., & McNally, T. S. (2000). Coping with technological disaster: An application of the Conservation of Resources model to the *Exxon Valdez* oil spill. *Journal of Traumatic Stress, 13*, 23–39.

Arata, C.M., Saunders, B.E., & Kilpatrick, D.G. (1991). Concurrent validity of a crime-related post-traumatic stress disorder scale for women within the Symptom Checklist-90-Revised. *Violence and Victims, 6,* 191–199.

Baum, A., & Fleming, R. (1993). Implications of psychological research on stress and technological accidents. *American Psychologist, 48,* 665–672.

Baum, A., Gatchel, R.J., & Schaeffer, M. (1983). Emotional, behavioral and psychophysiological effects of chronic stress at Three Mile Island. *Journal of Consulting and Clinical Psychology, 51,* 565–572.

Bogard, W. (1989). *The Bhopal tragedy.* Boulder, CO: Westview.

Brewin, C., Andrews, B., & Valentine, J. (2000). Meta-analysis of risk factors for posttraumatic stress disorder in trauma-exposed adults. *Journal of Consulting and Clinical Psychology, 68,* 748–766.

Bromet, E.J., Gluzman, S., Schwartz, J.E., & Goldgaber, D. (2002). Somatic symptoms in women 11 years after the Chornobyl accident: Prevalence and risk factors. *Environmental Health Perspectives, 110*(Suppl. 4), 625–629.

Bromet, E., Parkinson, D., Schulberg, H. C., & Dunn, L. (1980). *Three Mile Island: Mental health findings.* Pittsburgh, PA: Western Psychiatric Institute and Clinic and the University of Pittsburgh.

Brown, G.W., & Harris, T. (1979). *Laying waste: Love canal and the poisoning of America.* New York: Random House.

Brown, P., & Mikkelsen, E.J. (1989). *No safe place: Toxic waste, leukemia, and community action.* Berkeley, CA: University of California Press.

Bui, B.G., Sharr, S., & Seeb, J.E. (1998). Evidence of damage to pink salmon populations inhabiting Prince William Sound, Alaska, two generations after the *Exxon Valdez* oil spill. *Transaction of the American Fisheries Society, 127,* 35–43.

Cohen, M.J. (1995). Technological disaster and natural resource damage assessment: An evaluation of the *Exxon Valdez* oil spill. *Land Economics, 71,* 65–82.

Cohen, S., & Hoberman, H. (1983). Positive events and social supports as buffers of life change stress. *Journal of Applied Social Psychology, 13,* 99–125

Davidson, J.R.T., & Foa, E.B. (1993). Epilogue. In J.R.T. Davidson & E.B. Foa (Eds.), *Posttraumatic stress disorder: DSM-IV and beyond.* Washington, DC: American Psychiatric Press.

Davidson, L.M., & Baum, A. (1991). Victimization and self blame following a technological disaster. In S. R. Couch & J.S. Kroll-Smith (Eds.), *Communities at risk: Collective responses to technological hazards.* New York: Peter Lang.

Davis, N.Y. (1996). The *Exxon Valdez* oil spill, Alaska. In J.K. Mitchell (Ed.), *The long road to recovery: Community responses to industrial disaster.* New York: United Nations University Press.

Donald, R., Cook, R., Bixby, R.F., Benda, R., & Wolf, A. (1990). *The stress related impact of the Valdez oil spill on the residents of Cordova and Valdez, Alaska. A comparative study conducted by the Valdez Counseling Center.* Valdez, AK: Valdez Counseling Center.

Dyer, C.L. (1993). Tradition loss as secondary disaster: Long-term cultural impacts of the *Exxon Valdez* oil spill. *Sociological Spectrum, 13,* 65–88.

Dyer, C.L., Gill, D.A., & Picou, J.S. (1992). Social disruption and the Valdez oil spill: Alaskan Natives in a natural resource community. *Sociological Spectrum, 12,* 105–126.

Erikson, K. (1991). A new species of trouble. In S.R. Couch & J.S. Kroll-Smith (Eds.), *Communities at risk. Collective responses to technological disaster.* New York: Peter Lang.

Erikson, K.T. (1976). *Everything in its path: Destruction of community in the Buffalo Creek flood.* New York: Simon & Shuster.

Feng, S., Tan, H., Benjamin, A., Wen, S., Liu, A., Zhou, J., et al. (2007). Social support and posttraumatic stress disorder among flood victims in Hunan, China. *Annals of Epidemiology, 17,* 827–833.

Fontana, A., & Rosenheck, R. (1994). Posttraumatic stress disorder among Vietnam theater veterans: a causal model of etiology in a community sample. *Journal of Nervous and Mental Disease, 182,* 677–684.

Frederick, C.J. (1987). Psychic trauma in victims of crime and terrorism. In G.R. VandenBos & B.K. Bryant (Eds.), *Cataclysms, crises, and catastrophes: Psychology in action.* Washington, DC: American Psychological Association.

Freudenberg, W.R., & Jones, T.R. (1991). Attitudes and stress in the presence of technological risk: A test of the Supreme Court hypothesis. *Social Forces, 69,* 1143–1168.

Friedman, M.J., Schneiderman, C., & West, A. (1986). Measurement of combat exposure, posttraumatic stress disorder, and life stress among Vietnam combat veterans. *American Journal of Psychiatry, 143,* 537–539.

Galea, S., Resnick, H., Ahern, J., Gold, J., Bucuvalas, M., Kilpatrick, D., et al. (2002). Posttraumatic stress disorder in Manhattan, New York City, after the September 11th terrorist attacks. *Journal of Urban Health, 79,* 340–353.

Gill, D.A. (1994). Environmental disaster and fishery co-management in a natural resource community: Impacts of the *Exxon Valdez* oil spill. In C.L. Dyer & J.R. McGoodwin (Eds.), *Folk management in the world fisheries: Implications for fishery managers.* Boulder, CO: University of Colorado Press.

Gill, D. A., & Picou, J. S. (1997). The day the water died: Cultural impacts of the *Exxon Valdez* oil spill. In J. S. Picou, D. A. Gill, & M. J. Cohen (Eds.), *The Exxon Valdez disaster: Readings on a modern social problem*. Dubuque, IA: Kendall-Hunt.

Green, B. L., Grace, M. C., & Gleser, G. (1985). Identifying survivors at risk: Long-term impairment following the Beverly Hills Supper Club fire. *Journal of Consulting and Clinical Psychology, 53*, 672–678.

Hirsch, W. B. (1996). *The Exxon Valdez litigation justice delayed: Seven years later with no end in sight.* San Francisco, CA (September, 2007); http://www.lieffcabraser.com/wbh_Exxart.htm.

Hobfoll, S. E. (1988). *The ecology of stress*. Washington, DC: Hemisphere.

(1989). Conservation of resources: A new attempt at conceptualizing stress. *American Psychologist, 44*, 513–524.

Horowitz, M. J., Milner, N., & Alvarez, W. (1979). Impact of event scale: A measure of subjective stress. *Psychosomatic Medicine, 41*, 209–218.

Houts, P. S., Cleary, P. D., & Hsu, T. (1988). *The Three Mile Island crisis*. Hershey, PA: The Pennsylvania State University Press.

Impact Assessment, Inc. (1990). *Economic, social, and psychological impact assessment of the Exxon Valdez oil spill. Final report.* Prepared for Oiled Mayors Subcommittee, Alaska Conference of Mayors. La Jolla, CA: Impact Assessment, Inc.

Kaniasty, K., & Norris, F. (2004). Social support in the aftermath of disasters, catastrophes, and acts of terrorism: Altruistic, overwhelmed, uncertain, antagonistic, and patriotic communities. In R. Ursano, A. Norwood, & C. Fullerton (Eds.), *Bioterrorism: Psychological and public health interventions*. Cambridge: Cambridge University Press.

Keane, T. M., Marshall, A. D., & Taft, C. T. (2006). Posttraumatic stress disorder: Etiology, epidemiology, and treatment outcome. *Annual Review of Clinical Psychology, 2*, 161–197.

Kilpatrick, D. G., & Resnick, H. S. (1993). Posttraumatic stress disorder associated with exposure to criminal victimization in clinical and community populations. In J. R. T. Davidson & E. B. Foa (Eds.), *Posttraumatic stress disorder: DSM-IV and beyond.* Washington, DC: American Psychiatric Press.

King, D. W., King, L. A., Foy, D. W., Keane, T. M., & Fairbank, J. A. (1999). Posttraumatic stress disorder in a national sample of female and male Vietnam veterans: Risk factors, war-zone stressors, and resilience–recovery variables. *Journal of Abnormal Psychology, 108*, 164–170.

Kinzie, J. D., Boehnlein, J. K., Leung, P. K., Moore, L. J., Riley, C., & Smith, D. (1990). The prevalence of posttraumatic stress disorder and its clinical significance among Southeast Asian refugees. *American Journal of Psychiatry, 147*, 913–917.

Kroll-Smith, J. S., & Couch, S. R. (1991). Technological hazards, adaptation and social change. In S. R. Couch & J. S. Kroll-Smith (Eds.), *Communities at risk: Collective responses to technological hazards.* New York: Peter Lang.

(1993). Symbols, ecology, and contamination: Case studies in the ecological-symbolic approach to disaster. *Research in Social Problems and Public Policy, 5*, 47–73.

Lieff, Cabraser, Heimann, & Bernstein, LLP. (2008). *Exxon Valdez Oil disaster and class action lawsuit.* San Francisco, CA (January 2008); http://wwwlieffcabraser.com/wbh_Exxart.htm

Levine, A. (1982). *The love canal: Science, politics, and people*. Lexington, MA: Lexington Books.

Lindy, J., Green, B. G., & Grace, M. C. (1987). Commentary: The stressor criterion and posttraumatic stress disorder. *Journal of Nervous and Mental Disease, 175*, 269–272.

Lord, N. (1997). Oil in the sea: Initial biological impacts of the *Exxon Valdez* oil spill. In J. S. Picou, D. A. Gill & M. J. Cohen (Eds.), *The Exxon Valdez disaster: Readings on a modern social problem*. Dubuque, IA: Kendall-Hunt.

McLees-Palinkas, T. (1994). *Psychosocial impacts of disasters on families and children: The Exxon-Valdez oil spill.* Master's Thesis. San Diego, CA: Department of Child Development, San Diego State University.

McNabb, S. (1991). *Comparative analysis of spill impacts in ten communities.* Presented at the 50th annual meeting of the Society for Applied Anthropology, Charleston, SC, March 17.

Minerals Management Service. (1993). *Social indicators study of Alaskan coastal villages*. IV. Technical Report No. 155. Schedule C Communities, Part 1. Human Relations Area Files. Alaska OCS Region. Anchorage: Minerals Management Service, US Department of the Interior.

Murphy, S. A., & Keating, J. P. (1995). Psychological assessment of postdisaster class action and personal injury litigants: A case study. *Journal of Traumatic Stress, 8*, 473–482.

Neff, J. M., Bence, A. E., Parker, K. R., Page, D. S., Brown, J. S., & Boehm, P. D. (2006). Bioavailability of polycyclic aromatic hydrocarbons from buried shoreline oil residues thirteen years after the *Exxon Valdez* oil spill: A multispecies assessment. *Environmental and Toxicological Chemistry, 25*, 947–961.

Neria, Y., Nandi, A., & Galea, S. (2007). Post-traumatic stress disorder following disasters: A systematic review. *Psychological Medicine*, Sept 6, epub ahead of print.

Norris, F. H. (1992). Epidemiology of trauma: Frequency and impact of different potentially traumatic events on different demographic groups. *Journal of Consulting and Clinical Psychology, 60*, 409–418.

Norris, F. H., Baker, C. K., Murphy, A. D., & Kaniasty, K. (2005). Social support mobilization and deterioration after Mexico's 1999 flood: Effects of context, gender, and time. *American Journal of Community Psychology, 26*, 15–28.

Palinkas, L. A., Downs, M. A., Petterson, J. S., & Russell, J. (1993). Social, cultural and psychological impacts of the Exxon Valdez oil spill. *Human Organization, 52*(1), 1–13.

Palinkas, L. A., Petterson, J. S., Downs, M. A., & Russell, J. (2004). Ethnic differences in symptoms of posttraumatic stress after the *Exxon Valdez* oil spill. *Prehospital and Disaster Medicine, 19*, 102–112.

Palinkas, L. A., Petterson, J. S., Russell, J., & Downs, M. A. (1993). Community patterns of psychiatric disorders after the *Exxon Valdez* oil spill. *American Journal of Psychiatry, 150*, 1517–1523.

Palinkas, L. A., Russell, J., Downs, M. A., & Petterson, J. S. (1992). Ethnic differences in stress, coping, and depressive symptoms after the *Exxon Valdez* oil spill. *Journal of Nervous and Mental Disease, 180*, 287–295.

Peterson, C. H., Rice, S. D., Short, J. W., Esler, D., Bodkin, J. L., Ballachey, B. E., et al. (2003). Long-term ecosystem response to the *Exxon Valdez* oil spill. *Science, 302*, 2082–2086.

Picou, J. S., & Gill, D. A. (1996) The *Exxon Valdez* oil spill and chronic psychological stress. *American Fisheries Society Symposium, 18*, 879–893.

Picou, J. S., Gill, D. A., & Cohen, M. J. (Eds.) (1997). *The Exxon Valdez disaster: Readings on a modern social problem*. Dubuque, IA: Kendall-Hunt.

Picou, J. S., Gill, D. A., Dyer, C. L., & Curry, E. W. (1992). Disruption and stress in an Alaskan fishing community: Initial and continuing impacts of the *Exxon Valdez* oil spill. *Industrial Crisis Quarterly, 6*, 235–257.

Picou, J. S., Marshall, B. K., & Gill, D. A. (2004). Disaster, litigation, and the corrosive community. *Social Forces, 82*, 1493–1522.

Picou, J. S., & Rosebrook, D. R. (1993). Technological accident, community class-action litigation, and scientific damage assessment: A case study of court-ordered researcher. *Sociological Spectrum, 13*, 117–138.

Radloff, L. S. (1977). The CES-D Scale: A new self-report depression scale for research in the general population. *Applied Psychological Measurement, 1*, 385–401.

Robins, L. N., Fischbach, R. L., Smith, E. M., Cottler, L. B., Solomon, S. D., & Goldring, E. (1986) Impact of disaster on previously assessed mental health. In J. H. Shore (Ed.), *Disaster stress studies: New methods and findings*. Washington, DC: American Psychiatric Press.

Robins, L. N., Helzer, J. E., Cottler, L., & Goldring, E. (1989). *The NIMH diagnostic interview schedule, version III, Revised*. St. Louis, MO: Washington University.

Robins, L. N., Helzer, J. E., Croughan, J., & Ratcliff, K. S. (1981). National Institute of Mental Health Diagnostic Interview Schedule: Its history, characteristics, and validity. *Archives of General Psychiatry, 38*, 381–389.

Rodin, M., Downs, M., Petterson, J., & Russell, J. (1992). Community impacts resulting from the *Exxon Valdez* oil spill. *Organization & Environment, 6*, 219–234.

Russell, J. C., Downs, M. A., Petterson, J. S., & Palinkas, L. A. (1996). Psychological and social impacts of the *Exxon Valdez* oil spill and cleanup. *American Fisheries Society Symposium, 18*, 867–878.

Schnurr, P. P., Lunney, C. A., & Sengupta, A. (2004). Risk factors for the development versus maintenance of posttraumatic stress disorder. *Journal of Traumatic Stress, 17*, 85–95.

Shore, J. H., Tatum, E. L., & Vollmer, W. M. (1986). Psychiatric reactions to disaster: The Mount St. Helens experience. *American Journal of Psychiatry, 143*, 590–595.

Shore, J. H., Vollmer, W. M., & Tatum, E. L. (1989). Community patterns of posttraumatic stress disorders. *Journal of Nervous and Mental Disease, 177*, 681–685.

Short, J. W., Irvine, G. V., Mann, D. H., Maselko, J. M., Pella, J. J., Lindeberg, M. R., et al. (2007). Slightly weathered *Exxon Valdez* oil persists in Gulf of Alaska beach sediments after 16 years. *Environmental Science and Technology, 15*, 1245–1250.

Shrivastava, P. (1987). *Bhopal: An anatomy of a crisis*. Cambridge, MA: Harper & Row.

Smith, E. M., North, C. S., McCool, R. E., & Shea, J. M. (1990). Acute postdisaster psychiatric disorders: Identification of persons at risk. *American Journal of Psychiatry, 147*, 202–206.

Spies, R. B., Rice, S. D., Wolfe, D. A., & Wright, B. A. (1996). The effects of the *Exxon Valdez* oil spill on the Alaskan environment. *American Fisheries Society Symposium, 18*, 1–16.

Tomb, D. A. (1994). The phenomenology of post-traumatic stress disorder. *Psychiatric Clinics of North America, 17*, 237–250.

Vyner, H. M. (1988). *Invisible trauma: The psychological effects of invisible environmental contaminants*. Lexington, MA: Heath.

Young, A. (1995). *The harmony of illusions: Inventing post-traumatic stress disorder*. Princeton, NJ: Princeton University Press.

28 Enschede Fireworks Disaster

PETER. G. VAN DER VELDEN, C. JORIS YZERMANS, AND LINDA GRIEVINK

28.1. INTRODUCTION

That day seemed a very normal day. It was nice weather. My son and daughter-in-law had gone to the market. I was sitting out in the garden with my wife and our daughter. In the afternoon, we saw a large cloud of smoke. I also saw fireworks shooting up into the air. We said to each other, "Those are nice colors." I did find it strange, however, to just see this on a normal day. My wife and daughter wanted to go and look. I stayed at home to look after our grandchild. He was in the playpen. After having sat in the garden for approximately 10 minutes I got up and went inside. When I looked outside I could see lots of people walking down the street. I didn't quite understand where they had come from. What on earth were all these people doing here? Suddenly I heard an enormous bang. A large cloud of black smoke rose above the houses. I ran outside to see what had happened. I forgot to put on my shoes. I didn't realize yet what was going on. I saw lots of people standing in the road. When the next bang came I saw them all running away. I myself fled into the house. In the living room, all the photos had dropped off the walls. They lay broken on the floor. The windows were smashed. Some of the ceiling had collapsed. I quickly took my grandson out of the playpen and fled out of the house again. Outside, debris was falling out of the sky and there was glass everywhere. I still had no shoes on my feet.

My daughter and wife came running toward me along the street. My wife suffers from asthma; she can't really run fast at all. I could see she had been crying. She said she'd nearly been hit on the head with a lump of concrete on the way. Someone had called out just in time, so fortunately she'd been able just to jump out of the way. Right next to her, the debris had landed on a car. Someone had given her a glass of water and tried to calm her. Shortly afterward, a police officer came to our door. He told us to leave our home. It was too dangerous to stay inside. The house could collapse. I gave my son a quick ring to see if he could come and help us. Then we walked to the Oldenzaalsestraat. We stood there for quite some time. There were people crying everywhere. Some of them were wounded. I heard sirens and saw police, fire engines, and ambulances. We made sure we kept to the center of the road. We were afraid that otherwise a wall might collapse on top of us. I was really on my guard. After a while, we were quite keen to go back home, but that wasn't possible because the street had been cordoned off. I wasn't allowed to go and fetch my wife's medicine from our house either. So I went to get new medicine from a pharmacy that evening.

Our son and my brother let us stay with them because we weren't allowed to go home for 2 weeks. They did let us inside our house briefly after 4 days, to sort some clothes out. Every night we slept badly, and every day we peered at our house through a fence. Many houses in our street were declared uninhabitable. The windows and doors were nailed up in connection with the danger of asbestos. Since May 13, my wife's bronchitis has returned and she is often ill. (Van der Ploeg, Dorresteijn, Van der Velden, & Kleber, 2001).

The aforementioned narrative was told to researchers in an interview a few months after a major fireworks disaster occurred on Saturday, May 13, 2000, in the city of Enschede (152,000 inhabitants), the Netherlands, near the border with Germany. The disaster started with exploding fireworks at 2:24 p.m. in a fireworks storage and trade company. At 3:22 p.m., one of the concrete storage bunkers was on fire, and at 3:35 p.m., a massive and fatal explosion took place, destroying the central storage facilities and causing the explosion of several metal containers full of fireworks.

The company was located in the middle of a residential area and the explosion and ensuing fire severely damaged or destroyed approximately 500 houses (approximately 40 hectares in area). Consequently, 19 residents and four firefighters were killed, and approximately 1,000 people were injured (Commissie Onderzoek Vuurwerkramp Enschede, 2001). An estimated 10,000 or more residents of the affected area were evacuated for one or more days, while over 1,200 people lost their homes completely. Directly after the disaster a sports complex was used for temporary housing of affected residents who could not return to their homes. In addition, it is estimated that between 5,000 and 8,000 rescue workers provided help during the first days after the event, such as immediate aid to victims, beginning initial clearance, and surveillance of the affected area. The rescue workers were from the Enschede region, other parts of the Netherlands, and from neighboring countries (Germany and Belgium) (Roorda, Van Stiphout, & Huijsman-Rubingh, 2004).

Environmental measurements of the National Institute for Public Health and the Environment (RIVM) shortly after the disaster indicated that in general it was highly improbable that people were exposed to dangerous concentrations of various fireworks and firework-related substances, such as cadmium, strontium, and lead (Mennen, Kliest, & Van Bruggen, 2001). However, based on earlier experiences in the Netherlands (e.g., the Bijlmermeer disaster, see Section 28.2) the government decided to launch a health survey into the short- and long-term effects of the Enschede fireworks disaster. Blood and urine samples were analyzed for trace elements indicative of exposure to firework-related substances (barium, cadmium, chrome, copper, nickel, lead, antimony, strontium, titanium, and zinc), but results showed no systematic increases of heavy metal levels in the residential group (including children) or in the relief workers. In total, 22 people had relatively high levels that warranted clinical toxicological follow-up, but these were considered chance observation since there was no indication that the elevated levels were associated with exposures related to the disaster (Projectteam Gezondheidsonderzoek Vuurwerkramp Enschede, 2001).

A second purpose of the study was to make a rapid assessment of the immediate health effects and personal experiences (what people had heard, seen, done, and felt), by means of a large questionnaire, to prevent possible bias in the recollection of disaster experiences and emotions during and immediately after the disaster. In addition, the survey aimed to communicate acknowledgment of mental and physical health problems and to contribute to a sense of social support and a "caring government" (Roorda et al., 2004; Van Kamp et al., 2006).

28.2. RESEARCH AFTER THE ENSCHEDE FIREWORKS DISASTER IN PERSPECTIVE: LESSONS LEARNED FROM THE BIJLMERMEER DISASTER

The rapid assessment, developed and conducted under enormous time pressure, was profoundly influenced by a disaster 8 years earlier and its aftermath. On October 4, 1992, an El Al Boeing 747 cargo jet lost two engines from its right wing without being noticed by the crew. The captain, with his airplane out of control, decided to return to Schiphol Airport, but the plane crashed onto two apartment buildings in Amsterdam's densely populated Bijlmermeer district. Buildings were obliterated and human beings perished in the towering flames that arose from the tanks of the jumbo jet. Some 39 residents and four crewmembers lost their lives.

In the period immediately following the event, a media campaign was launched and leaflets were distributed in many languages to inform people about possible psychological after effects. General practitioners and mental health care professionals were instructed about potential disaster-related problems. The slogan "a normal reaction to an abnormal event" was coined to prepare people for the impending psychological after effects and simultaneously to reassure them that such effects were normal. The combined effect of all these efforts was that several hundred adults and children received some form of trauma intervention. Although a majority of survivors did make use of mental health care at some time, treatments were often terminated prematurely, notably because of financial constraints or perceived ineffectiveness of the treatments.

The first period postdisaster was dominated by posttraumatic symptoms and psychosocial problems. The second period was no longer characterized by determinations of the causes of the accident or the number of victims, but by growing suspicions about the plane's cargo and the potentially harmful physical effects this might have had on victims and rescue workers. The two black boxes, containing cockpit voice recorders and data flight recorders, were never found, which is very unusual in an accident on the ground. The initial information on the cargo – flowers, computers, and perfume – had been on the basis of an incomplete list. The plane also had been fitted with depleted uranium in its tail, as a counterweight. Action groups were set up, which launched their own investigation of toxic substances and radioactivity. Some of the worried residents and rescue workers publicly aired their physical complaints, such as skin rashes, respiratory problems, and fatigue, linking these to their presence at the disaster scene. A virtually unstoppable, tragic chain of events ensued, in which the public authorities responded too slowly and were too uncoordinated, at times even supplying incorrect information (Yzermans & Gersons, 2002).

It was not until almost 6 years after the disaster that the ministry of health launched a study on the possible health effects. Family physicians (FPs) in the Bijlmermeer were interviewed to see whether they had noticed an increase in disaster-related illnesses, and a toll-free call center was opened for 2 months to enable people to report their health symptoms. The Symptom Checklist-90 (SCL-90) was sent to all people who presented their complaints to the call center. As an additional precaution, after obtaining informed consent, the medical files of the people who called the toll-free center and completed the SCL-90 were checked to determine whether the FPs were informed about the health complaints (every Dutch citizen has a family physician who registers all reasons for encounter and diagnoses electronically). The nature of the health problems included posttraumatic stress disorder (PTSD) to medically unexplained physical symptoms, and a doctor had been consulted for the majority of the reported health problems. According to the medical files, 13% of the health problems were already known to the FP before the crash in 1992. However, 15% of the health problems originated in the period 5 to 6 years postdisaster. The results of the SCL-90 showed a large burden of distress (two standard deviations higher than a Dutch reference population on average).

At the same time as the study, a parliamentary inquiry committee presented their results in which, finally, the complete cargo list was published: No unknown toxic substances were aboard the plane. The inquiry committee implicitly acknowledged that psychological factors were behind the health complaints, but shied from actually stating thus. Rarely has such an abrupt line been drawn between body and mind in a public debate (Yzermans & Gersons, 2002). Despite this, continued intense political pressure induced the Minister of Health to conduct a large-scale physical examination of the affected population and an epidemiological study among the rescue workers. One year after the report of the parliamentary inquiry committee these results of the investigation were published amidst media hype (Vasterman, Yzermans, & Dirkzwager, 2005). When the Enschede fireworks disaster occurred in May 2000, the authorities tried to put in practice the lessons learned from the Bijlmermeer disaster.

28.3. AIM AND DESIGN OF HEALTH STUDIES AFTER THE ENSCHEDE FIREWORKS DISASTER

The main objective of the studies after the fireworks disaster was to obtain relevant information on the adverse effects on health in the short-, intermediate-, and long-term for use by health care providers and policy makers. In this way, FPs, mental health services (MHS), and the special Information and Advice Centre (IAC), which was set up after the disaster for affected residents and rescue workers, could target possible interventions and organize care aimed at the needs of victims. Also after the disaster, a special Mental After Care unit was organized to offer treatment and help for affected people; much public attention was given to the existence of this unit.

A secondary aim of postdisaster research after this event was, as described, to offer necessary recognition for negative consequences of the disaster. In addition, the health studies also had a scientific purpose, although the first series of reports (in Dutch) were aimed at providing relevant information for health care providers and policy makers. Although all participants received information about the outcomes and conclusions of the conducted studies, the purpose of the studies was not to provide individual-level feedback on health problems. Reports and summaries were available (summaries in Dutch, English, German, Arabic, and Turkish) via a special Internet site until the end of 2007 and the media also reported on the results to a wide audience (Roorda et al., 2004; van Kamp et al., 2006).

28.3.1. Longitudinal Comparative Health Study

In the disaster literature, there are very few longitudinal comparative studies postdisaster where control subjects are assessed at more than one wave in the intermediate and long term (Yzermans, Dirkzwager, & Breuning, 2005). For the Enschede disaster, the first wave of the study among affected adult residents, passers-by, and rescue workers (police, firefighters, and ambulance personnel) was conducted 2 to 3 weeks postevent (between May 31 and June 7, 2000). For the first wave a research center at Twente Air Force Base (close to the Enschede) was built especially for this project. Individuals were invited by mail or, in the case of rescue workers, via their employers to participate in the study. Furthermore, the survey was given much public attention to reach as many survivors as possible.

Participants were bussed from the town to the Air Force base and were given a verbal introduction (which was available in five languages) to the study procedures. Following that, they registered and signed informed consent forms. Next, blood and urine samples were collected, and a comprehensive questionnaire was completed by all participants who were 18 years of age and older. As some rescue workers came from Germany and many immigrants (approximately 25% of the population) lived in the affected area, the questionnaire was available in four different languages (Dutch, Turkish, English, and German) and (native speaking) interpreters were present to clarify questions or to assist in completing the questionnaire. A medical ethics committee approved all surveys. Main topics of the questionnaires are presented in Table 28.1. The first results with respect to health consequences were presented in meetings with affected residents, rescue workers, and policy makers 6 weeks after the disaster (van der Velden, Kleber, & Oostrom, 2000).

The second wave of the study took place at the end of October 2001 (approximately 18 months postdisaster). All respondents of the first survey received a letter describing the design of the survey (language depending on the respondent's country of origin). To stimulate participation, respondents were called at home within 2 weeks after the announcement. If the respondent agreed to participate, a questionnaire with a cover letter in the preferred language and a prepaid envelope were sent to their home address. Those who could not be reached after five phone call attempts or who did not have a known telephone number were sent a Dutch questionnaire with a cover letter. This personal approach was

Table 28.1. Summary main topics questionnaire in three-wave longitudinal study

Topics	At 2–3 Weeks	At 18 Months	At 4 Years
Informed consent	•	•	•
Demographics (gender, marital status, education, etc.)	•	•	•
Experiences during disaster (heard, seen, felt, done)	•		
Peri-traumatic dissociation (PDEQ) and emotions (PEL)	•		
Substance use (GGD/MORGEN) and use of medicines	•	•	•
Quality of life (RAND-36)		•	•
General physical health (VOEG)	•	•	•
Psychological problems (SCL-90-R) and burnout (MBI[T2, T3])	•	•	•
Disaster-related intrusions and avoidance reactions (IES)	•	•	•
Disaster-related PTSD (SRS-PTSD)		•	•
Medical illness		•	•
Life events		•	•
Postdisaster critical incidents at work (PAS, only rescue workers)		•	•
Social support (SSL)		•	•
Mental health services utilization and unmet needs (NEMISIS)		•	•
Utilization of other health care (FP, social work, etc.)		•	•
Dispositional optimism (LOT) and state anger (SSTAS)		•	•
Sick leave		•	•

Notes: FP, Family physician; GGD, Dutch Local and National Public Health Monitor GGD, standardized questions for smoking (GGD, 2003); IES, Impact of Event Scale (Horowitz, Wilner, & Alvarez, 1979); LOT, Life Orientation Test (LOT) (Scheier & Carver, 1985); MBI, sub scale of the Maslach Burnout Inventory (Maslach & Jackson, 1986); MORGEN, Dutch Monitoring Project on Risk Factors for Chronic Diseases: standardized questions for alcohol (MORGEN-project, Blokstra, Seidell, Smit, Bueno de Mesquita, & Verschuren, 1998); NEMISIS, Unmet needs question from NEMISIS study (Bijl & Ravelli, 1998); PAS, Acute Stress List (Van der Velden & Kleber, 1994); PEL, Peritraumatic Emotions List (Van der Velden, Van den Burg, Steinmetz, & van den Bout, 1992); PDEQ, Peritraumatic Dissociation Expericiences Questionnaire (Marmar, Weiss, & Metzler, 1997); PTSD, posttraumatic stress disorder; RAND-36, RAND-36-item Health Survey; Van der Zee & Sanderman, 1993); SCL-90-R, Symptom Checklist 90-R (Derogatis, 1977); SRS-PTSD, The Posttraumatic Stress Disorder Self-Rating Scale (Carlier, Lamberts, Van Uchelen, & Gersons, 1998); SSL, Social Support List (Van Sonderen, 1993); STASS, Spielberger State-Trait Anger Scale (Van der Ploeg, Defares, & Spielberger, 1982); VOEG, Questionnaire Research Perceived Health (Van Sonsbeek, 1990).

supported by extensive publicity before the start of the study. Those residents who needed help filling in the questionnaire could come to one of the two community centers during the daytime for 2 weeks. If the questionnaire was not returned within 3 weeks, the respondents were reminded by phone or by letter when the telephone number was unknown or the person could not be reached by telephone. Data collection ended in January 2002.

The third wave of the study was conducted in January and February of 2004 (almost 4 years postdisaster). All respondents who participated in the first wave, whether or not they had participated in the second wave, were asked to participate again. The same design was used as in the second wave. Participants in the second and third survey received a €12 (U.S. $15.00) gift.

Nonresponse was analyzed in three separate papers (Dijkema, Grievink, Stellato, Roorda, & Van der Velden, 2005; Grievink, Van der Velden, Yzermans, Roorda, & Stellato, 2006; Van den Berg, Van der Velden, Stellato, & Grievink, 2007). The main conclusion was that prevalence rates of self-reported symptoms were hardly or only slightly affected by selective response.

28.3.2. Comparison Groups

The best method to gain reliable insight into the effects of a disaster on health is comparing nonretrospectively collected data on preevent health and prospectively collected data on postdisaster health (see Section 28.3.4). A good alternative is comparing health of victims with a comparable group of nonaffected persons. owing to the sudden nature of the event and time constraints it was not possible to arrange a comparison groups 2 to 3 weeks postdisaster (first wave), but comparison groups were included for the second and third wave.

The city of Tilburg, located in another part of the Netherlands, was chosen as a reference city because both cities had comparable histories (rise and fall of textile industries). From Statistics Netherlands, four districts (postal areas) in Tilburg were chosen as comparison groups on the basis of age and gender composition, educational level, and country of origin. General health status of residents of these four districts was compared with Enschede survivors, using figures from the Dutch Public Health Status and forecast report. Within each of the districts, a sample of 400 adults, stratified on gender, age, and country of origin, was drawn from the Registry Office. Since this office does not have information on educational background, four districts were preselected that had comparable socioeconomic backgrounds to the affected area in Enschede through Statistics Netherlands. The stratification on age, gender, and country of origin was used to make the sample comparable to the affected residents in the first survey (Drogendijk et al., 2003; Grievink, Van der Velden, et al., 2006; Van der Velden, Grievink, Olff, Gersons, & Kleber, 2007; Van der Velden, Kleber, et al., 2007).

In addition, comparison groups of police, firefighters, and ambulance personnel from other parts of the Netherlands, not involved in this or another disaster in the Netherlands, were identified. They participated in the second survey and were approached via their employers. As analyses showed that self-reported general health problems between affected and nonaffected rescue workers hardly differed at the second survey, they were not asked to participate in the third survey; mental health problems also hardly differed from the affected sample and comparison groups of rescue workers. In addition, 0.7% of all groups of affected rescue workers met the criteria for PTSD 18 months postdisaster (range 0%–3.2%). Though significant, disaster exposure and postdisaster critical incidents explained little variance of disaster-related avoidance, anxiety and depression symptoms, sleeping problems, and somatic symptoms (Dirkzwager, Yzermans, & Kessels, 2004; Morren, Yzermans, Van Nispen, & Wevers, 2005; Van der Velden, Christiaanse, et al., 2006). A later prospective comparative study showed that sick leave – identified through electronic medical records – among rescue workers increased during the 18 months after the explosions. For example, the prevalence of absences attributed to psychological problems increased from 2.5% of workers during the 6 months before the disaster to 4.6% during the first 6-month period after the explosions and 5.1% during the second period (Morren, Dirkzwager, Kessels, & Yzermans, 2007).

28.3.3. Prospective Comparative Surveillance, Using Existing Registries of Family Physicians

Longitudinal studies measuring health before and after disaster are rarely executed. In the Netherlands we had the opportunity to implement a cohort study with inclusion of predisaster data, using the electronic medical records of FPs. From an exploratory study conducted 6 years after the Bijlmermeer plane crash, it appeared that FPs are well aware of the health problems survivors attribute to experiencing a disaster (Yzermans & Gersons, 2002). When disaster struck again in the Netherlands, authorities decided to launch longitudinal surveillance using the existing registry of FPs. Initially the length of the cohort study was 3 years postdisaster but later was extended to 5 years, and it appeared feasible to reconstruct 16 months predisaster.

As mentioned previously, in the Dutch health care system, every citizen is enrolled in the practice of just one FP. When a patient moves, the medical patient record is transferred to another FP. The FP acts as a gatekeeper to secondary care. More than 90% of the patients' problems are addressed by the FPs themselves; the remaining 10% or less are referred to a specialist. Over 75% of the Dutch population sees their FP at least once a year, and more than 96% at least once every 3 years (Schellevis, Westert, & De Bakker, 2005).

It was critical to recruit as many FPs as possible to participate in the study. Thus, the research coordinator and an FP who had participated in another postdisaster study attended a meeting in Enschede to motivate FPs to take part. The objectives and procedures of the study were presented, and the researchers explained that longitudinal surveillance would give insight into the course of postdisaster morbidity and the possible relationship to the disaster. Of the 44 FP practices in the disaster area, 30 decided to participate. Of the 14 practices who refused to participate, 4 anticipated an increased workload in times of pressure due to the disaster, and 9 did not have any survivors in their patient rolls. One practice had to be excluded because paper records were used. Overall, two-thirds of FP practices participated, including 89% of all registered survivors.

Surveillance using FPs' records was possible due to the existing framework of the National Information Network of General Practice (LINH) in the Netherlands. Data on the complete morbidity of the practice population (both exposed and unexposed persons) of the participating FPs was collected. Nonexposed individuals were used as a reference group after matching for age, gender, socioeconomic status, and family practice. Patient medical records include patient and contact information (Fleming, Schellevis, & Paget, 2004). Dutch FPs use the ICPC to register symptoms, problems, and/or diagnoses, and in the electronic medical record the evaluation of the patient (the diagnosis) is registered as an ICPC-code (Lamberts & Wood, 1987).

To make sure that FPs classified and registered the postdisaster morbidity similarly, two training sessions were arranged, in which the use of the ICPC was thoroughly explained and practiced using paper cases. Moreover, the software was built so that registration of at least one diagnosis per contact was made obligatory. In the beginning of the study some FPs had to invest substantial extra time to learn the methodology, but in the course of the study it became routine (Chauvin & Valleron, 1997). It was crucial that participating practices maintain a high-quality level of registration; therefore, each practice had to fulfill two registration requirements: (1) The mean number of contacts per patient per year per practice had to be a minimum of 3.0 because the mean number of contacts in Dutch general practice was 3.5 at the time, and (2) at least 80% of the contacts needed to contain an ICPC-code.

One of the main problems of this longitudinal study was keeping FPs motivated. Therefore, they received a practice feedback report every 3 months for all of their patients – survivor or not – including the number of ICPC-codes they had registered in their practice, the number of contacts a day, the total number of ICPC-codes per employee, the number of consultations per employee, and the top ten new symptoms and diseases. Additionally, regular meetings were organized for all participating FPs to maintain engagement in the study. In only one practice, the surveillance was terminated as the FP retired (Yzermans, Donker, et al., 2005).

A specific procedure was developed to protect the privacy of the survivors and still allow the ability to trace them. Linking of the database of the municipal Information and Advice Center (IAC), where all survivors were registered, and the patient records of the FPs was necessary for tracing data to the individual survivor in case of relocation within city borders. One person – who was stationed outside and acted independently of the research institute – was responsible for linking the IAC records with the FP records (only patient and no medical information), and a unique number was given to each survivor. The research institute analyzed completely anonimized data but still could make necessary adjustments when survivors relocated or died. This privacy procedure was made public in local newspapers and through posters and flyers in the waiting room of each FP. Moreover, announcements of the study and its procedures were made in a bulletin specially published for the survivors. People had the opportunity to call the research institute if they had any question; they could also refuse inclusion in the project, but nobody did (Roorda et al., 2004).

One of the major problems in conducting research postdisaster is determining who was a victim or survivor. About 12,000 persons were registered at the IAC, including all residents of the affected area (identified through the municipal identity register) and passers-by and rescue workers (identified through self-report). Thirteen percent of all survivors registered at the IAC – passers-by and rescue workers – could not be included because they lived outside town. The remaining 10,398 patients were all listed in general practices. Of this group, 11% could not be included because they were enlisted in nonparticipating practices.

28.3.4. Combining Both Studies

Disasters are mostly sudden and unexpected by nature. Therefore, relatively few researchers have been able to assess the predictive value of actual prior mental health problems among adult victims. Those that have had this opportunity have found that preceding depressive symptoms or depression (Alexander & Wells, 1991; Bravo, Rubio, Stipec, Canino, & Woodbury, 1990; Gignac, Cott, & Badley, 2003; Ginexi, Weihs, Simmens, & Hoyt, 2000; Knight, Gatz, Heller, & Bengtson, 2000; Nolen-Hoeksema & Morrow, 1991; Phifer, 1990), general health (Gignac et al., 2003), alcohol abuse (Bravo et al., 1990), psychological problems (Yzermans, Donker, et al., 2005; Dirkzwager, Grievink, Van der Velden, & Yzermans, 2006), and insomnia (Lin et al., 2002) were associated with more mental health problems after the disaster. Problems were predicted on the short term (within 3 months) (e.g., Ginexi et al., 2000), intermediate term (approximately 1–2 years) (e.g., Gignac et al., 2003) or long term (2 years or more) (e.g., Bravo et al., 1990). One recent study by Bromet and colleagues (2005) found that predisaster lifetime mental health/substance use disorder predicted PTSD 6 months postdisaster.

The prospective nature of the health surveillance data (16 months preevent) enabled us to assess the association between pre- and postdisaster problems as presented to the FP and self-reported health problems after the disaster (no electronic medical records were available for the Tilburg sample). Thus, the data of the three-wave longitudinal study among the affected residents was linked with the electronic medical records of the FPs. In agreement with the Dutch Data Protection Authority, an external party using numerical identification codes linked the data of the two studies. However, as could be expected, for several respondents in the longitudinal health study, no electronic records were available; a record was available for 649 out of the 813 participants who participated in all three surveys (Van der Velden, Yzermans, Kleber, & Gersons, 2007). In Figure 28.1 a flowchart is presented for the number of affected residents (18 years or older) in the main studies.

28.4. MAIN FINDINGS

Results of both studies have been published in peer-reviewed journals (approximately 40 as of the end of 2007). In the following paragraphs, we focus on the main results of our studies with respect to PTSD and other mental health disturbances, physical problems, and predictors of disturbances that were of special interest. In addition, some results of studies examining MHS utilization are presented. With respect to the adverse effect of the disaster on children

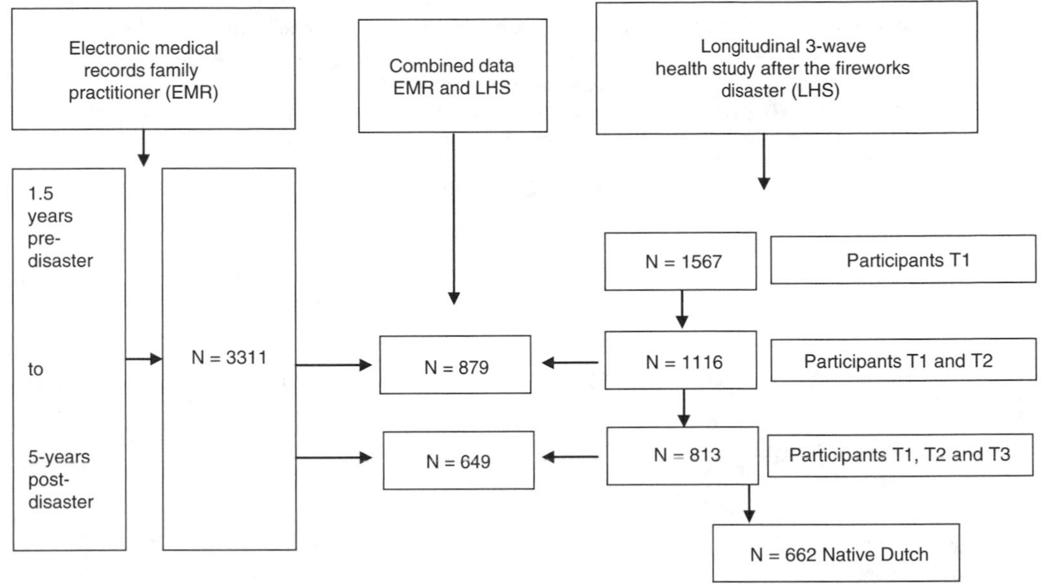

Figure 28.1. Flowchart for the number of affected residents (18 years or older) who participated in the different studies. T1, 2–3 weeks postdisaster; T2, 18 months postdisaster; T3, almost 4 years postdisaster.

we refer to the study of Dirkzwager, Kerssens, and Yzermans (2006).

28.4.1. Longitudinal Comparative Health Study

28.4.1.1. Self-Reported Mental Health Disturbances in Affected Residents and Control Subjects

In Table 28.2, a selection of self-reported mental health disturbances of affected natives ($N=662$) and comparison subjects ($N=526$) is presented. Both groups did not differ in relevant characteristics such as gender, age, education level, and life events. We did not examine PTSD at the first survey, since PTSD can only be diagnosed 1 month after a traumatic event (Drogendijk et al., 2003; Grievink, Van der Velden, Stellato, et al., 2007; Van der Velden, Grievink, et al., 2006; Van der Velden, Kleber, et al., 2007).

Results indicate a decline of mental health problems over the course of time. However, after 4 years, some symptoms were still elevated, and the same pattern was seen in other problems not presented in Table 28.2 (Van den Berg, Grievink, Stellato, Yzermans, & Lebret, 2005). According to the Impact of Event Scale (15-item version) the prevalences of severe intrusions and avoidance reactions (total score > 25) at 2 to 3 weeks, 18 months, and almost 4 years postdisaster were 70.6%, 36.8%, and 23.7%, respectively. According to the Self-Rating Scale for PTSD (SRS-PTSD), at 18 months 13.4% met the criteria of PTSD (DSM-IV) and 9.7% after 4 years (Van der Velden, Grievink, et al., 2006).

In a separate analysis, mental health problems 18 months postdisaster in affected native residents and in native control subjects were compared as well as mental health problems in affected and unaffected (Turkish) immigrant residents (Drogendijk et al., 2003). Results showed a much higher proportion of affected (Turkish) immigrants scored high or very high on all SCL-90-R subscales when compared with a control group of (Turkish) immigrants (ORs varied between 3.1 and 8.7). There were smaller significant differences in health problems between affected Dutch natives and a control group of Dutch origin (ORs varied between 1.7 and 3.2).

Table 28.2. Self-reported (Severe) mental health problems of survivors and controls at three waves

	Affected Native Residents (*N*=662)		**Comparison Group (*N*=526)**				
	Severe Symptoms/ PTSD		**Severe Symptoms**				
	No	**Yes**	**No**	**Yes**			
	%	%	%	%	χ^2	**df**	***p*-value**
Severe anxiety symptoms[a]							
at T1	58.2	41.8	–	–			
at T2	73.5	26.5	88.3	11.7	39.80	1	0.000
at T3	80.7	19.3	85.5	14.5	4.80	1	0.028
Severe depression symptoms[a]							
at T1	54.4	45.6	–	–			
at T2	69.6	30.4	77.8	22.2	9.87	1	0.002
at T3	74.7	25.3	79.1	20.9	3.18	1	ns.
Severe somatic problems[a]							
at T1	67.4	32.6	–	–			
at T2	72.4	27.6	82.6	17.4	16.69	1	0.000
at T3	81.0	19.0	83.8	16.2	1.57	1	ns
Severe sleeping problems[a]							
at T1	50.9	49.1	–	–			
at T2	69.0	31.0	82.6	17.4	28.60	1	0.000
at T3	71.0	29.0	82.3	17.7	20.44	1	0.000
Disaster-related PTSD							
at T2	86.6	13.4	–	–	–		
at T3	92.3	9.7	–	–			

Notes: ns., not significant; PTSD, posttraumatic stress disorder; SCL-90-R, Symptom Checklist 90-R.

T1, 2–3 weeks postdisaster; T2, 18 months postdisaster; T3 almost 4 years postdisaster.

[a] High or very high scores on the subscales of the SCL-90-R according to the Dutch norm tables (Arrindell & Ettema, 1986).

28.4.1.2. Self-Reported Use of Mental Health Services in Affected Residents and Control Subjects

Several studies after disasters have examined postevent MHS utilization. To the best of our knowledge, no longitudinal studies are available examining MHS utilization in the intermediate and long term or possible differences in MHS utilization between victims and nonexposed people. At the time of the second and third survey, participants were asked whether they have had contact with MHS in the year before the survey (e.g., Aftercare Unit, local mental health organizations, private psychiatrist, psychologist, and psychotherapist). Furthermore, in the third survey all participants were asked whether they had contact at any time with MHS in the period from May 13, 2000, to February 2004 (almost 4 years postdisaster) (Van der Velden, Grievink, Dorresteijn, et al., 2005; Van der Velden, Grievink, et al., 2006). Of the affected residents, 27.6% had used MHS in the period 6 to 18 months postdisaster in contrast to 9.0% of the control subjects (OR = 3.90, 95% CI = 2.75–5.52). In the 12 months before the last survey, these percentages were 17.9% and 8.3%, respectively (OR = 2.42, 95% CI = 1.66–3.52). In total, 45.0% of the affected residents used MHS since the disaster, and 17.2% of the control subjects used MHS in the same period (OR = 3.94, 95% CI = 2.99–5.18).

Interestingly, victims with severe depression and anxiety symptoms 18 months postdisaster had used MHS more often than control subjects with similar levels of these symptoms (OR 2.6 and 2.0); however, after 4 years, MHS utilization among participants in both groups with anxiety symptoms did not differ. In addition, no differences were found in MHS utilization between both groups in respondents with persistent symptoms, that is, having had symptoms at 18 months as well as 4 years postdisaster. The large majority of the affected residents with persistent PTSD (89.7%) had some contact with MHS in the period May 2000 to February 2004.

In separate papers we examined whether immigrants, among other risk groups, were less likely to use MHS than native affected residents. Results showed that they were not less likely to receive treatment (den Ouden et al., 2007; Van der Velden et al., 2005). In contrast, we found indications that more affected immigrants with mental health problems used MHS than affected natives with these problems (Van der Velden et al., 2005; Van der Velden, Yzermans, et al., 2007).

28.4.1.3. Risk Factors for Mental Health Disturbances

The design of the study enabled us to examine specific risk factors that have received relatively little attention in other longitudinal disaster research, in particular the independent predictive value of peritraumatic dissociation, dispositional optimism, and smoking (Breh & Seidler, 2007; Brewin, Andrews, & Valentine, 2000; Galea, Nandi, & Vlahov, 2005; Koenen et al., 2005; Ozer, Best, Lipsey, & Weiss, 2003). Of the longitudinal studies assessing the independent predictive value of peritraumatic dissociation (assessed within 1 month) for PTSD symptomatology 3 months or more after a traumatic event, one focused on disaster victims (see Van der Velden & Wittmann, 2008). Koopman and colleagues (1994) found an independent association between peritraumatic dissociation and PTSD. However, peritraumatic dissociation emerged as a significant predictor of posttraumatic avoidance, but not for intrusions, 7 to 9 months postevent. In our study we found no indications that – although associated on a bivariate level – peritraumatic dissociation is an independent predictor for intrusions and avoidance reactions and PTSD severity 18 months and almost 4 years postdisaster (Van der Velden, Kleber, et al., 2006). In the analyses we controlled for demographics, disaster experiences, intrusions, avoidance reactions, and psychological distress 2 to 3 weeks postevent. In accordance with other prospective studies on peritraumatic dissociation, these findings question whether peritraumatic dissociation, that is, a general construct of peritraumatic dissociation, is a relevant predictor of PTSD symptomatology after disasters (Bryant, 2007; Holeva & Tarrier, 2001; Marshall & Schell, 2002; Simeon, Greenberg, Nelson, Schmeidler, & Hollander, 2005; Wittmann, Moergeli, & Schnyder, 2006).

In a meta-analysis, Andersson (1996) concluded that dispositional optimism was statistically significantly associated with measures of coping, symptom reporting, and, most reliably, with negative affect. Dispositional optimism is the general tendency to believe that one will experience good outcomes in life, conceptualized as a relatively stable personality trait that determines the self-regulation of behavior (Scheier & Carver, 1985, 1992). However, few studies have assessed the association between dispositional optimism and PTSD symptomatology. Dougall and colleagues (2001) found that dispositional optimism was associated with less distress at 4 to 8 weeks and 6, 9, and 12 months after the disaster and with less avoidance coping. However, dispositional optimism at the first survey did not predict changes in overall symptoms of distress at each follow-up when controlling for distress at the first survey.

Benight and colleagues (1999) found that the impact of optimism – among other factors – on posttraumatic symptoms was entirely mediated through perceived coping self-efficacy. However, it is unknown whether the association between optimism and health problems among disaster victims has a similar magnitude as the association in a comparable group of nonexposed people. For this reason, we assessed the independent predictive value of dispositional optimism at 18 months postevent for mental health problems almost 4 yeast postdisaster. Results showed that pessimistic victims were only more at risk for severe depression symptoms (OR = 2.78, 95% CI = 1.37–5.65) and obsessive-compulsive symptoms (OR = 2.18, 95% CI = 1.08–4.39) than optimistic victims, when controlling for demographic characteristics, life events, smoking, and existing health problems 18 months postdisaster. However, pessimistic participants in the comparison group were also more at risk for severe anxiety symptoms, sleeping problems, somatic problems, and problems in social functioning than optimistic control participants ($2.76 \leq OR \leq 9.27$) (Van der Velden, Kleber, et al., 2007). Therefore, we concluded that professional helpers, such as general practitioners, psychologists, and psychiatrists, involved in postdisaster treatment programs in the intermediate and long term should not rely too much on optimistic views of disaster victims.

As discussed in Chapter 6, several studies have shown an association between trauma exposure, PTSD symptomatology, and smoking (Feldner, Babson, & Zvolensky, 2007). With respect to disasters, studies have shown that victims who increased smoking were more at risk for PTSD symptomatology than others (Joseph, Yule, Williams, & Hodgekinson, 1993; Nandi, Galea, Ahern, & Vlahov, 2005; Vlahov et al., 2004). Since smoking is also associated with subsequent mental health disturbances in nontrauma samples, we analyzed whether smoking is independently associated with a higher risk for mental health disturbances in affected residents compared with a control group. Victims who smoked 18 months postdisaster were more likely to have severe anxiety symptoms (OR = 2.32, 95% CI = 1.19–4.53), severe hostility symptoms (adjusted OR = 1.84, 95% CI = 1.06–3.22), and disaster-related PTSD (OR = 2.64, 95% CI = 1.05–6.62) 18 months postdisaster than nonsmokers. In the comparison group, smoking was not an independent risk factor. Interestingly, smokers in the control group who were confronted with stressful life events had a higher chance of having severe anxiety symptoms at the third survey than nonsmokers (OR = 4.11, 95% CI = 1.03–16.47) (Van der Velden, Grievink, Olff, Gersons, & Kleber , 2007).)

In addition, in affected ambulance personnel we examined the independent predictive value of cigarette consumption 2 to 3 weeks postevent for severe intrusions, avoidance, hostility, and depression symptoms 18 months postdisaster (Van der Velden, Kleber, & Koenen, 2008). We controlled for pre- (age, gender, education), peri- (disaster exposure, peritraumatic dissociation) and postdisaster variables (intrusions, avoidance, psychological distress, and alcohol consumption 2 to 3 weeks postdisaster). Results showed that cigarette consumption independently predicted these posttraumatic stress symptoms. These findings raise the question of whether victimized smokers can reduce the risk of PTSD symptomatology by quitting or reducing smoking after disaster. Finally, in subsamples of survivors we examined the relationships between PTSD, posttraumatic major depressive disorder, smoking, and levels of circadian cortisol 2 to 3 years postdisaster (Olff et al., 2006), and the relationship between sustained attention and PTSD symptoms 2 to 3 years postdisaster (Meewisse et al., 2005).

28.4.2. Psychological Problems as Presented in Family Practice

As previously mentioned, we were able to analyze health problems after the fireworks disaster using existing registries. Here we restrict ourselves to the surveillance in family practice. Because all FPs in the city of Enschede used electronic medical records and the International

Classification of Primary Care (ICPC) it was feasible to use predisaster data. Moreover, we could create a reference group of people from the same family practices who were not struck by the disaster, matched for age, gender, insurance type, and family practice. It was decided to use this reference group instead of a control group from another city to rule out interdoctor variation and culture as potential confounders.

In Figure 28.2 the mean numbers of contacts (per 3 months) in general practice are shown for survivors and their reference group. Despite the matching between survivors and their references, differences between both groups were already present before the disaster, presumably caused by differences in socioeconomic status; insurance type appeared to be an inaccurate proxy. Compared to both predisaster utilization and to the references, survivors had more contacts with the FP during the first 2 postdisaster years, especially bereaved survivors and those with mental health problems (den Ouden, Dirkzwager, & Yzermans, 2005; Dorn, Yzermans, Kerssens, Spreeuwenberg, & Van der Zee, 2006). In the fifth year postdisaster, differences between both groups are still statistically significant. Interestingly, people who were not struck by the disaster (the reference group) seemed to show some solidarity with the survivors and their FPs by less contact with their doctors in the first weeks postdisaster.

At the end of the study period the prevalence rate was still higher than predisaster. For psychological problems we summed the codes in the ICPC for feeling anxious/nervous, acute and chronic stress reactions, feeling depressed, feeling angry/irritable, sleeping problems/insomnia, disorders of memory and concentration, generalized anxiety disorder, and major depression. PTSD is not often diagnosed in family practice, but in general, patients with two or more of the problems and disorders mentioned, especially when they were persistent, would be referred to mental health care (Yzermans et al., 2006). Before the disaster no differences appeared between survivors and references for prevalences of psychological problems. In the first 3 months after the disaster (June to August 2000), an enormous increase (sixfold) occurred, followed by a fast decrease and a plateau, which lasted for almost 3 years (Figure 28.3). In the first year postdisaster more survivors presented psychological problems than before the disaster (OR = 4.51, 95% CI = 3.89–5.24), and this applied all the more for survivors who lost their house and personal belongings (OR = 5.92, 95% CI = 4.64–7.55) but to a lesser extent for women (OR = 1.18, 95% CI = 1.04–1.35). No differences were found for age, insurance type, or ethnicity: Differences between these groups postdisaster can be explained by existing predisaster differences. Five years postdisaster, survivors still presented more psychological problems to the family physician than predisaster (OR = 1.33, 95% CI = 1.14–1.57).

From multivariate logistic regression analyses, psychological problems, and disorders presented to the family physician during the

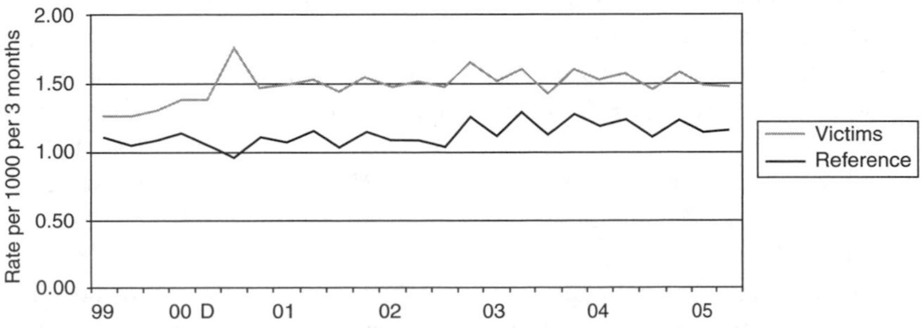

Figure 28.2. Utilization in family practice in the period 16 months predisaster till 5 years postdisaster, for victims and references in rates per 1,000 per 3 months. D, disaster date.

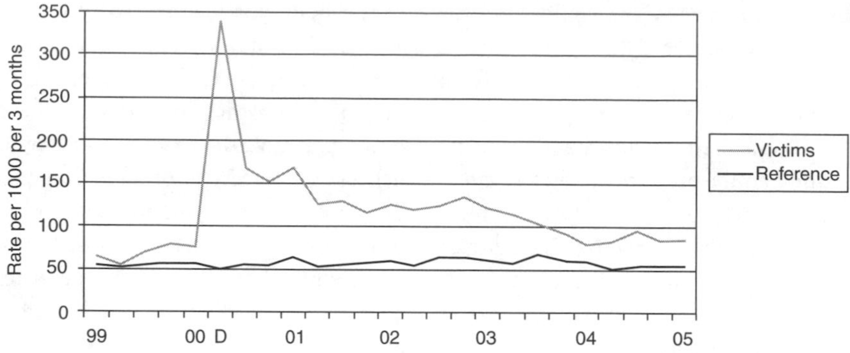

Figure 28.3. Prevalence rates of psychological problems as presented in family practice in the period 16 months predisaster till 5 years postdisaster, for victims and references in rates per 1,000 per 3 months. D, disaster date.

first year after the disaster were associated with predisaster psychological problems (OR = 3.37, 95% CI = 2.14–5.31), being injured by the disaster (OR = 2.27, 95% CI = 1.26–4.11), immigrant status (OR = 2.03, 95% CI = 1.37–3.00), female gender (OR = 1.82, 95% CI = 1.37–2.42), forced relocation (OR = 1.83, 95% CI = 1.24–2.70), and a higher degree of exposure (OR = 1.25, 95% CI = 1.08–1.44) (Dirkzwager, Grievink, et al., 2006; Soeteman et al., 2007). The most important predictor for psychological problems postdisaster appeared to be psychological problems predisaster. Even controls with predisaster psychological problems present more postdisaster psychological problems compared with survivors without predisaster psychological problems (Soeteman et al., 2006).

Considering individual psychological problems and disorders roughly two types of time courses are apparent: (1) an immediate increase, followed by a decrease, leveling off to a plateau for some time (see the course for all psychological problems and disorders, Figure 28.3) and (2) slowly increasing prevalence rates, which reach a peak after several years. Examples of the first course in time are "sleeping problems/ insomnia" (Figure 28.4), "feeling anxious/ nervous" (Figure 28.5), and "feeling depressed" (Figure 28.6), while the latter course is illustrated by "fatigue" (Figure 28.7) and "major depression" (Figure 28.8). Remarkable differences are seen in these figures between the problem as registered by the FP (feeling anxious, feeling depressed) and the disorders (anxiety disorder and major depression) (Figure 28.9). While FPs classified a lot of problems as anxiousness, anxiety disorder was hardly diagnosed (although more than in the reference group). On the other hand, "feeling depressed" was hardly registered, while "major depression" appeared in the top ten most frequently registered diagnoses among the survivors. Survivors also appeared to be at an increased risk of becoming an incident benzodiazepine user after the disaster. However, prolonged use was not often observed (Dorn, Yzermans, & Van der Zee, 2007; Fassaert et al., 2007).

In Chapter 6 this detailed evidence is presented for how mental and physical health problems (after disaster) are strongly intertwined. Therefore, here we will only describe the burden of health problems overall (for survivors and references together) as presented in family practice in the study period of 6 years postdisaster. Table 28.3 shows that 11.0% of all health problems (N = 371,680) were psychological and those problems were presented by 51.4% of all patients (N = 13,842), with a mean of 6.0 psychological problems per practice. In the postdisaster period survivors presented more medically unexplained symptoms (MUS) (especially immediately in the first months, but statistically significant in the

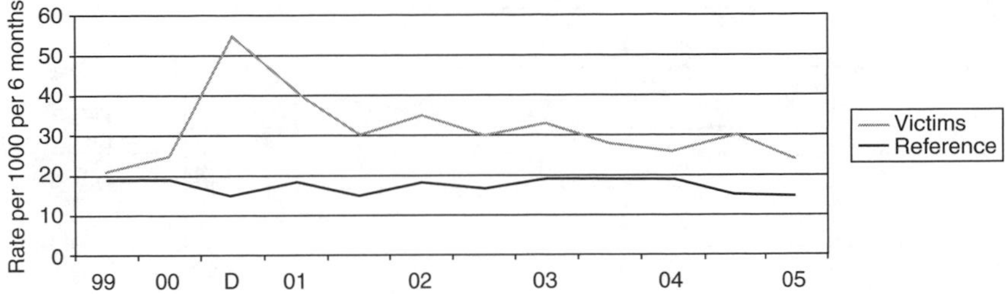

Figure 28.4. Sleeping problems as presented in family practice in the period 1-year before till 5 years after the fireworks disasters (D), expressed as prevalence rates per 1,000 per 6 months for survivors (upper line) and references (lower line). D, disaster date.

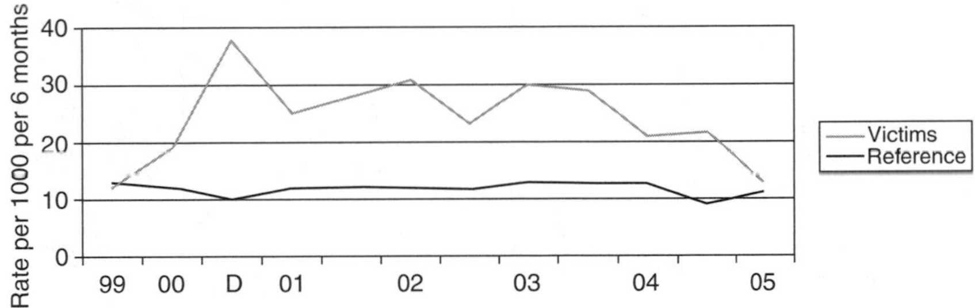

Figure 28.5. Feeling anxious/nervous as presented in family practice in the period 1-year before till 5 years after the fireworks disasters (D), expressed as prevalence rates per 1,000 per 6 months for survivors (upper line) and references (lower line). D, disaster date.

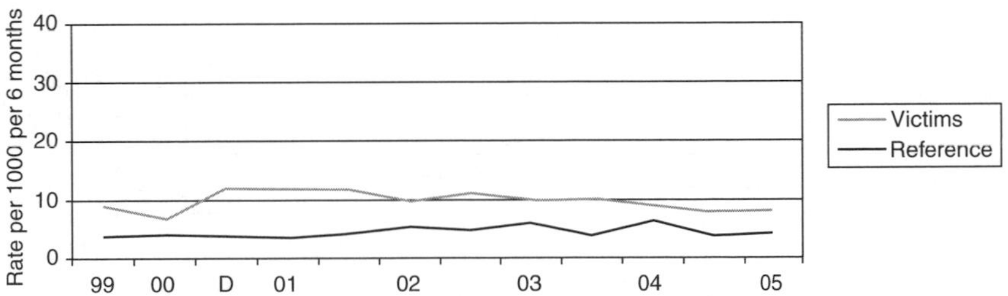

Figure 28.6. Feeling down, depressed as presented in family practice in the period 1 year before till 5 years after the fireworks disasters (D), expressed as prevalence rates per 1,000 per 6 months for survivors (upper line) and references (lower line). D, disaster date.

first 2 years, compared to the predisaster period and to the references) and more chronic diseases (faster increase and more among survivors than among references). Moreover, clear differences between survivors and references were seen for musculoskeletal symptoms (during the first 3 years postdisaster), gastrointestinal symptoms (whole period), and neurological symptoms (first 3 years). Individual symptoms and diseases that were more often seen in survivors included back pain, especially lower back pain without radiation symptoms (with a peak in the third and

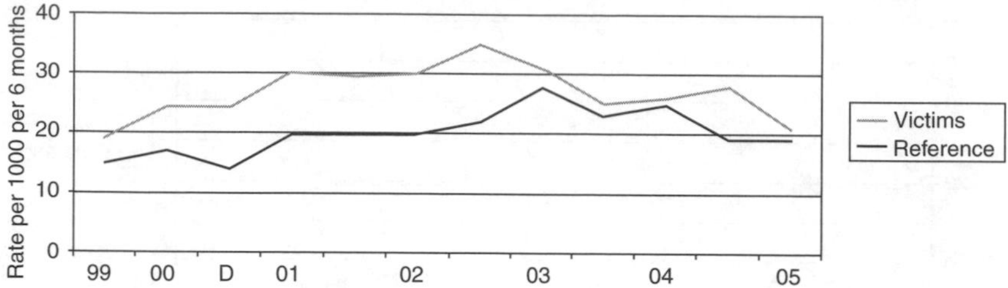

Figure 28.7. Fatigue as presented in family practice in the period 1 year before until 5 years after the fireworks disasters (D), expressed as prevalence rates per 1,000 per 6 months for survivors (upper line) and references (lower line). D, disaster date.

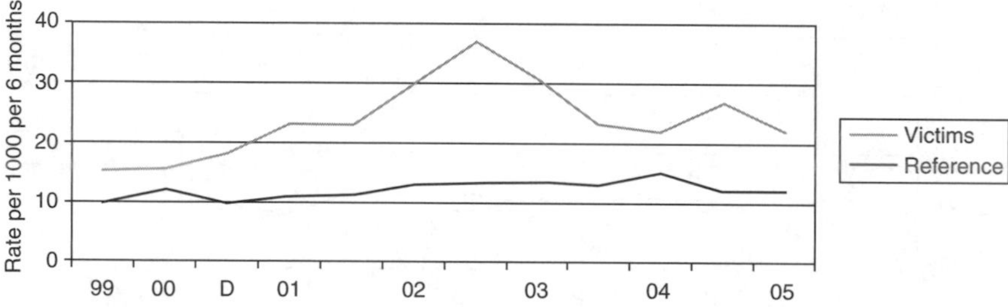

Figure 28.8. Major depression as diagnosed in family practice in the period 1-year before till 5 years after the fireworks disasters (D), expressed as prevalence rates per 1,000 per 6 months for survivors (upper line) and references (lower line). D, disaster date.

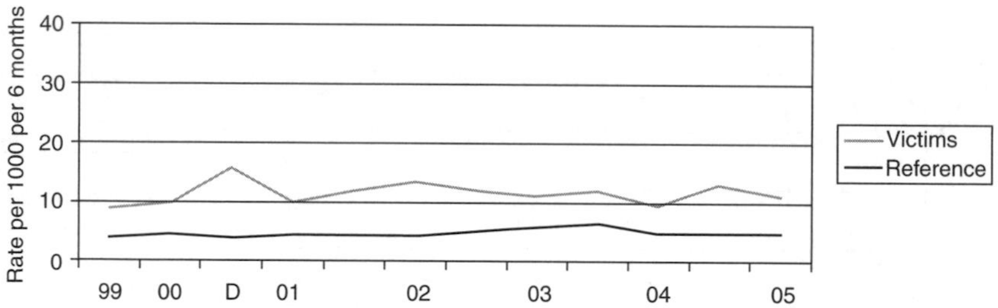

Figure 28.9. Generalized anxiety disorder as diagnosed in family practice in the period 1-year before till 5 years after the fireworks disasters (D), expressed as prevalence rates per 1,000 per 6 months for survivors (upper line) and references (lower line). D, disaster date.

the fourth year postdisaster), pain in the neck and/or the shoulder (first 2 years), hypertension, diabetes mellitus (both faster increase and higher prevalences), headache (whole period), and pain in stomach and abdomen (stomach latter years and abdomen first year) (Yzermans et al., 2006).

28.5. PREDISASTER HEALTH PROBLEMS AND POSTDISASTER FUNCTIONING: COMBINING TWO DATA SETS

In the next paragraphs three examples of the relationship between predisaster health issues

Table 28.3. Burden of health problems postdisaster presented in general practice (victims as well as references)

	% of All Problems	% of All Patients	Mean
Psychological	11.0	51.4	6.0
Musculoskeletal	8.5	59.8	4.0
Gastrointestinal	6.4	44.3	8.5
Respiratory	5.9	52.3	3.2
Skin	5.8	55.9	2.9
Ear	1.7	22.5	2.1
Eye	1.3	20.4	1.8
Neurological	1.4	16.4	2.5
MUS	*23.7*	*82.7*	*8.1*
Chronic	*25.0*	*69.7*	*10.2*
Other	9.3	–	–

Note: Medically unexplained symptoms (MUS) and chronic diseases are typed in italic because overlapping is possible between these two categories and the other eight mentioned.

and postdisaster outcomes are presented from the combined their data sets as described in Section 28.3.4. With respect to the association between predisaster psychological problems and postdisasters MHS utilization we refer to Van der Velden, Yzermans, and colleagues (2007) and Den Ouden and colleagues (2007).

28.5.1. Predisaster Psychological Problems as Presented to Family Physician and Postdisaster Self-Reported Health Problems

Gender, age, marital status, public health insurance (as an indicator for relatively low socioeconomic status), predisaster psychological problems, immigrant status, educational level, degree of disaster exposure, and disaster-related outcomes including sustained injuries, death of a significant other, and forced relocation are associated with postdisaster psychological problems (see Brewin et al., 2000; Galea et al., 2005). We examined whether these variables were independent predictors of very severe anxiety and depression symptoms, sleeping problems, somatization, and hostility (Dirkzwager et al., 2006). All variables were independently associated with one or more of these symptoms 2 to 3 weeks and/or 18 months postevent, except death of a significant other. For example, predisaster psychological problems as presented to the FP were independently associated with a higher risk for very severe symptoms of anxiety (OR = 2.44, 95% CI = 1.45–4.13), depression (OR = 2.08, 95% CI = 1.22–3.56), sleeping problems (OR = 2.44, 95% CI = 1.51–3.96), and hostility (OR = 2.38, 95% CI = 1.42–3.99) 2 to 3 weeks postdisaster. In addition, predisaster mental health issues were independently associated with a higher risk for feeling depressed (OR = 3.84, 95% CI = 2.15–6.86), sleeping problems (OR = 3.07, 95% CI = 1.76–5.38), somatization (OR = 2.39, 95% CI = 1.27–4.50), and hostility (OR = 1.91, 95% CI = 1.03–3.56) at 18 months postdisaster. Thus, our study further substantiates the previous findings that predisaster psychological problems are an independent risk factor.

28.5.2. Predisaster Chronically Ill as a Group at Risk

Chapter 6 presents findings of our combined studies with respect to physical symptoms (Dirkzwager, Van der Velden, Grievink, Yzermans, 2007; Van den Berg, Grievink, et al., 2008; Van den Berg, Grievink, Yzermans, et al., 2007; van den Berg, Yzermans, et al., 2007); therefore, for a detailed overview we refer to that chapter. As thus far no prospective studies have been conducted examining chronic illness as a possible risk factor (Van den Berg, Van der Velden, et al., 2006), here we highlight one study looking at predisaster chronic disease(s) (e.g., hypertension, asthma, chronic obstructive pulmonary disease, diabetes, heart diseases) identified in the electronic medical records as a predictor of postdisaster functioning. Results indicate that the course of postdisaster functional impairment and mental health symptoms (e.g., anxiety, depression, PTSD) until 4 years postdisaster did not consistently differ between survivors with chronic disease and survivors without chronic disease. Although chronically ill survivors had somewhat more problems with social functioning and bodily pain, they had fewer emotional role limitations 18 months postdisaster. The main conclusion is therefore that chronically ill are not more at risk for functional impairment and mental health symptoms.

28.5.3. Presentation of Self-Reported Symptoms to Family Physician

Finally, in two studies we examined the correspondence between postdisaster self-reported physical and psychological symptoms and symptoms presented to the FP after the disaster. Results indicate that survivors did not present the majority of self-reported physical symptoms (such as stomachache, back pain, fatigue, headache, pain in bones and muscles, shortness of breath, dizziness) to the FP, and survivors were most likely to present persistent symptoms to the FP in the 18 months postdisaster. For example, victims with persistent stomachache (reported at first and second survey) were more likely to report stomachache to their FP (28%) than survivors who reported stomachache 2 to 3 weeks (6%) postdisaster or 18 months postdisaster (13%). Remarkably, the presentation of individual symptoms to the FP was not consistently associated with functional impairment and psychological distress (Van den Berg, Yzermans, et al., 2007).

The same pattern was seen regarding several severe psychological problems, although the correspondence rates were much higher. For example, approximately 73% of the victims with persistent general psychological problems (SCL-90-R total score) and 60% of the victims with persistent severe disaster-related intrusions and avoidance reactions were identified as such by the FP. Of the victims only reporting with severe psychological problems 2 to 3 weeks or 18 months postdisaster, 53% and 61%, respectively, were identified. For severe disaster-related intrusions and avoidance reactions these rates were 34% and 42%, respectively. Immigrants, female survivors, and the elderly with psychological problems were not more likely to report these problems or be identified by the FP than their counterparts. Interestingly, relocated survivors and those with high disaster exposure were more likely to be identified by the FP as having general psychological problems and severe disaster-related intrusions and avoidance reactions than nonrelocated persons and survivors with lower exposure (relocated: OR = 2.33, 95% CI = 1.48–3.97 and OR = 2.23, 95% CI = 1.28–3.87, respectively; high exposure: OR = 1.43, 95% CI = 1.18–1.71 and OR = 1.40, 95% CI = 1.14–1.71, respectively) (Drogendijk et al., 2007). Therefore, we concluded that the FP diagnosis was partly affected by the survivor's status. However, it is unknown whether this can be attributed to bias in the FP (e.g., because the FP was aware of this status and therefore was more sensitive to these problems), reluctance of survivors who were less exposed to the disaster to speak about their postdisaster mental health problems or an interaction between both.

Finally, in another paper we demonstrated that victims who visited their physician relatively infrequently had a lower prevalence of psychological problems pre- and postdisaster than frequent attenders (Donker, Van der Velden, Kerssens, & Yzermans, 2008).

28.6. EPILOGUE

As Rubonis and Bickman (1991) have shown, studies using retrospectively collected data and having no comparison groups tend to overestimate adverse effects on health (also see Bravo et al., 1990). The design of the health studies after the Enschede fireworks disaster, with preevent measures, comparison groups, the use of self-reported health problems, medical records of FPs, and long-term assessments, enabled us to provide reliable estimates of the health effects of this technological disaster. Our results showed that adult victims had more health problems than nonexposed people, particularly during the first 1.5 years postdisaster. However, the course of health problems after the disaster differed between several subgroups. For instance, immigrants, those who lost their home and were forced to relocate, victims with psychological problems before the disaster, smokers, affected residents with severe posttraumatic stress symptoms during the first weeks after the disaster, and pessimists were more at risk for (later) posttraumatic stress symptoms after the disaster. Additional analyses (not presented in the chapter) showed that the large majority of those suffering from mental health problems 4 years postdisaster were victims with persistent problems. Compared with other studies (Galea et al., 2005), the prevalence of PTSD in native residents was relatively low at both 18 months and 4 years postdisaster, although a large majority of the affected residents reported severe intrusions and avoidance reactions 2 to 3 weeks postdisaster.

Unfortunately, our studies do not allow firm conclusions about the effects of the professional care provided by FPs, the IAC, MHS (including the specific After Care unit), and our studies themselves. After disasters a rigorous study design, with randomly selected intervention and nonintervention groups, cannot be implemented. Therefore, it is uncertain to what extent the care provided and our studies contributed to the recovery of mental health problems or to the relatively low prevalence of disaster-related PTSD, especially in native affected residents. Nevertheless, in this study the use of MHS in affected residents with mental health problems tends to be higher compared to MHS utilization after other disasters (Van der Velden, Grievink, et al., 2006). More than 99% visited their FP in the 5 years postdisaster and MHS utilization was still elevated 4 years postevent. We even found clear indications that victims with mental health problems used MHS more often than a comparable group of nonexposed people. These findings suggest that the mental health policy after the Enschede disaster facilitated recovery.

In contrast to the Bijlmermeer disaster, the Enschede Fireworks disaster was not characterized by continuous reports in the media and speculations about possible toxic exposure. We assume that the early measures of fireworks-related elements and the blood and urine assessments prevented this kind of negative aftermath ("the disaster after the disaster"), which might have delivered additional stress for the survivors. In addition, conducting health studies and supplying summaries of all studies to the respondents and the media may have provided the recognition and information necessary to forestall this situation. Notably, in cooperation with the relocated residents, the destroyed area was rebuilt in the past years.

ACKNOWLEDGMENTS

Finally, many persons and organizations contributed to the studies presented in this chapter. We gratefully thank all respondents and family physicians for their time, effort, and cooperation. All studies were facilitated by the GGD Regio Twente (the local health authority in Enschede) and conducted on behalf of the Dutch Ministry of Health, Welfare, and Sports. We thank the steering group for supervising the research process during the 5 years after the disaster. We especially thank Dr. R.R.R. Huijsman-Rubingh, chair of the steering group, for her continuous support, enthusiasm, and valuable comments during the past years.

REFERENCES

Alexander, D. A., & Wells A. (1991). Reactions of police officers to body handling after a major disaster: A before and after comparison. *British Journal of Psychiatry*, *159*, 547–555.

Andersson, G. (1996). The benefits of optimism: A meta-analytic review of the life orientation test. *Journal of Personality and Individual Differences*, *21*, 719–725.

Arrindell, W. A., & Ettema, J. H. M. (1986). *Handleiding bij een multidimensionele psychopathologie-indicator SCL-90* [Manual for a multidimensional psychopathology indicator SCL-90]. Lisse: Swets&Zeitlinger/Swets Test Publishers, The Netherlands.

Benight, C. C., Ironson, G., Klebe, K., Carver, C., Wynings, C., Greenwood, D., et al. (1999). Conservation of resources and coping self-efficacy predicting distress following a natural disaster: A causal model analyses where the environment meets the mind. *Anxiety, Stress & Coping*, *12*, 107–126.

Bijl, R. V., & Ravelli, A. (1998). Psychiatrische morbiditeit, zorggebruik en zorgbehoefte. Resultaten van de Netherlands Mental Health Survey and Incidence Study (NEMISIS) [Psychiatric morbidity, service utilization, and needs: Results of the Netherlands Mental Health Survey and Incidence Study]. *Tijdschrift voor Gezondheidswetenschappen*, *76*, 446–457.

Blokstra, A., Seidell, J. C., Smit, H. A., Bueno de Mesquita, H. B., & Verschuren, W. M. M. (1998). Het project Monitoring Risicofactoren en Gezondheid Nederland (MORGEN-project) Jaarverslag 1997 [The Monitoring Project on Risk Factors for Chronic Diseases (MORGEN project) Annual Report 1997]. Bilthoven: National Institute for Public Health and the Environment.

Bravo, M., Rubio, Stipec M., Canino, G. J., & Woodbury, M. A. (1990). The psychological sequelae of disaster stress prospectively and retrospectively evaluated. *American Journal of Community Psychology*, *18*, 661–680.

Breh, D. C., & Seidler, G. H. (2007). Is peritraumatic dissociation a risk factor for PTSD? *Journal of Trauma and Dissociation*, *8*, 53–69.

Brewin, C. R., Andrews, A., & Valentine, J. D. (2000). Meta-analysis or risk factors for posttraumatic stress disorder in trauma-exposed adults. *Journal of Clinical and Consulting Psychology*, *68*, 748–766.

Bromet, E. J., Havenaar, J. M., Glutzman, S. F., & Tintle N. L. (2005). Psychological aftermath of the Lviv air show disaster: A prospective controlled study. *Acta Psychiatrica Scandinavica*, *112*, 194–200.

Bryant, R. (2007). Does dissociation further our understanding of PTSD? Does dissociation further our understanding of PTSD? *Journal of Anxiety Disorders*, *21*, 183–191.

Carlier, I. V. E., Lamberts, R. D., Van Uchelen, A. J., & Gersons, B. P. R. (1998). Clinical utility of a brief diagnostic test for posttraumatic stress disorder. *Psychosomatic Medicine*, *60*, 42–47.

Chauvin, P., & Valleron, A. (1997). Monitoring the compliance of sentinel family physicians in public health surveillance: Which FPs persevere? *International Journal of Epidemiology*, *26*, 166–172.

Commissie Onderzoek Vuurwerkramp Enschede. (2001). Deel A. De vuurwerkramp: SE Fireworks, De Overheid, De ramp [Part A. The fireworks disaster: SE Fireworks, The Dutch Government, The disaster]. The Netherlands: Enschede/Den Haag.

Ouden, D. J. Den, Dirkzwager, A. J. E., & Yzermans, C. J. (2005). Health problems presented in general practice by survivors before and after a fireworks disaster: Associations with mental health care. *Scandinavian Journal of Primary Health Care*, *23*, 137–141.

Ouden, D. J. Den, Velden, P. G. Van der, Grievink, L., Morren, M., Dirkzwager, A. J. E., & Yzermans, C. J. (2007). Use of mental health services among disaster survivors: Predisposing factors. *BMC Public Health*, *7*(147), 173.

Derogatis, L. R. (1977). *SCL-90-R: Administration, scoring and procedures manual-I for the revised version*. Baltimore: Johns Hopkins University School of Medicine, Clinical Psychometrics Research Unit.

Dijkema, M., Grievink, L., Stellato, R., Roorda, J., & Velden, P. G. Van der (2005). Determinants of response in a longitudinal health study following the firework-disaster in Enschede, the Netherlands. *European Journal of Epidemiology*, *20*, 839–847.

Dirkzwager, A. J. E., Grievink, L., Velden, P. G. Van der, & Yzermans, C. J. (2006). Risk factors for psychological and physical health problems after a man-made disaster. *British Journal of Psychiatry*, *189*, 144–149.

Dirkzwager, A. J. E, Kerssens, J. J., & Yzermans, C. J. (2006). Health problems in children and adolescents before and after a man-made disaster. *Journal of the American Academy of Child and Adolescent Psychiatry*, *45*, 94–103.

Dirkzwager, A. J. E., Velden, P. G. Van der, Grievink, L., & Yzermans, C. J. (2007). Disaster-related posttraumatic stress disorder and physical health. *Psychosomatic Medicine*, *69*, 435–440.

Dirkzwager, A. J. E., Yzermans, C. J., & Kessels, F. J. M. (2004). Psychological, musculoskeletal, and respiratory problems and sickness absence before and after involvement in a disaster: A longitudinal study among rescue workers. *Occupational Environmental Medicine*, *61*, 870–872.

Donker, G., Velden, P. G. Van der, Kerssens, J., & Yzermans, J. (2008). Infrequent attendance in general practice after a major disaster: A problem? A longitudinal study using medical records and self-reported distress and functioning. *Family Practice*, *25*, 92–97.

Dorn, T., Yzermans, C. J., Kerssens, J. J., Spreeuwenberg, P. M. M., & Van der Zee, J. (2006). Disaster and subsequent healthcare utilization. A longitudinal study among victims, their family members, and control subjects. *Medical Care, 44*, 581–589.

Dorn, T., Yzermans, C. J., & Van der Zee, J. (2007). Prospective cohort study into postdisaster benodiazepine use demonstrated only short-term increase. *Journal of Clinical Epidemiology, 60*, 795–802.

Dougall, A. L., Hyman, K. B., Hayward, M. C., McFeeley, S., & Baum, A. (2001). Optimism and traumatic stress: The importance of social support and coping. *Journal of Applied Social Psychology, 31*, 223–245.

Drogendijk, A. N., Dirkzwager, J. E., Grievink, L., Velden, P. G. Van der, Marcelissen, F. G. H., & Kleber, R. J. (2007) The correspondence between persistent self-reported post-traumatic problems and general practitioners' reports after a major disaster. *Psychological Medicine*, 37, 193–202.

Drogendijk, A. N., Velden, P. G. Van der, Kleber, R. J., Christiaanse, B. C., Dorresteijn, S. M., Grievink, L., et al. (2003). Turkse getroffenen Vuurwerkramp Enschede: een vergelijkende studie [Turkish victims of the Enschede Fireworks Disaster: A comparative study]. *Gedrag & Gezondheid, 31*, 145–162.

Fassaert, T., Dorn, T., Spreeuwenberg, P. M. M., van Dongen, M. C. J. M., van Gool, C. J. A. W., & Yzermans, C. J. (2007). Prescription of benzodiazepines in general practice in the context of a man-made disaster: A longitudinal study. *European Journal of Public Health, 17*(6), 612–617.

Feldner, M. T., Babson, K. A., & Zvolensky, M. J. (2007). Smoking, traumatic event exposure, and post-traumatic stress: A critical review of the empirical literature. *Clinical Psychological Review, 27*, 4–45.

Fleming, D. M., Schellevis, F. G., & Paget, W. J. (2004). Health monitoring in sentinel practice networks. *European Journal of Public Health, Supplement, 3*, 80–84.

Galea, S., Nandi, A., & Vlahov, D. (2005). The epidemiology of posttraumatic stress disorder after disasters. *Epidemiologic Reviews, 27*, 78–91.

GGD Nederland (Health Authority Netherlands). 2003. Standaard vraagstelling roken (Standardized questions for smoking). Utrecht, The Netherlands: GGD Nederland.

Gignac, M. A. M., Cott, C. A., & Badley, M. (2003). Living with a chronic disabling illness and then some: Data from the 1998 ice storm. *Canadian Journal on Aging, 22*, 249–259.

Ginexi, E. M., Weihs, K., Simmens, S. J., & Hoyt, D. R. (2000). Natural disaster and depression: A prospective investigation of reactions to the 1993 Midwest floods. *American Journal of Community Psychology, 28*, 495–518.

Grievink, L, Velden, P. G. Van der, Stellato, R. K., Dusseldorp, A., Gersons, B. P. R., Kleber, R. J., et al. (2007). A longitudinal comparative study of the physical and mental health problems of affected residents of the firework disaster Enschede, the Netherlands. *Public Health, 121*, 367–374.

Grievink, L., Velden, P. G. Van der, Yzermans, C. J., Roorda, J., & Stellato, R. K. (2006). The importance of estimating selection bias on prevalence estimates shortly after a disaster. *Annals of Epidemiology, 16*, 782–788.

Holeva, V., & Tarrier, N. (2001). Personality and peritraumatic dissociation in the prediction of severity in victims of road traffic accidents. *Journal of Psychosomatic Research, 51*, 687–692.

Horowitz, M. J., Wilner, N., & Alvarez, W. (1979). Impact of Event Scale: A measure of subjective stress. *Psychosomatic Medicine, 41*, 209–218.

Joseph, S., Yule, W., Williams, R., & Hodgekinson, P. (1993). Increased substance use in survivors of the Herald of Free Enterprise Disaster. *British Journal of Medical Psychology, 66*, 185–191.

Knight, B. G., Gatz, M., Heller, K., & Bengtson, V. L. (2000). Age and emotional response to the Northridge earthquake: A longitudinal analysis. *Psychology and Aging, 15*, 627–634.

Koenen, K. C., Hitsman, B., Lyons, M. J., Niaura, R., McCaffery, J., Glodberg, J., et al. (2005). A twin registry study of the relationship between post-traumatic stress disorder and nicotine dependence in men. *Archives of General Psychiatry, 62*, 1258–1265.

Koopman, C., Classen, C., & Spiegel, D. (1994). Predictors of posttraumatic stress symptoms among survivors of the Oakland/Berkeley, Calif., firestorm. *American Journal of Psychiatry, 151*, 888–894.

Lamberts, H., & Wood, M. (1987). *International classification of primary care*. Oxford: Oxford University Press.

Lin, M. R., Huang, W., Huang, C., Hwang, H. F., Tsai, L. W., & Chiu, Y. N. (2002). The impact of the Chi-Chi earthquake on quality of life among elderly survivors in Taiwan: A before and after study. *Quality of Life Research, 11*, 379–388.

Marmar, C. R., Weiss, D. S., & Metzler, T. J. (1997). The peritraumatic dissociation experiences questionnaire. In J. P. Wilson & T. M. Keane (Eds.), *Assessing psychological trauma and severity*. New York: Guilford Press.

Marshall, G. N., & Schell, T. L. (2002). Reappraising the link between peritraumatic dissociation and severity symptom severity: Evidence from a longitudinal study of community violence. *Journal of Abnormal Psychology, 111*, 626–636.

Maslach, C., & Jackson, S.E. (1986). *Maslach burnout inventory: Manual research edition.* Palo Alto, CA: University of California, Consulting Psychologist Press.

Meewisse, M.L., Nijdam, M.J., de Vries, G.J., Gersons, B.P.R., Kleber, R.J., Velden, P.G. Van der, et al. (2005). Disaster-related posttraumatic stress symptoms and sustained attention: Evaluation of depressive symptomatology and sleep disturbances as mediators. *Journal of Traumatic Stress, 18*, 299–302.

Mennen, M.G., Kliest, J.J.G., & Bruggen, M. van (2001). *Fireworks disaster in Enschede, The Netherlands: Measurements for concentrations, dispersion and deposition of harmful substances: Report of the environment study. National institute of public health and environment (RIVM) [report in Ducth].* Bilthoven, The Netherlands: RIVM.

Morren, M., Dirkzwager, A.J., Kessels, F.J., & Yzermans, C.J. (2007). The influence of a disaster on the health of rescue workers: A longitudinal study. *Canadian Medical Association Journal, 176*, 279–283.

Morren, M., Yzermans, C.J., Nispen, R.M.A. van, & Wevers, S.J.M. (2005).The health of volunteer firefighters three years after a technological disaster. *Journal of Occupational Health, 47*, 523–532.

Nandi, A., Galea, S., Ahern, J., & Vlahov, D. (2005). Probable cigarette dependence, PTSD, and depression after an urban disaster: Results from a population survey of New York City residents 4 months after September 11, 2001. *Psychiatry, 68*, 299–310.

Nolen-Hoeksema, S., & Morrow, J. (1991). A prospective study of depression and posttraumatic stress symptoms after a natural disaster: The 1989 Loma Prieta earthquake. *Journal of Personality and Social Psychology, 61*, 115–121.

Olff, M., Meewisse, M., Kleber, R.J., Velden, P.G. Van der, Drogendijk, A.N., Van Amsterdam, J.G.C., et al. (2006). Tobacco usage interacts with post-disaster psychopathology on circadian salivary cortisol. *International Journal of Psychophysiology, 59*, 251–258.

Ozer, E.J., Best, S.R., Lipsey, T.L., & Weiss, D.S. (2003). Predictors of posttraumatic stress disorder and symptoms in adults: A meta-analysis. *Psychological Bulletin, 129*, 52–73.

Phifer, J.F. (1990). Psychological distress and somatic symptoms after natural disaster: Differential vulnerability among older adults. *Psychology and Aging, 5*, 412–420.

Projectteam Gezondheidsonderzoek Vuurwerkramp Enschede. (2001). *Fireworks disaster Enschede: Measurements of elements in blood and urine. Health impact assessment. National institute of public health and environment (RIVM) [report in Ducth].* Bilthoven, The Netherlands: RIVM.

Roorda, J., van Stiphout, W.A., & Huijsman-Rubingh, R.R.R. (2004). Post-disaster health effects: Strategies for investigation and data collection. Experiences from the Enschede firework disaster. *Journal of Epidemiology and Community Health, 58*, 982–987.

Rubonis, A., & Bickman, L. (1991). Psychological impairment in the wake of disaster: The disaster–psychopathology relationship. *Psychological Bulletin, 109*, 384–399.

Scheier, M.F., & Carver, C.S. (1985). Optimism, coping and health: Assessment and implications of generalized outcome expectancies. *Health Psychology, 4*, 219–247.

(1992). Effects of optimism on psychological and physical well-being: Theoretical overview and empirical update. *Cognitive Therapy Research, 16*, 201–228.

Schellevis, F.G., Westert, F.P., & de Bakker, D.H. (2005). The actual role of general practice in the Dutch health-care system: Results of the Second Dutch National Survey of General Practice. *Journal of Public Health, 13*, 265–269.

Simeon, D., Greenberg, J., Nelson, D., Schmeidler, J., & Hollander, E. (2005). Dissociation and posttraumatic stress 1 year after the World Trade Center disaster: Follow-up of a longitudinal survey. *Journal of Clinical Psychiatry, 66*, 231–237.

Soeteman, R.J.H., Yzermans, C.J., Kerssens, J.J., Dirkzwager, A.J.E., Donker, G.A., Veen, P.M.H. ten, et al. (2007). Health problems presented to family practices in the Netherlands 1 year before and 1 year after a disaster. *Journal of the American Board of Family Medicine, 20*, 548–556.

Soeteman, R.J.H., Yzermans, C.J., Kerssens, J.J., Dirkzwager, A.J.E., Donker, G.A., Bosch, W.J.H.M. van den, et al. (2006). The course of post-disaster health problems of victims with pre-disaster psychological problems as presented in general practice. *Family Practice, 23*, 378–384.

Berg, B. Van den, Grievink, L., Stellato, R.K., Yzermans, C.J., & Lebret, E. (2005). Symptoms and related functioning in a traumatized community. *Archives of Internal Medicine, 165*, 2402–2407.

Berg, B. Van den, Grievink, L., Velden, P.G., Van der Yzermans, C.J., Stellato, R.K., Lebret, E., et al. (2008). Risk factors for physical symptoms after a disaster: A longitudinal study. *Psychological Medicine, 38*(4), 499–510.

Berg, B. Van den, Grievink, L., Yzermans, J., & Lebret, E. (2005). Medically unexplained physical symptoms in the aftermath of disasters. *Epidemiological Reviews, 27*, 92–106.

Berg, B. Van den, Velden, P.G. Van der, Stellato, R.K., & Grievink, L. (2007). Selective attrition and bias in a longitudinal health survey among survivors of a disaster. *BMC Medical Research Methodology, 7*, 8.

Berg, B. Van den, Velden, P. G. Van der, Yzermans, C. J., Stellato, R.K., & Grievink, L. (2006). Health-related quality of life and mental health problems after a disaster: Are chronically ill survivors more vulnerable to health problems? *Quality of Life Research, 15*, 1571–1576.

Berg, B. Van den, Yzermans, C.J., Velden, P.G. Van der, Stellato, R.K., Lebret, E., & Grievink, L. (2007). Are physical symptoms among survivors of a disaster presented to the general practitioner? A comparison between self-reports and GP data. *BMC Health Services Research, 7*, 150.

Ploeg, E. Van der, Dorresteijn, A.M., Velden, P.G. Van der, & Kleber, R.J. (2001). *Abiding memories of the day of fireworks disaster May 31, Enschede* (text in five languages). Den Haag/ Enschede: Ministry of Health, Welfare and Sports/The Counsel of Enschede, The Netherlands.

Ploeg, H.M. Van der, Defares, P.B., & Spielberger, C.D. (1982) *Handleiding bij de Zelf-Analyse Vragenlijst. Een vragenlijst voor het meten van boosheid en woede, als toestand en als dispositie. Een nederlandse bewerking van de Spielberger State-Trait Anger Scale* [Manual Dutch Version Spielberger State-Trait Anger Scale]. Lisse: Swets & Zeitlinger, The Netherlands.

Velden, P.G. Van der, Christiaanse, B., Kleber, R.J., Marcelissen, F.M.G., Dorresteijn, A.M., Drogendijk, A.N., et al. (2006). The effects of disaster exposure and post-disaster critical incidents on intrusions, avoidance reactions and health problems among firefighters: A comparative study. *Stress, Trauma, and Crisis, 9*, 73–93.

Velden, P.G. Van der, Grievink, L., Dorresteijn, A.M., van Kamp, I., Drogendijk, A.N., Christiaanse, B., et al. (2005). Psychische klachten en het gebruik van de Geestelijke Gezondheidszorg na de vuurwerkramp Enschede: een longitudinale vergelijkende studie [Psychological problems and the use of mental health services after the fireworks disaster Enschede: A longitudinal comparative study]. *Tijdschrift voor Psychiatrie, 47*, 571–582.

Velden, P.G. Van der, Grievink L., Kleber, R.J., Drogendijk, A.N., Roskam, A.J.R., Marcelissen, F.G.H., et al. (2006). Post-disaster mental health problems and the utilization of mental health services: a four-year longitudinal comparative study. *Administration and Policy in Mental Health and Mental Health Services Research, 33*, 279–288.

Velden, P.G. Van der, Grievink, L., Olff, M., Gersons, B.P.R., & Kleber, R.J. (2007). Smoking as a risk factor for mental health disturbances after a disaster: A prospective comparative study. *Journal of Clinical Psychiatry, 69*, 87–92.

Velden, P.G. Van der, & Kleber, R.J. (1994). *Peilingslijst Acute Stress* [Acute Stress List]. Utrecht, The Netherlands: Instituut voor Psychotrauma.

Velden, P.G. Van der, Kleber, R.J., Christiaanse, B., Gersons, B.P.R., Marcelissen, F.G.H., Drogendijk, A.N., et al. (2006). The predictive value of peritraumatic dissociation for post-disaster intrusions and avoidance reactions and PTSD severity: A four-year prospective study. *Journal of Traumatic Stress, 19*, 493–506.

Velden, P.G. Van der, Kleber, R.J., Fournier, M., Grievink, L., Drogendijk, A.N., & Gersons, B.P.R. (2007). The association between dispositional and mental health problems among disaster victims and a comparison group: A prospective study. *Journal of Affective Disorders, 102*, 35–45.

Velden, P.G. Van der, Kleber, R.J., & Koenen, K.C. (2008). Smoking predicts posttraumatic stress symptoms among rescue workers: A prospective study of ambulance personnel involved in the Enschede Fireworks Disaster. *Drugs and Alcohol Dependence, 94*, 267–271.

Velden, P.G. Van der, Kleber, R.J., & van Oostrom, I. (2000). *Eerste rapportage Gezondheidsonderzoek Enschede. Deelrapportage (geestelijke) gezondheid van de bewoners, passanten en hulpverleners van de vuurwerkramp in Enschede* [First report Enschede Fireworks Disaster Study: Report on (mental) health of the affected residents, passers-by, and rescue workers]. Zaltbommel, The Netherlands: Instituut voor Psychotrauma.

Velden, P.G. Van der, Van der Burg, S., Steinmetz, C.H.D., & van den Bout, J. (1992). *Slachtoffers van bankovervallen* [Victims of bankrobberies]. Houten, The Netherlands: Bohn Stafleu Van Loghem.

Velden, P.G. Van der, & Wittmann, L. (2008). The independent predictive value of peritraumatic dissociation for PTSD symptomatology after type I trauma: A systematic review of prospective studies. *Clinical Psychology Review, 28*, 1009–1020.

Velden, P.G. Van der, Yzermans, C.J., Kleber, R.J., & Gersons, B.P.R. (2007). Correlates of mental health services utilization 18 months and almost 4 years postdisaster among adults with mental health problems. *Journal of Traumatic Stress, 20*, 1029–1039.

Zee, K.I. Van der, & Sanderman, R. (1993). *Het meten van de algemene gezondheidstoestand met de RAND-36: een handleiding* [Measuring general health with the RAND-36: A manual]. Groningen: Noordelijk Centrum voor Gezondheidsvraagstukken, Rijksuniversiteit Groningen.

van Kamp, I., Velden, P. G. Van der, Stellato, R., Roorda, J., van Loon, J., Kleber, R. J., et al. (2006). Physical and mental health shortly after a disaster: First results from the Enschede Fireworks Disaster Study. *European Journal of Public Health, 16*, 252–258.

Sonderen, E. van. (1993). *Het meten van sociale steun met de Sociale Steun Lijst - Interacties (SSL-I), en Sociale Steun Lijst - Discrepancties (SSL-D). Een handleiding* [The measurement of social support with the Social Support List-Interactions (SSL-I) and Social Support List-Discrepancies (SSL-D). A manual]. Groningen: Noordelijk Centrum voor Gezondheidsvraagstukken Rijksuniversiteit Groningen, The Netherlands.

Sonsbeek, L. J. A. van. (1990). *De VOEG, klaaglijst of lijst met gezondheidsklachten.* [The VOEG: list with complaints or instrument for health problems]. Statistische onderzoekingen M37. Heerlen, The Netherlands: The Hague Dutch Office for Statistics.

Vasterman, P., Yzermans, C. J., & Dirkzwager, A. J. E. (2005). The role of the media and media hypes in the aftermath of disasters. *Epidemiologic Reviews, 27*, 107–114.

Vlahov, D., Galea, S., Resnick, H., Ahern, J., Resnick, H., Boscarino, J. A., et al. (2004). Consumption of cigarettes, alcohol and marijuana among New York city residents six months after the September 11 terrorist attacks. *American Journal of Drug and Alcohol Abuse, 30*, 385–407.

Wittmann, L., Moergeli, H., & Schnyder, U. (2006). Low predictive power of peritraumatic dissociation for PTSD symptoms in accident survivors. *Journal of Traumatic Stress, 19*, 639–651.

Yzermans, C. J., Dirkzwager, A. J. E., & Breuning, E. (2005). Long-term health consequences of disaster; a bibliography. Utrecht: Netherlands Institute for Health Services Research (NIVEL).

Yzermans, C. J., Dirkzwager, A. J. E., Kerssens, J. J., Cohen-Bendahan, C. C. C., & ten Veen, P. M. H. (2006). *Gevolgen van de vuurwerkramp in Enschede voor de gezondheid* [Health effects of the Enschede fireworks disaster]. Utrecht: Netherlands Institute for Health Services Research.

Yzermans, C. J., Donker, G. A., Kerssens, J. J. Dirkzwager, A. J., Soeteman, R. J., & ten Veen, P. M. (2005). Health problems of victims before and after disaster: A longitudinal study in general practice. *International Journal of Epidemiology, 34*, 810–819.

Yzermans, C. J., & Gersons, B. P. R. (2002). The chaotic aftermath of an airplane crash in Amsterdam. In J. M. Havenaar, J. G. Cwikel, E. J. Bromet (Eds.), *Toxic turmoil: Psychological and societal consequences of ecological disasters*. New York: Kluwer Academic/Plenum Publishers.

29 Eyewitness to Mass Murder: Findings from Studies of Four Multiple Shooting Episodes

CAROL S. NORTH AND RICHARD V. KING

29.1. INTRODUCTION

Mass shootings or "shooting massacres" were once considered rare occurrences in the United States. Unfortunately, that is no longer the case. On August 1, 1966, a man who had already shot and killed his mother and wife opened fire at passersby from his sniper position at the top of a 27-story tower on the campus of the University of Texas in Austin, killing 17 people and wounding another 30. Mass shooting incidents occurred well before 1966, such as in the 1949 case of a mentally ill war veteran who, using a Luger pistol, shot and killed 13 people on the streets of Camden, New Jersey (Fox, 2007). However, the Austin Tower shootings was considered a turning point; since that time, the occurrence of mass shooting episodes has increased, and now such incidents occur with alarming frequency. More than 100 Americans have "gone on shooting sprees" in the past 40 years (Crenson, 2007).

Certain kinds of settings have attracted a number of mass shooting incidents, especially workplaces, schools or university campuses, restaurants, shopping centers or malls, and even places of worship. After a number of U.S. Postal Service employees shot their coworkers at worksites during the 1980s and early 1990s, the term "going postal" was coined to signify going berserk and shooting people. The latest postal incident occurred in 2006 when a former employee shot and killed six people at a letter-sorting facility in California (Crenson, 2007).

School shootings averaged two to four incidents per year nationally in the 1960s, 1970s, and 1980s. However, in the 1990s there were 13 such incidents, and since 2000 there have already been 21 (Virginia Tech Review Panel, 2007). According to a government report prepared jointly by the U.S. Department of Education and the Secret Service (Fein, Vossekuil, & Holden, 1995), "highly publicized school shootings have created uncertainty about the safety and security of this country's schools and generated fear that an attack might occur in any school, in any community." The Columbine High School massacre (near Littleton, CO, April 1999), in which 13 students were killed, is among the most tragic. Three mass shootings at educational institutions occurred in 2007, including the worst mass shooting in American history (32 fatalities), perpetrated by a mentally ill student at Virginia Tech (Blacksburg, VA, April 2007).

Examples of restaurant shootings are incidents at McDonald's (Ysidro, CA, July 1984; Wilkinsburg, PA, March 2000), Luby's (Killen, TX, October, 1991), and Burger King (Wilkinsburg, PA, March 2000). Notable instances of shooting episodes at malls and shopping centers include incidents at the Hudson Valley Mall (Kingston, NY, Feb 2005), Tacoma Mall (Tacoma, WA, Nov 2005), Trolley Square Mall (Salt Lake City, UT, Feb 2007), Ward Parkway Mall, (Kansas City, MO, April 2007), and Westroads Mall (Omaha, NE, Dec. 2007). Shooting massacres at places of worship include an incident at a Baptist prayer service in Fort Worth, TX (Sept. 1999), and a religious service of the Living Church of God in Brookfield, WI (March 2005).

Despite the increasing frequency of mass shooting episodes, surprisingly few studies have provided data on mental health outcomes of the survivors of these incidents (Norris, 2007). Variation in important elements of the events, small sample sizes, and inconsistent research methods have greatly hindered comparison of different mass shooting studies and generalization from them (Norris, 2007). This chapter will present combined data from longitudinal research on four separate studies of mass shooting episodes conducted with consistent assessment tools and time frames.

29.2. METHODS

29.2.1. Events and Samples

The four mass shooting incidents described in this report occurred between 1987 and 1992. Research methods and findings from these incidents have been presented in greater detail in previous publications (Johnson, North, & Smith, 2002; North, McCutcheon, Spitznagel, & Smith, 2002; North, Smith, McCool, & Shea, 1989; North, Smith, Spitznagel, 1994, 1997; North, Spitznagel, Smith, 2001). Table 29.1 summarizes the characteristics of each incident and the numbers of study participants at each site.

29.2.2. Data Collection

Index interviews were completed at approximately 1 month for the shooting episodes in Russelville, AR, and Iowa City, IA, and at approximately 2 months for the episodes in Killeen, TX, and Clayton, MO. All individuals exposed to the episodes were invited to participate in the Russelville, Killeen, and Iowa City research, but the sample in the Clayton Courthouse study was a volunteer sample of employees who had business at the courthouse at the time of the shooting episode. Follow-up interviews were completed at approximately 3 years (37 months) for Killeen, Clayton, and Iowa City and at 45 months for Russelville. Index and follow-up interviews utilized the Diagnostic Interview Schedule/Disaster Supplement (DIS/DS) (Robins & Smith, 1983), which provided full DSM-III-R assessment of lifetime, predisaster, and postdisaster psychiatric diagnoses and information on variables of relevance to disaster experience.

Institutional Review Board approval for these studies was provided by the sponsoring institution (Washington University School of Medicine in St. Louis). All study participants provided informed consent before participating in the research.

29.2.3. Data Analysis

Data analysis was conducted using SAS (2004). Descriptive data are presented with raw numbers and percentages. Comparisons of prevalence were made using chi-square analyses, substituting Fisher's exact tests when expected cell sizes were less than five. Comparisons of numerical variables were made with Student's t-tests, using Satterthwaite analyses for cases of unequal variances. Multiple regression models were constructed to control for the effects of multiple variables simultaneously in prediction of outcomes. Multiple logistic regression models were used for prediction of dependent variables representing dichotomous diagnosis, and multiple linear regression models were used for prediction of dependent variables representing numerical symptom counts. Significant alpha was set at $p < 0.05$, and two-sided probability values were reported.

On the basis of available descriptions of the events and the high rates of injury and extensive exposure to carnage in the Killeen and Russelville shooting episodes, a dichotomous variable was created to signify these two events as relatively "high-impact" and the Clayton and Iowa City shooting episodes as of lesser impact. This impact variable was used to represent episode type in multiple regression models rather than using the specific site variable, because of cell size limitations in the site variable.

29.3. RESULTS

29.3.1. Sample Characteristics

Table 29.2 summarizes characteristics of the study sample. The combined sample was slightly

Table 29.1. Description of the four mass shooting incidents

Place/Date	Description of Incident	Index Study Sample	Follow-up Number (*N*) (% of index)
Russelville, AR Local businesses December 28, 1987	After murdering 14 people in his rural mobile home, a man went on a 35-minute shooting rampage involving four local businesses. Two fatalities, four injuries	72% of the employees of two affected businesses *N* = 11	10 (91%)
Killeen, TX Restaurant October 16, 1991	A gunman drove his pickup truck through the front window of Luby's cafeteria and held 150 patrons and employees captive while shooting people at close range for 15 minutes. 24 fatalities (including gunman), 20 injuries	82% of individuals present during the shooting *N* = 123	105 (85%)
Iowa City, IA University campus November 2, 1991	After being passed over for an award, a disgruntled physics graduate student went on a shooting rampage on the campus of the University of Iowa. Six fatalities (gunman, university professors, students, and staff), one serious injury	77% of all individuals who encountered the gunman in the Physics Building, where most of the shooting occurred *N* = 9	6 (67%)
Clayton, MO Courthouse June 5, 1992	In court on divorce proceedings, a man shot at his wife, lawyers, and judge and then stalked hallways with guns for 10 minutes. One fatality (gunman's wife), five injuries (including both parties' lawyers)	Volunteer sample of courthouse employees, lawyers, judges, and law enforcement personnel in courthouse during shooting *N* = 79	76 (96%)
Total *N*		**222**	**197 (89%)**

over one-half female, average age in the mid-to-upper thirties, with nearly 2 years of college on average. Less than one-fifth of the sample had ethnic/racial minority status; African Americans accounted for most of the minorities. Nearly two-thirds of the combined sample were currently married, with higher rates in the Killeen sample compared with all the rest ($\chi^2 = 16.23$, df = 1, $p < 0.001$). The Clayton sample had more separated and divorced members compared with the rest of the combined sample ($\chi^2 = 11.51$, df = 1, $p < 0.001$). Over one-fourth of the entire sample reported having sustained an injury in the shooting incident. Nearly two-thirds of survivors of the Killeen and Russelville incidents reported feeling that they might die during the shooting episode.

At index, the Iowa City mass shooting survivor group had an overrepresentation of males

Table 29.2. Characteristics of the sample

Variable	Russelville (N=11)	Killeen (N=123)	Iowa City (N=9)	Clayton (N=79)	All (N=222)
Sex					
Male *n* (%)	5 (45.4)	60 (48.8)	[a]8 (88.9)	[a]28 (35.4)	101 (45.5)
Female *n* (%)	6 (54.6)	63 (51.2)	1 (11.1)	51 (64.6)	121 (54.5)
Years of age					
Mean (SD)	33.6 (6.5)	39.5 (14.3)	36.4 (14.2)	38.8 (11.0)	38.8 (12.9)
Median	36	37	30	37	36
Range	23–43	18–83	24–62	18–62	18–83
Years of education					
Mean (SD)	13.8 (1.3)	13.5 (2.1)	16.3 (1.3)	13.9 (2.1)	13.8 (2.1)
Median	14	13	17	13	13
Range	12–16	8–17	13–17	11–17	8–17
College graduate *n* (%)	1 (9.1)	298 (24.6)	[b]8 (88.9)	27 (34.2)	65 (30.0)
Race/ethnicity					
Caucasian *n* (%)	11 (100.0)	97 (78.9)	7 (77.8)	67 (84.8)	182 (82.0)
African American *n* (%)	0 (0.0)	14 (11.4)	2 (22.2)	12 (15.2)	26 (11.7)
Hispanic *n* (%)	0 (0.0)	10 (8.1)	0 (0.0)	0 (0.0)	10 (4.5)
Asian *n* (%)	0 (0.0)	0 (0.0)	0 (0.0)	0 (0.0)	2 (0.9)
Other *n* (%)	0 (0.0)	2 (1.6)	0 (0.0)	0 (0.0)	2 (0.9)
Marital status					
Currently married	7 (63.6)	[b]93 (75.6)	4 (44.4)	[b]38 (48.1)	142 (64.0)
Previously married	3 (27.3)	[b]7 (5.7)	0 (0.0)	[b]18 (22.8)	28 (12.6)
Single (never married)	1 (9.1)	23 (18.7)	[a]5 (55.6)	23 (29.1)	52 (23.4)
Injured in incident n (%)	2 (18.2)	[b]56 (45.5)	0 (0.0)	[b]8 (10.1)	66 (29.7)
"Thought I might die"	7 (63.6)	[a]78 (65.0)	3 (33.3)	40 (51.3)	128 (58.7)

Notes:
Compared with the rest of the combined sample:
[a] $p<0.05$
[b] $p<0.001$

(Fisher's exact $p=0.012$) and those from the Clayton Courthouse mass shooting disaster had an overrepresentation of females ($\chi^2=5.00$, df=1, $p=0.025$), compared with the rest of the sample. A higher proportion of the survivors of the Iowa City shootings had a college education (Fisher's exact $p<0.001$). Nearly one-half of the Killeen sample were injured ($\chi^2=32.95$, df=1, $p<0.001$), and fewer from the Clayton mass shooting ($\chi^2=22.56$, df=1, $p<0.001$) were injured, compared with the rest of the sample.

29.3.2. Psychopathology

Overall, 40.1% ($N=89$) were diagnosed with a predisaster lifetime mental illness: 11.3% ($N=25$) with posttraumatic stress disorder (PTSD), 9.9% ($N=22$) with major depression, 0.9% ($N=2$) with panic disorder, 1.8% ($N=4$) with generalized anxiety disorder, 25.2% ($N=56$) with alcohol use disorder, and 6.3% ($N=14$) with other drug use disorder. The samples of the four sites did not differ from one another in prevalence of predisaster lifetime diagnosis.

Table 29.3 presents prevalences of postdisaster diagnoses at index and prevalence of current (6-month) diagnoses at the 3-year follow-up assessment. Figure 29.1 illustrates the event impact-related postdisaster prevalences of PTSD and all psychiatric disorders at index. Figure 29.2 illustrates the combined sample prevalences for specific postdisaster diagnoses and total diagnosis at index and for current diagnoses (present in the last 6 months) at follow-up.

At index assessment, nearly one-third (32.0%) of the combined sample had a postdisaster

Table 29.3. Postdisaster diagnoses at index and 3-year follow-up

Variable	**Russelville (*N*=11)**	**Killeen (*N*=123)**	**Iowa City (*N*=9)**	**Clayton (*N*=79)**	**All (*N*=222)**
Index					
Any postdisaster diagnosis	4 (36.4)	45 (36.6)	1 (11.1)	21 (26.6)	71 (32.0)
Shooting-related PTSD	1 (9.1)	[c]36 (29.3)	0 (0.0)	[c]4 (5.1)	41 (18.5)
Other event-related PTSD	2 (18.2)	[a]1 (0.8)	0 (0.0)	5 (6.3)	8 (3.6)
Major depression	1 (9.1)	13 (10.6)	0 (0.0)	3 (3.8)	17 (7.7)
Panic disorder	0 (0.0)	3 (2.4)	0 (0.0)	1 (1.3)	4 (1.8)
Generalized anxiety disorder	0 (0.0)	1 (0.8)	1 (11.1)	0 (0.0)	2 (0.9)
Alcohol abuse/ dependence	2 (18.2)	10 (8.1)	0 (0.0)	8 (10.1)	20 (9.0)
Other drug abuse/ dependence	0 (0.0)	0 (0.0)	0 (0.0)	0 (0.0)	0 (0.0)
3-Year follow-up	*N*–10	*N*–105	*N*–6	*N*–76	*N*–197
Any current (6-months) diagnosis	3 (30.0)	[b]32 (30.5)	0 (0.0)	[a]10 (13.2)	45 (22.8)
Shooting-related PTSD	2 (20.0)	[b]20 (19.1)	0 (0.0)	[b]2 (2.6)	24 (12.2)
Major depression	0 (0.0)	95 (8.6)	0 (0.0)	3 (4.0)	12 (6.1)
Panic disorder	[a]2 (20.0)	25 (0.9)	0 (0.0)	1 (1.3)	5 (2.5)
Generalized anxiety disorder	0 (0.0)	45 (3.8)	0 (0.0)	0 (0.0)	4 (2.0)
Alcohol abuse/ dependence	0 (0.0)	85 (7.6)	0 (0.0)	3 (4.0)	11 (5.6)
Other drug abuse/ dependence	0 (0.0)	14 (0.0)	0 (0.0)	0 (0.0)	0 (0.0)

Notes:
Compared with the rest of the combined sample:
[a] $p<0.05$
[b] $p<0.01$
[c] $p<0.001$

diagnosis, the most prevalent being PTSD (18.5%), followed by major depression (7.7%). Of 41 cases of PTSD at index, 21 (51.2%) had suffered from a psychiatric disorder before the disaster and 16 (39.0%) were comorbid with another active postdisaster diagnosis (12 cases of major depression and four of alcohol use disorder). Two of the 222 study participants met criteria for a new alcohol use disorder with onset after the disaster, but there were no new drug use disorder cases. Survivors of the two "high-impact" incidents had higher combined rates of shooting-related PTSD compared with survivors of the other two events combined (27.6% vs. 4.6%, $\chi^2=18.77$, df=1, $p<0.001$).

At 3 years, nearly one-fourth (22.8%) of the sample had a current (6-month) diagnosis. The current (6-month) prevalence of PTSD in the combined sample was nearly two-thirds of its index value. As indicated in Table 29.3, the prevalence of current PTSD among Killeen survivors remained higher than among the survivors of the other sites together (19.1% vs. 4.4%,

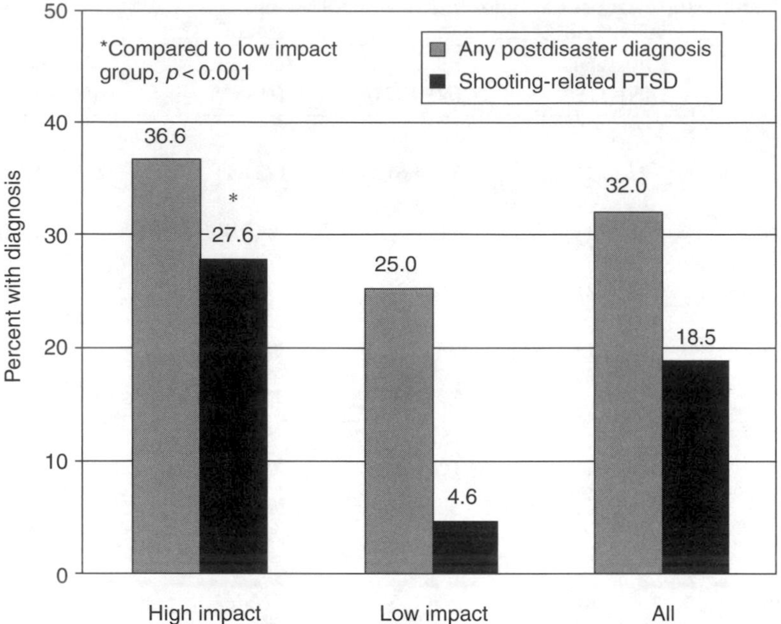

Figure 29.1. Prevalence of shooting-related PTSD and any postdisaster diagnosis at index, by shooting site.

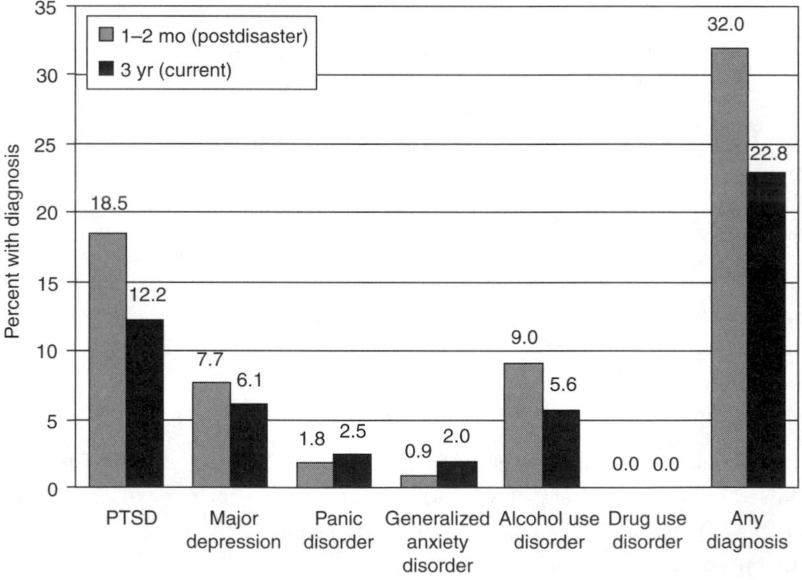

Figure 29.2. Prevalence of postdisaster diagnoses at index and current (6-month) diagnoses at follow-up, in the combined sample.

$\chi^2 = 9.90$, df = 1, $p = 0.002$). The current prevalence of PTSD at 3 years represents combined effects of both remission from PTSD and additional cases found to meet criteria after the index assessments. Between index and 3 years, another 20 cases of PTSD were diagnosed in addition to the 34 cases identified at index. Of all 54 of these PTSD cases diagnosed during the study, just over one-half (55.6%, $N = 30$) were no longer symptomatic at follow-up.

Table 29.4. Multiple regression model for prediction of shooting-related PTSD at index (dependent variable)

						Odds Ratio Estimates		
Parameter	**DF**	**Slope**	**Standard Error**	**Wald χ^2**	***P***	**Point Estimate**	**95% Wald CL**	
Intercept	1	−3.64	0.88	16.94	<0.001			
High-impact group membership[a]	1	1.99	0.60	11.06	<0.001	7.30	2.26	23.57
Gender (male)	1	−1.01	0.44	5.32	0.021	0.36	0.15	0.86
Age	1	0.00	0.02	0.15	0.701	0.99	0.96	1.03
College graduate	1	−0.25	0.48	0.27	0.603	0.78	0.31	1.99
Ethnic minority group member	1	0.51	0.49	1.09	0.296	1.67	0.64	4.34
Predisaster diagnosis	1	0.87	0.40	4.67	0.031	2.38	1.08	5.23
Currently married	1	1.33	0.54	6.10	0.014	3.79	1.32	10.92
Injured in event	1	−0.17	0.44	0.15	0.696	0.84	0.35	2.01

Note: [a]Denotes member of Killeen or Russelville samples

Table 29.5. Multiple regression model for prediction of number of postdisaster shooting-related PTSD symptoms at index (dependent variable) among individuals without a diagnosis of PTSD

Variable	**DF**	**Parameter Estimate**	**Standard Error**	***t* Value**	***P***
Intercept	1	6.42	0.89	7.24	<0.001
High-impact group membership[a]	1	0.91	0.54	1.68	0.095
Gender (male)	1	−0.88	0.53	−1.67	0.097
Age	1	−0.06	0.02	−2.90	0.004
College graduate	1	−1.03	0.55	−1.87	0.063
Ethnic minority group member[a]	1	1.18	0.62	1.91	0.058
Predisaster diagnosis	1	0.05	0.49	0.11	0.193
Currently married	1	1.16	0.58	1.99	0.048
Injured in event	1	0.37	0.59	0.62	0.536

Note: [a]Denotes member of Killeen or Russelville samples.

29.3.2.1. Predictors

In terms of predictors of PTSD diagnosis, most (78.9%) of those meeting Group C criteria for PTSD at index were diagnosed with PTSD (41/52), but few of those meeting Group B (24.3%, 41/169) or Group D (24.3%, 41/162) criteria were diagnosed with PTSD. Table 29.4 presents a multiple regression model for prediction of PTSD related to the shooting episode. In this model, vulnerability factors for PTSD were severity of the event (Killeen and Russelville samples), female gender, having a predisaster diagnosis, and being currently married. Table 29.5 presents a multiple regression model for prediction of a number of postdisaster shooting-related PTSD symptoms at index among survivors without PTSD from variables pertaining to characteristics of the sample and the incident. Youthfulness and married status both predicted PTSD symptoms

Table 29.6. Multiple regression model for prediction of recovery from PTSD at 3 years (dependent variable)

						Odds Ratio Estimates		
Parameter	**DF**	**Slope**	**Standard Error**	**Wald χ^2**	***P***	**Point Estimate**	**95% Wald CL**	
Intercept	1	5.27	4.88	1.17	0.280			
High-impact group membership[a]	1	−0.24	1.04	0.05	0.819	0.79	0.10	6.09
Gender (male)	1	0.53	0.86	0.37	0.542	1.69	0.31	9.05
Age	1	0.03	0.03	0.97	0.325	1.03	0.97	1.09
College graduate	1	−0.33	1.49	0.05	0.827	0.72	0.04	13.51
Ethnic minority group member	1	0.98	1.13	0.75	0.387	2.66	0.29	24.47
Predisaster diagnosis	1	−0.17	0.38	0.21	0.645	0.84	0.40	1.76
Currently married	1	0.49	0.94	0.27	0.600	1.63	0.26	10.23
Injured in event	1	−2.11	0.87	5.93	0.015	0.12	0.02	0.66

Notes: [a]Denotes member of Killeen or Russelville samples.

in people not meeting criteria for a PTSD diagnosis. Finally, Table 29.6 presents a multiple regression model for prediction of recovery from PTSD. In this model, only one variable – having been injured in the shooting incident – predicted nonrecovery.

29.4. DISCUSSION

A review of shooting episodes by Norris (2007) noted that research on mass shooting episodes is not extensive but that the available data provide enough information to permit some preliminary conclusions, namely the range of PTSD prevalence and the nearly universal presence of symptoms. The Norris review identified PTSD in 10% to 36% of survivors of these incidents. The lower statistic is derived from our team's report on the Clayton, Missouri, Courthouse shooting episode (Johnson et al., 2002), and the higher statistic is from a study of PTSD among 11 Hasidic yeshiva students subjected to a shooting attack on a van transporting them over New York City's Brooklyn Bridge (Trappler & Friedman, 1996). Previous attempts to compare and generalize from studies of shooting episodes have been limited by inconsistencies in research methods, such as variation in outcomes reported (diagnoses, symptoms, and other aspects of postdisaster experience). For example, only 4 of the 15 studies reviewed by Norris provided estimates of PTSD diagnosis (two of which were conducted by our research team). Elements intrinsic to each incident may further hinder generalization to other events and comparison of events (Norris, 2007).

This report has presented data on the experience of directly exposed survivors of four separate mass shooting episodes, two with a large number of survivors studied ($N=123$ in Killeen, Texas, Luby's Cafeteria, and $N=79$ at the Clayton Courthouse) and two with study samples that were relatively small ($N=11$ in the Russelville, Arkansas, incident and $N=9$ at the University of Iowa incident). Consistency of assessment tools used to assess survivors of the four shooting episodes in this report and uniformity of the timing of index assessment (1–2 months postdisaster) allowed comparison across these different events. Other strengths of these data and their analyses are the systematic assessment of full diagnostic criteria for psychiatric disorders, size of the combined sample, prospective longitudinal design, and measurement of simultaneous effects of multiple important variables. Limitations include unavailability of current symptom counts at follow-up, retrospective nature of the predisaster data, and absence of the follow-up assessment needed for detailed exploration of delayed-onset PTSD, defined at onset after 6 months (American Psychiatric Association, 2000). An additional limitation of this study is the volunteer nature of the Clayton Courthouse shooting sample, although the other three shooting samples represent a successfully selected majority of the universe of individuals known to be directly exposed to the incident.

Owing to the small numbers of survivors in two of the four samples in the current report, many specific comparisons across the four events lacked statistical power. To manage this situation, a "high-intensity event" variable was created to represent the combined experience of the Killeen and Russelville shooting incidents based on severity of the events, permitting cross-event comparisons by event severity. Two of the four shooting incidents studied (the Killeen, Texas, Luby's Cafeteria episode and the Russelville, Arkansas, shooting episode at local businesses) seemed to be of greater intensity for the exposed groups, judging by the rates of injuries sustained and acknowledgment of confrontation of the potential for death in the incident. Most of the survivors exposed to the other two disasters (the University of Iowa and the Clayton, Missouri, Courthouse shooting episodes) had less contact with the gunman. This variable was found to be a strong predictor of psychopathology, and its inclusion as a covariate among multiple independent variables helped to illuminate the roles of personal characteristics such as gender, age, and predisaster psychopathology in the prediction of general outcomes in the combined sample.

These studies revealed a range of prevalence of postdisaster psychiatric disorders among the four groups of survivors. PTSD was the most prevalent postdisaster diagnosis, and it was far more prevalent in the "high-impact" event groups than in the other two groups. Psychiatric comorbidity, both predisaster and postdisaster, was common in association with PTSD. Only slightly more than one-half of PTSD cases were in remission by the 3-year mark. Recovery from PTSD was less likely among those who were injured.

Predictors of posttraumatic symptoms differed from predictors of PTSD. Event severity, female gender, preexisting psychopathology, and being married predicted PTSD, while youthfulness and married status, but not event severity, gender, or prior psychopathology, predicted PTSD symptoms. These predictive differences support the notion that subdiagnostic symptoms, sometimes regarded as "distress" (National Academy of Sciences Institute of Medicine, 2003; Norris et al., 2002; North et al., 1999), represent a phenomenon divergent from PTSD. Methodological differences in research studies hinging on measurement of symptoms rather than well-defined syndromes or disorders may perhaps account for some of the apparent inconsistencies in predictors of posttraumatic outcomes reported in the existing disaster literature, as comprehensively documented in a monumental review by Norris and colleagues (Norris et al., 2002; Norris, Friedman, & Watson, 2002).

The prevalence of PTSD varied considerably across the four shooting incidents studied. The range of PTSD prevalence from 5% after the two less severe incidents to 28% in the "high-impact" groups is, however, generally within the ranges reported by our team for other disasters studied using similar methods: terrorism (the Oklahoma City bombing, 34%) (North et al., 1999), technological accidents (5%–36%) (Robins et al., 1986; Smith, North, McCool, & Shea, 1990), and natural disasters (3%–24%) (McMillen, North, & Smith, 2000; North, Kawasaki, Spitznagel, & Hong, 2004; North, Smith, McCool, & Lightcap, 1989). These comparisons suggest that the severity of the incident may be more influential than its disaster typology for predicting mental health outcomes.

The apparent differences in prevalence across the four shooting episodes compared in this study cannot be explained by variability of assessment tools. The Clayton sample, however, represented a volunteer sample rather than a universal sample, which may have introduced sampling biases into and blurred the comparison of findings from this particular group. Such difficulties in obtaining representative samples are well known in conducting disaster research. Even when representative sampling is not possible, researchers can still minimize methodological confounding of cross-disaster comparisons by using consistent methods of assessment.

29.5. CONCLUSION

Mass shooting incidents have been increasing in frequency, and there are no indications that research is close to developing the means to prevent these episodes. Therefore, mental health effects of such events can be expected to represent continuing problems for clinicians, researchers, and policy makers to address. The incidence, rapidity of onset, and chronicity of PTSD among the survivors of these events, as well as the high levels of distress (Group B and D posttraumatic symptoms), indicate need for access to early and long-term psychiatric assessment and treatment as well as availability of psychological first aid for these individuals.

Future research on mental health effects of mass shootings would benefit from focus on systematic and comparable measurement of psychiatric diagnoses and distress among highly exposed survivors. Consistent constructs for measurement of broader psychosocial effects on communities affected will facilitate comparison of findings and generalization to other settings. Finally, findings from the studies presented here suggest that important differences between psychiatric illness and symptoms of other distress merit greater attention in future disaster research.

REFERENCES

American Psychiatric Association. (2000). *Diagnostic and statistical manual of mental disorders 4th ed. Text Revision*. Washington, DC: American Psychiatric Association.

Crenson, M. (2007). *Mass shootings more common since 1960s*. New York (January, 2008); http://www.christianpost.com/article/20070422/27028_Mass_Shootings_More_Common_Since_1960s.htm.

Fein, R.A., Vossekuil, B., & Holden, G. (1995). *Threat assessment: An approach to prevent targeted violence*. Washington, DC: U.S. Department of Justice, Office of Justice Programs, National Institute of Justice.

Fox, J.A. (2007). *Rise in mass shootings linked to societal changes*. Salt Lake City (January, 2008); http://findarticles.com/p/articles/mI_qn4188/is_20070422/aI_n19035957

Johnson, S.D., North, C.S., & Smith, E.M. (2002). Psychiatric disorders among victims of a courthouse shooting spree: A three-year follow-up study. *Community Mental Health Journal, 38*(3), 181–194.

McMillen, J.C., North, C.S., & Smith, E.M. (2000). What parts of PTSD are normal: Intrusion, avoidance, or arousal? Data from the Northridge, California earthquake. *Journal of Traumatic Stress, 13*(1), 57–75.

National Academy of Sciences Institute of Medicine. (2003). *Preparing for the psychological consequences of terrorism: A public health strategy*. Washington, DC: National Academy Press.

Norris, F.H. (2007). Impact of mass shootings on survivors, families, and communities. *PTSD Research Quarterly, 18*(3), 1–7.

Norris, F.H., Friedman, M.J., & Watson, P.J. (2002). 60,000 disaster victims speak: Part II. Summary and implications of the disaster mental health research. *Psychiatry, 65*(3), 240–260.

Norris, F.H., Friedman, M.J., Watson, P.J., Byrne, C.M., Diaz, E., & Kaniasty, K. (2002). 60,000 disaster victims speak: Part I. An empirical review of the empirical literature, 1981–2001. *Psychiatry, 65*(3), 207–239.

North, C.S., Kawasaki, A., Spitznagel, E.L., & Hong, B.A. (2004). The course of PTSD, major depression, substance abuse, and somatization after a natural disaster. *Journal of Nervous and Mental Disease, 192*(12), 823–829.

North, C.S., McCutcheon, V., Spitznagel, E.L., & Smith, E.M. (2002). Three-year follow-up of survivors of a mass shooting episode. *Journal of Urban Health, 79*(3), 383–391.

North, C.S., Nixon, S.J., Shariat, S., Mallonee, S., McMillen, J.C., Spitznagel, E.L., et al. (1999). Psychiatric disorders among survivors of the Oklahoma City bombing. *Journal of the American Medical Association, 282*(8), 755–762.

North, C.S., Smith, E.M., McCool, R.E., & Lightcap, P.E. (1989). Acute post-disaster coping and adjustment. *Journal of Traumatic Stress, 2*(3), 353–360.

North, C.S., Smith, E.M., McCool, R.E., & Shea, J.M. (1989). Short-term psychopathology in eyewitnesses to mass murder. *Hospital and Community Psychiatry, 40*(12), 1293–1295.

North, C. S., Smith, E. M., & Spitznagel, E. L. (1994). Posttraumatic stress disorder in survivors of a mass shooting. *American Journal of Psychiatry, 151*, 82–88.

(1997). One-year follow-up of survivors of a mass shooting. *American Journal of Psychiatry, 154*(12), 1696–1702.

North, C. S., Spitznagel, E. L., & Smith, E. M. (2001). A prospective study of coping after exposure to a mass murder episode. *Annals of Clinical Psychiatry, 13*(2), 81–87.

Robins, L. N., Fishbach, R. L., Smith, E. M., Cottler, L. B., Solomon, S. D., & Goldring, E. (1986). Impact of disaster on previously assessed mental health. In J. H. Shore (Ed.), *Disaster stress studies: New methods and findings*. Washington, DC: American Psychiatric Association.

Robins, L. N. & Smith, E. M. (1983). *The diagnostic interview schedule/disaster supplement*. St. Louis, MO: Washington University.

SAS Institute. (2004). *SAS 9.1.3. Procedures guide volume 4*. Cary, NC: SAS Institute.

Smith, E. M., North, C. S., McCool, R. E., & Shea, J. M. (1990). Acute postdisaster psychiatric disorders: Identification of persons at risk. *American Journal of Psychiatry, 147*(2), 202–206.5

Trappler, B., & Friedman, S. (1996). Posttraumatic stress disorder in survivors of the Brooklyn Bridge shooting. *American Journal of Psychiatry, 153*(5), 705–707.

Virginia Tech Review Panel. (2007). *Mass shootings at Virginia Tech. Appendix L. Fatal school shootings in the United States: 1966–2007*. The Commonwealth of Virginia, http://www.governor.virginia.gov/TempContent/techPanelReport-docs/FullReport.pdf.

30 The Oklahoma City Bombing

BETTY PFEFFERBAUM, PHEBE TUCKER, AND CAROL S. NORTH

30.1. INTRODUCTION

Though now eclipsed by more devastating national and international disasters, the 1995 bombing of the Alfred P. Murrah Federal Building in Oklahoma City was, at the time, the deadliest act of terrorism on U.S. soil. The bombing resulted in 168 deaths, including 19 children and one responder. Eight hundred fifty people were injured, 30 children were orphaned, 462 people were left homeless, 7,000 people lost their workplace, and over 300 buildings were damaged or destroyed (Oklahoma City National Memorial Institute for the Prevention of Terrorism, n.d.). In addition to causing injury, death, sorrow, and grief, terrorism generates fear and intimidation and the impetus for changed attitudes and behavior. It creates disruption and chaos, and as we saw after the September 11th attacks, it can trigger wide-reaching and enduring socioeconomic and political change.

A major sentiment emerging in the days and weeks after the Oklahoma City bombing was the desire on the part of individuals, organizations, and the community to learn from this horrific event. Recognizing the potential for both personal and community effects, clinicians and scholars involved in the Oklahoma City bombing response focused on a range of issues, populations, and outcomes. Distinguishing this incident from natural disasters, clinicians and researchers recognized the importance of examining a number of groups that might be affected and a variety of outcomes that might result. Attention focused first on those most directly exposed, including people in the Federal Building and surrounding areas. Family members and associates of directly exposed individuals were included in intervention efforts and in some research samples. Studies also assessed community residents whose lives were disrupted, remotely affected populations in other communities in the region and across the country, and rescuers and responders and their families. This chapter describes the emotional and behavioral consequences of the bombing and the service delivery system established to respond. We conclude by reflecting on some of the important gains made in disaster mental health research as a result of Oklahoma City investigations.

30.2. DIRECTLY EXPOSED SAMPLES

A major impediment to disaster research is gaining access to the individuals most directly exposed to an event. This was facilitated in Oklahoma City by a registry established and maintained by the Oklahoma Department of Health after bombing morbidity and mortality were declared reportable (Quick, 1998). To understand the effects on those who were in or near the Federal Building or other damaged buildings at the time of the attack, North and colleagues (1999) used rigorous methodology and comprehensive assessments to study 182 survivors 6 months after the bombing. Most (87%) of the individuals in this representative sample sustained injuries, 82% witnessed the death or injury of others, 43% lost a family member or friend, and 92% knew someone killed or injured. In the first 6 months after the bombing, 45% met criteria for at least one psychiatric diagnosis, over one-third met criteria for bombing-related posttraumatic stress disorder (PTSD), and over 60% of those with PTSD met criteria for another disorder. Major depression was diagnosed in 23% of the sample. The onset of PTSD symptoms was acute, occurring on the day of the bombing for most.

To determine the time course of PTSD, North and colleagues (2004) reassessed most of the individuals in their index study 1 year later (75%). The group prevalence of PTSD between index and follow-up suggested stability of the disorder with rates just over 30% at both times. A careful analysis, tracking individual cases from index to follow-up and including subthreshold cases at index, cases not identified at follow-up, and the majority of PTSD cases that were diagnosed at both times, revealed a combined index and follow-up PTSD incidence of 41%. The index assessment alone failed to identify 16% of the total cases, and the follow-up assessment alone failed to identify 15% of the cases.

The 12 PTSD cases first identified at follow-up were not delayed-onset PTSD but rather subthreshold PTSD at index. These survivors had developed most of their PTSD symptoms quickly in the first days and weeks postbombing, with symptoms not reaching diagnostic threshold until after 6 months postbombing. For the most part, those who did not qualify for a diagnosis of PTSD until follow-up had milder symptoms, and they continued to report significantly fewer symptoms than those whose PTSD diagnosis was first identified at index. Thus, a small proportion of (mostly milder) PTSD cases may not be fully diagnosable until later in the postdisaster course. In addition to demonstrating the transition from subthreshold to diagnosis, the Oklahoma City follow-up revealed that no PTSD cases had remitted by 3 months, the temporal demarcation for chronic PTSD. Meeting avoidance and numbing (Group C) criteria was highly associated with illness and functional impairment at both index and follow-up, associations that were not observed with intrusive reexperiencing (Group B) or hyperarousal (Group D) symptoms in the absence of meeting Group C criteria. Thus, the presence of avoidance and numbing symptoms may identify individuals likely to develop PTSD (North et al., 2004).

Even longer-term follow-up of part of the sample $6^1/_2$ to 7 years after the bombing revealed continuing low levels of posttraumatic stress symptoms and greater physiologic reactivity in survivors than among community controls (Tucker et al, 2007). The survivor group had significantly higher resting heart rate and greater heart rate and blood pressure reactivity to an interview about the bombing than matched community controls. Only those who were free of cardiovascular or psychotropic medications that could confound results of the physiologic assessment participated, however. Thus, these participants were not representative of the full survivor sample. The levels of posttraumatic and depressive symptoms on research assessment in this relatively healthy group were below levels considered pathological, but despite their emotional resilience, the survivor group retained long-term autonomic sensitivity and subjective distress responses to reminders of their bombing experiences.

The longitudinal study conducted by North's group (North et al., 1999, 2004; Tucker et al., 2007) has yielded important findings to guide disaster mental health services. Taken together, the studies indicate that services should begin immediately and continue for those with persistent PTSD and other conditions. Those with subthreshold PTSD may benefit from PTSD prevention efforts and continued observation for additional symptoms over time (North et al., 2004). Survivors whose posttraumatic stress levels are not clinically elevated may have lasting physiologic reactivity and subjective distress in response to reminders of the bombing for many years (Tucker et al., 2007), but it remains unclear what, if any, long-term public health or mental health interventions are indicated for those who do not develop clinically elevated levels of stress.

A second study drew participants from individuals receiving mental health services at Project Heartland, the federally funded crisis counseling program established by the state's mental health authority (Tucker, Pfefferbaum, Nixon, & Foy, 1999). Eighty-six of the 170 individuals seen at Project Heartland during the sixth month of operation participated in the assessment. Most had been in close proximity to the Federal Building at the time of the bombing. Over 50% were evacuated from the building they were in at the time, and almost

80% reported damage to nearby buildings. Most (82%) had not been injured themselves, nor had their family members (95%) or friends (79%), but many knew someone who had been injured (47%) or killed (31%). Retrospectively reported acute anxiety reactions at the time of the bombing were related to the development of posttraumatic stress reactions (Tucker, Dickson, Pfefferbaum, McDonald, & Allen, 1997; Tucker, Pfefferbaum, Nixon, & Dickson, 2000) and injury (Pfefferbaum et al., 2003; Tucker et al., 2000), and most (75%) of the participants in this treatment-seeking sample experienced some difficulty functioning at the time of the study (Pfefferbaum, Call, et al., 2001). Sampling bias may have influenced the results, however. For example, individuals in this treatment-seeking sample may have experienced greater distress than victims who did not seek services, and those with the most severe reactions may have sought more traditional psychiatric services than were provided by Project Heartland, which delivered support counseling.

Approximately 20% of the participants in the Project Heartland sample reported increased drinking, and 15% reported increased smoking since the bombing (Pfefferbaum, Vinekar, et al., 2002). While no causal relationship can be assumed, the study revealed a relationship between increased substance use and injury, acute reactions at the time of the bombing, grief, posttraumatic stress reactions, worry about safety, and trouble functioning at home, work, and/or other places (Pfefferbaum, Vinekar, et al., 2002). This study did not examine substance use disorders, and the clinical significance of increased substance use remains in question. In their diagnostic study of Oklahoma City survivors, North and colleagues (1999) found no new bombing-related substance use disorders, and most predisaster substance use disorders were inactive after the incident. Their study did not report substance use behaviors, however, focusing instead on diagnoses. North's team did find that 16% of survivors and 32% of those who developed PTSD and comorbid disorders reported use of alcohol as a means of coping. Avoidance and numbing symptoms were related to the use of alcohol and medication to cope, while intrusion and arousal symptoms alone (without avoidance/numbing) were not associated with coping through use of substances (North et al., 1999).

It was widely believed that the day care center in the Federal Building was a target in the Oklahoma City attack, which left 19 children among the dead, including 15 children in the day care center and four children who were visiting the building. Five children in the day care center survived; all were injured and hospitalized (Pfefferbaum, 2003). Preschool children attending the day care at the nearby YMCA felt the impact of the bomb blast. No children or staff in the YMCA facility died or were seriously injured, but most (Gurwitch, Pfefferbaum, & Leftwich, 2002; Gurwitch, Sitterle, Young, & Pfefferbaum, 2002) suffered minor injuries with multiple cuts and bruises resulting from falling debris and glass (Gurwitch, Pfefferbaum, et al., 2002). The children experienced intense media attention during the evacuation and in the aftermath of the event (Gurwitch, Pfefferbaum, et al., 2002).

Adding to a sparse literature on the effects of disasters on very young children, Gurwitch and colleagues (Gurwitch, Pfefferbaum, et al., 2002; Gurwitch, Sitterle, et al., 2002) studied 11 of these children by interviewing their mothers, observing the children during unstructured play, and documenting staff observations. The children evidenced trauma reactions including extensive posttraumatic play and peer discussions about the bombing, increased arousal, regressive behaviors, and functional problems (Gurwitch, Sitterle, et al., 2002), but the extent to which these findings differed from children without this exposure was not determined. Interestingly, the children did not appear to avoid interactions or games reminiscent of the event, and restricted range of affect and foreshortened future were relatively absent (Gurwitch, Sitterle, et al., 2002). The professionals working with the children echoed the concern of others (Scheeringa, Zeanah, Drell, & Larrieu, 1995) about the ability of young children to accurately appraise and verbalize their emotions (Gurwitch, Pfefferbaum, et al., 2002; Gurwitch, Sitterle, et al., 2002).

30.3. COMMUNITY SAMPLES

A pervasive sense of horror and loss filled the Oklahoma City community after the attack, with close to 40% of community residents reporting that they knew someone killed or injured in the event (Smith, Christiansen, Vincent, & Hann, 1999). In conjunction with the Oklahoma Department of Health and the University of Oklahoma Health Sciences Center (OUHSC), the Gallup Organization fielded three surveys of Oklahoma City residents and comparable samples in Indianapolis. In the first survey, conducted 3 to 4 months after the bombing, Oklahoma City residents reported significantly higher rates of traumatic reminders, intrusive thoughts, dreams, avoidance, and stress than their Indianapolis counterparts. In the Oklahoma City group, overall stress was related to exposure, including injury, time off work, and relationship to an injured or killed victim. Oklahoma City residents also reported higher rates of increased alcohol use and smoking and higher rates of starting smoking (Smith et al., 1999).

Similar population-based surveys using newly drawn samples were conducted in 1996 and 1998. The results of the three studies demonstrated a consistent decrease in differences in the two communities over time. Differences in intrusive reexperiencing between Oklahoma City and Indianapolis persisted across all three time periods, findings likely representing normative distress (Pfefferbaum, Pfefferbaum, et al., 2006). In a representative national sample surveyed in 2002, Oklahoma City respondents were no different from the rest of the nation on most psychological responses to the September 11th attacks (Pfefferbaum, Pfefferbaum, et al., 2006). These results and similar findings in studies of New York City (Galea et al., 2003) and the nation (Silver, Holman, McIntosh, Poulin, & Gil-Rivas, 2002) after the September 11 attacks suggest optimism regarding psychological resilience and recovery from terrorism in affected communities.

Sprang (1999) also conducted telephone interviews of a random sample of Oklahoma City households representing the general community 6 months after the bombing. Unlike the Oklahoma City Gallup sample, individuals were not eligible to participate in this study if they had been exposed to another traumatic event in the preceding 5 years or if a family member or friend was injured or killed in the bombing. The comparison sample in Sprang's study was from Lexington, Kentucky, a city of similar size, situated approximately 800 miles from Oklahoma City (Sprang, 1999). Sprang (1999) divided her sample into three groups – a "high-exposure" Oklahoma City group (those who heard or felt the explosion), a "low-exposure" Oklahoma City group (those who lived in Oklahoma City but did not experience the explosion), and the Lexington group. The two Oklahoma City groups reported significantly greater current distress and victimization (measured as subjugation, vulnerability, attribution, and grief symptoms) than the Lexington group. Most of the respondents used informal interventions associated with church, family, and friends to cope, with no significant differences across groups (Sprang, 1999). When the groups were reassessed 2 years after the bombing, there were no significant differences in coping styles between the two Oklahoma City groups, but both of these groups reported higher use of task- and emotion-oriented coping than the Lexington group (Sprang, 2000). Participants who used avoidance coping reported higher levels of victimization and perception of future risk than those who used emotion-oriented and task-oriented coping, and they were less likely to seek services (Sprang, 2000).

In response to concerns about the reactions of Oklahoma City children, a survey of over 3,000 Oklahoma City middle and high school students was conducted 7 weeks after the bombing (Pfefferbaum, Nixon, et al., 1999). Most of the children in this convenience sample were at school on the day of the bombing and not physically present at the disaster site, though many heard and/or felt the explosion. More than 40% of the students surveyed knew injured survivors, and more than one-third knew deceased victims, though few of these relationships were with family members. Two-thirds of the participating children reported that most or all of their television viewing in the aftermath of the event was bombing-related. Posttraumatic stress reactions at the time of the assessment, measured with the Impact of Event Scale-Revised (Horowitz, Wilner, & Alvarez, 1979; Weiss & Marmar, 1997), were associated with female gender, interpersonal exposure through relationship with someone directly affected, initial fear and arousal, and bombing-related television viewing.

Children who reported knowing deceased victims were more likely than children who did not to endorse initial fear and arousal, changes at home and school, and posttraumatic stress reactions at 7 weeks. Bereaved children also reported greater bombing-related television viewing than those who were not bereaved. Proximity in relationship to the deceased correlated with self-report of difficulty calming down after watching bombing-related television coverage at 7 weeks. More than 60% of the nonbereaved children and over one-third of those who lost an immediate family member reported no such difficulty, however. Children reporting the greatest arousal at 7 weeks also reported the highest levels of exposure to television coverage of the bombing. Some undoubtedly turned to television coverage for information, and television viewing may have increased arousal in susceptible children. However, it is also possible that heightened states of arousal may increase a child's attention to media images, which, in turn, may maintain heightened reactivity to reminders (Pfefferbaum, Nixon, Tucker, et al., 1999). Thus, it is a mistake to assume a causal relationship between exposure to television coverage and acute or later symptoms.

Further, though Oklahoma City responders recognized that in some sense the federal government was the target of this terrorist incident, there was no systematic assessment of remotely affected individuals except individuals in the comparison samples from Indianapolis and Lexington in the Gallup study (Pfefferbaum, Pfefferbaum, et al., 2006; Smith et al., 1999) and the study by Sprang (1999, 2000), respectively. Owing to what appeared to be unrelenting media attention to the bombing, the criminal investigation, and the McVeigh trial, Pfefferbaum and colleagues (2000) studied 69 sixth-grade children 100 miles from Oklahoma City 2 years after the bombing at about the time activities related to the trial were beginning. Many children reported posttraumatic stress reactions at 2 years, reactions that correlated with exposure to media coverage. None of the children met the exposure criterion for PTSD, few children acknowledged deleterious effects on their functioning, and functional impairment was not associated with exposure to broadcast or print coverage.

The relationship between media exposure and posttraumatic stress in these studies should be interpreted with caution. Media coverage alone does not qualify as a stressor for the purpose of a PTSD diagnosis as defined by *DSM-IV-TR*. The mean PTSD reaction scores were relatively low in the Oklahoma City middle and high school samples and in the sample of children residing 100 miles away; for the most part, the children reported minimal impact on functioning. Furthermore, media exposure explained only a small amount of the outcome in the middle school study by Pfefferbaum and colleagues (Pfefferbaum, Nixon, et al., 2001). Thus, the clinical significance of the media findings in these studies is unclear; there is no evidence that exposure to media coverage caused PTSD or that it adversely affected children's mental health. The children's reactions were likely to have been normal reactions to community reminders.

30.4. RESCUERS AND RESPONDERS

The rescue and recovery efforts extended from days to weeks, exposing the men and women who participated in the work to horrific scenes. Two studies investigated the experiences and the reactions of Oklahoma City firefighters who served as first responders. The first, a survey of 325 responding firefighters conducted approximately 1 year after the bombing, revealed a generally positive outcome, which was measured by perceived effect, perceived recovery, and job satisfaction (Nixon, Schorr, Boudreaux, & Vincent, 1999a, 1999b). Firefighters reported substantial support from spouses or significant others, coworkers, and their faith (Nixon et al., 1999b). Those who reported more faith-based support also reported more positive outcomes; thus, a strong faith base may influence the perception of the effect of an event, the course of recovery, and the interpretation of the work environment during a stressful period, though causality should not be assumed (Nixon et al., 1999a, 1999b). These findings support the postdisaster role of chaplains and other faith-based professionals for those who report that faith is a comfort. Survivors who suffer serious emotional consequences may also need formal psychiatric services. With proper training and assistance, those with the strongest faith may be effective in delivering peer support, an approach that may be preferred by firefighters (Nixon et al., 1999a, 1999b).

A study of a convenience sample of 181 firefighters conducted 3 years after the bombing (North, Tivis, McMillen, Pfefferbaum, Cox et al., 2002; North, Tivis, McMillen, Pfefferbaum, Spitznagel, et al., 2002) used the same research instruments employed in the assessment of directly exposed survivors (North et al., 1999). Most of the firefighters who participated were male (97%) and Caucasian (89%). They described positive social adjustment (North, Tivis, McMillen, Pfefferbaum, Cox, et al., 2002) and few enduring problems in interpersonal relationships except marital disruption. Increases in the divorce rate had begun before the bombing, however (North, Tivis, McMillen, Pfefferbaum, Cox, et al., 2002). Overall, good adjustment of the firefighters was indicated by satisfaction with work, satisfactory or better self-assessed performance, and relatively little interference with daily functioning (North, Tivis, McMillen, Pfefferbaum, Cox, et al., 2002).

Only 13% of the firefighter sample met criteria for bombing-related PTSD, while 38% met criteria for any postdisaster psychiatric disorder. PTSD was associated with reduced job satisfaction and functional impairment, and more than one-half of those with bombing-related PTSD met criteria for another postdisaster disorder. Firefighters experienced less PTSD than male direct victims, which may reflect less intense exposure and lower injury rates in the firefighter sample, selection of the firefighter workforce, training and preparedness, experience, and attention to mental health needs through education and pre- and post-bombing support services (North, Tivis, McMillen, Pfefferbaum, Spitznagel, et al., 2002).

Alcohol abuse or dependence was the most prevalent disorder in this first responder sample, with 24% meeting criteria for current abuse or dependence and 47% meeting criteria for lifetime abuse or dependence. Only 2% of the alcohol abuse or dependence disorders were new cases emerging after the bombing. Most postdisaster psychiatric disorders were alcohol-related, and most of those with postbombing psychiatric disorders had preexisting psychopathology. The use of alcohol to cope was second only to seeking interpersonal support in identified coping strategies (North, Tivis, McMillen, Pfefferbaum, Cox, et al., 2002), and despite the high rates of alcohol use disorders among the firefighters, their use of alcohol to cope was no higher than in the male bombing survivors (North et al., 1999). Postdisaster alcohol use disorders and drinking to cope were significantly associated with indicators of poor functioning (North, Tivis, McMillen, Pfefferbaum, Cox, et al., 2002). The high prevalence of alcohol problems in this sample predating the bombing suggests the need for programs related to these problems in general, not just after disasters (North, Tivis, McMillen, Pfefferbaum, Spitznagel, et al., 2002).

Both firefighter studies examined reactions to debriefing, which was used during rescue and recovery. The findings are of interest especially in light of the controversy about this technique in recent years (National Institute of Mental Health, 2002; Rose, Bisson, Churchill, & Wessely, 2006). Most of the firefighters in the study conducted by North and colleagues (North, Tivis, McMillen, Pfefferbaum, Cox, et al., 2002) had participated in defusings or debriefing interventions. Two-thirds of the participants in the study were satisfied and one-third were dissatisfied with the intervention, though almost 90% said they would recommend it for colleagues. Less than one-fifth of the participants received any mental health services beyond the defusings and debriefings at work. Over one-fifth of the participants in the study by Nixon and colleagues (1999b) reported that debriefing was not helpful, while over 60% reported that it was either somewhat or very helpful, and almost 15% said they could not judge the helpfulness. Those who reported greater perceived effect of the bombing endorsed the usefulness of debriefing (Nixon et al., 1999a, 1999b). The sizeable number of participants who were dissatisfied with the intervention (North, Tivis, McMillen, Pfefferbaum, Cox, et al., 2002) or who found the intervention unhelpful (Nixon et al., 1999b) suggests the need for selective use of debriefing.

A small pilot sample of 24 female partners of the firefighters who participated in the study by North's team was studied 3½ years after the bombing (Pfefferbaum, North, et al., 2002; Pfefferbaum, Tucker, et al., 2006). Most of the partners with postbombing disorders suffered from preexisting conditions. One participant met all bombing-related PTSD symptom group criteria, and 40% met both intrusive reexperiencing (Group B) and hyperarousal (Group D) criteria (Pfefferbaum, Tucker, et al., 2006). Many of the women continued to exhibit physiological reactivity to reminders of the bombing when measured in the context of a trauma-cue interview, though it is unclear how representative these findings are of firefighter partners in general, how their reactions might compare with others in Oklahoma City at the time, or if these reactions were related to other anxiety or depressive conditions or to other life events experienced by the participants. Larger representative samples and studies in closer temporal proximity to the traumatic event will be needed to fully understand the effects of exposure through interpersonal relationships with disaster responders (Pfefferbaum, Tucker, et al., 2006).

A limited number of trained and experienced medical examiners and pathologists were available to identify the remains of the 168 people who died in the bombing (Jordan, 1999). Thus, volunteers of multiple medically related disciplines from the community assisted in these activities. Two-thirds of the participants in a convenience sample of 51 body handlers studied 2 years after the disaster had no disaster experience (Tucker et al., 2002). Many knew someone killed in the bombing. Nonetheless, retrospectively reported posttraumatic stress reactions and depressive symptoms at the time of the disaster were few, and numbers decreased significantly 1 year later. In addition to individual coping techniques, onsite critical incident stress management and debriefing, "esprit de corps," a strong sense of community, positive management style, and the participants' relatively high educational level and experience may have contributed to their resilience (Tucker et al., 2002) though these factors were not examined in this study. Ten percent of the sample said they increased their use of alcohol in the first 2 months after the disaster; 14% sought mental health services to cope with their distress. Greater symptomatology was related to increased alcohol use, new physical problems, and seeking mental health services (Tucker et al., 2002).

30.5. SERVICES

The emotional needs of survivors and family members were of immediate concern after the bombing. A family assistance program, which came to be known as the Compassion Center, was established by the medical examiner's office to collect information about the missing and to provide support for family members in a safe and protected environment (Jordan, 1999; Sitterle & Gurwitch, 1998). In the first 2 weeks after the bombing, the families of some 300 individuals thought to be missing gathered at the center. Regular briefings were held, and a well-organized, coordinated effort of professionals and volunteers representing many organizations delivered support services for families and participated in death notification. A children's corner, staffed with child mental health experts, provided activities and services for children and a respite for parents (Sitterle & Gurwitch, 1998).

Oklahoma City professionals responsible for organizing the system of care and the clinicians who delivered services were guided and supported by the federal government, which funded the Oklahoma Department of Mental Health and Substance Abuse Services to create a crisis counseling program, Project Heartland. Through subcontracts and other relationships, Project Heartland established a network of public and private partners to address the needs of various subpopulations including ethnic minorities, individuals with preexisting emotional disorders, the elderly, and children. This structure facilitated access to care and fostered integration within existing programs. Interventions included support groups and client advocacy; programmatic activities such as consultation, education and training, system support, and treatment team meetings; outreach services including door-to-door visits and mailings; emergency services and crisis intervention; counseling and therapy; and screening, evaluation, and referral services. In keeping with the crisis counseling program mandate, Project Heartland was not intended to provide traditional services for those with serious emotional problems or to provide comprehensive psychological assessment. Instead, those needing more intensive intervention were referred to professionals in the community (Call & Pfefferbaum, 1999).

To enhance access, normalize reactions, and decrease stigma associated with mental health services, an array of outreach, crisis intervention, and support services for children were delivered in local schools. The Oklahoma City public school district appointed a district-wide steering committee to screen requests from various public and private groups for school-based clinical and educational programs as well as media inquiries and research. Decisions about what to include were determined through consideration of the appropriateness of the programs for the school setting while balancing the goals of support and normalization. Individual schools also established their own priorities and could override decisions of the district-wide committee (Pfefferbaum, Call, & Sconzo, 1999). One intervention, a classroom exercise to assess the emotional status of children and foster adaptive coping, was used to screen over 6,000 children during the academic year after the bombing (Allen & Dlugokinski, 2002; Allen, Dlugokinski, Cohen, & Walker, 1999). Approximately 9% of the children assessed were considered at-risk for emotional problems because of their relationships with directly affected individuals or responders or because of other real or fabricated losses. Approximately one-third of these children received counseling (Allen et al., 1999).

The American Psychological Association's (1997) review of mental health services raised questions about the effectiveness of the school-based programs because few children were referred; however, absent an assessment of need, such conclusions must be tentative. It may be that the school-based programs were so effective that referral was not indicated. While less than 7% of the children studied by Pfefferbaum and colleagues (Pfefferbaum, Nixon, Tucker, et al., 1999) had sought counseling at 7 weeks, more than 40% of those who lost an immediate family member and approximately 15% of those who lost another relative had sought counseling. These figures suggest that children who needed services actually did receive them. On the other hand, for children with the highest levels of posttraumatic stress there was no correlation between posttraumatic stress reactions and seeking counseling (Pfefferbaum, Sconzo, et al., 2003). Therefore, some symptomatic children may not have been detected by screening, and other measures may have been necessary to identify them.

Disaster mental health professionals have noted that terrorist incidents may differ in substantive ways from other disasters (Pfefferbaum, North, Flynn, Norris, & DeMartino, 2002). For example, the potential for greater psychopathology in events that produce mass casualties, like the bombing, suggest the need for more traditional psychiatric services in such disasters. At the same time, terrorist goals of generating social disruption and fear in the larger society create concern about the broader range of victims who are likely to need reassurance, public education, accurate risk communication, and support services rather than formal psychiatric care. In the case of the Oklahoma City bombing, construing the bombing as an attack on the government led to questions about the appropriate division of authority and responsibility in response to the event (Pfefferbaum, North, Flynn, et al., 2002).

Oklahoma City professionals also called for program evaluation (Pfefferbaum, North, Flynn, et al., 2002), which was examined in a broad context years later (Norris, Watson, Hamblen, & Pfefferbaum, 2005), though unfortunately no intervention effectiveness or efficacy studies were conducted. The study by Norris and colleagues (2005) revealed disparity among providers in their opinions about credentials, the quality of services provided, the appropriateness of the crisis counseling model, and the failure to conduct ongoing needs assessment and service evaluation. Criticisms of Project Heartland reflected concerns about the federal crisis counseling model more generally. The study identified the need to balance local control with access to national expertise and to strengthen relationships between the public and private sectors. It also revealed the need to provide training about longer-term issues, standardized interventions, and program evaluation and to clarify issues related to referrals, fees, record keeping, the appropriate roles of paraprofessionals and licensed professionals, and the appropriate venues for services. The investigators identified the potential benefit of greater flexibility in structuring crisis counseling programs to provide traditional psychiatric services for those who need them while also providing crisis support for the majority who do not. They noted, however, that the lack of assessment data made it difficult to determine the extent to which traditional services actually were needed. The failure to obtain empirical data evaluating the available services also made it difficult to determine the quality of the services provided.

30.6. SUMMARY OF RESEARCH FINDINGS

Research after the Oklahoma City bombing advanced our understanding of the effects of major disasters in several ways. Key among them was the recognition of qualitative distinctions in disaster exposure. Thus, Oklahoma City studies included samples of directly exposed survivors and indirectly and remotely affected individuals. Comprehensive diagnostic studies examining directly exposed Oklahoma City survivors confirmed high rates of psychiatric disorders (North et al., 1999, 2004). Those studies also revealed the importance of avoidance and numbing in the diagnosis of PTSD at index and follow-up (North et al., 1999, 2004). As yet, similar comprehensive diagnostic studies of the most directly exposed survivors of subsequent major disasters have not been published.

Forerunners of the post–September 11th research with heterogeneous samples of individuals with a range of exposure (Galea et al., 2002; Pfefferbaum et al., 2008; Schlenger et al., 2002; Schuster et al., 2001; Silver et al., 2002; Vlahov et al., 2002), Oklahoma City studies also used survey methodology to examine posttraumatic stress responses, drinking, smoking, and coping in indirectly and remotely affected individuals (Pfefferbaum, Pfefferbaum, et al., 2006; Smith et al., 1999; Sprang, 1999, 2000). Investigators also studied indirect and remote effects in school children and documented a relationship between posttraumatic stress and exposure to bombing-related television coverage (Pfefferbaum, Nixon, Krug, et al., 1999; Pfefferbaum, Nixon, et al., 2001; Pfefferbaum, Nixon, Tucker, et al., 1999; Pfefferbaum, Seale, McDonald, Brandt, Rainwater, Maynard, Meierhoefer, Miller, 2000). The clinical significance of findings in indirectly and remotely affected populations is unclear, and the relationship between posttraumatic stress and exposure to media coverage should be interpreted with caution, avoiding causation attribution.

Oklahoma City bombing studies also advanced our understanding of the reactions of rescuers and responders. North and colleagues (North, Tivis, McMillen, Pfefferbaum, Cox, et al., 2002; North, Tivis, McMillen, Pfefferbaum, Spitznagel, et al., 2002) found good adjustment in firefighters with low rates of bombing-related PTSD but high rates of any postdisaster psychiatric disorder. Alcohol abuse or dependence was the most prevalent disorder, though this pathology predated the bombing in most who reported it.

Finally, Oklahoma City professionals raised a number of service delivery issues associated with the federally funded crisis counseling program (Norris et al., 2005; Pfefferbaum, North, Flynn, et al., 2002). Empirical studies focused specifically on service utilization, and investigations around barriers to care by-and-large were lacking, as were investigations examining the effectiveness of treatment interventions. Fortunately, there is now strong impetus to conduct such research.

30.7. ORGANIZING RESEARCH

Establishing and delivering services in Oklahoma City took precedence over research, and some in the community were suspicious about research, even research related to needs assessment, program evaluation, and the effectiveness of services and interventions (Pfefferbaum & Stein, 2006). Nonetheless, a concerted effort was made to establish a systematic approach to clinical research regarding the emotional consequences of the bombing on directly exposed survivors, community residents, and rescuers and responders. The Commissioner of Health declared bombing-related injuries to be reportable events, thus enabling the creation of a registry of victims that facilitated the research on survivors (Nixon, Vincent, Krug, & Pfefferbaum, 1998; Quick, 1998).

In addition to designating the Oklahoma Department of Mental Health and Substance Abuse Services as the responsible state authority to address mental health clinical needs, the Governor designated the OUHSC as the lead institution overseeing bombing-related research (North, Pfefferbaum, & Tucker, 2002; Quick, 1998). The OUHSC Institutional Review Board (IRB) assisted colleagues in other institutions and provided local oversight. The intent was for the OUHSC IRB to serve as a clearinghouse and to provide full, expedited review to bombing-related studies, with attention to study design, timing, participant confidentiality, and methods for contacting potential participants (Quick, 1998). Of particular concern was the protection of participants and their referral to services should that be indicated (North, Pfefferbaum, Tucker, 2002; Quick, 1998). While this edict had appeal in that, theoretically at least, it facilitated attention to clinical needs, it may also have discouraged or precluded involvement of national experts and researchers. However, the arrangement for local review did follow one of the disaster mental health research field's principal axioms – that disasters being local, their management is the responsibility of local authorities, and services and research should include and rely on local professionals. Furthermore, the position did not prevent a number of studies led by researchers from outside of Oklahoma City.

30.8. CONCLUSIONS AND FUTURE DIRECTIONS

Clinicians and researchers who responded to the bombing were aware that the event was unique in a number of ways. An understanding of the goals of terrorism led researchers to study a wider range of potential victims than in many prior disaster studies, and with increasing sophistication, this eventually resulted in the recognition of the need to identify salient research questions related to exposure and experiences and to select appropriate research methodologies and instruments. Oklahoma City bombing research set a high standard for methodologic rigor in studies of both directly affected populations (North et al., 1999, 2004; Tucker et al., 2007) and community samples (Pfefferbaum, Pfefferbaum, et al., 2006; Smith et al., 1999; Sprang, 1999, 2000). Not only were these Oklahoma City studies able to circumvent obstacles to access, they established important foundations for longitudinal work still greatly needed to advance our understanding of disaster effects.

We know that studies of directly exposed individuals warrant attention to PTSD and other psychiatric disorders that develop in the aftermath of a disaster, while studies of those without direct exposure cannot identify disaster-related PTSD because of the diagnostic requirement of exposure to a qualifying traumatic event. Differentiating types of exposure and outcomes is essential to determining appropriate interventions. Posttraumatic stress symptoms in affected populations without the requisite trauma exposure constitute emotional distress rather than PTSD. These symptoms may represent normative reactions and may even require mental health attention, though the interventions appropriate for these populations would include reassurance, psychoeducation, and supportive measures while directly exposed individuals with PTSD and other disorders such as major depression need formal psychiatric care (North & Pfefferbaum, 2004).

Studies of both directly exposed groups and groups that are either indirectly exposed or only remotely affected should also assess distress, fear, and other normative reactions rather than assuming purely pathological outcomes. In addition, more attention is needed in terms of defining and measuring exposure and in elucidating the differential effects of various forms of exposure. For example, few researchers to date have addressed bereaved individuals and the relationship between grief and trauma reactions. Comprehensive longitudinal evaluations of directly exposed children and responders (including mental health care providers, the media, and community leaders) are lacking. Research is also needed to illuminate the community structures and activities that promote recovery.

One major challenge for future disaster mental health research is establishing procedures for more rapid access to affected populations for early data collection without compromising the integrity of sampling and quality of measurement. Additional longitudinal disaster mental health studies using diagnostically sensitive measures to examine the course of recovery are also needed, and careful interpretation of results is vital to generate public and political will to allocate the necessary resources for continued work in this area (North & Pfefferbaum, 2002). Empirical data on the effectiveness of various interventions, to guide the development and refinement of services across all phases of disaster, are essential in establishing an evidence base for clinical interventions. Finally, concerns remain about disaster mental health service delivery issues, the federally funded disaster mental health system, populations needing services, and what those services should include (Norris et al., 2005; Pfefferbaum, North, Flynn, et al., 2002).

REFERENCES

Allen, S. F., & Dlugokinski, E. L. (2002). Assisting children in recovering from a traumatic community event. *Directions in Clinical and Counseling Psychology, 12*(1), 1–11.

Allen, S. F., Dlugokinski, E. L., Cohen, L. A., & Walker, J. L. (1999). Assessing the impact of a traumatic community event on children and assisting with their healing. *Psychiatric Annals, 29*(2), 93–98.

American Psychological Association. (July 1997). *Final report: American Psychological Association Task Force on the mental health response to the Oklahoma City bombing.* Retrieved October 2007, http://taxa.epi.umn.edu/~mbmiller/APA-Oklahoma/

Call, J. A., & Pfefferbaum, B. (1999). Lessons from the first two years of Project Heartland, Oklahoma's mental health response to the 1995 bombing. *Psychiatric Services, 50*(7), 953–955.

Galea, S., Ahern, J., Resnick, H., Kilpatrick, D., Bucuvalas, M., Gold, J., et al. (2002). Psychological sequelae of the September 11 terrorist attacks in New York City. *The New England Journal of Medicine, 346*(13), 982–987.

Galea, S., Vlahov, D., Resnick, H., Ahern, J., Susser, E., Gold, J., et al. (2003). Trends of probable posttraumatic stress disorder in New York City after the September 11 terrorist attacks. *American Journal of Epidemiology, 158*(6), 514–524.

Gurwitch, R. H., Pfefferbaum, B., & Leftwich, M. J. T. (2002). The impact of terrorism on children: Considerations for a new era. *Journal of Trauma Practice, 1*(3/4), 101–124.

Gurwitch, R. H., Sitterle, K. A., Young, B. H., & Pfefferbaum, B. (2002). The aftermath of terrorism. In A. M. La Greca, W. K. Silverman, E. M. Vernberg, & M. C. Roberts (Eds.), *Helping children cope with disasters and terrorism.* Washington, DC: American Psychological Association.

Horowitz, M., Wilner, N., & Alvarez, W. (1979). Impact of Event Scale: A measure of subjective stress. *Psychosomatic Medicine, 41*(3), 209–218.

Jordan, F. B. (1999). The role of the medical examiner in mass casualty situations with special reference to the Alfred P. Murrah Building bombing. *Journal of the Oklahoma State Medical Association, 92*(4), 159–163.

National Institute of Mental Health. (2002). *Mental health and mass violence: Evidence-based early psychological intervention for victims/survivors of mass violence. A workshop to reach consensus on best practices*. NIH Publication No. 02-5138. Washington, DC: U.S. Government Printing Office.

Nixon, S. J., Schorr, J., Boudreaux, A., & Vincent, R. D. (1999a). Perceived effects and recovery in Oklahoma City firefighters. *Journal of the Oklahoma State Medical Association, 92*(4), 172–177.

(1999b). Perceived sources of support and their effectiveness for Oklahoma City firefighters. *Psychiatric Annals, 29*(2), 101–105.

Nixon, S. J., Vincent, R., Krug, R. S., & Pfefferbaum, B. (1998). Structure and organization of research efforts following the bombing of the Murrah Building. *Journal of Personal and Interpersonal Loss, 3*, 99–115.

Norris, F. H., Watson, P. J., Hamblen, J. L., & Pfefferbaum, B. J. (2005). Provider perspectives on disaster mental health services in Oklahoma City. *Journal of Aggression, Maltreatment & Trauma, 10*(1/2), 649–661.

North, C. S., Nixon, S. J., Shariat, S., Mallonee, S., McMillen, J. C., Spitznagel, E. L., et al. (1999). Psychiatric disorders among survivors of the Oklahoma City bombing. *The Journal of the American Medical Association, 282*(8), 755–762.

North, C. S., & Pfefferbaum, B. (2002). Research on the mental health effects of terrorism. *The Journal of the American Medical Association, 288*(5), 633–636.

(2004). The state of research on the mental health effects of terrorism. *Epidemiologia e Psichiatria Sociale, 13*(1), 4–9.

North, C. S., Pfefferbaum, B., Tivis, L., Kawasaki, A., Reddy, C., & Spitznagel, E. L. (2004). The course of posttraumatic stress disorder in a follow-up study of survivors of the Oklahoma City bombing. *Annals of Clinical Psychiatry, 16*, 209–215.

North, C. S., Pfefferbaum, B., & Tucker, P. (2002). Ethical and methodological issues in academic mental health research in populations affected by disasters: Oklahoma City experience relevant to September 11, 2001. *CNS Spectrums, 7*(8), 580–584.

North, C. S., Tivis, L., McMillen, J. C., Pfefferbaum, B., Cox, J., Spitznagel, E. L., et al. (2002). Coping, functioning, and adjustment of rescue workers after the Oklahoma City bombing. *Journal of Traumatic Stress, 15*(3), 171–175.

North, C. S., Tivis, L., McMillen, J. C., Pfefferbaum, B., Spitznagel, E. L., Cox, J., et al. (2002). Psychiatric disorders in rescue workers after the Oklahoma City bombing. *American Journal of Psychiatry, 159*(5), 857–859.

Oklahoma City National Memorial Institute for the Prevention of Terrorism (n.d.). *Murrah Building bombing* – A look at numbers. Retrieved October 2007, http?//www.oklahomacitynationalmemorial.org/secondary.php?section=5&catid=145

Pfefferbaum, B. (2003). The children of Oklahoma City. In R. J. Ursano, C. S. Fullerton, & A. E. Norwood (Eds.), *Terrorism and disaster*. New York: Cambridge University Press.

Pfefferbaum, B., Call, J. A., Doughty, D. E., Traxler, W. T., Pai, M. N., Borrell, G. K., et al. (2003). Impact of injury on posttraumatic stress in survivors seeking counseling after the 1995 bombing in Oklahoma City. *Journal of Trauma Practice, 2*(2), 1–17.

Pfefferbaum, B., Call, J. A., Lensgraf, S. J., Miller, P. D., Flynn, B. W., Doughty, D. E., et al. (2001). Traumatic grief in a convenience sample of victims seeking support services after a terrorist incident. *Annals of Clinical Psychiatry, 13*(1), 19–24.

Pfefferbaum, B., Call, J. A., & Sconzo, G. M. (1999). Mental health services for children in the first two years after the 1995 Oklahoma City terrorist bombing. *Psychiatric Services, 50*(7), 956–958.

Pfefferbaum, B., Nixon, S. J., Krug, R. S., Tivis, R. D., Moore, V. L., Brown, J. M., et al. (1999). Clinical needs assessment of middle and high school students following the 1995 Oklahoma City bombing. *American Journal of Psychiatry, 156*(7), 1069–1074.

Pfefferbaum, B., Nixon, S. J., Tivis, R. D., Doughty, D. E., Pynoos, R. S., Gurwitch, R. H., et al. (2001). Television exposure in children after a terrorist incident. *Psychiatry, 64*(3), 202–211.

Pfefferbaum, B., Nixon, S. J., Tucker, P. M., Tivis, R. D., Moore, V. L., Gurwitch, R. H., et al. (1999). Posttraumatic stress responses in bereaved children after the Oklahoma City bombing. *Journal of the American Academy of Child and Adolescent Psychiatry, 38*(11), 1372–1379.

Pfefferbaum, B., North, C. S., Bunch, K., Wilson, T. G., Tucker, P., & Schorr, J. K. (2002). The impact of the 1995 Oklahoma City bombing on the partners of firefighters. *Journal of Urban Health: Bulletin of the New York Academy of Medicine, 79*(3), 364–372.

Pfefferbaum, B., North, C. S., Flynn, B. W., Norris, F. H., & DeMartino, R. (2002). Disaster mental health services following the 1995 Oklahoma City bombing: Modifying approaches to address terrorism. *CNS Spectrums, 7*(8), 575–579.

Pfefferbaum, B., North, C. S., Pfefferbaum, R. L., Christiansen, E. H., Schorr, J. K., Vincent, R. D., et al.

(2008). Change in smoking and drinking after September 11, 2001, in a national sample of ever smokers and ever drinkers. *The Journal of Nervous and Mental Disease, 196*(2), 113–121.

Pfefferbaum, B., Pfefferbaum, R.L., Christiansen, E.H., Schorr, J.K., Vincent, R.D., Nixon, S.J., et al. (2006). Comparing stress responses to terrorism in residents of two communities over time. *Brief Treatment and Crisis Intervention, 6*(2), 137–143.

Pfefferbaum, B., Sconzo, G.M., Flynn, B.W., Kearns, L.J., Doughty, D.E., Gurwitch, R.H., et al. (2003). Case finding and mental health services for children in the aftermath of the Oklahoma City bombing. *The Journal of Behavioral Health Services & Research, 30*(2), 215–227.

Pfefferbaum, B., Seale, T.W., McDonald, N.B., Brandt, E.N., Jr., Rainwater, S.M., Maynard, B.T., et al. (2000). Posttraumatic stress two years after the Oklahoma City bombing in youths geographically distant from the explosion. *Psychiatry, 63*(4), 358–370.

Pfefferbaum, B., & Stein, B.D. (2006). Disasters in the 21st century: Lessons from Project Liberty. *Psychiatric Services, 57*(9), 1251.

Pfefferbaum, B., Tucker, P., North, C.S., Jeon-Slaughter, H., Kent, A.T., Schorr, J.K., et al. (2006). Persistent physiological reactivity in a pilot study of partners of firefighters after a terrorist attack. *The Journal of Nervous and Mental Disease, 194*(2),128–131.

Pfefferbaum, B., Vinekar, S.S., Trautman, R.P., Lensgraf, S.J., Reddy, C., Patel, N., et al. (2002). The effect of loss and trauma on substance use behavior in individuals seeking support services after the 1995 Oklahoma City bombing. *Annals of Clinical Psychiatry, 14*(2), 89–95.

Quick, G. (1998). A paradigm for multidisciplinary disaster research: The Oklahoma City experience. *The Journal of Emergency Medicine, 16*(4), 621–630.

Rose, S., Bisson, J., Churchill, R., & Wessely, S. (2006). Psychological debriefing for preventing post traumatic stress disorder (PTSD). *The Cochrane Collaboration, 4*, 1–61.

Scheeringa, M.S., Zeanah, C.H., Drell, M.J., & Larrieu, J.A. (1995). Two approaches to the diagnosis of posttraumatic stress disorder in infancy and early childhood. *Journal of the American Academy of Child and Adolescent Psychiatry, 34*(2), 191–200.

Schlenger, W.E., Caddell, J.M., Ebert, L., Jordan, B.K., Rourke, K.M., Wilson, D., et al. (2002). Psychological reactions to terrorist attacks: Findings from the National Study of Americans' Reactions to September 11. *The Journal of the American Medical Association, 288*(5), 581–588.

Schuster, M.A., Stein, B.D., Jaycox, L.H., Collins, R.L., Marshall, G.N., Elliott, M.N., et al. (2001). A national survey of stress reactions after the September 11, 2001, terrorist attacks. *The New England Journal of Medicine, 345*(20), 1507–1512.

Silver, R.C., Holman, E.A., McIntosh, D.N., Poulin, M., & Gil-Rivas, V. (2002). Nationwide longitudinal study of psychological responses to September 11. *The Journal of the American Medical Association, 288*(10), 1235–1244.

Sitterle, K.A., & Gurwitch, R.H. (1998). The terrorist bombing in Oklahoma City. In E. S. Zinner & M. B. Williams (Eds.), *When a community weeps: Case studies in group survivorship*. Philadelphia, PA: Taylor & Francis.

Smith, D.W., Christiansen, E.H., Vincent, R., & Hann, N.E., (1999). Population effects of the bombing of Oklahoma City. *Journal of the Oklahoma State Medical Association, 92*(4), 193–198.

Sprang, G. (1999). Post-disaster stress following the Oklahoma City bombing. *Journal of Interpersonal Violence, 14*(2), 169–183.

(2000). Coping strategies and traumatic stress symptomatology following the Oklahoma City bombing. *Social Work & Social Sciences Review, 8*(2), 207–218.

Tucker, P., Dickson, W., Pfefferbaum, B., McDonald, N.B., & Allen, G. (1997). Traumatic reactions as predictors of posttraumatic stress six months after the Oklahoma City bombing. *Psychiatric Services, 48*(9), 1191–1194.

Tucker, P.M., Pfefferbaum, B., North, C.S., Kent, A., Burgin, C.E., Parker, D.E., et al. (2007). Physiologic reactivity despite emotional resilience several years after direct exposure to terrorism. *American Journal of Psychiatry, 164*(2), 230–235.

Tucker, P., Pfefferbaum, B., Doughty, D.E., Jones, D.E., Jordan, F.B., Vincent, R.D., et al. (2002). Body handlers after terrorism in Oklahoma City: Predictors of posttraumatic stress and other symptoms. *American Journal of Orthopsychiatry, 72*(4), 469–475.

Tucker, P., Pfefferbaum, B., Nixon, S.J., & Dickson, W. (2000). Predictors of post-traumatic stress symptoms in Oklahoma City: Exposure, social support, peri-traumatic responses. *The Journal of Behavioral Health Services & Research, 27*(4), 406–416.

Tucker, P., Pfefferbaum, B., Nixon, S.J., & Foy, D.W. (1999). Trauma and recovery among adults highly exposed to a community disaster. *Psychiatric Annals, 29*(2), 78–83.

Vlahov, D., Galea, S., Resnick, H., Ahern, J., Boscarino, J. A., Bucuvalas, M., et al. (2002). Increased use of cigarettes, alcohol, and marijuana among Manhattan, New York, residents after the September 11th terrorist attacks. *American Journal of Epidemiology, 155*(11), 988–996.

Weiss, D. S., & Marmar, C. R. (1997). The Impact of Event Scale-Revised. In J. P. Wilson & T. M. Keane (Eds.), *Assessing psychological trauma and PTSD*. New York: Guilford Press.

31 The Terrorist Attacks of September 11, 2001, in New York City

CHARLES DIMAGGIO AND PAULA MADRID

31.1. THE ATTACK

The early autumn morning of September 11, 2001, dawned cloudless and blue in New York City. It ended with images of debris-covered, panic-stricken individuals fleeing down the man-made canyons of lower Manhattan. The exact numbers differ slightly by report, but nearly 3,000 people died that morning as two hijacked jet liners smashed into the iconic twin towers of the World Trade Center (WTC) complex, while a third dropped into the Pentagon in Washington, DC, and a fourth crashed in a rural Pennsylvania field.

The traumas of that day and of those following now seem hazy, but they were startlingly clear at the time. One of the world's greatest transportation systems came to a sudden, jarring halt, forcing a mass migration of all ages across bridges under the perceived threat of renewed attacks. Communication became nearly impossible as millions attempted to reach out to loved ones. A fog of rumor and fear settled on the city and the surrounding area.

The reality of the following weeks was no less traumatizing. Thousands of photos of the missing fluttered from fences surrounding hospitals and morgues. Funeral processions, particularly for firefighters and police officers, became a sadly evocative and almost daily event in some communities surrounding New York City. Internal calculations of potential death from a bridge collapse or tunnel implosion factored into commuting decisions. Through it all was the pervasive daily sensory reminders of an altered visual landscape and the scent of the dying embers of the once massive buildings.

Terrorists aim to affect behavioral change through fear, and echoes of the fear planted 5 years ago in New York City continue to reverberate. A tourist's photographic flash bulb near a bridge (in a city of gracefully soaring bridges) may result in a police response; a forgotten handbag on the subway will prompt worried glances. The challenge to researchers and mental health professionals is to determine where normal adaptive behavior ends and unreasonable responses and pathology begin.

Amid the swirl of confusion and shock, mental health experts began to ask questions. Did the attacks have unique and quantifiable mental and behavioral health consequences? What were those consequences and how long might they last? Who was at risk and what put them at risk? In a city that large (and with constant and reported images of terror beaming into homes), what, in fact, constituted exposure to the attacks? Were the effects limited to New York City, and could one's community be expected to modify those effects? What services were needed and how could they best be delivered to a wounded city?

Some of the questions have yet to be answered. In this chapter, we hope to "tell the story" of the terrorist attacks of September 11, 2001, in New York City by presenting and discussing the accumulated efforts of some of the many clinicians, researchers, and mental health professionals who responded in the weeks and months following the attacks. We also hope to touch on some of the unique research and practical issues they confronted. Through this process we hope to paint a portrait of how New York City's mental health community responded to the attacks and, 7 years later, what lessons we have learned.

31.2. THE IMMEDIATE AFTERMATH

Up until the September 11th terrorist attacks – with the notable exception of the Oklahoma City bombings – research into terrorism was notably scant. This was due in part to the fact that most terrorist incidents occurred in poorer regions of the world. However, evidence from the bombing of the Murrah Federal Building in Oklahoma City indicated that over a third of those directly exposed had symptoms consistent with posttraumatic stress disorder (PTSD) 6 months after the event (North, 1999). This finding led to fears of a potential massive mental health crisis in the immediate aftermath of the September 11th terrorist attacks.

There also was concern that the effects of the WTC attack might extend beyond those traditionally defined as exposed (survivors, rescuers, family members) into the densely populated tri-state region of approximately 15 million residents. The New York State Office of Mental Health estimated that three million people in New York City and the surrounding region could experience substantial emotional distress (Felton, Donahue, Lanzara, Pease, & Marshall, 2006). Others estimated that 422,000 individuals could meet the criteria for PTSD and that 129,000 would seek treatment (Herman, Felton, & Susser 2002). For the general population, the direct measurable impacts of the disaster came in many forms, including loss of home, employment, and schooling. More than 50,000 people lived in lower Manhattan, and over 30,000 residents were temporarily displaced because of the event (Crow, 2001).

In this context it is no surprise that a number of efforts were immediately undertaken to determine the extent of potential mental and behavioral health outcomes and to mitigate the consequences of the event. These endeavors drew on the existing expertise of disaster preparedness professionals, mental health practitioners, epidemiologists, and scientists, as well as the fervor of well-intentioned volunteers. Owing to the diverse backgrounds of the researchers, the work varied from methodologically world class to scientifically suspect, and the results have been somewhat scattershot in nature. However, if we concentrate on the more reliable and valid research, the different pieces begin to fit together and the outlines of a picture emerge.

31.3. EARLY PATTERNS

In the first weeks following the September 11th terrorist attacks, one in ten New York area residents met the criteria for PTSD (Marshall & Galea, 2004). Approximately 7.6% of New York City's eight million residents reported using mental health services in the 30-day period given months after September 11th (Boscarino et al., 2004). Studies indicated that 7.5% of all Manhattan residents had symptoms consistent with PTSD in the first month after the terrorist attacks (Galea et al., 2002), and 20% of residents living in close proximity to the events met criteria for PTSD during the same time period (Galea, Resnick, et al., 2002). Other studies reported that the prevalence of anxiety-related diagnoses in the population of New York City's Chinatown, which is located in the immediate vicinity of the WTC, may have been as high as 50% (Chen, Chung, Chen, Fang, & Chen, 2003). It was estimated that New York City residents who lived closest to the WTC site had three times greater risk of developing PTSD than those who did not (Galea et al., 2002).

There were notable efforts to further quantify the prevalence of posttraumatic stress in the general population and identify those most at risk so as to guide interventions. Galea and colleagues initially sought to establish a cohort that could be followed over time to better elucidate the time course of PTSD, but in an example of the particular difficulties attendant on postdisaster research, they could not establish institutional review board approval for such a cohort in a timely fashion. They eventually settled on a series of prevalence studies conducted via random digit dial (Ahern et al., 2002; Boscarino, Galea, Ahern, Resnick, & Vlahov, 2002; Galea, Ahern, et al. 2002; Vlahov, Galea, & Frankel, 2002).

A number of results arose from this series of studies. The overall prevalence of PTSD in NYC in the immediate aftermath of the attack was approximately 6%, dropping to 1% 6 months later. The risk of developing PTSD following the terrorist attacks was twice as great among Hispanics and unmarried or divorced individuals and was directly correlated with social status as measured through yearly income. Experiencing previous traumatic events increased the risk of PTSD as high as six times. Controlling for these and other covariates, the researchers ascribed a risk of over three times for those directly exposed to the attacks compared with those unexposed. Surprisingly, there were conflicting data on the importance of proximity to the events in the subsequent development of PTSD. Residents of areas outside of Manhattan (notably Brooklyn, Staten Island, and the Bronx) were at high risk of PTSD. Various factors could account for this and highlight some of the issues attendant in defining spatial "exposure" in the setting of terrorism. Many residents of Brooklyn commute to lower Manhattan, many firefighters and police officers live on Staten Island, the Bronx has a large population of Hispanics. These factors all act as potential confounders of the effect of residence.

This series of studies also called into question the very definition of PTSD, which requires direct "exposure" to a trauma. What, in the context of this event, constituted such exposure? Does, perhaps, watching horrific televised images of individuals hurling themselves to their deaths from a high-rise building meet the criteria (Ahern et al., 2002)?

31.4. TRAJECTORIES AND LONG-TERM EFFECTS

Noji and Sivertson (1987) noted, "many health effects of a disaster do not occur immediately, but may be increased months or years afterwards." Silver and colleagues (2002) sought to document the behavioral and mental health effects of the terrorist attacks on a nationally representative sample of U.S. residents and found evidence of persistently elevated prevalence of psychological distress many months after and at long distances from the events of September 11, 2001. By casting a broad net, identifying a large enough group early after the event, and following them over an adequate amount of time, the researchers hoped to more firmly establish the causal role of such variables as preexisting traumas, the social environment, and coping mechanisms on mental and behavioral health outcomes associated with the terrorist attacks of September 11th. Early results indicated substantial variability in responses.

Silver and colleagues conducted a Web-based survey of a nationally representative sample of individuals 1, 3, 6, 12, 18, 24, and 36 months after the attacks. Nationally, high levels of stress symptoms were present in 11.7% of Americans 1 month after the attack (Silver, Holman, McIntosh, Poulin, & Gil-Rivas, 2002). The progression of PTSD symptoms nationwide was particularly instructive. Such symptoms were reported by 17% of respondents 3 months after the attacks, 5.2% of respondents 6 months after the attacks, and approximately 4% of respondents thereafter. Those who reported direct exposure to the attacks and those who reported exposure to stressful life events following the attacks were at highest risk (Silver et al., 2006). Other researchers found that a year after September 11th, New York City residents continued to be "very concerned" about future terrorist attacks (Boscarino, Figley, & Adams, 2003).

Among the results of long-term studies of the attack on New York City (Bonanno, Papa, Lalande, Westphal, & Coifman, 2004) were reiterations of findings that most people cope quite effectively with the traumas that frequently arise in their lives (Neria et al., 2000), and they in fact convert them to positive experiences (Dohrenwend et al., 2004). For some though, trauma, such as that experienced in New York City in September 2001, results in long-lasting and debilitating conditions such as PTSD, depression, anxiety and panic attacks, and substance abuse. The risk of developing these serious conditions is tied to the type, severity, and duration of exposure to the precipitating event, previous history of psychiatric disorders, age, gender, and socioeconomic status. (Norris et al., 2002; Norris, Friedman, & Watson, 2002)

31.5. SPECIAL POPULATIONS

31.5.1. Effects on Children

While research into the mental health effects of terrorism was at an early stage before September 11th, research into its effects on children was even more scarce (Markenson & Ryenolds, 2006), though early evidence suggested that its role could be significant. Children are known to be uniquely sensitive to their environments. Adverse childhood experiences have been linked to a nearly three-fold increased risk of depressive illness in adulthood (Chapman et al., 2004). Childhood exposure to family dysfunction, such as witnessing maternal violence, has a dose–response relationship to adverse mental health outcomes (Edwards, Holden, Felitti, & Anda, 2003).

In terms of disaster or larger traumatic events beyond the domestic environment, natural disasters have long been recognized to have an effect on children. Fifty-one percent of children exposed to Hurricane Andrew were reported to have a new-onset behavioral disorder; 33% had PTSD, a majority of who remained impaired half a year after the event (Norris, Friedman, et al., 2002). Other traumatic events also have been shown to have negative impacts; following a 1987 school shooting, 60.4% of exposed children experienced PTSD symptoms(Pynoos, Nader, Frederick, Gonda, & Stuber, 1987). After the terrorist bombing of the Murrah Building in Oklahoma City, nearly half of exposed children had PTSD reactions (Pfefferbaum, Moore, et al., 1999). Indirect exposures, such as viewing media images (Pfefferbaum, Nixon, et al., 1999), knowing someone who was affected (Pfefferbaum, Gurwitch, et al., 2000), or hearing about traumatic events such as school shootings (Brener, Simon, Anderson, Barrios, & Small, 2002), have been demonstrated to influence children's post-traumatic reactions.

Parental response and developmental competency have been cited as key mediators of behavioral vulnerabilities (Hagan, 2005) In a study of 7,000 children 7 weeks after the bombing in Oklahoma City, interpersonal and television exposure accounted for 12% of the variance associated with the diagnosis of PTSD. The authors concluded that a child's subjective response to trauma is a key predictor of PTSD and should be included in the diagnostic criteria for PTSD in children (Pfefferbaum, Doughty, et al., 2002). Another study of 69 sixth-graders geographically distant from Oklahoma City concluded that "children geographically distant from disaster who have not directly experienced an interpersonal loss report PTSD symptoms and functional impairment associated with increased media exposure and indirect loss" (Pfefferbaum, Seale, et al., 2000).

In the aftermath of the September 11th attacks, the impact on the children of New York City became a pressing issue. The effect of the terrorist attacks on students in schools close to the WTC site was an especial concern as these children were evacuated under hazardous conditions and were caught up in the general transportation shutdown of the day. To help define and address the potential mental health effects of the event on the city's children, a large multidisciplinary, multiinstitutional group of practitioners and scientists conducted a city-wide assessment of the mental health consequences of the attacks on New York City's public school population (Hoven, Duarte, & Mandell, 2003; Hoven et al., 2005; Hoven, Mandell, & Duarte, 2003). Six months after the attacks, investigators used an 8,236 member probability sample of New York City school children in grades 4 to 12 to determine how many children in New York City had a "probable psychiatric reaction" to the terrorist attacks. Exposures were determined to be either direct (e.g., witnessing the attacks) or indirect (e.g., having a family member who was a first responder to the attacks).

Many of the findings were consistent with those from Oklahoma City bombing. Rates of PTSD, depression, anxiety, agoraphobia, conduct disorder, and alcohol use were all elevated compared to previous community assessments (Hoven et al., 2005). The investigators expected that on average 3% to 5% of children could be expected to suffer from mental health complaints, but the study found levels of symptomatology at approximately 15%. The researchers found that all eight of the disorders screened were at higher levels than expected in the normal population and noted that younger children appeared to be more vulnerable overall (Hoven, 2003). Among the most common mental health disorders in New York City children following the terrorist attacks were agoraphobia (14.8%) and separation anxiety (12.3%) (Hoven, Duarte, et al., 2005). PTSD diagnosis increased 46% in children in New York City in the months following September 11th, compared with the previous months (Hoven, Duarte, et al. 2003); the comparable increase for adults was 12% (Hoge, Pavlin, & Milliken, 2002).

In terms of exposure groups, the studies indicated that children nowhere near Ground Zero that day had the same rates of disorder as those that witnessed the attacks first hand. Exposure also came in the form of interpersonal relationships; New York City school children who had an emergency medical technician as a member of their family had a PTSD prevalence of 18.9% 6 months following the attacks (Duarte et al., 2006).

31.5.2. Low Socioeconomic Status and Minority Populations

Before the attacks, thousands of New Yorkers were already struggling with unmet psychological issues. For the many New York City communities already burdened with community violence, domestic abuse, poverty, and homelessness, the events of September 11 resulted in life-changing stress and trauma. New Yorkers of lower socioeconomic status were two and half times more likely to develop PTSD (Galea, Resnick et al., 2002), and reports of increased alcohol and tobacco use were particularly widespread among drug users (Factor et al., 2002).

As noted earlier, the impact of the terrorist attacks reached far beyond those in close physical proximity of the WTC. As such, researchers set out to increase their understanding of the traumatic impact of September 11th on inner-city high school students living twenty miles north of Ground Zero, focusing on the presence and prevalence of PTSD 8 months postdisaster (Calderoni, Alderman, Silver, & Bauman, 2006). The sample consisted of 1,214 ethnically diverse students (56% Hispanic, 36% African-American, 6% Asian American, 2% Caucasian) studied at a Bronx community high school. In 2001, Bronx County had the highest incidence per 100,000 of murder, rape, and felonious assault in New York City in 2001; 30% of the students lived below the poverty level, more than twice the U.S. average.

In contrast with other studies demonstrating that the majority of adolescents exposed to the trauma of that day did not display symptoms that would lead to a diagnosis of PTSD, results of this study indicated that 7.4% of the surveyed students had PTSD symptom cluster 8 months after the attacks. Only one "personal exposure" variable – financial difficulties – was significantly associated with PTSD (at a rate five times more than those without financial difficulties). By contrast, knowing someone who died or was injured in the attacks was not strongly associated with PTSD. Students reporting current loss of psychosocial resources because of terrorist events were significantly more likely to have PTSD. Those reporting feeling less safe were 3.6 times more likely to have PTSD, and those who reported feeling less protected by the government were 4.04 more likely to display symptoms of PTSD. Students who reported using medication for emotional/behavioral problems were nearly four times more likely to have PTSD cluster, but seeing a mental health provider previously did not seem to have a connection with PTSD.

In contrast with this sample, a study of physical and psychological stress-related responses in African-American adolescents in Georgia 3 months after the attacks found the majority of the students not overly stressed (Barnes, Treiber, & Ludwig, 2005). Those adolescents who did report greater negative impact described higher levels of current anger and exhibited elevated expressions of anger. There were no significant gender differences in these anger reactions, and the small variance between males and females in regard to stressful feelings and emotions was attributed to the male tendency to underreport stress.

31.5.3. Rescuers and First Responders

Three hundred and forty three New York City firefighters and paramedics and 60 police officers lost their lives on September 11th. Despite heightened concern, attempts to understand the experience of their surviving colleagues remain preliminary at best. Significant gaps remain in the literature on the medical, social, and psychological impact of the events of September 11, 2001, and its aftermath on various categories of service personnel who were present and/or summoned to assist in the immediate rescue and recovery process.

In one study, researchers administered the Impact of Events scale to a convenience sample of 261 firefighters from the Pacific Northwest attending a series of conferences (Beaton, Murphy, Johnson, & Nemuth, 2004). Data analysis indicated temporal cohort group differences on measures of secondary traumatic stress symptoms; the group completing the instrument in the weeks following the terrorist attacks demonstrated acute stress reactions. Other studies have documented increased PTSD symptomology among cleanup and construction workers who had traumatic onsite experiences and respiratory problems (Gross et al., 2006).

A questionnaire administered to a random cross-sectional sample of 269 New York City transit employees who were working the morning of September 11th sought to identify the physical and mental health symptoms $7^{1}/_{2}$ months after the attacks (Tapp et al., 2005). Twenty-four percent reported having been in the dust cloud, and 88% reported having participated in Ground Zero activities; 21% witnessed the collapse of one of both towers; 17% witnessed one or both planes crashing into the towers; 10% witnessed people jumping from the towers, and 9% saw body parts among the debris. There was a strong relationship between having witnessed the attack in some way and depressive symptomatology (OR = 2.31, 95% CI = 1.04–5.15). Participants who reported having been impacted by a traumatic event before September 11th proved to be at increased risk for depressive symptoms.

31.6. HEALTH SERVICES UTILIZATION

In the aftermath of September 11th, New York City's already taxed social and mental health services were called upon to service an entire city in crisis. A community needs assessment in Lower Manhattan conducted by the New York City Department of Health and Mental Hygiene in October 2001 found that almost 40% of the residents interviewed reported symptoms suggestive of PTSD, but less than a third of those interviewed had received any supportive counseling (NYCDOH, 2002).

The city mobilized in a number of ways. Project Liberty was established as New York State's federally funded disaster mental health crisis-counseling program (Felton, 2002). As part of this effort, LifeNet, the city's existing 24-hour behavioral health hotline was expanded and mobilized to respond to the crisis (Wunsch-Hitzig, Plapinger, Draper, & del Campo, 2002). Before the terrorist attacks, LifeNet averaged 3,173 monthly calls; during 2002, the program averaged 7,086 calls. Mental health benefits were administered to 3,889 evacuees, 2,604 displaced residents, and 2,781 family members of the deceased (Draper, McCleery, & Schaedle, 2006). Funding through *The New York Times* 9/11 Neediest Fund established the New York Consortium for Effective Trauma Treatment at the areas four largest hospitals. Together they provided training to a cadre of 60 clinicians who then provided treatment and counseling at schools near Ground Zero, at firehouses, and to bereavement groups (*The New York Times*, 2002). Other nonprofit organizations also rose to the challenge, such as the Resiliency Program for underserved children and families (National Center for Disaster Preparedness, 2006).

Beyond these extraordinary efforts, studies of general mental health service utilization following the attack were conflicting. Surveys of self-reported health service utilization documented increased need for psychiatric and emergency care following the events (Boscarino et al., 2004; Fagan, Galea, Ahern, Bonner, & Vlahov, 2003). Data from Veteran's Healthcare Administration facilities in New York and New Jersey showed greater than expected mental health service utilization (Weissman, Kushner, Marcus, & Davis, 2003), and several other papers documented the high rate of utilization of mental health services through Project Liberty. (Felton, 2002; Moynihan, Levine, & Rodriguez, 2005; Rudenstine, Galea, Ahern, Felton, & Vlahov, 2003; Siegel, Wanderling, & Laska 2004).

In contrast, other researchers demonstrated that there was no significant increase in the utilization of mental health services for the treatment of PTSD among military veterans in the New York City area and that a national sample of those admitted to a specialized intensive PTSD treatment program for military veterans during that period did not have significantly worse symptomatology than in previous years (Rosenheck & Fontana, 2003). Another study found that most people in the metropolitan area did not, in fact, seek mental health care in the aftermath of September 11th (Stein et al., 2004).

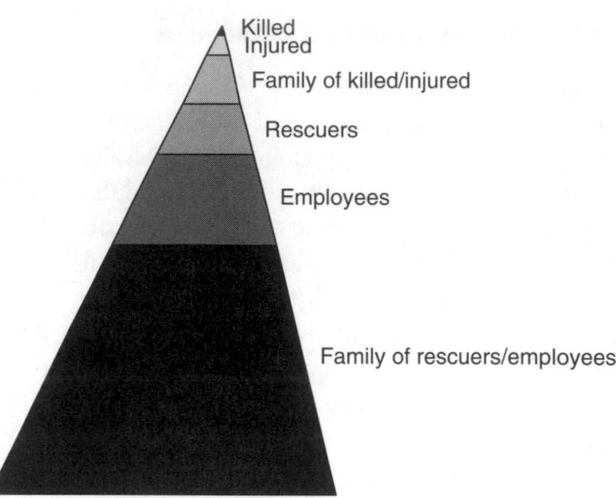

Figure 31.1. Relative proportion of people affected by trauma of September 11, 2001, New York City World Trade Center terrorist attacks (DiMaggio and Galea, 2006).

In response to this conflicting evidence, there arose an increasing appreciation for the role that the primary care setting plays in providing mental and behavioral health services (Fifer et al.,1994; Samson, Bensen, Beck, Price, & Nimmer, 1999). A study of the psychological sequelae of the terrorist attacks among a group of urban primary care patients was perhaps the first of its kind. (Neria, Gross, et al., 2006) Over a quarter (27.1%) of patients enrolled in the study said they knew someone killed in the attack. Approximately 1 year after the attacks, 4.7% of the sample had current PTSD related to the attacks; the majority of these patients had comorbid major depression. A family history of psychiatric disorder and pre–September 11th trauma exposure were associated with current attack-related PTSD.

Research on medications and prescriptions was similarly conflicting. One report indicated an approximately 5% statistically significant increase in national psychotropic drug use in the weeks following September 11th (Kettl & Bixler, 2002), while another study reported only small, nonsignificant increases in antidepressant use among employed members of a private insurance plan impacted by the events (McCarter & Goldman, 2002). A time series analysis compared New York State Medicaid prescription fills for selective serotonin reuptake inhibitors (used to treat depression, anxiety disorders, and PTSD) for the 8-month period before the attack to the 4-month period following the attack (DiMaggio, Galea, & Madrid, 2006) (Figure 31.1). For individuals living within three miles of the WTC site, there was a statistically significant 18.2% increase in prescription rates for selective serotonin reuptake inhibitors (Figure 31.2). The model fit to these data indicated a sudden temporary increase in such prescriptions starting in November 2001 (Figure 31.3).

31.7. OTHER POST-SEPTEMBER 11TH EFFECTS

Other postattack behavioral disturbances were assessed to varying degrees. There were a reported 99 hate crimes against middle easterners in the United States in the month following the September 11th terrorist attacks compared to 93 such crimes in all of 2001 and 12 in 2000 (Swahn et al., 2003). Some of this increase may be attributed to increased surveillance. There were conflicting reports on the

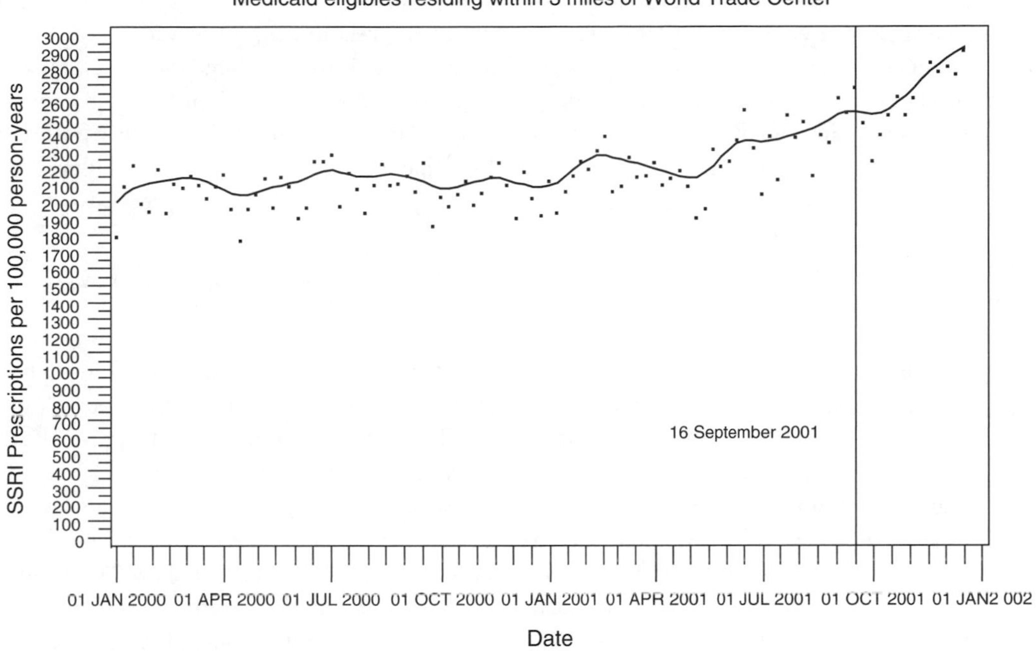

Figure 31.2. Time series plot, weekly selective serotonin reuptake inhibitor diagnoses, New York State Medicaid recipients residing within three miles of World Trade Center site.

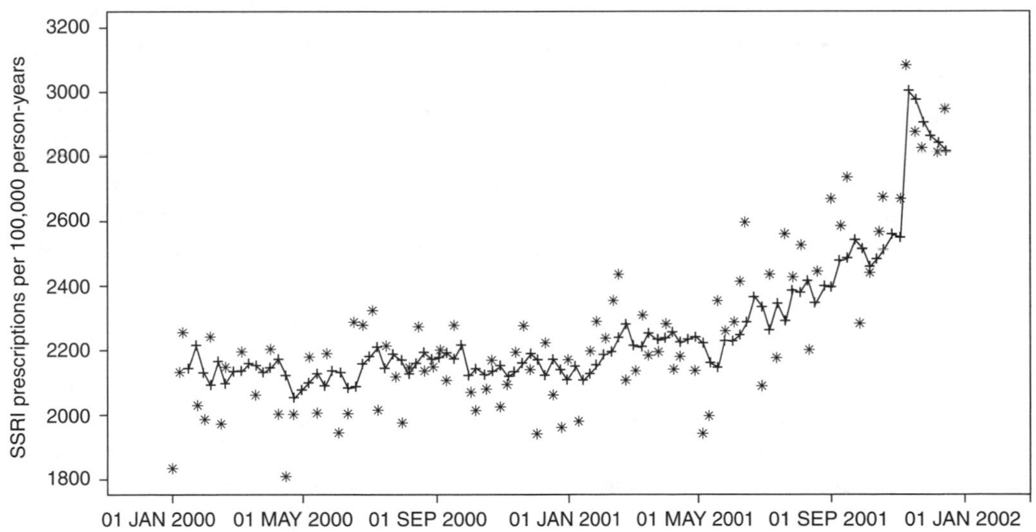

Figure 31.3. Interrupted times series model, serotonin reuptake inhibitor (SSRI) prescription rate, New York State Medicaid recipients residing with 3 miles of WTC site.

effect of September 11th on suicide rates with some investigators documenting an increase and others documenting nil effect (De Lange & Neeleman 2004; Salib, 2003).

31.7.1. Substance and Alcohol Use

In contrast to the ample evidence on psychopathology such as PTSD, the existing preattack literature on substance and alcohol use disorder following mass trauma such as terrorist attacks was less clear (Factor et al., 2002; Vlahov, Galea, Ahern, Resnick, & Kilpatrick, 2004). There were, however, early indications of an increase in drug seeking behavior among Manhattan residents following the attacks. Studies suggested greater use of cigarettes, alcohol, and marijuana (Vlahov et al., 2002; Vlahov et al., 2004) in the general population, and there were reports of increased alcohol and tobacco use among drug users (Factor et al., 2002). Some researchers concluded that evidence of persistently elevated prevalence of psychological distress many months after and at long distances from the events of September 11th (Silver et al., 2002) may have "contributed to symptom severity and the utilization of urgent health care services…in the NYC metropolitan area,"(Fagan et al., 2003) as well as to nonadherence to medication regimens (Halkitis, Kutnick, Rosof, Slater, & Parsons, 2003).

More recently, there have been reports of increased cigarette use in the months following September 11th (Nandi, Galea, Ahern, & Vlahov, 2005), a finding that was echoed in a study of a cohort of military personnel (Moore, Cunradi, & Ames, 2004). A recent survey of substance abuse treatment program administrators indicates continuing concerns about the need to update disaster planning to include responses to behavioral health and substance/alcohol abuse (Frank, Dewart, Schmeidler, & Demirjian, 2006).

Where a person lived in New York City appears to have contributed a measurable effect on their chances of exhibiting substance or alcohol related symptoms. In an analysis of New York State Medicaid recipients, controlling for gender, race, age, income, and employment-related exposure to the attack, the distance of an individual's residence from the WTC site was a statistically significant indicator of substance-use related diagnoses in both the 2000 and 2001 post–September 11th time periods. Each two-mile increment in distance away from the WTC was associated with 18% more substance or alcohol use-related diagnoses in the population studied. This inverse relation between distance from the WTC and substance or alcohol-use-related disorder was the opposite of the relationship observed 1 year before the attacks. Zip-code tabulation areas in the outer boroughs of New York City had elevated drug-related standardized mortality ratios in 2001 that were not present in 2000 (Figure 31.4) (DiMaggio, Galea, Vlahov, in press).

31.7.2. Cardiac and Respiratory Effects

Among the more important nonbehavioral health aspects considered in the wake of the September 11th in New York City were potential population-based postattack respiratory and cardiac effects. Much of the literature on respiratory disease following the collapse of the WTC towers has focused primarily on first responders and volunteers (Ault, 2004; Banauch et al., 2005; Banauch, Dhala, & Prezant, 2005; Herbstman et al., 2005). Press reports have highlighted the issue of respiratory-related disease and death among rescue workers and volunteers at the WTC site, with concern focusing on an apparent cluster of sarcoidosis in firefighters (DePalma, 2006). Indeed, New York firefighters' exposure to the WTC site has been shown to be associated with decreased pulmonary function as measured by decline in forced expiratory volume in one second (FEV1), equal to 12 years of aging (Banauch et al., 2006).

While no large-scale, comprehensive, population-based analysis of the effects of the terrorist attacks of September 11th on the respiratory and cardiac health of New Yorkers has been conducted, studies of respiratory symptoms in individuals residing close to the disaster site have raised concerns. One survey-based, self-report study reported a greater than two-fold increase in new-onset respiratory symptoms among residents of the area near the WTC (Lin et al., 2005); this increase may be related to increased bronchial hyper-responsiveness as measured by spirometry (Reibman et al., 2005). A survey of Medicaid enrollees reported a doubling of respiratory-related emergency department visits in individuals who lived near the WTC site (Wagner, Radigan, Roohan, Anarella, & Gesten, 2005).

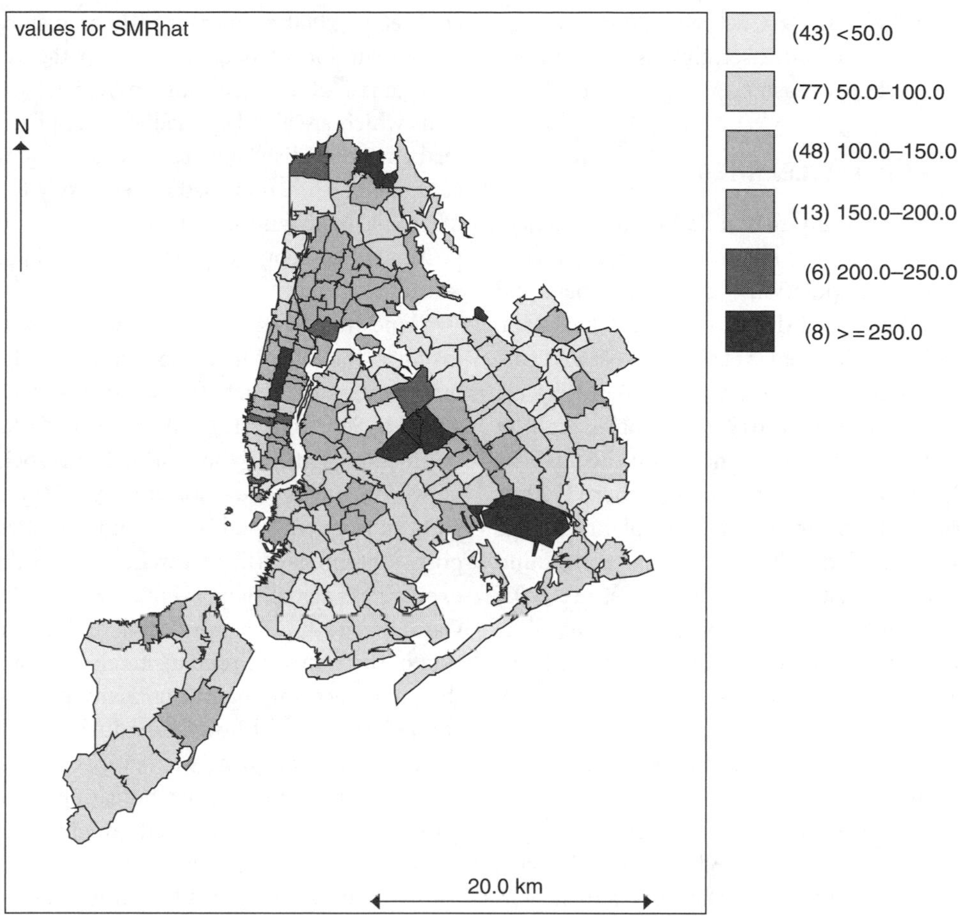

Figure 31.4. Post-September 11th New York City zip-code level substance-use SMRs.

While the physical health effects of the September 11th attacks have been considered separate from the behavioral, acute stress has been linked physiologically to cardiac ischemia and arrhythmias in susceptible individuals, as well as to increases in arterial blood pressure and coagulation abnormalities. This has been attributed to increased hematocrit, fibrinogen, and other coagulation factors, with the elderly perhaps most at risk (Qureshi, Merla, Steinberg, & Rozanski, 2003). In animal models, acute stress decreases the arrhythmia threshold by up to 40%. This effect has been shown to be interrupted by the administration of beta blockers (Qureshi, 2003).

Israeli researchers have reported a rise in acute myocardial infarctions during the first days of missile attacks during the 1991 Gulf War (Meisel et al., 1991). Further, although the same researchers could not document a statistically significant increase in sudden cardiac death among the Israeli civilian population during the same period (Weisenberg, Meisel, & David, 1996), U.S. researchers demonstrated an almost five-fold increase in sudden cardiac death among Los Angeles on the day of a 1994 California earthquake (Leor, Poole, & Kloner, 1996). The average daily rate of sudden cardiac death declined to baseline over the following week. There was a similar three-fold increase in myocardial infarctions in Japan following the Honshin Awerjuu earthquake (Qureshi et al., 2003).

Reports from New York City have documented increased emergency department diagnoses of myocardial infarction among nearby residents of New Jersey in the 3-month period following September 11 (Allegra, Mostashari,

Rothman, Milano, & Cochrane, 2005), though few studies have addressed this issue on a population level postdisaster.

31.8. LESSONS LEARNED

The behavioral and mental health consequences of mass trauma have long been a subject of concern among population health researchers and epidemiologists (DiMaggio & Galea, 2006; Galea, Ahern, et al., 2002; Galea et al., 2005; Norris et al., 2002; Norris, Friedman, Watson, Byme, et al., 2002; Pfefferbaum, 2001; Pfefferbaum, Call, et al., 2001). The lessons learned from the terrorist attacks on New York City on September 11, 2001, contribute to the growing body of knowledge that suggests that terrorism also has a profound effect on population health (Chen et al., 2003; DiMaggio et al., 2006; Galea, Ahern, et al., 2002; Galea et al., 2005; Galea, Resnick, et al., 2002; Norris et al., 2002; Norris, Friedman, Watson, Byme, et al., 2002).

Highlighted in these studies were factors that have consistently been shown to be associated with risk of psychological disorder after exposure to traumatic events, such as gender (Norris, Friedman, et al. 2002), particularly female gender for PTSD (North, 2004) and male gender for alcohol abuse (Norris, Friedman, et al., 2002), the unique risk to children and the need for effective interventions for them (Olness, Sinha, Herran, Cheren, & Pairojkul, 2005; Pfefferbaum, Call, & Sconzo, 1999), and the role of socioeconomic status in determining exposure (Norris, Friedman, et al. 2002).

Additionally, some of these risks were further clarified. Minority and lower socioeconomic status were clearly associated with increased risk of postdisaster mental health disorders (Galea, Resnick, et al. 2002), with reports of increased alcohol and tobacco use among drug users following mass trauma (Factor et al., 2002). As in natural disasters, the poor, the disenfranchised, and the vulnerable are more likely to bear the brunt of terrorism-related mental health disorders. They appear to be at greater risk of losing psychosocial resources, such as family, friends, and jobs, (Martin, Rosen, Durand, Knudson, & Stretch, 2000), more at risk of dislocation and disruption of neighborhood patterns, and more at risk of the preexisting psychiatric conditions which are also key mediators of postdisaster behavioral disturbances. (Norris, Friedman, et al. 2002) They may also be less likely to have the social and familial supports crucial to the postdisaster recovery process (Foy, Sipprelle, Rueger, & Carroll, 1984).

Some new insights were also garnered. For instance, the role of media exposure was thrown into particular relief following the terrorist attack of September 11, 2001, in New York City, the media capital of the world. The association between viewing television images of the event and subsequent pathology motivated some post–September 11th researchers to posit such exposure as a qualifying event for PTSD (Ahern, Galea, Resnick, & Vlahov 2004). Still, the direction of the exposure remains unclear because of the cross-sectional nature of many posttrauma studies. Where and how individuals seek mental health care following such events also gained greater appreciation, results indicating that communities facing such incidents might be better served by shoring up the mental health capacity of their primary health clinics and emergency departments, at least for the short term (Dimaggio, Galea, & Richardson, 2006; Neria et al., 2006).

Spatial analyses may play an increasingly important role in understanding patterns and trajectories of outcomes after such incidents (Marshall et al., 2007). There clearly were complex spatial patterns of mental and behavioral health in New York City after September 11th (DiMaggio, Galea, Emch, under review; DiMaggio, Galea, Vlahov, in press), likely reflecting both differential exposure to the WTC collapse throughout New York City and the geographic distributions of other population characteristics (e.g., race/ethnicity) that are known to be associated with psychopathology in the aftermath of disasters. Additionally, changes in social ties postdisaster may have been differentially spatially distributed in New York City (Adams & Boscarino, 2006), and as such, the mitigating effect of positive social ties and norms manifested in the different spatial patterns of disorders that were documented. The observed spatial patterns also may have reflected underlying patterns of mental health, which is true for any effect of the attacks.

Some of the more intriguing mental health lessons from the September 11th terrorist attacks may lie in the limitations to and gaps in our knowledge. Among these are the need to better determine what constitutes exposure to trauma, the requirement for uniform definitions among the multiple sources of health information (Noji, 1993), the difficulty of collecting data in post-terrorist environments, the necessity to frame questions in appropriate geographic contexts that account for varying levels of direct exposure and the imperative to address the clinical needs of socially and economically vulnerable populations across the life span while attempting to conduct valid and reliable research.

In sum, this suggests that ultimately the full explanation of the patterns of physical, mental, and behavioral health after terrorist attacks such as those of September 11, 2001, in New York City require computational models that can take into account the diverse factors that go beyond typical risk factor models and consider space, time, and the interrelation of risk factors at both the individual and societal level that contribute to population behavior.

REFERENCES

Adams, R. E., & Boscarino, J. A. (2006). Predictors of PTSD and delayed PTSD after disaster: The impact of exposure and psychosocial resources. *Journal of Nervous and Mental Disease, 194*(7), 485–493.

Ahern, J., Galea, S., Resnick, H., Kilpatrick, D., Bucuvalas, M., Gold, J., et al. (2002). Television images and psychological symptoms after the September 11 terrorist attacks. *Psychiatry, 65*(4), 289–300.

Ahern, J., S. Galea, Resnick, H., & Vlahov, D. (2004). Television images and probable posttraumatic stress disorder after September 11: the role of background characteristics, event exposures, and perievent panic. *Journal of Nervous and Mental Disorders, 192*(3), 217–226.

Allegra, J. R., Mostashari, F., Rothman J., Milano, P., & Cochrane, D. G. (2005). Cardiac events in New Jersey after the September 11, 2001, terrorist attack. *Journal of Urban Health, 82*(3), 358–363.

Ault, A. (2004). World Trade Center rescuers face lung distress. *Lancet, 363*(9421), 1614.

Banauch, G. I., Dhala, A., Alleyne, D. Alva, R., Santhyadka, G., Krasko, A., et al. (2005). Bronchial hyperreactivity and other inhalation lung injuries in rescue/recovery workers after the World Trade Center collapse. *Critical Care Medicine, 33*(Suppl. 1), S102–S106.

Banauch, G. I., Dhala, A., & Prezant, D. J. (2005). Pulmonary disease in rescue workers at the World Trade Center site. *Current Opinions in Pulmonary Medicine, 11*(2), 160–168.

Banauch, G. I., Hall, C., Weiden, M., Cohen, H. W., Aldrich, T. K., Christodoulou, V., et al. (2006). Pulmonary Function After Exposure to the World Trade Center in the New York City Fire Department. *American Journal of Respiratory and Critical Care Medicine, 174*(3), 312–319

Barnes, V. A., Treiber, F. A., & Ludwig, D. A. (2005). African American adolescents' stress responses after the 9/11/01 terrorist attacks. *Journal of Adolescent Health, 36*(3), 201–207.

Beaton, R. D., Murphy, S. A., Johnson, L. C., & Nemuth, M. (2004). Secondary traumatic stress response in fire fighters in the aftermath of 9/11/2001. *Traumatology, 10*(1), 7–16.

Bonanno, G. A., Papa, A., Lalande, K., Westphal, M., & Coifman, K. (2004). The importance of being flexible: The ability to both enhance and suppress emotional expression predicts long-term adjustment. *Psychological Science, 15*(7), 482–487.

Boscarino, J. A., Figley, C. R., & Adams, R. E. (2003). Fear of terrorism in New York after the September 11 terrorist attacks: Implications for emergency mental health and preparedness. *International Journal of Emergency Mental Health, 5*(4), 199–209.

Boscarino, J. A., Galea, S., Adams, R. E., Ahern, J., Resnick, H., & Vlahov, D. (2004). Mental health service and medication use in New York City after the September 11, 2001, terrorist attack. *Psychiatric Services, 55*(3), 274–283.

Boscarino, J. A., Galea, S., Ahern, J., Resnick, H., & Vlahov, D. (2002). Utilization of mental health services following the September 11th terrorist attacks in Manhattan, New York City. *International Journal of Emergency Mental Health, 4*(3), 143–155.

Brener, N. D., Simon, T. R., Anderson, M., Barrios, L. C., & Small, M. L. (2002). Effect of the incident at Columbine on students' violence- and suicide-related behaviors. *American Journal of Preventive Medicine, 22*(3), 146–150.

Calderoni, M. E., Alderman, E. M., Silver, E. J., & Bauman, L. J. (2006). The mental health impact of

9/11 on inner-city high school students 20 miles north of Ground Zero. *Journal of Adolescent Health, 39*(1), 57–65.

Chapman, D. P., Whitfield, C. L., Felitti, V. J., Dube, S. R., Edwards, V. J., & Anda, R. F. (2004). Adverse childhood experiences and the risk of depressive disorders in adulthood. *Journal of Affective Disorders, 82*(2), 217–225.

Chen, H., Chung, H., Chen, T., Fang, L., & Chen, J.P. (2003). The emotional distress in a community after the terrorist attack on the World Trade Center. *Community Mental Health Journal, 39*(2), 157–165.

CROW, K. (2001). As a neighborhood rebuilds, an ex-gadfly gets some clout. *New York Times* (New York, New York Times).

De Lange, A. W., & Neeleman, J. (2004). The effect of the September 11 terrorist attacks on suicide and deliberate self-harm: A time trend study. *Suicide and Life Threatening Behavior, 34*(4), 439–447.

DePalma, A. (2006). Tracing lung ailments that arose with 9/11 dust. *The New York Times*. New York. 155(53,578), A1, B5.

DiMaggio, C., & Galea, S. (2006). The mental health and behavioral consequences of terrorism. In R. Davis, A. Lurigio & S. Herman, (Eds.), *Victims of crime*. London, Sage.

DiMaggio, C., Galea, S., & Emch, M. (Accepted for publication). Spatial proximity and the risk of psychopathology after a terrorist attack. *Psychiatry Research*. 2008

DiMaggio, C., Galea, S., & Madrid, P. (2006). Changes in Selective Serotonin Reuptake Inhibitor prescription rates following a terrorist attack. *Psychiatric Services. 57*(11), 1656–1657.

DiMaggio, C., Galea, S., & Madrid, P. (2006). SSRI prescription rates after a terrorist attack. *Psychiatric Services, 57*(11), 1656–1657.

DiMaggio, C., Galea, S., & Richardson, L. D. (2006). Emergency department visits for behavioral and mental health care after a terrorist attack. *Annals of Emergency Medicine, 50*(3), 327–334.

DiMaggio C., Galea S., & Vlahov, D. (In press). Bayesian hierarchical spatial modeling of substance abuse patterns following a mass trauma: The role of time and place. *Substance Use and Misuse.*

Dohrenwend, B. P., Neria, Y., Turner, J. B., Turse, N., Marshall, R., Lewis-Fernandez, R., et al. (2004). Positive tertiary appraisals and posttraumatic stress disorder in U.S. male veterans of the war in Vietnam: The roles of positive affirmation, positive reformulation, and defensive denial. *Journal of Consulting and Clinical Psychology, 72*(3), 417–433.

Draper, J., McCleery, G. M., & Schaedle, R. (2006). Mental health services support in response to September 11: The central role of the Mental Health Association of New York City. Y. Neria, R.,R. Marshall, E. Susser, (Eds.), *9/11 Mental health in the wake of terrorist attacks*. Cambridge: Cambridge University Press.

Duarte, C. S., Hoven, C. W., Wu, P., Bin, F., Cotel, S., Mandell, D. J., et al. (2006). Posttraumatic stress in children with first responders in their families. *Journal of Trauma Stress, 19*(2), 301–306.

Edwards, V. J., Holden, G. W., Felitti, V. J., & Anda, R. F. (2003). Relationship between multiple forms of childhood maltreatment and adult mental health in community respondents: Results from the adverse childhood experiences study. *American Journal of Psychiatry, 160*(8), 1453–1460.

Factor, S. H., Wu, Y., Monserrate, J., Edwards, V., Cuevas, Y., Del Vecchio, S., et al. (2002). Drug use frequency among street-recruited heroin and cocaine users in Harlem and the Bronx before and after September 11, 2001. *Journal of Urban Health, 79*(3), 404–408.

Fagan, J., Galea, S., Ahern, J., Bonner, S., & Vlahov, D. (2003). Relationship of self-reported asthma severity and urgent health care utilization to psychological sequelae of the September 11, 2001 terrorist attacks on the World Trade Center among New York City area residents. *Psychosomatic Medicine, 65*(6), 993–996.

Felton, C., Donahue, S. A., Lanzara, C. B., Pease, E. A., & Marshall, R. D. (2006). Project Liberty: Responding to mental health needs after the World Trade Center terrorist attacks. In Y. Neria, R. R. Marshall, & E. Susser, (Eds.), *9/11 Mental health in the wake of terrorist attacks*. Cambridge: Cambridge University Press.

Felton, C. J. (2002). Project Liberty: A public health response to New Yorkers' mental health needs arising from the World Trade Center terrorist attacks. *Journal of Urban Health, 79*(3), 429–433.

Fifer, S. K., Mathias, S. D., Patrick, D. L., Mazonson, P. D., Lubeck, D. P., & Buesching, D. P. (1994). Untreated anxiety among adult primary care patients in a Health Maintenance Organization. *Archives of General Psychiatry, 51*(9), 740–750.

Foy, D. W., Sipprelle, R. C., Rueger, D. B., & Carroll, E. M. (1984). Etiology of posttraumatic stress disorder in Vietnam veterans: Analysis of premilitary, military, and combat exposure influences. *Journal of Consulting and Clinical Psychology, 52*(1) 79–87.

Frank, B., Dewart, T., Schmeidler, J., & Demirjian, A. (2006). The impact of 9/11 on New York City's substance abuse treatment programs: A study of program administrators. *Journal of Addictive Diseases, 25*(1), 5–14.

Galea, S., Ahern J., Resnick, H., Kilpatrick, D., Bucuvalas, M., Gold, J., et al. (2002). Psychological sequelae of the September 11 terrorist attacks in New York City. *New England Journal of Medicine, 346*(13), 982–987.

Galea, S., Nandi, A., & Vlahov, D. (2005). The epidemiology of post-traumatic stress disorder after disasters. *Epidemiologic Reviews, 27*(1), 78–91.

Galea, S., Resnick, H., Ahern, J., Gold, J., Bucuvalas, M., Kilpatrick, D., et al. (2002). Posttraumatic stress disorder in Manhattan, New York City, after the September 11th terrorist attacks. *Journal of Urban Health, 79*(3), 340–353.

Gross, R., Neria, Y., Tao, X. G., Massa, J., Ashwell L., Davis, K., et al. (2006). Posttraumatic stress disorder and other psychological sequelae among world trade center clean up and recovery workers. *Annals of the New York Academy of Science, 1071*, 495–499.

Hagan, J. F., Jr. (2005). Psychosocial implications of disaster or terrorism on children. A guide for the pediatrician. *Pediatrics, 116*(3), 787–795.

Halkitis, P. N., Kutnick, A. H., Rosof, E., Slater, S., & Parsons, J. T. (2003). Adherence to HIV medications in a cohort of men who have sex with men: Impact of September 11th. *Journal of Urban Health, 80*(1), 161–166.

Herbstman, J. B., Frank, R., Schwab, M., Williams, D. L., Samet, J. M., Breysse, P. N., et al. (2005). Respiratory effects of inhalation exposure among workers during the clean-up effort at the World Trade Center disaster site. *Environmental Research, 99*(1), 85–92.

Herman, D., Felton, C., & Suuser, E. (2002). Mental health needs in New York state following the September 11th attacks. *Journal of Urban Health, 79*(3), 322–331.

Hoge, C. W., Pavlin, J. A., & Milliken, C. S. (2002). Psychological sequelae of September 11. *New England Journal of Medicine, 347*(6), 443–445.

Hoven, C., Duarte, C., & Mandell, D. J. (2003). Children's mental health after disasters: The impact of the World Trade Center attack. *Current Psychiatry Reports, 5*(2), 101–107.

Hoven, C. W., Duarte, C. S., Lucas, C. P., Wu, P., Mandell, D. J., Goodwin, R. D., et al. (2005). Psychopathology among New York city public school children 6 months after September 11. *Archives of General Psychiatry, 62*(5), 545–552.

Hoven, C. W., Mandell, D. J., & Duarte, C. S. (2003). Mental health of New York City Public School children after 9/11: An epidemiologic investigation. In S.W. Coates J. L. Rosenthal, & D. S. Schecter (Eds.) et al *September 11: Trauma and human bonds relational perspectives book series*. Hillsdale, NJ: Analytic Press, Inc.

Kettl, P., & Bixler, E. (2002). Changes in psychotropic drug use after September 11, 2001. *Psychiatric Services, 53*(11), 1475–1476.

Leor, J., Poole, W. K., & Kloner, R. A. (1996). Sudden cardiac death triggered by an earthquake. *New England Journal of Medicine, 334*(7), 413–419.

Lin, S., Reibman, J., Bower, J. A., Hwang, S. A., Hoerning, A., Gomez, M. J., et al. (2005). Upper respiratory symptoms and other health effects among residents living near the World Trade Center site after September 11, 2001. *American Journal Epidemiology, 162*(6), 499–507.

Markenson, D., & Reynolds, S. (2006). The pediatrician and disaster preparedness. *Pediatrics, 117*(2), e340–e362.

Marshall, R. D., Bryant, R. A., Amsel, L., Suh, E. J., Cook, J. M., & Neria, Y. (2007). The psychology of ongoing threat: Relative risk appraisal, the September 11 attacks, and terrorism-related fears. *American Psychologist, 62*(4), 304–316.

Marshall, R. D., & Galea, S. (2004). Science for the community: Assessing mental health after 9/11. *Journal of Clinical Psychiatry, 65*(Suppl 1), 37–43.

Martin, L., Rosen, L. N., Durand, D. B., Knudson, K. H., & Stretch, R. H. (2000). Psychological and physical health effects of sexual assaults and non-sexual traumas among male and female United States Army soldiers. *Behavioral Medicine, 26*(1), 23–33.

McCarter, L., & Goldman, W. (2002). Use of psychotropics in two employee groups directly affected by the events of September 11. *Psychiatric Services, 53*(11), 1366–1368.

Meisel, S. R., Kutz, I., Dayan, K. I., Pauzner, H., Chetboun, I., Arbel, Y., et al. (1991). Effect of Iraqi missile war on incidence of acute myocardial infarction and sudden death in Israeli civilians. *Lancet, 338*(8768), 660–661.

Moore, R. S., Cunradi, C. B., & Ames, G. M. (2004). Did substance use change after September llth? An analysis of a military cohort. *Military Medicine, 169*(10), 829–832.

Moynihan, P. J., Levine, J. M., & Rodriguez, O. (2005). The experiences of Project Liberty crisis counselors in the Bronx. *Community Mental Health Journal, 41*(6), 665–673.

Nandi, A., Galea, S., Ahern, J., & Vlahov, D. (2005). Probable cigarette dependence, PTSD, and depression after an urban disaster: Results from a population survey of New York City residents 4 months after September 11, 2001. *Psychiatry, 68*(4), 299–310.

National Center for Disaster Preparedness. (2006). *The reiliency program*. (January, 2008); http://www.ncdp.mailman.columbia.edu/program_resiliency.htm.

Neria, Y., Gross, R., Olfson, M., Gameroff, M.J., Wickramaratne, P., Das, A., Pilowsky, D., et al. (2006). Posttraumatic stress disorder in primary care one year after the 9/11 attacks. *General Hospital Psychiatry*, *28*(3), 213–222.

Neria, Y., Solomon, Z., Ginzburg, K., Dekel, R., Enoch, D., & Ohry, A. (2000). Posttraumatic residues of captivity: A follow-up of Israeli ex-prisoners of war. *Journal of Clinical Psychiatry*, *61*(1), 39–46.

New York Times. (2002). New York Consortium for Effective Trauma Treatment New York Times 9/11 Neediest Fund 12 Month Report. (January, 2008); http://www.nytco.com/company/foundation/neediest/trauma_a.html.

Noji, E.K. (1993). Analysis of medical needs during disasters caused by tropical cyclones: Anticipated injury patterns. *Journal of Tropical Medicine and Hygiene*, *96*(6), 370–376.

Noji, E.K., & Sivertson, K.T. (1987). Injury prevention in natural disasters: A theoretical framework. *Disasters*, *11*(4), 290–296.

Norris, F.H., Friedman, M.J., & Watson, P.A. (2002). 60,000 disaster victims speak: Part II. Summary and implications of the disaster mental health research. *Psychiatry*, *65*(3), 240–260.

Norris, F.H., Friedman, M.J., Watson, P.A., Byme, C.M., Diaz, E., & Kaniasty, K. (2002). 60,000 disaster victims speak: Part I. An empirical review of the empirical literature, 1981–2001. *Psychiatry*, *65*(3), 207–239.

North, C.S. (2004). Psychiatric effects of disasters and terrorism: Empirical basis from study of the Oklahoma City bombing. In Gorman, J.M. (Ed.), *Fear and anxiety: The benefits of translational research*. Washington D.C.; London: American Psychiatric.

North, C. S., Nixon, S. J., Shariat, S., Mallonee, S., Mcmillen, J. C., Spitznagel, E. L. et al. (1999). Psychiatric disorders among survivors of the Oklahoma City bombing, *Jama*, *282*, 755–562.

NYCDOH. (2002). Community needs assessment of lower Manhattan residents following the World Trade Center attacks – Manhattan, New York City, 2001, *MMWR Morb Mortal Wkly Rep*, *51* Spec No, 10–13.

Olness, K., Sinha, M., Herran, M., Cheren, M., & Pairojkul, S. (2005). Training of health care professionals on the special needs of children in the management of disasters: Experience in Asia, Africa, and Latin America. *Ambulatory Pediatrics*, *5*(4), 244–248.

Pfefferbaum, B. (2001). The impact of the Oklahoma City bombing on children in the community. *Military Medicine*, *166* (Suppl. 12), 49–50.

Pfefferbaum, B., Call, J.A., Lensgraf, S.J., Miller, P.D., Flynn, B.W., Doughty, D.E., et al. (2001). Traumatic grief in a convenience sample of victims seeking support services after a terrorist incident. *Annals of Clinical Psychiatry*, *13*(1), 19–24.

Pfefferbaum, B., Call, J.A., & Sconzo, G.M. (1999). Mental health services for children in the first two years after the 1995 Oklahoma City terrorist bombing. *Psychiatric Services*, *50*(7), 956–958.

Pfefferbaum, B., Doughty, D.E., Reddy, C., Patel, N., Gurwitch, R.H., Nixon, S.J., et al. (2002). Exposure and peritraumatic response as predictors of posttraumatic stress in children following the 1995 Oklahoma City bombing. *Journal of Urban Health*, *79*(3), 354–363.

Pfefferbaum, B., Gurwitch, R.H., McDonald, N.B., Leftwich, M.J., Sconzo, G.M., Messenbaugh, A.K., et al. (2000). Posttraumatic stress among young children after the death of a friend or acquaintance in a terrorist bombing. *Psychiatric Services*, *51*(3), 386–388.

Pfefferbaum, B., Moore, V.L., McDonald, N.B., Mayanrd, B.T., Gurwitch, R.H., & Nixon, S.J. (1999). The role of exposure in posttraumatic stress in youths following the 1995 bombing. *Journal of the Oklahoma State Medical Association*, *92*(4), 164–167.

Pfefferbaum, B., Nixon, S.J., Tucker, P.M., Trivis, R.D., Moore, V.L., Gurwitch, R.H., et al. (1999). Posttraumatic stress responses in bereaved children after the Oklahoma City bombing. *Journal of the American Academy of Child and Adolescent Psychiatry*, *38*(11), 1372–1379.

Pfefferbaum, B., Seale, T.W., McDonald, N.B., Brandt, E.N. Jr., Rainwater, S.M., Maynard, B.T., et al. (2000). Posttraumatic stress two years after the Oklahoma City bombing in youths geographically distant from the explosion. *Psychiatry: Interpersonal & Biological Processes*, *63*(4), 358–370.

Pynoos, R.S., Nader, K., Frederick, C., Gonda, L., & Stuber, M. (1987). Grief reactions in school age children following a snipe attack at school. *Israel Journal of Psychiatry and Related Sciences*, *24*(1–2), 53–63.

Qureshi, E.A., Merla, V., Steinberg, J., & Rozanski, A. (2003). Terrorism and the heart: Implications for arrhythmogenesis and coronary artery disease. *Cardiac Electrophysiology Review*, *7*(1), 80–84.

Reibman, J., Lin, S., Hwang, S.A., Gulati, M., Bowers, J.A., Rogers, L., et al. (2005). The World Trade Center residents' respiratory health study: New-onset respiratory symptoms and pulmonary function. *Environmental Health Perspectives*, *113*(4), 406–411.

Rosenheck, R.A., & Fontana, A. (2003). a Post-september 11 admission symptoms and treatment response among veterans with posttraumatic stress disorder. *Psychiatric Services*, *54*(12), 1610–1617.

Rudenstine, S., Galea, S., Ahern, J., Felton, C., & Vlahov, D. (2003). Awareness and perceptions of a communitywide mental health program in New York city after September 11. *Psychiatric Services, 54*(10), 1404–1406.

Salib, E. (2003). Effect of 11 September 2001 on suicide and homicide in England and Wales. *British Journal of Psychiatry, 183*, 207–212.

Samson, A. Y., Bensen, S., Beck, A., Price, D., & Nimmer, C. (1999). Posttraumatic stress disorder in primary care. *Journal of Family Practice, 48*(3), 222–227.

Siegel, C., Wanderling, J., & Laska, E. (2004). Coping with disasters: Estimation of additional capacity of the mental health sector to meet extended service demands. *Journal of Mental Health Policy and Economics, 7*(1), 29–35.

Silver, R. C., Holman, E. A., McIntosh, D. N., Poulin, M., & Gil-Rivas, V. (2002).Nationwide longitudinal study of psychological responses to September 11. *JAMA, 288*(10), 1235–1244.

Silver, R. C., Holman, E. A., McIntosh, D. N., Poulin, M., Gil-Rivas, V, & Pizarro, J. (2006). Coping with a national trauma: A nationwide longitudinal study of responses to the terrorist attacks of September 11. In Y. Neria, R. Gross, R. D. Marshall, & E. Susser, (Eds.), *9/11 Mental health in the wake of terrorist attacks*. Cambridge: Cambridge University Press.

Stein, B. D., Elliott, M. N., Jaycox, L. H., Collins, R. L., Berry, S. H., Klein, D. J., & Schuster, M. A. (2004). A national longitudinal study of the psychological consequences of the September 11, 2001 terrorist attacks: Reactions, impairment, and help-seeking. *Psychiatry, 67*(2), 105–117.

Swahn, M. H., Mahendra, R. R., Paulozzi, L. J., Winston, R. L., Shelley, G. A., Taliano, J., et al. (2003). Violent attacks on Middle Easterners in the United States during the month following the September 11, 2001 terrorist attacks. *Injury Prevention, 9*(2), 187–189.

Tapp, L. C., Baron, S., Bernard, B., Driscoll, R., Mueller, C., & Wallingford, K. (2005). Physical and mental health symptoms among NYC transit workers seven and one-half months after the WTC attacks. *American Journal of Industrial Medicine, 47*(6), 475–483.

Vlahov, D., Galea, S., Ahern, J., Resnick, H., & Kilpatrick, D. (2004). Sustained increased consumption of cigarettes, alcohol, and marijuana among Manhattan residents after september 11, 2001. *American Journal of Public Health, 94*(2), 253–254.

Vlahov, D., Galea, S., & Frankel, D. (2002). New York City, 2001: Reaction and response. *Journal of Urban Health, 79*(1), 2–5.

Vlahov, D., Galea, S., Resnick, H., Ahern, J., Boscarino, J. A., Bucuvalas, M., et al. (2002). Increased use of cigarettes, alcohol, and marijuana among Manhattan, New York, residents after the September 11th terrorist attacks. *American Journal of Epidemiology, 155*(11), 988–996.

Wagner, V. L., Radigan, M. S., Roohan, P. J., Anarella, J. P., & Gesten, F. C. (2005). Asthma in Medicaid managed care enrollees residing in New York City: Results from a post-World Trade Center disaster survey. *Journal of Urban Health, 82*(1), 76–89.

Weisenberg, D., Meisel, S. R., & David, D. (1996). Sudden death among the Israeli civilian population during the Gulf War – incidence and mechanisms. *Israel Journal of Medical Sciences, 32*(2), 95–99.

Weissman, E. M., Kushner, M., Marcus, S. M., & Davis, D. F. (2003). Volume of VA patients with posttraumatic stress disorder in the New York metropolitan area after September 11. *Psychiatric Services, 54*(12), 1641–1643.

Wunsch-Hitzig, R., Plapinger, J., Draper, J., & del Campo, E. (2002). Calls for help after September 11: A community mental health hot line. *Journal of Urban Health, 79*(3), 417–428.

32 The Psychological Consequences of the London Bombings

NEIL GREENBERG, G. JAMES RUBIN, AND SIMON WESSELY

32.1. INTRODUCTION

The terrorist attacks on the Central London transport network on July 7, 2005, killed 52 commuters and caused approximately 700 injuries. The attacks marked the first major attack on the U.K. mainland since the Provisional Irish Republican Army (IRA) had ceased its bombing campaign nearly 10 years previously. The initial attacks happened at 8:50 a.m. on a busy Thursday morning as commuters were rushing about their daily business or finishing their journey to work. At first it was unclear what had happened; initial reports suggested there might have been a power surge before the explosions on London's underground railway system, which is known as the Tube. However, when a London commuter bus exploded in Tavistock Square, just north of the center of the city, at 9:47 a.m., it became clear it was the work of terrorists.

Emergency services responded rapidly across all five incident sites; in most cases resources arrived on scene within minutes of the first calls being received. The London Ambulance Service (LAS) deployed almost 200 vehicles and 400 staff simultaneously across the five sites, completing the handling of casualties within approximately 3 hours, by which time 404 patients had been moved to seven hospitals. The response by the police and fire services was equally effective.

Almost immediately after the attacks, there was considerable interest in how ordinary Londoners, not directly involved in the attacks themselves, had responded to the crisis. Our research group, based in the Department of Psychological Medicine at King's College London, were requested by the Home Office and the Health Protection Agency (the U.K. body with overall responsibility for public health and disaster management) to carry out a study of psychological responses within the general population of London. The King's team was aware of research carried out shortly after the September 11, 2001, attacks in the United States, which had shown that approximately 90% of U.S. adults reported symptoms of stress, and 44% had reported substantial symptoms (Schuster et al., 2001). After September 11th, emotional reactions had been noted across the United States and as far away as Italy (Apolone, Mosconi, La & Vecchia, 2002; Silver, Holman, McIntosh, Poulin, & Gil-Rivas, 2002), and we decided that an epidemiological investigation into the reaction of the London population to the bombings would fulfill both a useful academic and public health agenda.

Following the July 7th attacks, many commentators had suggested that terrorism would not have a major emotional impact on Londoners because of the city's history of dealing with IRA terrorism and the Blitz (Anonymous, 2005). Others, including many officials within the government, also argued that Londoners were not unprepared for these attacks: British politicians and security officials had warned on many occasions that acts of terrorism in London were probable, if not inevitable. The U.K. government had tried to prepare the British population for terrorism by sending a leaflet to every household in the country in August 2004 providing practical advice about what to do in the event of a major incident. For instance, it stated that if a bomb had gone off outside your building, then you should stay inside (away from windows, elevators, and outer doors) in case there is a second bomb in the area.

Whether these experiences and preparations had served to minimize short-term psychological effects of the recent attacks remained to be seen and were part of the focus of the research carried out by the King's-led research team.

32.2. THE LONDON BOMBINGS RESEARCH

32.2.1. The Initial Survey

As the research into the bombings required rapidly implementing a large-scale survey, the research team decided that both face to face and questionnaire survey methods were inappropriate. Instead, a market research company, MORI, conducted a telephone survey using a random-digit dialing method for all London telephone numbers on behalf of the research team. The survey used proportional quota sampling, a standard methodology for opinion polls in the United Kingdom that involves setting quotas for participants based on a range of demographic factors. Proportional quota sampling is a way of ensuring that the sample interviewed is demographically representative of the population of interest. Although not a commonly used method of survey in academic research, proportional quota sampling has been used for many years by market research companies in cases where data need to be collected very quickly and to ensure that accurate data is obtained that will be of commercial or political utility. In this survey, quotas were set with regard to sex, age, working status, residential location, housing tenure, and ethnicity to make our sample representative of the demographic distribution of London as revealed in the most recent Census data. Researchers made considerable efforts to both prepare documents for and liaise with the South London and Maudsley NHS Trust Research Ethics Committee; approval was granted in record time.

People aged 18 or over who spoke English were invited to participate in a survey about "issues facing Londoners." The 20-minute interviews were conducted in the evenings from Monday July 18 to Wednesday July 20, 2005. The timing was fortuitous as data collection was completed only hours before a second failed attack on London's transport network on Thursday July 21.

32.2.1.1. Primary Outcomes

We had two primary outcomes of interest. First, we wanted to assess whether "as a result of the London bombings" participants had experienced "substantial stress." This was defined as responding "quite a bit" or "extremely" to one or more of the five symptoms: feeling upset when reminded of what happened; repeated disturbing memories, thoughts, or dreams about what happened; difficulty concentrating; trouble falling or staying asleep; and feeling irritable or angry (Schuster et al., 2001). Other possible responses were "not at all," "a little bit," and "moderately." The measure was identical to that used in a similar study of the impact of the September 11th attacks on the adult U.S. population (Schuster et al., 2001). Second, we wanted to assess whether, once the transport system had returned to normal, participants intended to travel "more often," "less often," or with "no difference" on the Tube and overland trains or buses travelling into Central London. Those who did not normally travel by these means where excluded for the relevant items. For comparison, we also asked about travel intentions concerning cars and travel elsewhere in the United Kingdom.

32.2.1.2. Secondary Outcomes

We were also interested in whether the bombings had affected Londoner's sense of safety for self and for friends or relatives. To measure this construct we used identical questions to those used in a survey of reactions to terrorism in Israel (Bleich, Gelkopf, & Solomon, 2003). We were also interested in the perceived likelihood of another attack on London in "the near future" and Londoner's current sense of safety in relation to travelling by Tube, train, bus, car, into central London, or elsewhere in the United Kingdom.

Apart from measuring psychological health outcomes, we wished to study how people had coped with the effects of the bombings; other authors had also examined this topic in relation to terrorism (Bleich et al., 2003). We asked participants whether they had talked to someone about their thoughts and feelings regarding the bombing or if they had spoken to either a mental health specialist or a religious leader/advisor since the bombings. Given that many media articles mention "counseling" when covering a traumatic event, we also gathered views on the possible need to speak to a mental health specialist in the future.

Finally, we were also keen to examine a number of other issues frequently mentioned by the media in relation to disaster situations, including gaining an understanding of whether the bombings might have affected parents differently than those who did not have children. We therefore asked those with children whether they had attempted to check on their children's safety or went to the school earlier than usual to see or collect their children.

32.2.1.3. Predictor Measures

One of the goals of much of the psychosocial research on the impact of terrorism is to try and identify those most at risk of psychological reactions to trauma. Such knowledge might help target any public health response for those most at need. In addition to risk factors for distress, we were also interested in factors associated with psychological resilience. Given that experience is often useful in preparing for crisis, we wished to assess whether Londoners' previous exposure to terrorism might have affected outcomes or whether having read the government's 2004 leaflet concerning emergency preparedness had made any difference. Finally, it has been suggested that loss of contact within social networks can cause distress and panic in scenarios ranging from house fires to frontline combat (Mawson, 2005). Londoners rely heavily on their mobile phones to maintain contact with their loved ones, and intense overload on the mobile phone network resulted in widespread loss of service for large periods of July 7th. Thus, we asked participants whether they had attempted to contact their friends or family by mobile phone on the day of the attacks and how easy that had been on a four point scale from "very difficult" to "very easy."

32.2.1.4. Analysis

Because quota sampling rarely achieves a sample that is exactly representative of the target population, we first weighted our data to improve its representativeness. However, because our quota sampling worked well the effects of this weighting were small. We calculated odds ratios to assess the association between each predictor variable and substantial stress or reduced travel intentions. Informed by the considerable literature about possible confounders for psychological distress, we also controlled for age, sex, and social class.

32.3. RESULTS

Quota sampling involves contacting a large number of people (in this case $N = 11{,}072$) and accepting that a number will be over the quota with regards to their demographics ($N = 1{,}059$) and that others will not want to participate. Of the 10,013 eligible respondents, 1,207 agreed to participate and 1,010 completed the interview (10.1%). This response rate is standard for telephone based "cold calling" quota samples, and readers should note that response rates are not as valid an indication of nonparticipation in quota surveys as they are in random probability surveys. There were numerous reasons for nonparticipation among the 197 who began an interview but withdrew before completion; 21 were unhappy discussing the bombings, 8 did not believe the survey was relevant, 64 did not have time to continue, 36 refused to supply a reason, and 68 were dropped for technical or other reasons. Responses to the primary outcomes are given in Tables 32.1 and 32.2. Overall, approximately 31% of the sample reported substantial

Table 32.1. Primary outcomes: stress and travel intentions following the bombings

Variable	Number of Positive Responses (%)	Results for September 11th Study (%)[b]
Feeling upset when something reminds you what happened[a]	256/1,010 (25.3)	30
Repeated disturbing memories, thoughts, or dreams about what happened[a]	77/1,010 (7.6)	16
Having difficulty concentrating[a]	42/1,010 (4.2)	14
Trouble falling or staying asleep[a]	41/1,010 (4.1)	11
Feeling irritable or having angry outbursts[a]	92/1,010 (9.1)	9
Substantial stress on at least one item	311/1,010 (30.8)	44
Intending to travel less by tube	231/781 (29.6)	–
Intending to travel less by overground train	96/744 (12.9)	–
Intending to travel less by bus	114/797 (14.3)	–
Intending to travel less by car	27/838 (3.2)	–
Intending to travel less into Central London	181/920 (19.7)	–
Intending to travel less elsewhere in the U.K.	37/920 (4.0)	–
Intending to travel less for at least one item	318/1,010 (31.5)	–

Notes:

[a] Response of "quite a bit" or "extremely" taken as a positive response.

[b] Response in U.S. population to identical items immediately following September 11th (Schuster et al., 2001).

Source: Table reproduced with kind permission of the *British Medical Journal*.

Table 32.2. Alterations in travel intentions following the July 7th bombings among a representative sample of Londoners

Once the London Transport System Is Back to Normal, Do You Think You Will Travel More Often or Less Often in The Following Ways, or Will the London Bombings Make No Difference to How Often You Travel in the Following Ways	No difference (%)	More often (%)	Less often (%)
By tube	526/781 (67)	15/781 (2)	231/781 (30)
On an overground train	608/744 (82)	32/744 (4)	96/744 (13)
By bus	639/797 (80)	41/797 (5)	114/797 (14)
By car	712/838 (85)	92/838 (11)	27/838 (3)
Going into central London	719/920 (78)	17/920 (11)	181/920 (20)
Going elsewhere in the U.K.	28/920 (3)	28/853 (93)	37/920 (4)
Intending to travel less often by one of tube, train, bus or into central London	–	–	318/1,010 (32)

Notes: Numbers may not sum to the denominator due to a small number (<1%) of "don't know" responses.

Source: Table reproduced with kind permission of the *British Medical Journal*.

stress symptoms, and 32% reported that once the London transport system had returned to normal they intended to travel less by at least one of the methods. Tables 32.3 and 32.4 show data for the secondary outcomes.

When we controlled for age, sex, and social class, we found a number of significant correlates of substantial stress (see Table 32.5 for comparison groups), including being female, being from lower social class, not owning your

Table 32.3. Immediate responses to the July 7th bombings among a representative sample of Londoners

Variable	Number of Positive Responses (%)
Did you, your partner, or another member of your family attempt to contact your children or the school to check their safety[a]	42/174 (24)
Did you, your partner, or another member of your family go to school earlier than usual to collect or to see your children[a]	45/174 (26)
Did you try to check the safety of any immediate family members or friends	771/1,010 (76)

Note:

[a] Only asked of respondents with children in a London school on the day of the bombings.

Source: Table reproduced with kind permission of the *British Medical Journal*.

Table 32.4. Perceived sense of safety, self-efficacy and need to talk to someone about emotions among a representative sample of Londoners following the July 7th bombings

Variable	Number of Positive Responses (%)	Results for Israel Terrorism Study (%)[a]
Do you feel your life is in danger from terrorism	560/1,010 (55)	60.4
Do you feel the lives of your close family members or those dear to you are in danger from terrorism	588/1,010 (58)	67.9
Do you think another attack on London is likely in the near future	870/1,010 (86)	–
Do you feel unsafe when travelling by tube	361/781 (46)	–
Do you feel unsafe when travelling by overground train	174/744 (23)	–
Do you feel unsafe when travelling by bus	200/797 (25)	–
Do you feel unsafe when travelling by car	30/838 (4)	–
Do you feel unsafe when going into Central London	300/710 (33)	–
Do you feel unsafe when going elsewhere in the U,K.	91/966 (9)	–
Before the bombings, did you believe you would know what best to do if you were caught in a terrorist attack	544/1,010 (54)	–
How much have you talked with someone else about your thoughts and feelings about what happened[b]	721/1,010 (71)	–
As a result of the bombings, have you spoken to a psychiatrist, psychologist, counsellor of other mental health specialist	8/1,010 (1)	–
As a result of the bombings, do you think you need to speak to a psychiatrist, psychologist, counsellor of other mental health specialist	12/1,010 (1)	–
As a result of the bombings, have you spoken to a religious advisor or leader	43/1,010 (4)	–

Notes:

[a] Response in Israeli population to identical items during the ongoing intifada (Bleich et al., 2003).

[b] Responses of "a great deal" or "a fair amount" were classified as positive responses.

Source: Table reproduced with kind permission of the *British Medical Journal*.

Table 32.5. Predictors of the presence of substantial distress following the London bombings

Variable	Variable Levels	N (%)	% with Substantial Stress	Unadjusted Odds Ratio (95% CI)	Adjusted Odds Ratio (95% CI)[a]
Sex	Female	529 (52)	37	1.9 (1.4–2.4)	–
	Male	481(48)	24	–	–
Age	18–24	126 (13)	34	1.1 (0.7–1.9)	–
	25–44	476 (47)	30	0.9 (0.6–1.4)	–
	45–64	259 (26)	29	0.9 (0.6–1.4)	–
	65+	149 (15)	32	–	–
Social class[b]	Top	281 (29)	24	0.4 (0.3–0.6)	–
	Middle	483 (50)	30	0.6 (0.4–0.9)	–
	Lower	208 (21)	42	–	–
Working status	Working full-time	463 (46)	25	0.6 (0.5–0.8)	0.8 (0.6–1.1)
	Not full time	547 (54)	36	–	–
Residential location	Inner London	394 (39)	31	1.0 (0.7–1.3)	1.0 (0.7–1.3)
	Outer London	616 (61)	31	–	–
Housing tenure	House owner	562 (56)	26	0.6 (0.5–0.8)	0.6 (0.5–0.8)
	Rents / other	448 (44)	37	–	–
Ethnicity	White	718 (71)	24	0.3 (0.3–0.5)	0.3 (0.2–0.4)
	Other	292 (29)	48	–	–
Religion	Muslim	86 (9)	62	3.5 (2.2–5.5)	4.0 (2.5–6.6)
	None	218 (22)	17	0.4 (0.3–0.7)	0.5 (0.3–0.7)
	Other faith	704 (70)	31	–	–
Income[b]	Under £30,000	508 (57)	36	2.5 (1.9–3.5)	2.3 (1.6–3.4)
	Over £30,000	376 (43)	18	–	–
Parental status	Children under 18	313 (31)	32	1.1 (0.8–1.4)	1.0 (0.7–1.3)
	No children	697 (69)	30	–	–
Location at time[b]	Central London	218 (22)	33	1.2 (0.8–1.6)	1.4 (1.0–2.0)
	Elsewhere	783 (78)	30	–	–
Felt I might be injured or killed	Yes	80 (8)	60	3.7 (2.3–6.0)	3.8 (2.4–6.2)
	No	930 (92)	28	–	–
Felt family/close friend might be hurt/killed	Yes	606 (60)	36	1.9 (1.4–2.5)	1.8 (1.4–2.5)
	No	404 (40)	23	–	–
Saw an injured or killed person	Yes	27 (3)	44	1.8 (0.9–3.9)	1.8 (0.8–3.9)
	No	983 (97)	30	–	–
Family/close friend injured/ killed	Yes	35 (4)	54	2.7 (1.3–5.3)	2.7 (1.3–5.4)
	No	975 (97)	30	–	–
Prior terror experience	Yes	299 (30)	23	0.6 (0.4–0.8)	0.6 (0.5–0.9)
	No	711 (70)	34	–	–
Read government leaflet	Yes	375 (37)	30	0.8 (0.6–1.0)	0.8 (0.6–1.0)
	No	635 (63)	33.1	–	–
Certainty about others[b]	Very or fairly sure	425 (47)	25	0.6 (0.4–0.8)	0.6 (0.5–0.8)
	Very or fairly unsure	482 (53)	36	–	–
	Very or fairly easy	124 (23)	26	–	–

Notes:

[a] Controlling for sex, age, and social class using logistic regression.

[b] Base for analysis is not 1010 due to missing data, "don't know" responses, or previous screening questions.
CI, confidence intervals.

Source: Table reproduced with kind permission of the *British Medical Journal*.

own home, being non-White, being Muslim or from another faith, having a household income of under £30,000, believing that you or a close friend or relative might have been injured or killed, having a close friend or relative who was injured or killed, having no previous experience of terrorism, being unsure about the safety of others, and having had difficulty reaching contacts by mobile phone. In addition, Muslims were significantly more distressed than people of other faiths.

Similarly, we found a number of significant associations with reduced intention to travel by either Tube, train, bus, or into central London, including being female, being younger, being non-White, being religious, having a household income of less than £30,000, believing that you or a close friend or relative might have been injured or killed, having a close friend or relative who was injured or killed, not having read the government advice leaflet, having been unsure about the safety of others, having substantial stress, and feeling unsafe while travelling.

32.4. DISCUSSION

Eleven to thirteen days after the London attacks we found that 31% of respondents reported substantial levels of stress. Although no equivalent measure was taken before the attack, as participants were specifically asked about stress-related symptoms experienced "as a result of the London bombings," it seemed reasonable to ascribe the majority of this stress to the effects of terrorism. Direct exposure to the bombings was limited, with 8% of the sample having thought they might be injured or killed and 3% having seen someone injured or killed. In terms of indirect exposure, 60% had been concerned that a friend or relative might have been injured or killed and 4% reported knowing someone who was injured or killed. Unsurprisingly, levels of distress were highest amongst these participants.

Overall, the prevalence of distress was less than that reported in the general adult U.S. population following September 11th (Schuster et al., 2001). There may be several reasons for this difference, including the considerably greater loss of life and dramatic imagery and live television coverage of September 11th. The longer delay between the London attacks and our survey (11–13 days) compared to that between September 11th and the U.S. survey (3–5 days), may also be important as distress tends to rapidly decrease after a traumatic incident. An additional factor suggested by our results may be previous experience of IRA terrorism in London, with significantly reduced short-term emotional responses being observed amongst Londoners who had previously been exposed to terrorism or a terrorist false alarm. We also found some evidence consistent with the idea that preparation for terrorism can reduce its impact, with respondents who had read the government's advisory leaflet being less likely to have altered their travel intentions than those who had not read it. Thus, shortly after the bombings it appeared that those who had either coped with previous terrorist events or had read about what to do in an incident fared better than those who were inexperienced or unprepared.

Given that the attacks disrupted London's transport network for several weeks after the incidents, we could not measure the psychological effects of the bombings in terms of actual alterations in travel behavior. Instead, we assessed travel intentions. The majority of Londoners reported that the bombings would have no impact on their travel plans; indeed, the newspapers at the time reported that the so called "Blitz Spirit" – that is, the resilience of Londoners to the Luftwaffe's bombing campaign in World War II – still existed. However, a substantial minority (32%) reported that they intended to reduce the amount they used the Tube, trains, or buses or went into central London. Several factors probably mediate the impact of terrorism on such behavior. Londoners use public transport for numerous reasons, and it seems logical that whether someone uses public transport for leisure or is compelled to use it for work is probably an important factor in deciding how they might alter their travel plans in the future. As shown by our results, the perception of safety is also a significant factor: 46% of Londoners reported not feeling safe travelling by Tube, and 33% did not feel safe in central London. Personal safety concerns were also high; 55% believed that their lives were threatened, and 58% believed the same of their close family and friends. These are similar levels of concern to those expressed by the Israeli population in response to the current Intifada (Bleich et al., 2003).

Interestingly, we found that belonging to any religious group was associated with significantly higher levels of stress than belonging to none. The highest rates were found in Muslim respondents, with 62% reporting substantial stress. As has been found with previous terrorist attacks (Schuster et al., 2001), ethnic minorities suffered significantly worse emotional effects than White respondents. This increased prevalence of distress is not readily explainable by any preexisting vulnerability among these groups; there is little evidence that ethnic minorities in the United Kingdom have consistently higher rates of minor mental disorder (Meltzer, Gill, Petticrew, & Hinds, 1995; Weich et al., 2004). Perhaps these results partly reflect a response bias, with Muslim respondents attempting to emphasize to our interviewers the distinction between themselves and the bombers, or perhaps they reflect a genuine fear of reprisals or increased discrimination. Alternately, perhaps religious beliefs are sustaining during periods of day to day stress, but traumatic events, which have the potential to shatter an individual's life beliefs, may be harder to understand and come to terms with for those who believe that some higher, beneficent authority is looking after them.

We also found associations with many well-documented demographic predictors of stress, including female gender (Bleich et al., 2003; North et al., 1999; Schlenger et al., 2002), lower income (Bleich et al., 2003), and younger age (Schlenger et al., 2002). These risk factors are not just associated with postincident distress but also with more routine day to day stressors.

What, if any, were the therapeutic implications of our results? First, a common sense conclusion was that the psychological needs of those intimately caught up in the bombings through direct exposure or bereavement would need to be assessed after a reasonable time had passed. Indeed, such a response was being planned by four mental health trusts that provided services to the main hospitals that had dealt with the injured. However, as our results showed, most people were not ill or even exhibiting symptoms of distress. This likely accounted for the finding that less than 1% of respondents had sought professional help for their negative emotions, and only 12 respondents felt they needed such help. On the other hand, 71% had spoken to friends or relatives about the attacks "a great deal" or "a fair amount." Our results therefore confirmed those of previous studies that suggest that most people turn to peer support networks following traumatic events (Greenberg et al., 2003). Given that psychological debriefing in the immediate aftermath of a major incident is at best ineffective and at worst counterproductive (Rose, Bisson, & Wessely, 2003), we found our results reassuring. Our results thus supported the high level decision made after the bombings not to follow the example of large-scale public mental health interventions such as Project Liberty in New York following the September 11th attacks. Instead, the U.K. response was very much in keeping with the national policy exemplified by what we call the NICE[1] Guidelines, which advocate a policy of "watchful waiting" for the first four weeks after a traumatic incident.

Our findings shed some light on communication behavior after disasters. We found that 76% of respondents attempted to contact others in the immediate period following the bombings, which was similar to that in New York following September 11th (Schuster et al., 2001). Israelis also frequently check on the whereabouts of family and friends after attacks, with 83% of those who do finding it to be a helpful coping strategy (Bleich et al., 2003). The significant association we found between being unsure about the safety of others and the presence of substantial stress demonstrates the importance of reassuring oneself about friends

[1] NICE (National Institute for Clinical Excellence) is a U.K. body that sanctions particular treatments. In 2005 it issued guidance on the management of PTSD, which included some information of what should be done in the aftermath of traumatic incidents.

and relatives. On July 7th, uncertainty about others was fueled by the inability of the mobile phone networks to cope with demand; 78% of our sample reported that using their mobile was fairly or very difficult that day. Again, those who experienced difficulty contacting others on their mobile were also significantly more stressed. We concluded that although there is no doubt that priority should be given to emergency service use of the mobile network in the event of a major incident, ordinary people still need ways to communicate with each other (Wessely, 2005).

Our initial study had its limitations including, in particular, the low response rate. Although the quota sampling and weighting ensured that our sample was demographically representative of London, we could not be sure that bias had not affected our data. For example, individuals who were unaffected by the attacks may have been less interested in participating, as too might have individuals with high levels of distress. These effects could potentially result in under or overestimates of the true prevalence of distress. To mitigate this, interviewers were instructed to introduce the survey as concerning "issues facing Londoners," the bombings themselves not mentioned until part way through the interview. The fact that relatively few of those who withdrew from the study after beginning the interview stated that the survey was irrelevant to them or they were too upset to talk about the attacks provides some reassurance that these biases were limited.

32.5. FOLLOW-UP SAMPLE

Although the results of our initial survey provided considerable reassurance that Londoners had not been overly affected by the bombings, we remained interested in examining possible long-term effects. Given that it is well accepted that symptoms do not correspond well with disorder, although we had found that approximately one-third of Londoners were distressed, we anticipated that this would fade over time and that most would not be left with any disability as a result of the bombings. Therefore, approximately 7 to 8 months after the initial survey we attempted to contact the 815 Londoners who completed the first survey and who had given permission for us to follow-up with them at a later date (Rubin, Brewin, Greenberg, Simpson, & Wessely, 2007).

Attempts to recontact these 815 were made by telephone between February 3 and March 5, 2006; we traced respondents who had moved using directory enquiries and leads from the new occupants. As with the first study, ethical approval for this study was granted by the South London and Maudsley NHS Trust Research Ethics Committee.

32.5.1.1. Outcome Variables

As in the initial survey, we asked about the same five stress symptoms that might have been experienced in the preceding 3 weeks as a result of the London bombings (see previous text). We again defined the presence of "substantial stress" as an answer of "quite a bit" or "extremely" to any of these items.

London had remained at risk of sustaining another terrorist attack since the initial surveys, so we thought it prudent to find out whether participants felt that their own life or the lives of close friends or relatives were in danger because of terrorism. We used a scale from zero ("not at all") to four ("a lot") and coded responses of two, three, or four as indicating a high perceived threat. Participants were also asked how likely it was that London would experience another terrorist attack in the near future ("very likely" or "somewhat likely" versus "not very likely" or "not at all likely"). We also asked again about participants' sense of safety while traveling. Changes in the way respondents viewed the world or themselves were assessed by two new items asking whether they now saw the world differently or whether they felt different as a person since the bombings ("no difference," "a little difference," "a lot of difference"). Participants who responded "a little difference" or "a lot of difference" were asked whether these differences were positive, negative, or both.

In the initial surveys we had asked about travel intentions, but in the follow-up survey we were able to enquire about what behavioral alterations participants had actually made. Our questions related to respondents' travel patterns in the past month compared to their travel during the month before the bombings. We also asked whether adjustments were mainly because of the bombings or for another reason; people might have changed jobs or moved house and we wished to determine whether any change in travel was bombing-related. We also asked whether they now spent more time, less time or the same amount of time shopping in central London; performing private leisure activities such as reading, gardening, or walking alone; and performing social leisure activities such as going to parties, entertaining at home, or visiting others. Finally, a single open-ended question asked participants to report any other changes made to their daily routine because of the bombings.

32.5.1.2. Definition of "Persistent" Effects

Although it is accepted that, in most cases, distress decreases over time (National Institute for Clinical Excellence, 2005), we deemed it important to be able to estimate the possible treatment burden on London's mental health services due to the bombings. We therefore decided to classify those who exhibited substantial stress sense in both surveys as suffering from "persistent" effects. We applied the same definition in relation to a persistent sense of threat to self or lack of safety while traveling: Effects were categorized as short term if they gave positive answers in 2005 only. For travel alterations, effects were categorized as persistent if participants reported intending to reduce any travel behaviors in 2005 and actually reduced any travel behavior in 2006: Effects were categorized as short term if participants intended any reduction in travel in 2005 but did not actually reduce travel in 2006.

32.5.1.3. Analyses

One problem that affects any follow-up study is that of nonresponders. It is always difficult to make assumptions as to whether nonresponse might be due to illness, such as avoidance behavior as a result of posttraumatic stress disorder (PTSD) or lethargy because of clinical depression, or simply because of a lack of interest in the study or a busy lifestyle. Therefore, to try to account for missing data (Kristman, Manno, & Cote, 2005), we applied weights based on the presence of substantial stress in 2005 and the probability of a 2005 stress case or noncase responding to the 2006 survey. However, the use of weights resulted in an increase in substantial stress prevalence of only 1%, and therefore all final prevalence estimates were unweighted.

Changes in prevalence over time were assessed using McNemar's χ^2 test, and where appropriate, we again calculated odds ratios for associations between predictor variables. For the purposes of the analyses, participants who reported change that was both positive and negative were included in the "no change" category.

32.6. RESULTS OF THE FOLLOW-UP

Of the 815 people who gave consent for follow-up, we successfully interviewed 574 (70.4%) by telephone. Of the remainder, 125 could not be located, 40 were unavailable for interview during the month allocated for fieldwork, and 76 declined to be interviewed. Compared to nonrespondents, respondents were significantly older, of higher social class, were more likely to own their own home, more likely to be White, less likely to be Muslim, and less likely to have household incomes under £30,000. They were also significantly less likely to have reported substantial stress in 2005, to have felt that their life was in danger from terrorism in 2005, or to have had a low sense of safety while traveling in 2005. Thus, in general our follow-up sample was overrepresented with individuals who, demographically, were the least likely to exhibit stress.

32.6.1. Prevalence of Outcome Variables and Changes over Time

Just over 10% reported experiencing substantial stress in the past 3 weeks, which was a significantly lower proportion than in our 2005

Table 32.6. Prevalence of stress symptoms seven to eight months following the July 7, 2005, London bombings. Values are number (%) of respondents

As A Result Of the London Bombings, in the Last Three Weeks to What Extent have you Been Bothered by	Not at All	A Little Bit	Moderately	Quite a Bit	Extremely	Substantial Stress[a]	Results 11–13 Days after Bombing (%)[b]
Feeling upset when something reminds you of what happened	375 (65)	102 (18)	43 (7)	34 (6)	20 (3)	54/574 (9)	25
Repeated disturbing memories, thoughts, or dreams about what happened	525 (91)	24 (4)	13 (2)	10 (2)	2 (0)	12/574 (2)	8
Difficulty concentrating	553 (96)	16 (3)	2 (0)	3 (1)	0 (0)	3/574 (1)	4
Trouble falling or staying asleep	552 (96)	14 (2)	3 (1)	4 (1)	1 (0)	5/574 (1)	4
Feeling irritable or having angry outbursts	526 (92)	20 (3)	10 (2)	12 (2)	6 (1)	18/574 (3)	9
Substantial stress on at least one item	–	–	–	–	–	66/574 (11)	31
Substantial stress on at least one item, excluding "feeling upset"	–	–	–	–	–	30/574 (5)	–

Notes:

[a] Response of "quite a bit" or "extremely" taken as substantial stress.

[b] Response in this sample to identical questions asked 11 to 13 days after the bombings (Rubin et al., 2005).

Source: Table reproduced with kind permission of the *British Medical Journal.*

survey (27%) (see Table 32.6). Similarly, significantly fewer people in 2006 (43%) than in 2005 (52%) believed that their own life was in danger from terrorism. This change was not, however, reflected in a reduction in the perceived threat to loved ones or the perceived likelihood of another imminent attack on London. As described later, both of these concerns were frequently mentioned to the interviewers.

People's sense of safety while traveling had significantly improved, with 19% of respondents in 2005 feeling very unsafe while traveling, compared to just 12% in 2006. Similarly, while 30% of respondents originally said they intended

Table 32.7. Altered travel behaviors seven to eight months following the July 7, 2005, London bombings. Values are number (%) of respondents

Comparing the Way You Have Been Traveling in the Past Month to How You Used to Travel in the Month Before the Bombings, Do You Now Travel More Often or Less Often in the Following Ways, or Have You Made no Changes to How Often You Travel in the Following Ways. If More or Less Often: Is This Mainly Because of the London Bombings, or For Another Reason?	Less Often, Mainly Because of the Bombings (%)	More Often, Mainly Because of the Bombings (%)
By tube	89/574 (16)	0/574 (0)
On an overground train	16/574 (3)	7/574 (1)
By bus	21/574 (4)	14/574 (2)
By car	2/574 (0)	22/574 (4)
Going into Central London	60/574 (10)	0/574 (0)
Going elsewhere in the U.K.	3/574 (1)	0/574 (0)
Traveling differently by one or more of tube, train, bus or into Central London	107/574 (19)	19/574 (3)

Source: Table reproduced with kind permission of the *British Medical Journal*.

to travel less often, significantly fewer (19%) reported actually traveling less often in 2006 as a result of the bombings (see Table 32.7). In addition, 100 respondents (17%) reported shopping less often in central London, 17 (3%) reported reductions in private leisure activities, 31 (5%) reported reductions in social leisure activities, and 22 (4%) reported other behavioral changes as a result of the bombings. In total, 162 participants (28%) reported some form of behavior change, which indicated either a reduction in certain activities or increased cautiousness. However, respondents' behavioral changes was not, in general, seen as an important enough issue to seek help; only five participants (1%) reported having sought advice or treatment from a mental health specialist as a result of the bombings.

It is perhaps understandable that the process of coming to terms with living in a city that has suffered a serious and successful terrorist incident might change the way that Londoners view the world. Indeed, we found that 350 respondents (61%) reported that the bombings had altered their view of the world, and 151 (26%) reported feeling different as a person since the bombings.

32.6.2. Predictors of persistent effects

Forty-three participants (7%) were categorized as experiencing persistent substantial stress and 110 (19%) as short-term stress cases. Only two predictor variables significantly differentiated these groups, with participants from poorer households (OR = 3.2, 95% CI = 1.2–8.5) and those who initially feared that a family member or close friend might have been injured or killed (OR = 2.6, 95% CI = 1.0–6.9) being most at risk of persistent stress. The sample also included 198 people with persistent and 102 people with short-term sense of threat to self, and 42 people with persistent and 66 with short-term low sense of safety. However, the data we collected in 2005 were unable to predict these outcomes. This may be because the prediction of future risk perception is complex or because that there are numerous other factors that affected people views. We cannot be sure, for example, that those in the sample had not suffered further traumas or adverse life events since the bombings that would have influenced our results. Seventy-six participants were categorized as having made persistent travel alterations, compared with 97 short-term cases. Only parental status significantly differentiated between these groups, with parents of children under 18 being most likely to report continued alterations (OR = 1.9, 95% CI = 1.0–3.4).

No significant predictors were found for the small number (N = 22) who reported improvements in their perceptions of the world. Significant associations with negative changes to perceptions of the world (N = 191) were being a home owner (OR = 1.5, 95% CI = 1.0–2.3), having previous experience of terrorism (OR = 0.6, 95% CI = 0.4–0.9), having felt that they might be injured or killed (OR = 2.3, 95% CI = 1.0–5.1) and having felt that a close friend or relative might have been injured or killed (OR = 1.5, 95% CI = 1.0–2.1). Significant associations for positive changes to one's view of oneself (N = 44) were working full-time (OR = 2.1, 95% CI = 1.1–4.1), being White (OR = 0.4, 95% CI = 0.2–0.7), and having had previous experience of terrorist incidents (OR = 2.5, 95% CI = 1.3–4.7). Significant predictors of negative changes in one's view of oneself (N = 33) were being Muslim compared to being from any other faith (OR = 3.7, 95% CI = 1.3–9.8), having children under 18 (OR = 2.1, 95% CI = 1.0–4.3), having felt that they might be injured or killed (OR = 5.3, 95% CI = 2.0–14.3), having a friend or relative who was injured or killed (OR = 4.0, 95% CI = 1.1–15.1), and having consulted a mental health specialist for any reason before the bombings (OR = 2.2, 95% CI = 1.0–4.7).

32.6.3. New Cases

For completeness, we note that a minority of respondents to this survey could also be categorized as "new cases" for substantial stress (N = 23 (4%)), threat to self (N = 48 (8%)), low sense of safety (N = 26 (5%)), and changes in travel behavior (N = 32 (6%)). These new cases described effects that were present in 2006 but not 2005.

32.7. DISCUSSION

Approximately 11 to 13 days after the London bombings we found that 31% of Londoners reported one or more symptoms of "substantial stress" relating to the attacks (Rubin, Brewin, Greenberg, Simpson et al., 2005). The results of the follow-up survey show that after 7 to 8 months this figure had fallen to 11%. Although levels of substantial stress had considerably reduced, 11% is still not a trivial figure. Equally, while perceived threat to self had also reduced, the prevalence figures for the various threat variables remained relatively high, with 52% of people believing that the lives of loved ones were in danger, 43% believing their own life was in danger, and 90% believing that another attack on London was very or somewhat likely. Meanwhile, although perceived safety on transport had improved, substantial numbers of people continued to alter their travel behaviors in response to the bombings. In summary, although many of the psychological and behavioral repercussions of the July 7th attacks had diminished by the time of our seven-month follow-up, effects attributed to these attacks by respondents remained clearly observable.

Reductions in stress symptoms over time were expected, with several studies having shown that stress in the community abates in the months following an attack (Galea et al., 2003; Stein et al., 2004). There are relatively few comparable studies for our other main outcomes. Changes in perceived threat have been studied previously in one sample of U.S. adults who were questioned on the probability of their being hurt as a result of terrorism in the coming year (Fischhoff, Gonzalez, Lerner, & Small, 2005). The mean probability given by this sample remained almost constant from November 2001 (2 months after the September 11th attacks) to November 2002. Changes in behavior as a result of terrorism have been studied in more detail, although typically only within the first 2 or 3 months following an incident (Gigerenzer, 2006; Grieger, Fullerton, Ursano, & Reeves, 2003; Huddy, Feldman, Capelos, & Provost, 2002; Lopez-Rousseau, 2005; Stein et al, 2004). However, at least one survey has produced results suggesting that behavioral changes can last for some time, with 20% of U.S. adults reporting in December 2003 that they avoided travel in response to the threat of terrorism, despite the last major incident in the United States having been the Washington, DC, sniper attacks of over a year previously (Widmeyer Research and Polling, 2004). While stress symptoms normally recede following a terrorist attack, these results and those from our own survey suggest that other psychosocial responses may be more persistent. That is to say, although people may well change their views of the world and their behavior as a result of terrorism, it does not necessarily follow that these changes are due to illness or persistent high levels of distress. In many cases the changes may, in fact, represent adaptive coping to an ever-changing level of threat.

32.7.1. Predictors of Change

On an individual level, why do some people experience more persistent effects than others following an attack against their community? Several previous studies have attempted to answer this question for victims of traumatic events who have developed PTSD, though often with limited success (Breslau & Davis, 1992; North, Smith, & Spitznagel, 1992; Schnurr, Lunney, & Sengupta, 2004). Some evidence suggests that variables that relate to the type and severity of the trauma are important in predicting chronicity of PTSD, for example the degree of threat to one's life (Schnurr et al., 2004). In our study, feeling that one's friends or relatives might have been injured or killed was significantly associated with persistent stress, while this variable together with feeling that you yourself might have been injured or killed and having a friend or relative who actually was injured or killed were associated with negative changes to one's view of the world and one's view of oneself. Thus, our results suggest that how an individual views the various threats present at the time of an incident can predict the chronicity of psychological responses.

Other variables identified as predictors of chronicity in PTSD, such as preexisting emotional disorder (Dunmore, Clark, & Ehlers, 2001) and demographics (Breslau & Davis, 1992; Schnurr et al., 2004), also showed some limited associations with outcomes in our research. These variables included having consulted a mental health specialist for any reason before the bombings (associated with negative change in perception of self), having children under 18 (associated with both negative changes in self perception and persistent reductions in travel behaviors), having a low income (associated with persistent substantial stress), and owning a home (associated with negative changes in one's world view). Interestingly, while being Muslim was the most important risk factor for the development of substantial stress in our original survey (Rubin, Brewin, Greenberg, Hughes et al., 2005), religion did not predict the persistence of substantial stress in our follow-up. Being Muslim was a significant risk factor for experiencing negative changes in one's view of oneself; however, possibly due to the perceived negative portrayal of Muslims in the media and wider society following the July 7th attacks.

In our initial survey, having been unable to contact others by mobile phone and having been uncertain about the safety of loved ones on July 7th were both significant predictors of the development of substantial stress (Rubin, Brewin, Greenberg, Hughes et al., 2005). The need for individuals to maintain contact with others during stressful incidents to prevent negative cognitions – in disaster situations it is easy to assume the worst – and reduce distress has been noted before for scenarios ranging from building fires to military engagements (Mawson, 2005). According to our results, however, the relevance of these effects may be limited to the initial development of distress. Once effects had developed for our respondents, whether they were certain about the safety of loved ones on the day of the incident had little bearing on their subsequent chances of medium-term recovery. However, we found it interesting that several of the significant predictors of ongoing bombing-related effects were family related, involving parental status or fear that a family member or close friend might have been injured or killed. Similarly, although levels of perceived threat to self reduced during the period between our two surveys, perceived threat to "close family members or those dear to you" was more persistent. Amongst members of the wider community, therefore, it is possible that the medium-term psychological impact of a terrorist incident is largely mediated by the perceived risk to one's family, rather than to oneself; this may be a form of cognitive bias. This is perhaps understandable as after an event individuals can be surer of their own actions during a future event than their family members'. Our results can also be interpreted altruistically as evidence that people place the safety of their loved ones above their own.

Before July 7th, attempts had been made to prepare the U.K. population for a possible major incident. As part of this effort, in 2004 the Government had sent to every household leaflets containing advice on what to do during an emergency. While we found that reading this leaflet was associated with reduced likelihood of intending to alter travel behaviors immediately following the bombings, we found no evidence that having read the leaflet had any effect on subsequent duration of psychological or behavioral changes. Similarly, although having had experience with previous terrorist incidents or false alarms appeared to have had a protective effect against the development of substantial stress following the attacks, it did not predict persistence of substantial stress in this survey. One reason for this second finding may be that our predictor variable did not capture some important element underlying the relationship between prior experience and reactions to a subsequent event. For example, how an individual coped with a prior traumatic incident may be the crucial element in determining distress following a subsequent event. Previous experience did, however, predict reduced likelihood of perceiving the world more negatively, possibly because any preconceptions of the world as being fair or benign had already been tarnished for respondents with previous experience of terrorism.

The outcomes discussed so far have all been negative, yet there is growing recognition that traumatic events can also have positive effects for some people (Tedeschi & Calhoun, 1996). For example, nearly 80% of participants who reported changes in self-perception in this study reported that these changes were at least partially positive, and 45% of those who said they now saw the world differently saw it at least somewhat more positively than before. Interestingly, significant predictors of negative changes did not also predict positive changes, suggesting that the positive and negative aspects of self- and world-perception are qualitatively different and do not simply represent opposite ends of the same spectrum. Although no significant predictors of positive changes to worldview were identified, predictors of positive changes to self perception included working full time, being from an ethnic minority, and having had previous experience with terrorism. Other research has also shown that as well as positive changes in self perception, views about others can also change, including an increase in respect for family members (Shalev, Tuval, Frenkiel-Fishman, Hadar, & Eth, 2006).

32.7.2. Some Words of Caution

A degree of caution may be required in interpreting the results of the follow-up survey. While the 2005 survey was based on a demographically representative sample of adult Londoners, some bias likely occurred in the 2006 results as a result of differential attrition. Most problematically, as stated previously, respondents to the 2006 survey were significantly less likely than nonrespondents to have experienced substantial stress in 2005, to have felt their life was in danger, and to have felt unsafe while traveling. These biases suggest that our 2006 prevalence figures for these outcomes are, if anything, underestimates.

At the same time, it is reasonable to question whether our measure of substantial stress might have produced an artificially inflated prevalence estimate for this outcome. The scale was primarily chosen to enable comparison with previous studies in this field (Schuster et al., 2001; Vazquez, Perez-Sales, & Matt, 2006), but critics have pointed out that responses to one of its five items account for most of the stress cases it identifies (Vazquez, 2005). Should responses of "quite a bit" or "extremely" to an item that reads "have you been bothered by feeling upset when something reminds you of what happened" be taken as indicating "substantial stress," or could they equally be expressions of sorrow or displeasure at the attacks? Excluding responses to this single item would have reduced our prevalence estimate for substantial stress from 11% to 5%.

It is also possible that so-called demand characteristics may have inflated our estimates of the attack's medium-term impact. Previous studies have demonstrated that the way a survey is presented can influence its results, with participants tending to respond to questions in a way that is consistent with the perceived purpose of the survey (LaGuardia, Smith, Francois, & Bachman, 1983). Whether such priming effects influenced the responses of our own participants is unknown, but in the context of a 15-minute interview asking respondents to recall in detail the emotive events of July 7th, this possibility cannot be overlooked, and participants may have overemphasized the extent to which the attacks had affected them.

The large number of significance tests we performed, together with the small number of participants included in some of them, also present a problem in the interpretation of our results. Not only is it possible that some of the significant associations we found were type one errors, the large confidence intervals for some of the nonsignificant results suggest that these data were sometimes consistent with relatively large effects, which we did not have the power to detect.

Caution might also be warranted with regards to our analyses of positive and negative changes in self and world perception. In particular, how participants who reported both positive and negative changes should be handled in these analyses remains something of an open question. Placing these participants in the reference category, as we have done, might be seen as assuming that positive and negative changes somehow cancel each other out. On the other hand, including them in the same categories as those who reported entirely positive and entirely negative changes would have introduced substantial overlap between these groups, blurring any differences between them in terms of predictor variables. In practice, reanalyzing our data according to the second method of categorization altered few of the results for change in worldview, although it did have more of an impact on the results for feeling different as a person. Further research to characterize the exact nature of the changes reported by members of the community following acts of terrorism might help to clarify this issue in the future.

Finally, it should also be noted that, apart from the change in views about world and self variables, this study only attempted to identify predictors of persistent effects, comparing respondents reporting effects in 2005 and 2006 against those reporting effects in 2005 only. Another group of interesting participants who we did not study in detail were those who did not report problems in 2005 but who had developed them by 2006. Whether these "new" cases were indeed experiencing delayed-onset effects as a direct result of the bombings is unclear. Even before July 7th, some Londoners were reporting heightened perceptions of threat from terrorism and were making behavioral alterations in response (Goodwin, Wilson, & Gaines Jr., 2005; Schmocker, Fonzone, Quddus, & Bell, 2006). Since July 7th, continuing debate about the risk from terrorism in the United Kingdom combined with news from Iraq and Afghanistan and several false alarms and failed attacks have contributed to the elevated sense of disquiet felt by Londoners. It may be that the behavioral changes, perceptions of threat, reduced sense of safety, and stress symptoms described by our new cases were actually the result of these broader concerns but were attributed to the events of July 7th given their particular salience.

32.8. CONCLUSIONS OF THE STUDIES AND IMPLICATIONS FOR PRACTICE AND FUTURE RESEARCH

One of the first points to note is that, in spite of numerous difficulties in putting together questionnaires in haste in the aftermath of disasters, it is possible to carry out a substantial epidemiological survey shortly after a serious incident. That this was both achievable and useful suggests that emergency planning for disaster should ensure that funding and expertise for research be part of all disaster management plans. Personnel who plan disaster response require sufficiently robust data about the psychological consequences of major disasters, including terrorism, to move from doing what seems helpful to making management plans based on evidence. For instance, our data suggests that whilst sending out a "how to deal with emergencies" leaflet might be useful in the short term; it does not appear to help in the longer term. Using this information, it might be possible to design more effective educational methods to get essential information to the general population.

Distress is not the same as illness, and although our data suggest that, 7 to 8 months later, a residual level of disquiet remained among Londoners in relation to the July bombings, it is important to emphasize that residual levels of distress are unlikely to represent a clinical problem requiring treatment. The issue will only be resolved by using formal measures of trauma-related psychopathology as part of a direct clinical interview instead of questionnaires, which invariably overestimate the burden of illness.

To overcome the difficulties that result from the use of questionnaire surveys and the use of unqualified telephone interviewers, as was the case with the research presented in this chapter, a "rapid response research team" consisting of qualified mental health professionals who could formally assess those who might have psychological disorder and assign psychiatric diagnoses where applicable could be useful. However, it is worth considering some of the difficulties with such an approach. First, given the usually unpredictable nature of disaster, having sufficient, professionally trained staff available for "rapid response" might be problematic. Also, one of the ethical considerations for epidemiological research is that the outcome of one's response should not influence the answers to the questions. Put another way, if you know that you are going to be treated or diagnosed, then you may answer the questions differently. It is not clear that even assurances of confidentiality would address these possible biases; as in all epidemiological psychological research, answers are influenced by context – who is doing the asking, why are they asking, and when are they asking? In other studies we conduct at King's, we go some way toward addressing the ethical issues by signposting interviewees to services if they want to voluntarily access them.

Another potential difficulty in improving the quality of the research carried out in the aftermath of disasters is deciding how to decide what should be measured and at what point treatment should be started. For instance, our studies relied on the measurement of "substantial stress," perceived lack of safety, changes to behavior, and altered perceptions, all of which could be seen as normal responses to what is perceived by many to be an ongoing threat. Changing one's view of the world in the face of an ongoing threat of terrorism may indeed be a very adaptive response. Our studies also did not really explore important societal questions, such as when individuals would be prepared to reuse bombed infrastructure or reenter an area that has been deemed "clean" after a biological weapon had been used. We suggest that it is important that future psychological research does not only concern itself with the presence or absence of PTSD; there are other important variables which should be investigated to determine how a society responds to coming under attack.

Turning to the timing of treatment, while some studies have suggested that early treatment of acute stress disorder may be associated with good clinical outcomes, such studies are of clinical populations that have presented to a health care provider. The benefits, if any, of early treatment for "cases" identified by questionnaire or even early assessment by a professional mental health provider are unclear and would need to be subjected to scrutiny, preferably by a randomized controlled trial. The history of professional attempts at early intervention/prevention after trauma suggest that some caution and humility is justified, and that one should beware of succumbing to the "something must be done" mentality, even in the face of political pressure (Rose et al., 2003). Even seemingly "harmless" interventions, such as the provision of psychoeducation after routine trauma, can sometimes give rise to paradoxical and unexpected effects (Turpin, Downs, & Mason, 2005).

Our own results are supportive of the decision not to offer early psychological interventions to ordinary Londoners not directly involved in the four incidents, even if deemed to be experiencing short-term stress reactions. Although we were able to find several significant associations for some outcomes, it was striking how few consistent predictor variables for longer-term ill health could be identified in this general population sample. This finding underscores the impression of many clinicians that the group most in need of intervention are likely to be found among those with the greatest direct personal exposure to injury and death. Thus, another relevant message to be considered by emergency planners is that it is hard to predict who may have long-term problems. Therefore, it might be sensible to adhere to the U.K. National Institute of Clinical Excellence's view of watchful waiting for a month or so followed by a more formal assessment of psychological needs after that time if required. This might be facilitated, for instance, by a Web-based resource or other form of educational package, available to both those exposed to the traumatic event and their friends and family to ensure that they are aware of signs that someone might benefit from a more formal assessment of need.

The July 7th bombing affected Londoners in a similar manner to other communities impacted by terrorism. A substantial minority were distressed in the initial weeks, and many months later only a small proportion continued to show signs of distress. Our data suggests that it is difficult to predict those who might be especially at risk of developing psychological difficulties after terrorist activity; however, established risk factors (such as proximity to the incident) were found to be valid. We recommend that emergency planners should be cognizant of the limited psychological evidence available to them and include research as part of their postdisaster management planning. We also suggest that even more priority should be given toward maintaining communication not just with those affected (always a priority and concern for governments in this age of instant media) but between those affected, since the latter is important for both short- and long-term resilience. It is far more effective, and cost-effective, to mobilize people's existing social networks and resources than to provide alternative ones. Lastly, although there is much that is known about how communities are affected by disaster, there is much more that remains to be investigated. As it is inevitable that disasters and terrorism will continue around the world, it is essential that we ensure opportunities for research are not missed.

REFERENCES

Anonymous. (2005). London under attack. *The Economist, 9.*

Apolone, G., Mosconi, P., & La Vecchia, C. (2002). Post-traumatic stress disorder. *New England Journal of Medicine, 346,* 1495–1498.

Bleich, A., Gelkopf, M., & Solomon, Z. (2003). Exposure to terrorism, stress-related mental health symptoms, and coping behaviors among a nationally representative sample in Israel. *JAMA, 290*(5), 612–620.

Breslau, N., & Davis, G. C. (1992). Posttraumatic stress disorder in an urban population of young adults: Risk factors for chronicity. *American Journal of Psychiatry, 149,* 675.

Dunmore, E., Clark, D. M., & Ehlers, A. (2001). A prospective examination of the role of cognitive factors in persistent posttraumatic stress disorder (PTSD) after physical or sexual assault. *Behavioral Research and Therapy, 39,* 1063–1084.

Fischhoff, B., Gonzalez, R. M., Lerner, J. S., & Small, D. A. (2005). Evolving judgements of terror risks: Foresight, hindsight, and emotion. *Journal of Experimental Psychology: Applied, 11,* 124–139.

Galea, S., Vlahov, D., Resnick, H., Ahern, J., Susser, E., Gold, J., et al. (2003). Trends of probable post-traumatic stress disorder in New York City after September 11 terrorist attacks. *American Journal Epidemiology, 158,* 514–524.

Gigerenzer, G. (2006). Out of the frying pan into the fire: Behavioral reactions to terrorist attacks. *Risk Analysis, 26,* 347–351.

Goodwin, R., Wilson, M., & Gaines Jr., S. (2005). Terror threat perception and its consequences in contemporary Britain. *British Journal of Psychology, 96,* 389–406.

Greenberg, N., Thomas, S. L., Iversen, A., Unwin, C., Hull, L., & Wessely, S. (2003). Do military peacekeepers want to talk about their experiences? Perceived psychological support of UK military peacekeepers on return from deployment. *Journal of Mental Health, 12,* 565–573.

Grieger, T. A., Fullerton, C. S., Ursano, R. J., & Reeves, J. J. (2003). Acute stress disorder, alcohol use, and perception of safety among hospital staff after the sniper attacks. *Psychiatric Services, 54*, 1383–1387.

Huddy, L., Feldman, S., Capelos, T., & Provost, C. (2002). The consequences of terrorism: Disentangling the effects of personal and national threat. *Political Psychology, 23*, 485–509.

Kristman, V. L., Manno, M., & Cote, P. (2005). Methods to account for attrition in longitudinal data: Do they work? A simulation study. *European Journal of Epidemiology, 20*, 657–662.

LaGuardia, R. L., Smith, G., Francois, R., & Bachman, L. (1983). Incidence of delayed stress disorder among Vietnam era veterans: The effect of priming on response set. *American Journal of Orthopsychiatry, 53*(1), 18–26.

Lopez-Rousseau, A. (2005). Avoiding the death risk of avoiding a dread risk: The aftermath of March 11 in Spain. *Psychological Science, 16*, 426–428.

Mawson, A. R. (2005). Understanding mass panic and other collective responses to threat and disaster. *Psychiatry, 68*, 95–113.

Meltzer, H., Gill, B., Petticrew, M., & Hinds, K. (1995). *The prevalence of psychiatric morbidity among adults living in private households*. London: The Stationery Office.

National Institute for Clinical Excellence. (2005). National Collaborating Centre for Mental Health: Post-Traumatic stress disorder: The management of PTSD in adults and children in primary and secondary care. London, National Institute for Clinical Excellence.

North, C. S., Nixon, S. J., Shariat, W., Mallonee, S., McMillen, J. C., Spitznagel, E. L., et al. (1999). Psychiatric disorders among survivors of the Oklahoma City Bombing. *JAMA, 282*, 755–762.

North, C. S., Smith, E. M., & Spitznagel, E. L. (1992). One year follow-up of survivors of a mass shooting. *American Journal of Psychiatry, 154*, 1696–1702.

Rose, S., Bisson, J., & Wessely, S. (2003). A systematic review of single-session psychological interventions ('debriefing') following trauma. *Psychotherapy and Psychosomatics, 72*, 176–184.

Rubin, G. J., Brewin, C. R., Greenberg, N., Hughes, J. H., Simpson, J., & Wessely, S. (2007). Enduring consequences of terrorism: 7-month follow-up survey of reactions to the bombings in London on 7 July 2005. *British Journal of Psychiatry, 190*, 350–6.

Rubin, G. J., Brewin, C. R., Greenberg, N., Simpson, J., & Wessely, S. (2005). Psychological and behavioural reactions to the bombings in London on 7 July 2005: Cross sectional survey of a representative sample of Londoners. *BMJ, 331*(7517), 606.

Schlenger, W. E., Caddell, J. M., Ebert, L., Jordan, B. K., Rourke, K. M., Wilson, D., et al. (2002). Psychological reactions to terrorist attacks. Findings from the national study of Americans' reactions to September 11. *JAMA, 288*, 581–588.

Schmocker, J. D., Fonzone, A., Quddus, M., & Bell, M. G. H. (2006). Changes in the frequency of shopping trips in response to a congestion charge. *Transport Policy, 13*, 217–228.

Schnurr, P. P., Lunney, C. A., & Sengupta, A. (2004). Risk factors for the development versus maintenance of posttraumatic stress disorder. *Journal of Traumatic Stress, 17*, 85–95.

Schuster, M. A., Stein, B. D., Jaycox, L. H., Collins, R. L., Marshall, G. N., Elliott, M. N., et al. (2001). A national survey of stress reactions after the September 11, 2001, terrorist attacks. *New England Journal of Medicine, 345*, 1507–1512.

Shalev, A. Y., Tuval, R., Frenkiel-Fishman, S., Hadar, H., & Eth, S. (2006). Psychological responses to continuous terror: A study of two communities in Israel. *American Journal of Psychiatry, 163*, 667–673.

Silver, R. C., Holman, E. A., McIntosh, D. N., Poulin, M., & Gil-Rivas, V. (2002). Nationwide longitudinal study of psychological responses to September 11. *JAMA, 288*, 1235–1244.

Stein, B. D., Elliott, M. N., Jajcox, L. H., Collins, R. L., Berry, S. H., Klein, D. J., et al. (2004). A national longitudinal study of the psychological consequences of the September 11, 2001 terrorist attacks: Reactions, impairment, and help-seeking. *Psychiatry, 67*, 105–117.

Tedeschi, R. G., & Calhoun, L. G. (1996). The posttraumatic growth inventory: measuring the positive legacy of trauma. *Journal of Traumatic Stress, 9*, 455–471.

Turpin, G., Downs, M., & Mason, S. (2005). Effectiveness of providing self-help information following acute traumatic injury: Randomised controlled trial. *British Journal of Psychiatry, 187*, 76–82.

Vazquez, C., Perez-Sales, P., & Matt, G. (2006). Posttraumatic stress reactions following the March 11, 2004 terrorist attacks in a Madrid community sample: A cautionary note about the measurement of psychological trauma. *The Spanish Journal of Psychology, 9*, 61–74.

Vazquez Valverde, C. (2005). Stress reactions of the general population after the terrorist attacks of S11, 2001 (USA) and M11, 2004 (Madrid, Spain): Myths and realities. *Annuary of Clinical and Health Psychology, 1*, 9–25.

Weich, S., Nazroo, J., Sproston, K., McManus, S., Blanchard, M., Erens, B., et al. (2004). Common mental disorders and ethnicity in England: the EMPIRIC study. *Psychological Medicine*, *34*, 1543–1551.

Wessely, S. (2005). Don't panic!: Short and long term psychological reactions to the new terrorism: the role of information and the authorities. *Journal of Mental Health*, *14*, 1–6.

Widmeyer Research & Polling. (2004). Public Perspectives on the Mental Health Effects of Terrorism: a National Poll. www.nmha.org/newsroom/surveys.cfm

33 Psychological Responses to Terrorism in Israel: 2000–2004

ARIEH Y. SHALEV AND YAEL L. E. ERRERA

33.1. INTRODUCTION

Proper appraisal of the psychological effect of terrorism requires a good understanding of the changing social and geopolitical context within which it occurs. One proposition comes to mind when one tries to describe the context of terrorism in Israel: it seems to have always existed. Deliberate attacks against civilians were recorded throughout the State's 60 years of history – and before. The most prominent among them have left indelible marks. For instance, the 1929 Hebron massacre was remembered for decades, it eventually accelerated the re-creation of a Jewish settlement in Hebron (1968) and may have indirectly inspired a bloody retaliation in 1994 (Cave of Patriarchs Massacre). The legal ramifications of this event (i.e., who owns the houses abandoned in 1929) are still debated in Israeli courts, today.

Moreover, terrorism is not the only threat to Israel's peace and existence. Six military confrontations have shaken the country between 1948 and 2006, each taking its toll of death and destruction, and each leaving widows, orphans, traumatized survivors, and sediments of bitter memories. The recent and daunting prospect of nuclear threat and the reemergence of overt declarations of intent to annihilate the State of Israel enhance these existential worries. Such worries should be taken into account in any attempt to understand Israelis' reactions to terror. The latter range from stoically endorsing the burden as part of the cost of having an independent Jewish state, to periods of profound anguish and uncertainties.

Importantly, Israel is not just war- or terror-prone, nor is it perceived as such by its inhabitants. Israel is a country of rapid development and thriving economy, a stable Western democracy, a hub of literary and artistic creation, a land of informal relationships and close-knit social networks. Israel is also a country of profound social divides, cultural divergences, and power struggles. War and terror are but part of Israelis' total experience. Casualty lists are but a portion of the country's vital statistics.

For example, during the 2000 to 2004 wave of terror, which is the core of this chapter, Israel absorbed 181,500 new immigrants. At the same time the number of Israelis leaving the country rose from a yearly average of 19,500 (2.7 per thousand) to approximately 27,000 in 2002 and 2003 (approximately three per thousand). It returned, however, to its decades long average as the hostilities abated in 2004 (Israel Bureau of Statistics, 2008). The number of Israeli citizens returning to Israel, every year, remained a stable 10,000 throughout the events.

This brief illustration can convey the account of threats and achievements that is the true background of the psychological responses to terror in Israel. We offer the term "stability within instability" to describe both Israel's geopolitical position and the psychological matrix of Israeli's responses to terror. Accordingly, the psychological responses to terrorism in Israel sometimes reflect profound anxieties and other times express boldness and defiance. The two extremes are often mixed.

Within this context, the relative weight of terrorism in Israel's global security burden has been growing steadily-and the toll of straight military confrontations decreasing. Reflecting the growing threat of terror, the magnitude of anti-terror operations by Israel increased, progressively, and their harshness became acceptable as a means of

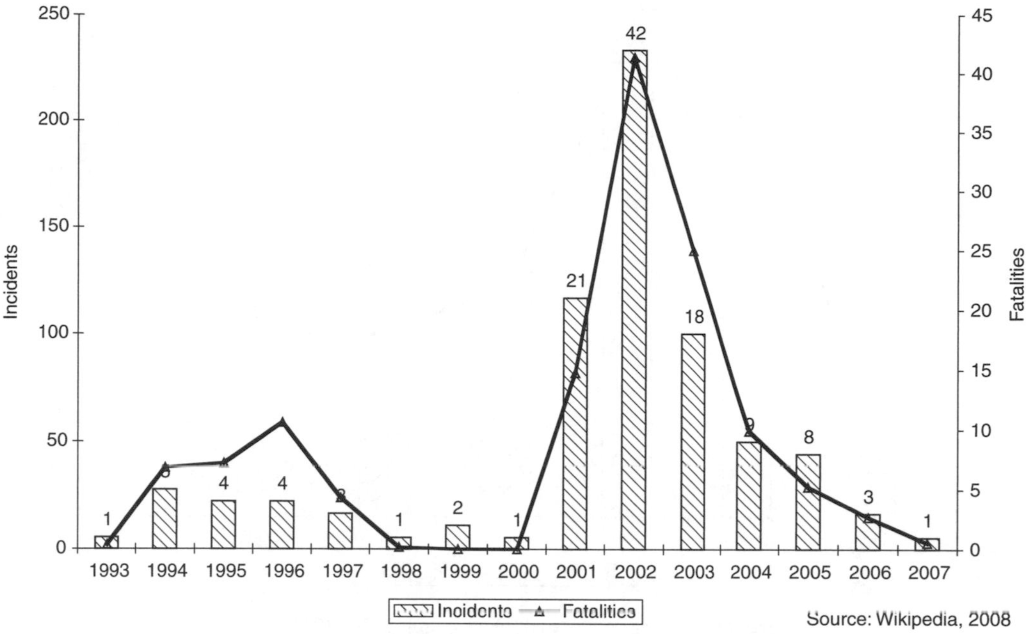

Figure 33.1. Incidence of suicide attacks in Israel, 1993–2007.

protecting lives and security. Terror and the fight against terrorism are, currently, the central expressions of the ongoing Israeli–Arab enmeshment.

Looking at an even larger picture, terrorism, which for decades enjoyed a degree of legitimacy (e.g., as a "weapon of the poor" or means of achieving worthy national goals), has been falling into disgrace since the September 11th terrorist attacks in New York and subsequent attacks Madrid, London or Belsan. In the Middle East, however, the boundary between terror, national struggle, and, recently, religious wrath is blurred.

Despite the constant presence of terrorism, its tactics keep changing. For example, a wave of major hostage taking events started with the deadly attack on the Israeli delegation to the Munich Olympics (1972) and culminated in the hijacking of Air France Airbus to Entebbe in 1976. This wave was, essentially, replaced by suicide bombing attacks that started in 1993, and became the deadliest and most horrifying form of terror between 2000 and 2004. The years 2005 to 2008 have seen an increasing use of rockets and missiles against civilians. Illustrating these changes, Figure 33.1 depicts the yearly occurrence of suicide attacks in Israel – clearly showing a major increase until 2002 and a decrease between 2002 and 2004.

This chapter addresses the events of the years 2000 to 2004, otherwise known as the "Second" or "Al-Aksa" *Intifada* (a term that translates to "uprising" or "shaking off"). This series of events was the deadliest and the longest wave of terror experienced by Israel. Starting in late September 2000, the events quickly escalated into a full-fledged, semi-organized campaign. Terrorist acts spread into the heart of Israel. The casualty toll grew monthly, reaching a peak of 77 in the "Black March" of 2002. Previously assumed boundaries to violence were breached, as exemplified by the January 17, 2002, attack on a Bar Mitzva celebration in the small town of Hadera, the March 17, 2002, suicide bomb attack of the public Passover Seder in Park Hotel, Netania (which left 22 dead and 140 injured), or the July 31, 2002, bombing of a presumed sanctuary of learning and research: the Frank Sinatra cafeteria at Hebrew University in Jerusalem.

The chapter reviews the published literature on terror and reactions to terror in Israel during the second intifada. It presents facts concerning terrorist attacks and their immediate victims. It

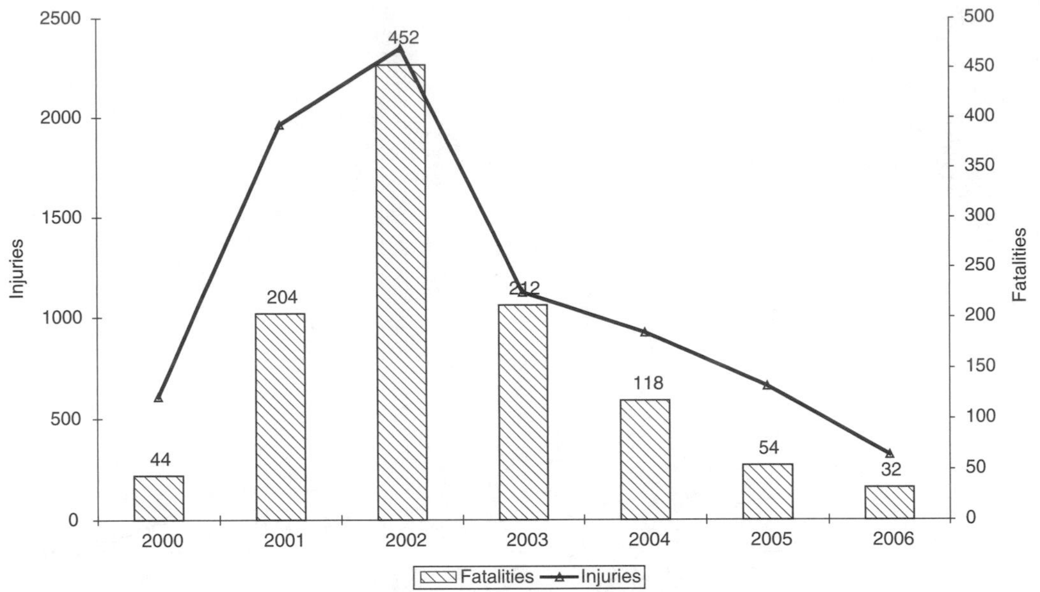

Figure 33.2. All terror casualties in Israel, 2000–2006.

then reviews the range of psychological reactions to terrorism, putative moderators of these reactions, and the effect of terror on different segments of the population. We conclude by considering resiliency, endurance, and growth under threat. Included in this chapter are publications found by PubMed and PsycINFO(R) search, using "terror" and "Israel" as keywords and the years 2000 to 2007 as the date range.

Whilst summarizing the literature, it became clear to us that the published research did not provide a full historical account of the second intifada. It often missed the context of events and people's reactions – as well as important response modulators. We attempted to fill the gap with a narrative pertaining to that which everyone in Israel knew – or took for granted – and no empirical study captured (e.g., timely and accurate media reporting of terrorist attacks, their casualties and sites of evacuation; quick repair of the physical damage caused by explosions, etc.). As we write this chapter, the ethnography of Israelis' experiences during the Intifada is being researched (e.g., Ochs Dweck, forthcoming). Publications emanating from such studies should complement our attempt not to neglect the larger picture.

33.2. AL AKSA INTIFADA: FACTS AND STATISTICS

Israeli chronicles assign the first victim of Al Aksa Intifada – an Israeli Border Police Officer – to a September 29, 2000, event. The troubles quickly escalated, leaving a total of 1,031 fatalities and 5,600 injuries by September 2004 (approximately 0.1% of the Israeli population). Seventy percent of those injured and 82% of those killed were civilians, and 54 were foreign residents – mostly temporary workers. Sixty-nine percent of the casualties were males. The year 2002 constituted the peak of the Intifada (Figure 33.2), with 2,309 Israelis injured and 452 killed, including 77 during the "Black March." Suicide attacks accounted for 60% of all fatalities; an additional 30% were caused by gunshots (e.g., shooting sprays, roadside ambushes, drive-by shooting), 5% to bombs, including car bombs, and approximately 5% followed other incidents such as stabbing, lynching ($N = 17$), or rock throwing. Estimates of the total number of incidents vary (e.g., $N = 13{,}700$ in the Ministry of Foreign Affairs report), but even the very conservative sources mention thousands of incidents, which translate to *an almost daily occurrence*.

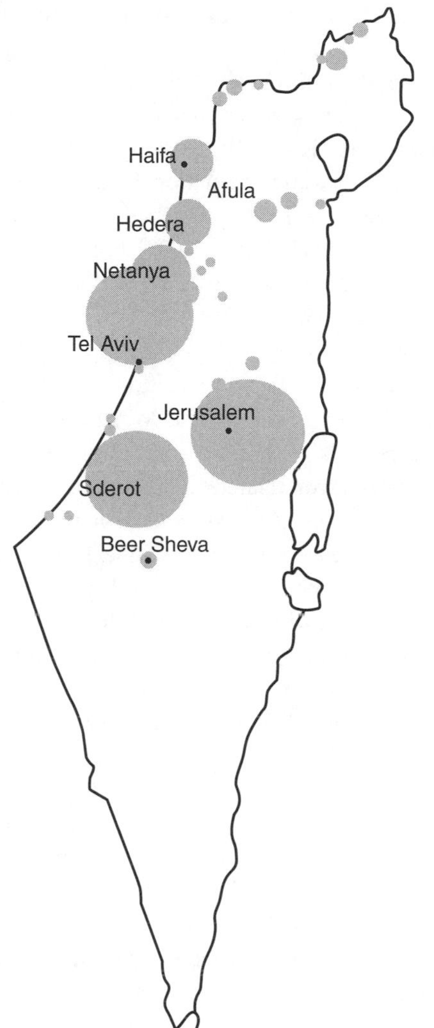

Figure 33.3. Geographical spread of terrorist attacks during Al Aksa Intifada The bullets' size is proportional to the number of attacks.
Source of data: Global Terrorism Database; http://209.232.239.37/gtd2

Another important aspect of the events in this time period was their geographical dispersion. Terrorist attacks occurred in all major cities and many small towns (see Figure 33.3). Suicide bombers reached schools, recreation areas, shopping malls, open markets and celebrations. Shooting incidents regularly blocked the roads leading to Jerusalem suburbs on the West Bank. Violence carried by individuals (e.g., stabbing, shooting) could occur in workplaces, gas stations, or crowded intersections. By their frequency and spread, terrorist acts have created, on the one hand, a feeling of unpredictable and pervasive threat and, on the other hand, a sense of common fate and vital struggle.

Contrasting with the reports of population responses to the September 11th attacks in the United States, there has been no real "secure geographical distance" from the events in Israel. Considering the size of the Israeli population (approximately 6.5 million) and the many interwoven layers of acquaintances, relationships, and group identities (e.g., having served in the same military unit; coming from the same small town, school, or youth movement; having a son in the military – approximately 100,000 families at any given time; belonging to the same wave of immigration; or coming from the same country of origin) there was little *psychological* distance available. Virtually everyone knew someone who was directly impacted by a terrorist attack, and each major attack caused personal concern to very large number of people. The events of 2000 to 2004 were personally meaningful to most Israelis.

Finally, the events caused significant disruption of daily activities (e.g., hours of going to work, ease of transportation, accompanying children to schools, searches in super-markets, delays on highways). In terror prone areas, such as Jerusalem and vicinity, the disruption of daily routines became a serious stressor, often more disturbing than direct exposure to terrorist acts (Shalev et al., 2006). Israelis have experienced terror not just as a sequence of discrete events but also as a continuous disruption of routines, activities, services, and resources.

33.3. TERROR'S DIRECT VICTIMS

As seen previously, the majority of casualties between 2000 and 2004 came from suicide bomb attacks. Suicide bomb attacks are characterized by the simultaneous occurrence of many physical casualties and by the exposure of those uninjured – and bystanders to sights of horror, body parts, agony and devastation. Injured family members could be separated during rescue and evacuation. Bombs containing metal fragments (e.g., screws, bolts) were used in many incidents, increasing their lethality and the total casualty rate. With transportation blocked, media flooded by hasty reports, and key services (police, ambulances, hospitals) shifting to emergency operation, every suicide bomb attack affected an entire city.

Because of the difficulty to distinguish, at the site of explosion, states of emotional shock from physical shock (e.g., from blunt or blast injury), stress casualties were evacuated to general hospitals' emergency rooms (ERs) along with the physically injured. These evacuees often outnumbered those physically injured. For example, noninjured casualties constituted 60% of ER admissions from sites of terrorist bomb attacks to Jerusalem's Hadassah University Hospital. These numbers replicate, in fact, the reported 72% rate of psychological casualties (stress responses plus unnecessary self-injections of atropine) in ERs during the Gulf War missile attacks (Bleich, Dycian, Koslowsky, Solomon, & Wiener, 1992). Exposed to horror, numerous rescuers and lay first-responders developed severe stress reactions and trickled into receiving ERs only slightly after the direct victims.

33.3.1. Evacuation and hospital care

From the perspective of caregivers in hospitals, recurring bomb attacks resulted in repeated experiences of utmost emergency. Though seldom happening in reality, the expected need to perform "triage" and thereby be unable to optimally treat all incoming patients created unusual challenges – and pressures. Sights of severely injured children could overwhelm experienced ER nurses – particularly those with young children – to the point of subsequently developing nightmares (Shalev – unpublished – self-support groups to ER nurses at Hadassah). A focus group of nursing staff (Riba & Reches, 2002) identified specific instances of stressful experiences during the response to terrorist attacks: the sudden call up to report for duty, the anxious waiting for casualties to arrive, caring for the victims, and closure of the event. Each of those created its particular challenges.

Several studies evaluated the prevalence and the extent of physical injury in suicide bomb attacks (e.g., Kluger et al 2004; Singer et al., 2005), often using the national trauma registry as a resource. A study published in the midst of the Intifada (Peleg et al, 2003) found that 70% of those admitted to ERs were younger than 29 years, 75% were male, 26% were admitted to intensive care units, and 6% died during hospital admission. Shapira, Adatto-Levi, Avitzour, Rivkind, Gertsenshtein, and Mintz (2006) evaluated records of 2,328 casualties pertaining to 28 major terror-related incidents in Jerusalem between September 2002 and September 2003. Injury scores were much higher than those observed in other incidents, and higher injury complexity was also noted. The overall mortality rate of the attacks was 11.7%, and approximately 83% of the deaths occurred immediately, at the site of the attacks. Half of the remaining 17% died in the hospital, within 4 hours of arrival. One quarter died within 5 to 24 hours, and one quarter later. Most of the patients operated on during the first 2 hours of hospital admission required multidisciplinary teams (Einav, Aharonson-Daniel, Weissman, Freund, & Peleg, 2006). Aschkenasy-Steuer and colleagues (2004) report:

> The hallmark of the injuries was a combination of blunt trauma and penetrating injuries due to bolts. Commonly, victims suffered injuries originating from more than one mechanism of injury. Moreover, victims commonly had injuries to several parts of the body (86 of 101 patients), the most frequently injured region being the head, neck and facial area.

A study of recovery from injury (Schwartz et al., 2007) compared 72 terror victims with complex ("multiple") trauma with 72 survivors of other incidents with similar injury. Terror victims ($N=27$) had longer rehabilitation periods but regained their activity of daily living as effectively as did other trauma survivors ($N = 72$). Despite higher rates of posttraumatic stress disorder (PTSD) in the former, there was no difference in the rate of return to previous occupations between the two groups.

For health professionals who lived through the Intifada, this period is remembered as extremely demanding and tense. Emergency calls could come every hour of the day, and few of them were false alarms. On the other hand, emergency medicine and ER psychiatry could have a tremendously gratifying effect, as many patients recovered from states of emotional shock with very simple intervention. Together, the pressure, the horror, and the professional challenges created mixed emotions and confusing memories.

33.3.2. First-Helpers' Responses, ER Symptoms, and ER Interventions

Weiniger and colleagues (2006) explored the psychological effect of repeated exposures to terror victims on hospital physicians. They compared three Jerusalem hospitals' physicians with either high exposure to terror victims ($N = 100$; mainly surgeons and anesthesiologists) or lower exposure ($N = 102$; internists, pediatricians, administrators). The rate of probable PTSD (per the PTSD Symptom Scale – Self Report) was similar in both groups (respectively 16% and 15%). Importantly, the likelihood of developing PTSD was related to (1) nonadaptive coping strategies and (2) higher exposure to terror in one's private life, not in the hospital. A follow-up paper (Einav et al., in press) revealed high levels of burnout, somatization, and depression in physicians who had PTSD symptoms. Remarkably, the prevalence of PTSD among hospital physicians was quite high, possibly reflecting a common experience of living in Jerusalem and the personal relevance of shared experiences.

As mentioned earlier, receiving hospitals provided early interventions to psychological casualties. In most cases, these interventions consisted of soothing and orienting the patient, reducing secondary stressors (e.g., uncertainty about relatives or about one's own health), recruiting family or friends' support, alleviating extreme emotional reactions (e.g., dissociation) and creating a link with community resources. Medications were seldom used. Few receiving hospitals provided debriefing – with no documented outcome for those that did. Indeed, little is known about the effect of the ER interventions. A study of 129 terror survivors admitted to a Tel Aviv hospital's ER (Schreiber et al., 2007) failed to show a long-term advantage of a memory-structuring intervention, relative to routine supportive treatment. A preliminary study of ER interventions in child survivors of terrorist attacks in Jerusalem similarly showed no advantage of professional intervention relative to usual care (see Galili-Weisstub & Benaroch, 2004).

Looking at the predictive power of PTSD symptoms in the ER, Shalev and Freedman (2006) prospectively evaluated terror victims and survivors of road traffic accidents. The prevalence of PTSD 4 months after the traumatic event was twice as high in terror survivors (38% vs. 19%). However, the intensity of early dissociation, ER heart rate, and early PTSD symptoms explained the entire difference between the groups. In other words, the excess of PTSD among terror survivors was entirely accounted for by higher levels of initial distress.

33.3.3. Population Studies

Questions regarding the prevalence of PTSD in the general populations have been asked in all recent national disasters. Studies of the aftermath of the September 11th terrorist attack in New York revealed an intriguing pattern of traumatic stress reactions in remotely exposed areas of the United States, significant but mostly transient rise in the prevalence of PTSD in more proximal areas (e.g., among residents of New York City), significant effects of proximity to the site of the attacks, an increase in smoking and use of psychotropic medication, and a positive relationship between exposure to the media and reported symptoms. A prospective study of the July 2005 London terrorist attacks revealed substantial stress and perceived threat for life in, respectively, 11% and 43% of responders 7 months after the attacks (Rubin et al., 2007).

Studies of responses to Al Aksa Intifada (Table 33.1) followed many of these paths, but some of their findings differ. As expected, the exposure to terrorist acts was much more prevalent in Israel (e.g., 16% of a representative sample of the population in a study by Bleich et al., 2003; 15.4% in Gidron et al., 2004; and 11% in Bleich, Gelkopf, Melamed, & Solomon, 2006). Indirect exposure, via personal friends and relatives, concerned twice as many subjects (28%, 36.5%, and 20.2% in the aformentioned studies, respectively). Studies also converge to show a population prevalence of PTSD of 9%, and 26.9% among residents of the highly exposed West Bank settlements (Shalev et al., 2006; see Figure 33.4.). The prevalence of PTSD among 11.5- to 15-year-old children was 12.4% in Jerusalem and 27.6% among those living in the West Bank settlements (Solomon & Lavi, 2005).

Attempts to better identify "true cases" of PTSD by taking into account DSM IV PTSD "F" criterion (clinically significant distress or impairment) reduced the population prevalence of PTSD to approximately one-third of that defined by symptom criteria alone, for example, from 9.4% to 2.4% in the Bleich et al. (2003) study, from 26.9% to 9.6% among residents of highly exposed areas in Shalev et al. (2006). Thus, despite the very broad exposure to terrorist acts, only 1 in 40 Israeli adults (2.4%) and approximately 1 in 10 of those living in highly exposed communities reported "clinically relevant" PTSD.

Why have so many Israelis reported qualifying PTSD symptoms without significant functional impairment? Possibly several PTSD "symptoms" describe components of normal behavior under threat (e.g., avoiding places and situations, reacting emotionally to threat-related signals, being unusually vigilant). People anticipating hostilities may, accordingly, endorse PTSD-like symptoms without being ill. The rapid decline of the prevalence of reported "PTSD" once adversities are over (e.g., Galea et al., 2004 is in line with this explanation.

From another perspective, this discrepancy emphasizes an often-neglected distinction between "exposure" and "trauma." Exposure may either traumatize or confer immunity. Moreover, some degree of exposure is a prerequisite for developing resilience (e.g., Masten 2001; Rutter, 1987). For example, prior combat exposure among the participants of the aforementioned study (Shalev et al., 2006) reduced the intensity of PTSD symptoms under terror threat. Laufer and Solomon's (2006) survey of 2,999 children in seventh to ninth grade during the Intifada showed a positive correlation between objective and subjective exposure to terror and both posttraumatic symptoms and posttraumatic growth. A study of repeated exposure to combat documented both "immunizing" and "sensitizing" effects (e.g., Solomon & Mikulincer, 2006; Solomon, Mikulincer, & Jakob, 1987). Compared with soldiers with first combat exposure during the 1982 Lebanon War, combat veterans of a previous war (the 1973 Yom Kippur War) who had not developed combat stress reaction (CSR) in 1973 had lower rates of CSR in 1982, whereas those who had a CSR in 1973 had higher rates of CSR in the later war. Higher combat exposure in the 1982 war only increased the gap between the groups. Thus, exposure's long-term effect seems to reside in its resolution, that is, whether one gains experience and mastery or one loses self-confidence and emotional balance.

In this context it is not at all surprising to see, in a study by Bleich and colleagues (2003), 58% of the participants reporting that they are depressed whilst at the same 82% of the sample expresses optimism about the future. Similarly, in a large sample of adolescents a 41.1% prevalence of mild to severe PTSD symptoms coexisted with 74.4% of the sample reporting an experience of growth (Laufer & Solomon, 2006). These numbers somehow anchor, in empirical findings, the Israeli ethos of "thriving within constraints," indeed, the Biblical ethos of growing stronger despite persecution: (e.g., "But the more they afflicted them, the more they multiplied and grew"; Exodus 1:12; King James version). These apparent paradoxes also resonate with an often forgotten generic lesson about resilience, namely the frequent combination of resilience in one domain (e.g., keep fighting)

Table 33.1. Population prevalence of PTSD

Study	Participants	Measure(s)	Results/Conclusions
Bleich et al. (2003)	Telephone survey, nationally representative sample ($N = 512$)	• Exposure levels • Appraisal of threat • PTSD and PTSD symptoms	• 16% personally exposed • 28% exposed through friends and relatives • 60% feel that their lives are in danger • 58% report being depressed • 82% express optimism about the future • 9.4% PTSD by symptom criteria • 2.4% PTSD by symptoms and distress/impairment • PTSD in women five fold higher than in men
Gidron et al. (2004)	Adults living in five cities ($N = 149$)	• Exposure • Perceived control • Control attributed to the government/ military • Frequency of listening to the news	• 15.4% was directly exposed to a terrorist attack • 36.5% knew someone who had been exposed • "Clinically significant" PTSD-like symptoms were reported by 10.1% • PTSD-like symptoms inversely correlate with perceived control in men, government control, and education in women and positively correlate with news-listening frequency in women
Bleich et al. (2005)	Old-old (>74), young-old (65–74) and younger (18–64) adults Telephone survey Stratified nationally representative sample	• Exposure • Traumatic stress symptoms • Coping: disengagement, optimism	• No difference between age groups
Shalev et al. (2006)	Adults living in two suburbs of Jerusalem with (a) Direct/high exposure ($N = 167$) (b) Indirect/low exposure levels ($N = 89$)	• Exposure to terror-related incidents • Disruption of daily living • PTSD symptoms general distress (Brief Symptom Inventory)	• Similar prevalence of PTSD rates in high and low exposure communities (26.95% vs. 21.35%). • PTSD criterion F reduces the prevalence of PTSD to 9.58% and 6.74%. • Women and men had equal rates of PTSD. • Exposure to discrete events does not affect PTSD symptom severity.

(continued)

Table 33.1 *(continued)*

Study	Participants	Measure(s)	Results/Conclusions
			• Disruption of daily routines significantly affects PTSD symptoms • Most of the variance in PTSD symptoms remains unexplained
Bleich et al. (2006)	Stratified national sample of Adults ($N = 501$)	• Level of exposure • PTSD and PTSD symptoms • Traumatic Stress Resiliency	• 11.2% directly exposed to a terrorist incidents • 20.2% have family members or friends exposed • 9% met symptom criteria for PTSD • 29.5% felt depressed, 10.4% anxious, 57% felt life-threatening • 9.7% endorsed a need for professional help • 14.4% traumatic stress resilient
Laufer & Solomon (2006)	Adolescents living in areas with different levels of exposure ($N = 2{,}999$)	• Posttraumatic symptoms • Psychological growth	• 41.1% reported mild to severe PTSD symptoms • 74.4% reported an experience of growth
Pat-Horenczyk (2007)	High school students ($N = 695$)	• Exposure • UCLA PTSD (Index for Adolescent Version) • Diagnostic Interview Schedule for Children • Beck Depression Inventory	• 7.6% prevalence of probable PTSD • Greater PTSD symptom severity in girls • Greater functional impairment in social and family domains in boys
Cohen & Eid (2007)	Israeli and Arab adolescents ($N = 346$)	• Exposure to terrorist attacks • Avoidance • Sharing of feelings Stress symptoms	• Mild to low levels of stress symptoms • No significant differences between Jews and Arabs • Being female, knowing someone injured, having parents who discuss terrorist attacks, and sharing of feelings positively correlated with stress symptoms

and withdrawal in another (become emotionally numb).

Another difference between findings in Israel and those reported in the United States is the inconsistency of the "proximity effect." In adults, both Bleich and colleagues (2003) Shalev and colleagues (2006) and Somer et al., (2005; 2007) have failed to demonstrate a relationship between

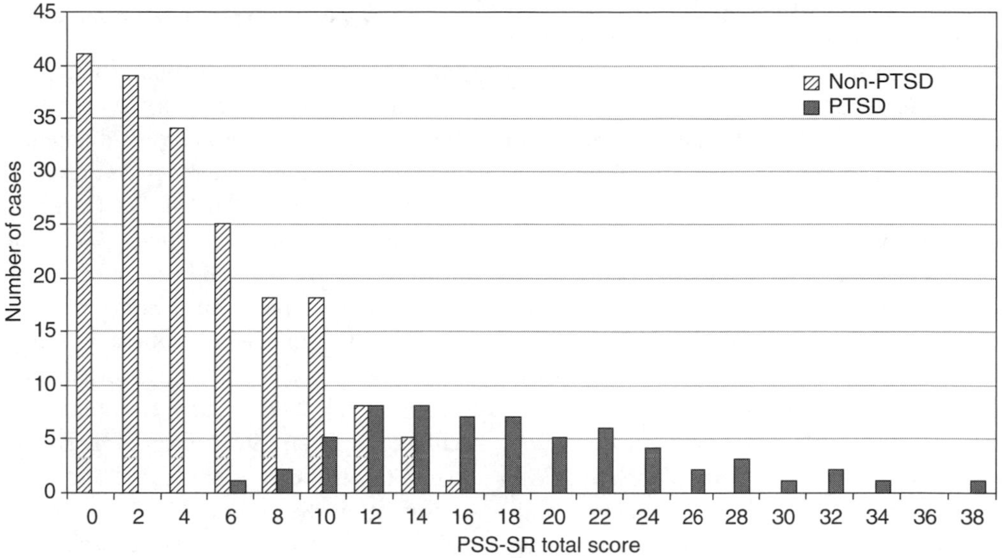

Figure 33.4. Distribution of PTSD symptom severity scores among residents of Jerusalem suburbs during Al Aksa Intifada (from Shalev et al., 2006).

levels of psychological distress and proximity to sites of the traumatic events, though a proximity effect has been documented in studies of children and adolescents (reviewed subsequently). How can one make sense of the lack of proximity effect in adults? The spread and the unpredictability of terror during the second Intifada provide a parsimonious explanation. Accordingly, the wave of terror of 2000 to 2004 effectively defied people's perception of safe territory. The ever-present sense of worry, the constant flow of media broadcast of terrorist acts, and the sense of personal relevance of events and situations may have created *psychological* proximity, despite geographical distances. The second Intifada differed in that sense from other waves of hostility (e.g., the shelling of the North of Israel before the Lebanon war or the 1969–1970 war of attrition on the Suez canal) during which large segments of the population continued to lead a normal life.

Given the widespread exposure to terrorism, differences between vulnerable and less vulnerable individuals became more salient. Figure 33.4 illustrates the distribution of PTSD symptom scores among residents of two suburbs of Jerusalem. Community residents who met PTSD symptom criteria are represented in dotted bars and those who did not in hatched bars. As can be seen, residents with full PTSD had higher levels of symptoms. However, those without PTSD were virtually symptom-free. Indeed, the Derogatis' Brief Symptom Inventory (BSI) scores of those without PTSD were within peacetime population norms (Shalev et al., 2006). In other words, exposure seriously affects a segment of the population, leaving most others untouched.

33.4. RESPONSE MODULATORS AND MODERATORS

Several studies have explored putative moderators of the relationship between exposure and psychological responses, such as gender, age, or religious belief. Studies conflict over the effect of gender (Cohen & Eid, 2007; Kimhi & Shamai, 2006; Shalev et al., 2006; Solomon et al., 2005; Strous et al., 2007), but most of the evidence supports a greater vulnerability in females (e.g., Zeidner, 2006). In a carefully stratified telephone survey, age was not found to have a major effect (Bleich et al., 2005). Several studies compared Jewish and Arab residents of Israel. Cohen and Eid (2007) found no significant difference in stress symptoms between Jewish and Arab adolescents; the levels of stress symptoms in both groups were mild to low. Hobfoll and colleagues (2006; 2008) found higher levels of PTSD and depressive symptoms in Palestinian residents of Israel than in Israeli Jews (18.0% vs. 6.6%), possibly related to greater trauma-related resource loss in the former.

Among Jews, traditional religiosity, lower social support, and greater economic resource loss predicted PTSD; low education and resource loss predicted PTSD among Arab residents of Israel. Arab ethnicity, lower household income, lower social support, economic loss from terrorism, higher levels of psychosocial resource loss, and meeting criteria for PTSD were significantly associated with increased severity of depressive symptoms in the same cohort (Tracy, Hobfoll, Canetti-Nisim, & Galea, 2008).

The extent to which religiousness, religious beliefs, or religious practices moderated the effect of stress was examined by several authors. Kaplan and colleagues (2005) compared residents of Tel Aviv with those of settlements in the West Bank and Gaza and found that religiousness, ideological convictions, and social cohesion were associated with substantial resilience among settlers. Laufer and Solomon (2006) have failed to show a relationship between religiosity and posttraumatic symptoms in adolescents living in areas of Israel with different exposure to terror. Religiosity, however, was strongly associated with psychological growth. Schiff (2006) compared religious and nonreligious adolescents living in Jerusalem (N = 600) and found lower rates of probable PTSD among religious adolescents; problem-solving coping mediated the protective effect of religiousness. Shalev and colleauges (2006) similarly found little protective effect of religiosity with regard to PTSD symptoms, yet psychological (or perhaps moral) assistance was more frequently sought in rabbis than in doctors and mental health providers. Along these lines, Levav and colleagues (2006) did not find an increase in the number of visits to psychiatric clinics in Jerusalem – nor a change in the proportion of ICD-10 diagnoses of mental disorders.

33.5. CHILDREN AND ADOLESCENTS

Table 33.2 summarizes the main studies of children and adolescent responses. As can be seen, children's reactions are not very different from those seen in adults: The reported prevalence of probable PTSD (e.g., 7.6% in Pat-Horenzcykm, Abramovitz et al., 2007; but 42% moderate to severe PTSD in Laufer & Solomon, 2006) may strongly depend on samples and instruments used. There seems to be a clearer proximity effect in children and adolescents (e.g., Cohen & Eid, 2007; Laufer & Solomon, 2006; Schiff et al., 2006) Stress symptoms are associated with an increase in alcohol and cannabis consumption (Schiff et al., 2007) and also with risk-taking behavior (Pat-Horenzcykm, Peled, et al., 2007). Girls are somewhat more symptomatic than boys (Pat-Horenzcykm, Abramovitz, et al., 2007). Vulnerable children (e.g., those with learning disabilities) have higher levels of PTSD symptom than nonclinical controls.

Several studies reflect an unexpected degree of resilience among children and adolescents: The majority of 2,999 adolescents in a study by Laufer and Solomon (2006) reported posttraumatic growth. Sharlin, Moin, and Yahav (2006) and Cohen and Eid (2007) find only mild to low levels of stress symptoms in both Jewish and Arab Israeli adolescents. Galili-Weisstub and Benarroch (2004) found uncontrollable reactions or dissociation in children seen in ERs immediately following terrorist attacks.

Sociodemographic factors and personal resources explained significant proportions of children's stressful reactions (Laufer & Solomon 2006; Solomon & Laufer 2004), and parents' reactions affected children's responses (e.g., Galili-Weisstub, Benarroch, 2004). Galili-Weisstub, (personal communication) found that an exposure to terrorist attacks could exacerbate the expression of previously existing or undiagnosed disorders among survivors (e.g., learning disability, OCD, or other anxiety disorders). Accordingly, child survivors of traumatic events should be evaluated for both trauma related and other symptoms and treatment tailored to the clinical findings.

Table 33.2. Responses of children and adolescents

Study	Participants	Measure(s)	Results/Conclusions
Solomon & Laufer (2004)	Adolescents aged 13–16. (*N* = 2,999)	• Exposure to terror • World Assumptions	• Personal and social resources make higher contribution to world assumptions than exposure to terror
Solomon & Lavi (2005)	Boys and girls aged 11.5–15 years from Jerusalem; settlements (*N* = 2,999)	• Exposure to terror • Posttraumatic stress reactions • Future orientation Trust in peace talks	• Higher prevalence of posttraumatic symptoms in more exposed areas • Children's future orientation is moderately optimistic. • Exposure related to both PTSD symptoms and attitudes toward peace - not to future orientation
Sharlin, Moin, & Yahav (2006)	Junior high school students in three Israeli cities. (*N* = 747)	• Children's reaction to terror • Child Behavioral Checklist	• Relatively low intensity of fear • Reactions to terror consistent with other personality dimensions • A new terrorist attack does not produce additional fears
Schiff et al. (2006)	High and junior high school students (*N* = 1,150)	• Physical and psychological proximity to terrorist attacks • Posttraumatic symptoms • Depressive symptoms Alcohol use	• Physical and psychological proximity to terrorist attacks associated with more posttraumatic symptoms, depression, and alcohol consumption
Finzi et al. (2006)	Adolescents (14–18) with learning disabilities (LD) Healthy controls (*N* = 56/*N* = 48)	• Posttraumatic stress disorder • Exposure to terror • Prior exposure to threatening life events • Avoidant and anxious attachment	• Higher PTSD symptoms in children with LD • All prior variable (current and past) exposure to avoidant and anxious attachment contributed significantly PTSD. • Past exposure increases both current anxious attachment and current PTSD upon exposure
Laufer & Solomon (2006)	Adolescents from four geographical areas with different exposure levels. (*N* = 2,999)	• Personal data • Exposure to terror • posttraumatic symptoms • posttraumatic growth	• Only 29.9% not exposed • Significant association between exposure and fear • Moderate to severe PTSD in 42% • Report of posttraumatic growth in 74% • Posttraumatic growth and posttraumatic symptoms correlate • Objective and subjective exposure positively correlates with both symptoms and growth. • Sociodemographic variables explained a greater portion • Religiosity not related to posttraumatic symptom; strongly associated with growth

(*continued*)

Table 33.2 *(continued)*

Study	Participants	Measure(s)	Results/Conclusions
Pat-Horenczyk (2007)	High school students (*N* = 695)	• Exposure to terrorist attacks • Posttraumatic symptoms Depression	• Probable PTSD in 7.6% of the sample. • Girls have greater severity of posttraumatic symptoms • Boys exhibit greater functional impairment in social and family domains
Pat-Horenzcyk (2007)	Israeli adolescents (*N* = 409)	• Risk-taking behavior • PTSD symptoms • Functional impairment	• Positive relationship between symptom severity, impairment, and risk taking behavior
Schiff et al. (2007)	10th and 11th grade students (*N* = 960)	• Physical proximity to terror • Cannabis and alcohol utilization	• Proximity to act of terror increased alcohol and cannabis consumption • The relationship remained significant after controlling for PTSD and depression
Cohen & Eid (2007)	Jewish and Israeli Palestinian adolescents (*N* = 346)	• Direct and indirect exposure to terror • Avoidance of public centers • Sharing feelings with significant others • Stress reaction symptoms	• Mild to low levels of stress symptoms • No significant differences between Jews and Arabs • Proximity and exposure explain 39% of the variance of symptoms • Being female, knowing someone injured, having parents who discuss terrorist attacks or forbid going out, and more sharing of feelings significantly related to higher stress symptoms • For Jewish adolescents, greater levels of sharing of feelings were related to higher distress
Kimhi & Shamai (2006)	Teenagers (*N* = 353) and Adults (*N* = 890)	• Gender • Cognitive appraisal of stress • Coping styles • Psychological symptoms • Life satisfaction	• In teenagers, gender differences were found only in cognitive appraisal and psychological symptoms • Among adults, gender differences were found in all the studied variables

33.6. FEAR, RESILIENCE, AND DEFIANCE

The term resilience is poorly defined in the literature. Nonetheless, several studies of the Second Intifada have addressed various aspects of resilience, and others can be read as reflecting a resilient, or even defiant attitude.

More frequently exposed than other Israelis, ZAKA volunteers have been at every scene of bomb attack where they meticulously collected body remains to get them properly buried as dictated by the Jewish Halacha. The name ZAKA is an abbreviation for the Hebrew Zihuy Korbanot Ason, literally "Disaster Victim Identification." Better named by its volunteers as Chesed Shel Emet or "True Kindness" (the meaning of the Hebrew word Chesed is somewhere between kindness, charity, and grace), the organization was created in 1990, quickly acquired a place of honor, and systematically dispatched teams of volunteers to each disaster scene. Most ZAKA volunteers come from the orthodox community.

Solomon and Berger (2005) evaluated 87 ZAKA volunteers for PTSD symptoms, sense of danger, and self-efficacy. They found low sense of danger, considerable self-efficacy, and a prevalence of PTSD (2.4%) resembling that of the general population. Exposure to disfigured dead bodies and severed body parts is a traumatic stressor (e.g., McCarroll et al., 1993, 2001), and what protected ZAKA volunteers from showing higher levels of distress is a matter of interpretation. Nonetheless, by its persistence and dedication this group constitutes a salient example of resilience. Indeed, ZAKA's activities are a central component of an ongoing "rapprochement" between orthodox and nonorthodox communities in Israel.

From a different perspective, Strous and colleagues (2007) evaluated 97 restaurant attendees at sites of recent terrorist attacks, exploring knowledge about the previous event, participants' previous terror exposure, coping mechanisms, and state of anxiety and mood. Ninety-three percent of the respondents were aware of the previous terror attack, 70.3% reported no fear at revisiting, 20.9% some anxiety, and 5.5% moderate or severe anxiety. Over half of respondents (53%) reported that the current security climate affected their mood. Participants in this study found that "calling to be in touch with friends and relatives" was the most effective way to cope with stress following suicide bombing (also in Bleich et al., 2003). Older individuals and females were more seriously affected by terror events.

Notwithstanding these defying attitudes, restaurants and public places in the center of cities (particularly Jerusalem) were virtually empty during the height of the Intifada, and a few had to close. Hotel occupancy went down to 15%. Interestingly – though not truly documented – it took approximately 2 weeks for Jerusalemites to trickle back into the "death crossing" of Jerusalem's two main streets, where one suicide bomb attack seemed to be following another. When you went back to those streets (e.g., to your accountant's office) you bargained on time (just a few minutes) and on your observation skills. Getting back to safe territory was a small victory over fear. Every public place had guards. Body checks were regularly performed in shopping centers, cafes, restaurants, schools, hospitals, and government offices. Despite inconvenience and queues, the more thoroughly you were checked the safer it felt to enter.

Most importantly, life had to go on. Children were born, weddings celebrated, schools were open and exams, unfortunately, persisted. Diplomas were bestowed on meritorious and less meritorious candidates. Businesses and industries remained active and creative (e.g., Israel high-tech industry's exports declined by 10% in 2001 and 10.9% in 2002 – but this period parallels the world's high-tech crisis. Israel's overall export declined by 1.9% in 2002 [Ministry of Industry, Trade, and Labor]). Despite several bus bombing incidents, the transport system did not collapse. Other public services continued as well, virtually undisturbed. These facts may be hard to appraise from a perspective of a society based on spending and a service-based economy. Indeed, from such a perspective the Intifada was a major blow: Tourism virtually stopped, and the average family earning declined. The essentials, however, were far from being severely impacted by the events. Possibly, Israel was not too far from decades of major economic difficulties (e.g., the 1973 War was followed by over 200% yearly inflation). Else, one can parsimoniously assume that Israelis (as others around the world) adjust to trouble – rather than break. Whether adjustment should be confounded with resilience is a matter of theory.

33.7. THE FACTS BEHIND THE FACTS

Reading this chapter may leave an erroneous impression of a resilient society, where tremendous exposure creates moderate reactions, handling body parts does not increase the rate of PTSD beyond that of the general population (Solomon & Berger, 2005), the proportion of growth experiences surpasses that of stress symptoms (Laufer & Solomon, 2006), only 20% of child survivors of terrorist suicide attacks express "pathological" stress reaction in ERs (Galili-Wiesstub & Benarroch, 2004), and optimism prevails in a population otherwise reporting depressed mood (Bleich et al., 2003).

However, these are but shadows of reality. Reality as captured by preexisting templates, and analyzed to reveal presumed conjunctions. Notwithstanding the bravery that the numbers convey, those who lived through the 4 bad years of the Intifada have very different stories to tell. Underlying the seemingly smooth surface were layers of fear and rage. Almost everyone had experienced – at least for a moment – a disturbing mixture of fury and total helplessness: The kind of experience that one can repress but never forget. Thus, as a result of these and previous events, there might be enough in the underground of individual and collective memories to fuel the next slaughter, and the ones that will follow.

So, where are the potential errors of empirical explorations? They are, first, the averaging of large groups, second, confounding surface with depth, third, a misappraisal of human capacity for resilience, and forth, a flattening of the human group.

33.7.1. Top-Down and Bottom-Up Effects

Starting from the last error: Research on 1,000 individuals is not a research of a group of 1,000 individuals. It is a study of multiple single specimens, attempting to uncover the "typical" or average experience. The Intifada, however, was lived as large group. Group reactions and discourses, therefore, determined much of the unexplained variance of specific measures (see Shalev et al., 2006). There are many examples of such group effect: Israelis were glued to the radio or to TV broadcasts and, in that sense, have lived the events as one small village would have. Individuals were reactive to the news, activated by what they were told, skeptical about leadership, but in need of a "big" figure. Each terrorist attack resulted in an activation of attachment networks. For example, major attacks were followed by transient failure of cellular telephone systems due to excessive call volume; hence, the desire to reaffirm the safety of attachment networks was intense. Similarly, subjects in the Efrat study (Shalev et al., 2006) similarly expressed more apprehension about their relatives taking a risk (e.g., driving at night) than about themselves taking the same risk. Thus, the locus of the events was somewhere above the individual level.

Several other cohesion-fostering factors were not captured by the studies reviewed earlier. Medical care in Israel is free of charge at the point of delivery. In addition, the National Insurance Institute of Israel (NII), a government agency that provides a safety net to the old and the disabled, supports the medical, financial, and rehabilitation costs related to trauma emanating from terror. The NII provides extensive coverage of medical care, disability compensation, dependents benefits, and the vocational rehabilitation of those affected by terror. It also provides other forms of assistance, such as loans and grants for housing or tuition fees to survivors and those who lost a family member. These benefits extend to psychological casualties. Indeed, the NII has been very active in reaching out to people experiencing psychological effects of terror. It also follows widows and dependents starting from the first days of bereavement and continuing for some for years. Despite some survivors' complaints about red tape and slow process of recognition, the NII provides a safety network for all physical and psychological casualties of terrorism, such that, injury, including mental injury, is not followed by social drift.

Along with the NII's assistance, other "top-down" processes (i.e., processes initiated by authorities) helped reduce the effect of terror. These included the allocation of resources for immediate repair and rebuilding. Sites of bombing were tended to immediately; all gruesome reminders were carried away, and repair of buildings, windows, or even replacement of trees started within hours of an event. Consequently, throughout the *Intafada*, Israeli towns and cities did not bear traces of terrorism other than symbolic commemoration icons. As previously reported, ZAKA had a major share in these efforts, painstakingly collecting body parts from sites of explosions.

These "top-down" efforts were echoed by "bottom-up" responses, that is, action taken by business owners, transportation companies, and the public at large to return to streets, shopping malls, or buses were the attacks had taken place. The absence of visual evidence or paralyzed center-cities significantly reduced the reminders of terror. From our own clinical perspective, survivors who returned to the sites of their trauma as part of an in vivo exposure of cognitive-behavioral therapies could see that life was back.

Responding to the desirability of information, after each major attack, the receiving hospitals opened communication centers, staffed by trained workers. These centers had immediate access to comprehensive lists of casualties reflecting all those admitted to different hospitals and providing identifying details (e.g., age, gender, appearance), including survivors whose names were still unknown. Relatives could consequently access reliable and comprehensive information by one telephone call and did not have to wander between hospitals. Similarly, in deference to the Jewish requirement not to postpone burial, the Institute of Forensic Medicine had developed expertise in rapid identification of human remains (Hiss & Kahana, 2000) and implemented it throughout the events. This greatly alleviated individuals' agonizing pain of expectation and fostered the public's sense of nonanonymity of the dead: The names of victims and their photographs could be seen on the next day's newspaper. Similarly the media, the police, rescue organizations, and local officials sensed and were sensitive to the public's need for instantaneous, reliable, and accurate information. Within minutes of a terrorist act and throughout the following hours, these sources provided accurate descriptions of the event itself (i.e., which bus was bombed and where exactly), casualty rates, road access, receiving hospital, and so on. The public readily translated the information into concrete and necessary knowledge about routes to take or avoid, relatives to be worried or reassured about. Except for those directly affected, the very concrete consequence of this information was, in fact, calming: For most people it contained a safety signal (e.g., "This bus serves another part of the city – my son could not have been there.").

It is hard to say what was behind these converging forces. Possibly, the events never reached a disastrous dimension, that is, never truly overwhelmed society's core structures. Else, years of experience in low-intensity terror prepared people and infrastructures for the 2000 to 2004 events. Importantly, during the events Israelis were not assured of the strengths of their own society, and the general feeling was one of troubles without foreseeable end.

33.7.2. Human Capacity for Resilience

As repeatedly found elsewhere, responses to disaster inherently include elements of altruism and resilience. In a previous publication we suggested that "resilience is the default" and not to be missed (Shalev & Errera, in press). We have further argued that daily adjustment is possibly the strongest mechanism behind the prevalent resilience of individuals and groups (alias the "Ordinary Magic") (Masten, 2001). Similarly, Israelis progressively adjusted to the fact of terror. They did so by shifting expectations, changing routines of living, territorializing threat. We negotiated one apprehension against another – trusting our judgment regardless of full proof. For example, at the height of the Intifada, our group hosted a visitor from abroad and held an evening event to honor him. A psychologist who drove to Jerusalem that evening on one of the most dangerous roads did so with the lights of his car turned off. "It's a way of not being visible to snipers," he explained, forgetting, perhaps, that only during 2002 the number of terror casualties exceeded that of road traffic accidents.

The country's residents also adjusted to daily living through drawing virtual fear maps, that is, identifying those places to which one should never go. Jerusalemites' "maps of fear" included East Jerusalem, and, once in a while the center of town. For those living in Tel Aviv, however, visiting Jerusalem was unthinkably risky. The essence of those "fear maps" was, indeed, seeing oneself in a safe zone. This feeling that is just the opposite of what PTSD patients describe – that is – always being in the center of threat. Nondepressed, nontraumatized people always similarly calibrated their expectations to what was achievable (e.g., "If not in a movie in a theater, let's get a DVD and watch it at home"), and thus every day carried a small victory, and life remained rewarding. Others have powerfully described the sense of living a meaningful life within deadly constraints (specifically, Primo Levy, in "*This is the Man*" or "*Ecce Homo,*" an Auschwitz account). These dispositions are universal and are shared by others in other disaster areas.

33.7.3. Averaging Large Samples

One of the principal considerations in all population-based research pertains to the large number of persons reflected in even seemingly small prevalence. Specifically, a 2.4% prevalence of PTSD in the general population represents 160,000 Israelis. Even assuming 60% recovery (e.g., Kessler et al., 1995) these numbers suggest approximately 94,000 residual cases of PTSD. This strongly suggests that a minority, albeit a substantial minority, of the population carries the majority of the burden. Furthermore, the numbers underestimate the ancillary damage of the Intifada, not including PTSD orphans, widows, and the physically maimed or disabled. In that sense, the impact of the Intifada on a "population" is somewhat of a myth. We may have endured the events as a group, but their long-term consequences are carried by individuals and families. Therefore, the true challenge of mitigating the effect of these events is in keeping those who were personally afflicted in the midst of the social group and not marginalizing them.

33.7.4. Confounding Surface with Depth

Measuring events while they occur is limited by lack of true perspective, and an inability to apprehend the underlying processes and their progression. A sequence of traumatic events such as the one endured by Israelis during Intifada takes time to "percolate," or to shape people's attitudes and create a background for interpreting subsequent occurrences. Therefore, it may take many years to comprehend the true nature of this historical event and its ramifications.

33.8. THE LONG-TERM EFFECTS OF TERRORISM

Since terror has such a central part in the Arab–Israeli enmeshment, one has to wonder whether its accumulating sediments are going to sink the boat or balance it. On the one hand, one can hope that these terrible experiences are a painful road to somewhere. On the other hand, we might be spiraling around and around and not getting anywhere. Traumatic exposure that ends with a sense of mastery eventually immunizes against further trauma. Else, one trauma amplifies another. What are the exact qualities of the latent learning from the Intifada – on both sides – is unknown at this point. Several recent conflicts between nations, ethnic groups, or tribes have clearly shown that incipient hostilities can be exploited or burst into major carnage. It is too early, therefore, to entirely understand some of the long-term effects of the Second Intifada.

REFERENCES

Aschkenasy-Steuer, G., Shamir, M., Rivkind, A., Mosheiff, R., Shushan, Y., Rosenthal, G., et al. (2004). Hospital preparedness for possible non conventional casualties: An Israeli experience. *General Hospital Psychiatry 26*(5), 359–366.

Bleich, A., Dycian, A., Koslowsky, M., Solomon, Z., & Wiener, M. (1992). Psychiatric implications of missile attacks on a civilian population. Israeli lessons from the Persian Gulf War. *JAMA, 268*(5), 613–615.

Bleich, A., Gelkopf, M., Melamed, Y., & Solomon, Z. (2005). Emotional impact of exposure to terrorism among young-old and old-old Israeli citizens. *American Journal of Geriatric Psychiatry, 13*(8), 705–712.

(2006). Mental health and resiliency following 44 months of terrorism: A survey of an Israeli national representative sample. *BMC Medicine, 274*, 21.

Bleich, A., Gelkopf, M., Solomon, Z., (2003). Exposure to terrorism, stress-related mental health symptoms, and coping behaviors among a nationally representative sample in Israel." *JAMA 290*, 612–20.

Cohen, M., & Eid, J. (2007). The effect of constant threat of terror on Israeli Jewish and Arab adolescents. *Anxiety, Stress and Coping: An International Journal, 20*(1), 47–60.

Einav, S., Aharonson-Daniel, L., Weissman, C., Freund, H.R., & Peleg, K. (2006). In-hospital resource utilization during multiple casualty incidents. *Annals of Surgery*. *243*(4), 533–540.

Einav, S., Shalev, A. Y., Ofek, H., Freedman, S., Matot, I., & Wininger, C. (2008). Differences in psychiatric co-morbidities in hospital physicians with and without post traumatic stress disorder. *British Journal Of Psychiatry*, *193*(2), 165–166.

Finzi-Dottan, R., Dekel, R., Lavi, T., & Su'ali, T. (2006). Posttraumatic stress disorder reactions among children with learning disabilities exposed to terror attacks. *Comprehensive Psychiatry*, *47*(2), 144–151.

Galea, S., Vlahov, D., Resnick, H., Ahern J., Susser, E. Gold, J. Bucuvalas, M., Kilpatrick, D. (2003). "Trends of probable post-traumatic stress disorder in New York City after the September 11 terrorist attacks." *Am J Epidemiol 158*(6): 514–524.

Galili-Weisstub, E., & Benarroch, F. (2004). The immediate psychological consequences of terror attacks in children. *Journal of Aggression, Maltreatment and Trauma*, *9*(3–4), 323–334.

Gidron, Y., Kaplan, Y., Velt, A., & Shalem, R. (2004). Prevalence and moderators of terror-related post-traumatic stress disorder symptoms in Israeli citizens. *The Israel Medical Association Journal*, *6*(7), 387–391.

Hiss, J., & Kahana, T. (2000). Trauma and identification of victims of suicidal terrorism in Israel. *Military Medicine*, *165*(11), 889–893.

Hobfoll, S. E., Canetti-Nisim, D., & Johnson, R. J. (2006). Exposure to terrorism, stress-related mental health symptoms, and defensive coping among Jews and Arabs in Israel. *Journal of Consulting and Clinincal Psychology*, *74*(2), 207–218.

Hobfoll, S. E., Canetti-Nisim, D., Johnson, R. J., Palmieri, P. A., Varley, J. D., & Galea, S. (2008). The association of exposure, risk, and resiliency factors with PTSD among Jews and Arabs exposed to repeated acts of terrorism in Israel. *Journal of Traumatic Stress*, *21*, 9–21.

Israel Bureau of Statistics. (May, 2008). Retrieved from http://www.cbs.gov.il.

Kessler, R.C., Sonnega, A., Bromet, E., Hughes, M., Nelson, C.B. (1995). Posttraumatic stress disorder in the National Comorbidity Survey. *Arch Gen Psychiatry 52*(12): 1048–1060.

Kaplan, Z., Matar, M. A., Kamin, R., Sadan, T., & Cohen, H. (2005). Stress-related responses after 3 years of exposure to terror in Israel: Are ideological-religious factors associated with resilience? *Journal of Clinical Psychiatry*, *66*(9), 1146–1154.

Kimhi, S., & Shamai, M. (2004). Community resilience and the impact of stress: Adult response to Israel's withdrawal from Lebanon. *Journal of Community Psychology*, *32*(4), 439–451.

(2006). Are women at higher risk than men? Gender differences among teenagers and adults in their response to threat of war and terror. *Women and Health*, *43*(3), 1–19.

Kluger, Y., Peleg, K., Daniel-Aharonson, L., & Mayo, A. (2004). The special injury pattern in terrorist bombings. *Journal of the American College of Surgeons*, *199*(6), 875–879.

Laufer, A., & Solomon, Z. (2006). Posttraumatic symptoms and posttraumatic growth among Israeli youth exposed to terror incidents. *Journal of Social and Clinical Psychology*, *25*(4), 429–447.

Levav, I., Novikov, I., Grinshpoon, A., Rosenblum, J., & Ponizovsky, A. (2006). Health services utilization in Jerusalem under terrorism. *The American Journal of Psychiatry*, *163*(8), 1355–1361.

Masten AS. (2001). Ordinary magic: Resilience processes in development. *American Psychologist*, *56*, 227–238.

McCarroll, J. E., Ursano, R. J., & Fullerton, C. S. (1993). Symptoms of posttraumatic stress disorder following recovery of war dead. *The American Journal of Psychiatry*, *150*(12), 1875–1877.

McCarroll J. E., Ursano, R. J., Fullerton, C. S., Liu, X., Lundy, A. (2001). Effects of exposure to death in a war mortuary on posttraumatic stress disorder symptoms of intrusion and avoidance. J *Nerv Ment Dis 189*(1), 44–48.

Ochs Dweck, J. (Forthcoming). *Suspicious objects: Fear and security in Israel*, Philadelphia: University of Pennsylvania Press.

Pat-Horenczyk, R., Abramovitz, R., Peled, O., Brom, D., Daie, A., & Chemtob, C. M., (2007). Adolescent exposure to recurrent terrorism in Israel: Posttraumatic distress and functional impairment. *American Journal of Orthopsychiatry*, *77*(1), 76–85.

Pat-Horenczyk, R., Peled, O., Miron, T., Brom, D., Villa, Y., & Chemtob, C. M. (2007). Risk-taking behaviors among Israeli adolescents exposed to recurrent terrorism: Provoking danger under continuous threat? *The American Journal of Psychiatry*, *164*(1), 66–72.

Peleg, K., Aharonson-Daniel, L., Michael, M., & Shapira, S.C. (2003). Patterns of injury in hospitalized terrorist victims. *American Journal of Emergency Medicine*, *21*(4), 258–262.

Riba, S., & Reches, H. (2002). When terror is routine: How Israeli nurses cope with multi-casualty terror. *Online Journal of Issues in Nursing*, *7*(3), 6.

Rubin, G. J., Brewin, C. R., Greenberg, N., Hughes, J. H., Simpson, J., & Wessely, S. (2007). Enduring consequences of terrorism: 7-month follow-up survey of reactions to the bombings in London on 7 July 2005. *The British Journal of Psychiatry, 190*, 350–356.

Rutter, M. (1987). Psychosocial resilience and protective mechanisms. *American Journal of Orthopsychiatry, 53*, 316–331.

Schiff, M. (2006). Living in the shadow of terrorism: Psychological distress and alcohol use among religious and non-religious adolescents in Jerusalem. *Social Science & Medicine, 62*(9), 2301–2312.

Schiff, M., Benbenishty, R., McKay, M., DeVoe, E., Liu, X., & Hasin, D. (2006). Exposure to terrorism and Israeli youths' psychological distress and alcohol use: An exploratory study. *The American Journal on Addictions, 15*(3), 220–226.

Schreiber, S., Dolberg, O. T., Barkai, G., Peles, E., Leor, A., Rapoport, E., et al. (2007). Primary intervention for memory structuring and meaning acquisition (PIMSMA): Study of a mental health first-aid intervention in the ED with injured survivors of suicide bombing attacks. *American Journal of Disaster Medicine, 2*, 307–320.

Schwartz, I., Tsenter, J., Shochina, M., Shiri, S., Kedary, M., Katz-Leurer, M., et al. (2007). Rehabilitation outcomes of terror victims with multiple traumas. *Archives of Physical Medicine and Rehabilitation, 88*(4), 440–448.

Singer, P., Cohen JD, & Stein, M. (2005). "Conventional terrorism and critical care." *Crit Care Med 33*: S61–5.

Shalev, A. Y., & Freedman, S. (2005). PTSD following terrorist attacks: A prospective evaluation. *American Journal of Psychiatry, 162*(6), 1188–1191.

Shalev, A. Y., & Errera Y. L. E. (In press). Resilience is the default: How not to miss it? In M. Blummenfield & R. J. Ursano, *Intervention and resilience after mass trauma*. Cambridge University Press.

Shalev, A. Y., Tuval, R., Frenkiel-Fishman, S., Hadar, H., & Eth, S. (2006). Psychological responses to continuous terror: A study of two communities in Israel. *American Journal of Psychiatry, 163*(4), 667–673.

Shapira, S. C., Adatto-Levi, R., Avitzour, M., Rivkind, A. I., Gertsenshtein, I., & Mintz, Y. (2006). *World Journal of Surgery, 30*(11), 2071–2077.

Sharlin, S. A., Moin, V., & Yahav, R. (2006). When disaster becomes commonplace: Reaction of children and adolescents to prolonged terrorist attacks in Israel. *Social Work in Health Care, 43*(2–3), 95–114.

Solomon, Z., & Berger, R. (2005). Coping with the aftermath of terror: Resilience of ZAKA Body Handlers. *Journal of Aggression Maltreatment and Trauma, 10*(1–2), 593–604.

Solomon, Z., Gelkopf, M., & Bleich, A. (2005). Is terror gender-blind? Gender differences in reaction to terror events. *Social Psychiatry and Psychiatric Epidemiology, 40*(12), 947–954.

Solomon, Z., & Laufer, A. (2004). In the shadow of terror: Changes in world assumptions in Israeli youth. *Journal of Aggression, Maltreatment and Trauma, 9*(3–4), 353–364.

Solomon, Z., & Lavi, T. (2005). Israeli youth in the second Intifada: PTSD and future orientation. *Journal of the American Academy of Child and Adolescent Psychiatry, 44*(11), 1167–1175.

Solomon, Z., & Mikulincer, M. (2006). Trajectories of PTSD: A 20-year longitudinal study. *The American Journal of Psychiatry, 163*(4), 659–666.

Solomon, Z., Mikulincer, M., & Jakob, B. R. (1987). Exposure to recurrent combat stress: Combat stress reactions among Israeli soldiers in the Lebanon War. *Psychological Medicine, 17*(2), 433–440.

Somer, E., Ruvio, A., Sever, I., & Soref, E. (2007). Reactions to repeated unpredictable terror attacks: Relationships among exposure, posttraumatic distress, mood, and intensity of coping. *Journal of Applied Social Psychology, 37*(4), 862–886.

Somer, E., Ruvio, A., Soref, E., & Sever, I. (2005). Terrorism, distress and coping: High versus low impact regions and direct versus indirect civilian exposure. *Anxiety, Stress and Coping: An International Journal, 18*(3), 165–182.

Strous, R. D., Mishaeli, N., Ranen, Y., Benatov, J., Green, D., & Zivotofsky, A. Z. (2007). Confronting the bomber: Coping at the site of previous terror attacks. *Journal of Nervous and Mental Disease, 195*(3), 233–239.

Tracy, M., Hobfoll, S. E., Canetti-Nisim, D., & Galea, S. (2008). Predictors of depressive symptoms among Israeli Jews and Arabs during the Al Aqsa intifada: A population-based cohort study. *Annals of Epidemiology*. [Epub ahead of print]

Weiniger C.F., Shalev A.Y., Ofek, H., Freedman, S., & Weissman, C. (2006). Posttraumatic stress disorder among hospital surgical physicians exposed to victims of terror: a prospective, controlled questionnaire survey. *J Clin Psychiatry 67*(6), 890–896.

Zeidner, M. (2006). Gender group differences in coping with chronic terror: The Israeli scene. *Sex Roles, 54*(3–4), 297–310.

PART SEVEN

Questions and Directions

34 Methodological Challenges in Studying the Mental Health Consequences of Disasters

SANDRO GALEA AND ANDREA R. MAXWELL

34.1. INTRODUCTION

In this chapter we discuss the methodological challenges that researchers face when designing, implementing, and analyzing studies aimed at understanding the mental health consequences of disasters. To do so, we start by summarizing the general logistical challenges of postdisaster research that underlie the methodological issues that are our focus. We then turn our attention to these methodological issues. First, we discuss the problems that pertain to finding and sampling populations of interest after disasters. Second, we consider the challenges inherent in designing postdisaster research studies. Third, we discuss particular measurement issues that are important to this work. Fourth, we consider the analytic issues that are relevant to this research. Our goal in highlighting these challenges is to better inform inference from the extant body of postdisaster research and to help illuminate approaches that may be fruitfully applied in the future to strengthen work in the field.

34.1.1. Logistical Challenges in Establishing Postdisaster Research

Disasters are, by their very nature, largely unanticipated and disruptive. They create confusion and interfere with services – ranging from sophisticated services, such as hospitals, to more basic services, such as telephone availability. Postdisaster circumstances are hardly optimal situations under which to design or launch research studies. Indeed, research studies typically are long planned and implemented in a highly controlled environment; in addition, they make use of a variety of services to ensure success of the research project. In contrast, disaster research studies are typically launched in circumstances that are exactly the *opposite* of these. This divide between the postdisaster reality and the conditions under which research typically thrives creates a tension that is the basis for the logistical challenges that are faced by postdisaster research studies. In particular, there are four key logistical challenges faced by postdisaster researchers: organizing the research plan, organizing the research team, establishing relationships with the local community, and obtaining funding and approvals. We discuss each in turn.

Probably the first clear challenge in establishing research relating to disasters pertains to organizing the research plan. Research plans for most studies are predicated on an intimate knowledge of underlying conditions and on manipulating, or studying, specific aspects of these conditions. In the postdisaster situation, underlying conditions are rapidly changing, with scant data to suggest what conditions are like at any given moment. For example, in the aftermath of a hurricane, maps that suggest where populations are or are not still residing and estimates of population size remaining in each of these areas may be hard to procure. Without this information it is challenging for researchers to formulate a precise research plan, including specific sampling plans, strategies for most effectively reaching participants, and strategies for obtaining the desired data. Therefore, effective postdisaster research often must rely on an on-the-ground understanding of the postdisaster situation – including population placement and availability of resources – to be able to guide the development of a rational, feasible, and scientifically valid research plan.

The second key logistical challenge faced by researchers after disasters relates to organizing the research plan and the research team. For most kinds of research, plans take months, if not years, to develop. However, after disasters, urgent questions arise that researchers may wish to address. The research team itself also typically takes months or years to assemble. Unfortunately, researchers seldom have such luxury in the postdisaster context. As a result, postdisaster research typically involves either already established or hastily formed research teams. This has several implications. Preestablished research teams have a particular skill set and interests. Therefore, such teams will, by definition, tackle postdisaster research questions that are within their scope and interest, driven more by the researcher than by the exigencies of a particular postdisaster circumstance. Conversely, research teams that are assembled after an event to provide a range of interests and expertise to address particular questions of interest may not be cohesive and may find it challenging, in the long term, to be either as effective or as productive as established research teams might be.

A corollary to this challenge is the balance in postdisaster research teams between local investigators and those from another city or even another country. Disasters always feel "local." If a city is hit by a disaster, local residents are aware that another city, several hundred miles away, is still standing and unaffected. Therefore, local residents, not unexpectedly, often feel possessive about the disaster experience and may be leery of "outsiders" who are not in the local environment strictly to "help." This attitude extends to research teams: Local researchers may feel that they should be the first to implement postdisaster research, regardless of their experience or expertise in the area. In recent years, several projects funded by the National Institutes of Health have been implemented to provide researchers with an opportunity to learn the essentials of postdisaster research quickly and to partner with other, more experienced researchers in the field (see www.redmh.org and www.disasterresearch.org).

No matter the makeup of the research team, simple communication challenges still abound in many postdisaster areas, particularly those involving researchers from different sites. Limited telephone or E-mail connection may make normal communication laborious, as does the absence of local office resources and support staff. As a further complication to the establishment of research teams, researchers sometimes find themselves in the unfamiliar situation of effectively being part of the first wave of responders. Maintaining detachment under such circumstances can be difficult. Although this is seldom documented in the peer-reviewed literature, anecdotal evidence suggests that researchers – particularly those trained as clinicians – may identify with affected research participants, threatening the dispassionate objectivity that is essential in population-based research (Goenjian, 1993).

Along these lines, the third challenge centers more specifically on the establishment of relationships between researchers and the local community. Contact between members of the research team and community members is always better served by a good relationship between the two, which takes time to build. Typical research projects have the luxury of having had time to meet local leaders, to produce informational material about a research study for local residents, and to carefully consider the best ways to gain access to the populations of interest. Very few of these opportunities are available to the researcher interested in health after a disaster. In most postdisaster situations, research needs to be established quickly, leaving little opportunity for time-consuming engagement of all local community leaders and their constituencies. In addition, the difficulty of establishing community relations may be compounded, as noted earlier, by the heightened local sensitivity to community needs and the possible perception among local residents that they are being exploited. Despite these difficulties, an optimal researcher-community relationship is likely a *sine qua non* of viable postdisaster research.

Fourth, the establishment of successful postdisaster research requires interaction with agencies that provide funding and ethics approval to allow the research to proceed effectively. These approvals are never easy or quick to be granted under the best of circumstances and are perhaps more challenging than ever after disasters. Mechanisms do exist to rapidly fund postdisaster research, such as the RAPID grant mechanism at the National Institutes of Health; however, even these mechanisms take many months to deliver funding after successful grant application. Many researchers who wish to implement investigations in the short term after disasters must rely on other, typically more ad hoc, nongovernmental sources of funding (Galea, et al., 2002). These funding sources typically depend on preexisting relationships and may be subject to particular idiosyncratic interests of the funder that may or may not be congruent with the most relevant research question.

Ethics approval, a must for all research, is also quite idiosyncratic, with the speed of approval being highly dependent on the effectiveness of Institutional Review Boards (IRBs) at different institutions. One of the challenges facing researchers seeking ethics review after disasters is dealing with IRBs that are unfamiliar with research in the area. IRBs, sensitive to the heightened awareness typically surrounding a particular disaster event, frequently worry about the potential for iatrogenic harm to research participants, even though this is likely unfounded. A substantial body of evidence has recently shown that research participation is not associated with adverse consequences among research participants (Boscarino, Adams, Stuber, & Galea, 2005; Galea, Nandi, Stuber, et al., 2005; Newman, Walker, & Gefland, 1999), and rather, most research participants make favorable cost–benefit appraisals of their participation in such research (Newman & Kaloupek, 2004). However, researchers interested in establishing postdisaster research frequently must educate their local IRBs about the risks and benefits of this type of research before obtaining the necessary review and approval to carry out the proposed work. Including this volume, several new books in the area (Norris, Galea, Friedman, & Watson, 2006; Ursano, Fullerton, Weisaeth, & Raphael, 2007) provide summaries of the research in the field and may be useful resources to efficiently educate IRBs about the nature of iatrogenic harm relating to postdisaster research.

34.2. DEFINING A POPULATION OF INTEREST AND FINDING PARTICIPANTS

It is the central goal of all human-based research to clearly identify a target population and to sample persons from that population as effectively as possible. This brings up one of the key challenges particular to postdisaster research design: defining the population of interest and finding these persons in a postdisaster circumstance.

34.2.1. Defining Populations

Defining the population of interest may be a relatively easy question in most nondisaster research, but it is substantially harder in the unpredictable, and frequently chaotic, postdisaster circumstance. For example, consider a situation where a town is hit by a hurricane. Researchers may be interested in assessing all those who were affected by this event. Who are those persons? Are all persons in the town through which the hurricane passed "affected"? Or would the affected be only persons who saw the hurricane? Or those who had property damage as a result of the hurricane? If the latter is the desired group, how much property damage is sufficient for a person to be considered to be part of the sampling frame? A further complication in defining the relevant sampling frame of interest pertains to mobile populations. For example, in southern Mississippi before Hurricane Katrina hit in 2005, a substantial (and still unknown) proportion of the population was migrant workers, frequently undocumented, who worked in the southern Mississippi casinos. These persons almost certainly left the area after Hurricane Katrina, literally leaving very little trace that they had been there. The extant studies that aimed to characterize mental health of persons in the gulf coast area after Hurricane Katrina almost indisputably undercounted these persons (Galea, et al., 2007). Such challenges in sampling frame definition have long bedeviled postdisaster research, making comparisons between postdisaster studies challenging (Galea, Nandi, & Vlahov, 2005). Central to handling this issue, a clear definition of the sampling frame of interest is needed for each postdisaster research study; careful indication of the range of persons who should be in the sampling frame (by specifying, for example, the exact nature of "exposure" that is an eligibility criterion for a particular study) and, if at all possible, an enumeration of the size of this population must be incorporated.

It is worth noting here that the challenge of defining the relevant population of interest pertains both to general population studies and also to studies of particular populations, such as persons injured in a disaster or rescue workers. While at first glance it may seem easy to define persons injured after a disaster, this is simply not the case. Extending our hurricane example, let us suppose that a particular research project was interested in documenting whether persons who were injured after a hurricane had substance use problems in the long term. Researchers would then be interested in studying all those injured. However, who would be considered injured? Persons who were hospitalized? Perhaps, but hospitalization is a function both of injury severity and of hospital access. Factors such as socioeconomic status and race/ethnicity influence the likelihood of hospitalization; these factors may confound the potential relations of interest, making hospitalization – when used as an eligibility criterion – a potential source of selection bias. What if all persons who had at least some physical injury were considered eligible? After some events, minor injuries, such as corneal abrasions or smoke inhalation, are the most typical injury (Feeney, Goldberg, Blumenthal, & Wallack, 2005). Would all these persons then be eligible? If such minor injuries are considered as part of the eligibility criteria, how might we find such persons, since those with relatively minor injuries are likely never to present to care?

We can extend these observations to studies that are concerned with the mental health of rescue workers after disasters. While the notion of "rescue workers" might suggest fire fighters or police officers, in fact, after many disasters, it is construction workers or maintenance and sanitation workers who spend an inordinate amount of time in disaster areas cleaning up after these events and being exposed to their realities and horrors (Perrin et al., 2007). Clearly, omitting these persons from sampling frames that are concerned with rescue workers would substantially undermine the ability of these sampling frames to represent the population of interest.

34.2.2. Finding Persons

While a central difficulty in designing robust postdisaster research is a clear definition of the population of interest, ancillary and inextricably linked to this conceptual challenge is the logistical challenge of finding persons who may be defined within a sampling frame of interest. There are several reasons why reaching participants may be challenging after disasters. Large disasters may result in population dispersal, scattering potential participants not only throughout the affected disaster area but also potentially throughout the state or country, as was the case after Hurricane Katrina (Galea, et al., 2007; Kessler et al., 2006). Also, the breakdown of typical communication mechanisms, including telephone communication or Internet communication, may make typical means of assessing participants available only in a limited way. Persons affected by disasters may also be busy handling its aftermath. Procuring services, reestablishing homes and employment, and, in large disasters, searching for loved ones are pressing needs of persons in postdisaster situations. These needs leave little time for research participation. Apart from their lack of time, persons in disaster-affected areas may be reluctant to participate in research that is not directly linked to service provision. Nonetheless, as noted earlier, available reports suggest that the vast majority of persons who do participate in such research find their participation rewarding (Newman & Kaloupek, 2004).

Ultimately, once the population of interest is defined, research studies must overcome these hurdles to appropriately sample, find, and collect information from research participants.

Unfortunately, the challenges inherent in doing so have resulted in a preponderance of disaster-related research that has used convenience (purposive) samples (Norris et al., 2002; Norris & Elrod, 2006). Convenience samples typically rely on participants to volunteer for a study, making no attempt to represent all persons who may be eligible. While necessary in some circumstances, particularly in highly unusual events where no other means of accessing participants is possible (North et al., 2005; Perrin et al., 2007), purposive samples have substantial limitations. Potential selection biases – the persons who volunteer to participate may well be different, frequently in unknown ways, from those who do not – limit their usefulness in describing the underlying population of interest. As a consequence, comparison across convenience samples both within the same disaster and across disasters is difficult, making these samples of limited use for scientific generalization and inference.

Several methods have been used to identify persons of interest after disasters and to facilitate sampling that better represents the underlying populations of interest. Each of these methods has their own strengths and weaknesses. Perhaps the most traditional method of finding research participants involves door-to-door sampling and in-person interviews (Bromet & Havenaar, 2006). Door-to-door sampling has the advantage of ensuring that all extant dwellings can be included in a sampling frame, which can be extended to include temporary dwellings, such as mobile homes, if necessary. Furthermore, it does not depend on functioning technology such as telephones. When used in conjunction with in-person interviewing, it can help establish diagnoses through the use of structured diagnostic interviews (Maes, Mylle, Delmeire, & Altamura, 2000). In some instances, it can also facilitate complicated research designs such as assessments of multiple family members or mixed methods designs that include qualitative and quantitative interviews. However, door-to-door sampling is expensive, slow, and dependent on the timely hiring and training of research personnel at the disaster site. It requires in-person access to areas that are frequently inaccessible to all but local residents; in addition, it is not an effective means of reaching persons in areas that have been devastated by disaster and from where local residents have essentially fled.

More recently, postdisaster research studies have used methods such as telephone interviewing and web-based interviewing to reach persons of interest after disasters. The central advantage of these methods is that they are substantially cheaper than in-person methods and that interviewers or researchers may implement them from a distance. These methods, however, have marked weaknesses. Both depend on functioning technology, which is in no way a certainty after disasters. While both telephone and Web-based survey methods were used effectively after the September 11, 2001, terrorist attacks in New York City (Galea, Ahern, Resnick, Kilpatrick, et al., 2002; Galea, et al., 2003; Schlenger et al., 2002; Silver, Holman, McIntosh, Poulin, & Gil-Rivas, 2002), telephone and Web service were very quickly restored in New York City after the terrorist attacks. Therefore, researchers could operate with some confidence that access to these modes of communication was not hindered. Nonetheless, even if postdisaster service is restored to normal levels, both these methods remain limited to persons who actually make use of these modes of communication. While nearly all residents in the United States have phones, Americans are increasingly using only cell phones, which are much harder to access than traditional land lines (see Galea, et al., 2006 for a review of the issues related to telephone sampling postdisasters). In regard to the Internet, a substantial proportion of Americans still do not have access, although this number is decreasing. Those who lack Web access differ from the general population on important characteristics such as age, race/ethnicity, and socioeconomic position (less access among older persons, poorer persons, and minorities). Hence, while both these methods may have utility, their effectiveness is very much dependent upon the particular postdisaster circumstance, and they must be deployed judiciously with these limitations carefully considered.

34.2.3. Special Populations

In our discussion thus far we have largely considered populations as undifferentiated wholes. However, particular populations may be of interest after disasters, each of which may pose specific challenges to researchers. By way of illustration, we consider here a few specific examples – children, marginalized populations, disabled and hospitalized persons, and global populations.

Researchers are beginning to appreciate that children are a particularly understudied group in the context of disasters (Pfefferbaum et al., 2003; Steinberg, Brymer, Steinberg, & Pfefferbaum, 2006), which is partially because of the challenges faced when sampling children. Studying children typically requires consent from both the parents as well as the children, essentially doubling the barrier to enlisting participant cooperation. In addition, children are typically cared for by institutions such as schools or day cares, whose cooperation also needs to be enlisted in order for children to be accessed. Illustrating these challenges, a population-based study of New York City public school children after the September 11th terrorist attacks involved a combination of active consent for older children and parental notification for younger children, together with school board participation (Hoven et al., 2005). Few studies are as well resourced or have the degree of cooperation from authorities as was the case with this study. As a result, relatively few studies have effectively sampled populations of affected children.

Particular challenges are also involved in reaching minority groups and marginalized populations. It is well established that minority populations mistrust authorities in general, which likely extends to researchers. For example, it has been shown that African Americans mistrust physicians' explanation of research more than other races, even after socioeconomic position is taken into account (Corbie-Smith, Thomas, & St George, 2002). Although we are not aware of explicit comparative evidence in postdisaster circumstances to this effect, it is plausible that this mistrust is heightened in these circumstances when social disadvantage and marginalization may be even more prominent, as was the case after Hurricane Katrina. In addition to trust, studies of minority populations must also contend with linguistic and cultural issues. In the context of studies that are being implemented against an immensely challenging logistical backdrop, as noted earlier, this adds an extra complexity to the investigation. In spite of these difficulties, extant work in the area suggests that there are important racial/ethnic differences in mental health consequences of disasters (Adams & Boscarino 2005; Galea et al., 2004). Other groups who may be difficult to recruit but are important to study include homeless persons, mobile populations, and transient young adults (Unger, Kipke, Simon, Montgomery, & Johnson, 1997).

Recent events such as Hurricane Katrina also have raised awareness of the particular challenges that disabled and hospitalized populations face after disasters. Although some studies have considered the particular mental health burden among persons in these groups (DeLisi, Cohen, & Maurizio, 2004), our understanding of well-being among these groups after disasters remains limited. Major difficulty inherent in studying these groups include the need for institutional involvement to gain permission for access and the potential ethical issues with studying persons affected by cognitive or other impairments.

A final point to consider in this area is the particular challenge of studying global populations affected by disasters. Although the focus of this book – and this chapter – is on Western populations broadly and U.S. populations specifically, it has been clearly shown that there is a glaring disparity between the burden of disasters worldwide and the preponderance of disaster research in wealthy countries (DiMaggio & Galea, 2006). For instance, little research was conducted in the aftermath of the Southeast Asian Tsunami of 2006 as compared to U.S.-based events such as the September 11th terrorist attacks. A multitude of reasons underlies this paucity of global work, with many parallels to the challenges discussed previously. In addition, as the majority of research continues to be conducted in wealthier countries, little research infrastructure exists or has been developed in many poorer countries, and what does exist is even further challenged in postdisaster circumstances. Linguistic barriers make the accessibility of populations even harder than after disasters in Western, English-speaking countries. Most measures that are routinely applied in the postdisaster situation were developed and validated in English. Researchers, therefore, must take extra steps to translate, adapt, and validate measures for use across the globe. Different local contexts also pose particular cultural barriers. For example, a series of studies after the Marmara earthquake in Turkey showed that the refusal rate of female potential study participants was higher when interviewees were male than when they were female (Başoğlu, Kilic, Salcıoglu, & Lıvanou, 2004).

34.3. STUDY DESIGN

34.3.1. The Problem of Post-Only Studies

Since most disasters are relatively unexpected, in almost all cases disaster research must contend with studies that are launched only after an event. Some exceptions do exist (Alexander & Wells, 1991; Asarnow et al., 1999; Knight, Gatz, Heller, & Bengtson, 2000), notably where disasters struck areas with preexisting studies that could then be extended postdisaster for a pre/post comparison. However, barring these exceptions, the vast majority of disaster-related mental health research has to rest on post-only designs. This is perhaps the central study design challenge in the field.

Having to rely on post-only designs means that researchers have limited ability to determine the extent to which disasters *caused* the mental health consequences being documented after these events. Although we do not provide a full discussion of causal thinking in this chapter, it is worth noting that modern epidemiologic thinking rests primarily on a counterfactual heuristic. Namely, we consider what might have happened if populations were, or were not, exposed to a full set of experiences present or absent in a putative cause. In many respects, then, disasters provide an ideal natural experiment for determining causation: They are population-based, relatively random events that incur changes likely brought on by the events themselves. However, absent an assessment of what the population of interest was like *before* the event, we are limited in our inference as to whether what we see after an event is truly a *change* or simply a reflection of the predisaster circumstances. Hence, postdisaster-only designs are limited in their assessments to prevalent cases of disease – which include ongoing psychopathology, regardless of the date of manifestation – rather than incident, or "new," cases of disease. Given this uncertainty surrounding disease onset, we can say very little about whether disease documented after disasters is caused by the disaster.

Studies in the field have adopted four central approaches to address this problem. First, most studies have obtained detailed history about the time course of symptoms of psychopathology to determine its onset relative to the disaster event (Bravo et al., 1990). Second, other studies have obtained explicit assessment of pre- and postdisaster behavior and psychological function (Vlahov et al., 2002). Third, some studies have compared postdisaster observations with preestablished estimates of baseline psychopathology in the population (Kessler et al., 2006). Fourth, studies have enrolled nondisaster affected communities to serve as controls, such as Smith, Christiansen, Vincent, and Hann (1999) who compared Indianapolis to Oklahoma City after the Oklahoma City bombing. These methods all have limitations. Retrospective historic assessment is limited to recall bias. Participants inevitably anchor their responses to the disaster event and may provide socially desirable responses, limiting inquiry into pre/post functioning. Comparisons to preexisting baseline estimates assume that these estimates are drawn from similar populations to the postdisaster samples. Similarly, comparisons to control communities are confounded by unmeasured differences between the case and control community that make inference from these studies challenging.

Ultimately, there is no easy solution to the challenge of the post-only study designs that are endemic in the field. Disaster research needs to be implemented with consideration of this challenge, and inference from its observations must be formulated carefully and judiciously, limited to that which can be drawn with confidence from such work.

34.3.2. Optimizing Study Design

Perhaps the key method to maximizing inference from postdisaster studies, bearing in mind the limitations noted here, is optimizing study design. Optimizing study design in the postdisaster context aims to find a balance between the most desirable study design and the study design that is feasible under less than ideal circumstances. Clearly an art underlies the science of research design, and it is one that benefits from the involvement of researchers from different disciplinary perspectives who are experienced in conducting studies after these events.

In an influential review of the postdisaster field, Norris and colleagues (Norris et al., 2002; Norris & Elrod, 2006) showed that nearly three-quarters of studies in the field make use of cross-sectional study design. Cross-sectional study designs are very appealing to those interested in the consequences of disasters because they provide a snapshot at one point in time, thereby producing a measure of the burden of mental health (e.g., Verger et al., 2004). Researchers and practitioners alike frequently seek this information after events. However, as has been noted elsewhere, the disaster mental health field is sufficiently mature that there is little need for more burden-of-disease studies (Galea et al., 2005). In addition, cross-sectional designs have a significant limitation: their inability to definitively establish temporal sequence between the variables being studied. Thus, for example, a cross-sectional study implemented 6 months after a disaster that assesses both depression symptoms and experience of traumatic events may be limited in its inference as to whether depression preceded these experiences or vice versa. Most cross-sectional studies attempt to overcome this limitation by carefully obtaining temporal histories of key experiences and the psychological symptoms assessed. This, however, remains limited by issues of recall bias as noted earlier in our discussion of post-only designs.

Longitudinal study designs overcome some of the challenges inherent in cross-sectional studies by allowing for the assessment of the course of psychopathology, an area of growing interest in the field. These studies are increasingly highlighting the complexity of psychopathology trajectories after disasters, suggesting new areas of both research and intervention (Beard, Tracy, Vlahov, & Galea, 2008; Carr et al., 1997; North, Smith, & Spitznagel, 1997). It is worth noting that postdisaster longitudinal designs do little to overcome the post-only challenge – determining causality – as previously noted. However, by broadening the time course of data collection and potentially assessing the explicit relationship between postdisaster experiences and psychological symptoms, they allow for greater inference to be drawn from postdisaster research. The central challenge with longitudinal studies is logistical: These studies are expensive and frequently bear costs that far exceed the resources available to rapidly develop postdisaster research. Other logistical challenges include the difficulty of tracking and following persons who may be transient, or at least in between residences, in the postdisaster period. Newer analytic methods that take into account follow-up loss may provide the means to deal with some of these limitations (Galea et al., 2008).

Two study designs – case-control and experimental – are seldom used in postdisaster research but may hold particular promise. Case-control study designs are conceptually equivalent to cohort studies but start with case identification; controls that are demographically matched to the cases are then selected. One advantage to case-control methods is the capacity to assess exposures historically since they are nested within the underlying life course of the cohort. This overcomes one of the limitations of cross-sectional studies noted earlier – recall bias. Case-control studies have two primary challenges. First, these methods are largely unfamiliar to the field of disaster mental health research and may require some notable examples before widespread acceptance. Second, case and control identification requires clear specification of the base population, raising all the challenges inherent in defining a sampling frame, noted previously.

The other study design that is underused in the field is the experimental study design. In some respects it is not surprising that there are very few experiments in the postdisaster situation. As noted earlier, sensitivity to potential exploitation of populations affected by disasters is always high after these events, and the notion of "experimenting" on these populations may seem untoward. However, in some respects, we suggest that the notion of *not* experimenting on these populations is much more problematic. Experiments on human populations are generally justified when it is not clear if a particular intervention is beneficial and when the benefit/risk ratio is favorable. Currently few examples of experimental interventional studies have been conducted in the postdisaster context (Başoğlu, Salcioglu, Livanou, Kalender, & Acar, 2005; Bryant, Moulds, & Nixon, 2003; Chemtob, Nakashima, & Carlson, 2002); as a result, evidence as to which interventions may successfully mitigate the consequences of these events is limited. Recent meta-analyses have shown that once common practices such as critical incident stress debriefing may actually do more harm than good (van Emmerik, Kamphuis, Hulsbosch, & Emmelkamp, 2002). These results further emphasize why new therapies, be they psychological or pharmacological, should be subject to rigorous experimental study designs to evaluate whether they are or are not effective in the postdisaster context.

34.4. MEASUREMENT

Research concerned with the mental health consequences of disasters must contend with key issues in measurement that frequently challenge the inferences that can be drawn from this work. We consider three key areas of measurement challenges in the field: measurement of disaster exposure, measurement of relevant covariates, and measurement of the health indicators of interest.

34.4.1. Disaster Exposure

Measurement of disaster exposure is a central part of all postdisaster research. Unfortunately, assessing "exposure" to a disaster is not as simple as it may first seem. Disasters are heterogeneous, and the population exposure within any given disaster may be heterogeneous. For example, the nature of the exposure to a hurricane may be quite different than that of a terrorist attack wherein a building is bombed. In the former, loss of a home and prolonged displacement from home and community may be key exposures; in the latter, loss of friends or family and disability may be key exposures. Hence, exposure to particular disasters is likely unique and must be considered on a disaster-by-disaster basis. Even assuming that the nature of exposure is dependent on broad categories of disaster-types may be problematic; for example, the exposure to one "natural disaster" may be quite different from another. Instead, it may be more fruitful to consider exposures to disaster events as being characterized by specific disaster dimensions, including intensity and duration. Thus, disasters that unfold slowly over time (e.g., Havenaar et al., 1997) may be characterized by prolonged exposure, in stark contrast to point events (e.g., Adams & Boscarino, 2005) wherein the exposure to the actual event may be short-lived. The challenge then is to adequately assess the nature of the exposure that was relevant to the participant in a particular event and to define the specific characteristics of this event. Ancillary to this challenge is the issue of drawing generalizable inference across several studies in the peer-reviewed literature. Given that both the types of exposure and the characteristics of disasters measured may vary amongst studies, comparison across studies must be done judiciously with consideration of these limitations.

Complicating the issue of measuring exposure is the emerging – and potentially important – issue of indirect exposure. Several studies have shown that after large disasters persons who were not directly affected by a disaster may still exhibit symptoms of psychopathology and changes in behavior (Salib, 2003; Schlenger et al., 2002). This raises important nosologic and conceptual challenges about the nature of exposure (Galea & Resnick, 2005). Researchers have suggested that phenomena such as widespread television watching (Ahern et al., 2002; Ahern, Galea, Resnick, & Vlahov, 2004) or perceived threat and relative risk appraisal (Marshall et al., 2007) may mediate the relation between indirect exposure to a disaster event and the consequences that have been typically associated with directly exposed persons only. Future postdisaster work that rigorously assesses the potential mechanisms that may mediate the relation between indirect disaster exposure and mental health would greatly strengthen the field.

34.4.2. Covariate Assessment

The challenge with covariate assessment in postdisaster research is not particularly different than the challenge faced by all studies in covariate assessment, but it is heightened by the relative paucity of research after any given disaster. Centrally, the covariates that are assessed in postdisaster studies frequently differ from study to study. While certain factors such as gender are measured quite reliably (Catapano et al., 2001), others such as peri-event emotional reactions are not (Pfefferbaum, Stuber, Galea, & Fairbrother, 2006). In addition, studies frequently operationalize covariates differently. The differential measurement and inclusion of covariates again results in challenges for cross-study comparability. This is best understood by reflecting on the reason for covariate assessment. Fundamentally, if postdisaster mental health research is concerned with understanding the relation between disasters and psychopathology, part of this work includes assessment of covariates that may be confounders (or alternate explanations), mediators, or modifiers of this relation of central interest. Hence, when a covariate set for a particular study is chosen, implicit assumptions are made about the structure of the relation between disasters and psychopathology, and the results may not be replicable for a study that assesses different covariates. In nondisaster research, the sheer number of comparable studies available overcomes this limitation. However, in postdisaster research, when there are typically only a handful of studies after any one particular event, this challenge is accentuated and frequently makes for noncomparability of studies of the same disaster event and across disaster events.

34.4.3. Health Indicators

The final measurement challenge pertains to measurement of the health indicators of interest. This book is concerned with the mental health consequences of disasters; therefore, the challenges inherent in all research assessment of mental health and function are also relevant in this area (Eaton 2002; Murphy 2002). For example, many approaches and measures are relevant to the assessment of posttraumatic stress disorder (PTSD), likely the sentinel disaster psychopathology (Brewin & Holmes, 2003; Brunello et al., 2001), but all are not equally valid. Perhaps the key measurement challenge of health indicators that is particular to postdisaster research is fully characterizing the range of psychopathology that may be present after these events. Although most postdisaster research is concerned with PTSD (Norris et al., 2002), it is increasingly recognized that this disorder seldom occurs in isolation and is often accompanied by comorbidity (Breslau, Chase, & Anthony, 2002; Goenjian et al., 1995). Thus, postdisaster studies need to consider a range of mental disorders to comprehensively assess mental health after these events. Unexplained medical symptoms and somatization pose further challenges to the accurate characterization of the full range of psychopathology after disasters (Foa, Stein, & McFarlane, 2006).

Finally, we note that we limit this discussion largely to postdisaster assessments that center around interview measures. Although the number remains small, studies in the field are increasingly incorporating biological measures in an attempt to assess the relationship between factors at all levels – genetic, molecular, and behavioral – and mental health and functioning after these events (Galea, Acierno, et al., 2006; Kilpatrick et al., 2007). Of course, inclusion of biological markers in these studies raises its own set of issues pertaining to the accuracy of these measures and to the challenges inherent in feasibly and reliably obtaining valid biological samples from the persons of interest. While a full discussion of the measurement issues that pertain to biological specimens is beyond the scope of this chapter, we suspect that in the coming years this will become an increasingly important area in the field.

34.5. ANALYSIS

A full consideration of the methodological challenges in postdisaster research must consider the analysis of these studies. Ultimately most of the analytic issues faced by this field arise from the challenges already discussed in this chapter in terms of population sampling, study design, and measurement.

34.5.1. Population Sampling

The particular challenges inherent in identifying and finding the population of interest in this work also lead to analytic challenges when data is collected. Study samples that are not representative of base populations may need to be suitably weighted, assuming that the characteristics of the base population are known. Low response rates, generally endemic in population-based samples (Galea & Tracy, 2007) despite efforts at incentivising participation (Bentley & Thacker, 2004), may also result in nonrepresentative samples that may need to be statistically adjusted. Studies that oversample special populations also may benefit from weighting. Importantly, however, no amount of statistical adjustment can correct for samples that are not representative and not adequately grounded in a clear understanding of the base population of interest.

34.5.2. Study Design

There are particular analytic concerns that pertain to all study designs. As noted earlier, cross-sectional designs, by far the most common study design in the field, are limited in their ability to establish temporality and to distinguish between prevalent and incident cases. This raises challenges for handling covariates within one cohesive analytic framework. The typical epidemiologic study design is concerned with dependent ("exposure") and independent ("outcome") variables, assuming a linear unidirectional relation that is then subjected to a regression-type mode to determine multivariate associations. However, in cross-sectional designs that measure variables that may not be temporally distinct, the assumptions underlying such analytic approaches – including independence of predictors and unidirectional relations between predictors and outcomes – are invalid, rendering the entire analytic exercise suspect. This concern is not particular to the field of disaster mental health but is rather an issue in all analyses that adopt these approaches. Alternate approaches to analyses that consider different interrelations between variables (e.g., multiagent based models) could have utility, but few such methods are in widespread use. Longitudinal designs can overcome these concerns and in theory may face fewer analytic challenges than cross-sectional designs. However, in practice, longitudinal designs in the postdisaster setting raise challenges for rigorous analysis. The difficulties inherent in following participants in these situations often result in a rate of loss to follow-up that requires data imputation procedures to account for potential biases (Galea et al., 2008). Work that moves toward understanding trajectories of mental health over time may benefit from latent class trajectory analyses and the use of analytic methods that take into account time-varying and time-to-event analyses.

34.5.3. Measurement

Two key analytic issues apply to measurement. First, a reliance on unidirectional models, in this field and in others, has frequently obscured complicated relationships and confused important mediators with confounders (Galea & Ahern, 2006). For example, the role of peri-event emotional reactions in determining posttraumatic stress after disasters remains largely unexplored. We suggest this in large part because peri-event emotional reactions are typically treated as confounders in unidirectional models applied to data from cross-sectional studies (Pfefferbaum et al., 2006). It is possible, and perhaps likely, that emotional reactions mediate the relation between traumatic event experiences and psychopathology. Therefore, this requires analytic approaches, such as structural equation models, that adequately assess different potential structural forms of this relation. Second, while the measurement of disaster exposure is becoming increasingly sophisticated, our analytic handling of this exposure remains limited to simple dichotomies (presence vs. absence of a particular exposure) or cumulative exposure scales that assign quantitative values to different types of exposure in a manner that almost certainly does not represent reality. To address some of these issues, researchers should consider using analyses, such as latent class analyses, that can more accurately characterize different exposure *types* and consider how these types influence mental health after disasters.

34.6. CONCLUSION

Substantial methodological challenges are inherent in the study of mental health consequences of disasters. These challenges arise primarily out of the difficulties in the establishment of research after disasters and out of the nature of disasters themselves. For example, the unexpectedness of disasters largely leads to postdisaster only designs being the only feasible research approach. While the logistical challenges that face researchers after disasters are not likely to change, we hope that their identification can serve to help researchers plan for postdisaster work and, through this planning, embark upon more productive and scientifically important research. Identifying and sampling the populations of interest after these events is frequently problematic, as is designing studies that sample and follow these populations forward in time. Future work may most fruitfully consider population-representative samples that include a longitudinal component to allow for the assessment of trajectories of psychopathology. Case-control studies and interventional designs also have tremendous potential in the field. Future work that addresses measurement issues of exposure and mental health indicators by considering dimensional measures of exposure, a range of health indicators to account for potential comorbidity, and covariates that may confound, mediate, or modify the central relations of interest has the potential to move the field forward substantially. Finally, key analytic issues include the need to statistically account for imperfect sampling and complicated nonlinear relations among variables; doing so may require the use of methods that extend beyond our current exposure-outcome paradigm. While challenging, such work holds promise in leading the way toward a greater understanding of the pathways that link disaster exposure to its mental health consequences.

REFERENCES

Adams, R. E., & Boscarino, J. A. (2005). Differences in mental health outcomes among Whites, African Americans, and Hispanics following a community disaster. *Psychiatry, 68*(3), 250–265.

Ahern, J., Galea, S., Resnick, H., Kilpatrick, D., Bucuvalas, M., Gold, J., et al. (2002). Television images and psychological symptoms after the September 11 terrorist attacks. *Psychiatry, 65* (4), 289–300.

Ahern, J., Galea, S., Resnick, H., & Vlahov, D. (2004). Television images and probable posttraumatic stress disorder after September 11: The role of background characteristics, event exposures, and perievent panic. *Journal of Nervous and Mental Disease, 192*(3), 217–226.

Alexander, D. A., & Wells, A. (1991). Reactions of police officers to body-handling after a major disaster. A before-and-after comparison. *British Journal of Psychiatry, 159*, 547–555.

Asarnow, J., Glynn, S., Pynoos, R. S., Nahum, J., Guthrie, D., Cantwell, D. P., et al. (1999). When the earth stops shaking: Earthquake sequelae among children diagnosed for pre-earthquake psychopathology. *Journal of the American Academy of Child and Adolescent Psychiatry, 38*(8), 1016–1023.

Başoğlu, M., Kiliç, C., Salcioğlu, E., & Livanou, M. (2004). Prevalence of posttraumatic stress disorder and comorbid depression in earthquake survivors in Turkey: An epidemiological study. *Journal of Traumatic Stress, 17*(2), 133–141.

Başoğlu, M., Salcioğlu, E., Livanou, M., Kalender, D., & Acar, G. (2005). Single-session behavioral treatment of earthquake-related posttraumatic stress disorder: Randomized waiting list controlled trial. *Journal of Traumatic Stress, 18*(1), 1–11.

Beard J, Tracy M, Vlahov D, & Galea S. (In press). Patterns and predictors of depression in a population-based prospective cohort study of urban residents. Annals of Epidemiology.

Beard, J. R., Tracy, M., Vlahov, D., & Galea, S. (In press). Trajectory and socioeconomic predictors of depression in a prospective study of residents of New York City. *Annals of Epidemiology*.

Bentley, J. P., & Thacker, P. G. (2004). The influence of risk and monetary payment on the research participation decision making process. *Journal of Medical Ethics, 30*(3), 293–298.

Boscarino, J. A., Adams, R. E., Stuber, J., & Galea, S. (2005). Disparities in mental health treatment following the World Trade Center Disaster: Implications for mental health care and health services research. *Journal of Traumatic Stress, 18*(4), 287–297.

Bravo, M., Rubio-Stipec, M., Canino, G. J., Woodbury, M. A., & Ribera, J. C. (1990). The psychological sequelae of disaster stress prospectively and retrospectively evaluated. *American Journal of Community Psychology, 18*(5), 661–680.

Breslau, N., Chase, G. A., & Anthony, J. C. (2002). The uniqueness of the DSM definition of post-traumatic stress disorder: Implications for research. *Psychological Medicine, 32*(4), 573–576.

Brewin, C. R., & Holmes, E. A. (2003). Psychological theories of posttraumatic stress disorder. *Clinical Psychology Review, 23*(3), 339–376.

Bromet, E. J., & Havenaar, J. M. (2006). Basic epidemiological approaches to disaster research: value of face-to-face procedures. In F. H. Norris, S. Galea, M. J. Friedman, & P. J. Watson (Eds.), *Methods for disaster mental health research*. New York: The Guilford Press.

Brunello, N., Davidson, J. R., Deahl, M., Kessler, R. C., Mendlewicz, J., Racagni, G., et al. (2001). Posttraumatic stress disorder: Diagnosis and epidemiology, comorbidity and social consequences, biology and treatment. *Neuropsychobiology 43*(3), 150–162.

Bryant, R. A., Moulds, M. L., & Nixon, R. V. (2003). Cognitive behaviour therapy of acute stress disorder: A four-year follow-up. *Behavior Research and Therapy, 41*(4), 489–494.

Carr, V. J., Lewin, T. J., Kenardy, J. A., Webster, R. A., Hazell, P. L., Carter, G. L., et al. (1997). Psychosocial sequelae of the 1989 Newcastle earthquake: III. Role of vulnerability factors in post-disaster morbidity. *Psychological Medicine, 27*(1), 179–190.

Catapano, F., Malafronte, R., Lepre, F., Cozzolino, P., Arnone, R., Lorenzo, E., et al. (2001). Psychological consequences of the 1998 landslide in Sarno, Italy: A community study. *Acta Psychiatrica Scandinavica, 104*(6), 438–442.

Chemtob, C. M., Nakashima, J., & Carlson, J. G. (2002). Brief treatment for elementary school children with disaster-related posttraumatic stress disorder: A field study. *Journal of Clinical Psychology, 58*(1), 99–112.

Corbie-Smith, G., Thomas, S. B., & St George, D. M. (2002). Distrust, race, and research. *Archives of Internal Medicine, 162*(21), 2458–2463.

DeLisi, L. E., Cohen, T. H., & Maurizio, A. M. (2004). Hospitalized psychiatric patients view the World Trade Center disaster. *Psychiatry Research, 129*(2), 201–207.

DiMaggio, C., & Galea, S. (2006). The behavioral con sequences of terrorism: A meta-analysis. *Academy of Emergency Medicine, 13*(5), 559–566.

Eaton, W. W. (2002). Studying the natural history of psychopathology. In M. T. Tsuang, & M. Tohen (Eds.), *Textbook in psychiatry epidemiology*. New York: Wiley-Liss, Inc.

Feeney, J. M., Goldberg, R., Blumenthal, J. A., & Wallack, M. K. (2005). September 11, 2001, revisited: A review of the data. *Archives of Surgery, 140*(11), 1068–1073.

Foa, E. B., Stein, D. J., & McFarlane, A. C. (2006). Symptomatology and psychopathology of mental health problems after disaster. *Journal of Clinical Psychiatry, 67* (Suppl. 2), 15–25.

Galea, S., Acierno, R., Ruggiero, K., Resnick, H., Tracy, M., & Kilpatrick, D. (2006). Social context and the psychobiology of posttraumatic stress. *Annals of the New York Academy of Science, 1071*, 231–241.

Galea, S., & Ahern, J. (2006). Invited commentary: Considerations about specificity of associations, causal pathways, and heterogeneity in multilevel thinking. *American Journal of Epidemiology, 163*(12), 1079–1082.

Galea, S., Ahern, J., Resnick, H., Kilpatrick, D., Bucuvalas, M., Gold, J., et al. (2002). Psychological sequelae of the September 11 terrorist attacks in New York City. *New England Journal of Medicine, 346*(13), 982–987.

Galea, S., Ahern, J., Tracy, M., Hubbard, A., Cerda, M., Goldmann, E., et al. (2008). Longitudinal determinants of posttraumatic stress in a population-based cohort study. *Epidemiology, 19*(1), 47–54.

Galea, S., Brewin, C. R., Gruber, M., Jones, R. T., King, D. W., King, L. A., et al. (2007). Exposure to hurricane-related stressors and mental illness after Hurricane Katrina. *Archives of General Psychiatry*, *64*(12), 1427–1434.

Galea, S., Bucuvalas, M., Resnick, H., Boyle, J., Vlahov, D., & Kilpatrick, D. (2006). Telephone-based research methods in disaster research. In F.H. Norris S. Galea, M.J. Friedman, & P.J. Watson (Eds.), *Methods for disaster mental health research*. New York: The Guilford Press.

Galea, S., Nandi, A., Stuber, J., Gold, J., Acierno, R., Best, C.L., et al. (2005). Participant reactions to survey research in the general population after terrorist attacks. *Journal of Traumatic Stress*, *18*(5), 461–465.

Galea, S., Nandi, A., & Vlahov, D. (2005). The epidemiology of post-traumatic stress disorder after disasters. *Epidemiologic Reviews*, *27*, 78–91.

Galea, S., & Resnick, H. (2005). Posttraumatic stress disorder in the general population after mass terrorist incidents: considerations about the nature of exposure. *CNS Spectrums*, *10* (2), 107–115.

Galea, S., & Tracy, M. (2007). Participation rates in epidemiologic studies. *Annals of Epidemiology*, *17* (9), 643–653.

Galea, S., Vlahov, D., Resnick, H., Ahern, J., Susser, E., Gold, J., et al. (2003). Trends of probable post-traumatic stress disorder in New York City after the September 11 terrorist attacks. *American Journal of Epidemiology*, *158*(6), 514–524.

Galea, S., Vlahov, D., Resnick, H., Kilpatrick, D., Bucuvalas, M.J., Morgan, M.D., et al. (2002). An investigation of the psychological effects of the September 11, 2001, attacks on New York City: Developing and implementing research in the acute postdisaster period. *CNS Spectrums*, *7*(8), 585–587, 593–596.

Galea, S., Vlahov, D., Tracy, M., Hoover, D.R., Resnick, H., & Kilpatrick, D. (2004). Hispanic ethnicity and post-traumatic stress disorder after a disaster: Evidence from a general population survey after September 11, 2001. *Annals of Epidemiology*, *14*(8), 520–531.

Goenjian, A. (1993). A mental health relief programme in Armenia after the 1988 earthquake. Implementation and clinical observations. *British Journal of Psychiatry*, *163*, 230–239.

Goenjian, A.K., Pynoos, R.S., Steinberg, A.M., Najarian, L.M., Asarnow, J.R., Karayan, I., et al. (1995). Psychiatric comorbidity in children after the 1988 earthquake in Armenia. *Journal of the American Academy of Child and Adolescent Psychiatry*, *34*(9), 1174–1184.

Havenaar, J.M., Rumyantzeva, G.M., van den Brink, W., Poelijoe, N.W., van den Bout, J., van Engeland, H., et al. (1997). Long-term mental health effects of the Chernobyl disaster: An epidemiologic survey in two former Soviet regions. *American Journal of Psychiatry*, *154*(11), 1605–1607.

Hoven, C.W., Duarte, C.S., Lucas, C.P., Wu, P., Mandell, D.J., Goodwin, R.D., et al. (2005). Psychopathology among New York city public school children 6 months after September 11. *Archives of General Psychiatry*, *62*(5), 545–552.

Kessler, R.C., Galea, S., Jones, R.T., Parker, H.A., & Hurricane Katrina Community Advisory Group. (2006). Mental illness and suicidality after Hurricane Katrina. *Bulletin of the World Health Organization*, *84*(12), 930–939.

Kilpatrick, D.G., Koenen, K.C., Ruggiero, K. J., Acierno, R., Galea, S., Resnick, H.S., et al. (2007). The serotonin transporter genotype and social support and moderation of posttraumatic stress disorder and depression in hurricane-exposed adults. *American Journal of Psychiatry*, *164*(11), 1693–1699.

Knight, B.G., Gatz, M., Heller, K., & Bengtson, V.L. (2000). Age and emotional response to the Northridge earthquake: A longitudinal analysis. *Psychology and Aging*, *15*(4), 627–634.

Maes, M., Mylle, J., Delmeire, L., & Altamura, C. (2000). Psychiatric morbidity and comorbidity following accidental man-made traumatic events: Incidence and risk factors. *European Archives of Psychiatry and Clinical Neuroscience*, *250*(3), 156–162.

Marshall, R.D., Bryant, R.A., Amsel, L., Suh, E.J., Cook, J.M., & Neria, Y. (2007). The psychology of ongoing threat: Relative risk appraisal, the September 11 attacks, and terrorism-related fears. *American Psychologist*, *62*(4), 304–316.

Murphy, J.M. (2002). Symptom scales and diagnostic schedules in adult psychiatry. In M. T. Tsuang & M. Tohen (Eds.), *Textbook in psychiatry epidemiology*. New York: Wiley-Liss, Inc.

Newman, E., & Kaloupek, D.G. (2004). The risks and benefits of participating in trauma-focused research studies. *Journal of Traumatic Stress*, *17*(5), 383–394.

Newman, E., Walker, E.A., & Gefland, A. (1999). Assessing the ethical costs and benefits of trauma-focused research. *General Hospital Psychiatry*, *21*(3), 187–196.

Norris, F.H., & Elrod, C.L. (2006). Psychosocial consequences of disaster: A review of past research. In F.H. Norris, S. Galea, M.J. Friedman, & P.J. Watson (Eds.), *Methods for disaster mental health research*. New York: The Guilford Press.

Norris, F.H., Friedman, M.J., Watson, P.J., Byrne, C.M., Diaz, E., & Kaniasty, K. (2002). 60,000 disaster victims speak: Part I. An empirical review of the empirical literature, 1981–2001. *Psychiatry*, *65*(3), 207–239.

Norris, F.H., Galea, S., Friedman, M.J., & Watson, P.J. (Eds.) (2006). *Methods for disaster mental health research*. New York: The Guilford Press.

North, C.S., Pfefferbaum, B., Narayanan, P., Thielman, S., McCoy, G., Dumont, C., et al. (2005). Comparison of post-disaster psychiatric disorders after terrorist bombings in Nairobi and Oklahoma City. *British Journal of Psychiatry, 186*, 487–493.

North, C.S., Smith, E.M., & Spitznagel, E.L. (1997). One-year follow-up of survivors of a mass shooting. *American Journal of Psychiatry, 154*(12), 1696–1702.

Perrin, M.A., DiGrande, L., Wheeler, K., Thorpe, L., Farfel, M., & Brackbill, R. (2007). Differences in PTSD prevalence and associated risk factors among World Trade Center disaster rescue and recovery workers. *American Journal of Psychiatry, 164*(9), 1385–1394.

Pfefferbaum, B., Pfefferbaum, R.L., Gurwitch, R.H., Nagumalli, S., Brandt, E.N., Robertson, M.J., et al. (2003). Children's response to terrorism: A critical review of the literature. *Current Psychiatry Reports*, 5(2), 95–100.

Pfefferbaum, B., Stuber, J., Galea, S., & Fairbrother, G. (2006). Panic reactions to terrorist attacks and probable posttraumatic stress disorder in adolescents. *Journal of Traumatic Stress, 19*(2), 217–228.

Salib, E. (2003). Effect of 11 September 2001 on suicide and homicide in England and Wales. *British Journal of Psychiatry, 183*, 207–212.

Schlenger, W.E., Caddell, J.M., Ebert, L., Jordan, B.K., Rourke, K.M., Wilson, D., et al. (2002). Psychological reactions to terrorist attacks: Findings from the National Study of Americans' Reactions to September 11. *Journal of the American Medical Association, 288*(5), 581–588.

Silver, R.C., Holman, E.A., McIntosh, D.N., Poulin, M., & Gil-Rivas, V. (2002). Nationwide longitudinal study of psychological responses to September 11. *Journal of the American Medical Association, 288*(10), 1235–1244.

Smith, D.W., Christiansen, E.H., Vincent, R., & Hann, N.E. (1999). Population effects of the bombing of Oklahoma City. *Journal of the Oklahoma State Medical Association, 92*(4), 193–198.

Steinberg, A.M., Brymer, M.J., Steinberg, J.R., & Pfefferbaum, B. (2006). Conducting research with children and adolescents after disaster. In F.H. Norris, S. Galea, M. J. Friedman, & P.J. Watson (Eds.), *Methods for disaster mental health research*. New York: The Guilford Press.

Unger, J.B., Kipke, M.D., Simon, T.R., Montgomery, S.B., & Johnson, C.J. (1997). Homeless youths and young adults in Los Angeles: Prevalence of mental health problems and the relationship between mental health and substance abuse disorders. *American Journal of Community Psychology, 25*(3), 371–394.

Ursano, R.J., Fullerton, C.S., Weisaeth, L., & Raphael, B. (Eds.) (2007). *Textbook of disaster psychiatry*. New York: Cambridge University Press.

van Emmerik, A.A., Kamphuis, J.H., Hulsbosch, A.M., & Emmelkamp, P.M. (2002). Single session debriefing after psychological trauma: A meta-analysis. *Lancet, 360*(9335), 766–771.

Vlahov, D., Galea, S., Resnick, H., Ahern, J., Boscarino, J.A., Bucuvalas, M., et al. (2002). Increased use of cigarettes, alcohol, and marijuana among Manhattan, New York, residents after the September 11th terrorist attacks. *American Journal of Epidemiology, 155*(11), 988–996.

Verger, P., Dab, W., Lamping, D.L., Loze, J.Y., Deschaseaux-Voinet, C., Abenhaim, L., et al. (2004). The psychological impact of terrorism: An epidemiologic study of posttraumatic stress disorder and associated factors in victims of the 1995–1996 bombings in France. *American Journal of Psychiatry, 161*(8), 1384–1389.

35 Disaster Mental Health Research: Current State, Gaps in Knowledge, and Future Directions

YUVAL NERIA, SANDRO GALEA, AND FRAN H. NORRIS

35.1. INTRODUCTION

Disasters affect many lives and reshape environments for years to come. This chapter aims to provide closing remarks about the evidence provided in this book, on what is known and not known about the impact of disasters on mental and physical health, the differential risk of certain populations and communities, and the determinants of vulnerability and resilience. We also look at lessons learned to date about intervention strategies that mitigate the mental health consequences of these events. Finally, we provide clear recommendations about critical gaps in knowledge and ways to address them going forward.

35.2. EXPOSURE

The mental health impact of disasters is strongly related to the scope of the disaster itself. In this book, Norris and Wind (Chapter 3) systematically review a host of factors that typically comprise exposure in disasters and categorize them into three groups: (1) traumatic stressors, such as loss of life, threats to life, injury, witnessing and horror; (2) loss of property, finances, or other resources, which may often follow floods, hurricanes, and fire; and (3) ongoing adversities, from lack of housing, displacement, and relocation to chronic stress. These potentially are involved in the development and persistence of mental and physical health outcomes, as well as in resilience and recovery processes (see Part Two and Three).

Importantly, a large body of research has documented the effects of indirect exposure to disasters, challenging previous definitions of exposure and leading to scientific debate about the accuracy of such findings and their meaning. Beyond the individual level, disasters negatively affect large communities (Norris, 2006) potentially through indirect routes such as media coverage (Ahern et al., 2002; Ahern, Galea, Resnick, & Vlahov, 2004; Neria et al., 2007). While a relationship between indirect exposure and psychopathology has been documented (e.g., Galea et al., 2002; Schlenger et al., 2002; Silver, Holman, McIntosh, Poulin, & Gil-Rivas, 2002), the question of whether indirect exposure is independently associated with adverse mental health consequences without confounding from other risk factors (e.g., prior trauma exposure; psychiatrist history) has yet to be fully answered (Neria et al., 2006).

35.3. PSYCHOPATHOLOGY

The emotional sequelae of disasters may be enduring and debilitating. The chapters in this book review the research that has documented a range of postdisaster mental health problems, including posttraumatic stress disorder (PTSD), depression and prolonged grief disorder, substance abuse, and physical illness. Subsequently, we highlight the key advances and future directions in each domain.

35.3.1. Posttraumatic Stress Disorder

PTSD is the psychiatric disorder most often studied in the aftermath of disasters. Across all types of disasters (natural, technological, human-made), PTSD has been found to be common and highly associated with exposure type and severity (Galea, Nandi, & Vlahov, 2005; Neria, Nandi, & Galea, 2008; Norris, Friedman, et al., 2002). Disaster type, duration, and severity may have differential impact on PTSD outcomes. For example, human-made disasters, characterized by large displays of violence, may cause a greater burden of psychopathology as compared to natural and technological incidents (Galea et al., 2005; Neria et al., 2008). Symptoms and disease burden generally decrease over time (e.g., Galea et al., 2003), but certain populations may maintain higher prevalence rates of PTSD over time (see Part Four).

35.3.2. Depression

Several disaster-related stressors may be particularly associated with depressive symptoms (Chapter 7). Loss of life and displacement (van Griensven et al., 2006), relocation (Kilic et al., 2006), lack of social support (Tak, Driscoll, Bernard, & West, 2007), or being alone (Ahern & Galea, 2006; Tak et al., 2007) have been found to exacerbate risk for depression among populations affected by disasters. However, our understanding of risk for depression postdisaster is limited by a paucity of predisaster data on prevalence rates and risk factors of this disorder. Moreover, only a few studies have examined trajectories of depression over time (Person, Tracy, & Galea, 2006). More thorough research on the course of depression following disasters will help to improve understanding of whether trajectories of PTSD and major depressive disorder postdisaster are differentially associated with risk factors.

35.3.3. Prolonged Grief

Loss of life is one of the most traumatic experiences associated with disaster and has been shown to be associated with a host of psychiatric disorders such as PTSD, depression, and other psychopathology domains (Chapter 3). However, grief-specific responses, their prevalence, and correlates have received only limited scientific attention. Prolonged grief disorder (PGD), also named complicated or traumatic grief, is a relatively new diagnosis, and different from normal grief in its lengthy duration and specific symptom profile (Horowitz et al., 1997). PGD also differs from PTSD and depression (Prigerson et al., 1996) in that it contributes to functional problems above and beyond these disorders (Bonanno, Neria, Mancini, Coifman, & Litz, 2007) and commonly results in severe functional impairment, decreased productivity, suicidality, and physical health problems (Lichtenthal, Cruess, & Prigerson, 2004). Studies conducted following the attacks of September 11th indicate a robust presence of PGD in people who had lost loved ones as a result of the attacks – 44% at 1.5 years after the attacks (Shear, Jackson, Essock, Donahue, & Felton, 2006) and 43% at 2.5 to 3.5 years afterward (Neria et al., 2007). While PGD is loss-specific, an important question yet to be answered is whether exposure to disaster trauma interacts with loss in exacerbating the response (Neria & Litz, 2004). More research is needed to fully understand the relations between trauma and loss, PTSD, and prolonged grief and whether they differ in their risk and protective factors.

35.3.4. Substance Use

Trauma exposure is often associated with increased substance abuse, either directly or indirectly through increased substance use associated with PTSD. Yet, research on substance use after disasters has received significantly less attention than either PTSD or depression. The available evidence, reviewed in this book by Van Velden and Kleber (Chapter 6), has mostly focused on human-made disasters and terrorism (e.g., Nandi, Galea, Ahern, & Vlahov, 2005; Vlahov et al., 2004; Vlahov et al., 2006). Though limited, existing research does not indicate that exposure to disasters results in a substantial increase in substance use; further, reported increases in substances, such as tobacco, alcohol, and drugs, are typically restricted to predisaster users, and the increase in the prevalence of substance use postdisaster generally declines over time.

While substance use can appear to be comorbid with PTSD and depression postdisaster, the true relationship with each of those disorders is unclear. Interestingly, emerging evidence suggests that smoking after disasters predicts later PTSD (Van der Velden, Kleber, & Koenen, 2008). In contrast, one study found that consuming alcohol during a disaster may be protective against the development of PTSD. The field would greatly benefit from well-designed, prospective examination of the relationships between different substances, different disaster-related disorders, and the temporal development of those relationships.

35.3.5. Physical Illness

There are consequences of disasters that extend beyond adverse mental illness. In Chapter 5, Yzermans and colleagues suggest that exposure to disaster is linked to one or more physical health effects including (1) exacerbation of predisaster health problems; (2) immediate health problems due to acute exposure (e.g., eye, hearing, and pulmonary problems); (3) short-term effects that are not related to injuries; (4) midterm effects (first year), which represents a chronic course, potentially comorbid with chronic psychiatric effects; and (5) long-term physical problems (e.g., fatigue, back pain, hypertension, diabetes mellitus). Also in their review, Yzermans and colleagues found that among healthy people, the prevalence of physical symptoms after disasters range widely between 3% and 78%, while symptoms of headache and fatigue appear to be more common than dyspnea or skin problems. Although much of the disparity in these estimates can be accounted for by timing and type of measurement used, type of disaster has a significant impact on these outcomes as well. For example when methyl isocynate, an element of pesticides, leaked from a plant in Bhopal, India, during the 1984 disaster, significant neurological, reproductive, and neurobehavioral effects were observed over time among exposed populations (Dhara & Dhara, 2002).

To accurately detect postdisaster effects on physical health, it is essential to assess individuals who already have physical illness when disaster strikes as compared with those who were healthy. For individuals with chronic diseases, disasters tend to aggravate the symptoms and conditions already present (Norris, Friedman, et al., 2002). In addition, studying the course of physical symptoms may significantly enhance the understanding of long-term effects of disasters. For example, the prevalence of symptoms indicating discomfort such as headaches and fatigue tend to decrease overtime in disaster-exposed populations (Chapter 5). It is not yet clear whether spikes in prevalence of physical symptoms shortly after the disaster are followed by decreases over time. More research is clearly needed on these issues to guide early recognition and treatment of physical morbidity resulting from disasters.

35.4. RESILIENCE AND RECOVERY

Remarkably, across most trauma types, including disasters, a significant proportion of the population is minimally affected and able to adapt to adverse circumstances. *Resilience* is defined as the human ability to maintain stable, healthy levels of psychological and physical functioning following a potentially highly disruptive event (Bonanno, 2004), and resilient individuals postdisaster manifest only transient, mild, stress reactions, which are not likely to significantly interfere with continued functioning and are typically of short duration (Bisconti, Bergeman, & Boker, 2006; Bonanno, Field, Kovacevic, & Kaltman, 2002; Bonnano, Moskowitz, Papa, & Folkman, 2005; Bonanno, Rennicke, & Dekel, 2005; Ong, Bergeman, Bisconti, & Wallace, 2006). *Recovery* from initial symptomatology occurs when individuals show elevated levels of psychological symptoms for several months before returning to a pretrauma baseline (Bonnano & Gupta, in press). The trend toward a decrease in symptomatology over time found for various outcomes, including PTSD (Carr et al., 1997; Galea et al., 2003), depression (Person et al., 2006), and somatic complaints (Foa, Stein, & McFarlane, 2006; Chapter 5), can be explained by this response pattern. When taken together, the net result of resilience and recovery is that only a small portion of the population will manifest long-term psychological difficulties.

Research has identified factors associated with effective coping during exposure and reduced psychopathology in its aftermath, including personality traits, such as attachment style and hardiness (Neria et al., 2001), cognitive attributional style (Dohrenwend et al., 2004), and a range of biological factors (Haglund, Nestadt, Cooper, Southwick, & Charney, 2007). A prospective study conducted by Neria and colleagues (2001) among 434 young Israeli adults recruited for an elite military unit may shed light on the role that personality traits can play under exposure to extreme stress. The study examined the complementary role of attachment style (Bowlby, 1980, 1982) and hardiness (Kobasa, Maddi, & Kahn, 1982) in exposure to stress and mental health outcomes. The findings suggest that individuals with secure attachment style manifest greater hardiness under stress (e.g., enhanced commitment and control), while avoidant and ambivalent attachment styles were negatively associated with these factors. In addition, secure attachment style and hardiness were positively associated with mental health and well-being and negatively associated with distress and general psychiatric symptomatology; avoidant and ambivalent styles were inversely related to mental health and well-being and positively related to distress and general psychiatric symptomatology. In a separate cross-sectional study of the role of those constructs play in postwar captivity mental health, the study team (Zakin, Solomon, & Neria, 2003) replicated the protective role of secure attachment style and hardiness in PTSD levels 18 years after war captivity.

Resilience to trauma may be further enhanced by the capacity to appraise the exposure as beneficial. Positive appraisals (e.g., "I was highly benefited by the experience of the war") recast the meaning of the experience in a positive light and may highlight a sense of mastery or control. In a study by Dohrenwend and colleagues (2004), the majority of the U.S. males who served in Vietnam suggested that their war time experiences affected their current lives in positive ways; however, those with negative appraisals had the highest rates of negative outcomes 15 years after the war, suggesting that the valence of the post-trauma cognitions may significantly mediate the impact of exposure to trauma on mental health.

Human beings possess an impressive capacity to adapt to adverse situations. Research with disaster victims and survivors of other traumas helps to illuminate our understanding of the factors that influence healthy outcomes in the majority of the population. Armed with this knowledge, professionals from multiple disciplines will be able to develop both prevention and intervention techniques that capitalize on innate strengths to overcome adverse situations.

35.5. SOCIAL AND COGNITIVE PROCESSES

In a critical review of the disaster literature, Benight, Cieslak, and Waldrep (Chapter 10) review prominent social and cognitive theoretical frameworks that have guided empirical examination of the mental health consequences of disaster. Among the most influential are studies on the role of the perceptions of self (Benight & Bandura, 2004) and collective efficacy (Benight, 2004), coping self-efficacy (Benight et al., 1999; Janoff-Bulmann, 1992), and the transactional theory of stress (Lazarus, 1966, Lazarus & Folkman, 1984). A central theory attempting to examine the factors involved in predicting exposure to stress is the conservation of resources (COR) theory (Hobfoll, 1989; 2001). COR, which has been repeatedly tested in the research context (see Chapter 10) has consistently captured the positive association between resource loss and an array of disaster outcomes.

During disasters, individuals commonly turn to their immediate social network for support. However, the increased need for social and material support during and after disasters may overwhelm available resources, and the ability to adapt to the postdisaster needs depends on ongoing cooperative action (see Chapter 11). Initially, remarkable patterns of "altruistic community" are expected (Barton, 1969), including outpouring of good will and material support from the immediate community as well as from national or international communities. Feelings of unity and solidarity are common in the initial stage, and the inflow of compassionate aide coupled with the prosocial behavior of community members promotes a sense of hope, solidarity (Chapter 11), and safety in a time when the world seems capricious, dangerous, or unjust (Lindy & Grace, 1986).

Sadly, after the initial "honeymoon" stage, those not involved directly in recovery efforts will return to their daily life, while affected individuals will soon experience physical fatigue, bereavment, and distress. Moreover, scarcity of resources will take its toll on local communities, resulting in a deterioration of social support, as well as increased interpersonal conflicts and social withdrawal (Chapter 11); relocation and job loss also contribute to the fracturing of social networks (Norris, 2006), and expectations are disappointed as the needs for support exceed its availability (Harvey et al., 1995; Kanaisty, Norris, & Murrell, 1990). Family, friends, and neighbors become emotionally exhausted in the face of these tangible and emotional stressors. A stress contagion effect can also occur, where hearing about the disaster experience of others begins to burden the listener, further escalating the loss of family and community support (Gil-Rivas, Silver, Holman, McIntosh, & Polin, 2007; Hobfoll & London, 1986; McFarlane, Polincansky, & Irwin, 1987). Fortunately, this deterioration is not entirely inevitable (see Chapter 11). If sustained resource mobilization infrastructures are established, material resources are provided, social ties are fostered, and care for medical problems – including mental health – is provided, community resilience and social connectedness are kept intact.

It is now known that resources provided to communities facing disasters are not equitably distributed across age, race, and income groups, and that this distribution is influenced by the rule of "relative advantage." Typically, survivors who are younger and have more years of education and higher income receive greater levels of assistance (Kaniasty, 2003; Kaniasty & Norris, 1995; Norris, Baker, Murphy, & Kaniasty, 2005; Tyler, 2006) while persons of lower socioeconomic status and ethnic minorities tend to face a pattern of neglect in the disbursement of aide. Kaniasty and Norris (1995) found, for example, that Black survivors consistently received less tangible or informational assistance in comparison with survivors who were White.

This unequal distribution of resources may carry strong implications for marginalized populations that are already at greater risk for poor postdisaster outcomes (Chapter 16). Besides an increased risk for death and severe damage resulting from the disaster itself (Norris, Stevens, Pfefferbaum, Wyche, & Pfefferbaum, 2007), these communities often have fewer economic or material resources available for the costly rebuilding process. There also tends to be a lack of adequate infrastructure to organize and distribute resources to lower income and minority groups, who tend to be more on the fringes of the established societal groups through which aide flows following disaster (Chapter 11). Armed with this insight, preparation and prevention efforts need to take into account the particular needs of these communities that are at elevated risk for poor long-term outcomes following disasters.

35.6. HIGH-RISK GROUPS

As emphasized earlier, disasters mental health impact is expected to vary across the exposed population. Different subgroups carry greater risk than others. While type and duration of exposure carry a lot of weight in risk for mental and physical health (see Chapter 3), additional factors, such as gender, age, disability status, race/ethnicity, income level, and profession (journalism and rescue and recovery), need to be considered. We consider some of these groups in the subsequent text.

35.6.1. Women

Increased risk for psychopathology among women has been widely reported in the aftermath of disasters across all disaster types and cultures (Norris, Friedman, et al., 2002). The wealth of data on gender differences in the post-disaster raises questions as to whether women may experience more and/or different risk factors than men (see Chapter 12). For example, in the wake of September 11th attacks in New York City, Pulcino and colleagues (2003) found that being the primary caretaker of children, past history of unwanted sexual contact, mental health problems in the past year, and more life stressors in the past year were all associated with greater PTSD among women. In a sample of 988 individuals who lived in close proximity to the WTC, women reported more perievent panic (17.4%) in comparison to men (7.3%) (Pulcino et al., 2003). Following a flood in Tobasco, Mexico, women also reported more perceptions of life threat (71.3% vs. 63.7% in men) (Norris et al., 2005). Such perceptions of threat and increased panic reactions produce feelings of fear, horror, or helplessness that may elevate disaster events to a trauma level in line with the A2 criterion for PTSD (Chapter 14). In addition, while no gender differences were found in received social support, Norris and colleagues (2005) found that women's perceptions of social support and embeddedness were lower than men's 6 months following floods and mudslides in Mexico. Interestingly, the differences in social support among women may be varied by exposure, suggesting that gender differences postdisaster may be greater in communities severely affected by disasters, as compared with communities less impacted.

While differences in predisaster risk factors, reported exposure, emotional distress, and various perceptions are helpful to illuminate gender differences in psychopathology, more research is needed to provide depth to our understanding of those differences. It is possible that some gender differences are confounded by other variables; for example, in a study conducted by Weissman and colleagues (2005) in a sample of patients from a primary care setting serving primarily low-income minorities, the researchers found that the elevated rates of PTSD among women were mediated by family context (e.g., living alone without a permanent relationship) and economic circumstances (e.g., little education or income). Moreover, researchers have only just begun to understand the complex differences between genders in social context, emotional reactivity to stress, and psychopathology.

35.6.2. Children

Despite substantial advances in the mental health research on children and adolescents postdisaster, the current research allows only limited understanding of the role of age in the relationships between exposure to high-impact trauma and psychopathology. As Hoven and colleagues suggest in their review (Chapter 13) current research is especially limited by insufficient focus on disaster type and developmental differences, as well as an acute lack of a scientific consensus among researchers with regard to instrumentation. Nevertheless, evidence on child disaster mental health outcomes, especially PTSD, has been accumulating in the last decade. Most studies have focused on natural and human-made disasters; only a few were longitudinal (e.g., La Greca, Silverman, Vernber, & Prinstein, 1996; Proctor et al., 2007; Terr et al., 1999; Thabet & Vostanis, 2000), and their findings are inconclusive with regard to duration of symptoms over time and recovery rates (see Chapter 13). Likewise, research on correlates of disaster impact also needs further exploration. Most studies lack data on predisaster mental health problems among parents and children and other predisaster risk factors. However, similar to findings from studies among adults (see Chapter 3), exposure to media was positively associated with PTSD among children in the aftermath of the Oklahoma City bombing (Pfefferbaum et al., 2002) and September 11th attacks (Hoven et al., 2000; Saylor, Cowart, Lipovsky, Jackson, & Finch, Jr., 2003).

As suggested by Hoven and colleagues (Chapter 13), despite impressive progress in studying the mental health consequences of exposure to disaster among children, both in the short (Hoven, 2002; La Greca, 2006; Pfefferbaum et al., 1999; Pynoos et al., 1987) and long term (La Greca et al., 1996; Proctor et al., 2007; Terr et al., 1997; Thabet & Vostanis, 2000), the lack of well-designed longitudinal studies across different type of disaster limit our understanding of the role of young age in long-term consequences of high-impact trauma.

35.6.3. Older Adults

As people age, they experience multiple life changes – changes in economic status, social support and relationships, and physical and mental health – and all may be associated with vulnerability to disasters among older adults (Elmore & Brown, in press; Fernandez, Byard, Lin, Benson, & Barbera, 2002; Norris, Kaniasty, Conrad, Inman, & Murphy, 2002). Yet, as Cook and Elmore (Chapter 14) suggest, despite those apparent vulnerabilities, older adults tend to report lower levels of distress and fewer impairments in psychological functioning than younger adults in postdisaster settings. For example, in a study of 831 subjects at 12, 18, and 24 months after Hurricane Hugo in 1989 (Thompson, Norris, & Hanacek, 1993), the highest symptom levels were found among middle-aged adults (age 40 to 59), as compared with young (age 19 to 39) and older adults (over age 60), suggesting a potential heightened burden due to caretaking responsibilities (Chapter 14), as well as the fact that older adults may be more sheltered from financial and other types of losses. While some older adults may report lower levels of distress as compared with young adults, they may still be vulnerable to a decline in physical health as a result of disaster exposure (e.g., fatigue, difficulty in daily tasks) (Norris, Phifer, & Kaniasty, 1994) and rapid depletion of their pre-event psychological resources.

Importantly, the trend for older adults to endorse lower levels of distress and emotional difficulties after disasters compared with other age groups does not hold true across cultures. Norris, Kaniasty, and colleagues (2002) evaluated PTSD symptoms in adults 12 months after the 1992 Hurricane Andrew in the United States (N = 270), the 1997 Hurricane Paulina in Mexico (N = 200), and the 1997 flood in Poland (N = 285). The American sample followed a curvilinear trend between age and PTSD, but in Mexico a linear relationship was found, with younger adults being the most distressed. In Poland the opposite trend was observed; as age increased, so did levels of PTSD symptoms. The authors suggested that Polish people had experienced several prior societal stressors, including war, oppression, and poor economic conditions.

As the field of disaster research continues to develop, paying greater attention to individual risk and protective factors will help to elucidate the effects of disaster on aging populations. Understanding capacities of resilience in this population – evidenced by lower reported levels of distress (Acierno, Ruggiero, Kilpatrick, Resnick, & Galea, 2006; Bolin & Klenow, 1982–1983; Thompson et al., 1993), and the mediating role of preexisting mental and physical health in elderly populations – will influence prevention efforts and enable disaster responders to target those with greater risk.

35.6.4. Individuals with Disabilities and Marginalized Populations

Few risk factors are more potent than predisaster medical and mental health problems, race/ethnicity, and socioeconomic status (Galea et al., 2005; Neria et al., 2008; Norris, Friedman et al., 2002). However, to date only a few efforts have been made to address the specific postdisaster needs of individuals with disabilities, the poor, or immigrant minorities (see Chapters 15 and 16).

Mobility impairments pose a substantial risk when disasters strike. A small but meaningful study conducted by Rooney and White (2007) among 56 individuals with mobility impairments, from 20 different states and 47 cities, suggests that while participants reported extensive exposure to different kinds of natural disasters, they experienced tremendous barriers to effective rescue and care stemming from lack of access to evacuation plans, shelters and temporary housing, public transportation systems, potable water, and elevators. Moreover they were often left behind when people without disabilities were evacuated. Anecdotal data on individuals with sensory (visually impaired or the blind;

auditorally impaired or deaf), cognitive, and psychiatric disabilities suggest a similar lack of attention with regards to preparedness and rescue plans (Chapter 15).

Compared to the role of the various disabilities on postdisaster outcomes, there is a more substantial body of research on racial/ethnic and socioeconomic determinants of mental health. As reviewed in the chapter by Hawkins and colleagues (Chapter 16) and in reviews by Norris and colleagues (Norris & Alegria, 2005; Norris, Friedman, et al., 2002), significant differences have been identified between racial/ethnic groups with regard to risk perception, cultural attitudes and beliefs, and acculturative stress, as well as help-seeking behaviors before, during, and after disaster. However, similar to disabled populations, marginalized, minority, and low-income populations experience significant disparities with regard to access to community, state, or federal resources. There are also significant inequalities in resources, predisaster preparation, and postdisaster care between socioeconomic groups.

35.6.5. Media and Rescue Personnel

According to Newman, Shapiro, and Voorhees (Chapter 17) no sector of civil society "bears more responsibility in times of disasters than the news media." In all stages of disasters, media personnel play a critical role in providing information to the public on the magnitude and scope of the disaster, the experiences of victims and survivors, and the quality of the role local and federal agencies play in preparedness before disasters and rescue and recovery efforts after the disaster. Consequently, journalists are continuously exposed to these events, both directly and indirectly (e.g., Newman, Simpson, & Handschuh, 2003; Pyevich, Newman, & Daleiden, 2003; Simpson & Boggs, 1999), which put them at risk for trauma-related outcomes. However, the little research that exists suggests only moderate to low effects (see Chapter 17) and impressive rates of resilience.

First responders to disaster include police, National Guard members, and fire fighters. McCaslin, Inslicht, Henn-Haase, Chemtob, Metzler, Neylan, and Marmar (Chapter 18) discussed the current literature on prevalences of and risk factors for mental health problems (e.g., PTSD depression, substance abuse, and other anxiety disorders) and comorbid physical symptoms (e.g., cough, wheezing, and asthma) among these populations. Although very few studies have examined disaster effects in these populations longitudinally (Marmar et al., 1999; Marmar, Weiss, Metzler, & Delucchi, 1996; McFarlane, 1986, 1988; McFarlane & Papay, 1992), McCaslin and colleagues (Chapter 18) highlight the critical role of training and experience in the outcome of exposure to trauma. Uniformed personnel stand to benefit greatly from systematic disaster preparation that aims to increase a sense of control and self-efficacy and to reduce uncertainty.

35.7. INTERVENTIONS AND MENTAL HEALTH SERVICE USE

Owing to their unpredictable nature and scope, disasters challenge ordinary models of mental health intervention and call for effective interventions ranging from preparedness efforts, to immediate, intermediate, and long-term programs. Moreover, a strategic approach is needed to address the heterogeneous impact of disasters. Key challenges for treating populations in the disaster context are (1) early identification and intervention for individuals who are at an elevated risk for developing long-term psychological difficulties; (2) treatment of existing mental health problems; and (3) long-term follow up to address delayed onset and possible relapse among remitted individuals.

Studies have shown that the majority of survivors who display acute stress symptoms will subsequently develop PTSD (Brewin, Andrews, Rose, & Kirk, 1999; Bryant, & Harvey, 1998; Difede & Eskra, 2002; Harvey & Bryant, 1998, 1999, 2000; Holeva, Tarrier, & Wells, 2001; Kangas, Henry, & Bryant, 2005; Murray, Ehlers, & Mayou, 2002). Nevertheless, testing evidence-based intervention models for individuals with early but severe symptomatology is only in the early stages (Chapter 19). Most work to date has been focused on derivations of psychological debriefing (Everly & Mitchell, 1999), a single-session intervention augmented with psychoeducation, conducted by nonprofessionals in the wake of trauma exposure with all people involved in the event, regardless of the level of distress or personal history. Most randomized control trials have not supported the efficacy of this approach (e.g., Rose, Bisson, Churchill, & Wessely, 2002), and a number of reviews suggested that debriefing may even be harmful to survivors (Carlier, Lamberts, van Ulchelen, & Gersons, 1998; Litz & Gray, 2002; McNally, Bryant, & Ehlers, 2003). Further, some have speculated that requiring individuals to discuss their disturbing experiences may heighten physiological and psychological arousal at a time when they need to restore equilibrium (Chapter 19; Bisson, Jenkins, Alexander, & Bannister, 1997; Hobbs, Mayou, Harrison, & Worlock, 1996; Solomon, Neria, & Witztum, 2000) and may impede the natural recovery process (Chapter 9; Solomon et al., 2000).

In a comprehensive discussion of what research is needed in this area, Bryant and Litz (Chapter 19) propose a useful distinction between short-term and intermediate-term interventions; short-term interventions should aim to promote safety, effective coping, and stabilization, while intermediate interventions are designed to prevent long-term chronic psychopathology by treating more stable psychopathological responses. In this same line, and in response to lack of a well-conceptualized model for disaster intervention in the short term, a consensus-based article by Hobfoll and colleagues (2007) has recently proposed five key areas for intervention in the early phase postdisaster: (1) promoting sense of safety, aiming to stabilize survivors and to enable gradual reduction of distress symptoms; (2) promoting sense of calming physiological arousal; (3) increasing feelings of self and collective efficacy; (4) encouraging social support and attachments with others; and (5) instilling hope to promote a sense of positive future. A similar approach was applied in the development of the short-term intervention Psychological First Aid (PFA), as described by Young (2006), aims to (1) facilitate adaptive coping and problem-solving skills that will allow survivors to obtain items necessary for daily life including food, water, and shelter; (2) ensure fulfillment of everyday needs and promote a sense of safety, the practice of relaxation skills, psychoeducation normalizing trauma reactions, and cognitive reframing techniques; and (3) locate additional resources that will aide in long-term coping, such as plans to rebuild and reestablish a normal mode of daily living. Importantly, in direct contrast with psychological debriefing, PFA does not encourage survivors to share their traumatic experiences unless the individual feels a need to discuss the event. This allows for a supportive environment where the main focus of intervention is the promotion of coping skills. Even though there is no empirical data evaluating the effectiveness of PFA, it appears to be a promising model for short-term interventions in the wake of disaster and has been endorsed at expert consensus meetings (National Institute of Mental Health, 2002). Any implementation of a short-term intervention should take into account the extent to which survivors may face threat and whether survivors have sufficient resources to manage the intervention (Chapter 19).

Cognitive-behavior therapy (CBT) models are particularly suited for the intermediate phase (Foa, 2000; Harvey, Bryant, & Tarrier, 2003). CBT modules mostly have been tested under research conditions with strict protocols and therefore may not be applied immediately for community samples in the aftermath of disasters; however, a small number of studies in earthquake survivors (see Chapter 24) provide promising data on the effectiveness of well-adapted, brief CBT methods for disaster survivors. For example, a single session intervention, comprised of self-exposure to fear-evoking situations with an emphasis on self-control, was found to be effective in decreasing PTSD and fear of subsequent earthquakes (Chapter 24).

Although numerous clinical trials in PTSD treatment have been conducted and reported (e.g., Institute of Medicine, 2006), only three studies have included disaster-exposed populations who suffer from chronic PTSD (Chapter 20). These studies successfully employed CBT protocols among survivors of a car bombing in Ireland (Gillespie, Duffy, Hackmann, & Clark, 2002) and the September 11th attacks (Difede, Cukor et al., 2007) and among disaster workers involved in the September 11th attacks (Difede, Malta, et al., 2007). There is a great need for more studies of pharmacotherapy and psychotherapy for different populations and needs to make sure enough efficacious, evidence-based treatments exist and can be used in the aftermath of disasters.

35.7.1. Interventions for Children

Despite the wide-reaching impacts of disasters on children (Chapter 13), interventions that target children's reactions have received only limited attention. To date, only three randomized controlled trials have been conducted with this population, and none of these studies included teenagers (Chapter 21). In the first trial, treatment for high levels of distress following Hurricane Andrew was tested among grade school children (grades one to five) (Field, Seligman, Scafidi, & Schanberg, 1996). In the second trial, eye movement desensitization and reprocessing therapy (EMDR) was tested in a group of 6- to 12-year-olds who met criteria for PTSD 1 year after Hurricane Iniki (Chemtob, Nakashima, & Carlson, 2002). The third trial evaluated the efficacy of a cognitive-behavioral intervention for 248 children with elevated trauma-related symptoms 2 years after Hurricane Iniki (Chemtob, Nakashima, & Hamada, 2002). While this research provides only partial answers to the question what is the best course of treatment for children with significant distress after disasters, the work that has been done indicates that focusing on combined cognitive and relaxation techniques may be beneficial. More well-designed randomized trials are needed to further elucidate which therapeutic mechanisms are the most beneficial for this group.

35.7.2. Treatment-Seeking

While evidence-based mental health treatments for disaster survivors and rescue groups are scarce in postdisaster settings (Part Five), high-need populations (e.g., those who develop PTSD) may seek treatments where they do exist (e.g., primary and specialty care). In their critical review of the literature, Elhai and Ford (Chapter 22) confirmed that the presence of psychopathology itself is more strongly associated with mental health treatment use postdisaster, as compared to enabling (e.g., access to care) and predisposing factors (e.g., age, race). Early research (e.g., Schwarz & Kowalski, 1992) suggested that patients with PTSD may avoid mental health treatment, possibly due to avoidance of trauma-related reminders (e.g., preferring not to discuss the trauma, becoming distressed when reminded of the trauma).

35.8. SUMMARY AND CONCLUSION

Disaster mental health research has become central to the field of traumatic stress (see Chapter 2). As reviewed in Part Six of this book, Natural (Chapters 23–25), technological (Chapters 26–28), and human-made (Chapters 29–33) events have received considerable scientific attention over the years from numerous research teams. The most studied psychiatric disorders are PTSD and depression, but there is emerging evidence on the effect of disasters on other health domains, such as physical symptoms and illness, substance abuse, and prolonged grief. Findings suggest substantial burden of illness among populations directly exposed to the mass trauma (e.g., evacuees, rescue workers, those in close proximity, bereaved). In addition, special groups such as minority and low-income populations, children, and women have consistently exhibited heightened risk for mental health problems.

To date, research has primarily focused on prevalence and risk factors of psychopathology postdisaster. Long-term, prospective studies are rare; thus, the full impact of disasters on both medical and mental health over time has yet to be described. There is greater knowledge with regard to the long-term effects of disasters on high-risk groups (e.g., low-income and minority populations; rescue workers), but the degree to which the general population is impacted remains unclear. Ample evidence of comorbidity between various mental health problems makes research on course of illness and its determinants quite challenging, but it nevertheless remains highly needed.

Previous research has consistently documented strong associations between type and severity of exposure disaster impact, and recent studies have begun to address the possibility that indirect exposure to trauma is a potent risk factor for psychopathology in the community. This is especially intriguing because it challenges existing consensus on the role of trauma as presented by the DSM and reflected in the literature since the early 1980s. Emerging evidence on associations between exposure to media and adverse outcomes in both the general population and specific groups suggests that humans are susceptible to trauma-related distress in ways previously not examined or expected.

In terms of data, up to this point most disaster research has relied primarily on self-report by disaster survivors, relief workers, and witnesses. Much less attention has been given to sources of hard data on exposure (e.g., proportions of injuries and fatalities) and its impact (e.g., economic and environmental effects). Data on physical destruction, devastation of natural environments and homes, displacement of populations, and economic damage should be utilized to better assess the nature, duration, and scope of the effects on mental and physical health. A recent study conducted by Dohrenwend and colleagues (2006) among Vietnam War veterans uses novel methods to verify self-report data on exposure with objective data on mortality figures and the likelihood of being killed. Immediately after the disaster, data on infrastructure destruction, loss of lives, and injuries can be incorporated to more reliably predict the physical and mental health needs of exposed populations. These predictions can serve in the process of policy making during the aftermath of the incident, enabling the deployment of mental health services as needed. This data can also be integrated into longitudinal models of risk for mental health problems.

While most studies on psychopathology after disaster have documented immediate distress, some studies have suggested that a significant minority of the cases with disaster-related PTSD may have a delayed onset, where individuals who do not meet PTSD criteria shortly after the disaster may meet criteria months or even years after the event (Adams & Boscarino, 2006; North et al., 2004). However, there is a dearth of evidence about the prevalence of different trajectories of disaster-related outcomes, including chronic course, remission from disorders, and delayed onset of disorders. Similarly, there is limited evidence about whether these trajectories are associated with different predictors and different patterns of medical comorbidity, psychiatric disorders, and functional impairment. Studying multiple trajectories and their determinants, while using well-ascertained data on mental health problems, is key to understanding the long-term sequelae of disasters.

Disaster mental health research has significantly advanced since its inception more than six decades ago. However, it has been mostly limited to epidemiological studies; treatment studies have been extremely scarce and have not systematically addressed the mental health needs of individuals postdisaster. Psychological debriefing has been central to disaster mental health practice for more than two decades; however, as it has not been found to be sufficiently beneficial, there is an urgent need for developing and testing postdisaster treatments in the short, intermediate, and long term. Hobfoll and colleagues' (2007) principles for early intervention, Bryant and Litz guidelines (Chapter 19) for the preferred timing for interventions, and the accumulating knowledge on the usefulness of CBT treatments (Chapters 19, 20, and 24) are all promising advances, and more research is urgently needed to test novel treatment modalities in both pharmacotherapy and psychotherapy in the wake of disasters.

Conducting mental health research in the wake of disasters is especially challenging. The postdisaster environment is unique due to its changing and uncontrollable nature. In all stages, from developing a research plan to data collection and data analysis, we must expect logistical and environmental challenges as inherent to this work (Chapter 34). To effectively operate in environments disrupted by disasters, research teams should be well trained, well funded, diverse, multidisciplinary, and respectfully network with local teams and affected communities (Chapter 34). Successful future research will be able to enhance knowledge on the longitudinal trajectories of illness and resilience; to educate clinicians and medical teams on the most efficacious, safe, and effective interventions to reduce mental health burden in the community; to improve lives soon after impact; and to facilitate recovery among those severely affected by traumatic events.

ACKNOWLEDGMENTS

We thank Rachel Fox for her input in the early versions of this chapter.

REFERENCES

Acierno, R., Ruggiero, K. J., Kilpatrick, D. G., Resnick, H. S., & Galea, S. (2006). Risk and protective factors for psychopathology among older versus younger adults following the 2004 Florida hurricanes. *American Psychologist, 59*, 236–260.

Adams, R. E., & Boscarino, J. A. (2006). Predictors of PTSD and delayed PTSD after disaster: The impact of exposure and psychosocial resources. *Journal of Nervous and Mental Diseases, 194*(7), 485–493.

Ahern, J., & Galea, S. (2006). Social context and depression after a disaster: The role of income inequality. *Journal of Epidemiology and Community Health, 60*, 766–770.

Ahern, J., Galea, S., Resnick, H., Kilpatrick, D., Bucuvalas, M., Gold, J., et al. (2002). Television images and psychological symptoms after the September 11 terrorist attacks. *Psychiatry, 65*(4), 289–300.

Ahern, J., Galea, S., Resnick, H., & Vlahov, D. (2004). Television images and probably posttraumatic stress disorder after September 11. *The Journal of Nervous and Mental Disease, 192*, 217–226.

Barton, A. M. (1969). *Communities in disaster*. Garden City, NJ: Doubleday.

Basoglu, M., Salcioglu, E., & Livanou, E. (2007). A randomized controlled study of single-session behavioral treatment of earthquake-related posttraumatic stress disorder using an earthquake simulator. *Psychological Medicine, 37*, 203–213.

Benight, C. (2004). Collective efficacy following a series of natural disasters. *Anxiety, Stress & Coping: An International Journal, 17*, 401–420.

Benight, C. C., & Bandura, A. (2004). Social cognitive theory of posttraumatic recovery: The role of perceived self-efficacy. *Behaviour Research and Therapy, 42*, 1129–1148.

Benight, C. C., Ironson, G., Klebe, K., Carver, C., Wynings, C., Greenwood, D., et al. (1999). Conservation of resources and coping self-efficacy predicting distress following a natural disaster: A causal model analysis where the environment meets the mind. *Anxiety, Stress, and Coping, 12*, 107–126.

Bisconti, T. L., Bergeman, C. S., & Boker, S. M. (2006). Social support as a predictor of variability: An examination of the adjustment trajectories of recent widows. *Psychology and Aging, 21*(3), 590–599.

Bisson, J. I., Jenkins, P. L., Alexander, J., & Bannister, C. (1997). Randomized controlled trial of psychological debriefing for victims of acute burn trauma. *British Journal of Psychiatry, 171*, 78–81.

Bolin, R., & Klenow, D. J. (1982–1983). Response of the elderly to disaster: An age-stratified analysis. *International Journal of Aging and Human Development, 16*, 283–296.

Bonanno, G. A., Field, N. P., Kovacevic, A., & Kaltman, S. (2002). Self-enhancement as a buffer against extreme adversity: Civil war in Bosnia and traumatic loss in the United States. *Personality and Social Psychology Bulletin, 28*(2), 184–196.

Bonanno, G. A., Moskowitz, J. T., Papa, A., & Folkman, S. (2005). Resilience to loss in bereaved spouses, bereaved parents, and bereaved gay men. *Journal of Personality and Social Psychology, 88*(5), 827–843.

Bonanno, G. A., Neria, Y., Mancini, A., Coifman, K. G., & Litz, B. (2007). Is there more to complicated grief than depression and posttraumatic stress disorder? A test of incremental validity. *Journal of Abnormal Psychology, 116*(2), 342–351.

Bonanno, G. A, Rennicke, C., & Dekel, S. (2005). Self-enhancement among high-exposure survivors of the September 11th terrorist attack: Resilience or social maladjustment? *Journal of Personality and Social Psychology, 88*(6), 984–998.

Bowlby, J. (1980). *Attachment and loss: Vol. 3. Loss.* New York: Basic Books.

(1982). Attachment and loss: Retrospect and prospect. *American Journal of Orthopsychiatry, 52*, 664–678.

Brewin, C. R., Andrews, B., Rose, S., & Kirk, M. (1999). Acute stress disorder and posttraumatic stress disorder in victims of violent crime. *American Journal of Psychiatry, 156*, 360–366.

Bryant, R. A., & Harvey, A. G. (1998). Relationship of acute stress disorder and posttraumatic stress disorder following mild traumatic brain injury. *American Journal of Psychiatry, 155*, 625–629.

Carlier, I.V., Lamberts, R.D., van Ulchelen, A.J., & Gersons, B.P. (1998). Disaster-related posttraumatic stress in police officers: A field study of the impact of debriefing. *Stress Medicine, 14,* 143–148.

Carr, V.J., Lewin, T.J., Webster, R.A., Kenary, J.A., Hazell, P.L., & Carter, G.L. (1997). Psychosocial sequelae of 1989 newcastle earthquake: II. Exposure and morbiditiy profiles during the first 2 years post-disaster. 27, 78.

Chemtob, C.M., Nakashima, J., & Carlson, J.G. (2002). Brief treatment for elementary school children with disaster-related posttraumatic stress disorder: A field study. *Journal of Clinical Psychology, 58,* 99–112.

Chemtob, C.M., Nakashima, J.P., & Hamada, & R.S. (2002). Psychosocial intervention for postdisaster trauma symptoms in elementary school children: A controlled community field study. *Archives of Pediatrics & Adolescent Medicine, 152,* 211–216.

Dhara, V.R., & Dhara, R. (2002). The Union Carbide disaster in Bhopal: A review of health effects. *Archives of Environmental Health, 57*(5), 391–404.

Difede, J., Cukor, J., Jayasinghe, N., Patt, I., Jedel, S., Spielman, L., et al. (2007). Virtual reality exposure therapy for the treatment of posttraumatic stress disorder following September 11, 2001. *Journal of Clinical Psychiatry, 68*(11), 1639–1647.

Difede, J., & Eskra, D. (2002). Adaptation of cognitive processing therapy for the treatment of PTSD following terrorism: A case study of a World Trade Center (1993) survivor. *Journal of Trauma Practice, 1*(3/4), 155–165.

Difede, J., Malta, L.S., Best, S., Henn-Haase, C., Metzler, T., Bryant, R., et al. (2007). A randomized controlled clinical treatment trial for World Trade Center attack-related PTSD in disaster workers. *Journal of Nervous Mental Disorders, 195*(10), 861–865.

Dohrenwend, B.P., Neria, Y., Turner, J.B., Turse, N., Marshall, R., Lewis-Fernandez, R., et al. (2004). Positive tertiary appraisals and posttraumatic stress disorder in U.S. male veterans of the war in Vietnam: The roles of positive affirmation, positive reformulation, and defensive denial. *Journal of Consulting and Clinical Psychology, 72*(3), 417–433.

Dohrenwend, B.P., Turner, J.B., Turse, N.A., Adams, B.G., Koenen, K.C., & Marshall, R. (2006). The psychological risks of Vietnam for U.S. veterans: A revisit with new data and methods. *Science, 313*(5789), 979–982.

Elmore, D.L., & Brown, L.M. (In press). Emergency preparedness and response: Health and social policy implications for older adults. *Generations.*

Everly, G.S., Jr., & Mitchell, J.T. (1999). *Critical incident stress management (CISM): A new era and standard of care in crisis intervention.* Ellicott City, MD: Chevron.

Fernandez, L.S., Byard, D., Lin, C.C., Benson, S., & Barbera, J.A. (2002). Frail elderly as disaster victims: Emergency management strategies. *Prehospital and Disaster Medicine, 17*(2), 67–74.

Field, T., Seligman, S., Scafedi, F., & Schanberg, S. (1996). Alleviating posttraumatic stress in children following Hurricane Andrew. *Journal of Applied Developmental Psychology, 17,* 35–50.

Foa, E.B. (2000). Psychosocial treatment of posttraumatic stress disorder. *Journal of Clinical Psychiatry, 61* (Suppl. 5), 43–48.

Foa, E.B., Stein, D.J., & McFarlane, A.C. (2006). Symptomatology and psychopathology of mental health problems after disaster. *Journal of Clinical Psychiatry, 67* (Suppl. 2), 15–25.

Galea, S., Ahern, J., Resnick, H., Kilpatrick, D., Bucuvalas, M., Gold, J., et al. (2002). Psychological sequelae of the September 11 terrorist attacks in New York City. *New England Journal of Medicine, 346*(13), 982–987.

Galea, S., Nandi, A., & Vlahov, D. (2005). The epidemiology of post-traumatic stress disorder after disasters. *Epidemiologic Reviews, 27*(1), 78–91.

Galea, S., Vlahov, D., Resnick, H., Ahern, J., Susser, E., Gold, J., et al. (2003). Trends of probable posttraumatic stress disorder in New York City after the September 11 terrorist attacks. *American Journal of Epidemiology, 158*(6), 514–524.

Gil-Rivas, V., Cohen, S.R., Holman, E.A., McIntosh, D., & Polin, M. (2007). Parental response and adolescent adjustment to the September 11, 2001 attacks. *Journal of Traumatic Stress, 20,* 1063–1068.

Gillespie, K., Duffy, M., Hackmann, A., & Clark, D.M. (2002). Community based cognitive therapy in the treatment of posttraumatic stress disorder following the Omagh bomb. *Behavioral Research and Therapy, 40*(4), 345–357.

Haglund, M.E.M., Nestadt, P.S., Cooper, N.S., Southwick, S.M., & Charney, D.S. (2007). Psychobiological mechanisms of resilience: Relevance to prevention and treatment of stress-related psychopathology. *Development and Psychopathology, 19,* 889–920.

Harvey, A.G., & Bryant, R.A. (1998). Relationship of acute stress disorder and posttraumatic stress disorder following motor vehicle accidents. *Journal of Consulting and Clinical Psychology, 66,* 507–512.

(1999). A two-year prospective evaluation of the relationship between acute stress disorder and posttraumatic stress disorder. *Journal of Consulting and Clinical Psychology*, *67*, 985–988.

(2000). A two-year prospective evaluation of the relationship between acute stress disorder and posttraumatic stress disorder following mild traumatic brain injury. *American Journal of Psychiatry*, *157*, 626–628.

Harvey, A.G., Bryant, R.A., & Tarrier, N. (2003). Cognitive behaviour therapy of posttraumatic stress disorder. *Clinical Psychology Review*, *23*, 501–522.

Harvey, J., Stein, S., Olsen, N., Roberts, R., Lutegendorf, S., & Ho, J. (1995). Narratives of loss and recovery from a natural disaster. *Journal of Social Behavior and Personality*, *10*, 313–330.

Hobbs, M., Mayou, R., Harrison, B., & Worlock, P. (1996). A randomized controlled trial of psychological debriefing for victims of road traffic accidents. *British Medical Journal*, *313*, 1438–1439.

Hobfoll, S.E. (1989). Conservation of resources: A new attempt at conceptualizing stress. *American Psychologist*, *44*, 513–524.

(2001). The influence of culture, community, and the nested-self in the process: Advancing conservation of resources theory. *Applied Psychology: An International Review*, *50*, 337–421.

Hobfoll, S.E., & London, P. (1986). The relationship of self-concept and social support to emotional distress among women during war. *Journal of Social and Clinical Psychology*, *12*, 87–100.

Hobfoll, S.E., Watson, P., Bell, C.C., Bryant, R.A., Brymer, M.J., Friedman, M.J., et al. (2007). Five essential elements of immediate and mid-term mass trauma intervention: Empirical evidence. *Psychiatry*, *70*(4), 283–315.

Holeva, V., Tarrier, N., & Wells, A. (2001). Prevalence and predictors of acute stress disorder and PTSD following road traffic accidents: Thought control strategies and social support. *Behavior Therapy*, *32*, 65–83.

Horowitz, M.J., Siegel, B., Holen, A., Bonanno, G.A., Milbrath, C., & Stinson, C.H. (1997). Diagnostic criteria for complicated grief disorder. *American Journal of Psychiatry*, *154*, 904–910.

Hoven, C.W. (2002). *Testimony: The United States Senate, hearing before the Committee on Health, Education, Labor and Pensions, (Chair, Hillary Rodham Clinton), children of September 11: The need for mental health services, June 10, 2002. Senate Hearing No. 107-540, Document No. 552-070-29-035-4.* U.S. Government Printing Office.

Hoven, C.W., Duarte, C.S., Lucas, C.P., Mandell, D.J., Cohen, M., Rosen, C., et al. (2002). *Effects of the World Trade Center Attack on NYC public school students: initial report to the New York City Board of Education.* New York: Columbia University Mailman School of Public Health-New York State Psychiatric Institute and Applied Research and Consulting, LLC, New York City.

Institute of Medicine. (2006). *Posttraumatic stress disorder: Diagnosis and assessment.* Washington DC. National Academics Press.

Janoff-Bulman, R. (1992). *Shattered assumptions: Toward a new psychology of trauma.* New York: Free Press.

Kaniasty, K. (2003). *Kleska zywiolowa czy katastrofa spoleczna? Psychospoleczne konsekwencje polskiej powodzi 1997 roku. (Natural disaster or social catastrophe? Psychosocial consequences of the 1997 Polish Flood).* Gdansk, Poland: Gdanskie Wydawnictwo Psychologiczne.

Kaniasty, K., & Norris, F.H. (1995). In search of altruistic community: Patterns of social support mobilization following Hurricane Hugo. *American Journal of Community Psychology*, *23*, 447–477.

Kaniasty, K., Norris, F., & Murrell, S. (1990). Percieved and recieved social support following natural disaster. *Journal of Applied Social Psychology*, *20*, 85–114.

Kangas, M., Henry, J.L., & Bryant, R.A. (2005). The relationship between acute stress disorder and posttraumatic stress disorder following cancer. *Journal of Consulting and Clinical Psychology*, *73*, 360–364.

Kilic, C., Aydin, I., Taskintuna, N., Ozcurumez, G., Kurt, G., Eren, E., et al. (2006). Predictors of psychological distress in survivors of the 1999 earthquakes in Turkey: Effects of relocation after the disaster. *Acta Psychiatrica Scandinavica*, *114*, 194–202.

Kobasa, S.C., Maddi, S.R., & Kahn, S. (1982). Hardiness and health: A prospective study. *Journal of Personality and Social Psychology*, *42*, 168–177.

La Greca, A.M. (2006). School-based studies of children following disasters. In F. Norris S. Galea M.J. Friedman, & P. Watson (Eds.), *Methods for disaster mental health research.* New York: Guilford Press.

La Greca, A.M., Silverman, W.K., Vernber, E.M., & Prinstein, M.J. (1996). Symptoms of posttraumatic stress in children after Hurricane Anderew: A prospective study. *Journal of Consulting and Clinical Psychology*, *64*, 712–723.

Lazarus, R.S. (1966). *Psychological stress and the coping process.* New York: McGraw–Hill.

Lazarus, R.S., & Folkman, S. (1984). *Stress, appraisal, and coping.* New York: Springer.

Lichtenthal, W.G., Cruess, D.G., & Prigerson, H.G. (2004). A case for establishing complicated grief as a distinct mental disorder in DSM-V. *Clinical Psychology Review*, *24*, 637–662.

Lindy, J., & Grace, M. (1986). The recovery environment: Continuing stressor versus a healing psychological space. In B. Sowder & M. Lystad. (Eds.), *Disasters and mental heatlh*. Washington, DC: American Psychiatric Press.

Litz, B. T., & Gray, M. J. (2002). Early intervention for mass violence: What is the evidence? What should be done? *Cognitive and Behavioral Practice*, *9*(4), 266–272.

Marmar, C., Weiss, D., Metzler, T. J., & Delucchi, K. L. (1996). Characteristics of emergency services personnel related to peritraumatic dissociation during critical incident exposure. *American Journal of Psychiatry*, *153*(7), 94–102.

Marmar, C. R., Weiss, D. S., Metzler, T. J., Ronfeldt, H. M., & Foreman, C. (1996). Stress responses of emergency services personnel to the Loma Prieta earthquake interstate 880 freeway collapse and control traumatic incidents. *Journal of Traumatic Stress*, *9*(1), 63–85.

McFarlane, A. C. (1986). Long-term psychiatric morbidity after a natural disaster. Implications for disaster planners and emergency services. *Medical Journal of Australia*, *145*(11–12), 561–563.

(1988). Relationship between psychiatric impairment and a natural disaster: The role of distress. *Psychological Medicine*, *18*(1), 129–139.

McFarlane, A. C., & Papay, P. (1992). Multiple diagnoses in posttraumatic stress disorder in the victims of a natural disaster. *Journal of Nervous and Mental Disease*, *180*(8), 498–504.

McFarlane, A. C., Polincansky, S., & Irwin, C. (1987). A longitundinal study of the psychological morbidity in children due to a natural disaster. *Psychological Medicine*, *17*, 727–738.

McNally, R. J., Bryant, R. A., & Ehlers, A. (2003). Does early psychological intervention promote recovery from posttraumatic stress? *Psychological Science in the Public Interest*, *4*(2), 45–79.

Murray, J., Ehlers, A., & Mayou, R. A. (2002). Dissociation and post-traumatic stress disorder: Two prospective studies of road traffic accident survivors. *British Journal of Psychiatry*, *180*, 363–368.

Nandi, A., Galea, S., Ahern, J., & Vlahov, D. (2005). Probable cigarette dependence, PTSD, and depression after an urban disaster: Results from a population survey of New York City residents 4 months after September 11, 2001. *Psychiatry*, *68*(4), 299–310.

National Institute of Mental Health. (2002). *Mental health and mass violence – Evidence based early psychological intervention for victims/survivors of mass violence: a workshop to reach consensus on best practices* (NIH Publication No. 02–5138). Washington, DC: U.S. Government Publishing Office.

Neria, Y., Guttmann-Steinmetz, S., Koenen, K., Levinovsky, L., Zakin, G., & Dekel, R. (2001). Do attachment and hardiness relate to each other and to mental health in real-life stress? *Journal of Social and Personal Relationships*, *18*(6), 844–858.

Neria, Y., Gross, R., Litz, B., Maguen, S., Insel, B., Seirmarco, G., et al. (2007). Prevalence and psychological correlates of traumatic grief among bereaved adults 2.5–3.5 years after September 11th attacks. *Journal of Traumatic Stress*, *20*, 251–262.

Neria, Y., Gross, R., Olfson, M., Gameroff, M. J., Wickramaratne, P., Das, A., et al. (2006). Posttraumatic stress disorder in primary care one year after the 9/11 attacks. *General Hospital Psychiatry*, *28*(3), 213–222.

Neria, Y., & Litz, B. (2004). Bereavement by traumatic means: the complex synergy of trauma and grief. *Journal of Loss and Trauma*, *9*, 73–87.

Neria, Y., Nandi, A., & Galea, S. (2008). Post-traumatic stress disorder following disasters: A systematic review. *Psychological Medicine*, *38*(4), 467–480.

Newman, E., Simpson, R., & Handschuh, D. (2003). Trauma exposure and post-traumatic stress disorder among photojournalists. *News Photographer*, *58*(1), 4–13.

Norris, F. H. (2006). Community and ecological approaches to understanding and alleviating postdisaster distress. In Y. Neria R. Gross R. Marshall, & E. Susser (Eds.), *9/11: Mental health in the wake of terrorist attacks*. New York: Cambridge University Press.

Norris, F. H., & Alegria, M. (2005). Mental health care for ethnic minority individuals and communities in the aftermath of disasters and mass violence. *CNS Spectrums*, *10*(2), 132–40.

Norris, F. H., Stevens, S. P., Pfefferbaum, B., Wyche, K. F., & Pfefferbaum, R. L. (2007). Community resilience as a metaphor, theory, set of capacities, and strategy for disaster readiness. *American Journal of Community Psychology*, *41*(1–2), 127–150.

Norris, F. H., Baker, C. K., Murphy, A. D., & Kaniasty, K. (2005). Social support mobilization and deterioration after Mexico's 1999 flood: Effects of contex, gender, and time. *American Journal of Community Psychology*, *36*(1–2), 15.

Norris, F. H., Friedman, M., Watson, P., Byrne, C., Diaz, E. & Kaniasty, K. (2002). 60,000 disaster victims speak. Part 1: An empirical review of the empirical literature, 1981–2001. *Psychiatry*, *65*, 207–239.

Norris, F. H., Kaniasty, K. Z., Conrad, M. L., Inman, G. L., & Murphy, A. D. (2002). Placing age difference in cultural contex: A comparison of the effects of age on PTSD after disasters in the United States, Mexico, and Poland. *Journal of Clinical Geropsychology*, *8*, 153–173.

Norris, F. H., Phifer, J. F., & Kaniasty, K. Z. (1994). Individual and community reactions to the Kentucky floods: Findings from a longitudinal study of older adults. In B. R. J. Ursano G. McCaughey, & C. S. Fullerton (Eds.), *Individual and community responses to trauma and disaster: The structure of human chaos*. Cambridge: Cambridge University Press.

North, C. S., Pfefferbaum, B., Tivis, L., Kawasaki, A., Reddy, C., & Spitznagel, E. L. (2004). The course of posttraumatic stress disorder in a follow-up study of survivors of the Oklahoma City bombing. *Annals of clinical psychiatry, 16*(4), 209–215.

Ong, A. D., Bergeman, C. S., Bisconti, T. L., & Wallace, K. A. (2006). Psychological resilience, positive emotions, and successful adaptation to stress in later life. *Journal of Personality and Social Psychology, 91*(4), 730–749.

Person, C., Tracy, M., & Galea, S. (2006). Risk factors for depression after a disaster. *Journal of Nervous and Mental Disease, 194*, 659–666.

Pfefferbaum, B., Gurwitch, R. H., McDonald, N. B., Leftwich, M. J., Sconzo, G. M., Messenbaugh, A. K., et al. (2000). Posttraumatic stress among young children after the death of a friend or acquaintance in a terrorist bombing. *Psychiatric Services, 51*, 386–388.

Pfefferbaum, B., Nixon, S. J., Krug, R. S., Tivis, R. D., Moore, V. L., Brown, J. M., et al. (1999). Clinical needs assessment of middle and high school students following the 1995 Oklahoma City bombing. *American Journal of Psychiatry, 156*(7), 1069–1074.

Prigerson, H. G., Bierhals, A. J., Kasl, S. V., Reynolds 3rd, C. F., Shear, M. K., Newsom, J. T., et al. (1996). Complicated grief as a disorder distinct from bereavement-related depression and anxiety: A replication study. *American Journal of Psychiatry, 153*(11), 1484–1486.

Proctor, L. J., Fauchier, A., Oliver, P. H., Ramos, M. C, Rios, M. A,. & Margolin, G. (2007). Family context and young children's responses to earthquake. *Journal of Child Psychology and Psychiatry, 48*, 941–949.

Pulcino, T., Galea, S., Ahern, J., Resnick, H., Foley, M., & Blahov, D. (2003). Posttraumatic stress in women after the September 11 terrorist attacks in New York City. *Journal of Women's Health, 12*(8), 809–820.

Pyevich, C., Newman, E., & Daleidan, R. (2003). The relationship among cognitive schemas, job-related traumatic exposure, and PTSD symptoms in journalists. *Journal of Traumatic Stress, 16*, 325–328.

Pynoos, R. S., Frederick, C., Nader, K., Arroyo, W., Steinberg, A., Eth, S., et al. (1987). Life threat and posttraumatic stress in school-age children. *Archives of General Psychiatry, 44*, 1057–1063.

Rooney, C., & White, G. W. (2007). Narrative analysis of a disaster preparedness and emergency response survey from persons with mobility impairments. *Journal of Disability Policy Studies, 17*(4), 206–215.

Rose, S., Bisson, J., Churchill, R., & Wessely, S. (2002). *Psychological debriefing for preventing post traumatic stress disorder (PTSD)* (Publication from Cochrane Database System); http://www.cochrane.org/reviews/en/ab000560.html.

Saylor, C. F., Cowart, B. L., Lipovsky, J. A., Jackson, C., & Finch, A. J., Jr. (2003). Media exposure to September 11: Elementary school students' experiences and posttraumatic symptoms. *American Behavioral Scientist, 46*, 1622–1642.

Schlenger, W. E., Caddell, J. M., Ebert, L., Jordan, B. K. M., Wilson, D., Thalji, L., et al. (2002). Psychological reactions to terrorist attacks: Findings of the National Study of Americans' Reactions to September 11. *Journal of the American Medical Association, 288*, 1235–1244.

Schwarz, E. D., & Kowalski, J. M. (1992). Malignant memories: Reluctance to utilize mental health services after a disaster. *Journal of Nervous and Mental Disease, 180*, 767–772.

Shear, K. M., Jackson, C. T., Essock, S. M., Donahue, S. A., & Felton, C. J. (2006). Screening for complicated grief among Project Liberty service recipients 18 months after September 11, 2001. *Psychiatric Service, 57*, 1291–1297.

Silver, R. C., Holman, E. A., McIntosh, D. N., Poulin, M., & Gil-Rivas, V. (2002). Nationwide longitudinal study of psychological responses to September 11. *Journal of the American Medical Association, 288*, 1235–1244.

Simpson, R. A., & Boggs, J. G. (1999). An exploratory study of traumatic stress among newspaper journalists. *Journalism and Communication Monographs, 1*(1), 1–26.

Solomon, Z., Neria, Y., & Witztum, E. (2000). Debriefing following combat exposure: the effectiveness of a therapeutic intervention. In B. Raphael & J. Wilson (Eds.), *Psychological debriefing: Theory, practice and evidence*. Cambridge University Press.

Tak, S., Driscoll, R., Bernard, B., & West, C. (2007). Depressive symptoms among firefighters and related factors after the response to Hurricane Katrina. *Journal of Urban Health, 84*, 153–161.

Terr, L. C., Bloch, D. A., Michel, B. A., Shi, H., Reinhardt, J. A., & Metayer, S. A. (1997). Children's thinking in the wake of Challenger. *American Journal of Psychiatry, 154*, 744–751.

(1999). Children's symptoms in the wake of Challenger: A field study of distant-traumatic effects and an outline of related conditions. *American Journal of Psychiatry, 156*, 1536–1544.

Thabet, A. A., & Vostanis, P. (2000). Post traumatic stress disorder reactions in children of war: a longitudinal study. *Child Abuse and Neglect, 24*, 291–298.

Thompson, M. P., Norris, F. H., & Hanacek, B. (1993). Age differences in the psychological consequences of hurricane Hugo. *Psychology and Aging, 6*, 606–616.

Tyler, K. (2006). The impact of support received and support provision on changes in perceived social support among older adults. *International Journal of Aging & Human Development, 62*, 21–38.

Van der Velden, P. G., Kleber, R. J., & Koenen, K. C. (2008). Smoking predicts posttraumatic stress symptoms among rescue workers: A prospective study of ambulance personnel involved in the Enschede Fireworks Disaster. *Drugs and Alcohol Dependence, 94*, 267–271.

van Griensven, F., Chakkraban, M. L., Thienkrua, W., Pengjuntr, W., Lopes Cardozo, B., Tantipiwatanaskul, P., et al. (2006). Rapid assessment of post-tsunami mental health problems among adults in southern Thailand. *JAMA, 296*, 537–548.

Vlahov, D., Galea, S., Ahern, J., Rudenstine, S., Resnick, H., Kilpatrick, D., et al. (2006). Alcohol drinking problems among New York residents after September 11 terrorist attacks. *Substance Use and Misuse, 41*, 1295–1311.

Vlahov, D., Galea, S., Ahern, J., et al. (2004). Consumption of cigarettes, alcohol, and marijuana among New York City residents six months after the September 11 terrorist attacks. *The American journal of drug and alcohol abuse, 30*(2), 385–407

Weissman, M. M., Neria, Y., Das, A., Feder, A. C., Lantigua, R., Shea, S., et al. (2005). Gender differences in posttraumatic stress disorder among primary care patients after the World Trade Center attack of September 11, 2001. *General Medicine*, 2(2), 77–87.

Young, B. H. (2006). The immediate pesponse ot disaster: Guidelines for adult psychological first aid. In E. C. Ritchie P. J. Watson, & M. J. Friedman (Eds.), *Interventions following mass violence and disasters: Strategies for mental health practice.* New York: Guilford.

Zakin, G., Solomon, Z., & Neria, Y. (2003). Hardiness, attachment style, and long term distress among Israeli POWs and combat veterans. *Personality and Individual Differences, 34*, 819–829.

Index